AF800956

Advances in Experimental Medicine and Biology

Volume 1232

Series Editors

Wim E. Crusio, *CNRS and University of Bordeaux UMR 5287, Institut de Neurosciences Cognitives et Intégratives d'Aquitaine, Pessac Cedex, France*
John D. Lambris, *University of Pennsylvania, Philadelphia, PA, USA*
Nima Rezaei, *Children's Medical Center, Tehran, University of Medical Sciences, Tehran, Iran*

More information about this series at http://www.springer.com/series/5584

Pan-Dong Ryu • Joseph C. LaManna
David K. Harrison • Sang-Suk Lee
Editors

Oxygen Transport to Tissue XLI

Springer

Editors
Pan-Dong Ryu
Department of Veterinary Pharmacology
College of Veterinary Medicine
Seoul National University
Seoul, Republic of Korea

Joseph C. LaManna
Department of Physiology and Biophysics
School of Medicine
Case Western Reserve University
Cleveland, OH, USA

David K. Harrison
Heilig-Kreuz-Strasse 19
St. Lorenzen, Italy

Sang-Suk Lee
Department of Oriental Biomedical Engineering
Sangji University
Wonju, Republic of Korea

ISSN 0065-2598 ISSN 2214-8019 (electronic)
Advances in Experimental Medicine and Biology
ISBN 978-3-030-34459-7 ISBN 978-3-030-34461-0 (eBook)
https://doi.org/10.1007/978-3-030-34461-0

© Springer Nature Switzerland AG 2020, Corrected Publication 2020
The chapters "Near-Infrared Spectroscopy Measured Cerebral Blood Flow from Spontaneous Oxygenation Changes in Neonatal Brain Injury", "Developing a Model to Simulate the Effect of Hypothermia on Cerebral Blood Flow and Metabolism" and "Broadband NIRS Cerebral Evaluation of the Hemodynamic and Oxidative State of Cytochrome-c-Oxidase Responses to +Gz Acceleration in Healthy Volunteers" are licensed under the terms of the Creative Commons Attribution 4.0 International License (http://creativecommons.org/licenses/by/4.0/). For further details see license information in the chapter.
This work is subject to copyright. All rights are reserved by the Publisher, whether the whole or part of the material is concerned, specifically the rights of translation, reprinting, reuse of illustrations, recitation, broadcasting, reproduction on microfilms or in any other physical way, and transmission or information storage and retrieval, electronic adaptation, computer software, or by similar or dissimilar methodology now known or hereafter developed.
The use of general descriptive names, registered names, trademarks, service marks, etc. in this publication does not imply, even in the absence of a specific statement, that such names are exempt from the relevant protective laws and regulations and therefore free for general use.
The publisher, the authors, and the editors are safe to assume that the advice and information in this book are believed to be true and accurate at the date of publication. Neither the publisher nor the authors or the editors give a warranty, expressed or implied, with respect to the material contained herein or for any errors or omissions that may have been made. The publisher remains neutral with regard to jurisdictional claims in published maps and institutional affiliations.

This Springer imprint is published by the registered company Springer Nature Switzerland AG
The registered company address is: Gewerbestrasse 11, 6330 Cham, Switzerland

The Heritage, Foundation, Mission and Legacy of ISOTT

Prior to the 1960s, it was almost unheard of for medical scientists and engineering scientists to collaborate on important medical research problems. It was during the 1960s that the concept of bioengineering was born. At that time, the research between Dr. Melvin H. Knisely's group at the Medical University of South Carolina and Dr. Duane F. Bruley's group at Clemson University focused on oxygen transport problems inspired the creation of ISOTT at the Clemson-Charleston founding meeting in 1973. In that same era, three of the traditional engineering disciplines, civil, mechanical, and electrical, were based primarily on physics and mathematics, and the fourth discipline, chemical engineering, was based on physics, chemistry, and mathematics. The fifth traditional discipline of engineering, bioengineering, was evolving and it was based on biology, in addition to the other basic sciences and mathematics.[1]

- The *heritage* of ISOTT lies directly in the established four traditional disciplines of engineering, the three basic sciences, the fundamental medical sciences, and mathematics. Until the 1960s, these disciplines were totally separate, except for rare instances, and not formalized as an approach to solving important medical problems.
- The *foundation* of our society was designed to bring teams of medical and engineering scientists together working on problems related to oxygen transport to tissues. The meetings were designed to promote inter- and cross-disciplinary research projects. Rather than break out into individual sessions, the meeting was to be held in one large venue that would hold all participants. This was done to enhance interactions and understandings of important medical issues related to oxygen transport to tissue.
- The mission of our society was conceived to promote collaboration between the medical sciences and engineering sciences to assemble more sophisticated teams

[1] Bruley, D.F., "Bioengineering: The Fifth Traditional Engineering Discipline," *Oxygen Transport to Tissue XIV*, Advances in Experimental Medicine and Biology, vol. 317, p. 3–6,1992, Plenum Press

to understand and solve medical problems related to oxygen supply and utilization in human tissue.
- The legacy of ISOTT will be its pioneering involvement in the formalization of the fifth traditional discipline of engineering, bioengineering. Secondly, its leadership as a focused and international research society to formulate and solve crucial medical problems related to oxygen transport in human health makes it important in reducing human suffering and mortality.

The author has prepared this document to inform our new as well as older members of the planning that went into establishing a meaningful society that enhances medical research. He hopes that ISOTT was and will continue to be a unique and high-level research organization that inspires and supports collaborative research on oxygen-related issues.

D. F. Bruley
Synthesizer, Inc.
Ellicott City, MD, USA

Preface

This volume is the publication of papers presented at the 46th annual meeting of the International Society on Oxygen Transport to Tissue (ISOTT) 2018 held in Seoul, Republic of Korea, from July 1 to July 5, 2018. It contains research results and perspectives on the transport of oxygen to tissues presented by the scientists in the multiple disciplines as did in the previous volumes. The papers in this book have been subjected to peer review by the leading experts in this area.

The meeting brought 122 participants including 30 students from 12 countries in Asia, Europe, and North America. The meeting was opened on Sunday July 1, 2018, with a welcome by Dr. Pan-Dong Ryu (President, ISOTT 2018), and followed by opening lecture of Dr. Kwang-Sup Soh, "Current Developments in the Primo Vascular System and Oxygen." He overviewed the research on the system and its relation to oxygen transport. The lecture was followed by the cultural event "Hidden Wonders of Korea" providing an opportunity for the participants to experience Korean culture.

In the scientific sessions, various key aspects of "oxygen transport to tissue" were addressed, as in previous meetings. The themes of the 11 oral presentation sessions were oxygenation theory and methods, NIRS methods, oximetry methods, brain disease, tumor 1 and 2, brain oxygenation 1 and 2, blood vessels, special topics (primo vascular system), and complementary and alternative medicine. In these sessions, there were 41 oral presentations, 9 keynote lectures, and 1 Peter Vaupel Lecture. Dr. G. Multhoff delivered the Peter Vaupel lecture under the title "Hypoxia Compromises Anti-cancer Immune Responses." A total of 56 posters were presented for two day sessions, and the contents of each poster were introduced in a 2-minute oral presentation in two poster flash sessions.

ISOTT 2018 hosted two evening get-togethers on the second and third days of the program. The July 2 event was held at Hoam Faculty House of Seoul National University, where various fusion dishes and beer and other refreshments were served. The July 3 get-together was held at a Korean food buffet restaurant (Nature Kitchen). This brought participants a time to mingle as well as a chance to sample various types of Korean foods popular among Seoulites. In addition, ISOTT 2018 offered two sight-seeing trips on the afternoon of July 4: one to visit historic sites, including UNESCO World Heritage sites, and another to see dynamic new locations, including Seoul Sky Observatory.

The conference concluded on July 5 with the Annual General Meeting of ISOTT and an awards ceremony and banquet. At the awards ceremony, the Melvin H. Knisely Award was presented to Anne Riemann, the Dietrich W. Lübbers Award to Hamoon Zohdi, and the Britton Chance Award to Jingjing Jiang. In addition, six Duane F. Bruley Travel Awards were presented to junior scientists: Andrei Belten, Dries Hendrikx, Yuki Komuro, Aldo Di Costanzo Mata, Joshua Russell-Buckland, and Shun Takagi. After the Awards Ceremony, the evening ended with a banquet where participants could enjoy food, drinks, and jazz played on a "Piri," a Korean traditional reed instrument, by crossover music group "Oriental Scholar."

We like to thank all the participants of ISOTT 2018. We acknowledge the great work done by the members of the local organizing and working committees (Sungchul Kim, So Yeong Lee, Ku Youn Baik, Ji Yoon Lee, Chae Jeong Lim), the session chairs, and the student supporters. We thank the ISOTT officers, including Dr. Oliver Thews and Harold M. Swartz, for their invaluable advice and support during the preparation of ISOTT 2018. Finally, we also thank those of our participants who submitted their manuscripts and the reviewers who improved the quality and significance of those papers. All these efforts made this volume come to its fruition.

Wonju, Republic of Korea Sang-Suk Lee
Seoul, Republic of Korea Pan-Dong Ryu

Acknowledgments

As the president of the 46th Annual Meeting of the International Society on Oxygen Transport to Tissue, held on July 1–5, 2018, in Seoul, Republic of Korea, I would like to gratefully acknowledge the generous support of our sponsors.

서울대학교 수의과대학
College of Veterinary Medicine
http://vet.snu.ac.kr

OBELAB
http://www.obelab.com

Scitech Korea Inc.
http://scitechkorea.com

BrainKorea21 PLUS
http://vetgrad.snu.ac.kr

KMPC 국가마우스표현형분석사업단 KOREA MOUSE PHENOTYPING CENTER
http://www.mousephenotype.kr

bio D
http://www.bio-d.co.kr

KANG STEM BIOTECH
http://www.kangstem.com

WONKWANG UNIVERSITY MEDICAL CENTER, GWANGJU
A.L.S CENTER
http://wkugh.com

KSPVS
Korean Society of Primo Vascular System

대한수의학회
The Korean Society of Veterinary Science
http://www.ksvs.or.kr

Panel of Reviewers

Reviewer	Affiliation
Ku Youn Baik	Kwangwoon University, Seoul, Republic of Korea
Gemma Bale	University College London, UK
Denis Bragin	University of New Mexico, Albuquerque, USA
Ann Flood	EPR Center at Dartmouth, Hanover, USA
Howard Halpern	University of Chicago, USA
David Harrison	Microvascular Measurements, St. Lorenzen, Italy
Peter Keipert	PAREXEL, San Diego, USA
Sungchul Kim	Wonkwang University Gwangju Korean Medical Hospital, Republic of Korea
Sung Joon Kim	Seoul National University, Republic of Korea
Joseph LaManna	Case Western Reserve University, Cleveland, USA
Fredéric Lange	University College London, UK
Ji Yoon Lee	CHA University, Seongnam, Republic of Korea
Sang-Suk Lee	Sangji University, Wonju, Republic of Korea
So Yeong Lee	Seoul National University, Republic of Korea
Lin Li	University of Pennsylvania, Philadelphia, USA
Timon Cheng-Yi Liu	South China Normal University, Guangzhou, China
Subhabrata Mitra	University College London, UK
Gabriele Multhoff	Technical University Munich, Germany
Edwin Nemoto	University of New Mexico, Albuquerque, USA
Daniel Ostojic	University of Zurich, Switzerland
Sally Pias	New Mexico Tech, Socorro, USA
Michelle Puchowicz	University of Tennessee Health Science Centre, Memphis, USA
Anne Reimann	University of Halle, Germany
Joshua Russell-Buckland	University College London, UK
Pan-Dong Ryu	Seoul National University, Republic of Korea
Gennadi Saiko	Oxilight Inc., Toronto, Canada
Kaoru Sakatani	Nihon University School of Medicine, Tokyo, Japan

(continued)

Reviewer	Affiliation
Felix Scholkmann	University of Bern and University of Zurich, Switzerland
Oxana Semyachkina-Glushkovskaya	Saratov State University, Russia
Harold Swartz	EPR Center at Dartmouth, Hanover, USA
Ilias Tachtsidis	University College London, UK
Shun Takagi	Doshisha University, Kyoto, Japan
Oliver Thews	University of Halle, Germany
Atsuhiro Tsubaki	Niigata University, Japan
Peter Vaupel	University Medical Center, Mainz, Germany
Martin Wolf	University of Zurich, Switzerland
Ursula Wolf	University of Bern, Switzerland
Sung-Joon Ye	Seoul National University, Republic of Korea

Technical Reviewer

Laraine Visser-Isles	Rotterdam, the Netherlands
Eileen Harrison	St. Lorenzen, Italy

ISOTT Participants at the Seoul National University

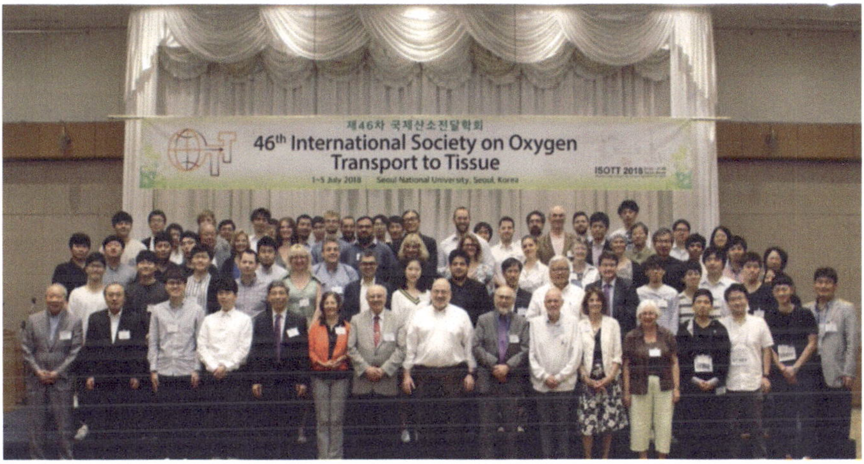

Local Organizing Committee

Pan-Dong Ryu
Hyeon-Min Bae
Ku Youn Baik
Hee Young Kim
Sungchul Kim
Sung Joon Kim
Sang-Suk Lee
So Yeong Lee
Ji Yoon Lee
Su Ho Park
Sung-Joon Ye
Chae Jeong Lim

Scientific Committee

Pan-Dong Ryu, Seoul National University, Republic of Korea
Sungchul Kim, Wonkwang University, Republic of Korea
Sang-Suk Lee, Sangji University, Republic of Korea
Terence Leung, University College London, UK
Lin Li, University of Pennsylvania, USA
Sally Pias, New Mexico Tech, USA
Eiji Takahashi, Saga University, Japan
Oliver Thews, Martin Luther University Halle-Wittenberg, Germany
Martin Wolf, University of Zurich, Switzerland

ISOTT Officers and Executive Committee

President
Name: Pan-Dong Ryu
Country: Republic of Korea
Telephone: (+82) 2-880-1254
Fax: (+82) 2-879-0378
Email: pdryu@snu.ac.kr

Past President
Name: Oliver Thews
Country: Germany
Telephone: (+49) 345 557-4048
Fax: (+49) 345 557-4019
Email: oliver.thews@medizin.uni-halle.de

Presidents-Elect
Name: Edwin M. Nemoto
Country: USA
Telephone: (+1) 505-272-5990
Fax: (+1) 505-272-6091
Email: Enemoto@salud.unm.edu

Secretary
Name: Oliver Thews
Country: Germany
Telephone: (+49) 345-557-4048
Fax: (+49) 345-557-4019
Email: oliver.thews@medizin.uni-halle.de

Treasurer

Name: Peter Keipert
Country: USA
Phone: (+1) 858-699-4789
Fax: (+1) 858-792-7489
Email: peterkeipert@gmail.com

Chairman, Knisely Award Committee

Name: Duane F. Bruley
Country: USA
Telephone: (+1) 410-313-9939
Fax: F: (+1) 410-313-9939
Email: bruley33@verizon.net

Executive Committee

Boris Epel (USA)
Edwin M. Nemoto (USA)
Sally Pias (USA)
Michelle A. Puchowicz (USA)
Anne Riemann (Germany)
Kaoru Sakatani (Japan)
Harold M. Swartz (USA)
Ursula Wolf (Switzerland)
Karen A. Yilmaz (USA)

ISOTT Award Winners

The Melvin H. Knisely Award

The Melvin H. Knisely Award was established in 1983 to honor Dr. Knisely's accomplishments in the field of the transport of oxygen and other metabolites and anabolites in the human body. Over the years, he has inspired many young investigators, and this award is to honor his enthusiasm for assisting and encouraging young scientists and engineers in various disciplines. The award is to acknowledge outstanding young investigators. It was first presented during the banquet of the 1983 annual conference of ISOTT in Ruston, Louisiana. The award includes a Melvin H. Knisely plaque and a cash prize.

Melvin H. Knisely Award Recipients

1983 Antal G. Hudetz (Hungary)
1984 Andras Eke (Hungary)
1985 Nathan A. Bush (USA)
1986 Karlfried Groebe (Germany)
1987 Isumi Shibuya (Japan)
1988 Kyung A. Kang (Korea/USA)
1989 Sanja Batra (Canada)
1990 Stephen J. Cringle (Australia)
1991 Paul Okunieff (USA)
1992 Hans Degens (the Netherlands)
1993 David A. Benaron (USA)
1994 Koen van Rossem (Belgium)
1995 Clare E. Elwell (UK)
1996 Sergei A. Vinogradov (USA)
1997 Chris Cooper (UK)
1998 Martin Wolf (Switzerland)

1999 Huiping Wu (USA)
2000 Valentina Quaresima (Italy)
2001 Fahmeed Hyder (Bangladesh)
2002 Geofrey De Visscher (Belgium)
2003 Mohammad Nadeem Khan (USA)
2004 Fredrik Palm (Sweden)
2005 Nicholas Lintell (Australia)
2006 –
2007 Ilias Tachtsidis (UK)
2008 Kazuto Masamoto (Japan)
2009 Rossana Occhipinti (USA)
2010 Sebastiano Cicco (Italy)
2011 Mei Zhang (USA)
2012 Takahiro Igarashi (Japan)
2013 Malou Friederich-Persson (Sweden)
2014 David Highton (UK)
2015 Alexander Caicedo Dorado (Belgium)
2016 Sally Pias (USA)
2017 Felix Scholkmann (Switzerland)
2018 Anne Riemann (Germany)

The Dietrich W. Lübbers Award

The Dietrich W. Lübbers Award was established in honor of Professor Lübbers' long-standing commitment, interest, and contributions to the problems of oxygen transport to tissue and to the society. This award was first presented in 1994 during the annual conference of ISOTT in Istanbul, Turkey.

Dietrich W. Lübbers Award Recipients

1994 Michael Dubina (Russia)
1995 Philip E. James (UK/USA)
1996 Resit Demir (Germany)
1997 Juan Carlos Chavez (Peru)
1998 Nathan A. Davis (UK)
1999 Paola Pichiule (USA)
2000 Ian Balcer (USA)
2001 Theresa M. Busch (USA)
2002 Link K. Korah (USA)
2003 James J. Lee (USA)

2004 Richard Olson (Sweden)
2005 Charlotte Ives (UK)
2006 Bin Hong (China/USA)
2007 Helga Blockx (Belgium)
2008 Joke Vanderhaegen (Belgium)
2009 Matthew Bell (UK)
2010 Alexander Caicedo Dorado (Belgium)
2011 Malou Friederich-Persson (Sweden)
2012 Maria Papademetriou (UK)
2013 Nannan Sun (China/USA)
2014 Felix Scholkmann (Switzerland)
2015 Shun Takagi (Japan)
2016 Gemma Bale (UK)
2017 Ben Jones (UK)
2018 Hamoon Zohdi (Switzerland)

The Britton Chance Award

The Britton Chance Award was established in honor of Professor Chance's long-standing commitment, interest, and contributions to the science and engineering aspects of oxygen transport to tissue and to the society. This award was first presented in 2004 during the annual conference of ISOTT in Bari, Italy.

Britton Chance Award Recipients

2004 Derek Brown (Switzerland)
2005 James Lee (USA)
2006 Hanzhu Jin (China/USA)
2007 Eric Mellon (USA)
2008 Jianting Wang (USA)
2009 Jessica Spires (USA)
2010 Ivo Trajkovic (Switzerland)
2011 Alexander Caicedo Dorado (Belgium)
2012 Felix Scholkmann (Switzerland)
2013 Tharindi Hapuarachchi (UK)
2014 Anne Riemann (Germany)
2015 Wenhao Xie (China)
2016 Linda Ahnen (Switzerland)
2017 Helene Isler (Switzerland)
2018 Jingjing Jiang (Switzerland)

The Duane F. Bruley Travel Awards

The Duane F. Bruley Travel Awards was established in 2003 and first presented by ISOTT at the 2004 annual conference in Bari, Italy. This award was created to provide travel funds for student researchers in all aspects of oxygen transport to tissue. The awards signify Dr. Bruley's interest in encouraging and supporting young researchers to maintain the image and quality of research associated with the society. As a cofounder of ISOTT in 1973, Dr. Bruley emphasizes cross-disciplinary research among basic scientists, engineers, medical scientists, and clinicians. His pioneering work constructing mathematical models for oxygen and other anabolite/metabolite transport in the microcirculation, employing computer solutions, was the first to consider system nonlinearities and time dependence, including multidimensional diffusion, convection, and reaction kinetics. It is hoped that receiving the Duane F. Bruley Travel Award will inspire students to excel in their research and will assist in securing future leadership for ISOTT.

The Duane F. Bruley Travel Award Recipients

2004 Helga Blockx (Belgium), Jennifer Caddick (UK), Charlotte Ives (UK), Nicholas Lintell (Australia), Leonardo Mottola (Italy), Samin Rezania (USA/Iran), Ilias Tachtsidis (UK), Liang Tang (USA/China), Iyichi Sonoro (Japan), Antonio Franco (Italy)

2005 Robert Bradley (UK), Harald Oey (Australia), Kathy Hsieh (Australia), Jan Shah (Australia)

2006 Ben Gooch (UK), Ulf Jensen (Germany), Smruta Koppaka (USA), Daya Singh (UK), Martin Tisdall (UK), Bin Wong (USA), and Kui Xu (USA)

2007 Dominique De Smet (Belgium), Thomas Ingram (UK), Nicola Lai (USA), Andrew Pinder (UK), Joke Vanderhaegen (Belgium)

2008 Sebastiano Cicco (Italy)

2009 Lei Gao (UK), Jianting Wang (USA), Obinna Ndubuizu (USA), Joke Vanderhaegen (Belgium)

2010 Zareen Bashir (UK), Tracy Moroz (UK), Mark Muthalib (Australia), Catalina Meßmer (USA), Takashi Eriguchi (Japan), Yoshihiro Murata (Japan), Jack Honeysett (UK), Martin Biallas (Switzerland)

2011 Catherine Hesford (UK), Luke S. Holdsworth (UK), Andreas Metz (Switzerland), Maria D. Papademetriou (UK), Patrik Persson (Sweden), Felix Scholkmann (Switzerland), Kouichi Yoshihara (Japan)

2012 Allann Al-Armaghany (UK), Malou Friederich-Persson (Sweden), Tharindi Hapuarachchi (UK), Benjamin Jones (UK), Rebecca Re (Italy), Yuta Sekiguchi (Japan), Ebba Sivertsson (Sweden), Andre´ Steimers (Germany)

2013 Allann Al-Armaghany (UK), Gemma Bale (UK), Alexander Caicedo Dorado (Belgium), Luke Dunne (UK)

2014 Geraldine De Preter (Belgium), Benjamin Jones (UK), Stefan Kleiser (Switzerland), Nassimsadat Nasseri (Switzerland), Marie-Aline Neveu (Belgium), Shinsuke Nirengi (Japan), Takuya Osawa (Japan)

2015 Nannan Sun (China), Gemma Bale (UK), Chenyang Gao (China), Guennadi Saiko (Canada), Kuangyu Shi (Germany), Phong Phan (UK), Chae Jeong Lim (Korea)
2016 Isabel De Roever (UK), Yuya Enokida (Japan), Jingjing Jiang (Switzerland), Frédéric Lange (UK), Andreas J. Metz (Switzerland), Shun Takagi (Japan)
2017 Luca Giannoni (UK), Jingjing Jiang (Switzerland), Alexander Kalyanov (Switzerland), Zuzana Kovacsova (UK), Nassim Nasseri (Switzerland), Maheen Faisal Siddiqui (UK), Shun Takagi (Japan), Yusuke Tsuruno (Japan), Lina Xu (Germany), Hamoon Zohdi (Switzerland)
2018 Andrei Belten (Canada), Dries Hendrikx (Belgium), Yuki Komuro (Japan), Aldo Di Costanzo Mata (Switzerland), Joshua Russell-Buckland (UK), and Shun Takagi (Japan)

Kovách Lecture

The Kovách Lecture is presented periodically to honor a career dedicated to oxygenation research. Arisztid Kovách was a world-renowned cardiovascular physiologist and one of the early leaders of ISOTT. This lecture is dedicated to his remarkable scientific and teaching career.

Kovách Lecture Recipients

2011 John Severinghaus
2012 Peter Vaupel
2014 Edwin Nemoto

Peter Vaupel Lecture

The Peter Vaupel Lecture is presented to honor a career dedicated to oxygenation research. Peter Vaupel is a world-renowned tumor pathophysiologist and one of the early leaders of ISOTT. This lecture is dedicated to his remarkable scientific and teaching career.

Peter Vaupel Lecture Recipients

2018 Gabriele Multhoff

Contents

Part I
Brain Oxygenation and Function

Near-Infrared Spectroscopy Measured Cerebral Blood Flow from Spontaneous Oxygenation Changes in Neonatal Brain Injury

Gemma Bale, Nathan Taylor, Subhabrata Mitra, Aleh Sudakou, Isabel de Roever, Judith Meek, Nicola Robertson, and Ilias Tachtsidis

Abstract Neonates with hypoxic-ischaemic (HI) brain injury were monitored using a broadband near-infrared spectroscopy (NIRS) system in the neonatal intensive care unit. The aim of this work is to use the NIRS cerebral oxygenation data (HbD = oxygenated-haemoglobin − deoxygenated-haemoglobin) combined with arterial saturation (SaO_2) from pulse oximetry to calculate cerebral blood flow (CBF) based on the oxygen swing method, during spontaneous desaturation episodes. The method is based on Fick's principle and uses HbD as a tracer; when a sudden change in SaO_2 occurs, the change in HbD represents a change in tracer concentration, and thus it is possible to estimate CBF. CBF was successfully calculated with broadband NIRS in 11 HIE infants (3 with severe injury) for 70 oxygenation events on the day of birth. The average CBF was 18.0 ± 12.7 ml 100 g^{-1} min^{-1} with a range of 4 ml 100 g^{-1} min^{-1} to 60 ml 100 g^{-1} min^{-1}. For infants with severe HIE (as determined by magnetic resonance spectroscopy) CBF was significantly lower ($p = 0.038$, $d = 1.35$) than those with moderate HIE on the day of birth.

Keywords Near-infrared spectroscopy · Cerebral blood flow · Neonatal brain injury · Hypoxic-ischaemic encephalopathy · Clinical

---

G. Bale (✉) · N. Taylor · I. de Roever · I. Tachtsidis
Medical Physics and Biomedical Engineering, University College London, London, UK
e-mail: g.bale@ucl.ac.uk

S. Mitra · J. Meek · N. Robertson
Institute for Women's Health, University College London, London, UK

A. Sudakou
Nalecz Institute of Biocybernetics and Biomedical Engineering, Polish Academy of Sciences, Warsaw, Poland

© The Author(s) 2020

P.-D. Ryu et al. (eds.), *Oxygen Transport to Tissue XLI*, Advances in Experimental Medicine and Biology 1232, https://doi.org/10.1007/978-3-030-34461-0_1

1 Introduction

Hypoxic ischaemic encephalopathy (HIE), which affects 1–2 full term newborns per 1000, is associated with severe neurodevelopmental problems and is the third leading cause of global child deaths [1]. HIE is an evolving process; after ischaemia during the injury, the brain is reperfused but the cerebral blood flow (CBF) can fluctuate between hypo-and hyper-perfusion in the first days after birth, and in some cases the injury can progress into a secondary energy failure [1]. Strategies to treat HIE focus on the maintenance of cerebral perfusion and preventing the cascade of events leading to further brain injury.

We have previously presented a broadband NIRS device called CYRIL (CYtochrome Research Instrument and appLication) to monitor cerebral haemodynamics and metabolism via cytochrome-c-oxidase in the newborn brain [2]. In this paper, we present a method to additionally monitor CBF changes with CYRIL in neonates with HIE. Previously, researchers have used NIRS to measure CBF by using the oxygen swing method; oxygenation changes in the brain can be used to calculate the CBF via Fick's law [3]. This states that the quantity of substance taken up by an organ per unit time (dQ/dt) is equal to the rate of arrival of the substance to an organ (arterial concentration (C_a) multiplied by the blood flow (F)), minus the rate of departure from the organ (venous concentration (C_v) multiplied by F):

$$dQ/dt = F\left(C_a - C_v\right) \tag{1}$$

If Q varies with time, then this equation can be integrated with respect to time to obtain blood flow in terms of the quantity of tracer within the organ, and its arterial and venous concentrations:

$$F = Q / \int \left(C_a - C_v\right) dt \tag{2}$$

Q is equivalent to the product of the concentration of tracer in the tissue (C_T) and the unit weight of the tissue (W). This relationship can be used to obtain CBF in the more commonly used units, ml per 100 g of brain tissue per minute. Furthermore, if the accumulation is measured within the minimum transit time of the organ, reported as around 8 s for the brain in neonates [4], then the venous concentration of the substance will be zero. CBF can then be calculated from the ratio of the tracer accumulated to the quantity of tracer introduced during time t:

$$F/W = C_T / \int C_a(t) dt = CBF \tag{3}$$

When applied to NIRS measurements of CBF, the arterial concentration of substance introduced over time t can be represented by the integral of the change in fractional arterial oxygen saturation (SaO_2) multiplied by the total concentration of haemoglobin in the blood. The accumulation of substance in the organ becomes the concentration of oxy-haemoglobin (HbO_2) in the brain, measured by NIRS, and CBF is then obtained from the equation:

$$CBF = K \cdot \Delta\left[HbO_2\right] / \left[tHb \cdot 10^{-2}\right] \cdot \int \Delta SaO_2 dt \tag{4}$$

with

$$K = MWHb \cdot 10^{-2} / Dt \cdot 10 \tag{5}$$

where MW_{Hb} is the molecular weight of haemoglobin (64,500 g mol^{-1}), tHb is the total haemoglobin concentration, and Dt is the tissue density, assumed to be 1.05 $g.ml^{-1}$ in the brain [3].

Haemoglobin difference (HbD = HbO_2 - HHb) is a measure of oxygen delivery that has a larger amplitude (and thus higher signal to noise) and is also more stable than either of the two individual signals as artefacts are subtracted. If total haemoglobin concentration remains stable throughout the measurement, the change in HbD can be expressed as twice the change in HbO_2 and therefore CBF is:

$$CBF = K \cdot \Delta\left[HbD\right] / 2\left[tHb \cdot 10^{-2}\right] \cdot \int \Delta SaO_2 dt \tag{6}$$

Here we demonstrate the use of this method not with controlled oxygen challenges, but on spontaneous desaturation events in newborns with brain injury undergoing intensive care. This allows non-invasive measurements of CBF at the cot side without intervention.

2 Methods

2.1 Data Collection

Ethical approval for the Baby Brain Study at University College London Hospitals (UCLH) Trust, London was obtained from the North-West Research Ethics Centre (REC reference: 13/LO/0106). Term infants born at or transferred to UCLH for treatment of acute brain injury were eligible for investigation; infants with congenital malformations were excluded. Informed consent was obtained before each study. Each subject was monitored continuously with EEG and treated with hypothermia which was initiated within 6 hours of birth; body temperature was lowered to 33.5 °C and was maintained for 72 hours before gradual rewarming.

Broadband NIRS measurements were collected with CYRIL continuously over a period ranging from 1–15 hours on the first day of life during therapeutic hypothermia. NIRS probes were placed over the left-side of the forehead (covering the left frontal lobe) with 3 cm optode separation and with a sampling frequency of 1 Hz. Changes in chromophore concentrations (HbO_2, HHb, and the oxidation state of cytochrome-c-oxidase, oxCCO) were calculated from the measured changes in light attenuation using the modified Beer-Lambert law. This was applied across 770-906 nm with a differential pathlength factor of 4.99 [5], which is corrected for the pathlength wavelength-dependency. Examples of obtained intensity spectra are published in Bale et al. [2].

Systemic data from the Intellivue Monitors (Philips Healthcare, UK) were collected using ixTrend (ixellence GmbH, Germany). Signals recorded include oxygen saturation (SaO_2) measured by pulse oximetry, heart rate (HR), respiratory rate (RR), and mean arterial blood pressure (MABP).

An MRI scan was performed after rewarming; this occurred on average on day 7 of life (range: day 5–15). MR scans included a measurement of thalamic Lac/NAA with proton (^{1}H) magnetic resonance spectroscopy (MRS); Lac/NAA score ≥ 0.3 has been shown to be associated with poor outcome [6].

2.2 Data Analysis

Data analysis was carried out in MATLAB (Mathworks, USA). Systemic data were down-sampled and interpolated to the NIRS data timeframe (1 Hz). Changes in SaO_2 of 2% or greater occurring in under 7 seconds (determined to be the transit time of the brain) were identified manually using a graphical user interface written in-house. Events were rejected if the initial SaO_2 was less than 70%, if there was a change in HR or RR of more than 10 bpm during the event, or if the HbD standard deviation was greater than 1 μM in the 10s before the event. An example of the pulse oximetry and broadband NIRS data used is shown in Fig. 1a and b). The gradient of the change in HbD and integral of SaO_2 with respect to time during the first 7 seconds of the event was used to calculate the CBF (see Fig. 1c) and Eq. 6). Data are presented as median and confidence interval, and statistical significance was assessed with the Mann-Whitney U test ($p > 0.05$ is significant) and the effect size was tested by Cohen's d ($d > 1.2$ is 'very large') [7].

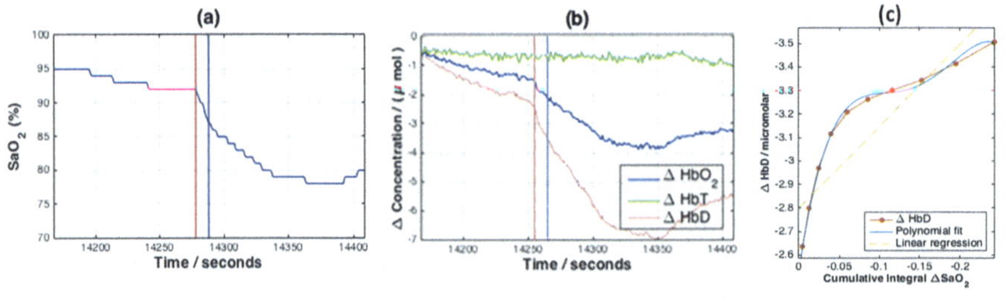

Fig. 1 Example of the CBF calculation method: (**a**) SaO_2 and (**b**) HbD. The vertical lines indicate the region of interest (10 seconds) used for the calculation. (**c**) The change in HbD plotted against the equivalent cumulative change in SaO_2 integral; with a fitted fourth order polynomial and a fitted linear regression. The CBF in this event is 22.1 ml 100 g^{-1} min

3 Results

CBF was calculated during 42 desaturation episodes noted in 11 infants with HIE on the day of birth. Of these infants, 3 were predicted to have a poor outcome by the MRS Lac/NAA biomarker. See Table 1 for clinical details, number of events and mean CBF for each neonate. The mean gestational age was 39.3 ± 1.2 weeks and the mean birth weight was 3262 ± 334 g. The median CBF was 12 ml 100 g^{-1} min^{-1} with a range of 4 ml 100 g^{-1} min^{-1} to 60 ml 100 g^{-1} min^{-1}. For infants with severe HIE, CBF was lower (8.5 (6.5–11.0) ml 100 g^{-1} min^{-1}) than moderate HIE infants (15.2 (4.0–60.0) ml 100 g^{-1} min^{-1}) on the day of birth ($p = 0.038$, $d = 1.35$, see Fig. 2).

4 Discussion

The NIRS measured CBFs are in line with those previously measured in newborns by the oxygen swing technique [4, 8], Xenon clearance [4, 9], dynamic contrast-enhanced NIRS with indocynanine green [10] and phase contrast MRI [11] which had means of 29.7 (range 11.4–62.1), 11.7 (range 5–26.1), 14.8 (range 5.1–30.4), 13 ± 7.4, 16.5 ± 2.1 and 9.6 (range 7.5–15.1) ml 100 g^{-1} min^{-1} respectively. This suggests that using the oxygen swing method on spontaneous desaturation events is a feasible way to measure CBF without intervention.

Neonates with severe HIE experienced hypoperfusion on the first day of life. This is consistent with a finding from an MRI arterial spin labelling study; infants with severe HIE had significantly lower CBF on the first two days of life than those with moderate HIE [12]. The decreased CBF in more severe injury could be caused by evolving pathophysiology of HIE - following HI, there is a period of hypoperfusion

Table 1 Clinical details and number of eligible desaturation events for neonates included. Unfavourable outcome was determined by MRS Lac/NAA > 0.3. Birth weight measured in grams, CBF measured in ml 100 g^{-1} min^{-1}

Neonate	Gender	GA (weeks)	Birth weight	Lac/NAA	Injury outcome	No of events	CBF
3	F	41.0	3800	0.2	Favourable	2	14 ± 4
9	M	38.9	2850	0.16	Favourable	6	10 ± 1
11	F	40.6	3580	0.08	Favourable	12	16 ± 5
14	M	37.7	3750	0.25	Favourable	4	47 ± 10
15	F	39.6	3240	0.15	Favourable	9	11 ± 4
17	F	37.4	3160	0.35	Unfavourable	2	7 ± 1
33	F	38.4	2900	0.43	Unfavourable	4	9 ± 2
35	F	38.7	3150	0.14	Favourable	4	21 ± 11
37	F	39.4	3330	0.2	Favourable	2	41 ± 2
56	M	40	3365	0.34	Unfavourable	1	11 ± 0
60	F	40.7	2754	0.15	Favourable	3	12 ± 3

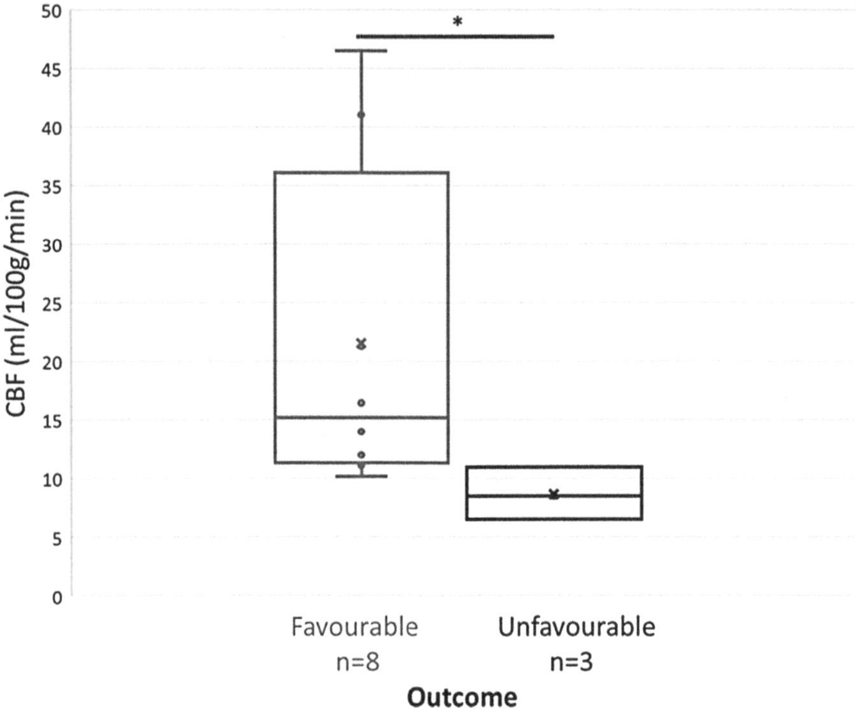

Fig. 2 Boxplot of CBF on first day of life per injury severity group (*p = 0.024)

associated with hypometabolism during the latent phase, followed by relative hyperperfusion in the secondary phase [1].

Therapeutic hypothermia itself can reduce CBF; an index of CBF measured by diffuse correlation spectroscopy has been shown to be reduced during cooling compared to after rewarming in a HIE group, as well as compared to a control group at normothermia [13]. However, this cannot account for the differences in CBF between the injury severity groups because all neonates were being treated with hypothermia during the measurement. It important to be aware of the impact of cooling on CBF, as an early study without hypothermia showed the opposite trend; there was a trend for higher CBF in infants with severe HIE [8]. This observation of hypoperfusion solely in the severe group suggests that the temporal progression of injury and/or the response to treatment is injury dependent.

We have demonstrated a method of calculating absolute CBF non-invasively and without any intervention using NIRS during spontaneous hypoxic events in HIE infants. This technique is advantageous because it can be performed at the cot side and does not require any intervention, but is limited because the spontaneous nature of the events. Indeed, desaturation episodes are not guaranteed in all infants during a study period. However, we could identify a difference in the level of perfusion between neonates with moderate and severe injury on the first day of life. This suggests that monitoring CBF during HIE will give important clinical information that may have further prognostic value.

Acknowledgments The authors would like to thank the parents who gave consent for their children to participate. This research was funded by The Wellcome Trust (1004580/Z/14/Z). NR, SM and JM acknowledge the support of the UCLH Biomedical Research Centre.

References

1. Hassell KJ, Ezzati M, Alonso-Alconada D, Hausenloy DJ, Robertson NJ (2015) New horizons for newborn brain protection: enhancing endogenous neuroprotection. Arch Dis Child Fetal Neonatal Ed 100(6):F541–F552
2. Bale G, Mitra S, Meek J, Robertson N, Tachtsidis I (2014) A new broadband near-infrared spectroscopy system for in-vivo measurements of cerebral cytochrome-c-oxidase changes in neonatal brain injury. Biomed Opt Express 5(10):3450–3466
3. Elwell CE, Cope M, Edwards AD, Wyatt JS, Reynolds EO, Delpy DT (1992) Measurement of cerebral blood flow in adult humans using near infrared spectroscopy--methodology and possible errors. Adv Exp Med Biol 317(4):235–245
4. Skov L, Pryds O, Greisen G (1991) Estimating cerebral blood flow in newborn infants: comparison of near infrared spectroscopy and 133Xe clearance. Pediatr Res 30(6):570–573
5. Duncan A et al (Feb. 1995) Optical pathlength measurements on adult head, calf and forearm and the head of the newborn infant using phase resolved optical spectroscopy. Phys Med Biol 40(2):295–304
6. Thayyil S et al (2010) Cerebral magnetic resonance biomarkers in neonatal encephalopathy: a meta-analysis. Pediatrics 125(2):e382–e395
7. Sawilowsky SS (2009) New effect size rules of thumb. J Mod Appl Stat Methods 8:597–599
8. Meek J, Elwell C (1999) Abnormal cerebral haemodynamics in perinatally asphyxiated neonates related to outcome. Arch Dis Child 81:F110–F115
9. Pryds O, Edwards AD (1996) Cerebral blood flow in the newborn infant. Arch Dis Child 74:F63–F69
10. Diop M, Tichauer KM, Elliott JT, Migueis M, Lee T-Y, St Lawrence K (2015) Comparison of time-resolved and continuous-wave near-infrared techniques for measuring cerebral blood flow in piglets. J Biomed Opt 15(5):057004
11. Jain V et al (2013) Cerebral oxygen metabolism in neonates with congenital heart disease quantified by MRI and optics. J Cereb Blood Flow Metab 34(3):380–388
12. Wintermark P, Hansen A, Warfield SK, Dukhovny D, Soul JS (2014) Near-infrared spectroscopy versus magnetic resonance imaging to study brain perfusion in newborns with hypoxic-ischemic encephalopathy treated with hypothermia. Neuroimage 85(1):287–293
13. Dehaes M et al (2014) Cerebral oxygen metabolism in neonatal hypoxic ischemic encephalopathy during and after therapeutic hypothermia. J Cereb Blood Flow Metab 34(1):87–94

Open Access This chapter is licensed under the terms of the Creative Commons Attribution 4.0 International License (http://creativecommons.org/licenses/by/4.0/), which permits use, sharing, adaptation, distribution and reproduction in any medium or format, as long as you give appropriate credit to the original author(s) and the source, provide a link to the Creative Commons license and indicate if changes were made.

The images or other third party material in this chapter are included in the chapter's Creative Commons license, unless indicated otherwise in a credit line to the material. If material is not included in the chapter's Creative Commons license and your intended use is not permitted by statutory regulation or exceeds the permitted use, you will need to obtain permission directly from the copyright holder.

Nonlinear Transfer Entropy to Assess the Neurovascular Coupling in Premature Neonates

Dries Hendrikx, Liesbeth Thewissen, Anne Smits, Gunnar Naulaers, Karel Allegaert, Sabine Van Huffel, and Alexander Caicedo

Abstract In the adult brain, it is well known that increases in local neural activity trigger changes in regional blood flow and, thus, changes in cerebral energy metabolism. This regulation mechanism is called neurovascular coupling (NVC). It is not yet clear to what extent this mechanism is present in the premature brain. In this study, we explore the use of transfer entropy (TE) in order to compute the nonlinear coupling between changes in brain function, assessed by means of EEG, and changes in brain oxygenation, assessed by means of near-infrared spectroscopy (NIRS). In a previous study, we measured the coupling between both variables using a linear model to compute TE. The results indicated that changes in brain oxygenation were likely to precede changes in EEG activity. However, using a nonlinear and nonparametric approach to compute TE, the results indicate an opposite directionality of this coupling. The source of the different results provided by the linear and nonlinear TE is unclear and needs further research. In this study, we present the results from a cohort of 21 premature neonates. Results indicate that TE values computed using the nonlinear approach are able to discriminate between neonates with brain abnormalities and healthy neonates, indicating a less functional NVC in neonates with brain abnormalities.

Keywords Neurometabolic Coupling (NMC) · Transfer Entropy (TE) · EEG · NIRS · Premature Neonates

D. Hendrikx (✉) · S. Van Huffel · A. Caicedo
Department of Electrical Engineering (ESAT), STADIUS, KU Leuven, Leuven, Belgium
e-mail: dries.hendrikx@esat.kuleuven.be

L. Thewissen · A. Smits · G. Naulaers
Department of Development and Regeneration, KU Leuven, Leuven, Belgium

Department of Neonatology, UZ, Leuven, Belgium

K. Allegaert
Department of Development and Regeneration, KU Leuven, Leuven, Belgium

Department of Pediatric Surgery and Intensive Care, Erasmus MC-Sophia Children's Hospital, Rotterdam, The Netherlands

Department of Neonatology, Erasmus MC-Sophia Children's Hospital, Rotterdam, The Netherlands

© Springer Nature Switzerland AG 2020

P.-D. Ryu et al. (eds.), *Oxygen Transport to Tissue XLI*, Advances in Experimental Medicine and Biology 1232, https://doi.org/10.1007/978-3-030-34461-0_2

1 Introduction

In the adult brain, increases in local neural activity trigger increases in regional blood flow, and thus changes in regional cerebral energy metabolism. We call this regulation mechanism between neural activity and hemodynamics neurovascular coupling (NVC). In practice, brain oxygenation levels can be assessed by means of near-infrared spectroscopy (NIRS), while brain function can be measured by means of EEG. In the neonatal brain, however, the presence and extent of the MVC is still unclear. Some neonatal fMRI and NIRS studies have reported adult-like NVC [1] [2], while other studies in both humans and rodent models have reported differences in hemodynamic responses in the early postnatal brain compared to adults [3] [4].

In this paper, we use nonlinear and nonparametric transfer entropy (TE) to compute the coupling between NIRS and EEG; we use this measure to assess the NVC in the premature brain. TE allows to quantify the directionality of information transfer between NIRS and EEG signals. In a previous study, we measured the coupling between NIRS and EEG using a linear model to compute TE [6]. The results indicated that changes in brain oxygenation were likely to precede changes in amplitude of EEG activity, indicating a NVC response that differs from the response commonly observed in adults. In this regard, however, it is important to mention that the coupling between neuronal activity and brain hemodynamics incorporates nonlinear effects, indicating that a nonlinear measure (such as the nonlinear TE presented in this paper) is more appropriate for NVC quantification [7].

Finally, we compare the NVC in a cohort of neonates that underwent sedation with propofol. We evaluated the prognostic value of TE in order to detect neonates that presented small brain hemorrhages.

2 Dataset

Concomitant measurements of brain oxygenation (brain tissue saturation), measured by means of NIRS (INVOS 5100, Covidien, neonatal probe), and raw EEG (Olympic CFM 6000, Natus) were acquired as part of a study to identify the optimal dose of propofol for procedural sedation in neonates [5]. The NIRS optode was located left frontoparietal and the EEG was measured between the C3 and C4 of the 10–20 system. The sampling frequency was equal to 1 Hz and 100 Hz for NIRS and EEG, respectively. All recordings were shortened to 6 h, with the start of the 6 h aligned to the moment of propofol administration.

The EEG signal was preprocessed in order to remove bad electrode contact artifacts (impedance exceeding 10 kΩ) and motion artifacts, observed as peaks in the EEG impedance. Due to the different temporal characteristics between the NIRS and EEG signal, we used the running root mean squared (RMS) of the EEG, which is a continuous estimate of EEG power. More specifically, the RMS value was computed using a window length of 5 s and an overlap of 4 s, producing a new value every second. The window length of 5 s was defined in order to assess EEG delta activity.

Table 1 Stratification of the original study group into two subgroups, based on the presence of brain abnormalities on a routine ultrasound scan. For each group characteristic, the median value is presented, together with the interquartile range (in brackets). The *p*-value was computed using the Wilcoxon rank-sum test

	Population		
	Without brain injury ($n = 15$)	With brain injury ($n = 6$)	*p*-value
Postmenstrual age (weeks)	30 (29–30.5)	29.5 (28.25–30)	0.5471
Postnatal age (days)	1 (1–1)	1 (1–1.75)	0.1247
Propofol dose (mg/kg)	1 (1–1.50)	1 (0.625–1.75)	0.6285

The study group consisted of 21 premature neonates, stratified into two groups based on the presence of brain abnormalities, observed on routine ultrasound scans. More information on the study group is presented in Table 1.

3 Methods

We use TE to assess the NVC. TE measures the amount of information transferred from one signal (process) to another. More specifically, the TE from one signal X to another signal Y is the amount of uncertainty that is reduced in future values of Y by knowing the past values of X given the past values of Y. Mathematically, if X and Y denote two discrete-time signals, the TE is defined as:

$$T_{X\to Y} = H\left(Y_n | Y_n^-\right) - H\left(Y_n |, X_n^- |, Y_n^-\right)$$

where Y_n, $Y_n^- = Y_{(n-1:n-L)}, X_n^- = X_{(n-1:n-L)}$ denote the signal Y at time n, the past of Y and the past of X, respectively, and H denotes the conditional Shannon entropy, which is defined as

$$H\left(Y_n | Y_n^-\right) = -\sum_{i,j} p\left(y_i, y_j^-\right) \log \frac{p\left(y_i, y_j^-\right)}{p\left(y_j^-\right)}$$

where $p\left(y_i, y_j^-\right)$ is the probability that $Y_n = y_i$ *and* $Y_n^- = y_j^-$.

In the present analysis, the TE is estimated by binning the original time series, which allows us to estimate the probability density functions (PDF) required to compute the TE. This approach is very general, since no model is assumed for the data. Therefore, this approach also takes into account nonlinear interactions. Moreover, uniform embedding with dimension $L = 10$ was used to capture the past of the signals. In order to assess the statistical significance ($p < 0.05$) of the TE values, we used surrogate data, obtained by randomly shuffling the original signals. Since the TE is a non-symmetric measure, two different thresholds were defined. The TE curves are computed using a window of 15 min with an overlap of 10 min, producing a new value every 5 min.

Two features are computed from the resulting TE curves in order to quantify the effect of propofol on the TE curves: the minimal value M and the maximal deviation Δ from baseline. These feature values are computed in the first 3 h of the analysis window. Baseline level is defined as the median value of the last 3 h of the analysis window. Since propofol is considered to be washed out after 3 h, we assume that the baseline level presents an indication for the background, reference NVC.

4 Results

In Fig. 1, the median TE curves are presented for the cohort of neonates without (solid circles) and with brain injury (open circles). The significance of the TE values is defined by a randomly shuffling of the data (Monte Carlo simulation), which leads to the significance thresholds depicted in Fig. 1. The Wilcoxon rank-sum test indicates that $T_{\mathrm{EEG} \rightarrow \mathrm{NIRS}}$ is significantly higher than $T_{\mathrm{NIRS} \rightarrow \mathrm{EEG}}$ ($p < 0.001$).

Figure 2 shows a comparison between the group of neonates without (white boxplots) and with (gray boxplots) brain injuries based on the features M and Δ. In addition, the baseline level is also compared between the two groups. Resulting p-values are equal to 0.259, 0.845 and 0.039 for features M, Δ and the baseline, respectively, which indicates that the response to propofol is comparable in both groups (features M and Δ), while background NVC (baseline) might be lower in neonates with brain injury.

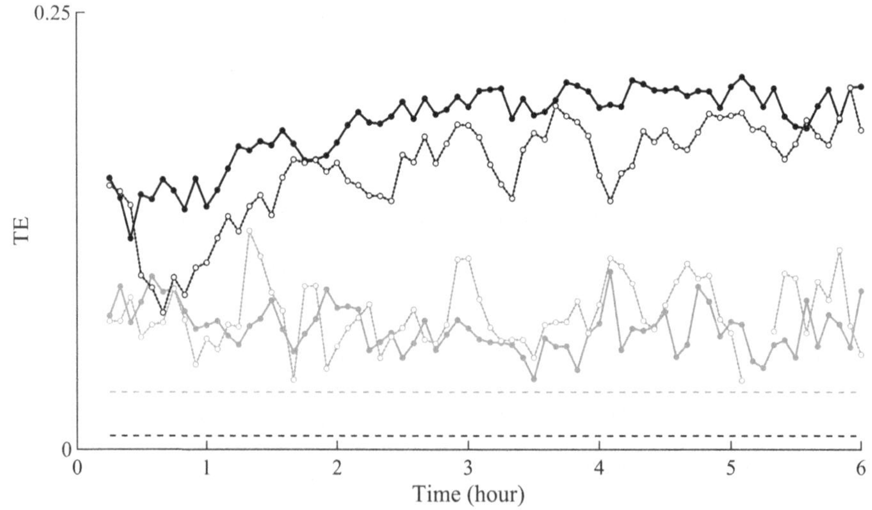

Fig. 1 TE curves after administration of propofol at $t = 0$; $T_{\mathrm{NIRS} \rightarrow \mathrm{EEG}}$ and $T_{\mathrm{EEG} \rightarrow \mathrm{NIRS}}$ are depicted in gray and black, respectively. The solid circles represent the median values for normal neonates, while the open circles indicate the abnormal group. The dashed lines indicate the significance levels ($p < 0.05$) for the TE values, obtained by surrogate data analysis

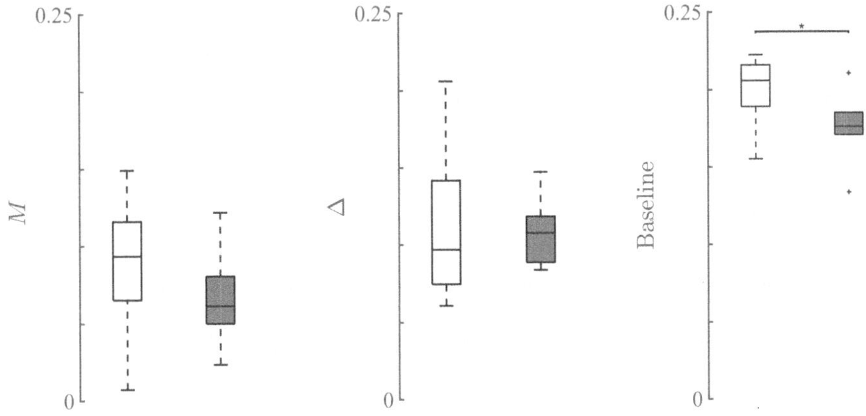

Fig. 2 Comparison of feature and baseline values between the normal and abnormal neonates; M, Δ, and baseline indicate the minimal value, the maximal deviation from baseline and baseline values, respectively. White and gray boxplot indicate the group without and with brain injury, respectively

5 Discussion and Conclusions

In this study, we found that the transfer of information, quantified by means of TE, is larger in the direction from EEG to NIRS than from NIRS to EEG. This indicates that changes in EEG amplitude are likely to precede changes in NIRS. In other words: changes in brain function trigger changes in brain hemodynamics and metabolism, which is in agreement with the NVC of the adult brain. It is however important to note that the transfer of information NIRS to EEG is not zero, indicating a flow of information also in this direction. This might be caused by the feedback mechanisms that are in charge of the regulation of brain metabolism, i.e. the delivery of nutrients and oxygen to meet the metabolic demand.

In a previous study, we measured the coupling between NIRS and EEG using a linear model to compute TE [6]. The results indicated that changes in brain oxygenation were likely to precede changes in amplitude of EEG activity. This contradicts the results we obtained in the present study. The non-parametric approach to compute TE, used in this study, estimates all the transfer of information from one process to another, including the linear and non-linear part. Taking this into account, and the results presented in [6], we can conclude that the linear model for TE is not able to model the nonlinear processes involved in NVC which, once taken into account, determine a different directionality in the flow of information. In addition, the nonlinear TE is able to capture the effect of propofol in the NVC, which was not observed using the linear model. These results indicate that it is possible that there are two different mechanisms affecting NVC, one acting on its linear part, and another one explained more by a non-linear process.

In Fig. 1, lowered values of EEG to NIRS coupling are observed, which consequently increase to a steady baseline value in all patients in the study group. Propofol induces a reversible state of diminished responsiveness behaviorally similar to quiet sleep, which is characterized by a more discontinuous EEG and is associated with lower fractional tissue oxygenation extraction (FTOE) values. This indicates lower brain oxygen consumption, which could explain the reduced EEG to NIRS interaction. Based on visual inspection of Fig. 1, it appears that the reduction in EEG to NIRS coupling is more severe for the cohort of abnormal neonates. A more in-depth study, based on the feature values of M and Δ, presented in Fig. 2, indicates that there is no significant difference in response between the healthy neonates and the neonates with brain injury. The NIRS to EEG coupling is not influenced by propofol.

The TE baseline values, presented in Fig. 2, were observed to be significantly lower in the cohort of neonates with brain injury. A lower TE indicates a less functional NVC. Thus, the cerebral vascular network in the neonates with brain injury is less able to compensate for increased metabolism resulting from neuronal activation. These results are in agreement with a study from Mahmoudzadeh et al., who observed a less functional NVC in preterm neonates with intraventricular hemorrhage (IVH) compared to healthy neonates [8]. In addition, Chalak et al. observed a significantly lower NVC in newborns with neonatal encephalopathy (NE) compared to a healthy control group, assessed by means of wavelet coherence [9]. These studies point out that brain abnormalities alter the NVC, and that this alteration in NVC can be captured using signal processing techniques combining NIRS and EEG measurements. Therefore, we have shown that the nonlinear TE can be used as a physiological marker to guide therapeutic decision-making or predict neurological outcome. However, further studies are needed in order to validate this methodology in a larger cohort of neonates, using a different clinical model.

Acknowledgments Dries Hendrikx is a SB PhD fellow at the Fonds voor Wetenschappelijk Onderzoek (FWO) Vlaanderen. This research was also supported by Bijzonder Onderzoeksfonds KU Leuven (BOF): SPARKLE – Sensor-based Platform for the Accurate and Remote monitoring of Kinematics Linked to E-health #: IDO-13-0358, The effect of perinatal stress on the later outcome in preterm babies #: C24/15/036 and TARGID – Development of a novel diagnostic medical device to assess gastric motility #: C32-16-00364. Fonds voor Wetenschappelijk Onderzoek-Vlaanderen (FWO): Hercules Foundation (AKUL 043) 'Flanders BCI Lab – High-End, Modular EEG Equipment for Brain Computer Interfacing'. Agentschap Innoveren en Ondernemen (IWT): O&O HBC 2016 0184 eWatch. imec funds 2017. imec ICO projects: ICON HBC.2016.0167, 'SeizeIt'. Belgian Foreign Affairs-Development Cooperation: VLIR UOS programs (2013-2019). EU: European Union's Seventh Framework Programme (FP7/2007-2013): The HIP Trial: #260777. ERAMUS+: INGDIVS 2016-1 SE01-KA203-022114. European Research Council: The research leading to these results has received funding from the European Research Council under the European Union's Seventh Framework Programme (FP7/2007-2013) / ERC Advanced Grant: BIOTENSORS (no 339804). This paper reflects only the author's views and the Union is not liable for any use that may be made of the contained information. EU H2020-FETOPEN 'AMPHORA' #766456.

References

1. Arichi T, Moraux A, Melendez A et al (2010) Somatosensory cortical activation identified by functional MRI in preterm and term infants. NeuroImage 49:2063–2071
2. Liao S, Gregg N, White B et al (2010) Neonatal hemodynamic response to visual cortex activity: high-density near-infrared spectroscopy study. J Biomed Opt 15:1–9
3. Kozberg M, Chen B, Deleo S et al (2013) Resolving the transition from negative to positive blood oxygen level-dependent responses in the developing brain. Proc Natl Acad Sci 110:4380–4385
4. Zehendner C, Tsohataridis S, Luhmann H et al (2013) Developmental switch in neurovascular coupling in the immature rodent barrel cortex. PLoS One 8:e80749
5. Smits A, Thewissen L, Caicedo A et al (2016) Propofol dose-finding to reach optimal effect for (semi-)elective intubation in neonates. J Pediatr 179:54–60
6. Caicedo A, Thewissen L, Smits A et al (2016) Changes in oxygenation levels precede changes in amplitude of the EEG in premature infants. Adv Exp Med Biol 923:143–149
7. Mahmoudzadeh M, Dehaene-Lambertz G, Kongolo G et al (2018) Consequence of intraventricular hemorrhage on neurovascular coupling evoked by speech syllables in preterm neonates. Dev Cog Neurosc 30:60–69
8. Chalak L, Fenghua T, Beverley A-H et al (2017) Novel wavelet real time analysis of neurovascular coupling in neonatal encephalopathy. Sci Rep 7:45958

Reference Value of Brain Tissue Oxygen Saturation in Newborns Immediately After Birth

Ryota Kato, Shigeharu Hosono, and Syori Takahashi

Abstract The Consensus on Resuscitation Science and Treatment Recommendations indicate the target SpO2 values during the first 10 min of life. There are a few studies of values of brain regional saturation of oxygen (rSO2) in newborns, conventional instruments are large and not suitable for measuring in the delivery room. The purpose of this study was to develop reference values for brain rSO2 up to 10 min after birth and to review the changes in cerebral oxygenation in late preterm and term newborn infants immediately after birth. **Method:** We evaluated both brain rSO2 and SpO2 at 1, 3, 5 and 10 min after birth in 100 neonates. rSO2, was measured at the forehead using a finger-mounted oximeter. This is 1/100 the size of conventional NIRS and can be carried. To measure SpO2, a Radical-7 was used. This study was approved by the institutional review board at our hospital. **Results:** The gestational age and birth weight were 37.9 ± 1.2 weeks and 2825 ± 429 g, respectively. Eighty-seven infants and 13 infants were term and late preterm infants, respectively, and there were 21 vaginal deliveries and 79 cesarean sections. In all cases, rSO2 levels were measured at 1, 3, 5, and 10 min after birth. For the SpO2 measurements, nine cases at 1 min, 40 cases at 3 min, 81 cases at 5 min and 93 cases at 10 min were available. The median rSO2 level was 43% at 1 min after birth, 48% at 3 min, 52% at 5 min and 57% at 10 min. **Conclusion**: We used a finger-mounted oximeter to observe changes in brain rSO2 values of 100 normal transition infants. It was easier to detect rSO2 in comparison to the peripheral oxygen saturation monitored by our pulse oximeter. Brain rSO2 values might be useful to evaluate oxygenation immediately after birth.

Keywords Neonatal cardio-pulmonary resuscitation · Near-infrared spectroscopy · Regional saturation of oxygen · SpO2 · Brain Oxygenation

R. Kato (✉) · S. Hosono · S. Takahashi
Department of Pediatrics and Child Health, Nihon University School of Medicine, Chiyoda, Japan

© Springer Nature Switzerland AG 2020

P.-D. Ryu et al. (eds.), *Oxygen Transport to Tissue XLI*, Advances in Experimental Medicine and Biology 1232, https://doi.org/10.1007/978-3-030-34461-0_3

1 Introduction

The Japan Society of Perinatal and Neonatal Medicine aims to establish a system that allows medical staff who have acquired neonatal resuscitation skills to attend all neonates as staff in charge of neonatal care. The society established the Japanese version of the Neonatal Cardio-Pulmonary Resuscitation (NCPR) dissemination project in July 2007. We have developed and implemented resuscitation guidelines in accordance with the International Resuscitation Liaison Committee Consensus 2005, and these are revised every 5 years; the current resuscitation guidelines conform to Consensus 2015. Target SpO_2 values are stated as 1 min 60%, 3 min 70%, 5 min 80%, and 10 min 90%. Since the arterial duct remains open in neonates immediately after birth, there is a possibility of measuring the SpO_2 of arteriovenous mixed blood in the limbs other than the right upper limb. Therefore, measurement of SpO_2 is to be performed on the right upper limb. However, it is unknown whether SpO_2 measured in the right upper limb reflects brain tissue oxygenation. Thus, an index of brain tissue oxygenation is considered necessary. Tissue oxygenation is typically assessed by measuring regional saturation of oxygen (rSO_2) using near-infrared spectroscopy (NIRS). Changes in SpO_2 during neonatal transition were reported by Dawson et al. Median SpO_2 values in 468 term infants were 68, 66, 81, 88, 92, 94, 95, and 96 for 1 min from 1 to 10 min after birth [1]. Devices using the spatial decomposition method are widely used in NIRS which is currently on sale, and various reports have been made using these. Changes in brain rSO_2 have been reported for several minutes after birth [2–4]. G Pichler, Zhou CL et al. have conducted several studies on rSO_2 levels in the brain immediately after birth [5, 6]. However due to the difference in measurement depth due to the difference in measurement equipment and the spread of NCPR, the reference value of rSO_2 immediately after birth has not been clearly defined since the resuscitation algorithm in the delivery room is different from before. In recent years, a diagnostic finger-mounted oximeter (Toccare KN-15; Astem Co., Kawasaki, Japan) was developed by Kanayama and Ninwahama [7]. The instrument has a probe with a small NIRS sensor attached to the finger of the operator and is 100th the size of a conventional device. The principle of measurement is the spatial resolution method, using near-infrared light at 770 nm and 830 nm. With this instrument, we measured the rSO_2 of the head of the fetus immediately before parturition and reported correlations with umbilical cord blood pH [7]. During neonatal resuscitation, the only index used for objective oxygenation assessment is SpO_2, and the relationship between SpO_2 and prognosis has not been studied. We clarified the rSO_2 changes for up to 10 min after birth in 100 neonates who did not need resuscitation, and developed reference values.

2 Methods

This is a prospective observational study of neonates of gestational age > 34 weeks and < 42 weeks between October 2015 and July 2017 at the Nihon University Itabashi Hospital. Exclusion criteria were (1) major anomaly (lethal malformation, chromosomal abnormality, congenital bone disease or visceral morphological abnormality such as intracranial, heart, or kidney, or diagnosis of fetal edema, (2) multiple pregnancy, (3) meconium-stained amniotic fluid or oligohydramnios, (4) neonatal asphyxia requiring resuscitation, and (5) infants with a disease affecting oxygen saturation at birth.

The examiner was placed independently from the person in charge of resuscitation, and the resuscitator performed resuscitation according to the current NCPR Consensus 2015. The SpO_2 probe was then attached to the right hand or right wrist and the heart rate was measured together with SpO_2. rSO_2 measurements were performed at 1, 3, 5, and 10 min after birth, at positions 2 cm each to the left and right from the center of the forehead of the infant. There was no left-right difference in the rSO_2 of the forehead in the preliminary test. The index finger-mounted oximeter Toccare KN-15 oximeter was used to obtain measurements of rSO_2. This is 1/100 the size of conventional NIRS and can be carried. In this device, the distance from the light source to the detector is set at 6, 8 mm. This position has the same sensitivity of the scalp and brain tissue, and the tissue oxygen saturation just below 5 mm from the body surface can be measured. The presence or absence and ratio of rSO_2, SpO_2 measurable examples at 1, 3, 5, and 10 min after birth, and the changes in each parameter for up to 10 min were evaluated. A regression curve was generated at the 3rd, 10th, 50th, 75th, 90th, and 97th percentile for rSO_2 of the term infants. This study was approved by the Institutional Review Board of the Nihon University Itabashi Hospital (RK-150714-1), and written informed consent was obtained from parents before the birth. Statistical analysis was performed with JMP14 (SAS Institute Japan Ltd.).

3 Results

Measurements were made on 100 subjects (59 boys, 41 girls); 88 and 12 were term infants and late preterm (34 weeks–36 weeks 6 days), respectively (Table 1). In 8 cases, oxygen administration was needed after resuscitation, and 12 cases were excluded from analysis because of meconium-stained amniotic fluid.

In all cases, rSO_2 was measurable at 1, 3, 5, and 10 min after birth, whereas SpO_2 was 9 at 1 min, 40 at 3 min, 81 at 5 min, and 93 at 10 min.

From 1 min after birth to 10 min after birth, $y = 1.23X + 23.03$ is shown in the primary regression equation, and rSO_2 and SpO_2 showed a positive correlation

Table 1 Characteristics of the study population

Full term	88 (88)
Male	59 (59)
Gestational age (weeks)	38.3 ± 1.2
Birth weight (g)	2812 ± 432
Vaginal delivery	21 (21)
Umbilical artery blood gas analysis	
pH	7.4 ± 0.4
PCO_2 (mmHg)	25.2 ± 6.2
Base excess (mmol/L)	22.8 ± 3.1
Apgar score	
1 min	8 (7–9)
5 min	9 (8–9)

Mean ± SD (%)

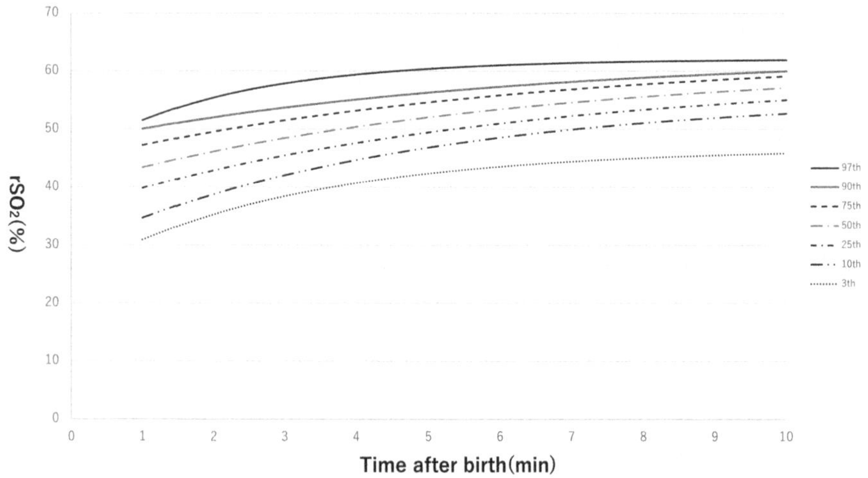

Fig. 1 rSO2 transition up to 10 min post-partum using logistic parametric analysis.

(R^2 = 0.53). Regression curves of the 3rd, 10th, 25th, 50th, 75th, 90th, and 97th percentile values of rSO_2 at 1–10 min after birth of one term infant are shown in Fig. 1. These percentile values were similar to the logarithmic regression curve as well as the quadratic regression curve (R^2 = 0.95–0.99).

4 Discussion

We examined the changes in postnatal rSO_2 in transitional neonates requiring no resuscitation by using the Toccare KN-15 finger-mounted oximeter. Changes in rSO_2 from 1 to 10 min after birth were examined in 100 cases; to our knowledge, this is the largest number of cases. In this study, rSO_2 on the forehead was in the range of 31–63%, the mean rSO_2 value was 43% in 1 min and 56% in 10 min. This value increased with time after birth and tended to reach a plateau at around 60% at 8–10 min after birth and was consistent with the values reported by Watanabe et al. [3], measured using similar equipment. G Pichler measured rSO2 in the brain from 2–15 min after birth of 381 healthy neonates using INVOS-5000 and reported a median of 79% (65–90) at 10 min after birth. In addition, Zhou CL et al. Measured the rSO2 of the brain from the first day to the third day of birth of 223 healthy neonates using NIRS called TSAH-100, and reported a normal range of 62 ± 2%. Both values were different from this study. It is conceivable that the measuring algorithm differs depending on the instrument, so that there is a difference in the measuring depth. Also, in this study, resuscitation treatment is being performed in compliance with the latest NCPR 2015. NCPR 2015 also refers to body temperature control that was not conventionally stated, and it is possible that changes in body temperature during resuscitation have also influenced cerebral blood flow.

In this study, it was difficult to measure SpO_2 in the majority of cases from 1 to 3 min after birth. Dawson et al. reported that 63% of neonates at 1 min, 43% at 3 min, and 40% at 5 min could not be measured [1]. In pulse oximetry, it is necessary to fix the probes of the light-emitting part and the light-receiving part so that the finger or the palm of the subject is sandwiched between the two, and the positions of the light emitting part and the light receiving part are adjusted so as not to shift. On the other hand, measurement of rSO_2 using a diagnostic finger-mounted oximeter was convenient because it only involved placing the probe on the forehead and was measurable in all cases. Although it is difficult to evaluate SpO_2 for up to 3 min after birth, rSO_2 was measurable from 1 min after birth, and rSO_2 was considered to be more useful for early postnatal evaluation. In this study, rSO_2 and SpO_2 showed a positive correlation up to 10 min after birth, and as a postnatal monitoring index, rSO_2 measurement using a diagnostic finger-mounted oximeter appeared to be useful. However, since the pulse oximeter measures arterial oxygen saturation around the limb, rSO_2 is representative of central tissue oxygen saturation and is completely different, so the relation between rSO_2 and SpO_2 after 10 min postnatally should be studied in the future. From this present study, measurement of frontal rSO_2 using the finger-mounted oximeter Toccare KN-15 can evaluate brain oxygenation more conveniently than SpO_2 and is a useful index for postnatal monitoring of neonates. It is measured in only healthy neonates, and cases where oxygenation is impaired, such as respiratory disorder, neonatal asphyxia, and in preterm infants before 34 weeks gestation; it is not measured in very low birth weight infants or less. It is therefore considered possible in the future to investigate the necessity of oxygen therapy and the optimal administration method by measuring rSO_2 trends after birth even at a gestational age of 34 weeks or earlier. Because rSO_2 measurements can theoretically be obtained, even in conditions such as peripheral circulatory insufficiency and cardiac arrest, unlike pulse oximetry, it is necessary to investigate the effects of resuscitation on rSO_2 in infants with neonatal asphyxia. The relationship between rSO_2 shown here and neurological prognosis from 1 to 10 min is unknown and requires future studies.

5 Limitation

Toccare KN-15 is smaller than the conventional NIRS, the measurement depth is shallow. Therefore, there is a possibility that the measurement site is not the brain tissue but only the surface layer.

6 Conclusion

In neonates immediately after birth, Measurement of rSO_2 using portable NIRS was positively correlated with SpO_2 and were measured more easily than pulse oximetry. SpO_2 measures arterial components and rSO_2 measures the oxygenation of tissues where venous components are predominant. In NIRS, brain oxygenation can be evaluated directly, which seemed to be more useful than SpO2 in this respect. Although this value is considered to be a useful reference in neonatal resuscitation, evaluation of long-term prognosis is indispensable for final determination of its adequacy.

References

1. Dawson JA, Kamlin CO, Vento M et al (2010) Defining the reference for oxygen saturation for infants after birth. Pediatrics 125:e1340–e1347
2. Isobe K, Kusaka T, Fujiwara Y et al (2002) Measurement of cerebral oxygenations in neonates after vaginal delivery and cesarean section using full-spectrum near infrared spectroscopy. Comp Biochem Physiol A Moi integr Physiol 132:133–138
3. Watanabe T, Ito M, Miyake F et al (2017) Measurement of brain tissue oxygen saturation in term infants using a new portable near-infrared spectroscopy device. Pediatr Inter 59:167–170
4. Mari M, Toshiyuki U, Hiroaki I et al (2017) Tissue oxygen saturation levels from fetus to neonate. J Obstet Gynaecol Res 43:855–859
5. Pichler G, Binder C, Avian A et al (2013) Reference ranges for regional cerebral tissue oxygen saturation and fractional oxygen extraction in neonates during immediate transition after birth. J Pediatr 163(6):1558–1563
6. Zhou CL, Liu YF, Zhang JJ et al (2009) Measurement of brain regional oxygen saturation in neonates in China: a multicenter randomized clinical trial. Zhonghua Er Ke Za Zhi 47:517–522
7. Kanayama N, Niwayama M (2014) Examiner's finger-mounted fetal tissue oximetry. J Biomed Opt 19:067008

Changes in Brain Tissue Oxygenation and Metabolism During Rewarming After Neonatal Encephalopathy are Related to Electrical Abnormality

Subhabrata Mitra, Gemma Bale, Isabel de Roever, Judith Meek, Nicola J. Robertson, and Ilias Tachtsidis

Abstract Hypoxic ischemic encephalopathy (HIE) leads to significant mortality and morbidity, and therapeutic hypothermia (TH) has become a standard of care following HIE. After TH, the body temperature is brought back to 37 °C. Early electroencephalography (EEG) is a reliable outcome biomarker following HIE. We hypothesized that changes in cerebral oxidative metabolism, measured as Δ[oxCCO], in relation to changes in brain tissue oxygenation (measured as Δ[HbD]) during rewarming will correlate with injury severity as evidenced on amplitude integrated EEG/EEG at initial presentation. Broadband near-infrared spectroscopy (NIRS) and systemic data were collected during rewarming from 14 infants following HIE over a mean period of 12.5 h. All infants were monitored with video EEG telemetry using a standard neonatal montage. aEEG and EEG background was classified into mild, moderate and severely abnormal groups based on the background pattern. Two infants had mild, 6 infants had moderate and another 6 infants had severe abnormality at presentation. The relationship between [oxCCO] and [HbD] was evaluated between two groups of infants with abnormal electrical activity (mild vs moderate to severe). A significant difference was noted between the groups in the relationship between [oxCCO] and [HbD] (as r^2) ($p = 0.02$). This result indicates that the mitochondrial injury and deranged oxidative metabolism persists in the moderate to severely abnormal group during rewarming.

Keywords Hypoxic ischaemic encephalopathy · Cerebral metabolism · Near-infrared spectroscopy · Cerebral metabolism · Cerebral oxygenation

S. Mitra (✉) · J. Meek · N. J. Robertson
Institute for Women's Health, University College London and Neonatal Unit, University College London Hospitals Trust, London, UK
e-mail: subhabrata.mitra.13@ucl.ac.uk

G. Bale · I. de Roever · I. Tachtsidis
Department of Medical Physics and Biomedical Engineering, University College London, London, UK

© Springer Nature Switzerland AG 2020

P.-D. Ryu et al. (eds.), *Oxygen Transport to Tissue XLI*, Advances in Experimental Medicine and Biology 1232, https://doi.org/10.1007/978-3-030-34461-0_4

1 Introduction

Perinatal hypoxic-ischaemic (HI) brain injury causes significant morbidity and mortality. TH is beneficial following HIE and has become the standard of care in recent years [1, 2]. During TH, body temperature is lowered to 33.5 °C and maintained over 72 h, followed by a slow rewarming that brings body temperature back to 37 °C over 14 h. Rewarming is an important physiological process. Early rewarming induces neuronal apoptosis following HIE [3]. Rebound seizures have been noted during rewarming period both in an animal model [5] and neonatal intensive care [4] and further 'cooling' with slower rewarming has been beneficial. Changes in cerebral metabolism and hemodynamics have been investigated in both a preclinical model and clinical studies during and after HI, but the dynamic effects of rewarming on newborn cerebral metabolism and hemodynamics have not yet been fully investigated. We earlier reported that the relationship between mitochondrial metabolism and cerebral oxygenation becomes more impaired with rising severity of injury [5].

Using a broadband NIRS system, we monitored changes in oxidised cytochrome-c-oxidase (Δ[oxCCO]), oxy-haemoglobin ($\Delta[HbO_2]$) and deoxy-haemoglobin (Δ[HHb]) in neonatal brain in a cohort of infants following HIE [6]. Cytochrome-c-oxidase (CCO) is the terminal electron acceptor in the electron transport chain (ETC) and changes in its redox state indicates the state of mitochondrial oxidative metabolism and ATP synthesis [7]. Changes in total haemoglobin ($HbT = HbO_2 + HHb$) and haemoglobin difference ($HbD = HbO_2 - HHb$) were derived. Changes in HbD and HbT reflect changes in cerebral oxygenation and changes in cerebral blood volume, respectively.

Following HIE, aEEG and EEG together are an early reliable early predictor of neurodevelopmental outcome [8].

The aim of this study was to assess the cerebral metabolic and haemodynamic changes during the rewarming period in a cohort of term infants following perinatal hypoxic-ischaemic brain injury, and compare with early injury severity assessed on aEEG and EEG. We hypothesized that the dynamic changes in cerebral oxygenation and metabolism during the rewarming period would relate to the injury severity assessed by aEEG/EEG.

2 Methods

This prospective observational study was approved by the research ethics committee of University College London Hospital and London Bloomsbury REC. Informed written consent was provided by parents before each study. Therapeutic hypothermia and subsequent rewarming were instituted with a servo-controlled cooling machine (Tecotherm Neo, Inspiration Healthcare, UK). Normally, the core temperature is increased by 0.5 °C over each 2-h period during rewarming. Rewarming data were collected from a cohort of 14 infants. Broadband NIRS monitoring was commenced as early as possible in the rewarming phase and was continued for the maximum possible period and data were collected at 1 Hz. The optode source-detector distance of 2.5 cm was chosen to ensure a good depth penetration [9] with a differential path length (DPF) of 4.99 [10] which was corrected for the wavelength-dependency of the pathlength. The changes in chromophore concentrations were calculated from the measured changes in broadband NIR light attenuation using the modified Beer-Lambert law as applied with the UCLn algorithm [11] across 136 wavelengths (770-906 nm). Systemic data were collected using ixTrend software (ixellence GmbH, Germany) and were synchronised with the broadband NIRS data.

3 Data Analysis

Systemic data were down-sampled and interpolated to the NIRS data timeframe (1 Hz). Artefacts from movement or changes in external lighting were removed and baseline shifts were corrected on MATLAB (Mathworks, USA). using the method suggested by Scholkmann et al. [12]. No significant difference was noted between the two sides in the broadband NIRS data and data from the left side was used for analysis. Linear regression analysis was performed to assess the relationship between Δ[oxCCO] and Δ[HbD] and an averaged regression coefficient (r^2) was created to compare this relationship between groups. All statistical analyses were performed using GraphPad Prism 6 (GraphPad Software, USA) (Fig. 1)

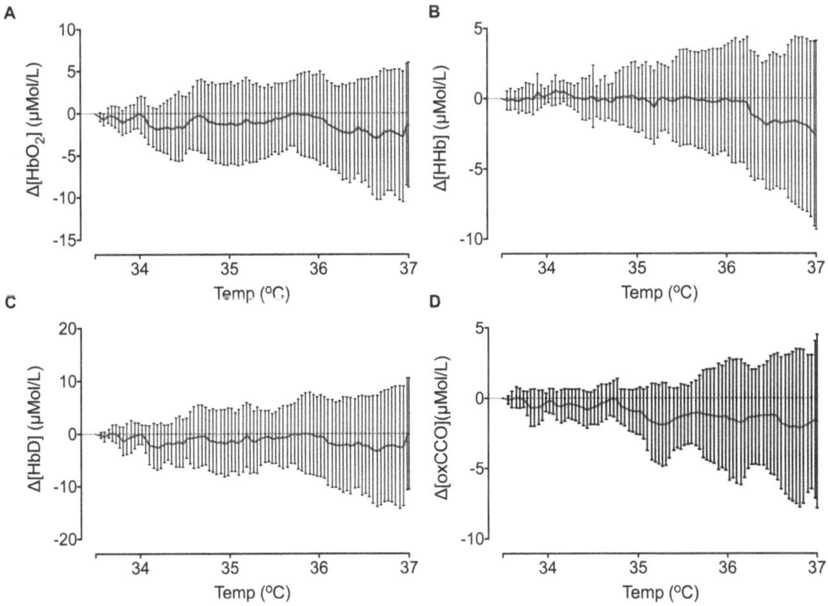

Fig. 1 Changes in [HbO_2] (**A**), [HHb] (**B**), [HbD] (**C**) and [oxCCO] (**D**) during rewarming period in all infants measured on the left side as mean ± s.d. Please note that the x-axis presents a time scale of 14 h over which the temperature was increased from 33.5 °C to 37 °C

4 Results

NIRS and systemic data were collected over a mean period of 12.5 (5–14) h. Active cooling was started at a mean of 3 h of age. All infants were ventilated during rewarming. During rewarming the heart rate gradually increased from a mean of 108/min (range 75–130/min) to 128/min (121–135/min). The peripheral oxygen saturation (SpO_2) fell briefly at the start of rewarming, but was mostly over 95%. Mean BP was stable through out the rewarming (45–55 mm Hg). The averaged regression coefficient (r^2) between Δ[oxCCO] and Δ[HbD] were calculated.

All infants had some degree of abnormal electrical activity in the initial recording. Two infants had mild abnormality (normal aEEG upper (>10 μV) and lower border (>5 μV), but low amplitude EEG), 6 infants had moderately abnormal background (abnormal aEEG upper and/or lower margin with EEG discontinuity) and another 6 infants had severe abnormality (abnormal aEEG voltage with discontinuous or flat EEG trace) (Table 1). Some of the moderate and severely abnormal traces recovered during therapeutic hypothermia. Relationships between [oxCCO] and [HbD] were evaluated between two groups of abnormal electrical activity (mild vs moderate to severe) measured in the first hour after starting active cooling. A significant difference was noted between the groups in the relationship between [oxCCO] and [HbD] (as r^2) ($p = 0.02$, Mann-Whitney test) (Fig. 2).

Table 1 Initial aEEG/EEG characteristics and relationship between [oxCCO] and [HbD] (r^2 values). (n = 14)

Study No	Initial electrical activity	[oxCCO] vs [HbD] (r^2)
1	Severely abnormal	0.0100
2	Severely abnormal	0.2100
3	Mildly abnormal	0.0018
4	Moderately abnormal	0.7900
5	Severely abnormal	0.0100
6	Severely abnormal	0.6400
7	Moderately abnormal	0.1500
8	Moderately abnormal	0.4800
9	Severely abnormal	0.5500
10	Moderately abnormal	0.4300
11	Mildly abnormal	0.0096
12	Severely abnormal	0.3700
13	Moderately abnormal	0.7000
14	Moderately abnormal	0.6900

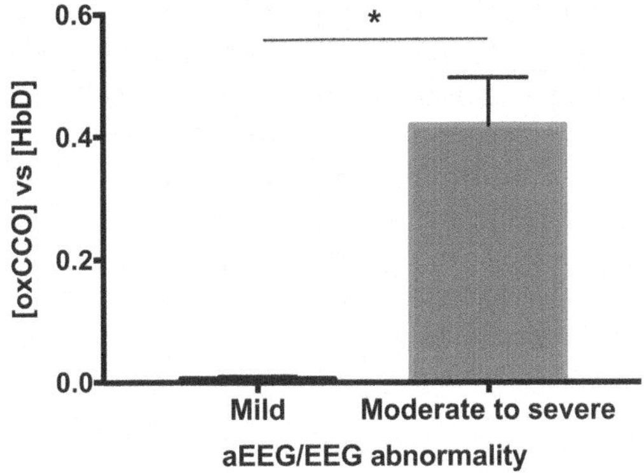

Fig. 2 Relationship between [oxCCO] and [HbD] (as r^2) differed between the two groups of abnormal electrical activity (mild vs moderate to severe) ($p = 0.02$)

5 Discussion

The relationship between cerebral metabolism and oxygenation measured during rewarming following TH in a group of infants with HIE became stronger with increasing degree of brain injury, measured as aEEG/EEG abnormality at presentation. This indicates a higher oxygen dependency of the cerebral metabolism with increasing severity of injury. Availability of oxygen has a considerable influence on the oxidation of CCO. The results imply a significant mitochondrial injury and low cerebral metabolic rate in neonatal brain following moderate to severe hypoxic ischaemic injury persists even after TH during rewarming in comparison to neonates with evidence of mild brain injury at presentation.

There was no significant pattern of changes in Δ[oxCCO] with change in temperature, nor did we notice any specific cut-off temperature point which indicated any change in the trend of cerebral metabolism during rewarming.

We recently showed that the degree of injury severity was not predictable with changes in cerebral oxygenation or haemodynamics alone [13]. In near-term foetal sheep, carotid artery blood flow (CaBF) and mean arterial blood pressure (MABP) changed only transiently during rewarming. No significant difference was noted from 6 h onwards [3]. Peng et al. also described that, asphyxiated newborn infants had stable regional cerebral oxygenation during rewarming [14]. Our data suggest that broadband NIRS-derived measurement of cerebral oxidative metabolism can be a useful cot-side indicator of changes in mitochondrial oxidative metabolism following HIE.

Bale et al. showed that a strong relationship exists between cerebral metabolism and oxygenation during spontaneous desaturation episodes in infants with severe HIE [15]. Impairment of cerebral energy metabolism following HIE is well documented and the degree of the metabolic disturbance is related to subsequent neurodevelopmental outcome [16]. Impairment of cerebral oxidative metabolism is also evidenced with increased cerebral lactate following perinatal HI during secondary energy failure and beyond [17]. A biphasic pattern of changes in the redox state of oxCCO has been documented in both clinical [16] and preclinical studies [18].

The point of change in this biphasic pattern has been described as the point when ETC becomes significantly suppressed leading to reduction and failure of ATP production. It is likely that in severe HIE, apoptotic changes and progressive cell death impairs the mitochondrial capacity resulting in the need for a higher tissue oxygenation or increased oxygen tissue gradient [15]. In infants with mild brain injury, mitochondria are likely to have a lower oxygen saturation threshold and the oxygen tension is above the value at which their redox state becomes oxygen dependent, thus the correlation (r^2) between oxCCO and HbD is low.

The limitation of this study is the small number of infants enrolled, as it is not possible to generalize our findings from this study before testing it in a larger cohort.

We noted that the mitochondrial metabolism-oxygenation coupling during rewarming was influenced by the severity of hypoxic ischemic brain injury. This has the potential to become a useful cot-side biomarker of outcome in infants with HIE.

Acknowledgments We thank all the families and neonatal staff in UCLH for their support. This project was supported by EPSRC (EP/G037256/1), The Wellcome Trust (088429/Z/09/Z and 104580/Z/14/Z) and UK Department of Health's NIHR BRC funding scheme.

References

1. NICE (2010) Therapeutic hypothermia with intracorporeal temperature monitoring for hypoxic perinatal brain injury. http://www.nice.org.uk/guidance/ipg347/chapter/1-guidance. Committee on fetus and newborn. American Academy of Pediatrics (2014) Hypothermia and Neonatal Encephalopathy. Pediatrics 133(6): 1146–1150
2. Gerrits LC, Battin MR, Bennet L et al (2005) Epileptiform activity during rewarming from moderate cerebral hypothermia in the near-term fetal sheep. Pediatr Res 57(3):342–346
3. Wang B, Armstrong JS, Lee JH et al (2015) Rewarming from therapeutic hypothermia induces cortical neuron apoptosis in a swine model of neonatal hypoxic-ischemic encephalopathy. J Cereb Blood Flow Metab 35(5):781–793
4. Kendall GS, Mathieson S, Meek J et al (2012) Recooling for rebound seizures after rewarming in neonatal encephalopathy. Pediatrics 130(2):e451–e455
5. Mitra S, Bale G, Meek J et al (2016) Relationship between cerebral oxygenation and metabolism during rewarming in newborn infantafter therapeutic hypothermia following hypoxic-ischemic brain injury. Adv Exp Med Biol 923:245–251
6. Bale G, Mitra S, Meek J et al (2014) A new broadband near-infrared spectroscopy system for in-vivo measurements of cerebral cytochrome-c-oxidase changes in neonatal brain injury. Biomed Opt Express 5(10):3450–3466
7. Richter OM, Ludwig B (2003) Cytochrome c oxidase—structure, function, and physiology of a redox-driven molecular machine. Rev Physiol Biochem Pharmacol 147:47–74
8. Murray DM, Boylan GB, Ryan CA et al (2009) Early EEG findings in hypoxic-ischemic encephalopathy predict outcomes at 2 years. Pediatrics 124(3):e459–e467
9. Grant PE, Roche-Labarbe N, Surova A et al (2009) Increased cerebral blood volume and oxygen consumption in neonatal brain injury. J Cereb Blood Flow Metab 29(10):1704–1713
10. Duncan A, Meek JH, Clemence M et al (1996) Measurement of cranial optical path length as a function of age using phase resolved near infrared spectroscopy. Pediatr Res 39:889–894
11. Matcher S, Elwell C, Cooper C (1995) Performance comparison of several published tissue near-infrared spectroscopy algorithms. Anal Biochem 227(1):54–68

12. Scholkmann F, Spichtig S, Muehlemann T et al (2010) How to detect and reduce movement artifacts in near-infrared imaging using moving standard deviation and spline interpolation. Physiol Meas 31(5):649–662
13. Mitra S, Bale G, Highton D et al (2017) Pressure passivity of cerebral mitochondrial metabolism is associated with poor outcome following perinatal hypoxic ischemic brain injury. Cereb blood flow Metab. https://doi.org/10.1177/0271678X17733639
14. Peng S, Boudes E, Tan X et al (2015) Does near-infrared spectroscopy identify asphyxiated Newborns at risk of developing brain injury during hypothermia treatment? Am J Perinatol 32(6):555–564
15. Bale G, Mitra S, de Roever I et al (2018) Oxygen dependency of mitochondrial metabolism indicates outcome of newborn brain injury. J Cereb blood flow Metab. https://doi.org/10.1177/0271678X18777928
16. Azzopardi D, Wyatt JS, Cady EB et al (1989) Prognosis of newborn infants with hypoxic-ischemic brain injury assessed by phosphorus magnetic resonance spectroscopy. Pediatr Res 25:445–451
17. Hassell KJ, Ezzati M, Alonso-Alconada D et al (2015) New horizons for newborn brain protection: enhancing endogenous neuroprotection. Arch Dis Child Fetal Neonatal Ed 100(6):F541–F552
18. Bainbridge A, Tachtsidis I, Faulkner SD et al (2014) Brain mitochondrial oxidative metabolism during and after cerebral hypoxia-ischemia studied by simultaneous phosphorus magnetic-resonance and broadband near-infrared spectroscopy. Neuroimage 102(Pt 1):173–183

Impact of Skull Thickness on Cerebral NIRS Oximetry in Neonates: An *in silico* Study

D. Ostojic, J. Jiang, H. Isler, S. Kleiser, T. Karen, M. Wolf, and F. Scholkmann

Abstract Monitoring of cerebral tissue oxygen saturation (StO_2) by near-infrared spectroscopy (NIRS oximetry) has great potential to reduce the incidence of hypoxic and hyperoxic events and thus prevent long-term disabilities in preterm neonates. Since the light has to penetrate superficial layers (bone, skin and cerebrospinal fluid) before it reaches the brain, the question arises whether these layers influence cerebral StO_2 measurement. We assessed this influence on the accuracy of cerebral StO_2 values. For that purpose, we simulated light propagation with 'N-layered medium' software. It was found that with a superficial layer thickness of ≤6 mm, typical for term and preterm neonates, StO_2 accurately reflects cerebral tissue oxygenation.

Keywords Cerebral oximetry · Tissue oxygenation · Superficial layer thickness · Neonates · NIRS

1 Introduction

Near-infrared spectroscopy enables to reduce the incidence of cerebral hypoxic and hyperoxic events in neonatal care [1]. This is likely to decrease long-term disabilities [1]. Although the brain is the actual organ of interest, StO_2 values might be influenced by superficial layers [skin, bone and cerebrospinal fluid (CSF)], as reported for adults [2]. Therefore, we aimed to assess the influence of typical neonatal superficial layer thicknesses [3] on 'cerebral' StO_2 by a multi-layered simulation.

D. Ostojic (✉) · J. Jiang · H. Isler · S. Kleiser · T. Karen · M. Wolf · F. Scholkmann
Biomedical Optics Research Laboratory (BORL), Department of Neonatology, University Hospital Zurich, University of Zurich, Zurich, Switzerland
e-mail: Daniel.Ostojic@usz.ch

© Springer Nature Switzerland AG 2020

P.-D. Ryu et al. (eds.), *Oxygen Transport to Tissue XLI*, Advances in Experimental Medicine and Biology 1232, https://doi.org/10.1007/978-3-030-34461-0_5

2 Methods

Software was employed to simulate the light propagation in the head of the neonates [4]. The simulated geometry also corresponds to a phantom for comparing different oximeters [5, 6] and assessing the influence of superficial layers [7, 8]. In these phantom experiments, we employed the OxiplexTS (ISS Inc., Champaign, IL, USA) as reference [5, 6], a frequency domain (FD) NIRS tissue oximeter, which in reflectance mode (Fig. 1) measures the attenuation and the phase shift ($\ln(r^2 I)$ and $\Delta\varphi$) at multiple source-detector-separations (SDS = 25, 30, 35 and 40 mm, rigid sensor). From the slopes of $\ln(r^2 I)$ and $\Delta\varphi$ (Fig. 2), the absorption coefficients (μ_a)

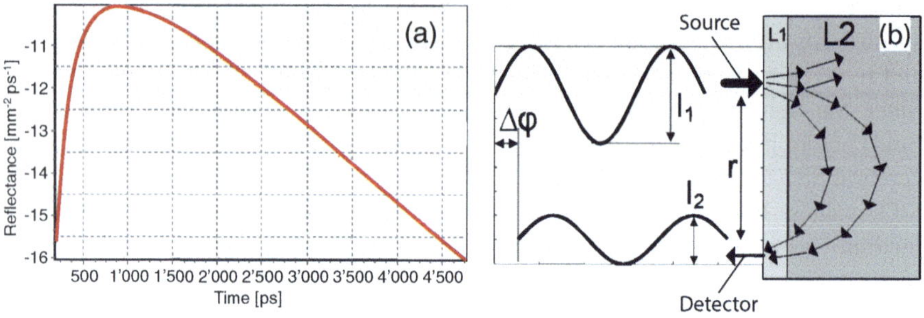

Fig. 1 (**a**) Point spread function at source detector separation of 40 mm and input parameters of Table 1. (**b**) Frequency-domain (FD-NIRS) measurement principle. There is a phase shift and attenuation of intensities

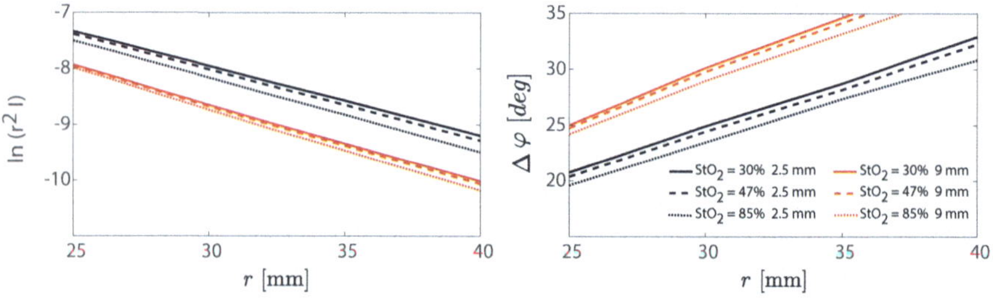

Fig. 2 Intensity and phase slopes at 834 nm (at 25, 30, 35 and 40 mm) and associated total hemoglobin concentration of 45 μM for three different tissue oxygenations (StO_2 = 30, 47 and 85%) with superficial layer thicknesses of 2.5 and 9 mm

Table 1 Set of typical input parameters for N-layered-medium simulation software at 834 nm. Number of layers: 2, position of detection: 40 mm

	L1	L2
$\mu_s'(\lambda)$ [mm^{-1}]	0.84	0.5
$\mu_a(\lambda)$ [mm^{-1}]	0.0101	0.0218
Refractive index	1.4	1.33
Thickness [mm]	12.0	50.0

were calculated (Eq. 1) as well as the clinically relevant oxy-, deoxy-and total hemoglobin concentrations [O_2Hb], [HHb] [tHb] and the StO_2 (Eqs. 2 and 3). For this OxiplexTS rigid sensor we simulated the $\ln(r^2I)$ and $\Delta\varphi$ for 9 different thicknesses of skull (0, 2.5, 4, 6, 9, 12, 15, 35 and 55 mm) by the 'N-layered medium' light propagation software [4]. While the superficial layer thickness varied, the thickness of the underlying layer, which imitated the brain, was kept constant at 50 mm. The superficial layer (Layer 1 in Fig. 1b) represented the optical properties of the skull bone [3, 9] with the neonatal term and preterm thickness ranging between 1.1 mm (lower quartile) and 2.8 mm (upper quartile) with a median of 2.2 mm [3]. The simulation was run for thicknesses above the neonatal Q_3 of 2.8 mm to compensate for the effects caused by the additional superficial layers of skin and CSF, which typically add up to an overall median superficial layer thickness of 6 mm for term and preterm infants [3]. Simulating above the thickness of 6 mm provides an insight into the influence the superficial layers have when the measurement is performed on adults [9]. Thicknesses above 20 mm were simulated out of scientific interest. The superficial layer's optical properties (Layer 1 of the Table 2) are equivalent to the corresponding values of [tHb] of 45.8 μM and StO_2 of 60.5%. They remain constant throughout all simulation steps and all simulations. The underlying layer (Layer 2 in Fig. 1b) has the optical properties of the brain tissue [3, 9]. We simulated three different StO_2 states: 30, 47 and 85% at a typical neonatal [tHb] of 45 μM. The corresponding $\mu_a(\lambda)$ and $\mu_s'(\lambda)$ for 692 nm and 834 nm employed in the simulations and the equations are given in Table 2. The OxiplexTS and its rigid sensor measure the $\ln(r^2I)$ and $\Delta\varphi$ for two wavelengths: 692 and 834 nm [6]. To obtain the $\ln(r^2I)$ and $\Delta\varphi$ from the point spread function (Fig. 1a) provided by the simulation software, a Fourier transform was performed (Matlab R2014a, Mathworks, Inc., Mass., USA). The results of the Fourier transform were band pass-filtered at the center frequency of 110 MHz (f_{low} = 109.8 MHz, f_{high} = 110.2 MHz, ideal rectangle), which is the frequency of OxiplexTS light modulation. The slope (S_{AC}) for $\ln(r^2I)$ and slope ($S\varphi$) of $\Delta\varphi$ are shown in Fig. 2. The $\mu_a(\lambda)$ was calculated from S_{AC} and S_φ (Fig. 2) according to Eq. 1 and we just took the $\mu_s'(\lambda)$ for L2 according to Table 2. The rationale was that the commercial NIRS oximeters used today in clinical application are continuous-wave (CW) instruments, which are unable to measure $\mu_s'(\lambda)$ and therefore have to assume a reasonable value. 2) The other way was to determine the $\mu_s'(\lambda)$ from the S_{AC} and $S\varphi$, i.e. the true $\mu_s'(\lambda)$, which is indeed measurable by frequency domain instruments such as the OxiplexTS. For both methods, [HHb], [O_2Hb] and StO_2 were calculated according to Eqs. 2 and 3 [10].

Table 2 Optical properties of the superficial (L1) and underlying (L2) layers [5, 9]

	L1	L2
$\mu_s'(\lambda = 692$ nm) [mm^{-1}]	0.97	0.59
μ_a ($\lambda = 692$ nm) [mm^{-1}]	0.0106	0.0062 to 0.0161
$\mu_s'(\lambda = 834$ nm) [mm^{-1}]	0.84	0.5
μ_a ($\lambda = 834$ nm) [mm^{-1}]	0.0101	0.0106 to 0.0123

$$\mu_a(\lambda) = \frac{-3\mu_s'(\lambda) + \sqrt{9\mu_s'(\lambda)^2 + 12\left(S_{AC}^2 - S_\varphi^2\right)}}{6} \quad (1)$$

$$\begin{bmatrix} \text{HHb} \\ \text{O}_2\text{Hb} \end{bmatrix} = \begin{bmatrix} \varepsilon_{\text{HHb}}(\lambda_1) & \varepsilon_{\text{O}_2\text{Hb}}(\lambda_1) \\ \varepsilon_{\text{HHb}}(\lambda_2) & \varepsilon_{\text{O}_2\text{Hb}}(\lambda_2) \end{bmatrix}^{-1} \begin{bmatrix} \mu_a(\lambda_1) \\ \mu_a(\lambda_2) \end{bmatrix} \quad (2)$$

$$\text{StO}_2 = \frac{[\text{HHb}]}{[\text{HHb}] + [\text{O}_2\text{Hb}]} \quad (3)$$

3 Results

The typical term and preterm range of skull bone thicknesses between 1.1 and 2.8 mm ($Q_1 - Q_3$ [3]) does not influence the measurements of the [HHb], [O_2Hb] and hence there is no influence on StO_2 estimation either (Fig. 3). If the skull bone thickness is extended to 6 mm to include the superficial layers of skin and the CSF, there is still no influence on the [HHb], [O_2Hb] and StO_2 as confirmed by the (Figs. 3 and 4). The errors in StO_2 due to hypothetical skull thickness of below 6 mm remain between 2.71% and 0.99% for the CW case (Fig. 5) and between 2.68% and 0.97% for the frequency domain case.

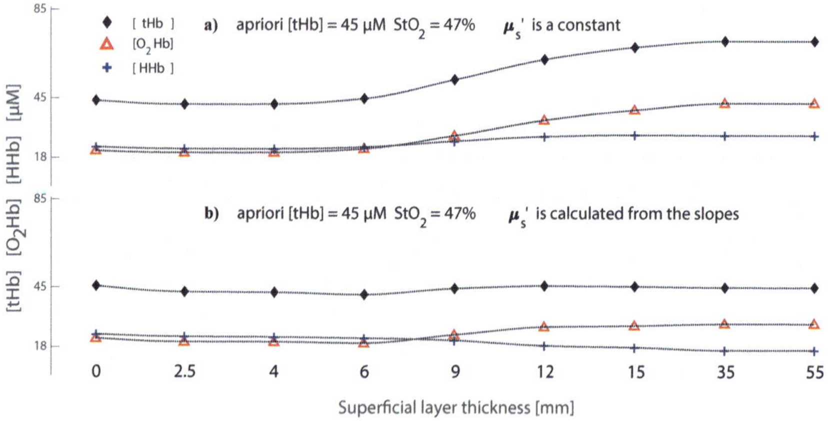

Fig. 3 (**a**) [O_2Hb], [HHb], [tHb] as they would be determined by a CW-NIRS-device with the rigid sensor geometry of the OxiplexTS at different superficial layer thicknesses. Since CW devices cannot measure the $\mu_s'(\lambda)$, here we assumed a reasonable $\mu_s'(\lambda)$ as reported in Table 2 (L2) yielding values for [tHb] that are representative of the underlying layer (brain) for L1-thicknesses ≤6 mm, but erroneous in concentrations for higher thicknesses. (**b**) The FD-NIRS-device in contrast is capable of measuring the $\mu_s'(\lambda)$. The measured [O_2Hb], [HHb], [tHb] values are representative of the underlying layer (brain) for superficial layer thickness ≤ 6 mm, while for L1 thicknesses >15 mm they correctly represent the superficial layer ([tHb] of 45.8 μM and StO_2 of 60.5%)

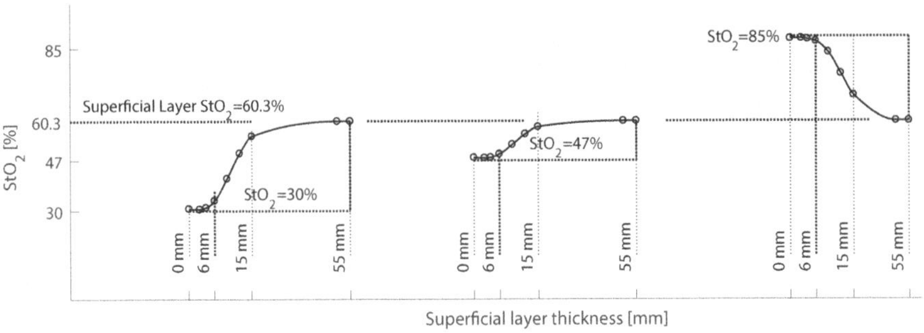

Fig. 4 Brain values for StO_2 of 30% (left), 47% (center) and 85% (right) are accurately determined for a superficial layer thickness of up to 6-mm for the CW case. For a thickness ≥ 35 mm the StO_2 of 60.3% represents the superficial layer. In-between there is a transient S-type function of StO_2 [7]

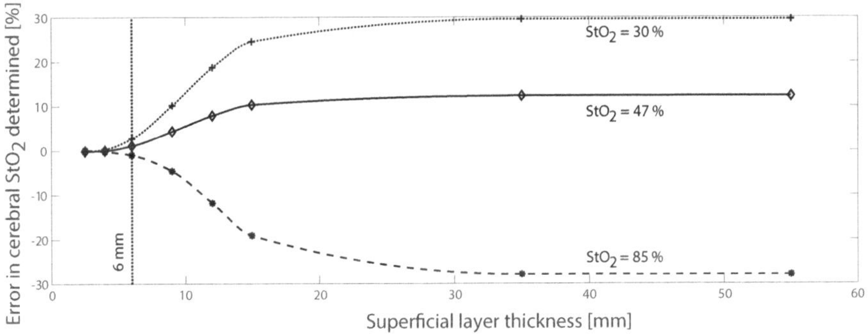

Fig. 5 Errors in StO_2 as a function of thickness of the skull for [tHb] = 45 μM for the CW case. For the error estimation, the brain StO_2 was subtracted from the simulated StO_2 value of the two-layered system

4 Discussion and Conclusions

We have chosen the two-layer model, because it is similar to the in vitro phantoms [5–8] and because it simulates the neonatal head. The results are consistent with the OxiplexTS measurements on two-layer media in [7], where it was found that the measured optical coefficients are representative of the underlying layer if the superficial layer is less than ~0.4 cm thick, whereas they are representative of the superficial layer if it is more than ~1.3 cm thick. The typical overall superficial layer thickness in term newborns is ≤6 mm [3] in a preterm, it is even less. Thus, the errors in StO_2 are below 2.71%, which is acceptable from the clinical point of view [11]. To conclude, NIRS is capable to provide accurate cerebral StO_2 values of preterm and term infants.

Acknowledgments This work was supported by the Nano-Tera RTD project NewbornCare, the Clinical Research Priority Programs (CRPP) Molecular Imaging Network Zürich (MINZ) of the University of Zurich and the Swiss Cancer Research grant KFS-3732-08-2015 and the Swiss National Science Foundation project 159490. We thank Dr. Salvador Sanchez Majos and Dr. Alexander Kalyanov for inspiring discussions on the topic.

References

1. Hyttel-Sorensen S, Pellicer A, Alderliesten T et al (2015) Cerebral near infrared spectroscopy oximetry in extremely preterm infants: phase II randomised clinical trial. BMJ 350:g7635
2. Strangman GE, Li Z, Zhang Q (2013) Depth sensitivity and source-detector separations for near infrared spectroscopy based on the Colin27 brain template. PLoS One 8:e66319
3. Demel A, Feilke K, Wolf M et al (2014) Correlation between skin, bone, and cerebrospinal fluid layer thickness and optical coefficients measured by multidistance frequency-domain near-infrared spectroscopy in term and preterm infants. J Biomed Opt 19:17004
4. Kienle A. PMS. https://www.ilm-ulm.de/forschung/foerderprojekte/material-und-gewebeoptik/software-zur-lichtausbreitung.html. 1997
5. Kleiser S, Nasseri N, Andresen B et al (2016) Comparison of tissue oximeters on a liquid phantom with adjustable optical properties. Biomed Opt Express 7:2973–2992
6. Kleiser S, Hyttel-Sorensen S, Greisen G et al (2016) Comparison of near-infrared oximeters in a liquid optical phantom with varying Intralipid and blood content. Adv Exp Med Biol 876:413–418
7. Franceschini MA, Fantini S, Paunescu LA et al (1998) Influence of a superficial layer in the quantitative spectroscopic study of strongly scattering media. Appl Opt 37:7447–7458
8. Nasseri N, Kleiser S, Ostojic D et al (2016) Quantifying the effect of adipose tissue in muscle oximetry by near infrared spectroscopy. Biomed Opt Express 7:4605–4619
9. Choi J, Wolf M, Toronov V et al (2004) Noninvasive determination of the optical properties of adult brain: near-infrared spectroscopy approach. J Biomed Opt 9:221–229
10. Spichtig S Multi-distance and multi-frequency domain near-infrared spectroscopy: Characterization and application, Doctoral Thesis ETH. 2010
11. Greisen G, Andresen B, Plomgaard AM et al (2016) Cerebral oximetry in preterm infants: an agenda for research with a clear clinical goal. Neurophotonics 3:031407

Resuscitation with Drag Reducing Polymers after Traumatic Brain Injury with Hemorrhagic Shock Reduces Microthrombosis and Oxidative Stress

Denis E. Bragin, Olga A. Bragina, Marina V. Kameneva, and Edwin M. Nemoto

Abstract Outcome after traumatic brain injury (TBI) is worsened by hemorrhagic shock (HS); however, the existing volume expansion approach with resuscitation fluids (RF) is controversial as it does not adequately alleviate impaired microvascular cerebral blood flow (mCBF). We previously reported that resuscitation fluid with drag reducing polymers (DRP-RF) improves CBF by rheological modulation of hemodynamics. Here, we evaluate the efficacy of DRP-RF, compared to lactated Ringers resuscitation fluid (LR-RF), in reducing cerebral microthrombosis and reperfusion mitochondrial oxidative stress after TBI complicated by HS. Fluid percussion TBI (1.5 ATA, 50 ms) was induced in rats and followed by controlled HS to a mean arterial pressure (MAP) of 40 mmHg. DRP-RF or LR-RF was infused to restore MAP to 60 mmHg for 1 h (pre-hospital period), followed by blood reinfusion to a MAP = 70 mmHg (hospital period). In vivo 2-photon laser scanning microscopy over the parietal cortex was used to monitor microvascular blood flow, nicotinamide adenine dinucleotide (NADH) for tissue oxygen supply and mitochondrial oxidative stress (superoxide by i.v. hydroethidine [HEt], 1 mg/kg) for 4 h after TBI/HS, followed by DiI vascular painting during perfusion-fixation. TBI/HS decreased mCBF resulting in capillary microthrombosis and tissue hypoxia. Microvascular CBF and tissue oxygenation were significantly improved in the DRP-RF compared to the LR-RF treated group ($p < 0.05$). Reperfusion-induced oxidative stress, reflected by HEt fluorescence, was 32 ± 6% higher in LR-RF vs. DRP-RF ($p < 0.05$). Post-mortem whole-brain visualization of DiI painted vessels

D. E. Bragin (✉) · O. A. Bragina · E. M. Nemoto
Department of Neurosurgery, University of New Mexico School of Medicine, Albuquerque, NM, USA
e-mail: dbragin@salud.unm.edu

M. V. Kameneva
McGowan Institute for Regenerative Medicine, University of Pittsburgh, Pittsburgh, NM, USA

© Springer Nature Switzerland AG 2020
P.-D. Ryu et al. (eds.), *Oxygen Transport to Tissue XLI*, Advances in Experimental Medicine and Biology 1232, https://doi.org/10.1007/978-3-030-34461-0_6

revealed multiple microthromboses in both hemispheres that were 29 ± 3% less in DRP-RF vs. LR-RF group ($p < 0.05$). Resuscitation after TBI/HS using DRP-RF effectively restores mCBF, reduces hypoxia, microthrombosis formation, and mitochondrial oxidative stress compared to conventional volume expansion with LR-RF.

Keywords Traumatic brain injury (TBI) · Hemorrhagic shock (HS) · Microthrombi · Superoxide · Resuscitation fluid (RF) · Drag reducing polymer (DRP)

1 Introduction

Outcome after traumatic brain injury (TBI) is significantly worsened by hemorrhagic shock (HS) due to increased severity of reduced cerebral blood flow (CBF) leading to capillary microthrombosis, hypoxia, reactive oxygen species formation due to mitochondrial dysfunction, neuronal death and a two-fold increase in contusion volume [1, 2]. The existing volume expansion approach with resuscitation fluids (RF) is controversial as it does not adequately alleviate impaired microvascular cerebral blood flow (mCBF) and is thus not neuroprotective. We previously reported that resuscitation fluid with drag-reducing polymers (DRP-RF) improved CBF and reduced cerebral hypoxia and neuronal necrosis by rheological modulation of hemodynamics. Here, we evaluate the efficacy of DRP-RF compared to lactated Ringers resuscitation fluid (LR-RF), in reducing cerebral microthrombosis and reperfusion mitochondrial oxidative stress after TBI complicated by HS.

2 Methods

Most of the procedures used in these studies have already been described [3]. Protocol #200640 was approved by the Institutional Animal Care and Use Committee of the University of New Mexico and the studies were conducted according to the NIH Guide for the Care and Use of Laboratory Animals.

Surgical Preparation Laboratory-acclimated male Sprague-Dawley rats (250–300 g) were mechanically ventilated on isoflurane (2%), nitrous oxide (69%) oxygen anesthesia (29%). Femoral vein and artery catheters were inserted. For imaging and TBI, a 5-mm craniotomy over the left parietal cortex was filled with 2% agarose in saline and sealed by a cover glass. The fluid percussion was used as a model of TBI and was induced by 1.5 atm 50 ms pulse from a custom-built Pneumatic Impactor connected to the brain through a pressure transducer filled with artificial cerebrospinal fluid. HS was performed in a way similar to that described by Robertson et al. [2].

Overall Design of the Study TBI was induced after baseline in-vivo 2-photon laser scanning microscopy (2PLSM) and followed by a 1-h hemorrhagic phase, where blood was slowly withdrawn through the femoral vein to reduce mean arterial pressure (MAP) to 40 mmHg. In the following 1-h pre-hospital care phase, resuscitation fluids (LR-RF or DRP-RF) were slowly infused i.v. to raise MAP to ~55 mmHg and CBF to ~65% of baseline. In a subsequent 3-h definitive hospital care phase, shed blood was re-infused to a MAP of 70 mmHg and CBF of ~75% of baseline. In vivo 2PLSM was done throughout the study over the peri-contusion area of the parietal cortex of the rat brain. Monitored variables included: cerebral microvascular blood flow velocity, number of perfused capillaries, tissue oxygen supply (NADH autofluorescence) and superoxide production by i.v. Hydroethidine (HEt, Sigma-Aldrich, USA). The laser Doppler flux was measured via a lateral temporal window using a 0.9-mm diameter probe (DRT4, Moor Inst., Axminster, UK) in the same region of the brain studied by 2PLSM. Brain and rectal temperatures were monitored and maintained at 38 ± 0.5 °C. Arterial blood gases, electrolytes, hematocrit and pH were measured hourly (epoc Blood Analysis System, Alere Inc., Waltham, MA, USA). At the end of experiments animals were subjected to perfusion with Vessel Painting.

Superoxide Production Evaluation 0.5 mg of HEt in a concentration of 1 mg/ml in 0.1 M phosphate buffer solution (PBS) containing 20% DMSO, was injected intravenously during surgical preparation [4]. Hydroethidine (HEt) is a fluorescent dye that is oxidized to ethidium (ET) by superoxide. ET fluoresces at a different wavelength (Em = 595 nm) than HEt (Em = 415 nm) and thus may be used to visualize superoxide production.

Animal perfusion and Vessel Painting Vessel painting was done during cardiac perfusion according to Hughes with 1,1′-dioctadecyl-3,3,3′,3′-tetramethylindo carbocyanine perchlorate (DiI, Invitrogen, USA) which binds directly and preferentially to endothelial cells [5]. The Vessel Painting included the following sequential order for delivery of perfusion solutions: a) PBS (150 ml), b) 50 ml of DiI (13 μg/ml), and c) paraformaldehyde (4%, 200 ml). After fixation and perfusion, the brain was extracted from the cranium and all meninges were removed with care. Imaging was done with 2PLSM in a custom-made fixed tissue imaging chamber.

DRP Preparation Polyethylene oxide (PEO, MW ~4000 kDa) was dissolved in saline to 0.1% (1000 ppm), dialyzed against saline using a 50 kD cutoff membrane, diluted in saline to 50 ppm, slow rocked for ~2 h and then sterilized using a 0.22 μm filter [6]. DRP-RF was prepared before infusion by adding DRP to Lactated Ringer to reach the final DRP concentration of 0.0005% (5 ppm).

Two-Photon Laser Scanning Microscopy Fluorescent serum (i.v. fluorescein isothiocyanate (FITS) dextran, 150 kDa in physiological saline, 5% wt/vol) was visualized using an Olympus BX 51WI upright microscope and water-immersion LUMPlan FL/IR 20X/0.50 W objective. Excitation was provided by a PrairieView Ultima multiphoton microscopy laser scan unit powered by a Millennia Prime 10 W diode laser source pumping a Tsunami Ti: Sapphire laser (Spectra-Physics,

Mountain View, CA, USA) tuned to 750 nm center wavelength. Band-pass-filtered epifluorescence (510–530 nm for FITS, 445–475 nm for NADH and 565–600 for ET) was collected by photomultiplier tubes of the Prairie View Ultima system. Images (512 x 512 pixels, 0.15 um/pixel in the x- and y-axes) or line scans were acquired using Prairie View software. Red blood cell flow velocity was measured in microvessels ranging from 3–50 μm diameter up to 500 μm below the surface of the parietal cortex, as described previously [5]. Tissue hypoxia was assessed by measurement of NADH autofluorescence. In offline analyses using NIH ImageJ software, a three-dimensional anatomy of the vasculature in areas of interest were reconstructed from two-dimensional (planar) scans of the fluorescence intensity obtained at successive focal depths in the cortex (XYZ stack).

Statistical analyses were done using GraphPad Prism software 6.0 (La Jolla, CA, USA) by Student's t-test or Kolmogorov-Smirnov test where appropriate. Differences between groups were determined using two-way analysis of variance (ANOVA) for multiple comparisons and post-hoc testing using the Mann-Whitney U-test.

3 Results

As in our previous studies, TBI followed by HS decreased mCBF resulting in capillary microthrombosis and tissue hypoxia. Microvascular CBF, the number of perfused capillaries and tissue oxygenation in peri contusion areas were significantly better in the DRP-RF compared to the LR-RF treated group.

Post-mortem whole-brain visualization of DiI painted vessels revealed multiple microthromboses and reduction of microvascular density in both hemispheres in rats after TBI with HS (Fig. 1A, B): i.e., in the injured hemisphere in DRP-RF, microvascular density was higher than in LR-RF (% vessel/total area∗100 was 4.9 ± 0.4 vs. 3.1 ± 0.3, respectively, $p < 0.05$) as opposed to 6.8 ± 0.4 in Sham rats

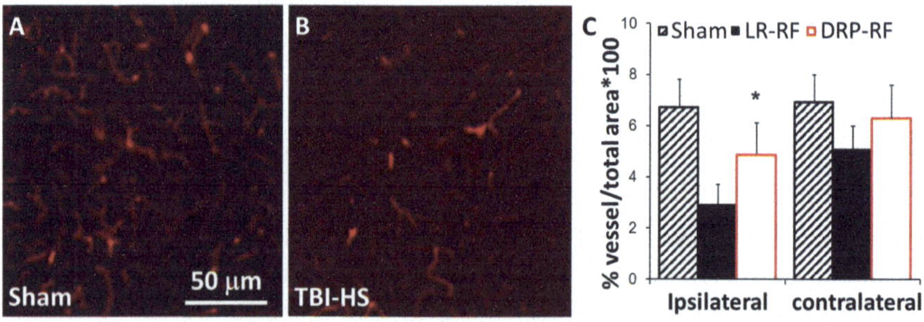

Fig. 1 Resuscitation with DRP-RF reduces microthrombosis in both hemispheres after TBI with HS as shown by post-mortem DiI vascular painting. (**a**) Cortical microvascular network in Sham mouse brain; and (**b**) after TBI with HS; (**c**) Graph showing reduced cortical microvasculature in LR-RF group and better-preserved microvasculature in DRP-RF group in both, traumatized and contralateral hemispheres. Mean ± SEM, N = 10 rats per group, ∗$P < 0.05$ from the LR-RF group

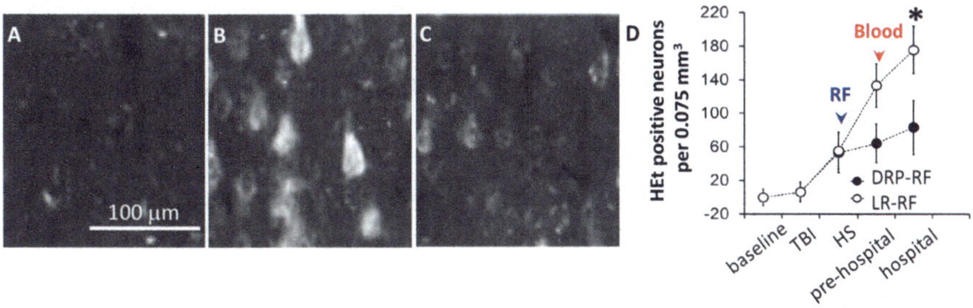

Fig. 2 Resuscitation with DRP-RF reduces superoxide production in cortical neurons after TBI with HS: (**a**) Representative image of a rat cortex at baseline without ET positive neurons; (**b**) Neurons with diffuse cytosolic ET fluorescence in a rat cortex from LR-RF group by the end of experiment; (**c**) and from DRP-RF group; The dynamics of the increase in ET positive cortical neurons. Mean ± SEM, n = 10 rats per group, $*P < 0.05$ from the LR-RF group

(Fig. 1C). In contralateral to the injury hemisphere, microvascular density was also reduced (% vessel/total area$*$100 was 6.1 ± 0.5 vs 5.2 ± 0.5, in DRP-RF, vs. LR-RF, respectively, $p < 0.09$) (Fig. 1C).

Superoxide production was determined by oxidation of HEt to ET. Under normal physiological conditions at baseline, ET fluorescence appeared as small particles in the cytosol, suggesting mitochondrial generation of superoxide (Fig. 2A). In pathological conditions, the ET fluorescent signal filled the cytosolic space and allowed clear visualization and differentiation of individual soma and dendritic processes. Neurons in which the accumulated fluorescence demonstrated the entire body of the soma and obscured the nucleus were considered positive for diffuse cytosolic ET fluorescence.

TBI with subsequent HS caused generation of superoxide; in both groups the number of Et positive neurons increased to 58.1 ± 5.2 per 0.075 mm^3 (Fig. 2D). In the pre-hospital phase, in the group in which the conventional LR-RF was slowly infused in the amount of 5.6 ± 2.2 ml, the number of Et positive neurons further increased to 137.9 ± 5.6 per 0.075 mm^3 (Fig. 2D). In the group in which DRP-RF was slowly infused in a smaller amount of 2.0 ± 0.3 ml, the number of Et positive neurons increased to only 62.3 ± 4.8 per 0.075 mm^3 (Fig. 2D). By the end of the hospital phase with re-infusion of blood, in the LR-RF group, the number of Et positive neurons further increased to 176.5 ± 6.2 per 0.075 mm^3 (Fig. 2B, D), reflecting active reactive oxygen species (superoxide) formation probably due to excessive oxidative phosphorylation in metabolically stressed mitochondria. In the DRP-RF group, the number of Et positive neurons increased to only 84.2 ± 5.3 per 0.075 mm^3 (Fig. 2C, D), reflecting lower oxidative stress.

4 Discussion

The most common free radical in TBI, responsible for tissue damage, is superoxide that is produced when oxygen molecules gain an electron from other molecules [7, 8]. The major source of superoxide in brain injury is the mitochondria [8, 9].

As demonstrated in this work, attenuation of oxidative stress by DRP-RF after TBI with HS is related to the mitigation of microthrombosis formation and hypoxia reduction. Hypoxia, induced by TBI and exacerbated by HS, causes mitochondrial impairment leading to excessive and altered oxidative phosphorylation in mitochondria and, as a result, superoxide hyperproduction [10]. Resuscitation re-perfusion exacerbates this process [11]. Attenuation of reduction of cerebral microvascular density by mitigation of microthrombosis formation by DRP-RF does not allow hypoxia to reach the critical level which, possibly, reduces mitochondrial injury and neuronal excitotoxicity and, as a result, reactive oxygen species overproduction. The mechanisms of hemorheological modulation by DRP include increasing the arteriolar blood volume flow via the increase of flow velocity by reduction of flow separations and vortices at vessel bifurcations and decreasing pressure loss across the arterial network due to the viscoelastic properties of DRP [11]. This leads to a rise in pre-capillary blood pressure thus enhancing capillary perfusion, countering capillary stasis, increasing the density of functioning capillaries and the number of red blood cells passing through capillaries to improve tissue oxygenation [11].

5 Conclusion

Rheological modulation of blood flow using advanced resuscitation fluid with DRP in nanomolar amounts effectively restores microvascular CBF, reduces hypoxia, microthrombosis formation and mitochondrial oxidative stress compared to conventional volume expansion with lactated Ringer.

Acknowledgments Supported by DOD DM160142.

References

1. Manley G, Knudson MM, Morabito D et al (2001) Hypotension, hypoxia, and head injury: frequency, duration, and consequences. Arch Surg 136(10):1118–1123
2. Navarro JC, Pillai S, Cherian L et al (2012) Histopathological and behavioral effects of immediate and delayed hemorrhagic shock after mild traumatic brain injury in rats. J Neurotrauma 29(2):322–334
3. Bragin DE, Kameneva MV, Bragina OA et al (2017) Rheological effects of drag-reducing polymers improve cerebral blood flow and oxygenation after traumatic brain injury in rats. J Cereb Blood Flow Metab 37(3):762–775
4. Hughes S, Dashkin O, Defazio RA (2014) Vessel painting technique for visualizing the cerebral vascular architecture of the mouse. Methods Mol Biol 1135:127–113
5. Peterson SL, Morrow D, Liu S et al (2002) Hydroethidine detection of superoxide production during the lithium-pilocarpine model of status epilepticus. Epilepsy Res 49(3):226–238
6. Kameneva MV, Wu ZJ, Uraysh A et al (2004) Blood soluble drag-reducing polymers prevent lethality from hemorrhagic shock in acute animal experiments. Biorheology 41(1):53–64
7. Abdul-Muneer PM, Chandra N, Haorah J (2015) Interactions of oxidative stress and neurovascular inflammation in the pathogenesis of traumatic brain injury. Mol Neurobiol 51(3):966–979

8. Hiebert JB, Shen Q, Thimmesch AR et al (2015) Traumatic brain injury and mitochondrial dysfunction. Am J Med Sci Aug 350(2):132–138
9. Yonutas H, Vekaria HJ, Sullivan PG (2016) Mitochondrial specific therapeutic targets following brain injury. Brain Res 1640:77–93
10. Fiskum G (2000) Mitochondrial participation in ischemic and traumatic neural cell death. J Neurotrauma 17(10):843–855
11. Kameneva MV (2012) Microrheological effects of drag-reducing polymers in vitro and in vivo. Int J Eng Sci 59:168–183

Anodal Transcranial Direct Current Stimulation Improves Impaired Cerebrovascular Reactivity in Traumatized Mouse Brain

Olga A. Bragina, Oxana V. Semyachkina-Glushkovskaya, Edwin M. Nemoto, and Denis E. Bragin

Abstract Cerebrovascular reactivity (CVR) is a compensatory mechanism where blood vessels dilate in response to a vasodilatory stimulus, and is a biomarker of vascular reserve and microvascular health. Impaired CVR indicates microvascular hemodynamic dysfunction, which is implicated in traumatic brain injury (TBI) and associated with long-term neurological deficiency. Recently we have shown that anodal transcranial direct current stimulation (tDCS) caused prolonged dilatation of cerebral arterioles that increased brain microvascular flow and tissue oxygenation in traumatized mouse brain and was associated with neurologic improvement. Here we evaluate the effects of tDCS on impaired CVR and microvascular cerebral blood flow (mCBF) regulation after TBI. TBI was induced in mice by controlled cortical impact (CCI). Cortical microvascular tone, mCBF, and tissue oxygen supply (by nicotinamide adenine dinucleotide, NADH) were measured by two-photon laser scanning microscopy before and after anodal tDCS (0.1 mA/15 min). CVR and mCBF regulation were evaluated by measuring changes in arteriolar diameters and NADH during hypercapnia test before and after tDCS. Transient hypercapnia was induced by 60-s increase of CO_2 concentration in the inhalation mixture to 10%. As previously, anodal tDCS dilated arterioles which increased arteriolar blood flow volume that led to an increase in capillary flow velocity and the number of functioning capillaries, thereby improving tissue oxygenation in both traumatized and sham animals. In sham mice, transient hypercapnia caused transient dilatation of cerebral arterioles with constant NADH, reflecting intact CVR and mCBF regulation. In TBI

O. A. Bragina
Department of Neurosurgery, University of New Mexico School of Medicine, Albuquerque, NM, USA

Department of Human and Animal Physiology, Saratov State University, Saratov, Russia

O. V. Semyachkina-Glushkovskaya
Department of Human and Animal Physiology, Saratov State University, Saratov, Russia

E. M. Nemoto · D. E. Bragin (✉)
Department of Neurosurgery, University of New Mexico School of Medicine, Albuquerque, NM, USA
e-mail: dbragin@salud.unm.edu

© Springer Nature Switzerland AG 2020

P.-D. Ryu et al. (eds.), *Oxygen Transport to Tissue XLI*, Advances in Experimental Medicine and Biology 1232, https://doi.org/10.1007/978-3-030-34461-0_7

animals, arteriolar dilatation response to hypercapnia was diminished while the NADH level increased (tissue oxygen supply decreased), reflecting impaired CVR and mCBF regulation. Anodal tDCS enhanced reactivity in parenchymal arterioles in both groups (especially in TBI mice) and restored CVR thereby prevented the reduction in tissue oxygen supply during hypercapnia. CVR has been shown to be related to nitric oxide elevation due to nitric oxide synthases activation, which can be sensitive to the electrical field induced by tDCS.

Keywords Traumatic brain injury (TBI) · Transcranial direct current stimulation (tDCS) · Cerebrovascular reactivity (CVR) · Microvascular dysfunction · Hypercapnia test

1 Introduction

Cerebrovascular reactivity (CVR), the compensatory mechanism where blood vessels dilate in response to a vasodilatory stimulus, is an essential element of cerebrovascular regulation and a biomarker of cerebrovascular reserve and microvascular health [1]. Past researches have demonstrated that CVR is impaired following traumatic brain injury (TBI) which indicates underlying microvascular dysfunction wherein the metabolically active regions of the brain will not be supplied adequately to meet demands. This impairment increases susceptibility to secondary injury following TBI and exacerbates long-term neurological deficiency [2, 3]. Since neurocentric approaches for the treatment of TBI have failed, the NIH suggested that the neurovascular unit and a larger microsystem of vessels and associated glial cells should be considered as the functional target for new therapeutic approaches [3]. Transcranial direct current stimulation (tDCS) that potentially modulates all polarizable brain cell types is a promising electroceutical therapy suggested for TBI [4]. However, due to a lack of pre-clinical studies, the mechanisms of tDCS are poorly understood. Recently we have shown that anodal transcranial direct current stimulation (tDCS) caused prolonged dilatation of cerebral arterioles that increased brain microvascular flow and tissue oxygen supply in traumatized mouse brain and was associated with neurologic improvement. Since CVR was also suggested as a therapeutic target for TBI [5], we evaluate here the effects of the anodal tDCS on impaired CVR and microvascular cerebral blood flow (mCBF) regulation in the traumatized mouse brain.

2 Methods

2.1 Experimental Design

Protocol #200247 was approved by the Institutional Animal Care and Use Committee of the University of New Mexico and the studies were conducted according to the NIH Guide for the Care and Use of Laboratory Animals. Two groups of 10 mice each were used in the study: TBI and Sham. TBI was induced by a Benchmark Controlled Cortical Stereotaxic Impactor (Leica Biosystems, Germany) through craniotomy (5 mm diam, centred at 3.5 mm posterior and left-lateral to bregma) using a 3-mm flat-tip impounder deployed at a velocity of 5 m/sec and depth of 2.0 mm from the cortical surface, as in our previous study [6]. Sham controls were subjected to craniotomy only. Anodal tDCS (0.1 mA/15 min) was done using an Animal DCS Stimulator 2100 (Soterix Medical, USA). The anode was placed around the craniotomy and the counter electrode on the thorax. Microvascular cerebral blood flow (mCBF) concurrently with NADH were measured *in vivo* by two-photon laser scanning microscopy (2PLSM) before and after stimulation. For imaging, mice were initially anesthetized with 2% isoflurane in 70% N_2O and 30% O_2. Later on, to preserve vasoreactivity, isoflurane was gradually reduced over a 10-min period to a range of 0.5–1%.

2.2 Two-Photon Laser Scanning Microscopy

Fluorescent serum (i.v. tetramethylrhodamine isothiocyanate (TAMRA) dextran, 150 kDa in physiological saline, 5% wt/vol) was visualized using an Olympus BX 51WI upright microscope and water-immersion LUMPlan FL/IR 20X/0.50 W objective of PrairieView Ultima multiphoton system. Excitation was provided by a PrairieView Ultima multiphoton microscopy laser scan unit powered by a Millennia Prime 10 W diode laser source pumping a Tsunami Ti: Sapphire laser (Spectra-Physics, Mountain View, CA, USA) tuned to 750 nm center wavelength. Band-pass-filtered epifluorescence (570–600 nm for TAMRA and 425–475 nm for NADH) was collected by photomultiplier tubes of the Prairie View Ultima system. Images (512 X 512 pixels, 0.15 um/pixel in the x- and y-axes) were acquired using Prairie View software as described previously [6]. Brain tissue oxygen supply was assessed by measurement of NADH autofluorescence. In offline analyses using NIH ImageJ software, the three-dimensional anatomy of the vasculature in areas of interest was reconstructed from two-dimensional (planar) scans of the fluorescence intensity obtained at successive focal depths in the cortex (XYZ stack).

2.3 Cerebrovascular Reactivity Test

Changes in arteriolar diameters and NADH autofluorescence were measured during hypercapnia test before and after tDCS (Fig. 1). Transient hypercapnia was induced by a 60-s increase in CO_2 concentration to 10% in the inhalation mixture through the face mask. Each trial consisted of 3 min of baseline data acquisition, 1 min of hypercapnia challenge, and 3 min during the post-hypercapnic surveillance period [7].

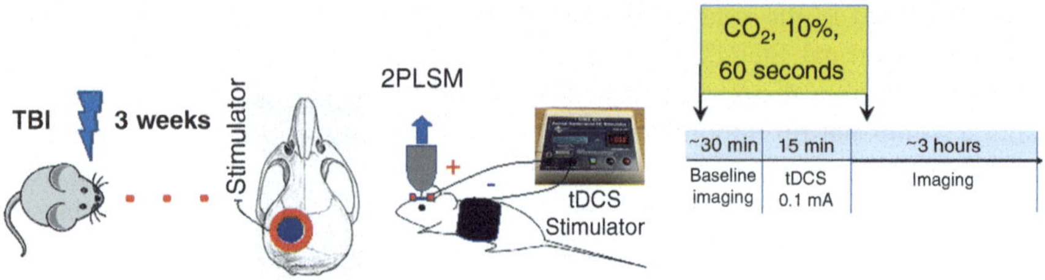

Fig. 1 Scheme of the experimental design. At 3 weeks after traumatic brain injury (TBI), anesthetized mouse underwent two-photon laser scanning microscopy before and after anodal transcranial direct current stimulation (tDCS). Hypercapnia test was performed at baseline and after tDCS

2.4 *Statistical Analyses*

Statistical analyses were done using GraphPad Prism software 6.0 (La Jolla, CA, USA) by Student's t-test or Kolmogorov-Smirnov test where appropriate. Differences between groups were determined using two-way analysis of variance (ANOVA) for multiple comparisons and post-hoc testing using the Mann-Whitney U-test.

3 Results

As in our previous study, controlled cortical impact caused a decrease in arteriolar diameters leading to a reduction in cerebral blood flow volume, capillary red blood cell flow velocity and tissue oxygen supply in the peri-contusion areas of cerebral cortex. Anodal tDCS dilated arterioles leading to an increase in blood flow volume, which increased blood flow velocity in capillaries. The improved perfusion in capillaries after tDCS caused a prolonged increase in tissue oxygen supply, as reflected by NADH autofluorescence decrease in TBI and Sham mouse brain.

Baseline hypercapnia test showed that, in sham mice, cerebral arterioles dilated during inhalation of 10% CO_2 (by 44.2 ± 4.6%) and constricted to the pre-hypercapnia diameter after CO_2 termination (Fig. 2a–b) reflecting intact CVR. In TBI mice, however, cerebral arterioles dilatation response to CO_2 inhalation was slower, reaching a plateau almost at the end of 1-min hypercapnia, was more gradual and had an amplitude twice as low as that in sham animals (Fig. 2a–b, 28.7 ± 5.1%). The decline in dilatation after CO_2 termination was twice as slow and was more gradual than in sham animals (Fig. 2a), both reflecting impaired CVR. Anodal tDCS enhanced the reactivity of cortical arterioles: their response to hypercapnia was faster and the dilatation was stronger in both the sham (57.6 ± 5.6%, $p < 0.05$) and TBI (39.6 ± 4.9%, $p < 0.01$) groups (Fig. 2a–b).

Simultaneous NADH autofluorescence imaging did not show any significant changes in tissue oxygen supply during hypercapnia in Sham animals as a result of arteriolar dilatation and increased RBC traffic, reflecting intact mCBF regulation (Fig. 2 c–d). In TBI animals, NADH autofluorescence during hypercapnia increased

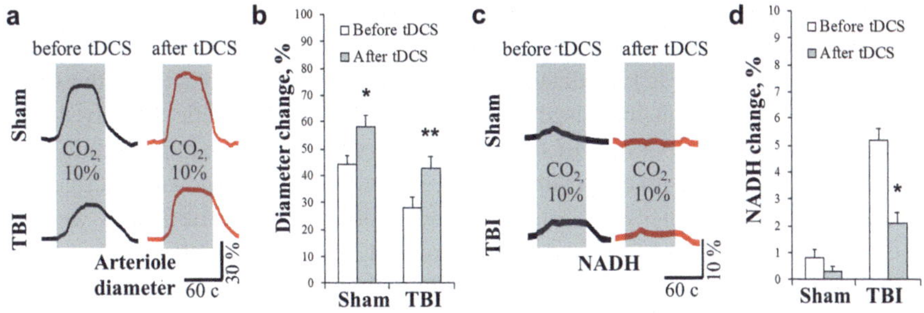

Fig. 2 Anodal tDCS improves cerebrovascular reactivity. (**a**) Change in the diameter of the arterioles during hypercapnia test, and (**b**) Cerebrovascular reactivity is better after tDCS; (**c**) NADH autofluorescence dynamics during the hypercapnia test, and (**d**) NADH autofluorescence before and after tDCS; n = 10, $* \ p < 0.05$. mean ± SEM

by 5.3 ± 0.5%, reflecting decreased tissue oxygen supply due to impaired CVR (Fig. c–d). Anodal tDCS in TBI mice abolished the reduction in tissue oxygen supply during hypercapnia by improving CVR (Fig. 2 c–d, 2.2 ± 0.4%, $p < 0.05$).

4 Discussion

Injury of microvasculature, blood flow, and blood flow regulation is a common complication in TBI, as reported in experimental TBI and in patients [2, 3, 8]. Our data also show that after TBI, the dilatation response of cerebral arterioles to hypercapnia was reduced, reflecting impaired CVR and an inability of the traumatized brain to adequately adjust blood flow and oxygen delivery according to metabolic demand. The decrease in tissue oxygen supply, reflected by NADH increase during hypercapnia, confirms a mismatch between cerebral blood flow and neuronal metabolism that may further damage the brain. Since CO_2 reactivity is dependent on the well-known vasodilator, nitric oxide (NO), generated by constitutive endothelial NOS (eNOS), our results suggest that NO concentration is low due to eNOS dysfunction, which has been shown in TBI [9, 10]. Anodal tDCS not only dilates cerebral arterioles thereby increasing cerebral microvascular flow and tissue oxygenation in mouse brain, as we shown in previous study [6], but also improves CVR and mCBF regulation. Because both dilatation of cerebral arterioles and CVR depend on the NO, it is highly-likely that anodal tDCS activates functional eNOS in normal brain and restores functionality of dysfunctional eNOS in the traumatized brain.

To our knowledge, this study is the first describing the influence of tDCS on CVR in cerebral parenchymal arterioles. Previous studies on human subjects reported decrease in vasomotor reactivity (VMR), the related to CVR index, of middle cerebral artery (MCA) after 15-minute 1-mA anodal tDCS [11, 12]. Vernieri et al. calculated VMR from measured blood flow velocity by Transcranial Doppler before and during hypercapnia, induced by the inhalation of a mixture of 7% CO2/

air [11]. Giorli et al. assessed VMR by Transcranial Color-Coded Sonography calculating through Breath Holding Index and Heart Rate Variability before and during 30-second breath hold [12]. Both suggested that anodal tDCS can activate the sympathetic system and that increased after anodal tDCS sympathetic activity could reduce the potential capability of further dilating vessels after a hypercapnia [11, 12]. This discrepancy with our results is only superficial, as it is known, that reactivity and reserve in parenchymal arterioles and middle cerebral arteries, as well as mechanisms involved, are sufficiently different [13]. Middle cerebral arteries are indeed regulated mainly by the adrenergic sympathetic system, while parenchymal arterioles and microvessels are innervated from within the brain tissue and tightly involved in neurovascular coupling [14]. Moreover, in our study, the maximal CVR and mCBF regulation increase were observed and traumatized brain with substantially impaired CVR and regulation, while Vernieri et al. and Giorli et al. studied healthy volunteers with intact VMR [11, 12].

5 Conclusion

Anodal tDCS restores cerebrovascular reactivity of parenchymal arterioles and regulation of mCBF in traumatized mouse brain that could contribute to neurologic improvement.

Acknowledgments Supported by NIH-NIGMS P20GM109089.

References

1. Yezhuvath US, Lewis-Amezcua K, Varghese R et al (2009) On the assessment of cerebrovascular reactivity using hypercapnia BOLD MRI. NMR Biomed 22:779–786
2. Enevoldsen EM, Jensen FT (1978) Autoregulation and CO_2 responses of cerebral blood flow in patients with acute severe head injury. J Neurosurg 48:689–703
3. Jullienne A, Obenaus A, Ichkova A et al (2016) Chronic cerebrovascular dysfunction after traumatic brain injury. J Neurosci Res 94:609–622
4. Clayton E, Kinley-Cooper SK, Weber RA et al (2016) Brain stimulation: Neuromodulation as a potential treatment for motor recovery following traumatic brain injury. Brain Res 1640(Pt A):130–138
5. Tully H (2018) Go with the flow: cerebrovascular reactivity as a therapeutic target for TBI symptoms. Sci Transl Med 10(433):eaat1643
6. Bragina OA, Lara DA, Nemoto EM et al (2018) Increases in microvascular perfusion and tissue oxygenation via vasodilatation after anodal Transcranial direct current stimulation in the healthy and traumatized mouse brain. Adv Exp Med Biol 1072:27–31
7. Balbi M, Koide M, Wellman GC et al (2017) Inversion of neurovascular coupling after subarachnoid hemorrhage in vivo. J Cereb Blood Flow Metab 37(11):3625–3634
8. Kenney K, Amyot F, Haber M et al (2016) Cerebral vascular injury in traumatic brain injury. Exp Neurol 275(Pt 3):353–366

9. Cherian L, Hlatky R, Robertson CS (2004) Nitric oxide in traumatic brain injury. Brain Pathol 14:195–201
10. Wada K, Chatzipanteli K, Busto R et al (1998) Role of nitric oxide in traumatic brain injury in the rat. J Neurosurg 89:807–818
11. Vernieri F, Assenza G, Maggio P et al (2010) Cortical Neuromodulation modifies cerebral vasomotor reactivity. Stroke 41:2087–2090
12. Giorli E, Tognazzi S, Briscese L et al (2015) Transcranial direct current stimulation and cerebral vasomotor reserve: a study in healthy subjects. J Neuroimaging 25(4):571–574
13. Cipolla MJ, Sweet J, Chan SL et al (2014) Increased pressure-induced tone in rat parenchymal arterioles vs. middle cerebral arteries: role of ion channels and calcium sensitivity. J Appl Physiol 117(1):53–59
14. Cipolla MJ (2009) The cerebral circulation. San Rafael (CA): Morgan & Claypool Life Sciences; Chapters 3–5. https://www.ncbi.nlm.nih.gov/books/NBK53081/toc/?report=reader

Comparative Analysis of Simultaneous Transcranial Doppler and Perfusion Computed Tomography for Cerebral Perfusion Evaluation in Patients with Traumatic Brain Injury

Alex Trofimov, Artem Kopylov, Michael Dobrzeniecki, Anatoly Sheludyakov, Dmitry Martynov, Kseniia Trofimova, Darya I. Agarkova, and Denis E. Bragin

Abstract The aim was to investigate the feasibility of simultaneous comparison of cerebral circulation in major vessels and microvasculature in patients suffering traumatic brain injury (TBI) with or without intracranial hematomas (IH). *Methods.* 170 patients were divided into two groups: Group 1 – diffuse TBI (75 patients); and Group 2 – TBI with IH (95 patients: 18 epidural, 65 subdural and 12 multiple). Perfusion computed tomography (PCT) for assessment of volumetric cerebral blood flow (CBF) was done 2–15 days after admission to hospital. Simultaneous assessment of cerebral blood flow velocity (CBFV) in both middle cerebral arteries was done by transcranial Doppler. *Results.* In patients with diffuse TBI, CBF had statistically valid correlations with CBFV ($r = 0.28$, $p = 0.0149$ on the left side; $r = 0.382$, $p = 0.00075$ on the right side). In patients with TBI and IH, the analysis did not reveal any reliable correlations between the CBFV and CBF velocity in the temporal lobes, either on the side of the removed IH or on the opposite side. *Conclusion.* The greatest linear correlation was noted in patients with diffuse TBI without the development of a coarse shift of the midline structures and dislocation syndrome. This correlation decreases with the increase in injury severity and development of secondary complications in the acute period, which probably reflects impairment of the coupling of oxygen consumption by brain tissue and cerebral microcirculation.

Keywords Traumatic brain injury · Perfusion computer tomography · Cerebral blood flow · Doppler · Cerebral blood flow velocity · Intracranial hematoma

A. Trofimov (✉) · A. Kopylov · M. Dobrzeniecki · A. Sheludyakov · D. Martynov
K. Trofimova · D. I. Agarkova
Department of Neurosurgery, Privolzhsky Research Medical University, Nizhny Novgorod, Russia

D. E. Bragin
Department of Neurosurgery, University of New Mexico School of Medicine, Albuquerque, USA

© Springer Nature Switzerland AG 2020

P.-D. Ryu et al. (eds.), *Oxygen Transport to Tissue XLI*, Advances in Experimental Medicine and Biology 1232, https://doi.org/10.1007/978-3-030-34461-0_8

1 Introduction

The common definition of cerebral autoregulation (CA) describes the brain's ability to maintain adequate microcirculation in the context of changes in mean arterial pressure [1, 2]. Cerebral autoregulation assessment techniques, used clinically, typically evaluate responses in cerebral blood flow (CBF) and cerebral blood flow velocity (CBFV) to changes in arterial blood pressure (ABP) alone [3]. Comparative studies have investigated the relationship between CBF and CBFV [2, 4, 5] during steady-state changes in mean arterial pressure (MAP); however, no comparison has been made between CBF and CBFV in traumatic brain injury (TBI). To provide insight into the utility of correlations between CBF and CBFV as a measure of autoregulation in this patient group, and to add to the body of comparative literature on this topic [6], we performed a comparison between CBF and CBFV in TBI patients without intracranial hematomas (IH) and after neurosurgical removal of developed IH.

The aim of our work was to investigate the feasibility of simultaneous comparison of the cerebral circulation in major vessels and microvasculature, using perfusion computer tomography (PCT) and transcranial Doppler in traumatized brain with and without IH.

2 Materials and Methods

This single-center prospective study complies with the Declaration of Helsinki and the protocol was approved by the local Ethics Committee. All the patients gave informed consent to participate in the study. All 170 patients with TBI were treated at the Nizhny Novgorod Regional Trauma Center Level I in 2012–2017. Mean age of the patients was 35.5 ± 14.8 (range 15–73) years; 65 women/105 men,). The patients were divided into two groups: Group 1 included 75 patients with diffuse TBI (Marshall II-III and Rotterdam 1–3) without hematomas; and Group 2 included 95 patients with TBI after neurosurgical removal of IH (18 epidural, 65 subdural, 12 multiple). These two groups were comparable in age and severity of TBI (GCS) and concomitant lesions (Injury Severity Score). All patients in Group 2 underwent surgery within the first 3 days. A complex of the neuromonitoring 'Centaurus' was used during the study (Ver. 2.0, Nizhny Novgorod State Medical Academy, Russia). The neuromonitoring system is shown in Fig. 1.

All patients were subjected to dynamic PCT by 64-slice tomograph Philips Ingenuity CT (Philips Medical Systems, Cleveland, USA). The tomography was performed 1–12 days after TBI (mean 4 ± 3 days) in Group 1 and 2–8 days (mean 4 ± 2 days) after surgical evacuation of the hematoma in Group 2. The perfusion examination report included an initial contrast-free CT of the brain. Extended scanning was further performed in 16 areas of interest, 160 mm in thickness, within 60 s, with a contrast agent (Perfusion JOG mode). The scanning parameters were 160 kVp, 160 mA, 70 mAs, 512×512. The contrast agent Ultravist 370 (Schering AG,

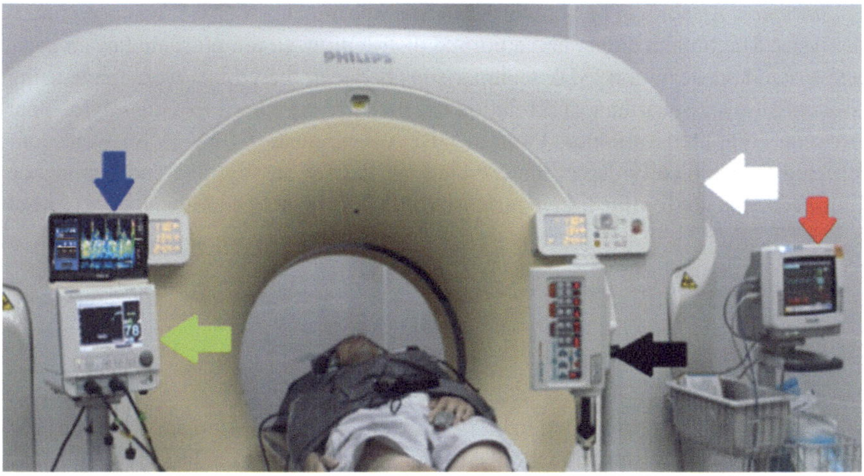

Fig. 1 The Neuromonitoring System: white arrow, CT; blue arrow, TCD; red arrow, ECG-ABP monitor; black arrow, syringe injector; and green arrow, cerebral oximeter

Germany) was administered with an automatic syringe injector (Stellant, Medrad, Indianola, USA) into a peripheral vein through a standard catheter (20 G) at a rate of 4–5 ml/sec in a dose of 30–50 ml per examination.

After scanning, data were transferred to a Philips Extended Brilliance Workspace workstation (Philips HealthCare Netherland B.V., Best, the Netherlands). Artery and vein marks were automatically recorded, followed by the manual control of indices in the time-concentration diagram. Regions of interest (ROI) were established in subcortical areas of the middle cerebral artery. Perfusion maps were derived from the tissue time-attenuation curve on the basis of the change in X-ray attenuation, which is linearly related to iodinated contrast concentration on a per-voxel basis with time. Errors introduced by delay and dispersion of the contrast bolus before arrival in the cerebral circulation were corrected by block-circulant deconvolution algorithm. Quantitative perfusion indices, including CBF, were calculated on a voxel-wise basis and were used to generate color-coded maps. The voxels with volumetric CBF >100 mL/100 g/min or cerebral blood volume (CBV) >8 mL100 g were assumed to contain vessels and removed from the ROI, using the Remote vessels' mode.

CBF velocity in the middle cerebral artery (Vav, cm/sec) was measured simultaneously and bilaterally by transcranial Doppler through the temporal window with a 2-MHz probe (Sonomed 300 M, Spectromed, Russia) according to the method developed by R. Aaslid [7]. The probe was positioned over the temporal bone window above the zygomatic arch and fixed. This procedure ensured that the angle and individual depth of insonation remained constant during investigation. The temporal ultrasound window and depth of the insonation provided the highest velocities were used for all measurements. The Doppler probe was fixed over the temple with a special headset.

Statistical Analysis. The Statistica 7.0 (StatSoft Inc., USA, 2004) was used for all analyses. The obtained data had a normal distribution, so are presented as an average ± standard deviation (SD). Comparisons between the groups were made using Student's t-test. Spearman's correlation coefficients were used to assess agreement between computed variables. Plots of CBF versus mean CBFV (Vav) were constructed to graphically depict the correlations. The regression line and confidence limits for each are for illustrative purposes only. The level of significance was preset to $p < 0.05$.

3 Results

Basic statistics for recorded parameters (Vav, CBF) and the comparison of the analyzed parameters are shown in Table 1. In patients with diffuse TBI the volumetric CBF had statistically valid, moderately expressed correlations with the cerebral blood flow velocity (Spearman's $r = 0.28$, $p = 0.0149$ on the left side (Fig. 2a); Spearman's $r = 0.382$, $p = 0.00075$ on the right side (Fig. 2b)).

In patients with TBI after surgical removal of IH, the performed correlation analysis did not reveal any statistically reliable correlations between the linear blood flow velocity in the MCA and the volumetric flow velocity in the temporal lobes, either on the side of the removed hematoma (perifocal zone) or on the opposite side (Fig. 3).

4 Discussion

In this study, we investigated patients with diffuse TBI and focal TBI (after surgery for hematomas) and did not find a statistically significant difference between CBF and CBFV on the left and right side in patients with diffuse TBI which is consistent with previous studies [1].

Table 1 Data on comparison of the analyzed parameters

		Vav (cm/sec)	CBF (ml/100 g × min)
1	Group 1 (left side)	46.1 ± 13.8	31.7 ± 10
2	Group 1 (right side)	45.7 ± 12.9	31.6 ± 10,2
3	Group 2 (ipsilateral side of former hematoma)	36.8 ± 12.8	32.3 ± 17.7
4	Group 2 (contralateral side of former hematoma)	48.7 ± 17.7	28.4 ± 11.1
	P (1–2)	0.983	0.994
	P (1–3)	<0.005[aa]	0.138
	P (1–4)	<0.5[a]	0.194
	P (3–4)	<0.001[aaaa]	0.247

[a]Significant difference ($p < 0.01$)

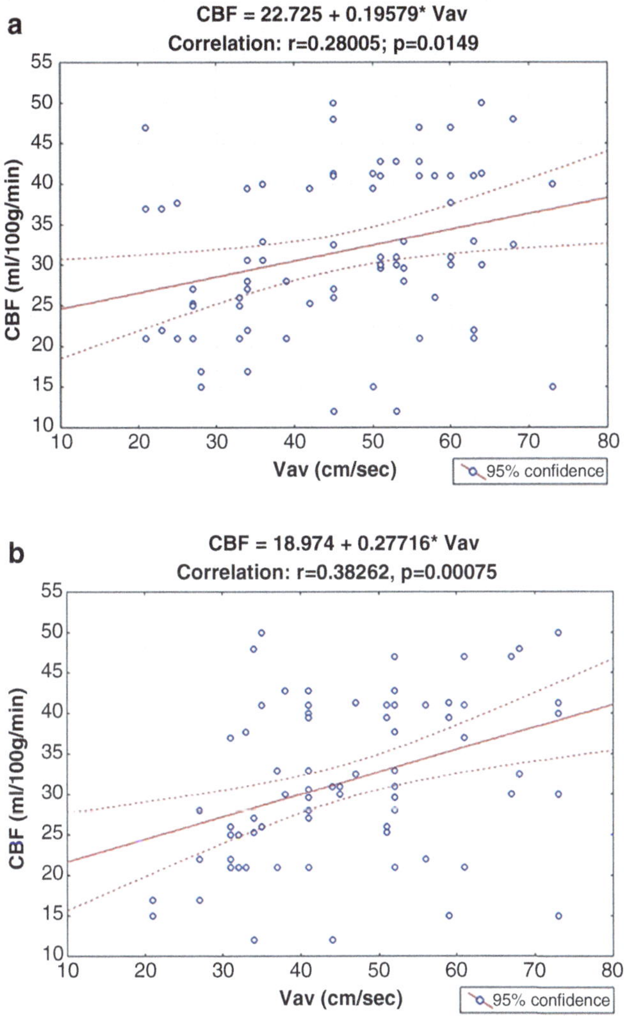

Fig. 2 Volumetric CBF plotted against Vav (CBFV) on the left side (**a**) and right side (**b**) in Group 1 with diffuse TBI. Dashed red lines represent 95% confidence intervals for the regression (solid red line)

Previous studies have shown statistically significant correlations between absolute values of flows and velocities were statistically significant in healthy volunteers, and the relationship between CBF and MV was described according to a linear model [4].

The most marked correlation was noted in TBI patients with diffuse lesions without the development of a coarse shift of the midline structures and dislocation syndrome. This correlation decreased with the increase in injury severity and development of secondary complications in the acute period, which probably

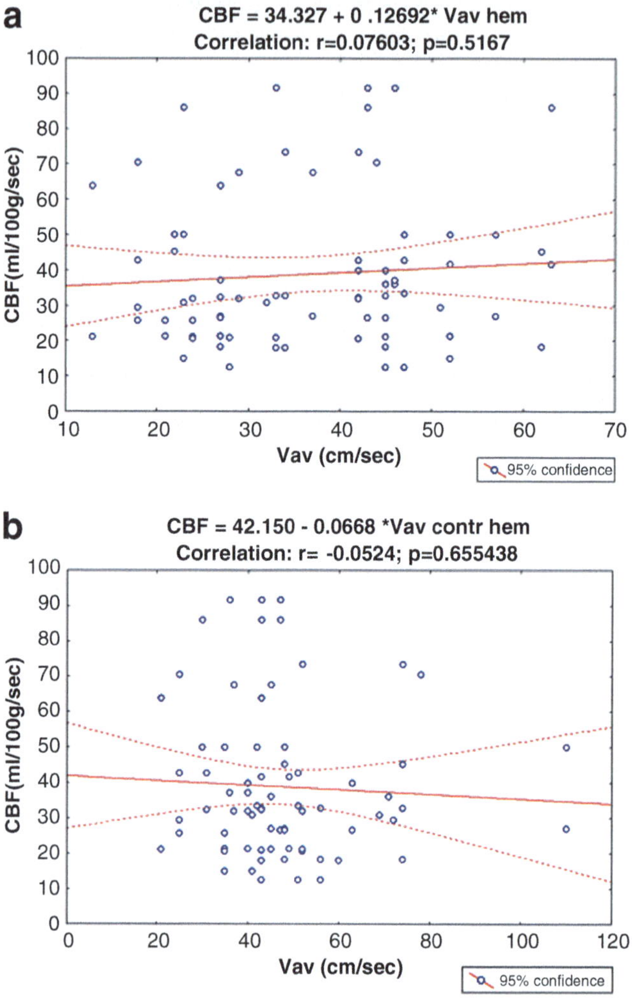

Fig. 3 Volumetric CBF plotted against Vav (CBFV) in group 2 after surgical removal of intracranial hematomas (**a**) on the side of the removed hematoma (**b**) on contralateral side. Dashed red lines represent 95% confidence intervals for the regression (solid red line)

reflects impairment of the coupling of oxygen consumption by brain tissue and cerebral microcirculation. We assume that the volumetric CBF depends on both the regional blood supply and the linear blood flow velocity.

The nonlinear correlation between the volumetric blood flow and regional blood supply in the damaged brain areas might be similar to Lassen's autoregulation curve [8, 9], which also shows the nonlinear dynamics of changes in volumetric blood flow in the case of brain injuries. We noted a similar pattern when studying patients in the acute phase after the removal of traumatic IH. Although comparison of the perfusion data in patients in Group 2 has not revealed any significant differences between the side of the removed hematoma and the opposite hemisphere, the correlations between these parameters of CBF were seriously disrupted. Thus, we have shown that in patients of this group the volumetric blood flow velocity did not reliably correlate with its linear velocity.

In our opinion, development of the disruption between linear and volumetric cerebral flow reflects a serious disturbance of CBF autoregulation, as an increase in linear blood flow velocity after surgery causes a reverse reaction, i.e. a drop in volumetric blood flow. In contradistinction to our data, in healthy individuals, no such differences have been identified [4]. It is possible that the disparity between the blood flow through the MCA and the capacity of the microvasculature may be one of the reason for the second progression of the parenchymal hemorrhages [1].

We believe that comparative correlation analysis of CBF and CBFV is necessary to specify the development of secondary brain damage and uncoupling between cerebral circulation and brain tissue oxygen consumption, to determine possible ways to prevent their formation during treatment [2]. The analysis of correlation between CBF and CBFV could help to predict efficiency or limitations of infusion therapy. In the case of the lack of correlation between CBF and CBFV, infusion therapy can provoke detrimental hyperemia or hyperperfusion [1].

5 Conclusion

In this study, the strongest linear correlation between CBF and CBFV was noted in TBI patients with diffuse lesions without the development of a coarse shift of the midline structures and dislocation syndrome. This correlation probably reflects impairment of the cerebral autoregulation and uncoupling of oxygen consumption by brain tissue and cerebral microcirculation. The reported study was funded by RFBR, project number 20-015-00110 and RSF 20-15-00037.

References

1. Payne S (2016) Cerebral autoregulation: control of blood flow in the brain. Springer, Berlin
2. Pries AR, Secomb TW, Gaehtgens P, Gross J (1990) Blood flow in microvascular networks. Experiments and simulation. Circ Res 67(4):826–834
3. Liu J, Zhu YS, Hill C, Zhang R (2013) Cerebral autoregulation of blood velocity and volumetric flow during steady-state changes in arterial pressure. Hypertension 62(5):973–979. https://doi.org/10.1161/HYPERTENSIONAHA.113.01867
4. Démolis P, Tran Dinh YR, Giudicelli JF (1996) Relationships between cerebral regional blood flow velocities and volumetric blood flows and their respective reactivities to acetazolamide. Stroke 27(10):1835–1839
5. Larsen FS, Olsen KS, Hansen BA, Paulson OB, Knudsen GM (1994) Transcranial doppler is valid for determination of the lower limit of cerebral blood flow autoregulation. Stroke 25:1985–1988

6. Mohrman DE, Heller LJ (2013) Cardiovascular physiology, 8th edn. McGraw-Hill, New York
7. Aaslid R, Markwalder TM, Nornes H (1982) Noninvasive transcranial Doppler ultrasound recording of flow velocity in basal cerebral arteries. J Neurosurg 57(6):769–774
8. Newell DW, Aaslid R, Lam A, Mayberg TS, Winn HR (1994) Comparison of flow and velocity during dynamic autoregulation testing in humans. Stroke 25:793–797
9. Lassen NA (1964) Autoregulation of cerebral blood flow. Circulation research 15. Supplement P201–204

Meningeal Lymphatic Pathway of Brain Clearing From the Blood After Haemorrhagic Injuries

O. Semyachkina-Glushkovskaya, N. Navolokin, A. Shirokov, A. Terskov, A. Khorovodov, A. Mamedova, M. Klimova, E. Rafailov, and J. Kurths

Abstract This seems to be the time to gain new knowledge about the meningeal lymphatic system and a deeper understanding of its anatomy and physiology. Although it is known that the meningeal lymphatics present in the layers of the brain, limited information is available about the role of this system in brain function. Here, for the first time we clearly demonstrate that the meningeal lymphatic pathway is involved in brain clearing from the blood after intracranial hemorrhage associated with hypoxia and forms a connective bridge between interstitial, cerebral spinal fluid and peripheral lymphatics. We also show that the development of methods to stimulate meningeal lymph flow after hemorrhagic evidence in the brain might be a neuroprotective strategy for effective recovery of the brain after a cerebrovascular catastrophe.

Keywords Intracranial hemorrhages · Hypoxia · Blood-brain barrier · Lymphatic system · Brain drainage and clearance

O. Semyachkina-Glushkovskaya (✉) · A. Terskov · A. Khorovodov · A. Mamedova
M. Klimova
Saratov State University, Saratov, Russia

N. Navolokin
Saratov State Medical University, Saratov, Russia

A. Shirokov
Russian Academy of Sciences, Institute of Biochemistry and Physiology of Plants and Microorganisms, Saratov, Russia

E. Rafailov
Saratov State University, Saratov, Russia

Optoelectronics and Biomedical Photonics Group, Aston University, Birmingham, UK

J. Kurths
Saratov State University, Saratov, Russia

Physics Department, Humboldt University, Berlin, Germany

Potsdam Institute for Climate Impact Research, Potsdam, Germany

© Springer Nature Switzerland AG 2020
P.-D. Ryu et al. (eds.), *Oxygen Transport to Tissue XLI*, Advances in Experimental Medicine and Biology 1232, https://doi.org/10.1007/978-3-030-34461-0_9

1 Introduction

The meningeal lymphatic system, as a network of transparent vessels in the layer of the brain, was discovered by the Italian anatomist Paulo Mascagni two centuries ago [1, 2]. However, because his experiments could not be repeated, the absence of a lymphatic system in the brain was reported in the late nineteenth century. However, in recent years the meningeal lymphatic system has received increasing interest [3–14]. The number of publications in this field has increased exponentially: e.g. only 3 years after the confirmation of Mascagni's discoveries by Louveau et al. and Aspelund et al. in 2015, 208 articles were included in PubMed.

Thus, it seems the right time for fundamental studies of the anatomic and functional pathways for the cerebrospinal fluid (CSF)-lymph connections.

Although the concept is accepted that the CSF draws from the brain to the deep cervical lymph nodes (dcLN) [3–9], there is a gap in our understanding regarding the pattern of the meningeal lymphatics in the CSF-lymph link.

Our earlier data on healthy rodents showed that tracers injected into the cisterna magna or directly into the brain tissues, as well as tracers which crossed the opened blood-brain barrier (BBB), are rapidly present in meningeal lymphatics and in dcLN [6, 7]. These results clearly demonstrate a relationship between BBB opening and activation of brain drainage via the meningeal lymphatics, which draws CSF-lymph into dcLN.

Taking these facts into account, we hypothesized that meningeal lymphatics play an important role in brain drainage and clearing function, which is activated by changes in cerebrovascular homeostasis. To test our hypothesis, we focus on investigation of meningeal lymphatic scenarios of brain clearing using an animal model of brain hemorrhage associated with opening of BBB and hypoxia, as the two main factors contributing to cerebrovascular disbalance.

2 Methods

The studies were carried out with 60 male mice (20–25 g) divided into two groups: i) a control group without brain hemorrhage (n = 30), and ii) an experimental group with brain hemorrhage (n = 30).

To induce brain hemorrhage, the protocol of the impact of sound stress adapted to adult mice was used (120 dB, 370 Hz, uninterrupted sound) [12, 13]. All mice were decapitated for histological study of brain tissue.

For analysis of BBB permeability, we used a confocal microscopy of FITC-dextran 70 kDa extravasation and a specific marker of the cerebral endothelium, SMI (Santa Cruz Biotechnology, Santa Cruz, CA, USA) [14].

The level of blood oxygen saturation (SpO2) in the brain was monitored using a pulse oximeter (model CMS60D, Contec Medical Systems Co., Ltd., Qinhuangdao, China). Oxy-hemoglobin saturation is presented as a percentage of HbO2 vs. the total Hb in the blood.

For visualization of the meningeal lymphatic vessels we used the protocol for immunohistochemical analysis with the specific marker lymphatic vessel endothelial hyaluronan receptor 1 (LYVE-1, eBioscience, clone ALY7, anti-LYVE1 antibody (1 : 1000). For analysis of the presence of blood products in the deep cervical lymph node (dcLN), we used the histological method of Perls' Prussian blue staining technique for hemosiderin, and atomic absorption spectroscopy (Thermo Scientific Inc., USA) for measurement of the level of iron in dcLN [6].

3 Results

3.1 *Brain Clearance from Blood after Brain Hemorrhage Associated with Hypoxia*

Figure 1B is an example of stress-induced brain hemorrhage that was close to the first lateral ventricle of the brain (Fig. 1A, normal brain tissue). All mice with brain hemorrhage showed a significant decrease in SpO_2 compared with controls (97 ± 3% vs. 64 ± 5%, $p < 0.001$)

Figure D shows that, within 1 h after brain hemorrhage, hemosiderin was present and diffusely distributed in dcLN (Fig. 1C, normal tissue of dcLN). These changes were accompanied by a high level of iron in dcLN vs. the control group (0.610 ± 0.031 μg/g vs. 0.0002 ± 0.0001 μg/g, $p < 0.001$).

These results clearly demonstrate the accumulation of products of denatured hemoglobin, such as hemosiderin in dcLN, that is the first anatomic station of the exit of CSF from the brain and the first connective lymph node between the meningeal and peripheral lymphatics [3, 4, 6, 7]. Taking these facts into account, we concluded that the brain is cleaned from the blood via the meningeal lymphatic system.

3.2 *Activation of Brain Drainage Via the Meningeal Lymphatics after Brain Hemorrhage*

To better understand changes in the meningeal lymphatic system after the development of brain hemorrhage, we then performed immunohistochemical analysis of the diameter of the meningeal lymphatic vessels. Figures 2A and B show that, 1 h after brain hemorrhage, the meningeal lymphatic vessels were 4.3-fold larger as compared to controls. The increased diameter of the meningeal lymphatic vessels after development of brain hemorrhage suggests activation of brain drainage that is accompanied by interstitial fluid influx into the lymphatic vessels. We assume that, after brain hemorrhage, the Virhow-Robin space might be a pathway for rapid removal of the interstitial fluid and the blood from the extracellular space into the subarachnoid space where the meningeal lymphatics draw off CBF/lymph in dcLN, i.e. to peripheral lymphatics, as discussed in our recent publications [6, 7].

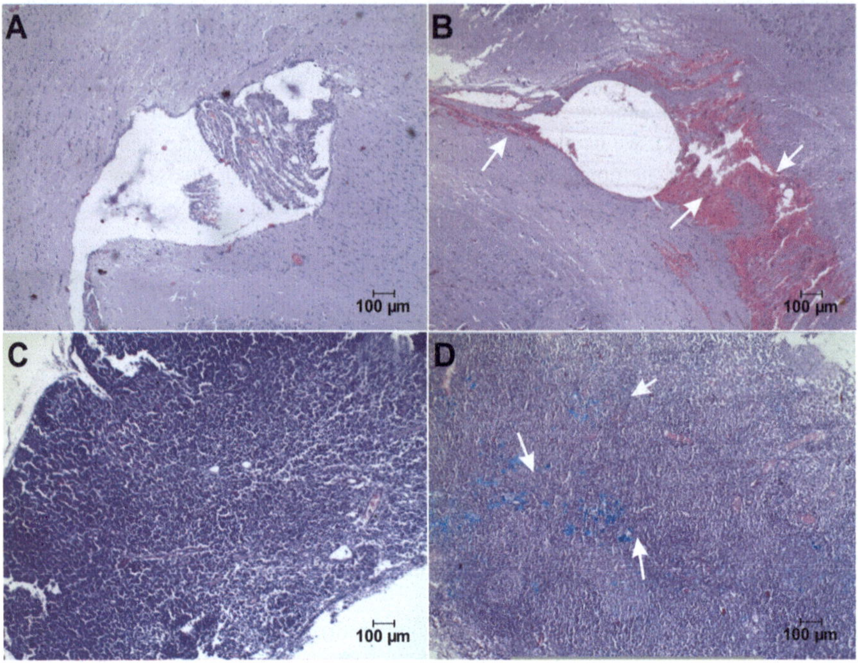

Fig. 1 Histological analysis of the brain tissues before and after brain hemorrhage: A, the control group, normal cerebral ventricle; B, brain bleeding (red, arrowed) close to the first lateral cerebral ventricles; C, control group, normal tissues of dcLN; D, tissues of dcLN at 1 h after brain hemorrhage with presence of hemosiderin (blue, arrowed) (n = 10 in each group). A and B, hematoxylin & eosin staining; C and D, Perls' Prussian blue staining. Bars represent 10 μm (magnification × 64.6)

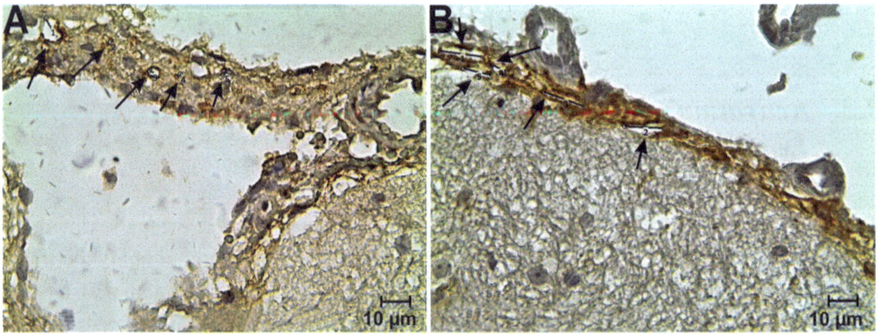

Fig. 2 Immunohistochemical analysis of changes in the diameter of the meningeal lymphatic vessels before and after brain hemorrhage: A, the control group; B, after brain hemorrhage. The average diameter of the meningeal lymphatic vessels (black, arrowed, labeled by specific marker, LYVE-1) was 4.3-fold higher in rats after brain hemorrhage vs. rats from the control group (without hemorrhage). Approximately 10 slices per animal were imaged. Bars represent 10 μm (magnification × 246.4)

3.3 Opening of BBB after Brain Hemorrhage Stimulates the Brain Drainage Function Via the Meningeal Lymphatics

Figure 3 shows the results of confocal imaging. Our data demonstrate strong FITC-dextran extravasation from the cerebral vessel into the brain parenchyma after development of brain hemorrhage. Extravasation of FITC-dextran was determined as a clear fluorescence visualized outside the vessel walls (Fig. 3B and C). No extravasation of FITC-dextran was observed in the control group (Fig. 3A and B)

Figure 3E and F illustrate presence of FITC dextran in the meningeal lymphatic vessels in mice with disrupted BBB after brain haemorrhage. We did not detected FITC-dextran in the meningeal lymphatics in the control group.

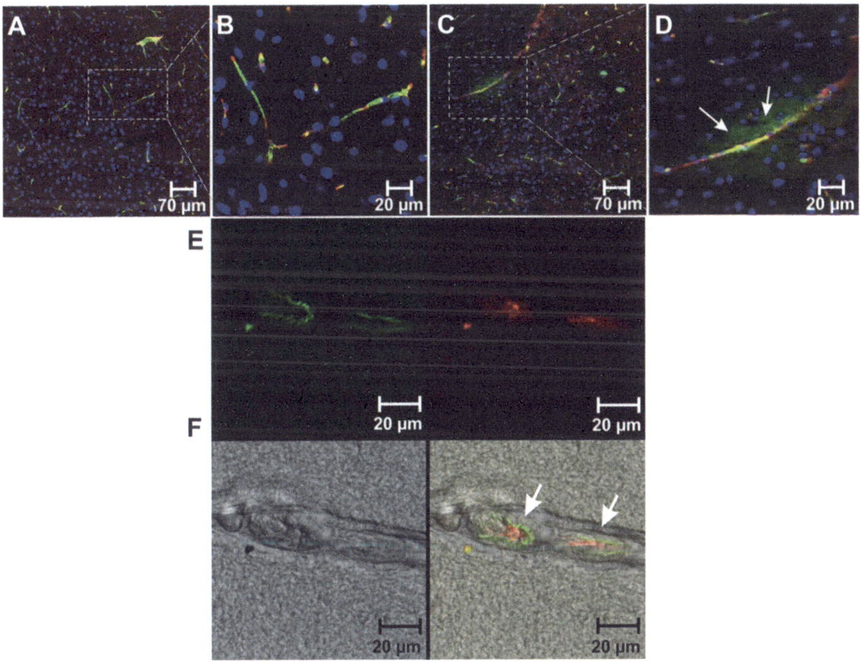

Fig. 3 Confocal microscopy of the BBB permeability for FITC-dextran 70 kDa (green; DAPI blue, arrowed) before and after brain hemorrhage using specific markers of cerebral vascular endothelium, SMI-71 (red). A, no FITC-dextran leakage in the control group; B, same area at higher magnification, from A; C, FITC-dextran extravasation from the cerebral vessel into the brain parenchyma; D, the same area at higher magnification, from C. Approximately 10 slices per animal from the cortical and subcortical regions were imaged (except for the hypothalamus and choroid plexus where the BBB is leaky); E, presence of FITC-dextran (red) in the meningeal lymphatic vessels (labeled by LYVE-1 conjugated with Alexa 488, green) after brain hemorrhage associated with opening of the BBB

4 Conclusions

In summary, our results demonstrate that brain hemorrhage associated with hypoxia is accompanied by high the BBB permeability to FITC-dextran, suggesting disruption of BBB. The presence of FITC-dextran in the meningeal lymphatics and hemosiderin/iron in dcLN after the BBB opening in mice with intracranial heamorrhages, indicates an important role of the meningeal lymphatic system in post-hemorrhagic activation of the brain drainage and clearing processes.

Acknowledgments This work was supported by grants from the Russian Science Foundation (18-15-00172): Visualization of the meningeal lymphatics, RFBR № 17-02-00358\18: SpO2 recording, grant from the Ministry of Science and Education № 17.1223.2017: Methods for BBB opening.

References

1. Mascagni P, Bellini GB. (1816) Presso Euse bio Pacinie Figlio: Florence. p 195
2. Lukić IK, Glunčić V, Ivkić G et al (2003) Virtual dissection: a lesson from the 18th century. Lancet 362:2110–2113
3. Louveau A, Smirnov I, Keyes T et al (2015) Structural and functional features of central nervous system lymphatic vessels. Nature 523:337–341
4. Aspelund A, Antila S, Proulx S et al (2015) A dural lymphatic vascular system that drains brain interstitial fluid and macromolecules. J Exp Med 212(7):991–999
5. Koh L, Zhaharov A, Jonston M (2005) Integration of the subarachnoid space and lymphatics: is it time to embrace concept of cerebrospinal fluid absorption? Cerebrospinal Fluid Res 2:6. https://doi.org/10.1186/1743-8454-2-6
6. Semyachkina-Glushkovskaya O, Chehonin V, Borisova E et al (2017) Photodynamic opening of the blood-brain barrier and pathways of brain clearing pathways. J Biophotonics. https://doi.org/10.1002/jbio.201700287
7. Semyachkina-Glushkovskaya O, Abdurashitov A, Dubrovsky A et al (2017) Application of optical coherent tomography for in vivo monitoring of the meningeal lymphatic vessels during opening of blood-brain barrier: mechanisms of brain clearing. J Biomed Opt 22(12):1–9. https://doi.org/10.1117/1.JBO.22.12.121719
8. Bradbury MWB, Cserr HF, Westrop RJ (1981) Drainage of cerebral intestinal fluid into deep cervical lymph of the rabbit. Am J Phys 240:329–336
9. Cserr HF, Harling-Berg CJ, Knopf PM (1992) Drainage of brain extracellular fluid into blood and deep cervical lymph and its immunological significance. Brain Pathol 2:269–276
10. Johnston M, Papaiconomou C (2002) Cerebrospinal fluid transport: a lymphatic perspective. News Physiol Sci 17:227–230
11. Weller R, Kida S, Zhang E-T (1992) Pathways of fluid drainage from the brain: morphological aspects and immunological significance in rat and man. Brain Pathol 2:277–284
12. Semyachkina-Glushkovskaya O, Borisova E, Avramov L et al (2016) The stress and vascular catastrophes in newborn rats: mechanisms preceding and accompanying the brain hemorrhages. Front Physiol. 14;7:210 | doi: https://doi.org/10.3389/fphys.2016.00210
13. Semyachkina-Glushkovskaya O, Pavlov A, Kurths J et al (2015) Optical monitoring of stress-related changes in the brain tissues and vessels associated with hemorrhagic stroke in newborn rats. Biomed Opt Express 6(10):4088–4097
14. Hoffmann A, Bredno J, Wendland M et al (2011) High and low molecular weight fluorescein isothiocyanate (FITC)-dextran to assess blood-brain barrier disruption: technical consideration. Transl Stroke Res 2(1):106–111

Relationship Between Cerebral Oxygenation and Skin Blood Flow at the Frontal Lobe during Progressive Hypoxia: Impact of Acute Hypotension

Masahiro Horiuchi, Junko Endo, and Yoko Handa-Kirihra

Abstract We investigated the relationship between cerebral oxygenation (COX) and skin blood flow (SkBF) at the left frontal lobes of 10 healthy young men during progressive hypoxia (~ −1 h at each of 21%, 18%, 15%, and 12% of inspired oxygen [FiO_2]). Acute hypotension was manipulated by a thigh-cuff-release technique, where a pressure of 220 mmHg was applied at both thigh muscles for 3 min and the cuff was immediately released to induce acute hypotension. While the resting baseline for COX before the thigh-cuff release manipulation decreased gradually with the reduction of FiO_2 ($P < 0.05$), the resting baseline for SkBF, mean arterial blood pressure (MAP), and cutaneous vascular conductance (CVC) were unaffected by FiO_2 ($P > 0.05$). The acute hypotension that was induced by the thigh-cuff release decreased COX, SkBF, MAP, and CVC; thereafter, these values recovered toward their baseline values. During the hypotension phase, while the time to the nadir values for COX slowed progressively with reductions in FiO_2 ($P < 0.05$), those for SkBF, MAP, and CVC were unaffected by FiO_2 ($P > 0.05$). These results suggest that COX may not be associated with SkBF for the protocol or with the subjects in the present study.

Keywords Acute hypotension · Blood pressure · Cerebral autoregulation · Near-infrared spectroscopy · Vascular conductance

1 Introduction

Several studies have demonstrated that cerebral oxygenation (COX) assessments with near-infrared spectroscopy (NIRS) are impacted by skin blood flow (SkBF). For example, studies have shown that tissue oxygenation at the frontal lobe is related to SkBF during dynamic exercise [1] and a phenylephrine-induced decrease in COX

M. Horiuchi (✉) · J. Endo · Y. Handa-Kirihra
Division of Human Environmental Science, Mt. Fuji Research Institute, Yamanashi, Japan
e-mail: mhoriuchi@mfri.pref.yamanashi.jp

© Springer Nature Switzerland AG 2020
P.-D. Ryu et al. (eds.), *Oxygen Transport to Tissue XLI*, Advances in Experimental Medicine and Biology 1232, https://doi.org/10.1007/978-3-030-34461-0_10

reflects vasoconstriction in the SkBF [2]. Thus, it is doubtful whether assessing COX with NIRS can truly reflect oxygen levels in the brain. Acute hypoxia reduces dynamic cerebral autoregulation, which helps maintain COX via blood flow to the brain. Since maintaining COX during hypoxia prevents certain high-altitude incidents, such as syncope [3], a proper evaluation of COX is needed. Additionally, from the viewpoint of the practical implications (e.g., mountain climbing), a full account of the effects of different levels of hypoxia is necessary. Nevertheless, it is unclear if COX is impacted by SkBF during progressive hypoxia.

Accordingly, we hypothesized that COX would be affected by SkBF during progressive hypoxia. To test this hypothesis, we used NIRS and laser Doppler flowmetry to monitor changes in regional COX and SkBF during progressive normobaric hypoxia (21%, 18%, 15%, and 12% fractions of inspired oxygen [FiO_2]). Further, we used a thigh-cuff release technique because observations during spontaneous cerebrovasculature responses in hypoxia appear less sensitive than assessments derived from the classical thigh-cuff release method, which imposes a larger and more abrupt change in blood pressure stimulus [4].

2 Methods

This study was approved by the ethical committee of the Mt. Fuji Research Institute in Japan and conducted according to the guidelines of the Declaration of Helsinki. The present report includes additional data from a previously published investigation [5]. Of the 11 subjects in the previous study, the data of 10 of the subjects were obtained for this study. Their mean age, height, and body weight were 23 ± 2 years, 174 ± 7 cm, and 71 ± 13 kg, respectively (values are mean ± standard deviation [SD]). Each subject sat on a comfortable chair in a semi-recumbent position. Subjects breathed room air (21% O_2), followed by three graded hypoxic gas mixtures containing 18%, 15%, and 12% O_2 for 60 min each. After 30 min of exposure to room air or each level of hypoxia, 2 min of baseline data were recorded. Subsequently, bilateral thigh-cuffs were inflated to a pressure of 220 mmHg for 3 min using a custom cuff inflator. To induce acute hypotension, the cuffs were then rapidly deflated. This protocol was repeated 2–3 times at 5 min intervals to allow for the recovery of resting values. After 1 h of exposure, subjects breathed the next graded level of O_2. Throughout all protocols, the subjects breathed hypoxic gas through a mask using a hypoxic generator (YHS-B05S; YKS, Nara, Japan).

COX was measured using NIRS (BOM-L1TRW; Omega Wave, Tokyo, Japan). Three laser-diodes (780, 810, and 830 nm) were used in this NIRS device and relative tissue levels of oxygenated hemoglobin (HbO_2) and deoxygenated hemoglobin (HHb) according to the modified Beer-Lambert-law were calculated. COX was expressed as $[HbO_2/(HbO_2 + HHb)] \times 100$ (i.e., as a percentage). NIRS optodes were placed on the left forehead and the light source was paired with two detectors set 2 cm and 4 cm apart. The hemoglobin concentrations received by detector 1 were subtracted from those received by detector 2 to minimize the influence of SkBF [6]. Additionally, SkBF at the frontal lobe was monitored using laser flowmetry (ATBF-LC1; Unique Medical, Tokyo, Japan) ~ 2 cm medial from the NIRS probes. To avoid crosstalk between NIRS and SkBF signals, we measured whether contamination NIRS and SkBF signals were recorded at 1 Hz (es8; TEAC, Tokyo, Japan). Heart rate (HR) was recorded using a lead II electrocardiograph. Partial pressure of end tidal CO_2 ($P_{ET}CO_2$) was measured by a breath-by-breath gas analyzer (AE-300; Minato Medical Science, Osaka, Japan). Beat-by-beat mean arterial pressure (MAP) was measured using finger photoplethysmography from the middle finger of the left hand (MUB-101; Medi-sens, Saitama, Japan). Peripheral arterial oxygen saturation (SpO_2) was monitored by finger pulse oximetry (PULSOX-300i; Konica Minolta, Tokyo, Japan). Based on an original study that have established thigh-cuff test [7], cutaneous vascular conductance (CVC) was calculated by dividing SkBF by MAP.

Data are presented as mean ± SD. One-way repeated ANOVAs (Sigma Stat version 3.5; Hulinks, Chicago, IL, USA) were conducted to compare the physiological responses among testing conditions with Bonferroni post-hoc tests. A paired t-test was also conducted to compare the time to nadir for COX and SkBF at each oxygen condition. A *P*-value less than 0.05 was considered statistically significant.

3 Results

The resting HR gradually increased with a reduction in FiO_2 (63 ± 9 bpm in 21% O_2 and 72 ± 9 bpm in 12% O_2, $P < 0.05$). By contrast, $P_{ET}CO_2$ (38.1 ± 3.6 mmHg in 21% O_2 and 35.3 ± 3.6 mmHg in 12% O_2, $P < 0.05$) and SpO_2 (96.9 ± 0.6% in 21% O_2 and 79.6 ± 11.0% in 12% O_2, $P < 0.05$) gradually decreased with a reduction in FiO_2. There were no significant differences in MAP between 21% O_2 (89 ± 5 mmHg) and 12% O_2 (91 ± 8 mmHg). Table 1 shows the resting baseline for the cerebrovascular variables across different oxygen conditions. COX decreased linearly with a reduction in FiO_2. Conversely, there were no differences in SkBF and CVC among conditions.

The time to nadir values in COX induced by the thigh-cuff test (acute hypotension) slowed with a reduction in FiO_2 ($P < 0.05$), while those in MAP, SkBF, and

Table 1 Resting baseline values of hemodynamic variables during progressive normobaric hypoxia

	21% O_2	18% O_2	15% O_2	12% O_2
Cerebral				
COX (%)	63.9 ± 4.8	63.1 ± 4.7*	59.7 ± 5.1*†	52.8 ± 8.6*†‡
SkBF (mV)	731 ± 320	786 ± 348	703 ± 309	696 ± 334
CVC (mV $mmHg^{-1}$)	8.28 ± 3.57	7.13 ± 2.38	6.78 ± 2.68	7.49 ± 2.41

Values are mean ± standard deviation (SD). COX, cerebral oxygenation; SkBF, skin blood flow; CVC, cutaneous vascular conductance. *$P < 0.05$ vs. 21%; †$P < 0.05$ vs. 18%; ‡$P < 0.05$ vs. 15%

Table 2 Hemodynamic responses to thigh-cuff test during progressive normobaric hypoxia

	21% O_2	18% O_2	15% O_2	12% O_2
MAP				
Maximal ΔMAP (%)	−22.4 ± 4.3	−21.7 ± 3.9	−21.4 ± 3.2	−22.4 ± 3.0
Time to nadir (s)	6.7 ± 1.3	6.6 ± 1.7	6.5 ± 1.3	7.1 ± 2.3
Time to baseline (s)	20.9 ± 4.0	19.0 ± 3.6	19.6 ± 5.4	20.9 ± 5.2
COX				
Maximal ΔCOX (%)	−2.3 ± 0.9	−2.3 ± 0.8	−2.9 ± 1.1	−2.7 ± 1.4
Time to nadir (s)	14.8 ± 11.0$^{\#}$	15.4 ± 9.5$^{\#}$	24.7 ± 18.2$^{*\dagger\#}$	28.5 ± 13.4$^{*\dagger\#}$
Time to baseline (s)	NA	NA	NA	NA
SkBF				
Maximal ΔSkBF (%)	−43.8 ± 14.3	−46.6 ± 16.2	−42.8 ± 11.6	−41.4 ± 11.0
Time to nadir (s)	7.3 ± 3.2	6.7 ± 2.0	6.2 ± 2.5	6.9 ± 2.3
Time to baseline (s)	17.1 ± 4.2	17.8 ± 4.2	16.3 ± 2.7	17.5 ± 4.2
CVC				
Maximal ΔCVC (%)	−28.5 ± 14.2	−27.8 ± 14.1	−33.2 ± 18.8	−31.2 ± 12.9
Time to nadir (s)	7.5 ± 2.4	6.8 ± 2.7	7.1 ± 2.4	8.3 ± 3.6
Time to baseline (s)	17.3 ± 5.4	17.1 ± 3.9	17.5 ± 4.2	18.3 ± 4.3

Values are mean ± SD. NA, not appreciable. $^{*}P < 0.05$ vs. 21%; $^{\dagger}P < 0.05$ vs. 18%; $^{\ddagger}P < 0.05$ vs. 15%; $\#P < 0.05$ in the time to nadir between COX and SkBF at each oxygen condition

CVC showed similar values (Table 2 and Fig. 1). Additionally, the time to nadir for COX at each oxygen condition was significantly slower than for SkBF. The % changes from the thigh-cuff test and the time to baseline before cuff release for MAP, SkBF, and CVC also showed similar values. However, a subset of subjects for COX did not recover to baseline values and, therefore, we did not calculate average values (i.e., not appreciable in Table 2).

4 Discussion

This study provides several important findings related to the assessment of COX during hypoxia. First, resting baseline for COX decreased progressively with a reduction in FiO_2, while SkBF, MAP, and CVC were unaffected by oxygen levels. Second, during hypotension, the time to nadir values for COX slowed progressively with a reduction of FiO_2 and did not recover within 30 s after thigh-cuff release, while the time to nadir values for SkBF, MAP, and CVC were unaffected by oxygen levels and recovered to baseline within 20 s after thigh-cuff release.

A previous study demonstrated that acute hypoxic exposure of ~ 20 min in 12% O_2, decreased middle cerebral artery blood flow velocity (MCA*v*), cerebral oxygenated hemoglobin, and $P_{ET}CO_2$, but MAP remained unchanged [8]. Our results are consistent with the previous study [8]. By contrast, it has been reported that hypoxic exposure causes cutaneous vasodilation [9], and our results showing no changes in SkBF before the thigh-cuff test are inconsistent. However, since the subjects in the

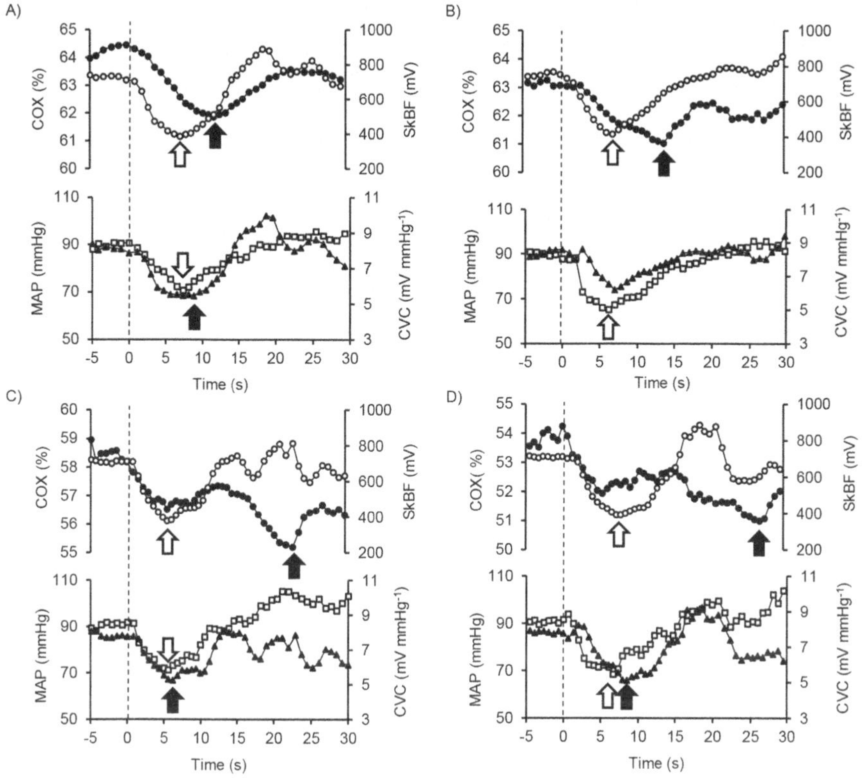

Fig. 1 Typical changes in cerebral oxygenation (COX; solid circles), skin blood flow (SkBF; open circles), mean arterial pressure (MAP; open squares), and cutaneous vascular conductance (CVC; solid triangles) under 21% O_2 (panel A), 18% O_2 (panel B), 15% O_2 (panel C), and 12% O_2 (panel D) before and following cuff release (single subject). Vertical lines (time = 0) indicate the point of thigh-cuff release. Arrows indicate the point showing nadir values in each variable

previous study was exposed to hypoxia for 20 min and the measurement site was forearm, and therefore, the study protocol was completely different between their study and our study [9], differences between study designs make it difficult to compare these discrepancies. In addition, possible explanation may be due to regional blood flow redistribution into the brain. A previous study demonstrated that face cooling with mist water at rest decreased SkBF at the forehead, resulting in increases in MCA*v* [10]. Anatomically, the external carotid artery (ECA) supplies blood to the face, and the MCA is supplied from the internal carotid artery (ICA). As our results showed, progressive reductions in COX with hypoxia and maintained SkBF (not vasodilation) may indicate sufficient oxygen delivery to the brain, but SkBF maintenance could not fully compensate for supplying oxygen into the brain.

During the acute hypotension phase, the responses for SkBF (i.e., thigh-cuff-induced reductions of magnitude levels, the time to nadir values and recovery time to the baseline) remained unchanged throughout progressive hypoxic exposure.

It has been reported that steady-state orthostatic stress (90° head-up tilt) failed to alter the ECA [11]. On the assumption that SkBF is an index that reflects the ECA, these results suggest that it is an unloading of cardiopulmonary baroreceptors that likely affects the SkBF rather than hypoxic exposure and dynamic arterial blood pressure changes via the arterial baroreflex. In the present study, MAP, SkBF, and CVC showed similar responses across four different oxygen conditions. For example, these metrics showed nadir ~10 s after cuff release and recovered after ~20 s; however, the time to nadir for COX extended with a reduction in FiO_2 and did not recover after 30 s past thigh-cuff release. These results suggest that the changes for COX were more passive in hypoxia than for MAP, SkBF, or CVC; moreover, COX may not be represented by SkBF. However, it should be noted that links between COX and SkBF existed as in the 21% O_2 trial because they were both able to recover in the subset of subjects and the difference in the time to nadir between COX and SkBF was only ~7 s yet more than 20 s in 12% O_2. It has been reported that MCA*v* regulation is not affected by sympathoexcitation with lower body negative pressure [12]. Similarly, sympathoexcitation via the unloading of the arterial baroreflex with the thigh-cuff release technique did not affect MCA*v* and ICA blood flow, but COX, ECA blood flow, and SkBF may not be affected during this acute hypotension period [13]. Thus, our results are not supported by these two studies [12, 13]. However, these two studies were conducted only in normoxia, and thus, it is uncertain whether the results of their study can be applied to our results. Moreover, another study demonstrated that changes in MCA*v* induced by thigh-cuff release were strongly correlated with changes in COX [14], indicating that a universal finding has not yet been obtained and the precise mechanisms are still unclear. Future studies are warranted.

It should be also considered the interaction between near-infrared light and tissues. For example, NIRS signals at the frontal lobe includes not only from the brain, but also from the scalp and skull. In this regard, a recent study reported that the distance between the probe and detector of <10 mm would be the optimum distance to derive only the extra-cerebral tissues (i.e., scalp and skull) using an anatomically informed multilayer models [15]. Thus, the distance between the probe and detector 1 that was used in the present study was rather large, i.e., 20 mm. Although the study design was different between their study and our study, we must acknowledge that potential effects of NIRS signals of extra-cerebral tissues on the COX in the present study.

In summary, COX response during acute hypotension periods induced by thigh-cuff release was more passive in hypoxia as compared to MAP, SkBF, and CVC response. Moreover, COX may not be associated with SkBF for the protocol or with the subjects in the present study. These results may help assess hypoxic-induced syncope and/or patients with hypoxic encephalopathia.

Acknowledgments The authors thank all participants for their time and effort. We also thank Prof. Katsuhiro Koyama, Mr. Masataka Kiuchi and Mr. Shohei Dobashi for their technical assistance. This study was supported by the Grant in JSPS (No. 26440268 to M.H.).

References

1. Miyazawa T, Horiuchi M, Komine H et al (2013) Skin blood flow influences cerebral oxygenation measured by near-infrared spectroscopy during dynamic exercise. Eur J Appl Physiol 113(11):2841–2848
2. Ogoh S, Sato K, Okazaki K et al (2014) A decrease in spatially resolved near-infrared spectroscopy frontal lobe tissue oxygenation by phenylephrine reflects reduced skin blood flow. Anesth Analg 118(4):823–829
3. Van Lieshout JJ, Wieling W, Karemaker JM et al (2003) Syncope, cerebral perfusion, and oxygenation. J Appl Physiol 94(3):833–848
4. Subudhi AW, Grajzel K, Langolf RJ et al (2015) Cerebral autoregulation index at high altitude assessed by thigh-cuff and transfer function analysis techniques. Exp Physiol 100(2):173–181
5. Horicuhi M, Endo J, Dobashi S et al (2016) Effects of progressive normobaric hypoxia on dynamic cerebral autoregulation. Exp Physiol 101(10):1276–1284
6. Ando S, Hatamoto Y, Sudo M et al (2013) The effects of exercise under hypoxia on cognitive function. PLoS One 8(5):e63630
7. Aaslid R, Lindegaard KF, Sorteberg W et al (1989) Cerebral autoregulation dynamics in humans. Stroke 20(1):45–52
8. Ainslie PN, Barach A, Murrell C et al (2007) Alterations in cerebral autoregulation and cerebral blood flow velocity during acute hypoxia: rest and exercise. Am J Physiol Heart Circ Physiol 292(2):H976–H983
9. Simmons GH, Minson CT, Cracowski JL et al (2007) Systemic hypoxia causes cutaneous vasodilation in healthy humans. J Appl Physiol 03(2):608–615
10. Miyazawa T, Horiuchi M, Ichikawa D et al (2012) Face cooling with mist water increases cerebral blood flow during exercise: effect of changes in facial skin blood flow. Front Physiol. https://doi.org/10.3389/fphys.2012.00308
11. Geinas JC, Marsden KR, Tzeng YC et al (2012) Influence of posture on the regulation of cerebral perfusion. Aviat Space Environ Med 83(8):751–757
12. LeMarbre G, Stauber S, Khayat RN et al (2003) Baroreflex-induced sympathetic activation does not alter cerebrovascular CO_2 responsiveness in humans. J Physiol 551:609–616
13. Ogoh S, Lericollais R, Hirasawa A et al (2014) Regional redistribution of blood flow in the external and internal carotid arteries during acute hypotension. Am J Physiol Regul Integr Comp Physiol 306(10):R747–R751
14. Miyazawa T, Horiuchi M, Ichikawa D et al (2012) Kinetics of exercise-induced neural activation; interpretive dilemma of altered cerebral perfusion. Exp Physiol 97(2):219–227
15. Brigadoi S, Cooper RJ (2015) How short is short? Optimum source-detector distance for short-separation channels in functional near-infrared spectroscopy. Neurophotonics 2(2):025005

Cerebral Autoregulation During Active Standing Test in Juvenile Patients with Instantaneous Orthostatic Hypotension

Wakako Ishii, Yukihiko Fujita, Tadayasu Kawaguchi, Kaori Kimura, Ayumi Fukuda, Tatsuo Fuchigami, and Ichiro Morioka

Abstract Instantaneous orthostatic hypotension (INOH) is one of the main types of orthostatic dysregulation in children and adolescents. In patients with INOH arterial pressure drops considerably after active standing and is slow to recover. We investigated changes in cerebral oxygenation in the bilateral prefrontal cortex during an active standing test in juvenile INOH patients to evaluate changes in cerebral oxygen metabolism. We enrolled 82 INOH patients (mean age 13.8 ± 2.2 years, 52 mild and 30 severe patients) at Nihon University Itabashi Hospital from October 2013 to April 2018. We measured cerebral oxygenated hemoglobin, deoxygenated hemoglobin, and total hemoglobin levels in the bilateral prefrontal cortex using near-infrared spectroscopy during an active standing test. In severe INOH patients, cerebral oxygenation of the right prefrontal cortex remained constant when blood pressure dropped; however, de-oxy-Hb significantly increased. These findings confirm that there is asymmetrical autoregulation between the right and left prefrontal cortex.

Keywords Orthostatic dysregulation · Instantaneous orthostatic hypotension (INOH) · Near-infrared spectroscopy (NIRS) · Cerebral autoregulation · Rapid recovery

---

W. Ishii · T. Kawaguchi · K. Kimura · A. Fukuda · T. Fuchigami · I. Morioka
Department of Pediatrics and Child Health, Nihon University School of Medicine, Tokyo, Japan

Y. Fujita (✉)
Department of Pediatrics and Child Health, Nihon University School of Medicine, Tokyo, Japan

Center for Institutional Research and Medical Education, Nihon University School of Medicine, Tokyo, Japan
e-mail: fujita.yukihiko@nihon-u.ac.jp

© Springer Nature Switzerland AG 2020
P.-D. Ryu et al. (eds.), *Oxygen Transport to Tissue XLI*, Advances in Experimental Medicine and Biology 1232, https://doi.org/10.1007/978-3-030-34461-0_11

1 Introduction

Orthostatic intolerance is caused by dysfunctions of the autonomic nervous system [1]. In Japan, it is well known as orthostatic dysregulation (OD) and has become a major health concern among school-aged children and adolescents. Various symptoms, including recurrent dizziness, chronic fatigue, headache, and syncope, are caused by the failure of the mechanisms that compensate for changes in cardiovascular hemodynamics due to active standing. OD is classified into four subsets according to Japanese clinical guidelines: instantaneous orthostatic hypotension (INOH), postural tachycardia syndrome (POTS), neutrally mediated syncope, and delayed orthostatic hypotension (Delayed OH).

It has recently become possible to measure oxygen metabolism in brain tissue safely and easily using near-infrared spectroscopy (NIRS). Previous studies indicate that in healthy people, cerebral blood flow remains constant even if the arterial pressure changes, which is referred to as 'cerebral autoregulation' [2]. In patients with OD, cerebral autoregulation is impaired as their oxygenated hemoglobin (oxy-Hb) levels significantly decrease under orthostatic load [3, 4]. Tanaka et al. studied the oxygen metabolism of chronic fatigue syndrome patients with OD under orthostatic load for each OD subset. They reported that in three subsets (INOH, Delayed OH, and POTS) of OD patients, the right prefrontal cortex showed no recovery after a transient decrease in oxy-Hb at the onset of standing, and the decrease persisted while the patients remained standing [5]. Furthermore, Kamiyama et al. reported asymmetric changes in cerebral blood oxygenation during active standing in children with POTS, with a significant decrease in the left compared with the right frontal cortex [6]. However, the laterality of the rapid recovery and cerebral oxygen metabolism during active standing in INOH patients remain unclear.

In this study, we used NIRS to measure the quantitative changes in the concentrations of cerebral oxy-Hb, deoxygenated hemoglobin (deoxy-Hb), and total hemoglobin (total-Hb) in the bilateral prefrontal cortex during an active standing test in pediatric patients with INOH.

2 Methods

The study enrolled 82 patients (mean age: 13.8 ± 2.2 years) with INOH diag-nosed in accordance with the Japanese clinical guidelines for juvenile OD [1]. INOH is classified as mild or severe according to the time taken to recover from a drop in arterial pressure. The criteria for diagnosing mild INOH are 1) recovery time for mean arterial pressure of ≥25 s or 2) recovery time of ≥20 s with an initial decrease of ≥60% in mean arterial pressure, and the severe form is diagnosed with the additional criterion of 3) a reduction in systolic arterial pressure of ≥15% during the later stage of standing (3–7 min after standing) [1]. All subjects were recruited from the outpatient clinic of the Department of Pediatrics and Child Health at Nihon University Itabashi

Table 1 Clinical characteristics of all patients with INOH

	Mild form (n = 52)	Severe form (n = 30)	*p*- value
Gender, male; n (%)	24 (46.2)	15 (50.0)	0.74[a]
Age (years), mean ± SD	13.9 ± 2.0	13.8 ± 2.6	0.53[b]
Body mass index (kg/m^2), mean ± SD	18.8 ± 3.1	19.0 ± 3.5	0.52[b]
Small heart (CTR $\leq$ 0.4) on chest X-ray findings; n (%)	24/50 (48.0)	13/29 (44.8)	0.79[a]

[a] Evaluated by chi-square analysis, [b] Evaluated by Mann-Whitney analysis

Hospital from October 2013 to April 2018. The subjects were classified as mild (52 patients) or severe (30 patients) using the active standing test described below. We excluded patients from whom we could not obtain appropriate cerebral blood oxygenation data. Table 1 shows the clinical characteristics of the subjects according to severity. There was no significant difference between mild and severe patients.

The subjects performed the active standing test between 9:00 a.m. and 11:00 a.m. After resting for 10 min in the supine position, subjects were instructed to stand up quickly by themselves and remain upright for 10 min. During the test, the subjects' blood pressure and heart rate were monitored with the following non-invasive beat-to-beat blood pressure monitors: BP-608 Evolution II CS (Omlon Colin Co., Ltd., Tokyo, Japan; October 2013~December 2016) and Task Force monitor TFM-3040 (Nihon-Kohden, Tokyo, Japan; January 2017 ~April 2018). Cerebral blood oxygenation in the bilateral prefrontal cortex was simultaneously measured using a NIRS 2-channel miniaturized wireless tool (Pocket NIRS Duo<TM>, Hamamatsu Photonics, Shizuoka, Japan). This instrument can continuously detect changes in oxy-Hb, deoxy-Hb, and total-Hb based on the modified Beer-Lambert law. The NIRS probes were symmetrically fitted on both sides of the subjects' foreheads.

Healthy individuals usually show rapid recovery in reaction to the initial drop in oxy-Hb at the onset of active standing [5]. We evaluated the detection of rapid recovery in the NIRS parameters of the bilateral prefrontal cortices. Subjects who showed a rapid recovery followed by a reduction in oxy-Hb in the later stage of standing were included among the rapid recovery positive subjects.

The experimental time was divided into three periods, as shown in Fig. 1 b: 10 min resting time, standing time from starting to 5 min, and standing time from 5 to 10 min. The average oxy-Hb, deoxy-Hb, and total-Hb levels in each period were calculated for the selected 60-second intervals (R, S1, S2) during which the variability rates were stable and oxy-Hb levels were lower. Arterial blood pressure decreased in all cases of mild and severe forms in S1. In all mild patients, recovery of arterial blood pressure was observed in S2, but such recovery was not observed in the cases of severe patients. Therefore, I divided the standing time into two groups to investigate the influence of arterial blood pressure.

The data were analyzed using Statcel 3 software (OMS Publishing Inc., Tokorozawa, Japan). Chi-square tests were used to compare the detection of rapid recovery in the left and right prefrontal cortices. Mann-Whitney U tests were used to compare the oxy-Hb changes associated with active standing between the left and right frontal cortices. Differences were considered statistically significant when the p-values were < 0.05. The average delta oxy-Hb concentrations were analyzed among three groups using the Friedman test. Differences with p-values <0.05 were considered statistically significant. Wilcoxon signed-rank test was used in addition to the Friedman test for analysis among each group. Differences with p-values <0.017 were considered statistically significant.

This study was approved by the ethical committee of Nihon University Itabashi Hospital and was in accordance with the revised version of the Declaration of Helsinki on October 3, 2008. Informed consent was obtained from all patients and their guardians.

3 Results

The increase in heart rate during standing was not significantly different between mild and severe patients (38.2 ± 13.6 vs. 39.7 ± 12.3, p = 0.78). Among the severe INOH patients, arterial pressure remained low during the active standing test.

The rate of rapid recovery detected by the NIRS parameters on the left and right sides following the initial drop in oxy-Hb at the onset of active standing was compared according to severity. The rapid recovery in bilateral prefrontal cortex of INOH patients is shown in Fig. 1 a The mild form patients showed a more significant rapid

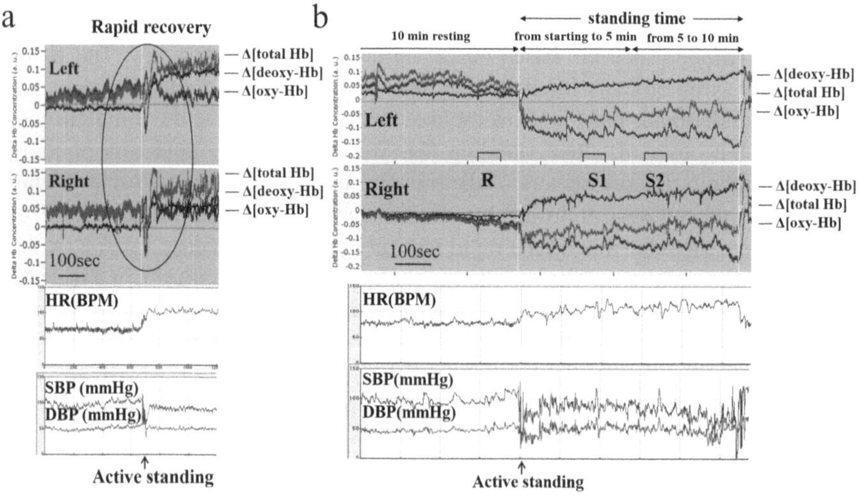

Fig. 1 (**a**) The rapid recovery in NIRS parameters of a 13-year-old girl with severe INOH. The delta Hb concentration changes on the left and right sides are shown in the upper and lower box, respectively. (**b**). The NIRS parameter changes in a 10-year-old girl with severe INOH. Interval R represents 60 s selected during the resting period. Interval S1 represents 60 seconds selected from the start of the standing period to 5 min. Interval S2 represents 60 s selected from the standing time between 5 and 10 min. "A.u" is an abbreviation for "arbitrary unit"

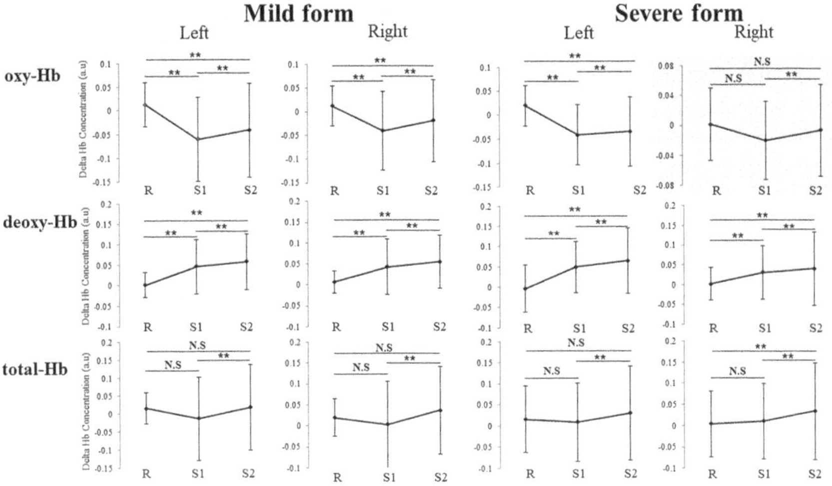

Fig. 2 Comparison of changes in NIRS parameters. There was no significant difference between the changes in oxy-Hb concentration in severe INOH patients' right prefrontal cortex during active standing tests. (**$p < 0.017$) "A.u" is an abbreviation for "arbitrary unit"

recovery on the right than the left side (46.2% vs. 22.2%, $p = 0.007$). Among the severe patients, there was no significant difference between the two sides ($p = 0.12$).

Figure 2 shows the changes in the NIRS parameters. Using each subject's average delta oxy-Hb concentration level in the R, S1, and S2 periods, the NIRS parameters tended to show a decrease in oxy-Hb and an increase in deoxy-Hb in the bilateral prefrontal cortex in both mild and severe INOH subjects after active standing. Furthermore, oxy-Hb showed a significant decrease ($p < 0.01$) in the left prefrontal cortices of both mild and severe patients after standing. Oxy-Hb also showed a significant decrease in the right prefrontal cortices of mild INOH patients, but the difference was not significant in severe INOH patients. Oxy-Hb in the right prefrontal cortices of severe patients showed a greater significant increase in S2 than in S1.

4 Discussion

The change in oxy-Hb measured by NIRS is closely correlated with local cerebral blood flow [7]. Although the absolute value of oxy-Hb measured by NIRS does not directly reflect cerebral blood flow, oxy-Hb is an important indicator of cerebral oxygen metabolism.

Our results clearly demonstrated that the detection rate of rapid recovery from the initial drop in oxy-Hb at the onset of active standing was more significant in the right than the left prefrontal cortex in mild INOH patients. Absence of rapid recovery caused by impaired cerebral autoregulation is recognized as a characteristic of OD patients. Our study is the first to reveal the asymmetry of this effect.

In addition, we revealed that the NIRS parameters tend to show a decrease in oxy-Hb and an increase in deoxy-Hb in the bilateral prefrontal cortex in mild and severe INOH patients after active standing. This change suggests that neuronal activation induces relative ischemia [8]. However, severe INOH patients did not show a significant decrease in the right prefrontal cortex. Furthermore, the delta oxy-Hb concentration in the right prefrontal cortex showed a significant increase from S1 to S2, although none of the severe patients showed any recovery of arterial pressure. Oxygen metabolism of the right prefrontal cortex was maintained only in severe INOH patients.

Recently, the central autonomic network has been revealed as the center of the autonomic nervous system [9]. The network includes the insular, prefrontal cortex, amygdala, hypothalamus, and ventrolateral medulla. Right prefrontal activity plays an important role in the autonomic nerve system, particularly in sympathetic control of the heart rate [10, 11]. In INOH patients, the decrease in cardiac output when arterial pressure drops is compensated by tachycardia, and the compensation is greater in severe than in mild INOH patients [12]. However, in this study, because we did not observe a significant difference in the increase in heart rate between mild and severe patients during active standing, we could not elucidate why right prefrontal oxygenation was maintained only in severe INOH patients during active standing. Because the arterial pressure of severe INOH patients tends to decrease in daily life, their brains might become tolerant to active standing, so that strong activation of the right prefrontal cortex can maintain the oxygen metabolism of the brain.

Comparisons with healthy controls and other subtypes are lacking in our study. In addition, handedness was not revealed in our study. Therefore, we could not clarify whether these findings were associated with a dominant hemisphere.

In conclusion, right prefrontal oxygenation tends to be maintained despite decreased arterial pressure during active standing in both mild and severe INOH patients. These findings confirm that there is asymmetrical cerebral autoregulation between the right and left prefrontal cortex.

References

1. Tanaka H, Fujita Y, Takenaka Y et al (2009) Japanese clinical guidelines for juvenile orthostatic dysregulation version 1. Pediatr Int 51:169–179
2. Lassen NA (1956) Cerebral blood flow and oxygen consumption in man. Physiol Rev 39:183–238
3. Kim YT, Tanaka H, Takaya R et al (2009) Quantitative study on cerebral blood volume determined by a near-infrared spectroscopy during postural change in children. Acta Paediatr 98:466–471
4. Endo A, Fujita Y, Fuchigami T et al (2014) Changes in cerebral blood oxygenation induced by active standing test in children with POTS and NMS. Adv Exp Med Biol 812:253–261
5. Tanaka H, Matsushima R, Tamai H et al (2002) Impaired postural cerebral hemodynamics in young patients with chronic fatigue with and without orthostatic intolerance. J Pediatr 140:412–417

6. Kamiyama Y, Fujita Y, Fuchigami T et al (2014) Asymmetrical changes in cerebral blood oxygenation induced by an active standing test in children with postural tachycardia syndrome. Adv Exp Med Biol 812:271–278
7. Holzschuh M, Woertgen C, Metz C et al (1997) Comparison of changes in cerebral blood flow and cerebral oxygen saturation measured by near infrared spectroscopy (NIRS) after acetazolamide. Acta Neurochir 139:58–62
8. Sakatani K, Xie Y, Lichty W et al (1998) Language-activated cerebral blood oxygenation and hemodynamic changes of the left prefrontal cortex in poststroke aphasic patients: a near-infrared spectroscopy study. Stroke 29:1299–1304
9. Wei L, Chen H, Wu GR (2018) Structural covariance of the prefrontal-amygdala pathways associated with heart rate variability. Front Hum Neurosci 12:1–11
10. Sakatani K (2012) Optical diagnosis of mental stress: review. Adv Exp Med Biol 737:89–95
11. Foster PS, Hubbard T, Yung RC et al (2013) Cerebral asymmetry in the control of cardiovascular functioning: evidence from lateral vibrotactile stimulation. Laterality 18:108–119
12. Tanaka H, Yamaguchi H, Matushima R et al (1999) Instantaneous orthostatic hypotension in children and adolescents: a new entity of orthostatic intolerance. Pediatr Res 46:691–696

Cerebral Blood Oxygenation Changes in Juvenile Patients with Delayed Orthostatic Hypotension During an Active Standing Test

T. Kawaguchi, Y. Fujita, W. Ishii, K. Kimura, A. Fukuda, T. Fuchigami, and I. Morioka

Abstract Delayed orthostatic hypotension (OH) is a minor subset of orthostatic dysregulation (OD). Cerebral blood oxygenation in juvenile patients with delayed OH has not been studied. We investigated the bilateral changes in cerebral oxygenation in the prefrontal cortex during an active standing test in 23 juvenile patients with delayed OH using near-infrared spectroscopy (NIRS). We measured the oxy-Hb, deoxy-Hb, and total-Hb during the active standing test. Four observations were made during the test: t1 in a resting supine position, t2 when maintaining blood pressure, and the remaining two (t3, t4) during hypotension. The concentration of oxy-Hb significantly decreased prior to satisfying the diagnostic criteria of delayed OH after standing and did not change thereafter. The concentration of deoxy-Hb increased gradually during the measurement periods. In addition, total-Hb increased from t2 to t3. There was no significant difference in the change in each Hb parameter between the left and right cerebral hemispheres. Our results indicate that NIRS parameters are more sensitive than blood pressure for the interpretation of cerebral autoregulation in juvenile patients with delayed OH.

Keywords Active standing test · Cerebral blood oxygenation · Delayed orthostatic hypotension · NIRS · Orthostatic dysregulation

---

T. Kawaguchi · W. Ishii · K. Kimura · A. Fukuda · T. Fuchigami · I. Morioka
Department of Pediatrics and Child Health, Nihon University School of Medicine, Chiyoda, Japan

Y. Fujita (✉)
Pediatrics and hospital director, Ashikaganomori Ashikaga Hospital, Ashikaga, Japan
e-mail: fujita.yukihiko@nihon-u.ac.jp

© Springer Nature Switzerland AG 2020

P.-D. Ryu et al. (eds.), *Oxygen Transport to Tissue XLI*, Advances in Experimental Medicine and Biology 1232, https://doi.org/10.1007/978-3-030-34461-0_12

1 Introduction

Orthostatic intolerance (OI), commonly known as orthostatic dysregulation (OD) in Japan, is a disorder of the autonomic nervous system seen mainly during childhood and adolescence. The symptoms of OD are diverse, including headache, dizziness, and fainting during standing. Near-infrared spectroscopy (NIRS) is a commonly used non-invasive technique. It can be used to measure the concentration change of oxy-Hb, deoxy-Hb, and total-Hb. However, it has been reported that oxy-Hb correlates with cerebral blood flow [1]. Kamiyama et al. reported a decrease in right cerebral blood oxygenation compared with the left side in children with postural orthostatic tachycardia syndrome (POTS) in an active standing test [2]. In addition, Endo et al. also examined cerebral blood oxygenation using quantitative NIRS and cerebral blood flow using transcranial Doppler sonography in patients with POTS and neurally mediated syncope [3].

Delayed orthostatic hypotension (OH) is a minor subset accounting for 5.0% of OD cases [4]. Delayed OH is diagnosed when the blood pressure after active standing is within the normal limit, but after 3 min, systolic blood pressure decreases by more than 20 mmHg or 15% of the value during a resting supine position. There are some reports on cerebral blood oxygenation in OD patients in childhood and adolescence.

The aim of this study was to investigate the bilateral changes in cerebral oxygenation in the prefrontal cortex during an active standing test in juvenile patients with delayed OH using NIRS.

2 Methods

2.1 Active Standing Test

After 10 min of resting in a supine position, patients stood up quickly and stayed upright for 10 min. NIRS monitors (Pocket NIRS Duo™, Hamamatsu Photonics, Shizuoka, Japan) were attached to the forehead on both sides, and changes in oxy-Hb, deoxy-Hb, and total-Hb were recorded. In addition, arterial blood pressure and heart rate were monitored using the following non-invasive beat-to-beat blood pressure monitors: BP-608 Evolution II CS; Omron Colin Co., Ltd., Tokyo, Japan (October 2013~December 2016) and Task Force monitor TFM-3040; Nihon-Kohden, Tokyo, Japan (January 2017~April 2017). We obtained measurements for i) a 1-min period in a stable supine position (t1), ii) for a 1-min period at 1 min after active standing (t2) with normal blood pressure, iii) for a 1-min period from the moment of satisfying the diagnostic criteria of delayed OH (t3), and iv) for a 1 min period at the end of active standing (t4). The average value of NIRS parameters in each period was evaluated (Fig. 1).

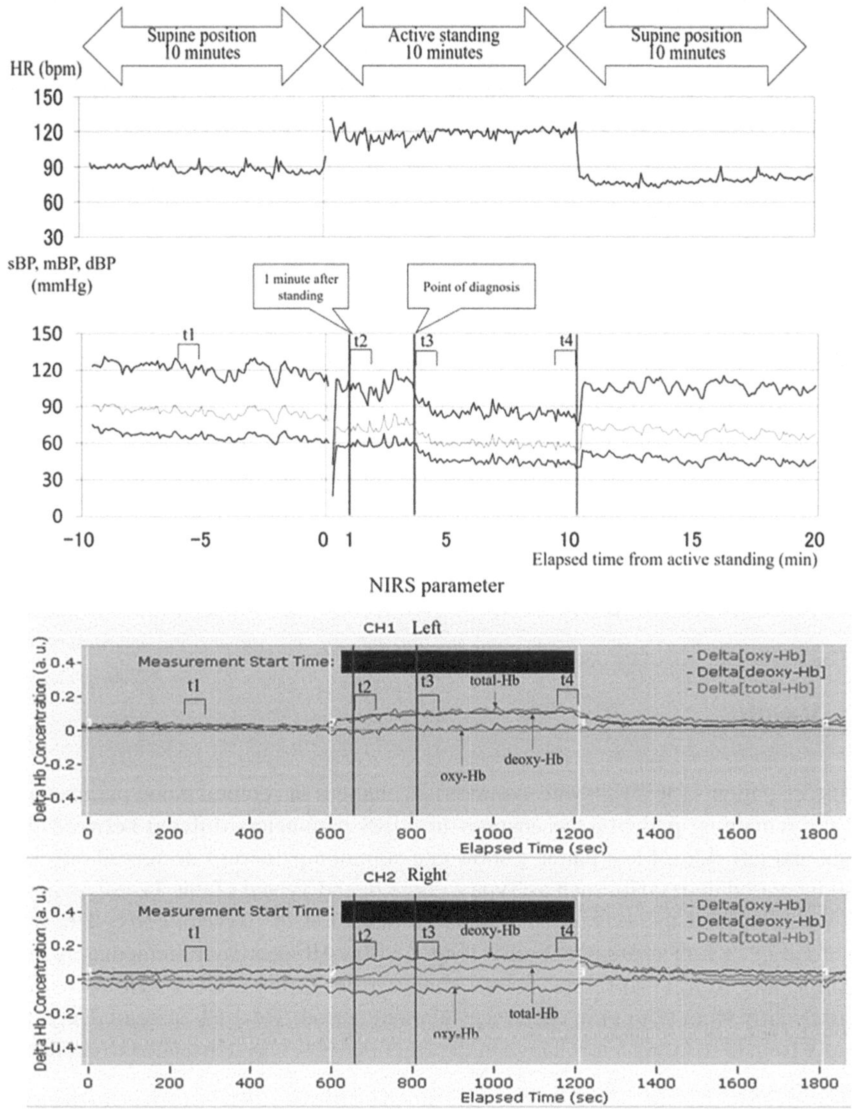

Fig. 1 Near-infrared spectroscopy results for a 14-year-old girl.t1: stable 1-min period in supine position, t2: 1-min period at 1 min after active standing, t3: 1-min period from moment of diagnosis of delayed orthostatic hypotension, t4: final 1-min period of active standing

2.2 Participants

We enrolled 23 patients (7 boys and 16 girls, aged 9–18 years) with delayed OH who were diagnosed at our outpatient section in accordance with the Japanese clinical guidelines for juvenile OD [3]. All subjects were recruited from the outpatient clinic of the Department of Pediatrics and Child Health at Nihon University Itabashi Hospital from October 2014 to April 2018. This study was approved by the ethical committee of Nihon University Itabashi Hospital, and informed consent was obtained from all patients and guardians.

2.3 Statistical Analysis

Statcel 3 software (OMS publishing Inc. Saitama, Japan) was used for statistical analysis. The Wilcoxon signed-ranks test was used for the analysis of each Hb measure over time. The Mann-Whitney U-test was used to test the difference between the left and right sides in each period. A p-value of less than 0.05 was considered an indicator of statistical significance.

3 Results

Thirteen patients (56%) showed symmetrical changes in cerebral blood parameters. In the remaining patients, the changes in NIRS parameters differed between the right and left sides. Most patients showed a common pattern of decreased oxy-Hb and increased deoxy-Hb, such as Type a, Type b, and Type d (Table 1).

We calculated the average and standard deviation of oxy-Hb, deoxy-Hb, and total-Hb in each measurement period (Fig. 2). Oxy-Hb decreased immediately and significantly from t1 to t2 but did not change from t2 to t4. Deoxy-Hb increased significantly from t1 to t4 in each measurement period. Total-Hb increased significantly from t2 to t3, with no change in the other periods. Oxy-Hb tended to decrease

Table 1 Patterns of changes in NIRS parameters and the number of cases

				Number of cases		
Type	oxy-Hb	deoxy-Hb	total-Hb	Left	Right	Total
a	↓↓	↑	↓	8	4	12
b	↓	↑	→	5	4	9
c	↑	↑	↑↑	2	1	3
d	↓	↑	↑	6	9	15
e	↓	↓	↓	0	1	1
f	→	→	→	2	3	5
b → d				0	1	1

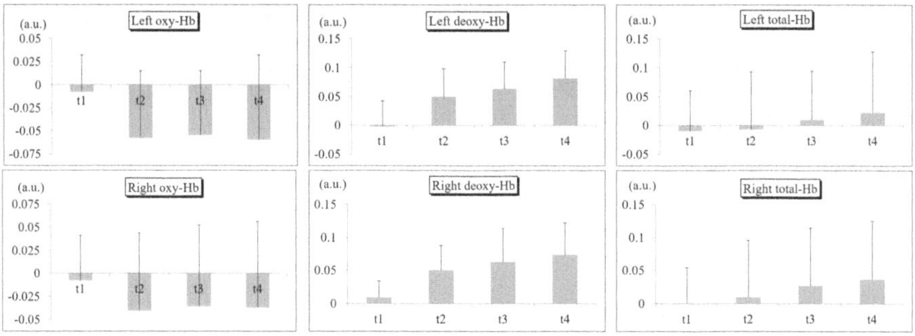

Fig. 2 Average and standard deviation of oxy-Hb, deoxy-Hb, and total-Hb in each period

Table 2 The p-value in each measurement period

	oxy-Hb			deoxy-Hb			total-Hb		
	t1-t2	t2-t3	t3-t4	t1-t2	t2-t3	t3-t4	t1-t2	t2-t3	t3-t4
Left	<.005	0.39	0.63	<.005	<.005	<.005	0.78	<.005	0.083
Right	<.005	0.29	0.81	<.005	<.005	<.005	0.43	<.005	0.052

in the left cerebral cortex from t1 to t2 (average variation: −0.029 in the right vs −0.064 in the left). However, none of the Hb parameters, including oxy-Hb, showed significant laterality in any period (Table 2).

4 Discussion

In this study, we made two new observations regarding changes in NIRS parameters in juvenile patients with delayed OH. First, oxy-Hb concentrations decrease prior to a drop in the systolic blood pressure, followed by oxy-Hb concentrations that are maintained at the same low levels, although the systolic blood pressure drops. Second, decreases in oxy-Hb concentrations do not show a significant difference between the right and left sides.

Kim et al. reported that 16 children with OD (including one with delayed OH) showed a significant reduction in oxy-Hb at the onset of standing compared with their normal counterparts [5]. In our study, oxy-Hb concentrations decreased before meeting the diagnostic criteria of delayed OH. Our results indicate that changes in oxy-Hb concentrations are more sensitive than blood pressure for interpreting cerebral autoregulation in juvenile patients with delayed OH.

The right cerebral hemisphere has a greater role in cerebral autoregulation. One study showed that oxy-Hb decreased significantly in the left cerebral hemisphere compared with the right in patients with POTS in an active standing test [2]. In the present study, oxy-Hb seemed to decrease in the left side rather than in the right. However, none of the Hb parameters, including oxy-Hb, showed significant laterality in any measurement period. This result suggests that the changes in cerebral blood flow and oxygenation are immediate and marked in patients with delayed OH. Therefore, cerebral autoregulation was impaired and cerebral oxy-Hb concentrations in both sides decreased simultaneously.

4.1 Study Limitations

NIRS is useful for evaluating cerebral circulation. However, frequency domain technique enables the measurement of absolute values and not only absolute values of changes. In addition, in this study, we enrolled 23 patients with delayed OH from a single institute. However, because the number of cases might be too small to achieve statistical power, a multicenter study involving more patients is necessary. And we need to investigate a gender difference and the physiological development within childhood and adolescence period in NIRS parameter.

5 Conclusions

NIRS parameters can be a helpful monitoring tool for the assessment of cerebral autoregulation in juvenile patients with delayed OH.

Acknowledgments We would like to express our gratitude to Mr. Shinichi Sekiguchi, Medical Electronics Laboratory of Medical Research Support Center at Nihon University School of Medicine who helped in the analysis of the clinical data.

References

1. Sibrand H, Jorge MS, Willy NJMC et al (2001) Changes in cerebral oxygenation and blood flow during LBNP in spinal cord-injured individuals. J Appl Physiol 91:2199–2204
2. Kamiyama Y, Fujita Y, Fuchigami T et al (2014) Asymmetrical changes in cerebral blood oxygenation induced by an active standing test in children with postural tachycardia syndrome. Adv Exp Med Biol 812:271–278
3. Endo A, Fujita Y, Fuchigami T et al (2014) Changes in cerebral blood oxygenation induced by active standing test in children with POTS and NMS. Adv Exp Med Biol 812:253–261
4. Tanaka H, Fujita Y, Takenaka Y et al (2015) The clinical guidelines on psychosomatic disease in childhood by the Japanese society of psychosomatic pediatrics, 2nd Edition Pediatr Int 51:169–179
5. Kim YT, Tanaka H, Takaya R et al (2009) Quantitative study on cerebral blood volume determined by a near-infrared spectroscopy during postural change in children. Acta Paediatr 98:466–471

Relationship Between Cognitive Dysfunction and Systemic Metabolic Disorders in Elderly: Dementia Might be a Systematic Disease

Y. Komuro, K. Oyama, L. Hu, and K. Sakatani

Abstract Vascular cognitive impairment (VCI) plays an important role in dementia in elderly people, and refers to the contribution of vascular pathology to the entire spectrum of cognitive disorders, ranging from mild cognitive impairment to severe dementia, as well as the pathological spectrum, from 'pure' Alzheimer disease through degrees of vascular comorbidity to 'pure' vascular dementia. In the present study, we investigated the relationship between cognitive dysfunction and systemic metabolic disorders, by employing deep learning (DL). We studied 202 patients (73.4 ± 13.0 years), 94.6% of whom were undergoing treatment for lifestyle diseases, and 68.8% of whom had a history of cerebrovascular disorder. We evaluated cognitive dysfunction by performing a Mini Mental State Examination (MMSE). We performed general blood examination, including Complete Blood Count and Basic Metabolic Panel, and measured cerebral blood oxygenation in the prefrontal cortex (PFC) using time-resolved near infrared spectroscopy (TNIRS). We then used deep neural networks to assess the MMSE scores of the subjects based on the TNIRS parameters and the blood examination data, independently. Next, we compared predicted MMSE scores based on the TNIRS and the blood examination. There was a significant positive correlation between the TNIRS parameters and the blood examination data ($r = 0.6$, $p < 0.01$). These observations suggest that cognitive dysfunction in patients with VCI may be caused by combinations of systemic metabolic disorders such as energy and oxygen metabolisms and cerebral circulatory disturbance due to arteriosclerosis resulting from lifestyle-related diseases.

Y. Komuro · L. Hu
Department of Electrical and Electronic Engineering, NEWCAT Research Institute, Koriyama, Japan

K. Oyama
Department of Computer Science, Nihon University, Koriyama, Japan

K. Sakatani (✉)
Department of Human and Engineered Environmental Studies, Universal Sports Health Science Laboratory, Graduate School of Frontier Sciences, The University of Tokyo, Kashiwanoha, Kashiwa-shi, Chiba, Japan
e-mail: k.sakatani@edu.k.u-tokyo.ac.jp

© Springer Nature Switzerland AG 2020
P.-D. Ryu et al. (eds.), *Oxygen Transport to Tissue XLI*, Advances in Experimental Medicine and Biology 1232, https://doi.org/10.1007/978-3-030-34461-0_13

Keywords Time-resolved near infrared spectroscopy · Vascular cognitive impairment · Deep learning · Arteriosclerosis · Dementia

1 Introduction

It has been recently proposed that vascular cognitive impairment (VCI), which is caused by arteriosclerosis resulting from lifestyle-related diseases, plays an important role in cognitive disorders ranging from mild cognitive impairment (MCI) to severe dementia [1–3]. Importantly, vascular pathology could contribute not only to vascular dementia, but also to Alzheimer's disease (AD) [4]. Other systemic disorders that could affect cognitive function are metabolic disorders, which include malnutrition [5], anemia [6], lipid metabolism disorders [7], purine metabolism disorders [8], and renal dysfunction [9]. These observations indicate that systemic disorders, such as arteriosclerosis due to lifestyle-related diseases and metabolic disorders, could affect cognitive function in patients with VCI. However, the relationship between systemic disorders and cerebral blood flow (CBF) and metabolism in VCI has yet to be elucidated.

In order to clarify this issue, we evaluated the relationship between cognitive function predicted by CBF/metabolism and systemic disorders in VCI. Recently, we have demonstrated that CBF and oxygen metabolism measured by a time-resolved spectroscopy (TNIRS) could predict cognitive functions in VCI employing deep learning (DL) [10]; DL is a subset of machine learning strategies that use deep neural networks, and allows the analysis of regularity and relevance from a large amount of data to make judgments and predictions [11]. In the present study, we first predicted cognitive dysfunctions in VCI based on general blood test data, which reflect the systemic disorders, including life-style diseases and metabolic disorders; we studied the same subjects in the TNIRS study [10]. Then, we evaluated the correlation between the cognitive function predicted using the TNIRS data and the blood data.

2 Methods

2.1 Subjects

We studied 202 subjects (87 males, 115 females; age 73.4 ± 13.0 years (mean ± SD) who had been admitted to Southern Tohoku Kasuga Rehabilitation Hospital (Fukushima, Japan) for rehabilitation. Of these subjects, 68.8% had cerebrovascular diseases and 94.6% had at least one life-style disease. The patients exhibited a variety of cognitive function between normal and dementia, with a mean MMSE score of 22.8 ± 6.3. In all subjects, we performed a blood test that included a complete blood count and a basic metabolic panel at the time of the experiment (Table 1).

Table 1 Blood test items for the prediction of cognitive function

Complete Blood Count	General Biochemical Examination	
WBC count	Total Protein	BUN
RBC count	Albumin	Creatinine
Hemoglobin	A/G ratio	Uric acid
Hematocrit	AST (GOT)	Glucose
MCV	ALT (GPT)	Na
MCH	r-GTP	K
MCHC	Total cholesterol	Cl
Platelet count	Triglyceride	

MCV = mean corpuscular volume, MCH = mean corpuscular hemoglobin
MCHC = mean corpuscular hemoglobin concentration
BUN = Blood urea nitrogen

The subjects provided written informed consent as required by the Human Subjects Committee of the Rehabilitation Hospital, or their family provided it when the subject had difficulty understanding due to cognitive dysfunction and were unable to do so themselves.

2.2 *Time-Resolved NIRS Measurement*

We measured the baseline concentrations of Hb in the bilateral PFC at resting condition employing TNIRS (TRS-21, Hamamatsu Photonics K.K., Hamamatsu, Japan). Details of this system have been described previously [12]. The TNIR parameters includes oxy-Hb, deoxy-Hb, t-Hb SO2, and optical pathlengths (61, 791, and 836 nm); the concentrations of Hb were expressed in μM.

The TNIRS probes were set symmetrically on the forehead with a flexible fixation pad so that the midpoint between the emission and detection probes was 3 cm above the centers of the upper edges of the bilateral orbital sockets; this positioning is similar to the midpoint between electrode positions Fp1/Fp3 (left) and Fp2/Fp4 (right) of the international electroencephalographic 10–20 system.

2.3 *Data Analysis*

We employed the deep neural network (DNN) to predict the mini mental state examination (MMSE) scores. The DNN examined for the data analysis was the H2O open source platform [13]. H2O uses the DNN model of multi-layer, feedforward neural networks for predictive modeling. The DNN tested in this study includes the neuron, and the input layer includes 24 neurons, i.e., the variables include age and 23 items from the blood test (Fig. 1); the variables included the same TNIRS data, blood test data and ages. Each hidden layer is placed with 400 neurons, and a

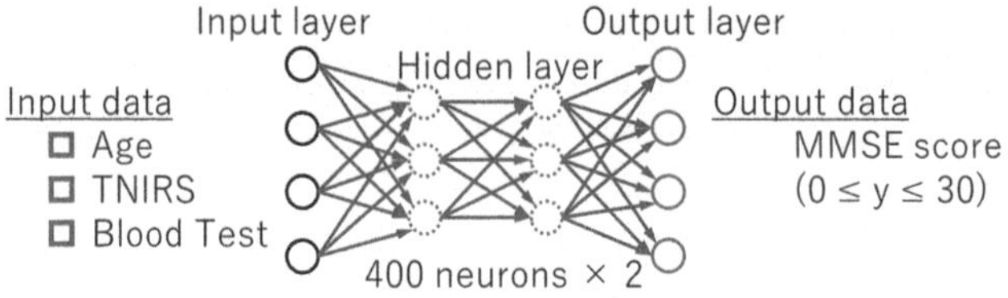

Fig. 1 Structure of the deep neural network for the data analysis. Input vectors include age and the blood test data or age and T-NIRS data. The output vector is regressed to estimate the MMSE score. The hidden layer contains no backward connections from downstream layers

total of two hidden layers. The weighted combination $\alpha = \sum_{i=1}^{n} w_i x_i + b$ aggregates input signals x_i in each layer to activate an output signal $f(\alpha)$ to the connected neuron in the next layer. The function f represents the nonlinear activation function used throughout the network, and the bias b accounts for the neuron's activation threshold. The output signals $f(\alpha)$ in each layer are thus determined using a weighted combination with the input signals x_i from upstream of the DNN. In the output layer, a loss function, $L(W,B \mid j)$, is measured using the mean square error between the estimated value and the actual MMSE score. The learning process updates the weights W and biases B until a loss function, $L(W,B \mid j)$, is minimized. Note that W is the collection $\{W_i\}_{1:N-1}$, where W_i denotes the weight matrix connecting layers i and $i + 1$ for a network of N layers. Similarly, B is the collection $\{b_i\}_{1:N-1}$, where b_i denotes the column vector of biases for layer $i + 1$.

In order to evaluate the correlation between the cognitive function predicted by the CBF/metabolism and the systemic disorders, we compared the MMSE scores predicted by the blood test data and the TNIRS data.

3 Results

The MMSE scores predicted using blood test data and age exhibited a significant positive correlation with the measured-MMSE scores ($r = 0.85$, $p < 0.001$) (Fig. 2A). The MMSE scores predicted using the TNIRS data and age also showed a significant positive correlation with the measured-MMSE scores ($r = 0.85$, $p < 0.001$) (Fig. 2B). Interestingly, the blood items related to nutrition (albumin) and anemia (RBC, Ht, Hb) were important variables for prediction in all cases [13].

In order to evaluate the relationship between cognitive function predicted by the CBF/metabolism and the systemic disorders, we compared the MMSE scores predicted by the blood test data and the TNIRS data. There was a significant positive correlation between the MMSE scores predicted using the blood test data and the TNIRS data (Fig. 3).

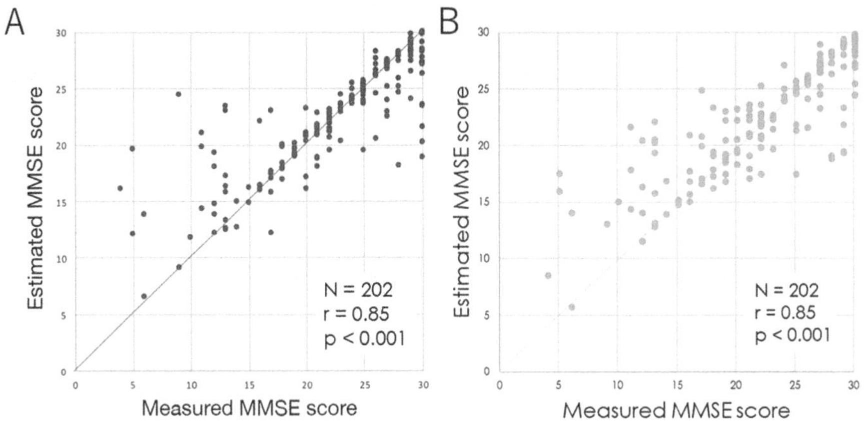

Fig. 2 (**A**) relationship between the predicted MSSE score using blood test data and the measured MMSE score, (**B**) relationship between the predicted MMSE score using TNIRS data and measured MMSE score

Fig. 3 The predicted MMSE score using TNIRS data versus the predicted MMSE score using blood test data

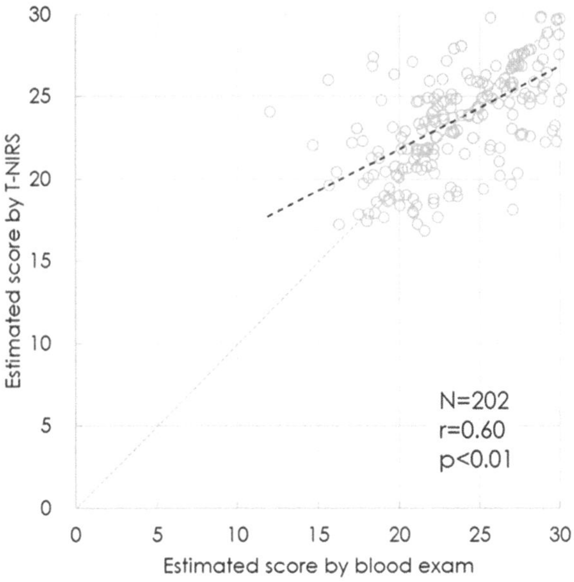

4 Discussion

The present study demonstrated that the DNN allowed the prediction of cognitive function expressed by MMSE scores with high accuracy based on the blood test data. In addition, the MMSE scores predicted using the basic blood test data exhibited a significant positive correlation with those predicted using the TNIRS data.

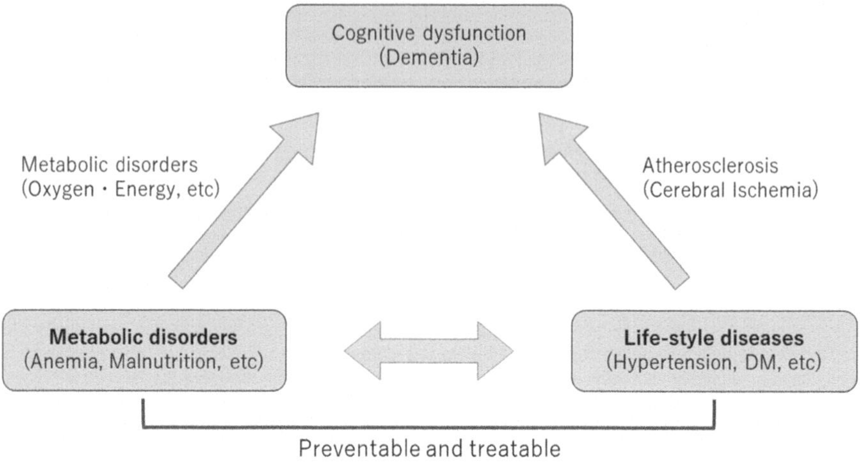

Fig. 4 Basic blood test data allow to estimate cognitive function, which is suggested to have two mechanisms

The underlying reason why the basic blood test data could predict cognitive function is not yet clear; however, the following two mechanisms should be considered. First, vascular factors due to arteriosclerosis might play an important role in the mechanism [3, 4]. In the present study, most of the subjects had a history of cerebrovascular disorders and lifestyle diseases, suggesting that the subjects suffered from VCI due to atherosclerosis. Another possible mechanism is the systemic metabolic disorders such as malnutrition [5] and anemia [6]. Indeed, the blood items related to nutrition (albumin) and anemia (RBC, Ht, Hb) were important variables for prediction in all cases.

Based on these observations, we hypothesize that cognitive dysfunction in VCI may be caused by a joint action of systemic metabolic disorders such as energy and oxygen metabolism disorder, as well as cerebral circulation disorder due to arteriosclerosis based on lifestyle-related diseases (Fig. 4). This paradigm suggests that VCI could be regarded as a systemic disease rather than a brain disease localized to the central nervous system. It should be noted that systemic metabolic disorders and lifestyle diseases can be prevented and treated, which would lead to the prevention of the clinical expression of dementia.

In summary, the results of the present study suggest that cognitive dysfunction in patients with VCI may be caused by a combination of systemic metabolic disorders, such as energy and oxygen metabolisms, and cerebral circulatory disturbance due to arteriosclerosis resulting from lifestyle-related diseases. Behavioral changes during middle age to ameliorate these systemic disorders such as exercise and diet therapy may be able to prevent dementia in the elderly.

Acknowledgments This work was supported in part by JSPS Grant-in-Aid for Young Scientists (B; 16 K16077), Strategic Research Foundation Grant-aided Project for Private Universities (S1411017) from the MEXT, Groundwork Project for Creating Industrial Models Using IoT from the NEDO, and grants from Iing Co., Ltd. (Tokyo, Japan) and Southern Tohoku General Hospital (Fukushima, Japan).

References

1. Van der Flider, Skoog I, Schneider JA et al (2018) Vascular cognitive impairment. Nat Rev Dis Primer 4:18003
2. Al-Oazzaz NK, Ali SH, Islam S et al (2014) Cognitive impairment and memory dysfunction after a stroke diagnosis: a post-stroke memory assessment. Neuro Dis Treat 10:1977–1991
3. Gorelick PB, Scuteri A, Black SE et al (2011) Vascular contributions to cognitive impairment and dementia: a statement for healthcare professionals from the American Heart Association/ American Stroke Association. Stroke 42:2672–2713
4. Provenzano FA, Muraskin J, Tosto G et al (2013) White matter hyperintensities and cerebral amyloidosis: necessary and sufficient for clinical expression of Alzheimer disease. JAMA Neurol 70:455–461
5. Broke J, Ojo O (2015) Enteral nutrition in dementia: a systematic review. Nutrients 7:2456–2468
6. Hong CH, Falvey C, Harris TB et al (2013) Anemia and risk of dementia in older adults: findings from the health ABC study. Neurology 81:528–533
7. Oizilbash N, Gregson J, Johnson ME et al (2015) BMI and risk of dementia in two million people over two decades: a retrospective cohort study. Lancet Diabetes Endocrinol 3:431–436
8. Delgado-Alvarado M et al (2016) Biomarkers for dementia and mild cognitive impairment in Parkinson's disease. Mov Disord 31:861–881
9. Miranda AS, Cordeiro TM, Dos Santos Lacerda Soares TM et al (2017) Kidney-brain axis inflammatory cross-talk: from bench to bedside. Clin Sci 131:1093–1105
10. Oyama K, Hu L, Sakatani K (2018) Prediction of MMSE score using time-resolved near-infrared spectroscopy. Adv Exp Med Biol. in press
11. Sze V, Chen YH, Yang TJ et al (2017) Efficient processing of deep neural networks: a tutorial and survey. Proc IEEE 105(12):2295–2329
12. Murayama Y, Sato Y, Hu L et al (2017) Relation between cognitive function and baseline concentrations of Hemoglobin in prefrontal cortex of elderly people measured by time-resolved near-infrared spectroscopy. Adv Exp Med Biol 977:269–276
13. Candel A, Parmar V, LeDell E et al. (2016) Deep learning with H2O. H2O. ai Inc

Relationship Between Cerebral Blood Oxygenation and Electrical Activity During Mental Stress Tasks: Simultaneous Measurements of NIRS and EEG

Y. Nagasawa, M. Ishida, Y. Komuro, S. Ushioda, L. Hu, and K. Sakatani

Abstract The incidence of stress-induced psychological and somatic diseases has been increasing rapidly, and it is important to clarify the neurophysiological mechanisms of stress response in order to establish effective stress management methods. We previously reported that the prefrontal cortex (PFC) plays an important role in stress response. In the present study, we employed near-infrared spectroscopy (NIRS) and electroencephalography (EEG) to investigate the characteristics of PFC activity during mental arithmetic tasks. A two-channel NIRS device was used to measure hemoglobin (Hb) concentration changes in the bilateral PFC during a mental arithmetic task (2 min) in normal adults. Simultaneously, EEG was used to also measure bilateral PFC activity during the same task. We evaluated concentration changes of oxy-Hb induced by the task while analyzing α wave changes using power spectrum analysis. It was observed that oxy-Hb in the bilateral PFC increased significantly during the task ($p < 0.05$), while α wave power in the PFC decreased significantly ($p < 0.01$). The present results indicate that mental stress tasks caused the activation of the bilateral PFC. Simultaneous measurements of NIRS and EEG are useful for evaluating the neurophysiological mechanism of stress responses in the brain.

Keywords Near infrared spectroscopy · Electroencephalography · Mental stress · Prefrontal cortex · Hemoglobin

Y. Nagasawa · M. Ishida · Y. Komuro · S. Ushioda · L. Hu
NEWCAT Research Institute, Department of Electrical and Electronic Engineering, College of Engineering, Nihon University, Tokyo, Japan

K. Sakatani (✉)
Department of Human and Engineered Environmental Studies, Universal Sports Health Science Laboratory, Graduate School of Frontier Sciences, The University of Tokyo, Kashiwanoha, Kashiwa-shi, Chiba, Japan
e-mail: k.sakatani@edu.k.u-tokyo.ac.jp

© Springer Nature Switzerland AG 2020
P.-D. Ryu et al. (eds.), *Oxygen Transport to Tissue XLI*, Advances in Experimental Medicine and Biology 1232, https://doi.org/10.1007/978-3-030-34461-0_14

1 Introduction

The prefrontal cortex (PFC) plays an important role in mediating behavioral and somatic responses to stress via projections to the neuroendocrine and autonomic centers in the medial hypothalamus [1]. Mental stress tasks induce an increase of neuronal activity in the PFC. Near-infrared spectroscopy (NIRS) was previously reported to demonstrate an increase of oxyhemoglobin (oxy-Hb) and total-Hb associated with a decrease of deoxy-Hb in the PFC during mental stress tasks [2–4]; this pattern of NIRS parameter changes reflects an increase in regional cerebral blood flow (rCBF) induced by neuronal activation [5].

NIRS measures blood oxygenation not only in the brain but also in extracranial tissue such as skin. Therefore, oxy-Hb changes measured using NIRS reflect blood flow in the brain and skin. Indeed, Takahashi et al. reported close correlations between oxy-Hb changes and skin blood flow during verbal fluency tasks, suggesting that a major part of the task-related changes in oxy-Hb in the forehead is due to skin blood flow [6].

In the present study, in order to evaluate whether the oxy-Hb measured in the forehead using NIRS mainly reflects skin blood flow or brain blood flow, we compared oxy-Hb changes with electrical activity measured by electroencephalography (EEG) which allows selective monitoring of the brain activity.

2 Methods

2.1 Subjects and Experimental Protocol

We studied 20 healthy subjects (18 males, two females, mean age 21.5 ± 0.5 years). To avoid the influence of environmental stress, the subjects were seated in a comfortable chair in a regular room with good air conditioning throughout the experiments. The subjects provided written informed consent as required by the Human Subjects Committee of Nihon University College of Engineering.

We employed mental arithmetic (MA) tasks to activate the PFC, since MA tasks previously been used in various activation studies on the PFC, including NIRS studies [2, 3]. The subjects were asked to serially subtract two-digit numbers from four-digit numbers (e.g. 1022–13) as quickly as possible for 120 s.

2.2 Simultaneous Measurements of NIRS and EEG

A two-channel NIRS device (Pocket NIRS Duo, DynaSense, Hamamatsu, Japan) was used for measurements of cerebral blood oxygenation (CBO) in the bilateral PFC. This system is wireless (Bluetooth®), which meant that the subject could move relatively freely. Each of the two channels uses light-emitting diodes with wavelengths 735, 810, and 850 nm as light sources, and one photo-detector. The device is powered by two AAA batteries, which can operate for up to 8 h of continuous measurement for the two-probe operation. The sampling rate was 61.3 Hz, and the concentration changes in hemoglobin were expressed as arbitrary units (a.u.). The NIRS probes were set symmetrically on the subject's forehead, so that the midpoint between the emission and detection probes was 3 cm above the centers of the upper edges of the bilateral orbital sockets; the distance between the emitter and the detector was set at 3 cm. This positioning was similar to positions Fp1 (left) and Fp2 (right) of the international electroencephalographic 10–20 system. Magnetic resonance imaging confirmed that the emitter-detector was located over the dorsolateral and front polar areas of the PFC.

A 14-channel EEG (Emotiv EPOC+, Emotiv Corporation, San Francisco, USA) was used to measure the electrical activity of the PFC. Two electrodes were set symmetrically on positions AF3 (left) and AF4 (right) of the international electroencephalographic 10–20 system. The NIRS probe and the EEG electrode were placed on the subject's forehead so as not to interfere with each other.

2.3 *Data Analysis*

Each subject performed the protocol under three kinds of experimental conditions during continuous measurement of NIRS and EEG: (1) control conditions for 120 s; (2) the MA task for 120 s; and (3) the recovery phase for 120 s. The oxy-Hb concentration changes were analyzed by subtracting the mean control values from the mean activation values induced by the MA task. The α wave power changes measured using EEG were analyzed using MwVisualizer software; alpha power is inversely related to regional brain activity, and decreased power values of the alpha band indicate an increase in cortical activation. In addition, in order to compare oxy-Hb changes measured using NIRS and the α wave power measured using EEG; we normalized both sets of changes. Furthermore, the minimum values during the recording period (1~3) were set to zero, while the maximum values were set to one.

3 Results

NIRS demonstrated an increase in oxy-Hb in the PFC during the MA task, while EEG demonstrated a decrease of the α wave power. Figure 1A, B show the normalized changes of oxy-Hb and α wave power during the task, respectively. Figure 2 shows the average changes of oxy-Hb and α wave power during the task; oxy-Hb increased significantly in the bilateral PFC ($p < 0.01$), while the α wave power decreased significantly during the task ($p < 0.01$). In addition, both oxy-Hb and α wave power returned to the control level after the task ($p < 0.01$).

Figure 3 is a scatter plot of the normalized changes of oxy-Hb and α wave power in the bilateral PFC during the task, demonstrating a significant correlation between these two parameters ($p < 0.01$).

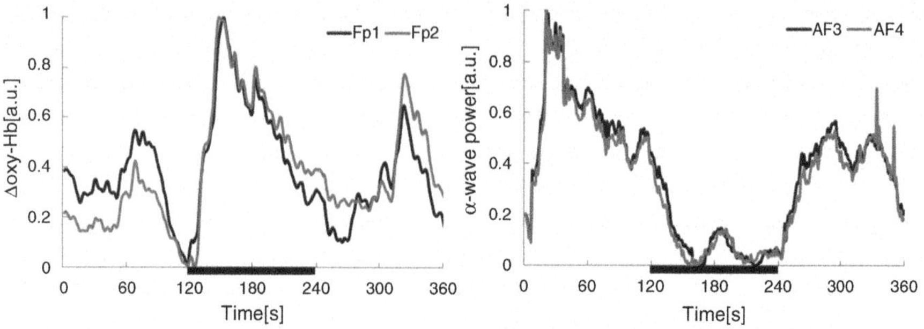

Fig. 1 Normalized changes of oxy-Hb (**A**) and α power (**B**) during the mental arithmetic task

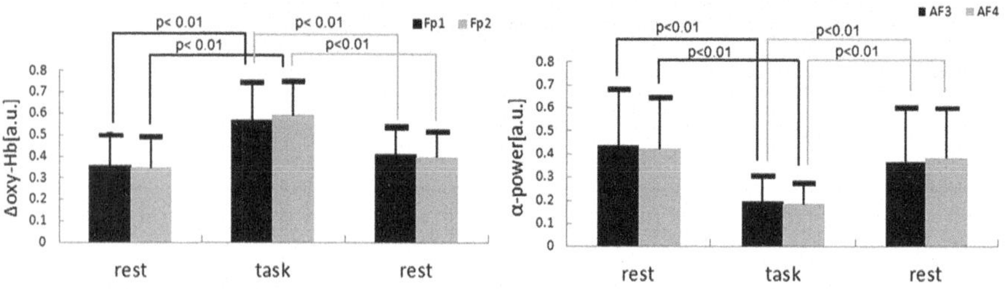

Fig. 2 Average changes of oxy-Hb (**A**) and α power (**B**) during the mental arithmetic task

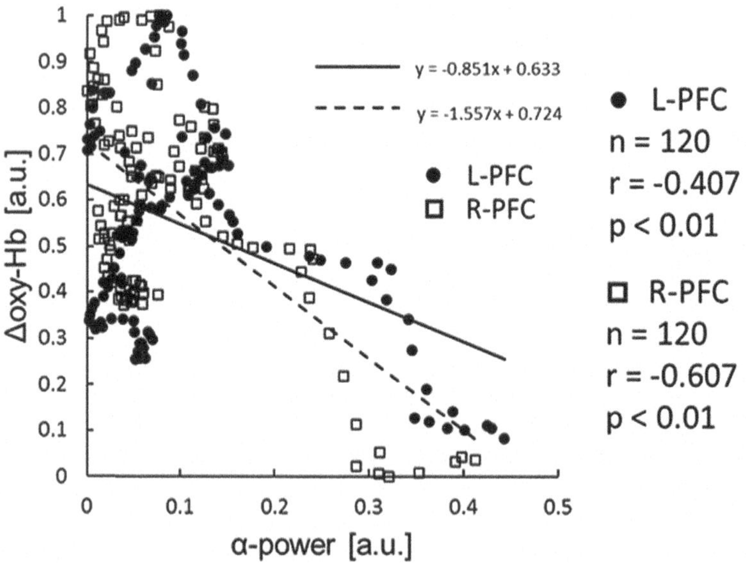

Fig. 3 Scatter plot of the normalized changes of oxy-Hb and αpower PFC during the mental arithmetic task; data of Fig. 1 were used for this scatter plot

4 Discussion

NIRS demonstrated an increase in oxy-Hb in the PFC during the MA tasks, indicating an increase of rCBF in the PFC. In contrast, EEG demonstrated a decrease of α wave power during the MA tasks. Additionally, there was a negative correlation between the changes in oxy-Hb and those in α wave power during the tasks. These observations suggest that increases in oxy-Hb measured using NIRS reflect brain activity in the PFC since α wave power is inversely related to regional brain activity, and decreases in α power indicate an increase in cortical activation [7]. It has been reported that mental stress causes skin blood flow by evoking sympathetic discharges in the supraorbital nerve which leads to a vasodilator response of the facial skin [8]. However, the present results suggest the increase in oxy-Hb measured by NIRS mainly reflect the PFC activity.

The present results are consistent with earlier studies on the comparison of optical signals and electrical signals during activation [8, 9]. For example, Rovati et al. compared changes in oxy-Hb and visual evoked potential amplitude with a black/white pattern at variable contrast; they also found a strong linear correlation between hemodynamic changes and evoked potential amplitude [10]. These results indicate that oxy-Hb changes in the visual cortex measured using NIRS are caused by neurovascular coupling.

Simultaneous measurements of NIRS and positron emission tomography (PET) support the hypothesis that NIRS signals reflect hemodynamic changes in the brain [11, 12]. For example, it was demonstrated that changes of oxy-Hb in the PFC measured using NIRS reflect changes of rCBF measured using PET [11]. In addition, Ohmae et al. compared pharmacologically-perturbed hemodynamic parameters, such as CBF, using acetazolamide administration with PET and time-resolved NIRS (TNIRS) simultaneously to investigate whether TNIRS could measure hemodynamics in the brain tissue quantitatively [12]. They compared changes in the PET and TNIRS parameters by changing optode spacing from 2 to 5 cm, and found that TNIR with 4-cm optode spacing could be used to measure cerebral hemodynamic responses optimally and quantitatively. In the present study, we set 3 cm for the distance between probes was that the S/N ration of NIRS signals at 3 cm is better than that at 4 cm. The present results indicate that the distance between probes of 3 cm allows measurements of the PFC activity.

The mental arithmetic task could activate the sympathetic nervous system, which might increase the systemic blood pressure by the beta-1 adrenergic receptor on cardiac muscle tissue. However, activation of the sympathetic nervous system also causes vasoconstriction by activation of the alpha-1 adrenergic receptor on smooth muscle cells of blood vessels in various organs including the skin. Therefore, changes of facial skin blood flow during the task are determined by the balance of activation of beta-1 and alpha-1 adrenergic receptors. In order to evaluate changes of the facial skin blood flow during the mental arithmetic task, our research group monitored the skin blood flow employing a thermography, and found no significant changes during the task [13]. These observations suggest that the effect of skin blood flow on the oxy-Hb changes measured by NIRS was limited. However, the effect of skin blood flow on NIRS signal cannot be removed completely, since irradiated NIR light and reflected NIR light must both pass through the skin. Further studies are necessary to evaluate the effect of skin blood flow and develop techniques to reduce its effect on NIRS parameters.

Acknowledgments This work was supported in part by the Strategic Research Foundation Grant-aided Project for Private Universities (S1411017) from the MEXT, Groundwork Project for Creating Industrial Models Using IoT from the NEDO, and grants from Iing Co., Ltd. (Tokyo, Japan) and Southern Tohoku General Hospital (Fukushima, Japan).

References

1. Buijs RM, van Eden CG (2000) The integration of stress by the hypothalamus, amygdala and prefrontal cortex: balance between the autonomic nervous system and the neuroendocrine system. Prog Brain Res 126:117–132
2. Tanida M, Sakatani K, Takano R et al (2004) Relation between asymmetry of prefrontal cortex activities and the autonomic nervous system during a mental arithmetic task: near infrared spectroscopy study. Neurosci Lett 369:69–74
3. Tanida M, Katsuyama M, Sakatani K (2007) Relation between mental stress-induced prefrontal cortex activity and skin conditions: a near infrared spectroscopy study. Brain Res 1184:210–216
4. Sakatani K (2012) Optical diagnosis of mental stress: review. Adv Exp Med Biol 737:89–95
5. Hoshi Y, Kobayashi N, Tamura M (2001) Interpretation of near-infrared spectroscopy signals: a study with a newly developed perfused rat brain model. J Appl Physio l90:1657–1662
6. Takahashi T, Takikawa Y, Kawagoe R et al (2011) Influence of skin blood flow on near-infrared spectroscopy signals measured on the forehead during a verbal fluency task. NeuroImage 57:991–1002
7. Allen JJ, Coan JA, Nazarian M (2004) Issues and assumptions on the road from raw signals to metrics of frontal EEG asymmetry in emotion. Biol Psychol 67:183–218
8. Nordin M (1990) Sympathetic discharges in the human supraorbital nerve and their relation to sudo- and vasomotor responses. J Physiol 423:241–255
9. Chiarelli AM, Zappasodi F, Di Pompeo F et al (2017) Simultaneous functional near-infrared spectroscopy and electroencephalography for monitoring of human brain activity and oxygenation: a review. Neurophotonics 4. https://doi.org/10.1117/1.NPh.4.4.041411
10. Rovati L, Salvatori G, Bulf L et al (2007) Optical and electrical recording of neural activity evoked by graded contrast visual stimulus. Biomed Eng Online:6–12
11. Hoshi Y, Onoe H, Watanabe Y et al (1994) Non-synchronous behavior of neuronal activity, oxidative metabolism and blood supply during mental tasks in man. Neurosci Lett 172:129–133
12. Ohmae E, Ouchi Y, Oda M et al (2006) Cerebral hemodynamics evaluation by near-infrared time-resolved spectroscopy: correlation with simultaneous positron emission tomography measurements. NeuroImage 29:697–705
13. Tanida M, Katsuyama M, Sakatani K (2008) Effects of fragrance administration on stress-induced prefrontal cortex activity and sebum secretion in the facial skin. Neurosci Lett 432:157–161

Right-Left Asymmetry of Prefrontal Cerebral Oxygenation: Does it Depend on Systemic Physiological Activity, Absolute Tissue Oxygenation or Hemoglobin Concentration?

Felix Scholkmann, Hamoon Zohdi, and Ursula Wolf

Abstract Background: We have repeatedly observed a right-left asymmetry (RLA) of prefrontal cerebral oxygenation of subjects during the resting state. Aim: To clarify if the RLA is a reliably observable phenomenon at the group level and whether it is associated with systemic physiology, absolute tissue oxygen saturation (StO_2) or total hemoglobin concentration ([tHb]). Material and Methods: StO_2 and [tHb] values at the right and left prefrontal cortex (PFC) were calculated for two 5- min resting phases based on data from 76 single measurements (24 healthy adults, aged 22.0 ± 6.4 years). StO_2 and [tHb] were measured with an ISS OxiplexTS frequency domain near-infrared spectroscopy device. In addition, end-tidal CO_2 ($P_{ET}CO_2$), heart rate (HR), respiration rate (RR) and the pulse-respiration quotient (PRQ = HR/RR) were measured and analyzed for the two phases. Results: On the group level it was found that i) StO_2 was higher at the right compared to the left PFC (for both phases), ii) RLA of StO_2 ($\Delta StO_2 = StO_2$ (right)–StO_2 (left) was independent of $P_{ET}CO_2$, HR and PRQ, and iii) ΔStO_2 was associated with absolute StO_2 and [tHb] values (positively and negatively, respectively). Discussion and Conclusion: This study shows that i) RLA of StO_2 at the PFC is a real phenomenon, and that ii) ΔStO_2 at the group level does not depend on $P_{ET}CO_2$, HR, RR or PRQ, but on absolute StO_2 and [tHb]. We conclude that the RLA is a real effect, independent of systemic physiology, and most likely reflects genuine properties of the brain, i.e. different activity states of the two hemispheres.

Keywords Cerebral oxygenation · Near-infrared spectroscopy · Cardiorespiratory system · Capnography

F. Scholkmann (✉)
Institute of Complementary and Integrative Medicine, University of Bern, Bern, Switzerland

Biomedical Optics Research Laboratory, Department of Neonatology, University Hospital Zurich, University of Zurich, Zurich, Switzerland
e-mail: Felix.Scholkmann@ikim.unibe.ch

H. Zohdi · U. Wolf
Institute of Complementary and Integrative Medicine, University of Bern, Bern, Switzerland

© Springer Nature Switzerland AG 2020

P.-D. Ryu et al. (eds.), *Oxygen Transport to Tissue XLI*, Advances in Experimental Medicine and Biology 1232, https://doi.org/10.1007/978-3-030-34461-0_15

1 Introduction

In several functional near-infrared spectroscopy (NIRS) studies performed by our group in recent years, we observed a tendency of a right-left asymmetry (RLA) of prefrontal cerebral oxygenation during the resting-state phases of the subjects. Since the aims of the studies were to investigate task and stimulus evoked cerebral brain activity [1–5], we did not analyze RLA in detail. Therefore, this study aimed to investigate these phenomena in detail based on a large dataset from one of our previous studies. In particular, we aimed to clarify if the RLA is a reliably observable phenomenon on the group level and if it is associated with cardiorespiratory activity, absolute tissue oxygenation (StO_2) or total hemoglobin concentration ([tHb]).

2 Materials and Methods

Resting-state StO_2 and [tHb] values were calculated for two baseline phases from a dataset of our previous study [1] comprising 76 single measurements performed on 24 healthy subjects (aged 22.0 ± 6.4 years). Median StO_2 and [tHb] values at the right and left prefrontal cortex (PFC) were calculated for two 5-min resting-state phases (one during the pre-task baseline and the other from the post-task phase). Only data of high signal quality (i.e. StO_2 in the range of 40–100%, no movement artifacts) were included.

StO_2 and [tHb] were measured with an ISS OxiplexTS frequency domain NIRS device enabling StO_2 measurements relatively immune against oxygenation and hemodynamics in the superficial tissue layers. In addition, systemic physiology variables were assessed by measuring end-tidal CO_2 ($P_{ET}CO_2$) (N1000 gas analyzer, Nellcor, Boulder, CO, USA), heart rate (HR) (Medilog AR12, Schiller AG, Baar, Switzerland), respiration rate (RR) and the pulse-respiration quotient (PRQ = HR/RR). The RR was determined from the capnography signal by extracting the instantaneous frequency based on wavelet time-frequency decomposition.

Data were analyzed with Bayesian statistics (JASP, v.0.8.6) to assess whether i) RLA of StO_2 was detectable (Bayesian *t*-test, Cauchy scale: 0.4, hypothesis: StO_2 (right) > StO_2 (left), and whether ii) ΔStO_2 was correlated with HR, RR, PRQ, $P_{ET}CO_2$, mean of absolute StO_2 ($\langle StO_2 \rangle$) or the mean of absolute [tHb] ($\langle [tHb] \rangle$) (Bayesian linear regression; Cauchy prior width 1; tested hypothesis: correlated, correlated positively, or correlated negatively, depending on visual inspection of the scatter plot). Furthermore, it was assessed how well the ΔStO_2 values from both phases agreed (Bayesian linear regression).

3 Results

The distributions of StO_2 values for the left and right PFC and for both phases are depicted in Fig. 1. Also shown is the correlation between StO_2 (phase 1) and StO_2 (phase 2) as well as the distribution of ΔStO_2 values for both phases. The results of the correlation analysis are shown in Figs. 2 and 3.

The results of the analysis can be summarized as follows:

- At the group level, StO_2 measured on the right PFC was higher compared to the left PFC. This was true for both measurement times (median, interquartile range (IQR), phase 1 StO_2 (right) = 68.9% (63.7–72.3%), StO_2 (left) = 57.5% (52.7–62.9%); phase 2 StO_2 (right) = 68.3% (63.1–73.3%), StO_2 (left) = 56.8% (53.4–63.8%), as well as for the combined data set (i.e., phase 1 and 2 combined): StO_2 (right) = 68.6% (63.5–72.4%) vs. StO_2 (left) = 56.8% (52.9–63.4%). All three right-left comparisons yielded Bayes factors (BF_{10}) higher than 100 (with a Cauchy prior width of 0.4), i.e. indicating extreme evidence for the hypothesis StO_2 (right) > StO_2 (left).
- ΔStO_2 (phase 1) and ΔStO_2 (phase 2) were correlated to a high degree ($r = 0.949$ (% confidence interval, CI 0.916–0.967), $BF_{10} = 4.29 \times 10^{34}$ for the hypothesis of a positive correlation), indicating that the RLA of StO_2 is a stable phenomenon for each subject during the whole experiment.
- For both phases, the correlation analysis between ΔStO_2 and HR, RR, PRQ and $P_{ET}CO_2$ ($|r| < 0.2$) delivered BF_{10} values associated with strong to substantial

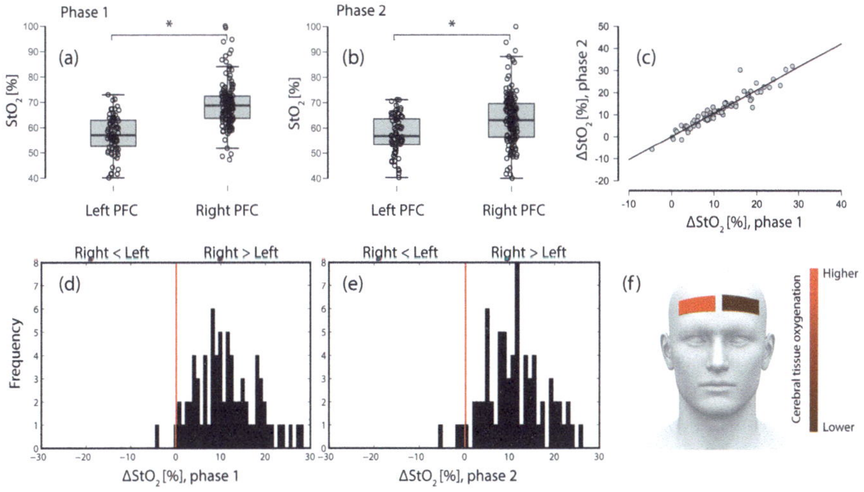

Fig. 1 (**a**, **b**) StO_2 for the right and left PFC measured at two different times (phase 1 and 2). (**c**) Correlation between ΔStO_2 (phase 1) with ΔStO_2 (phase 2). (**d**, **e**) Distribution of ΔStO_2 for both phases. (**f**) Visualization of the RLA of StO_2 observed in this study

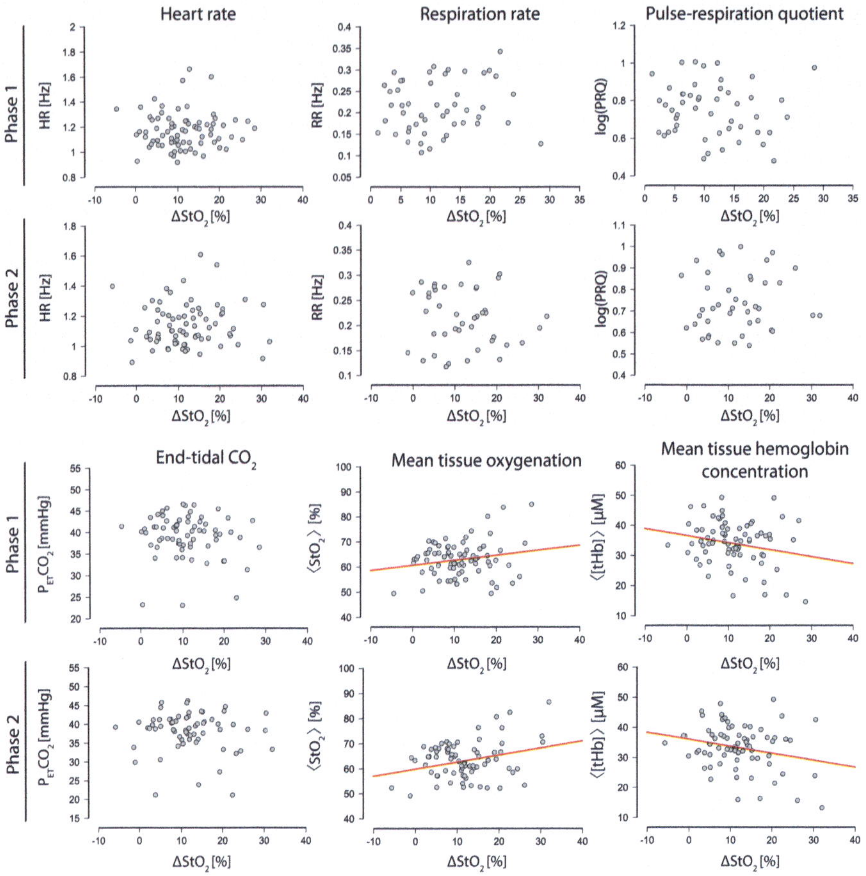

Fig. 2 Scatter plots showing ΔStO_2 vs. HR, RR, PRQ, $P_{ET}CO_2$, $\langle StO_2 \rangle$ and $\langle [tHb] \rangle$ for both phases of the resting-state time series. Correlations between the data are indicated by a linear fit

evidence (BF_{10} = 0.03–0.3) for the hypothesis of no correlation (see Table 1 for individual values and Fig. 2 for a visualization).

- ΔStO_2, was found to be correlated with absolute StO_2 and [tHb] (Table 1, Fig. 2). These correlations are most evident when analyzing the combined data (phase 1 and 2 combined), resulting in a positive correlation of ΔStO_2 with StO_2 (r = 0.247, BF_{10} = 19.40) and a negative correlation with [tHb] (r = −0.230, BF_{10} = 10.69) (Fig. 3). With $BF_{10} > 10$ there is strong evidence for the hypothesis that the variables are correlated. A Bayes factor robustness check (BF vs. Cauchy prior width) confirmed that the evidence of correlation does not change substantially when changing the Cauchy prior width from 0.25 to 1.5 (see Fig. 3).

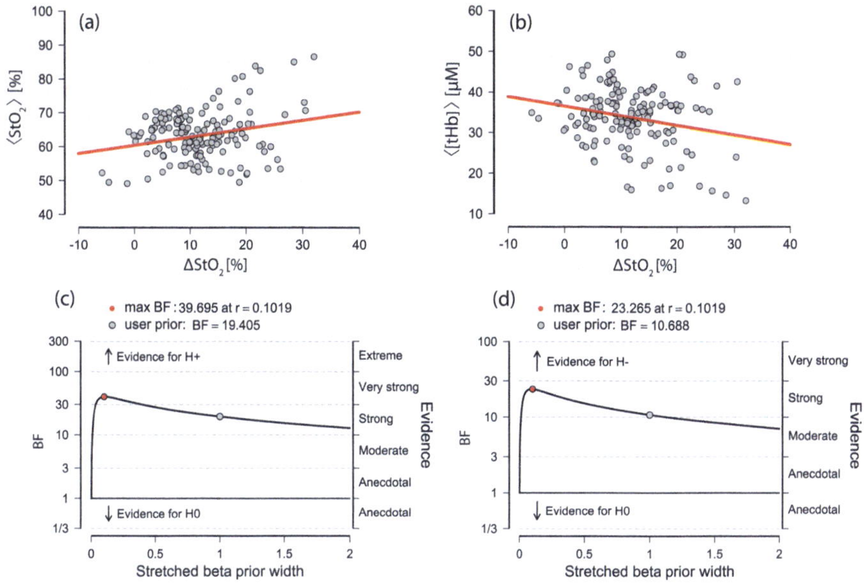

Fig. 3 Bayes factor robustness check (BF vs. Cauchy prior width) for the correlations ΔStO_2 vs. $\langle StO_2 \rangle$ and $\langle [tHb] \rangle$, respectively. For the analysis, the data from period 1 and 2 were combined to increase the robustness of the analysis

Table 1 Correlations between the right-left asymmetry of prefrontal cerebral oxygenation (ΔStO_2) and HR, RR, PRQ, $P_{ET}CO_2$, $\langle StO_2 \rangle$ and $\langle [tHb] \rangle$

Parameter 1	Parameter 1	Correlation coefficient (r), 95% CI	Bayes factor (BF_{10})
ΔStO_2 (phase 1)	HR (phase 1)	0.017 [-0.207, 0.238]	0.146
ΔStO_2 (phase 2)	HR (phase 2)	0.039 [-0.188, 0.260]	0.153
ΔStO_2 (phase 1)	RR (phase 1)	0.129 [-0.154, 0.385]	0.129
ΔStO_2 (phase 2)	RR (phase 2)	-0.084 [-0.367, 0.218]	0.220
ΔStO_2 (phase 1)	PRQ (phase 1)	-0.076 [-0.340, 0.204]	0.203
ΔStO_2 (phase 2)	PRQ (phase 2)	0.071 [-0.230, 0.355]	0.212
ΔStO_2 (phase 1)	$P_{ET}CO_2$ (phase 1)	-0.124 [-0.352, -0.10]	0.420
ΔStO_2 (phase 2)	$P_{ET}CO_2$ (phase 2)	-0.077 [-0.326, -0.007]	0.271
ΔStO_2 (phase 1)	$\langle StO_2 \rangle$ (phase 1)	0.196 [0.023, 0.400]	1.107
ΔStO_2 (phase 2)	$\langle StO_2 \rangle$ (phase 2)	0.289 [0.073, 0.478]	6.171
ΔStO_2 (phase 1)	$\langle [tHb] \rangle$ (phase 1)	-0.218 [-0.418, -0.031]	1.570
ΔStO_2 (phase 2)	$\langle [tHb] \rangle$ (phase 2)	-0.240 [-0.437, -0.040]	2.257
ΔStO_2 (combined)	$\langle StO_2 \rangle$ (combined)	0.247 [0.090, 0.389]	19.40*
ΔStO_2 (combined)	$\langle [tHb] \rangle$ (combined)	-0.230 [-0.374, -0.074]	10.69*

$*BF_{10} > 10$

4 Discussion and Conclusion

This study shows that i) RLA of StO_2 at the PFC is a real phenomenon, and that ii) ΔStO_2 at the group level does not depend on $P_{ET}CO_2$, HR, RR or PRQ, but on absolute StO_2 and [tHb].

The absolute StO_2 values at the human PFC measured in our study (StO_2 (right) = 68.6 (IQR 63.5–72.4), StO_2 (left) = 56.8% (IQR 52.9–63.4%), combined values for both phases) are in the range of values reported by previous studies, e.g. 64.5 ± 10% (Invos 3100; measurement avoiding contributions from the extracerebral layer, but obtained without using a frequency domain NIRS instrument) [6], or slightly lower, e.g., 75.19 ± 8.3% (Imagent, ISS; combined values for the right and left PFC; measurement avoiding contributions from the extracerebral layer) [7] and 75.5 ± 4.5% (NIRO300, 4 cm source-detector separation, average over 2 channels and left and right PFC) [8]. The reason for the differences in StO_2 values between studies might be a difference in the age or physiological state of the subjects and the measurement methodology. For example, according to the manufacturer, the Invos NIRS device is not intended for measuring absolute values, provides slightly lower values than the ISS instrument, and the StO_2 values depend on the tHb concentration [9].

Our finding that on the group level during rest the right PFC has a higher oxygenation than the left, i.e. a RLA of StO_2 at the PFC, has seldom been investigated with NIRS. The only NIRS studies that investigated this aspect found no difference (right vs. left PFC (extracerebral tissue): 71.7 ± 3.03% vs. 71.7 ± 3.86%, and right vs. left PFC (cerebral tissue): 74.8 ± 5.83% vs. 75.6 ± 5.86%; 15 subjects, aged 20–50 years, using an ISS Imagent device [7] and right vs. left PCF (cerebral and extracerebral tissue combined, 4 cm source-detector separation): 75.6 ± 4.2% vs. 75.4 ± 4.9%, 16 subjects, using a NIRO300 device [8]. In these studies, much larger distances were employed, which leads to a substantially lower SNR. The explanation for this difference may be that the SNR was not high enough to show the RLA. In addition, the measurements of Quaresima et al. [8] were also sensitive to the extracerebal tissue layer whereas our measurements avoided this confounding effect.

To exclude a simple artifact, we tested whether our NIRS measurements were dependent on the specific NIRS optode by switching the right optode with the left and vice versa. Since the StO_2 difference persisted (data not shown; for the test the ISS Imagent was used; also here the RLA was observed), we conclude that the StO_2 RLA measured is not simply due to a measurement error.

That task or stimulus evoked brain activity shows a laterality in the PFC has been shown by many electroencephalography (EEG) studies linking the asymmetry to side-specific activities of behavior regulation, especially reflecting the activity of a "moderator of emotional responding for both approach and withdrawal related emotions", as summarized in a recent review [10]. The right PFC in particular seems to be "crucially involved in a regulatory control system that supervises the motivational systems of approach and avoidance" [11].

Studies applying functional NIRS (fNIRS) to investigate the frontal asymmetry by Sakatani et al. are generally in line with these EEG studies and also with our finding of a RLA of StO_2: several studies showed a higher increase in the concentration of oxyhemoglobin ([O_2Hb]) in the right PFC during mental stress tasks, mediated by the individual psychological state (anxiety level) [12–14] and the age [15]. However, a decrease in [O_2Hb] in the right PFC, and a decrease in EEG activity at the same side, during a mental arithmetic task was reported in an fNIRS-EEG by others [16]. A stronger response (increase) in the left compared to the right PFC to a continuous colored light exposure (10 min) of the subjects was observed in a study by our group [17]. From this it can be concluded that the activity-dependent RLA of frontal NIRS-signal changes was observed by several fNIRS studies, and the magnitude and sign varied, probably depending on the task, individual subjects and differences in methodology.

Our study is the first to investigate whether the RLA of StO_2 during the resting state was dependent on the state of the cardiorespiratory system of the subjects; however, such a dependence was not observed in our study. This finding supports the notion that the degree of RLA of frontal oxygenation does not simply reflect systemic physiological (i.e. cardiorespiratory) activity, but rather constitutes real frontal asymmetry of brain activity (neurovascular coupling). The reason for the observed ΔStO_2 depends on absolute StO_2 and [HHb] and needs further research.

References

1. Scholkmann F et al (2013) End-tidal CO_2: an important parameter for a correct interpretation in functional brain studies using speech tasks. NeuroImage 66:71–79
2. Scholkmann F, Wolf M, Wolf U (2013) The Effect of Inner Speech on Arterial CO_2 and Cerebral Hemodynamics and Oxygenation: A Functional NIRS Study. Adv Exp Med Biol 789:81–87
3. Scholkmann F et al (2014) Cerebral hemodynamic and oxygenation changes induced by inner and heard speech: a study combining functional near-infrared spectroscopy and capnography. J Biomed Opt 19(1):017002
4. Metz AJ et al (2017) Physiological effects of continuous Colored light exposure on Mayer wave activity in cerebral Hemodynamics: a functional near-infrared spectroscopy (fNIRS) study. Adv Exp Med Biol 977:277–283
5. Scholkmann F et al (2017) Effect of short-term colored-light exposure on cerebral hemodynamics and oxygenation, and systemic physiological activity. Neurophotonics 4(04):1
6. Germon TJ et al (1995) Extracerebral absorption of near infrared light influences the detection of increased cerebral oxygenation monitored by near infrared spectroscopy. J Neurol Neurosurg Psychiatry 58(4):477–479
7. Choi J et al (2004) Noninvasive determination of the optical properties of adult brain: near-infrared spectroscopy approach. J Biomed Opt 9(1):221–229
8. Quaresima V et al (2000) Noninvasive measurement of cerebral hemoglobin oxygen saturation using two near infrared spectroscopy approaches. J Biomed Opt 5(2):201–205
9. Kleiser S et al (2017) Comparison of tissue oximeters on a liquid phantom with adjustable optical properties: an extension. Biomed Opt Express 9(1):86
10. Reznik SJ, Allen JJB (2018) Frontal asymmetry as a mediator and moderator of emotion: an updated review. Psychophysiology 55(1):e12965

11. Allen JJB et al (2018) Frontal EEG alpha asymmetry and emotion: From neural underpinnings and methodological considerations to psychopathology and social cognition. Psychophysiology 55(1):e13028
12. Tanida M, Katsuyama M, Sakatani K (2007) Relation between mental stress-induced prefrontal cortex activity and skin conditions: a near-infrared spectroscopy study. Brain Res 1184:210–216
13. Tanida M, Katsuyama M, Sakatani K (2008) Effects of fragrance administration on stress-induced prefrontal cortex activity and sebum secretion in the facial skin. Neurosci Lett 432(2):157–161
14. Ishikawa W et al (2014) Correlation between asymmetry of spontaneous oscillation of hemodynamic changes in the prefrontal cortex and anxiety levels: a near-infrared spectroscopy study. J Biomed Opt 19(2):027005
15. Sakatani K, Tanida M, Katsuyama M (2010) Effects of Aging on Activity of the Prefrontal Cortex and Autonomic Nervous System during Mental Stress Task. Adv Exp Med Biol 662:473–478
16. Al-Shargie F, Tang TB, Kiguchi M (2017) Assessment of mental stress effects on prefrontal cortical activities using canonical correlation analysis: an fNIRS-EEG study. Biomed Opt Express 8(5):2583–2598
17. Metz AJ et al (2017) Continuous coloured light altered human brain haemodynamics and oxygenation assessed by systemic physiology augmented functional near-infrared spectroscopy. Sci Rep 7(1):10027

Effect of Gum Chewing on PFC Activity During Discomfort Sound Stimulation

M. Konno, K. Nakajima, T. Takeda, Y. Kawano, Y. Suzuki, and K. Sakatani

Abstract The prefrontal cortex (PFC) is sensitive to the stress exposure and involved in stress coping. And the effects of gum chewing on the stress have been studied using NIRS. However, when measuring NIRS on PFC during gum chewing, blood flows in shallow tissues (scalp, skin, muscle) might be affected. A NIRS used in the present study first, which has a short distance (1 cm) and the usual (3 cm) source-detector (S-D) regression, can allow eliminating shallow tissues effect of gum chewing. The aim of this study was to investigate the hypothesis that gum chewing activates the right prefrontal cortex (PFC) in stress coping against negative sounds (NS) from the International Affective Digitized Sounds-2 (IADS) as a mental stress task. NS showed activation in the right PFC. There was a significant difference between NS, and NS with Gum, where NS with Gum showed an increased PFC activity, increased alpha wave appearance rate, a higher value in heart rate level, and a higher VAS score indicating 'pleasant'. Gum chewing activated right PFC activity while exposed to negative sounds from IADS as a mental stress task.

Keywords Prefrontal cortex · Near-infrared spectroscopy · International affective digitized sounds-2 · Electroencephalogram · Gum-chewing

M. Konno (✉) · K. Nakajima · T. Takeda · Y. Kawano · Y. Suzuki
Division of Sports Dentistry, Department Oral Health and Clinical Science, Tokyo Dental College, Tokyo, Japan
e-mail: mkonno@tdc.ac.jp

K. Sakatani
Department of Electrical and Electronics Engineering, Nihon University, NEWCAT Institute, College of Engineering, Fukushima, Japan

Department of Neurological Surgery, Nihon University, School of Medicine, Tokyo, Japan

© Springer Nature Switzerland AG 2020

P.-D. Ryu et al. (eds.), *Oxygen Transport to Tissue XLI*, Advances in Experimental Medicine and Biology 1232, https://doi.org/10.1007/978-3-030-34461-0_16

1 Introduction

In modern society, many people suffer from many kinds of stress. Although activation of the stress response system improves the ability of an organism to maintain homeostasis, persistent activation of this system may lead to psychological or somatic diseases [1]. Therefore, individuals may adopt different approaches to coping with stress. Stress coping is thought to be important for an individual's survival and wellbeing. In dental-related fields, many studies have investigated the effects of gum chewing as a stress coping measure [2–5]. These studies have mainly investigated the influence of chewing on the salivary glands and blood stress markers (alpha-amylase activity, cortisol level, and secretory immunoglobulin A secretion rate as indicators of mental stress using an arithmetic calculation as a stress loader. They suggested that gum chewing is effective for both physical and psychological stress coping in humans. In their fMRI study, Yu et al. studied how stress is relieved by a popular coping behavior, i.e. gum chewing [6].

Nevertheless, the neurophysiological mechanisms involved are still unclear. The prefrontal cortex (PFC) is the most sensitive to the effects of stress exposure [7]. The stress response involves activation of the PFC which stimulates the hypothalamic-pituitary-adrenal (HPA) axis and influences the autonomic nervous system (ANS), since neuronal networks exist between the PFC and the neuroendocrine centers in the medial hypothalamus [8], and the PFC has direct access to sympathetic and/or parasympathetic motor nuclei in the brainstem and the spinal cord. The PFC will set the endocrine/autonomic balance, depending on emotional status [8]. The left hemisphere specializes in the processing of positive emotions while the right hemisphere specializes in the processing of negative emotions [9–12].

Among many functional neuroimaging techniques, functional NIRS is a powerful, non-invasive imaging technique that offers many advantages, including compact size, no need for specially equipped facilities, and the potential for real-time measurement [11, 13]. However, when measuring NIRS on PFC during gum chewing, blood flows in shallow tissues (scalp, skin, muscle) might be affected. Hot-1000 (NeU Corporation, Tokyo, Japan) has dual source-detector (S-D) regression. The short distance S-D (1 cm) pair captures the shallow blood-flow signal. The deep signal from the usual S-D distance (3 cm) channel contains both the superficial and cortical (neural) blood-flow components. The neural signal is calculated automatically using these different distance S-D pair results [14]. Therefore, this first used NIRS can allow eliminating shallow tissues effect of gum chewing.

On the other hand, selection of a stress loading task is also an important factor in functional neuroimaging technique measurements. The International Affective Digitized Sounds-2 (IADS) is a standardized database of 167 naturally occurring sounds, which is widely used in the study of emotions. The IADS is part of a system for emotional assessment developed by the Center for Emotion and Attention [15–17].

The aim of this study was to investigate the hypothesis that gum chewing activates the right PFC in stress coping against negative sounds from IADS as a mental stress task.

2 Methods

Negative sounds (NS) were selected from the IADS, with fewer than 3.0 in pleasure value. Selected sounds of approximately 5-s length each were mixed and assigned as a task. The study followed a controlled, randomized design: two different conditions of not gum chewing and gum chewing during the negative sound task (hereafter, referred to as NS, and NS with Gum), both on the same day, with a 10-min rest period between experiments. Each task session was designed in a block manner; 4 rests: Brown Noise (30 sec) and 3 task blocks: NS or NS with Gum (30 sec) (Fig. 1).

A total of 12 healthy volunteers participated in the study (mean age 24.0 years, male/female 10:2). All participants had complete natural dentition. The study was conducted in agreement with the principles of the Declaration of Helsinki, and the protocol was approved by the Ethics Committee of Tokyo Dental College (Ethical Clearance No. 436). Written informed consent was obtained from all participants.

Participants were told to refrain from substances containing caffeine (e.g., coffee, etc.) and not to eat for 2 h before the test. They were also instructed to avoid drinking alcohol excessively and lack of sleep the night before the test. To prevent the influence of environmental stress, the participants were seated in a comfortable chair in an air-conditioned room with temperature and humidity maintained at approximately 25°C and 50%, respectively. After a 10-min rest, they then performed an auditory stimulation task with eyes closed. A piece of tasteless gum weighing 1.0 g (Lotte, Saitama, Japan) was used as a chewing sample. Chewing rate and force were determined by the subjects themselves. Activity in the right PFC was measured by a two-channel NIRS (HOT-1000, NeU, Japan). Two probes were placed at Fp1 and Fp2 (Fig. 2). The probe locations were determined according to the international 10–20 system. The region of interest was placed at Fp2 [11, 12]. HOT-1000 can also measure heart rate (HR). EEG (Muse Brain System, Syscom, Japan) was monitored simultaneously (Fig. 3). Alpha wave appearance rate was calculated by dividing the value of alpha by the sum of alpha, theta, and beta. The self-rated psychological measurement was evaluated using a 100-mm visual analogue scale (VAS) [18]. The VAS consisted of a single unmarked 100-mm line with end-points labeled 'very uncomfortable' on the left side and 'very comfortable' on the right side. We analyzed the total-Hb values during the task. Alpha wave (8–13 Hz)

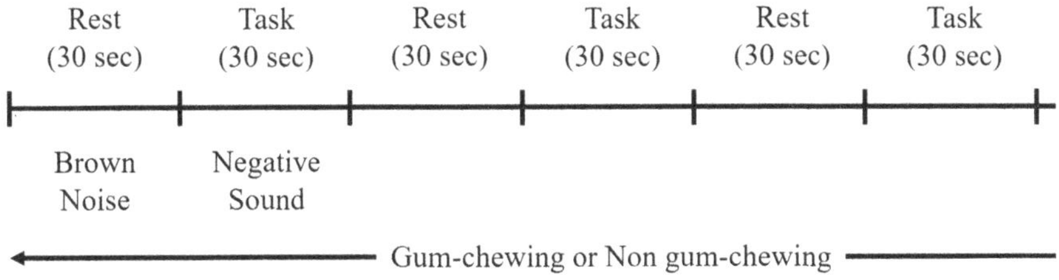

Fig. 1 Experimental protocol trial that consisted of four rests (Smoothed Brown Noise, 30 s) and three blocks of tasks: negative sounds from IADS

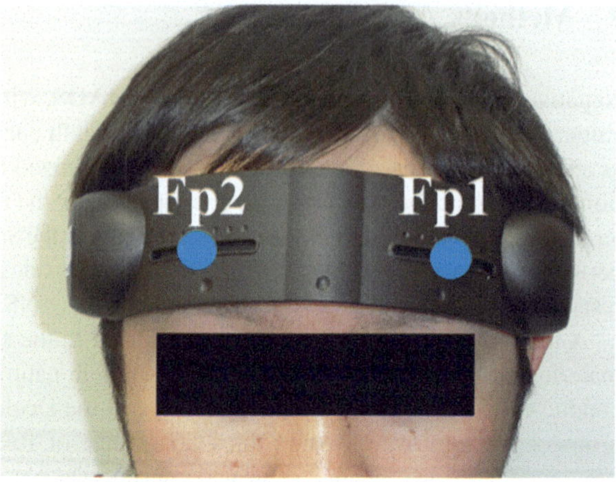

Fig. 2 Activity in the right PFC was measured by a two-channel NIRS (HOT-1000, NeU, Japan). The region of interest was placed at Fp2

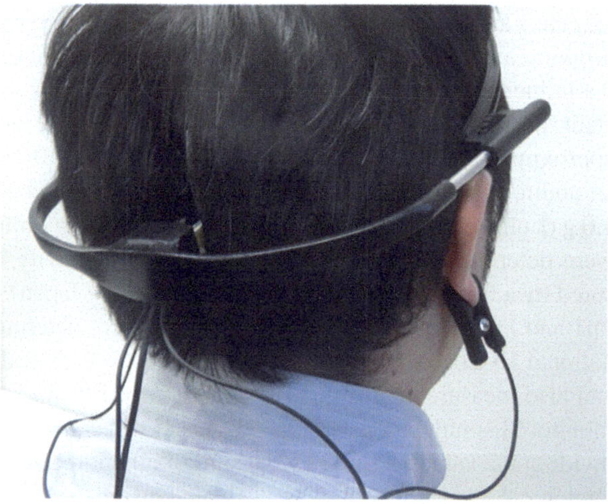

Fig. 3 We recorded and analyzed participans electroencephalogram (alpha wave appearance rate). EEG channel was installed in the back of the head

appearance rates in theta, alpha and beta waves were calculated. Statistical evaluation was performed using a paired Student's t-test (Excel Statistics 2010, Bell Curve, Japan).

3 Results

Results are summarized in Table 1. NS showed activation in the right PFC. There was a significant difference between NS and NS with Gum, where NS with Gum showed an increase in PFC activity (Fig. 4). Also, there was a significant difference between NS and NS with Gum, where NS with Gum showed an increase in the alpha wave appearance rate. NS with Gum showed a larger value in the HR level. In addition, there was a significant difference between NS and NS with Gum, where NS with Gum showed a larger VAS score indicating 'pleasant'.

Table 1 Psychological and physiological assessment (a lower VAS score indicates 'less pleasant')

			Stimuli of site	Mean (S.D.)	P-value	Cohen's d
Psychological assessment	VAS level (smaller figure indicates "more unpleasant")		NS	35.83 (8.10)	0.0084	0.92
			NS + Gum	43.75 (9.16)		
Physical assessment	Heart rate (bpm)		NS	73.65 (9.13)	00100	0.45
			NS + Gum	77.69 (8.79)		
	Alpha wave (%) (appearance rate in theta, alpha, and beta waves)		NS	42.78 (0.03)	0.0227	0.85
			NS + Gum	44.43 (0.03)		
	NIRS (mM·mm)	Right PFC	NS	0.027 (0.09)	0.0006	1.26
			NS + Gum	0.120 (0.08)		

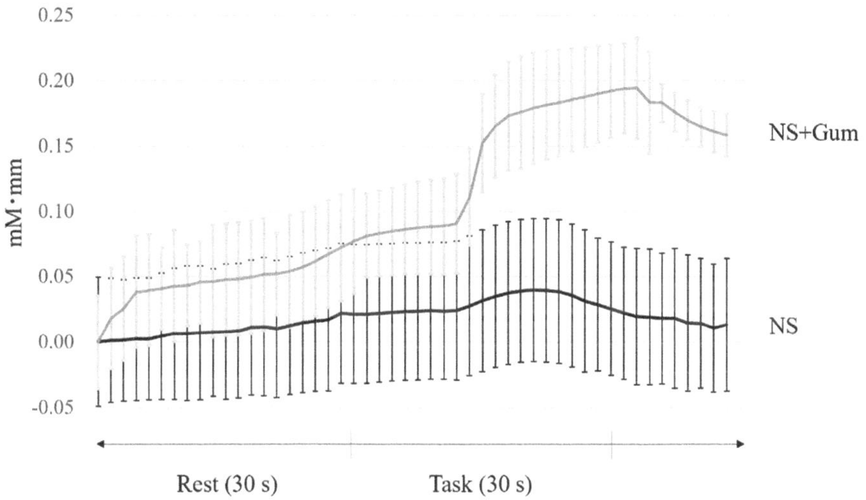

Fig. 4 Total-Hb hemodynamic responses (group averages with S.E.) in the right PFC

4 Discussion and Conclusion

Judged mainly by the psychological VAS result, the subjects felt discomfort during NS, which could cause acute stress responses in the brain. Indeed, NS increased total-Hb in the PFC, indicating that NS induced neural activation of the PFC [14]. This is in line with previous findings that used a noisy sound stress [19]. The unpleasant task-induced PFC activation could cause activation of the HPA axis and influence ANS, by the networks between the PFC and the medial hypothalamus and ANS [8].

EEG reflects the neuronal activities of a human brain that can be directly affected by emotional states. Especially an alpha wave appearance in the awaked EEG with an eyes-closed condition seems to indicate a relaxed state [20]. Listening to an unpleasant tone [21] and a loud siren reduced the alpha wave [22]. The increased alpha wave by gum chewing might indicate a reduction of the uncomfortable mood.

Gum chewing itself is reported to increase HR [23]. In the present study, NS with gum chewing increased HR. The increase in HR could be related to PFC blood flow. The change in blood supply might have an influence on emotional control.

Gum chewing reduced negative psychological scores on the VAS indicating relief of mental stress.

Gum chewing inhibited the connectivity between the brain stress network caused by the noise [6] and a possible interpretation for the gum chewing effect is that gum chewing might shield the organism from the external stressor through attention distraction. Gum chewing generates internal noise within the auditory system which may itself partially mask the impact of external noise or distract attention from external noise. This mechanism might be related to the result [19] that the gum chewing suppressed not only the stress-induced increase in BOLD signals in these two regions but also the stress-induced elevation in plasma levels of these catecholamines and ACTH.

The NIRS technique has some limitations: NIRS can detect only surface areas of the brain, NIRS measurement has possible confounders such as skin blood flow, respiration and blood pressure, and NIRS has a relatively low spatial resolution. Despite its shortcomings, NIRS is becoming increasingly useful in neuroscience for its advantages such as simplicity, small size, and the potential for real-time and natural condition measurement [11, 13].

Within the limitations of this study, the findings suggest that gum chewing reduced stress-related responses, and there was a gum chewing-induced change in the level of PFC activity. Gum chewing might have an effect on stress coping.

Gum chewing activated the right PFC activity while exposed to negative sounds from IADS as a mental stress task.

Acknowledgments This research was partly supported by Japan Science and Technology Agency, under Strategic Promotion of Innovative Research and Development Program, and a Grant-in-Aid from the Ministry of Education, Culture, Sports, Sciences and Technology of Japan(Grant-in-Aid for Scientific Research 22592162, 25463025, and 25463024, Grant-in-Aid for Exploratory Research 25560356).

References

1. Chrousos GP, Gold PW (1992) The concepts of stress and stress system disorders. Overview of physical and behavioral homeostasis. JAMA 267:1244–1252
2. Scholey A, Haskell C, Robertson B et al (2009) Chewing gum alleviates negative mood and reduces cortisol during acute laboratory psychological stress. Physiol Behav 97:304–312
3. Smith AP, Chaplin K, Wadsworth E (2012) Chewing gum, occupational stress, work performance and wellbeing. An intervention study. Appetite 58:1083–1086
4. Tahara Y, Sakurai K, Ando T (2007) Influence of chewing and clenching on salivary cortisol levels as an indicator of stress. J Prosthodont 16:129–135
5. Tasaka A, Takeuchi K, Sasaki H et al (2014) Influence of chewing time on salivary stress markers. J Prosthodont Res 58:48–54

6. Yu H, Chen X, Liu J et al (2013) Gum chewing inhibits the sensory processing and the propagation of stress-related information in a brain network. PLoS One 8:e57111
7. Arnsten AF (2009) Stress signalling pathways that impair prefrontal cortex structure and function. Nat Rev Neurosci 10:410–422
8. Buijs RM, Van Eden CG (2000) The integration of stress by the hypothalamus, amygdala and prefrontal cortex: balance between the autonomic nervous system and the neuroendocrine system. Prog Brain Res 126:117–132
9. Davidson RJ (2003) Affective neuroscience and psychophysiology: toward a synthesis. Psychophysiology 40:655–665
10. Coan JA, Allen JJ (2004) Frontal EEG asymmetry as a moderator and mediator of emotion. Biol Psychol 67:7–49
11. Tanida M, Sakatani K, Takano R et al (2004) Relation between asymmetry of prefrontal cortex activities and the autonomic nervous system during a mental arithmetic task: near infrared spectroscopy study. Neurosci Lett 369:69–74
12. Tanida M, Katsuyama M, Sakatani K (2007) Relation between mental stress-induced prefrontal cortex activity and skin conditions: a near-infrared spectroscopy study. Brain Res 1184:210–216
13. Shibusawa M, Takeda T, Nakajima K et al (2009) Functional near-infrared spectroscopy study on primary motor and sensory cortex response to clenching. Neurosci Lett 449:98–102
14. Nozawa T, Sasaki Y, Sakaki K et al (2016) Interpersonal frontopolar neural synchronization in group communication: an exploration toward fNIRS hyperscanning of natural interactions. NeuroImage 133:484–497
15. Soares AP, Pinheiro AP, Costa A et al (2013) Affective auditory stimuli: adaptation of the international affective digitized sounds (IADS-2) for European Portuguese. Behav Res Methods 45:1168–1181
16. Stevenson RA, James TW (2008) Affective auditory stimuli: characterization of the international affective digitized sounds (IADS) by discrete emotional categories. Behav Res Methods 40:315–321
17. Bradley MM, Lang PJ (2007) The international affective digitized sounds (2nd edition, IADS-2): affective ratings of sounds and instruction manual (technical report B-3). University of Florida, NIH Center for the Study of Emotion and Attention, Gainesville
18. Folstein MF, Luria R (1973) Reliability, validity, and clinical application of the visual analogue mood scale. Psychol Med 3:479–486
19. Niwa M, Hiramatsu I, Nakata F et al (2005) Functional significance of stress-relieving act of chewing and it effect on brain activation by stress (in Japanese). J Jpn Ass Rural Med 54:661–666
20. Davidson RJ, Jackson DC, Kalin NH (2000) Emotion, plasticity, context, and regulation: perspectives from affective neuroscience. Psychol Bull 126:890–909
21. Nishifuji S (2011) EEG recovery enhanced by acute aerobic exercise after performing mental task with listening to unpleasant sound. Conference proceedings: Annual International Conference of the IEEE Engineering in Medicine and Biology Society IEEE Engineering in Medicine and Biology Society Conference 2011:3837–3840
22. Horii A, Yamamura C, Katsumata T et al (2004) Physiological response to unpleasant sounds. J Int Soc Life Inf Sci 22:536–544
23. Suzuki M, Ishiyama I, Takiguchi T et al (1994) Effects of gum hardness on the response of common carotid blood flow volume, oxygen uptake, heart rate and blood presure to gum-chewing. J Masticat Health Soc 4:51–62

Effect of Mastication Muscle Activity on Prefrontal Cortex NIRS Measurement: A Pilot Study

Kazunori Nakajima, Tomotaka Takeda, Maho Saito, Michiyo Konno, Yoshiaki Kawano, Yoshihiro Suzuki, Masayasu Nishino, Yoshiaki Matsuda, Keiichi Ishigami, and Kaoru Sakatani

Abstract Changes in NIRS signals are related to changes in local cerebral blood flow or oxy-Hb concentration. On the other hand, recent studies have revealed the effect of chewing gum on cognitive performance, stress control etc. which accompanied brain activity in the prefrontal cortex (PFC). However, these relationships are still controversial. To evaluate the chewing effect on PFC, NIRS seems to be a suitable method of imaging such results. When measuring NIRS on PFC, blood volume in superficial tissues (scalp, skin, muscle) might have some affect. The aim of the present study was to clarify the effect of the anterior temporal muscle on NIRS signals during gum chewing. Eight healthy volunteers participated. Two-channel NIRS (HOT-1000, NeU, Japan), which can distinguish total-Hb concentrations in deep tissue and superficial tissue layers, was used. In addition to a conventional optode separation distance of 3.0 cm, Hot 1000 has a short distance of 1.0 cm (NEAR channel) to measure NIRS signals that originate exclusively from surface tissues. NIRS probes were placed at Fp1 and Fp2 in the normal probe setting. The headset was displaced to the left in order to allow the left probe to be placed over the left anterior temporal muscle. In the normal setting, the superficial signal curve shows no notable change; however, the neural (calculated and defined in HOT-1000) and deep curves show an increase during the gum chewing task. At the deviated setting, all three signals show marked changes during the task. Total-Hb concentration in the deviated probe setting is significantly large ($p < 0.05$) than that

K. Nakajima (✉) · T. Takeda · M. Saito · M. Konno · Y. Kawano · Y. Suzuki · M. Nishino
Y. Matsuda · K. Ishigami
Department of Oral Health and Clinical Science, Division of Sports Dentistry,
Tokyo Dental College, Tokyo, Japan
e-mail: knakaji@tdc.ac.jp

K. Sakatani
NEWCAT Institute, College of Engineering, Department of Electrical and Electronics Engineering, Nihon University, Tokyo, Japan

School of Medicine, Department of Neurological Surgery, Nihon University, Tokyo, Japan

© Springer Nature Switzerland AG 2020

P.-D. Ryu et al. (eds.), *Oxygen Transport to Tissue XLI*, Advances in Experimental Medicine and Biology 1232, https://doi.org/10.1007/978-3-030-34461-0_17

of in the normal probe setting. When using gum chewing as a task, it would be better to consider a probe position carefully so that the influence of muscle activity on NIRS signal can be distinguished.

Keywords Prefrontal cortex · Near-infrared spectroscopy · Gum-chewing · Muscle activity · Temporal muscle

1 Introduction

PFC plays an important role in the process of cognitive function. Many functional neuroimaging techniques, including positron emission tomography, functional MRI, magnetoencephalography and NIRS are thought to relatively evaluate human cranial nerve activity. NIRS measures the concentration changes of oxygenated hemoglobin (oxy-Hb), deoxygenated hemoglobin (deoxy-Hb) and total hemoglobin (total hemoglobin = oxy-Hb + deoxy-Hb) [1, 2]. Signal changes relate to changes in local cerebral blood flow and oxygen expenditure; and a synchronous increase in the oxy-Hb, with a decrease in the deoxy-Hb concentrations can be indicative of a brain activity [3]. Functional NIRS is a powerful, non-invasive imaging technique that offers many advantages, including its compact size, no need for specially equipped facilities, and the potential for real-time measurement [4, 5].

Recent gum chewing studies have reported the effects on cognitive performance [6–8], stress control [9–12] and others, together with brain activity in PFC. However, these relationships are still controversial. To evaluate the chewing effects on PFC, NIRS seems to be a suitable method of imaging such results.

To investigate the effect of gum chewing on these issues, two different kinds of study designs were employed. One such study focuses on the search for the gum chewing effect itself (the measurement observed while gum chewing); the other study focuses on the remaining gum chewing effect (the measurement which is observed immediately after gum chewing). Naturally, it would be better to employ the former method. However, when measuring NIRS on PFC while gum chewing, blood flows in superficial tissues (scalp, skin, muscle) might have some affect. The signal from the superficial tissues is thought to have no correlation with the signals of neural activity and, therefore, needed to be eliminated [13–17].

Among the many effective artifact reduction methods, the method using multi-distance optodes seems to be effective. As a marketed measuring device, Hot-1000 (NeU Corporation, Tokyo, Japan) [14] has dual source-detector (S-D) regression. It can measure both sides of the PFC simultaneously. Each of the two S-D pairs, with a distance of 1.0 cm and 3.0 cm, can measure the superficial and deep signals [14].

The aim of the present study is to clarify the influence of anterior temporal muscle activity on PFC NIRS signals while gum chewing.

2 Methods

The study design was approved by the Ethics Committee of Tokyo Dental College, Japan (No. 436).

Eight healthy volunteers (mean age 25.3 years) participated in this study after written informed consent had been obtained. Participants had no personal or family history of neuropsychiatric illness, were free of medication and all were right-handed. Subjects were told to refrain from substances containing caffeine (e.g., coffee, etc.) and not to eat for 2 h before the test. They were also instructed to avoid drinking alcohol excessively and avoid lack of sleep the night before the test. To prevent the influence of environmental stress, the subjects were seated in a comfortable chair in an air-conditioned room with the temperature and humidity maintained at approximately 25 °C and 50%, respectively. After a 30-min rest the test began. NIRS signals of total-Hb concentrations in the PFC were measured using the two-channel NIRS Hot-1000. The dual S-D regression method of the Hot-1000 has a short distance S-D pair in addition to a usual distance S-D pair (Fig. 1: left panel). NIRS probes were placed at Fp1 and Fp2 in the normal probe setting. The location of the probe was determined according to the international 10–20 system. The headset was displaced to the left in order to allow the left probe to be placed over the left anterior temporal muscle (deviated probe setting). (Figure 1: middle and right panel).

Each task session was designed in a block manner. For example, four periods of rest (30 s each) and three blocks of four tasks (30 s each). The task used was gum chewing for which a piece of xylitol gum (Citrus aurantifolia mint) (Lotte, Saitama, Japan) was provided. The chewing side was on the left side, and chewing rate and force were determined by the subjects themselves.

For the signals, moving average (10 samples) with a 10 Hz sampling frequency was used. A linear fitting function for baseline correction was employed. The pre-task baseline was determined as the mean across 20 s just before the active task period; the post-task baseline was determined as the mean across the last 20 s of the

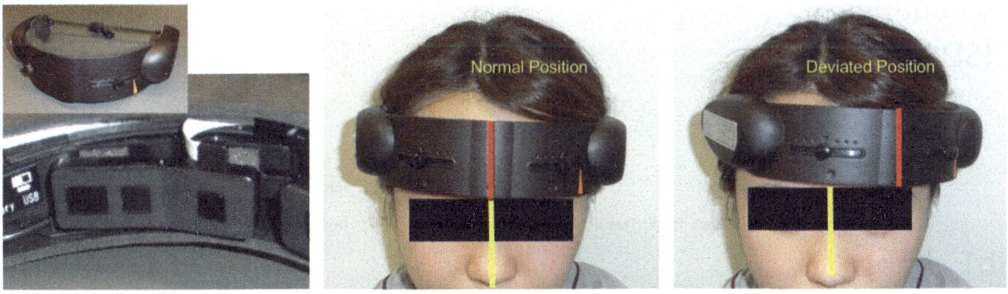

Fig. 1 The dual S-D regression method of the Hot-1000 has a short distance S-D pair in addition to a usual distance S-D pair (left panel). NIRS probes were placed at Fp1 and Fp2 in the normal probe setting. The headset was displaced to the left in order to allow the left probe to be placed over the left anterior temporal muscle (middle and right panel)

resting period; then, linear fitting was performed on the task data between these two baselines. Following this correction, data were averaged in each channel for each subject. Since the blood volume did not increase immediately after beginning the tasks, the Hb values between 10–30 s in each task were used for analysis.

The Mann-Whitney U test was used for statistical analysis of the Excel Statistics (Excel Statistics 2015, Social Survey Information Co., Ltd. Tokyo, Japan). A p-value of <0.05 was considered statistically significant.

3 Results

Figure 2 shows a representative subject's curves while gum chewing at the normal probe setting (left) and the deviated probe setting (right); from the top neural signal, superficial signal, and deep signal curves. In the normal setting, the superficial signal curve shows no notable change; however, the neural and deep curves show an increase during the gum chewing task. At the deviated setting, all three curves show marked changes during the task. Total-Hb concentration in the deviated probe

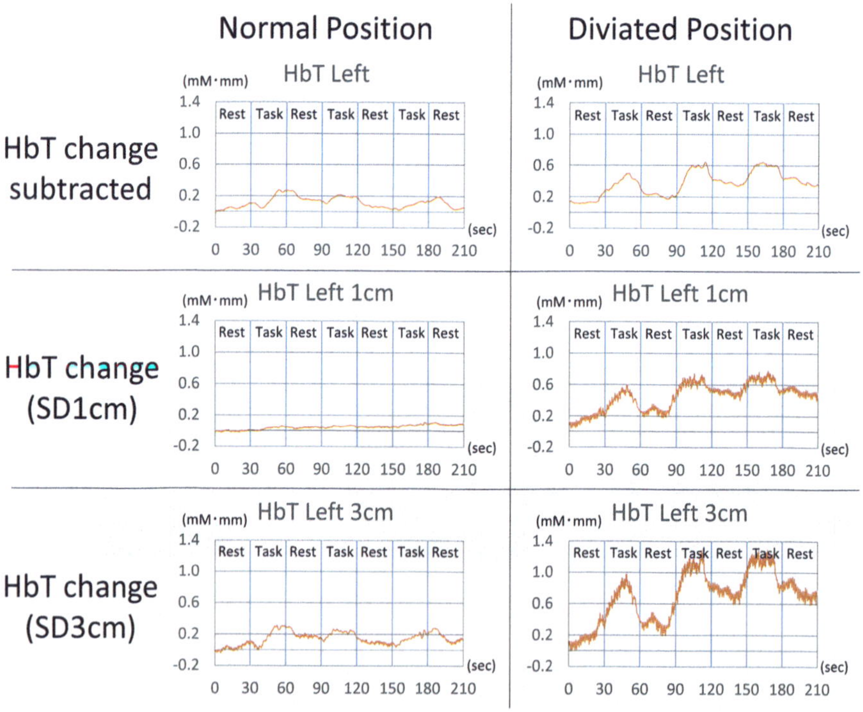

Fig. 2 A representative subject's signal curves during gum chewing at the normal probe setting (left) and the deviated probe setting (right)

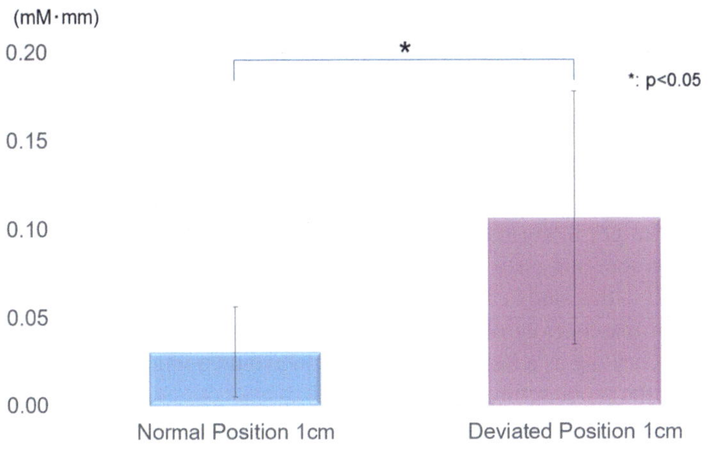

Fig. 3 Influence of the probe position on total-Hb changes on short distance S-D

setting is significantly large than that of in the normal probe setting. Namely, the NIRS signal of the total-Hb originated from the gum chewing was influenced by probe setting position (Fig. 3).

4 Discussion and Conclusions

The Hot 1000 NIRS device allows to measure detailed changes in cerebral blood volume rates related to brain activity and more. Usually, the short distance S-D (1.0 cm) pair captures the blood volume in the superficial tissues, which is dominated by the systemic components in the superficial layers of the scalp. The deep signal from the usual S-D distance (3.0 cm) channel contains both the superficial and cortical blood volume. The neural signal (defined in HOT-1000) is calculated automatically using two different distance S-D pairs results, motion sensor, and so on [14].

In the normal setting, the finding of NIRS signal during gum chewing task is in line with previous studies [18–20]. Namely, the short distance S-D pair signal curve showed very little change. This means the systemic components had a small effect on the superficial tissue blood volume. However, the neural and deep curves showed an increase during the gum chewing task. PFC is involved in the higher-order function such as a memory, attention, learning, monitoring of action, working memory, etc. While chewing, it is necessary to correspond to a change in hardness [21], size, etc. Further, PFC activation related to taste [22], smell [23] etc., might occur from an intake experience memory that might exist. When humans think about eating, higher-order mental activities are essential. For instance, while eating we have to recognize the features of the foods in the mouth and manipulate them adequately during mastication [19]. Therefore, PFC activation is necessary to control and perform an aimed action of chewing gum rhythmically [24].

On the other hand, in the deviated position, obtained signals differed from the normal position results. Namely, significantly increased signals were obtained in the gum chewing task. Increased signals of the short distance signal mean that skin and temporal muscle blood flow increases while gum chewing.

Gum chewing increased short distance signal of superficial tissues in the deviation position, but not in normal position. Namely, the NIRS signal of the total-Hb originated from the gum chewing was influenced by probe setting position. Since HOT-1000 used in this study can only evaluate total-Hb, it is possible that may have subtle different results from other NIRS devices. In future NIRS study involving PFC and gum chewing as a task, it is important to avoid an influence of the temporalis muscle at the probe setting.

References

1. Hoshi Y (2003) Functional near-infrared optical imaging: utility and limitations in human brain mapping. Psychophysiology 40:511–520
2. Jobsis FF (1977) Noninvasive, infrared monitoring of cerebral and myocardial oxygen sufficiency and circulatory parameters. Science 198:1264–1267
3. Scholkmann F, Kleiser S, Metz AJ et al (2014) A review on continuous wave functional near-infrared spectroscopy and imaging instrumentation and methodology. NeuroImage 85:6–27
4. Tanida M, Sakatani K, Takano R et al (2004) Relation between asymmetry of prefrontal cortex activities and the autonomic nervous system during a mental arithmetic task: near infrared spectroscopy study. Neurosci Lett 369:69–74
5. Shibusawa M, Takeda T, Nakajima K et al (2009) Functional near-infrared spectroscopy study on primary motor and sensory cortex response to clenching. Neurosci Lett 449:98–102
6. Kawakami Y, Takeda T, Konno M et al (2017) Relationships between gum chewing and stroop test: a pilot study. Adv Exp Med Biol 977:221–226
7. Takeda T, Kawakami Y, Konno M et al (2017) PFC blood oxygenation changes in four different cognitive tasks. Adv Exp Med Biol 977:199–204
8. Tucha L, Simpson W (2011) The role of time on task performance in modifying the effects of gum chewing on attention. Appetite 56:299–301
9. Yu H, Chen X, Liu J et al (2013) Gum chewing inhibits the sensory processing and the propagation of stress-related information in a brain network. PLoS One 8:e57111
10. Konno M, Takeda T, Kawakami Y et al (2016) Relationships between gum-chewing and stress. Adv Exp Med Biol 876:343–349
11. Scholey A, Haskell C, Robertson B et al (2009) Chewing gum alleviates negative mood and reduces cortisol during acute laboratory psychological stress. Physiol Behav 97:304–312
12. Johnson AJ, Jenks R, Miles C et al (2011) Chewing gum moderates multi-task induced shifts in stress, mood, and alertness. a re-examination. Appetite 56:408–411
13. Funane T, Atsumori H, Katura T et al (2014) Quantitative evaluation of deep and shallow tissue layers' contribution to fNIRS signal using multi-distance optodes and independent component analysis. NeuroImage 85(Pt 1):150–165
14. Nozawa T, Sasaki Y, Sakaki K et al (2016) Interpersonal frontopolar neural synchronization in group communication: an exploration toward fNIRS hyperscanning of natural interactions. NeuroImage 133:484–497

15. Takahashi T, Takikawa Y, Kawagoe R et al (2011) Influence of skin blood flow on near-infrared spectroscopy signals measured on the forehead during a verbal fluency task. NeuroImage 57:991–1002
16. Saager RB, Telleri NL, Berger AJ (2011) Two-detector corrected near infrared spectroscopy (C-NIRS) detects hemodynamic activation responses more robustly than single-detector NIRS. NeuroImage 55:1679–1685
17. Tak S, Ye JC (2014) Statistical analysis of fNIRS data: a comprehensive review. NeuroImage 85(Pt 1):72–91
18. Onozuka M, Fujita M, Watanabe K et al (2003) Age-related changes in brain regional activity during chewing: a functional magnetic resonance imaging study. J Dent Res 82:657–660
19. Takada T, Miyamoto T (2004) A fronto-parietal network for chewing of gum: a study on human subjects with functional magnetic resonance imaging. Neurosci Lett 360:137–140
20. Narita N, Kamiya K, Yamamura K et al (2009) Chewing-related prefrontal cortex activation while wearing partial denture prosthesis: pilot study. J Prosthodont Res 53:126–135
21. Toko S (2014) Changes in the physical properties of food bolus and mandibular movement during masticatory. Shikokushigakaizashi 27:1–13
22. Okamoto M, Matsunami M, Dan H et al (2006) Prefrontal activity during taste encoding: an fNIRS study. NeuroImage 31:796–806
23. Okamoto M, Dan H, Singh AK et al (2006) Prefrontal activity during flavor difference test: application of functional near-infrared spectroscopy to sensory evaluation studies. Appetite 47:220–232
24. Sakuma S (2014) Relation between mastication and prefrontal cortex activity. Health culture 49:1–8

Part II
Tumor Oxygenation and Metabolism

Hypoxia Compromises Anti-Cancer Immune Responses

Gabriele Multhoff and Peter Vaupel

Abstract Hypoxia, one of the hallmarks of cancer, is caused by an insufficient oxygen supply, mostly due to a chaotic, deficient tumor microcirculation. Apart from a hypoxia-mediated resistance to standard therapies, modulated gene and protein expression, genetic instability and malignant progression, hypoxia also plays a pivotal role in anti-cancer immune responses by (a) reducing survival, cytolytic and migratory activity of effector cells such as $CD4^+$ cells, $CD8^+$ cytotoxic T cells, natural killer-like T cells and natural killer cells, (b) reducing the production and release of effector cytokines, (c) supporting immunosuppressive cells such as regulatory T cells, myeloid-derived suppressor cells and M2 macrophages, (d) increasing the production and release of immunosuppressive cytokines, and (e) inducing the expression of immune checkpoint inhibitors. In this minireview, immunosuppressive effects of hypoxia- and HIF-1a-driven traits in cancers are described.

Keywords Tumor hypoxia · Anti-cancer immunity · Hypoxia · Immunosuppression · Tumor microenvironment HIF-1 alpha hypoxia · Immunosuppressive cells hypoxia · Immunosuppressive factors

1 Introduction

Sustained proliferative signaling, evasion of growth suppressors, resistance to apoptosis, replicative immortality, activation of invasiveness, metastasis and induction of angiogenesis have been postulated as hallmarks of cancer by Hanahan & Weinberg in 2000 [1]. Eleven years later, deregulated cellular energetics, genomic instability

G. Multhoff (✉)
Center for Translational Cancer Research (TranslaTUM), Radiation Immuno-Oncology Group, Klinikum rechts der Isar, TU Munich (TUM), München, Germany
e-mail: gabriele.multhoff@tum.de

P. Vaupel
Department of Radiation Oncology, Klinikum rechts der Isar, TU München (TUM), München, Germany

© Springer Nature Switzerland AG 2020

P.-D. Ryu et al. (eds.), *Oxygen Transport to Tissue XLI*, Advances in Experimental Medicine and Biology 1232, https://doi.org/10.1007/978-3-030-34461-0_18

and mutation, tumor-promoting inflammation and avoidance of immune destruction were added to the formerly postulated hallmarks by the same authors [2]. This paper discusses the effects of tumor hypoxia causing an adaptive metabolic re-programming of cancer and immune cells with respect to compromised anti-cancer immune responses.

The role of the immune system in immunosurveillance of cancer has a long history. Already in 1863, Rudolf Virchow detected infiltrating lymphocytes in regressing tumors. In 1909, Paul Ehrlich [3] for the first time described the "virulent" nature of tumors, and in 1957 MacFarlane Burnet postulated the cancer immunosurveillance hypothesis [4]. A large set of data reveals that immunodeficient patients have a significantly higher risk to develop cancer compared to immunocompetent individuals [5–8]. Furthermore, many groups, including ours, have demonstrated that a high tumor infiltration with $CD8^{+}$ cytotoxic T lymphocytes [9–11] can serve as a biomarker for favorable prognosis and beneficial clinical outcome [12].

It is well known that the induction of protective anti-tumor immunity depends on a complex interplay of different immune cell types and soluble mediators. Classically, the generation of a T cell mediated anti-tumor immune response involves the acquisition and processing of tumor antigens derived from dying tumor cells (e.g., after radiochemotherapy) to peptides that are phagocytosed by antigen-presenting cells including monocytes, macrophages and dendritic cells (DCs). Macrophages which are multifunctional cells with a high plasticity release a wide range of immunomodulatory cytokines. M1 macrophages secrete immunostimulatory cytokines such as IFN-γ or TNF-α, whereas immunosuppressive M2 macrophages, also termed tumor associated macrophages (TAMs), predominantly secrete IL-4, IL-5, IL-6 and IL-10. After migration to the draining lymph nodes and cross-presentation of tumor-derived peptides on MHC class II and class I molecules to $CD4^{+}$ helper T cells and $CD8^{+}$ cytotoxic T lymphocytes, respectively, T cells express T cell receptors with an appropriate anti-tumor specificity. Clonal expansion and activation of T cells occurs only in the presence of adequate co-stimulatory signals including CD80/CD86 on antigen presenting cells and CD28 on T cells. In the absence of co-stimulatory signals, T cells become anergic and undergo apoptosis. Adequately activated T cells are able to migrate, recognize and kill tumor cells that present tumor peptides on MHC molecules by using their clonogenic T cell receptor complex [13]. Natural killer (NK) cells, which are involved in the first line of immune defense against pathogens and cancer, are able to recognize stress-inducible danger associated molecular patterns (DAMPs) that are presented on the surface of stressed tumor cells without previous priming. The absence of MHC class I molecules, which occurs during immune escape of tumor cells, allows NK cells with immunoglobulin-like receptors to recognize and kill these tumor cells. NK cells express a large variety of different activatory and inhibitory receptors belonging either to the immunoglobulin, C-type lectin or natural cytotoxicity receptor families. The balance of these activatory (with immunoreceptor tyrosine-based activatory motif) and inhibitory (with immunoreceptor tyrosine-based inhibitory motif) receptors determines the activation status of an individual NK cell. In a best-case scenario, the adaptive and innate immune system recognizes and kills tumor cells via effector enzymes granzyme B and perforin. The induction of a T cell memory can mediate long-term protective anti-cancer immunity. Ongoing immune responses mediated by $CD8^+$ T cells or NK cells are regulated by regulatory T cells (Treg) formerly also termed 'veto cells' that are characterized by the expression of CD4 and the alpha chain of the IL-2 receptor CD25 and the intracellular transcription factor Forkhead Box p3 (FoxP3). Under physiological conditions, Treg cells regulate peripheral self-tolerance to avoid autoimmunity. Tumor cells have gained the capacity to attract Treg cells to protect them against the cytolytic attack mediated by T and NK cells and thereby escape immunosurveillance [14, 15].

2 Hypoxia

A major driver that favors an immunosuppressive tumor microenvironment (TME) is hypoxia (oxygen tensions <10 mmHg). Hypoxia is caused by an insufficient oxygen supply, mostly due to a chaotic, deficient tumor microcirculation. Due to a rapid tumor growth and high concentrations of proangiogenic factors, tumor vessels often remain immature and are leaky with dead ends where pericytes are only loosely attached [16]. It is well established that critically reduced oxygen levels found in most human tumors [17, 18] lead to the activation of a plethora of pro-tumorigenic transcription factors that promote tumor progression, angiogenesis, invasiveness, cancer stem cell renewal and metastasis. Hypoxia is able to mediate radiation resistance due to reduced fixation of DNA damage, cell cycle arrest, increased stemness [19, 20], decreased cell proliferation, modulated gene and protein expression and genetic instability [21]. A hypoxic TME is often associated with extracellular acidosis ($pH < 6.8$), high extracellular lactate (up to 40 mM), adenosine (up to 100 μM) and ammonium (2–5 mM) concentrations, externalization of phosphatidylserine (PS) to the outer membrane leaflet, increased heat shock protein (HSP) levels and nutrient deprivation [22]. More recently, it became obvious that hypoxia also can impair anti-cancer immune responses [23–28].

2.1 Hypoxia-/HIF-1a-Induced Immunosuppression

As mentioned above, tumor hypoxia is caused by an insufficient blood supply [16, 29–31]. The TME consisting *(inter alia)* of stromal and immune cells including $CD4^+$ T helper cells, $CD8^+$ cytotoxic T cells, FoxP3/$CD25^+$ regulatory T cells (Tregs), NK cells, NK-like T (NKT) cells, myeloid derived suppressor cells (MDSC), M1 and M2 macrophages are highly responsive to hypoxia. Hypoxia negatively affects anti-tumor immune responses by reducing survival, cytolytic and migratory activity of effector cells such as $CD4^+$, $CD8^+$ T cells, NKT and NK cells by (a) reducing the production and release of immunostimulatory cytokines, (b) supporting immunosuppressive activity of M2 macrophages, (c) increasing the production and release of immunosuppressive cytokines, and (d) inducing the expression of immune checkpoint inhibitors (Table 1). Hypoxia increases the recruitment of immunosuppressive Treg cells and decreases the motility of monocytes and DCs and thereby impairs T cell stimulation [32]. HIF-1 promotes MDSC accumulation in the tumor halo via an upregulated ectonucleoside triphosphate diphosphohydrolase 2 (ENT-PD2) expression that converts ATP to 5`-AMP [33]. Furthermore, the immune checkpoint inhibitor ligand PDL-1 on MDSC is a direct target of HIF-1 in hypoxic tumor cells [34].

2.2 Adenosine-Induced Immunosuppression

The HIF-driven downstream factor adenosine (ADO), a metabolite of ATP, is accumulated in the extracellular space of tumors (30–100 μM) due to several mechanisms such as an increased exocytosis, vesicular export, or pannexin-1 (Panx-1) channel-mediated release of ATP. ATP acts as an immunostimulatory factor, however, a HIF-1a-induced elevated expression of the ectonucleoside triphosphate diphosphohydrolase 1 CD39 and ecto-5`-nucleotidase CD73, via NAD^+ mediated CD38/CD203a/CD73 enzymes on tumor and Treg cells [35–38] results in a rapid conversion of ATP to ADO [39–43].

Furthermore, hypoxia/HIF-1α inactivates the equilibrative nucleoside transporter ENT-1 which, in turn, inhibits the re-uptake of ADO into tumor cells. Highly elevated extracellular ADO levels result in a decreased antigen presenting activity of M1 macrophages and DCs (Table 1). Furthermore, the immune effector cell function of NK, NKT cells and $CD4^+/CD8^+$ T cells is impaired, predominantly by an interaction of ADO with the A2A/A2 receptors [44] and by increased levels of immunosuppressive cAMP [45, 46].

2.3 VEGF-Induced Immunosuppression

The expression of the vascular endothelial growth factor (VEGF) which is increased upon activation of the VEGF-receptor (VEGF-R) is elevated in the tumor micromilieu of hypoxic tumors. High VEGF levels promote tumor evasion from the immune system [47, 48] via the release of other immunosuppressive and angiogenic factors, including CSF-1, MCP-1 and SDF1, CXCL2 that accelerate tumor growth and metastatic spread and thereby recruit immunosuppressive MDSCs, M2 macrophages and neutrophils into the TME. IL-4 and IL-6 induce the differentiation of monocytes into M2 macrophages which, in turn, further promote the production of hypoxia-regulated pro-tumorigenic factors. Furthermore, VEGF decreases the amount of immature DCs and thereby impairs T cell stimulation against tumor antigens (Table 1).

Table 1 Hypoxia-/HIF-1α-induced features of the tumor microenvironment (TME) compromising anti-tumor immune responses (selection). PS: phosphatidylserine

Feature	Main causative mechanism(s)	Immunostimulatory antigen presenting cells (APCs)	Immunostimulatory effector cells	Immunosuppressive cells/ factors	Refs.
↑HIF-1α activation	↑Hypoxia ↑Oncogenes ↓Suppressor genes	↓M1 ↓DC	↓$CD4^+$, $CD8^+$, NK, NKT ↓IL-2 release	↑M2, MDSC, Treg ↑Immune checkpoint inhibitors	[23–28]
↑Extracellular [ADO] (30-100 μM)	↑ATP export ↑CD39/CD73 activation ↑CD38/CD203a/CD73 ↓ENT1 (ADO re-uptake)	↓M1 (M1-M2 switch) ↓DC ↑TGF-β, VEGF production ↑IDO, COX-2 production	↓$CD8^+$, NK, NKT	↑M2, MDSC, Treg ↑IL-10 ↑TGF-ß ↑Immune checkpoint inhibitors	[24, 41–43]
↑VEGF	↑Hypoxia	↓DC	↓$CD8^+$, NK, NKT	↑M2	[47, 48]
↑Extracellular [lactate] (up to 40 mM)	↑Glycolysis ↑LDH-A ↑GLUT transporter ↑Glutaminolysis	↓M1 (M1-DC blockade) ↓T stimulation ↓IL-12 production ↓IFN-γ production	↓$CD8^+$, NK, NKT ↓Granzyme, perforin ↓IFN-γ ↓T growth ↑T apoptosis	↑M2, Treg, MDSC ↑Protumoral factors (IL1-β, IL-23, IL-17, ARG1) ↑Immune checkpoint inhibitors ↑Inflammasome activation	[55–58]

(continued)

Table 1 (continued)

Feature	Main causative mechanism(s)	Immunostimulatory antigen presenting cells (APCs)	Immunostimulatory effector cells	Immunosuppressive cells/ factors	Refs.
↑Extracellular acidosis (pH<6.8)	↑Hypoxia/HIF-1α	↓M1 (M1-M2 switch)	↓$CD8^+$, NK, NKT	↑M2	[54–59]
	↑Glycolysis	↓IFN-γ production	↓Granzyme, perforin production	↑Treg activation	
	↑Lactate accumulation	↓IL-12 production (by DC)	↓IFN-γ production	↑Inflammasome activation	
	↑Glutaminolysis ↑ATP hydrolysis ↑Ketogenesis ↑CO_2 generation by OXPHOS	↑T stimulation ↑antigen presentation	↓IL-2, IL-12 production ↓mTOR signaling ↑Angiogenesis (VEGF)	↑Immune checkpoint inhibitors	
↑Extracellular [ammonia] (2-5 mM)	↑Glutaminolysis	↑DC dysfunction ↓neutrophil activity (phagocytosis)	↓$CD8^+$	↑M2 ↑Immune checkpoint inhibitors	[64–66]
PS translocation to the outer membrane leaflet	↓PS assymetry in plasma membrane leaflets		↓Cytokine release (IFN-γ, TNFα)	↑MDSC ↑IL-4, IL-10, TGF-β	[68]
Exosomal HSP	↑Hypoxia (stress)	↓M1	↓$CD8^+$, NK, NKT	↑M2	[81]
↑IDO-1/kynurenine	↑Tryptophan uptake	↓DC	↓$CD8^+$,$CD4^+$, NK	↑Treg, MDSC	[82, 83]

2.4 *Lactate- and Acidosis-Induced Immunosuppression*

2.4.1 Lactate-Induced Immunosuppression

The hypoxia-/HIF-1α-driven upregulation of glycolysis (via increased expression of glucose transporters and key glycolytic enzymes) and the enhanced glutaminolysis result in elevated extracellular lactate levels in the TME [49–55]. High extracellular lactate concentrations lead to immunosuppression by decreasing the number of M1 macrophages, by blocking the M1 to DC switch and by a reduction in the release of immunostimulatory cytokines such as IL-12 and IFN-γ. Furthermore, high extracellular lactate levels decrease the activity of $CD8^+$ T and NK cells by a reduction of their effector enzymes granzyme B and perforin and pro-inflammatory cytokines such as IL-2 and IL-12. T cell proliferation is reduced and T cell apoptosis is increased by high extracellular lactate levels. In contrast, growth of immunosuppressive M2 macrophages and Treg cells appear to be increased and the protumorigenic inflammasome is activated (IL-1β, NFκB, TNFα, IL-6, CXCL1, CCL2). Moreover, the induction of expression of immune checkpoint inhibitors is associated with increased extracellular lactate levels (Table 1).

Upon export from tumor cells via $lactate^-/H^+$-transporters (MCT4) into the extracellular space, the major oncometabolite lactate acts as a 'signaling molecule' (ligand) that binds to the G-protein coupled receptor 81 (GPR81) to exert the abovementioned immunosuppressive actions of TME factors.

2.4.2 Acidosis-Induced Immunosuppression

Many effects described in the above section are also promoted by an acidic TME ($pH < 6.8$). Low pH values have been measured in the microenvironment of most tumor entities [29]. A major effect of low pH values is a delayed neutrophil apoptosis which promotes infections and stimulates tumor angiogenesis. Acidosis is known to inhibit T cell activity, proliferation and cytokine production, impairs the production of IFN-γ, TNFα, granzyme B and perforin by NK cells, reduces the INF-γ-release by M1 macrophages and induces the production of IL1-β [56–59] (Table 1).

Besides the upregulated anaerobic/aerobic glycolysis (Warburg effect) and glutaminolysis, intracellular ATP hydrolysis and CO_2 generation by OXPHOS, ketogenesis in cancer-associated fibroblasts (CAFs) is a further pathomechanism involved in tumor acidification. Mechanisms underlying H^+ sensing most probably include (a) G-protein coupled receptors (GPCRs, widely expressed in immune cells within a pH range of 6.4–6.8), (b) acid-sensing channels (ASICs, expressed in macrophages and dendritic cells), and (c) transient receptor potential channel vanilloid subfamily 1 (TRPV1, highly expressed in immune cells; receptor activation induces Ca^{2+}-influx) [60–63].

2.5 Ammonia-Induced Immunosuppression

The extracelluar HIF-driven downstream factor ammonia (2–5 mM), resulting from an upregulated glutaminolysis of tumor cells, impairs ROS-related pathways, induces the production of immature DCs with a reduced phagocytosis capacity and decreases the amount of neutrophils and mature DC counts [64–66]. The drastically reduced antigen presenting capacity of DCs to stimulate anti-tumor specific T cells results in a severe immunosuppression and induces a M2 switch (Table 1).

2.6 PS-Induced Immunosuppression

The negatively charged lipid component phosphatidylserine (PS) in the membrane of all mammalian cells is exclusively found in the inner membrane leaflet. This asymmetric localization is maintained in viable cells by the activity of ATP-dependent aminophospholipid translocases that permanently translocate PS from the outer to the inner membrane leaflet. Following stress, including hypoxia, PS can be externalized to the outer membrane leaflet via an activation of ATP- and Ca^{2+}-dependent phospholipid scramblases. PS on the outer membrane leaflet acts as an 'eat-me' and efferocytosis signal for macrophages expressing the PS receptors Mertk and Axl [67, 68]. These receptors are also expressed in stressed tumor cells. As a consequence, tumors can escape the immune cells by the induction of the immunosuppressive cytokine IL-10 which antagonizes anti-tumor immune responses by $CD8^+$ and NK cells. A concomitant induction of TGF-β increases the metastatic capacity of PS and PS-receptor expressing tumor cells [69] (Table 1).

2.7 Role of Intracellular, Membrane-Bound and Extracellular HSP of Tumor Cells for the Immune System

Reoxygenation after hypoxia is a strong stress signal for the induction of the synthesis of heat shock proteins (HSPs). HSPs are highly overexpressed in the cytosol of nearly all tumor types. Besides cytosolic HSPs, our group has identified a tumor-specific cell surface expression of the major stress-inducible 72 kDa Hsp70 on the plasma membrane of tumor cells [70] and in the extracellular milieu either as a free molecule derived from dying tumor cells or in exosomes that are actively released by viable tumor cells [71–74]. Membrane and extracellular Hsp70s can exert immunostimulatory and immune-suppressive functions. Elevated cytosolic Hsp70 levels are known to protect tumor cells from programmed cell death by interfering with apoptotic pathways [75–77], promote tumor cell proliferation and migration, mediate therapy resistance and thereby contribute to a highly aggressive tumor phenotype [78]. The role of exosomes derived from stressed tumor cells on the induction of anti-tumor immune responses is not yet completely understood: on the one hand exosomes derived from stressed tumor cells have been found to stimulate $CD8^+$ T cell responses [79] via the transfer of cGAS/STING DNA and silencing of TGF-ß in DCs [80]. On the other hand, exosomes of hypoxic (stressed) tumor cells also promote tumor progression [81] by immunosuppressive mechanisms such as the suppression of anti-tumor M1 macrophages, the inhibition of the activity of cytotoxic $CD8^+$ and helper $CD4^+$ T cells and NK cells and the support of pro-tumorigenic M2 macrophages (Table 1).

2.8 *Indoleamine-2,3-Dioxygenase-1/Kynurenine-Induced Immunosuppression*

Indoleamine-2,3-dioxygenase-1 (IDO) is known to catalyze the breakdown of tryptophan to kynurenine, and high levels of IDO positively correlate with tumor angiogenesis. Tumor cells, as well as TME cells such as DCs, endothelial cells and stromal cells, block anti-tumor immunity by suppressing the activity of T cells, NK cells and DCs, and by promoting immunosuppressive MDSCs and Tregs. Upon high uptake rates of tryptophan and the increase of the tryptophan metabolite kynurenine, the activity of effector T cells and DCs is blocked (Table 1).

A high microvascular density associated with high IDO-1 activities is associated with a negative tumor outcome. Wei et al. demonstrated that IDO-1 promotes growth of endothelial cells expressing CD105, a transmembrane glycoprotein marker on activated endothelial cells in breast cancer [82].

3 Conclusions

Hypoxia and HIF-1α *per se* as well as hypoxia-/HIF-1α-induced high extracellular levels of lactate, adenosine, and ammonia, extracellular acidosis, VEGF actions, exosomal HSPs and a high IDO-1 expression/kynurenine levels sabotage anti-tumor immune responses mediated by $CD8^+$ cytotoxic T cells, $CD4^+$ helper T cells, NK cells, M1 macrophages and DCs. Moreover, these detrimental traits favor immunosuppressive cells such as MDSC, M2 macrophages and Treg cells and promote the secretion of immunosuppressive cytokines [83].

Acknowledgments The authors thank Anett Lange for editorial support. Funded in part by DFG (SFB824; STA 1520/1-1), BMBF (01GU0823, 02NUK038A) and BMWi (ZF4320102CS7).

References

1. Hanahan D, Weinberg RA (2000) The hallmarks of cancer. Cell 100:57–70
2. Hanahan D, Weinberg RA (2011) Hallmarks of cancer: the next generation. Cell 144:646–674
3. Ehrlich P (1909) Über Immunität mit besonderer Berücksichtigung der Beziehung zwischen Verteilung und Wirkung der Antigene. Beiträge zur experimentellen Pathologie und Chemotherapie:3–49
4. Burnet M (1957) Cancer: a biological approach. III. Viruses associated with neoplastic conditions. IV. Practical applications. Br Med J 1:841–847
5. Thomas L (1982) On immunosurveillance in human cancer. Yale J Biol Med 55:329–333
6. Verhoeven D, Stoppelenburg AJ, Meyer-Wentrup F et al (2018) Increased risk of hematological malignancies in primary immunodeficeint disorders: opportunities for immunotherpay. Clin Immunol doi: 10.1016/j.clim2018.02.007
7. Gatti RA, Good RA (1971) Follow-up of correction of severe dual system immunodeficiency with bone marrow transplantation. J Pediatr 79:475–479
8. Penn I (2000) Post-transplant malignancy: the role of immunosuppression. Drug Saf 23:101–113
9. Balermpas P, Rödel F, Rödel C et al (2016) $CD8^+$ tumour-infiltrating lymphocytes in relation to HPV status and clinical outcome in patients with head and neck cancer after postoperative chemoradiotherapy: a multicentre study of the German Cancer consortium radiation oncology group (DKTK-ROG). Int J Cancer 138:171–181
10. Stangl S, Tontcheva N, Sievert W et al (2018) Heat shock protein 70 and tumor-infiltrating NK cells as prognostic indicators for patients with squamous cell carcinoma of the head and neck after radiochemotherapy: a multicentre retrospective study of the German Cancer consortium radiation oncology group (DKTK-ROG). Int J Cancer 142:1911–1925
11. Gunther S, Ostheimer C, Stangl S et al (2015) Correlation of Hsp70 serum levels with gross tumor volume and composition of lymphocyte subpopulations in patients with squamous cell and adeno non-small cell lung cancer. Front Immunol 6:556
12. Fridman WH, Pages F, Sautes-Fridman C et al (2012) The immune contexture in human tumours: impact on clinical outcome. Nat Rev Cancer 12:298–306
13. Dranoff G (2004) Cytokines in cancer pathogenesis and cancer therapy. Nat Rev Cancer 4:11–22
14. Schreiber RD, Old LJ, Smyth MJ (2011) Cancer immunoediting: integrating immunity's roles in cancer suppression and promotion. Science 331:1565–1570
15. Dunn GP, Old LJ, Schreiber RD (2004) The immunobiology of cancer immunosurveillance and immunoediting. Immunity 21:137–148
16. Vaupel P, Mayer A, Höckel M (2004) Tumor hypoxia and malignant progression. Methods Enzymol 381:335–354
17. Vaupel P, Hoeckel M, Mayer A (2007) Detection and characterization of tumour hypoxia using $p0_2$ histography. Antioxid Redox Signal 9:1221–1235
18. Vaupel P, Mayer A (2007) Hypoxia in cancer: significance and impact on clinical outcome. Cancer Metastasis Rev 26:225–239
19. Soeda A, Park M, Lee D et al (2009) Hypoxia promotes expansion of the CD133-positive glioma stem cells through activation of HIF-1alpha. Oncogene 28:3949–3959
20. Li P, Zhou C, Xu L et al (2013) Hypoxia enhances stemness of cancer stem cells in glioblastoma: an in vitro study. Int J Med Sci 10:399–407
21. Vaupel P, Multhoff G (2016) Commentary: a metabolic immune checkpoint: adenosine in tumor microenvironment. Front Immunol 7:332
22. Multhoff G, Vaupel P (2012) Radiation-induced changes in microcirculation and interstitial fluid pressure affecting the delivery of macromolecules and nanotherapeutics to tumors. Front Oncol 2:165
23. Rankin EB, Giaccia AJ (2016) Hypoxic control of metastasis. Science 352:175–180

24. Vaupel P, Multhoff G (2017) Accomplices of the hypoxic tumor microenvironment compromising antitumor immunity: adenosine, lactate, acidosis, vascular endothelial growth factor, potassium ions, and phosphatidylserine. Front Immunol 8:1887
25. Wang Y, Roche O, Xu C et al (2012) Hypoxia promotes ligand-independent EGF receptor signaling via hypoxia-inducible factor-mediated upregulation of caveolin-1. Proc Natl Acad Sci U S A 109:4892–4897
26. Kumar V, Gabrilovich DI (2014) Hypoxia-inducible factors in regulation of immune responses in tumour microenvironment. Immunology 143:512–519
27. Samanta D, Semenza GL (2018) Metabolic adaptation of cancer and immune cells mediated by hypoxia-inducible factors. Biochem Biophys Acta Rev Cancer. https://doi.org/10.1016/j.bbcan.2018.07.002
28. Hirschhaeuser F, Sattler UG, Mueller-Klieser W (2011) Lactate: a metabolic key player in cancer. Cancer Res 71:6921–6925
29. Vaupel P, Kallinowski F, Okunieff P (1989) Blood flow, oxygen and nutrient supply, and metabolic microenvironment of human tumors: a review. Cancer Res 49:6449–6465
30. Vaupel P (2004) Tumor microenvironmental physiology and its implications for radiation oncology. Semin Radiat Oncol 14:198–206
31. Vaupel P (2008) Hypoxia and aggressive tumor phenotype: implications for therapy and prognosis. Oncologist 13(Suppl 3):21–26
32. Ohta A (2016) A metabolic immune checkpoint: adenosine in tumor microenvironment. Front Immunol 7:109
33. Chiu DK, Tse AP, Xu IM et al (2017) Hypoxia inducible factor HIF-1 promotes myeloid-derived suppressor cells accumulation through ENTPD2/CD39L1 in hepatocellular carcinoma. Nat Commun 8:517
34. Noman MZ, Desantis G, Janji B et al (2014) PD-L1 is a novel direct target of HIF-1alpha, and its blockade under hypoxia enhanced MDSC-mediated T cell activation. J Exp Med 211:781–790
35. Narravula S, Lennon PF, Mueller BU et al (2000) Regulation of endothelial CD73 by adenosine: paracrine pathway for enhanced endothelial barrier function. J Immunol 165:5262–5268
36. Whiteside TL, Jackson EK (2013) Adenosine and prostaglandin E2 production by human inducible regulatory T cells in health and disease. Front Immunol 4:212
37. Deaglio S, Dwyer KM, Gao W et al (2007) Adenosine generation catalyzed by CD39 and CD73 expressed on regulatory T cells mediates immune suppression. J Exp Med 204:1257–1265
38. Alam MS, Kurtz CC, Rowlett RM et al (2009) CD73 is expressed by human regulatory T helper cells and suppresses proinflammatory cytokine production and helicobacter felis-induced gastritis in mice. J Infect Dis 199:494–504
39. Synnestvedt K, Furuta GT, Comerford KM et al (2002) Ecto-5′-nucleotidase (CD73) regulation by hypoxia-inducible factor-1 mediates permeability changes in intestinal epithelia. J Clin Invest 110:993–1002
40. Deaglio S, Robson SC (2011) Ectonucleotidases as regulators of purinergic signaling in thrombosis, inflammation, and immunity. Adv Pharmacol 61:301–332
41. Allard B, Longhi MS, Robson SC et al (2017) The ectonucleotidases CD39 and CD73: novel checkpoint inhibitor targets. Immunol Rev 276:121–144
42. Ben Addi A, Lefort A, Hua X et al (2008) Modulation of murine dendritic cell function by adenine nucleotides and adenosine: involvement of the a(2B) receptor. Eur J Immunol 38:1610–1620
43. Ryzhov S, Novitskiy SV, Zaynagetdinov R et al (2008) Host A(2B) adenosine receptors promote carcinoma growth. Neoplasia 10:987–995
44. Ohta A, Sitkovsky M (2014) Extracellular adenosine-mediated modulation of regulatory T cells. Front Immunol 5:304
45. Yaqub S, Tasken K (2008) Role for the cAMP-protein kinase a signaling pathway in suppression of antitumor immune responses by regulatory T cells. Crit Rev Oncogen 14:57–77

46. Vaupel P, Multhoff G (2016) Adenosine can thwart antitumor immune responses elicited by radiotherapy: therapeutic strategies alleviating protumor ADO activities. Strahlenther Onkol 192:279–287
47. Rivera LB, Bergers G (2015) Intertwined regulation of angiogenesis and immunity by myeloid cells. Trends Immunol 36:240–249
48. Chouaib S, Noman MZ, Kosmatopoulos K et al (2017) Hypoxic stress: obstacles and opportunities for innovative immunotherapy of cancer. Oncogene 36:439–445
49. Husain Z, Huang Y, Seth P et al (2013) Tumor-derived lactate modifies antitumor immune response: effect on myeloid-derived suppressor cells and NK cells. J Immunol 191:1486–1495
50. Brand A, Singer K, Koehl GE et al (2016) LDHA-associated lactic acid production blunts tumor immunosurveillance by T and NK cells. Cell Metab 24:657–671
51. Romero-Garcia S, Moreno-Altamirano MM, Prado-Garcia H et al (2016) Lactate contribution to the tumor microenvironment: mechanisms, effects on immune cells and therapeutic relevance. Front Immunol 7:52
52. Gottfried E, Lang SA, Renner K et al (2013) New aspects of an old drug-diclofenac targets MYC and glucose metabolism in tumor cells. PLoS One 8:e66987
53. Mendler AN, Hu B, Prinz PU et al (2012) Tumor lactic acidosis suppresses CTL function by inhibition of p38 and JNK/c-Jun activation. Int J Cancer 131:633–640
54. Nasi A, Fekete T, Krishnamurthy A et al (2013) Dendritic cell reprogramming by endogenously produced lactic acid. J Immunol 191:3090–3099
55. Seth P, Csizmadia E, Hedblom A et al (2017) Deletion of lactate dehydrogenase - in myeloid cells triggers antitumor immunity. Cancer Res 77:3632–3643
56. Dietl K, Renner K, Dettmer K et al (2010) Lactic acid and acidification inhibit TNF secretion and glycolysis of human monocytes. J Immunol 184:1200–1209
57. Pötzl J, Roser D, Bankel L et al (2017) Reversal of tumor acidosis by systemic buffering reactivates NK cells to express IFN-gamma and induces NK cell-dependent lymphoma control without other immunotherapies. Int J Cancer 140:2125–2133
58. Calcinotto A, Filipazzi P, Grioni M et al (2012) Modulation of microenvironment acidity reverses anergy in human and murine tumor-infiltrating T lymphocytes. Cancer Res 72:2746–2756
59. Lacroix R, Rozeman EA, Kreutz M et al (2018) Targeting tumor-associated acidity in cancer immunotherapy. Cancer Immunol Immunother 67:1331–1348. https://doi.org/10.1007/s00262-018-2195-z
60. Damaghi M, Wojtkowiak JW, Gillies RJ (2013) pH sensing and regulation in cancer. Front Physiol 4:370
61. Radu CG, Nijagal A, McLaughlin J et al (2005) Differential proton sensitivity of related G protein-coupled receptors T cell death-associated gene 8 and G2A expressed in immune cells. Proc Natl Acad Sci U S A 102:1632–1637
62. Tong J, Wu WN, Kong X et al (2011) Acid-sensing ion channels contribute to the effect of acidosis on the function of dendritic cells. J Immunol 186:3686–3692
63. Basu S, Srivastava P (2005) Immunological role of neuronal receptor vanilloid receptor 1 expressed on dendritic cells. Proc Natl Acad Sci U S A 102:5120–5125
64. Luo C, Shen G, Liu N et al (2014) Ammonia drives dendritic cells into dysfunction. J Immunol 193:1080–1089
65. Dang CV (2010) Rethinking the Warburg effect with Myc micromanaging glutamine metabolism. Cancer Res 70:859–862
66. Kroemer G, Pouyssegur J (2008) Tumor cell metabolism: cancer's Achilles' heel. Cancer Cell 13:472–482
67. Cook RS, Jacobsen KM, Wofford AM et al (2013) Mer TK inhibition in tumor leukocytes decreases tumor growth and metastasis. J Clin Invest 123:3231–3242
68. Birge RB, Boeltz S, Kumar S et al (2016) Phosphatidylserine is a global immunosuppressive signal in efferocytosis, infectious disease, and cancer. Cell Death Differ 23:962–978
69. Stanford JC, Young C, Hicks D et al (2014) Efferocytosis produces a prometastatic landscape during postpartum mammary gland involution. J Clin Invest 124:4737–4752

70. Multhoff G, Botzler C, Wiesnet M et al (1995) A stress-inducible 72-kDa heat-shock protein (HSP72) is expressed on the surface of human tumor cells, but not on normal cells. Int J Cancer 61:272–279
71. Schmitt E, Gehrmann M, Brunet M et al (2007) Intracellular and extracellular functions of heat shock proteins: repercussions in cancer therapy. J Leukoc Biol 81:15–27
72. Hantschel M, Pfister K, Jordan A et al (2000) Hsp70 plasma membrane expression on primary tumor biopsy material and bone marrow of leukemic patients. Cell Stress Chaperones 5:438–442
73. Pfister K, Radons J, Busch R et al (2007) Patient survival by Hsp70 membrane phenotype: association with different routes of metastasis. Cancer 110:926–935
74. Breuninger S, Erl J, Knape C et al (2014) Quantitative analysis of liposomal heat shock protein 70 (Hsp70) in the blood of tumor patients using an novel lipHsp70 ELISA. Clin Cell Immunol 5:2–10
75. Nylandsted J, Gyrd-Hansen M, Danielewicz A et al (2004) Heat shock protein 70 promotes cell survival by inhibiting lysosomal membrane permeabilization. J Exp Med 200:425–435
76. Nylandsted J, Rohde M, Brand K et al (2000) Selective depletion of heat shock protein 70 (Hsp70) activates a tumor-specific death program that is independent of caspases and bypasses Bcl-2. Proc Natl Acad Sci U S A 97:7871–7876
77. Jäättelä M (1999) Heat shock proteins as cellular lifeguards. Ann Med 31:261–271
78. Calderwood SK, Khaleque MA, Sawyer DB et al (2006) Heat shock proteins in cancer: chaperones of tumorigenesis. Trends Biochem Sci 31:164–172
79. Diamond JM, Vanpouille-Box C, Spada S et al (2018) Exosomes shuttle TREX1-sensitive IFN-stimulatory dsDNA from irradiated cancer cells to DCs. Cancer Immunol Res 6:910–920. https://doi.org/10.1158/2326-6066.CIR-17-0581
80. Bobrie A, Krumeich S, Reyal F et al (2012) Rab27a supports exosome-dependent and -independent mechanisms that modify the tumor microenvironment and can promote tumor progression. Cancer Res 72:4920–4930
81. Wei L, Zhu S, Li M et al (2018) High indoleamine 2,3-dioxygenase is correlated with microvessel density and worse prognosis in breast cancer. Front Immunol 9:724
82. Angajala A, Lim S, Phillips JB et al (2018) Diverse roles of mitochondria in immune responses: novel insights into immuno-metabolism. Front Immunol 9. https://doi.org/10.3389/fimmu.2018.01605
83. Sormendi S, Wielockx B (2018) Hypoxia pathway proteins as central mediators of metabolism in the tumor cells and their microenvironment. Front Immunol 9:40

'Oxygen Level in a Tissue' – What Do Available Measurements Really Report?

H. M. Swartz, P. Vaupel, B. B. Williams, P. E. Schaner, B. Gallez, W. Schreiber, A. Ali, and A. B. Flood

Abstract The aim of the paper is to discuss what currently is feasible clinically to measure the level of oxygen and how that measurement can be clinically useful. Because oxygen in tissues is quite heterogeneous and all methods of measurement can only provide an average across heterogeneities at some spatial and temporal resolution, the values that are obtained may have limitations on their clinical utility. However, even if such limitations are significant, if one utilizes repeated measurements and focuses on changes in the measured levels, rather than 'absolute levels', it may be possible to obtain very useful clinical information. While these considerations are especially pertinent in cancer, they also pertain to most other types of pathology.

Keywords Oxygen heterogeneity · Imaging · lEPR · Radiation therapy · Immunotherapy

---

H. M. Swartz (✉)
Department Radiology, Dartmouth Medical School, Hanover, NH, USA

Section Radiation Oncology, Dartmouth-Hitchcock Medical Center, Lebanon, NH, USA
e-mail: Harold.M.Swartz@dartmouth.edu

P. Vaupel
Department Radiation Oncology, University Medical Center, Mainz, Germany

B. B. Williams
Department Radiology, Dartmouth Medical School, Hanover, NH, USA

Section Radiation Oncology, Dartmouth-Hitchcock Medical Center, Lebanon, NH, USA

P. E. Schaner
Section Radiation Oncology, Dartmouth-Hitchcock Medical Center, Lebanon, NH, USA

B. Gallez
Louvain Drug Research Institute, Université catholique de Louvain, Brussels, Belgium

W. Schreiber · A. B. Flood
Department Radiology, Dartmouth Medical School, Hanover, NH, USA

A. Ali
Department Radiation Oncology, Emory School of Medicine, Atlanta, GA, USA

© Springer Nature Switzerland AG 2020

P.-D. Ryu et al. (eds.), *Oxygen Transport to Tissue XLI*, Advances in Experimental Medicine and Biology 1232, https://doi.org/10.1007/978-3-030-34461-0_19

1 Introduction

The penultimate purpose of a clinical measurement is to obtain information that can be used to advance the clinical care of the patient. The ultimate test of the usefulness of the information is whether it impacts clinical outcomes. The outcomes can be survival or other clinically desirable parameters such as quality of life, cost-effectiveness, reduction of side effects, etc. The mechanisms by which the outcomes may be impacted can include enhancing diagnosis or improving individualized radiotherapy plans and/or combined treatments, as well as direct impacts on outcomes. But the bottom line is that when we make a clinical measurement, the ultimate criterion for its usefulness should be: does it improve clinical efficacy to an extent that offsets the costs (monetary, time, discomfort etc.) for getting that result and/or provide information that in the future could enhance clinical outcomes. Therefore, in evaluating the usefulness of a clinical measurement such as the value of oxygen in a tissue, we should take into account the purpose of making that measurement. When we focus on these considerations, we may find that, while it is not very valuable to state that there is a particular level of oxygen in a tissue, measurements of oxygen if repeated can reveal changes, and even if the amount is not rigorously quantified, these may be very useful indeed.

2 Oxygen Levels in Tissues

Heterogeneity of oxygen in the tissues of interest exists over many dimensions, including time, and over a wide range of scales [1]. Any practical method of measurement to characterize the tissue oxygenation and the heterogeneity present will necessarily provide data that represent some average over space and time; hence, careful considerations of the impacts of the averaging must be made to generate clinically relevant information. This average may include complex weighting factors with spatial, temporal, and oxygen dependencies. In some cases, additional processing of these data may provide other statistical measures, such as median, mean, max/min, etc. These practical considerations hold true for historic polarographic electrode measurements, modern PET and MRI approaches, optical methods, and all EPR techniques either in development or clinical implementation, as well as all other techniques. Consequently, there may be high value in using multiple techniques that together can provide complementary information.

There are spatial variances in oxygen levels in normal tissues due to the longitudinal gradient in oxygen as the blood passes through the microcirculatory bed (decreasing from the arterial inlet to the outlet microvessels) [2]. After the oxygen leaves the microvascular networks the oxygen partial pressures decrease from the vessels into the tissue as it diffuses through the tissues, due to oxygen consumption by the cells (radial gradients). Within the cells the oxygen decreases in a microspatially complex manner as it is intracellularly consumed, with most of the consumption occurring in the mitochondria. There also is growing evidence that the diffusion of oxygen into the cell may be constrained, i.e., that oxygen does not freely and rapidly flow into cells across the membrane [3, 4]. As a result there are variations in oxygen levels from cell to cell (according to their distance from the microvessel) and then also within the cell. These variations of oxygen from micro vessels to dimensions that are smaller than cells currently cannot be measured; note as detailed below in discussing temporal variations, even if we could make such measurements of spatial heterogeneity, they would be inadequate to understand the full heterogeneity of oxygen. Also, in some normal tissues there is additional significant macroscopic heterogeneity of oxygen over space because of their physiology, e.g., macroscopic heterogeneity between grey and white matter of the brain, and between renal cortex and renal medulla as consequence of substantial differences in blood flow. There also are more minor heterogeneities in resting skeletal muscle or in the subcutis, due to low O_2 extraction rates.

There also are temporal changes in oxygen levels in normal tissues [5]. The supply of oxygen by arteries and arterioles can vary periodically due to rhythmic changes in microcirculatory blood flow, which is reflected at all levels from the inflow arteries to the microcirculation. Within the microcirculation there are variations in microvascular flow due to regional regulation in response to varying metabolic demands.

The presence of pathology often significantly increases the amount and extent of oxygen heterogeneity both spatially and temporally [6]. The presence of pathology often impacts the structure/morphology of the vessels. In tumors there often is a significant amount of neoangiogenesis which results in much less ordered and less functional blood vessels. These vessels are much less efficient in delivering blood and also tend to be much more prone to leak. The leakage from these vessels can cause variations in the interstitial pressure, which can reduce the effectiveness of the microcirculation due to reduction of the perfusion pressure in the tumor capillaries [7]. The pathological changes also can result in altered consumption of oxygen, potentially decreasing oxygen consumption due to poor oxygen delivery and because of a switch to glycolysis due to metabolic re-programming (i.e., the Warburg effect) as a consequence of HIF-overexpression, upregulation of oncogenes, downregulation of suppressor genes, activation of certain signaling pathways etc. The pathology can also impact the integrity of the blood vessels. For example, tumor growth may physically impinge on the integrity of the blood vessels, and the metabolic abnormalities in diabetes can impact the structure of blood vessels (microangiopathy, macroangiopathy). The results of these processes can produce very significant local variations in the availability of fully functional vascular structures, resulting in local hypoxic regions.

Pathology also can impact temporal changes of oxygen and the response to treatment, which can result in significantly greater variability in oxygen levels in the presence of pathology (especially shown in cancer and peripheral vascular disease). These include short term changes, especially associated with the structural abnormalities of the microcirculation resulting in increased local variability in flow and long-term changes over time, due to disease progression and responses to therapy [8]. There also is a potential for anemic hypoxia to be present in tumors due to the underlying anemia of the patient [9].

3 Use of EPR Oximetry to Illustrate the Thesis of the Paper

We first consider the measurement of oxygen levels in tumors by EPR, because it is one of the few (maybe only) specific techniques that is currently being used clinically to make direct measurements of oxygen in tissues [10]. We then consider how these conclusions apply to other pathophysiological processes and other available measurement techniques.

Using appropriate oximetric paramagnetic materials, EPR oximetry can provide direct measurements of oxygen, i.e., the EPR signal it is directly proportionate to the amount of oxygen. Most other clinically available techniques measure parameters that often are only indirectly related to oxygen levels in tissues, e.g., they assess oxygen in nearby microcirculatory units or measure blood flow. In contrast, EPR measurements are made in the tissues of interest, not in the vascular compartment; for example, compare EPR with NIRS of hemoglobin or BOLD MRI.

The measured parameter of an EPR spectrum that indicates the amount of oxygen present is the line width of the observed resonance peak. There usually is a fixed relationship between the line width and the amount of oxygen, with the relationship being specific for each type of paramagnetic material. Using particulate oximetric materials, the measurements can be continuous over any span of time and can be repeated indefinitely. The method does require that the sensing material be injected or implanted in one or more regions of interest, but thereafter all measurements can be made entirely non-invasively. Importantly the measurements can be carried out in a clinical setting and can fit into the workflow needed for patient care, etc.

The initial clinical EPR measurements of oxygen in tissues have used India Ink as the oxygen sensor [10]. The carbon particles are the components that respond to oxygen. After injection of 30–50 μl of the suspension through a small needle, the carbon particles disperse non-uniformly through the local region as small extracellular aggregates. They are often engulfed by macrophages. The resulting EPR spectra in the region probed by the resonator (i.e., the surface coil used for signal detection) are a composite of the oxygen-dependent line widths from each of the particles. In reality, because of the relatively broad lines from the India Ink particles, the range of 'oxygen levels' that are likely to be present in the tissue, and the limited number of particles in each subregion, it is a challenge to resolve directly even the major groups of similar line widths. So using the observed line width to provide a quantitative measure of oxygen would seem to have modest utility in itself.

The other method of clinical EPR oximetry is based on the use of micro-crystalline probes (e.g., LiPc, LiNc-BuO), encapsulated in biocompatible polymers [10]. Clinical measurements currently are being performed using the 'OxyChip' which consists of oxygen sensitive microcrystals of lithium octa-n-butoxynaphthalocyanine (LiNc-BuO) embedded in polydimethylsiloxane (PDMS) [11–13]. The dimensions currently used in humans are cylinders that are 5 mm long with a diameter of

0.6 mm. The EPR signal from the sensor (OxyChip) reflects the partial pressure of oxygen within the PDMS, which itself reflects an average of the partial pressure of oxygen in contact with the external surface of the cylinder. The dimensions of the OxyChip are much greater than those of a microcirculatory unit and therefore reflect many different such units. The microcirculatory networks sampled by the OxyChip are likely to include regions with quite different oxygen levels. The 'values' of oxygen that are obtained therefore do not, in themselves, provide any information on the heterogeneity of the sampled capillary networks.

Given the impacts of unavoidable averaging by any real method of oxygen measurements in tissues, one may question the value beyond that of more qualitative measures of absolute measurements (e.g., pO_2 in mm Hg). See Flood et al. [14] for details on statistical issues in this regard.

4 Examples of Circumstances in which Current Methods to Measure Oxygen Can Be Clinically Very Useful

4.1 Screening for Responsiveness to Hyperoxic Interventions

One of the clinical paradoxes in radiation oncology is that, although we have known for more than 100 years that the response of tumors to ionizing radiation would probably be very significantly enhanced if we could irradiate them at times of more favorable oxygenation status, this knowledge has not been able to be used directly in ways that are applicable to the usual clinical uses of radiation therapy. Although many techniques have been tried that were expected to increase the amount of oxygen present at the time of radiation therapy, their apparent ineffectiveness has not resulted in modifying clinical practice [15]. We and others have hypothesized that these clinical failures were due to the fact that a significant number of tumors do not respond to methods to increase oxygenation of the tumors; consequently, unless these intrinsic non-responders are identified and removed from the pool of patients in which the hyperoxic interventions are tested, their presence would make it very difficult to obtain statistically significantly improved outcomes in the sampled population [10, 16]. Therefore, if measurements of oxygen in tumors could provide information as to which tumors could respond to a particular hyperoxic intervention, it would allow targeting that subpopulation with attempts to change the tumor oxygenation during radiotherapy.

Now it is feasible to carry out proper tests of the efficacy of hyperoxic interventions in human subjects to change oxygen in individual tumors and determine if such interventions result in clinically significant improvements in outcomes. For example, EPR oximetry has been used in preclinical models to measure tumor pO_2 over time for strategies changing oxygen delivery [17], oxygen consumption [18], both oxygen delivery and oxygen consumption [19], or an allosteric modifier of hemoglobin [20]. Ideally such a set of measurements would be carried out only on the hypoxic cells whose oxygenation needs to be improved, but this seems impractical at this time because of the lack of clinically applicable methods to measure oxygen levels selectively in the hypoxic cells. But it may be reasonable to assume that repeated measurements in representative parts of the tumor before and during the hyperoxic treatment, could be a workable method to determine the effectiveness of the treatment to increase oxygen throughout the tumor including the hypoxic cells. It would be desirable to test this directly by using such screening for responsiveness and then observing the impact on outcomes. It may be reasonable, given unavoidable impacts of spatial and temporal averaging and/or the use of a limited number of discrete measurements, to use data that only indicate whether or not the treatment resulted in a repeatable increase in oxygen, and not to need to focus on the quantitative aspects of the increase.

4.2 Impact of Hypoxia on the Effectiveness of Immunotherapy

There is increasing evidence indicating that the level of oxygen is an important determinant of the efficacy of immunotherapy [21–23]. Understanding these relationships and then exploiting them could have a very significant impact on the efficacy of immunotherapy, enabling physicians to determine which patients are likely to benefit from immunotherapy, providing early indications of the likelihood of response, and potentially providing a mechanism to enhance the effectiveness by altering the oxygen levels. These developments would be greatly aided by the use of repeated measures to determine changes in oxygen levels.

4.3 Role of Radiation-Induced Hypoxia on Fibrosis

Following large doses of radiation (as used in therapy), some individuals have significant fibrotic responses which can be uncomfortable and sometimes disabling. Hypoxia is considered potentially to be an important factor in the pathogenesis of fibrosis, but data to test this hypothesis are limited. By carrying out serial measurements of oxygen, it should be feasible to obtain more definitive data on the role of radiation-induced hypoxia in the pathogenesis of fibrosis. Serial measurements also might be useful for identifying subjects at risk before the changes become clinically obvious. Repeated measurements in the same individual, perhaps augmented by observing changes associated with breathing enriched oxygen mixtures, are key to gaining insights into the adaptive capacity of the vasculature. Measurements of relative changes should be appropriate for this purpose.

4.4 *Quantitative Delineation of the Hypoxic Fraction*

In principle such measurements would be ideal for use in guiding radiation therapy. Certainly, even relatively crude, one-time estimates using the Eppendorf electrode demonstrated the predictive capability of such measurements [24]. The problem is the technical difficulty in now making such measurements. The Eppendorf and related types of devices are no longer available for clinical use. Attempts to provide equivalent information by other methods have not been successful. This remains an area of opportunity for future developments of imaging. But it also should be noted that, especially in preclinical models as well as clinical studies using the oxygen electrode, some clinically useful correlations have been found between a limited number of measurements and outcomes, even if the measurements could not provide absolute measures of pO_2 [25].

4.5 *Use of EPR Oximetry for Other Types of Pathology*

The applicability and challenges of EPR oximetry are similar regardless of the types of pathology. Two instances where repeated measurements of oxygen would be especially valuable for guiding therapy are peripheral vascular disease and wound healing [10]. Although absolute measurements remain challenging, serial measurements of *relative* changes should be quite sufficient to help guide therapy, providing indications of the success of interventions to improve local oxygenation.

5 Conclusions

The previous discussion of what types of EPR-generated information about tissue oxygen have practical utility for medical decision-making extends to all types of such measurements [26, 27]. Some techniques have the advantage of directly measuring oxygen, but even they cannot fully resolve spatial and temporal heterogeneities. Others have the additional limitation of not being able to make repeated measurements. It would appear that repetition is likely to be particularly important for solving these problems, since it allows characterization of both spatial and temporal *changes,* which may be the most valuable clinical information.

Although it does not seem practical for any clinically available technique to provide a meaningful single (or 'absolute') number for oxygen levels in tissues, that does not need to be a fatal flaw if these limitations are recognized and adaptations are made to use the information in conjunction with other techniques that, when combined, provide the information needed to solve the clinical problem and to obtain the goal of using oxygen measurements to improve patient outcomes.

Acknowledgments Major funding is from the National Cancer Institute, PPG Grant P01CA190193. We gratefully acknowledge all the other scientists, clinicians, engineers and coordinators on the PPG. Disclaimer: ABF and HMS are owners of Clin-EPR, LLC which manufacturers clinical EPR instruments for investigational use only.

References

1. Harrison D, Vaupel P (2014) Heterogeneity in tissue oxygenation: from physiological variability in normal tissues to pathophysiological chaos in malignant tumors. Adv Exp Med Biol 812:25–31
2. Erickson K, Braun RD, Yu D et al (2003) Effect of longitudinal oxygen gradients on effectiveness of manipulation of tumor oxygenation. Can Res 63(15):4705–4712
3. Khan N, Shen J, Chang TY et al (2003) Plasma membrane cholesterol: a possible barrier to intracellular oxygen in normal and mutant CHO cells defective in cholesterol metabolism. Biochemist 42:23–29
4. Kurokawa H, Ito H, Inoue M et al (2015) High resolution imaging of intracellular oxygen concentration by phosphorescence lifetime. Sci Rep 5:10657. https://doi.org/10.1038/srep10657
5. Griffith TM (1996) Temporal chaos in the microcirculation. Cardiovasc Res 3:342–358
6. Vaupel P, Mayer A (2016) Tumor hypoxia: causative mechanisms, microregional heterogeneities, and the role of tissue-based hypoxia markers. Adv Exp Med Biol 923:77–86
7. Fukumura D, Duda DG, Munn LL et al (2010) Tumor microvasculature and microenvironment: novel insights through intravital imaging in pre-clinical models. Microcirculation 17(3):206–225
8. Konerding MA, Fait E, Gaumann A (2001) 3D microvascular architecture of pre-cancerous lesions and invasive carcinomas of the colon. Brit J Cancer 84:1354–1362. https://doi.org/10.1054/bjoc.2001.1809
9. Vaupel P, Mayer A (2014) Hypoxia in tumors: pathogenesis-related classification, characterization of hypoxia subtypes, and associated biological and clinical implications. Adv Exp Med Biol 812:19–24
10. Swartz HM, Williams BB, Zaki BI et al (2014) Clinical EPR: unique opportunities and some challenges. Acad Rad 21(2):197–206
11. Hou H, Khan N, Gohain S et al (2018) Pre-clinical evaluation of OxyChip for long-term EPR oximetry. Biomed Microdevices 20(2):29
12. Jarvis LA, Williams BB, Schaner PE et al (2016) Phase 1 clinical trial of OxyChip, an implantable absolute pO_2 sensor for tumor oximetry. Int J Rad Onc Biol Phys 96(2):S109–S110
13. Hou H, Khan N, Nagane M et al (2016) Skeletal muscle oxygenation measured by EPR oximetry using a highly sensitive polymer-encapsulated paramagnetic sensor. Adv Exp Med Bio 923:351–357. https://doi.org/10.1007/978-3-319-38810-6_46
14. Flood AB, Schaner PE, Vaupel P et al (2019) Clinical and statistical considerations when assessing oxygen levels in tumors: illustrative results from clinical EPR oximetry studies. Adv Exp Med Bio. (In Press)
15. Overgaard J (2007) Hypoxic radiosensitization: adored and ignored. J Clin Oncol 10;25(26):4066–4074
16. Swartz HM, Williams BB, Hou H et al (2016) Direct and repeated clinical measurements of pO_2 for enhancing cancer therapy and other applications. Adv Exp Med Biol 923:95–104. https://doi.org/10.1007/978-3-319-38810-6_13
17. Ansiaux R, Baudelet C, Jordan BF et al (2005) Thalidomide radiosensitizes tumors through early changes in the tumor microenvironment. Clin Cancer Res 11:743–750
18. Gallez B, Neveu MA, Danhier P et al (2017) Manipulation of tumor oxygenation and radiosensitivity through modification of cell respiration: a critical review of approaches and imaging biomarkers for therapeutic guidance. Biochim Biophys Acta 1858(8):700–711

19. Jordan BF, Sonveaux P, Feron O et al (2004) Nitric oxide as a radiosensitizer: evidence for an intrinsic role in addition to its effect on oxygen delivery and consumption. Int J Cancer 109(5):768–773
20. Hou H, Khan N, O'Hara JA et al (2004) Effect of RSR13, an allosteric hemoglobin modifier, on oxygenation in murine tumors: an *in vivo* electron paramagnetic resonance oximetry and bold MRI study. Int J Radiat Oncol Biol Phys 59(3):834–843
21. Vaupel P, Multhoff G (2019) Fatal alliance of hypoxia-/HIF-1α-driven microenvironmental traits promoting cancer progression and resistance to therapy. Adv Exp Med Biol. (In press)
22. O'Hara JA, Blumenthal RD, Grinberg OY et al (2001) Response to radioimmunotherapy correlates with tumor pO_2 measured by EPR oximetry in human tumor xenografts. Radiat Res 155:466–473
23. Noman MZ (2015) Hypoxia: a key player in antitumor immune response. A review in the theme: cellular responses to hypoxia. Am J Physiol Cell Physiol 309(9):C569–C579
24. Vaupel P, Höckel M, Mayer A (2007) Detection and characterization of tumor hypoxia using pO_2 histography. Antioxid Redox Signal 9:1221–1235
25. Colliez F, Gallez B, Jordan BF (2017) Assessing tumor oxygenation for predicting outcome in radiation oncology: a review of studies correlating tumor hypoxic status and outcome in the preclinical and clinical settings. Front Oncol 25(7):10
26. Springett R, Swartz HM (2007) Measurements of oxygen *in vivo*: overview and perspectives on methods to measure oxygen within cells and tissues. Antioxid Redox Signal 9(8):1295–1301
27. Flood AB, Satinsky VA, Swartz HM (2016) Comparing the effectiveness of methods to measure oxygen in tissues for prognosis and treatment of cancer. Adv Exp Med Biol 923:113–112. https://doi.org/10.1007/978-3-319-38810-6_15.

Clinical and Statistical Considerations when Assessing Oxygen Levels in Tumors: Illustrative Results from Clinical EPR Oximetry Studies

A. B. Flood, P. E. Schaner, P. Vaupel, B. B. Williams, B. Gallez, E. Y. Chen, A. Ali, T. Liu, V. H. Lawson, W. Schreiber, and H. M. Swartz

Abstract The success of treatment for malignancies, especially those undergoing radiation therapy or chemotherapy, has long been recognized to depend on the degree of hypoxia in the tumor. In addition to the prognostic value of knowing the tumor's initial level of hypoxia, assessing the tumor oxygenation during standard therapy or oxygen-related treatments (such as breathing oxygen-enriched gas mixtures or taking drugs that can increase oxygen supply to tissues) can provide valuable data to improve the efficacy of treatments. A series of early clinical studies of tumors in humans are ongoing at Dartmouth and Emory using electron paramagnetic resonance (EPR) oximetry to assess tumor oxygenation, initially and over time during either natural disease progression or treatment. This approach has the potential for reaching the long-sought goal of enhancing the effectiveness of cancer therapy.

A. B. Flood (✉) · W. Schreiber
Department Radiology, Dartmouth Medical School, Hanover, NH, USA
e-mail: Ann.Barry.Flood@Dartmouth.edu

P. E. Schaner
Department Radiation Oncology, Dartmouth-Hitchcock Medical Center, Lebanon, NH, USA

P. Vaupel
Department Radiation Oncology, University Medical Center, Mainz, Germany

B. B. Williams · H. M. Swartz
Department Radiology, Dartmouth Medical School, Hanover, NH, USA

Department Radiation Oncology, Dartmouth-Hitchcock Medical Center, Lebanon, NH, USA

B. Gallez
Louvain Drug Research Institute, Université catholique de Louvain, Brussels, BE, Belgium

E. Y. Chen
Department Surgery, Dartmouth-Hitchcock Medical Center, Lebanon, NH, USA

A. Ali · T. Liu
Department Radiation Oncology, Emory School of Medicine, Atlanta, GA, USA

V. H. Lawson
Department Neurology, Dartmouth-Hitchcock Medical Center, Lebanon, NH, USA

© Springer Nature Switzerland AG 2020

P.-D. Ryu et al. (eds.), *Oxygen Transport to Tissue XLI*, Advances in Experimental Medicine and Biology 1232, https://doi.org/10.1007/978-3-030-34461-0_20

In order to effectively reach this goal, we consider the validity of the practical and statistical assumptions when interpreting the measurements made *in vivo* for patients undergoing treatment for cancer.

Keywords EPR oximetry · Measures of oxygen · Clinical applications

1 Introduction

Hypoxia in malignant tumors has been well established to be associated with poor prognosis due both to its association with more aggressive growth and with greater resistance to therapy, including radiation and chemotherapy [1]. Hypoxia's enhancement of tumor resistance is generally thought to be due to the physical/chemical effects that negate the process by which therapeutic interventions work to destroy tumors. For example, the sustainability of damage to malignant cells caused by ionizing radiation depends on the immediate presence of molecular oxygen (O_2) to block the tumor cell's ability to repair the damage [2, 3]. There is evidence of increased survival and reduced recurrence of tumors that are reasonably well-oxygenated, in comparison to those that are hypoxic at the time of treatment [1, 4–8]. Consequently, clinical studies have attempted to increase the O_2 available in tumor cells coincident with active therapy, with the goal of increasing the therapeutic effect. However, when various methods to increase the O_2 in the tumors have been used in clinical trials, the results have been surprisingly weak [9, 10] - one reason why hyperoxygenation during therapy has yet to be adopted into clinical practice.

Why doesn't adding oxygen to the microenvironment of tumor cells appear to improve outcomes? One explanation is that only hypoxic tumors may benefit from the attempt to increase the oxygen delivery, as shown in the ARCON study [11]. There is another large body of literature looking at the partial pressure of oxygen (pO_2) in tissues that provides strong evidence of the heterogeneity of pO_2 in tissues. Heterogeneity exists in normal tissues, i.e., there are large differences in 'average' pO_2 or concentration of oxygen by types of tissue [12, 13]. More to the point about tumors, there is a large variation within a given tumor at a given point in time [14–16]. To add to this complexity, other work has demonstrated the continual dynamics of the amount of O_2 present in tissues as a result of the ever-changing gradients of O_2 that evolve in the microenvironment of cells [17]. Two main processes drive this dynamic: metabolic consumption of oxygen and the resulting diffusion of O_2 into the tissues in response to the presence of lower pO_2. Finally, pathological processes introduce variability relating to *chronic* vs *acute* hypoxia [18, 19]) and serve to up-regulate *or* down-regulate these effects, depending on the microenvironment [20].

Nevertheless, to establish clinically meaningful diagnostic measurements of oxygen in relevant tissue and thereby improve outcomes, clinicians and researchers continue to try to unravel these dynamic and complex relationships between hypoxia and outcomes. Indeed, the potential for oximetry to become a useful diagnostic tool to improve clinical outcomes is expanding beyond tumors. For example, new studies are underway to try to understand the role of hypoxia in causing some of the debilitating side effects of cancer therapy such as radiation-induced fibrosis [21, 22] or chemotherapy-induced peripheral neuropathy or peripheral vascular disease [23, 24]. Likewise, studies are being designed to examine other pathologies related to hypoxia, e.g., peripheral vascular problems associated with diabetes or poor healing following surgery, with the ultimate goal of improving care, especially by personalizing the knowledge of each patient's hypoxic tissue and his/her responsiveness to hyperoxygenation to alter the outcomes.

For all these reasons, it is important to understand the promise and pitfalls of currently used methods to measure O_2 in tissues. Swartz et al. in a companion article [25] focus on the biological and clinical implications of measurement techniques, using electron paramagnetic resonance (EPR) oximetry as an illustrative technique. Here, we focus on the practical qualities and limitations of these same EPR techniques, especially those based on carbon particulates, and bear in mind the ability to carry out oximetry in a usual healthcare setting and a typical clinical workflow. We discuss the strengths and weaknesses of several statistical models to summarize EPR data into indicators of hypoxia or a response to hyperoxygenation.

2 Materials and Methods and What they Illustrate

In vivo EPR oximetry has a long history and is detailed elsewhere [26–29]. Briefly, the instrument used in this paper is an identical clone of the instrument developed and used at Dartmouth Medical School. The major difference between the ongoing studies is the type of oxygen sensor used, each of which requires being implanted or injected into the tissue of interest (see Table 1). After a sensor is implanted in the tissue (and after a suitable time for healing the minor wounds associated with this invasive step), EPR measurements can be made easily via a small sensor loop placed externally on the surface above the sensor. These non-perturbing EPR measurements can be repeated as long as the sensor remains in the body.

Table 1 compares and contrasts basic features for the three types of EPR sensors: oxygen-sensitive carbon particulates [30–32], crystals embedded in a polymer [33–35], and the implantable resonator [36]. The first two sensors are used in ongoing studies in humans; the implantable resonator is currently only in preclinical use.

The principal sensor focused on is composed of carbon particles suspended in a pharmaceutically appropriate base (principally water). The carbon is injected as a sterile 'ink' into the subcutaneous layer and thus is only applicable to superficial tumors [30–32]. Although the amount of ink in each injection is ~equal (30–50 μl), the dispersion of the carbon particulates in the tissue is variable when injected; the ink is made more viscous to try to minimize this dispersion; however, it can leak from some tumors, e.g., friable tumors at the surface may lose some ink during the pressure of the injection. Because the suspending ingredients subsequently dissipate leaving only the carbon particles, the particles are interspersed with tumor cells,

Table 1 Principal features of three types of EPR oximetry sensors

Types of sensor: Current status of sensor features:	Carbon particles[1] in solution (aka 'Printex and Carlo Erba ink') [28, 30–32]	LiNc-BuO crystals encapsulated in PDMS (aka 'OxyChip') [33, 34]	Multiple LiNc-BuO capsules (aka 'implantable resonator')[27, 28, 36]
Current use and max detection depth for measurements	In several clinical studies[2]; at ≤5mm in subcutaneous layer [27]	In Phase 1 safety trial in human tumors[3] [27, 35]	In preclinical studies; at any depth of tumor [27]
Physical condition and mode of implanting (invasive step)	30-50 μl pharmaceutical quality suspension that dissipates after injection; injected w 0.5 ml insulin syringe & 29½-gauge needle	Crystals encased in PDMS, formed into semi-rigid 'rod' (5.0 mm h x 0.6 mm diam); implanted w 18-gauge brachytherapy needle	Crystals encased in PDMS as ~spheroids with 0.7mm diam; 4 'spheres', separated by 7mm bio-wire coated w PDMS; implant mode TBD
Physical condition after recovering from implantation (allows non invasive measurements)	Carbon particles remain permanently in subcutaneous tissue, encapsulated in macrophage cells and macroscopic pockets	cylinder remains in tissue until scheduled surgery	Same as OxyChip
Ease of placing within tumor	Easy; applies to surface tumors so shallow; hard to control dispersion, esp if porous	May be difficult when tumor is below skin surface; location re tumor unsure until path	NA, implanted in animals during open surgery with anesthesia
Estimated volume of tissue that can be queried[4]	Variable, due to dispersion of carbon particles; surface[5] =220 mm^2; volume=158 mm^3 (max)	Immediate vicinity of the surface of cylinder (surface ~10 mm^2)	Four 0.7mm diam 'spheres', each independently sampling at 7 mm intervals
Visibility, for resonator placement	Easily visualizable on skin; intra-cavity use may not be easily seen	Not visible; improved w ultrasound or systemic movement of resonator or with metal fiducials to improve visibility	Coupling loop on wire is visible and easily accessible

[1]Printex ink uses fine carbon black particles; Carlo Erba ink uses fine charcoal; see Flood et al. 2016 for details of ingredients.

[2]Non treatment trials to assess O_2 and response to hyperoxygenation in tumors (skin, SCC, breast) [28 patients {2 in post surg bed only} and healthy tissue (14 healthy volunteers), to assess peripheral vascular oxygen (not yet enrolling), and to predict radiation-induced fibrosis (23 patients and chemo-induced neuropathy (3 patients); [total ink sensor enrollees to date=68].

3Current IDE Phase 1 safety trial of tumors requires surgical extraction; intended use is to remain in tissue permanently [total enrollees to date: 20].

[4]Estimates are expressed as the surface area of the shape of each sensor, assuming they each query only the immediate local environment of the surface area; ink is also expressed as 3D volume since interspersed w tumor

[5]See Fig. 1. Estimates on surface and 3D are based on a cylinder 2 mm deep and 1 cm diam. Note this is a large but actual typical specimen size so represents a likely maximum volume queried.

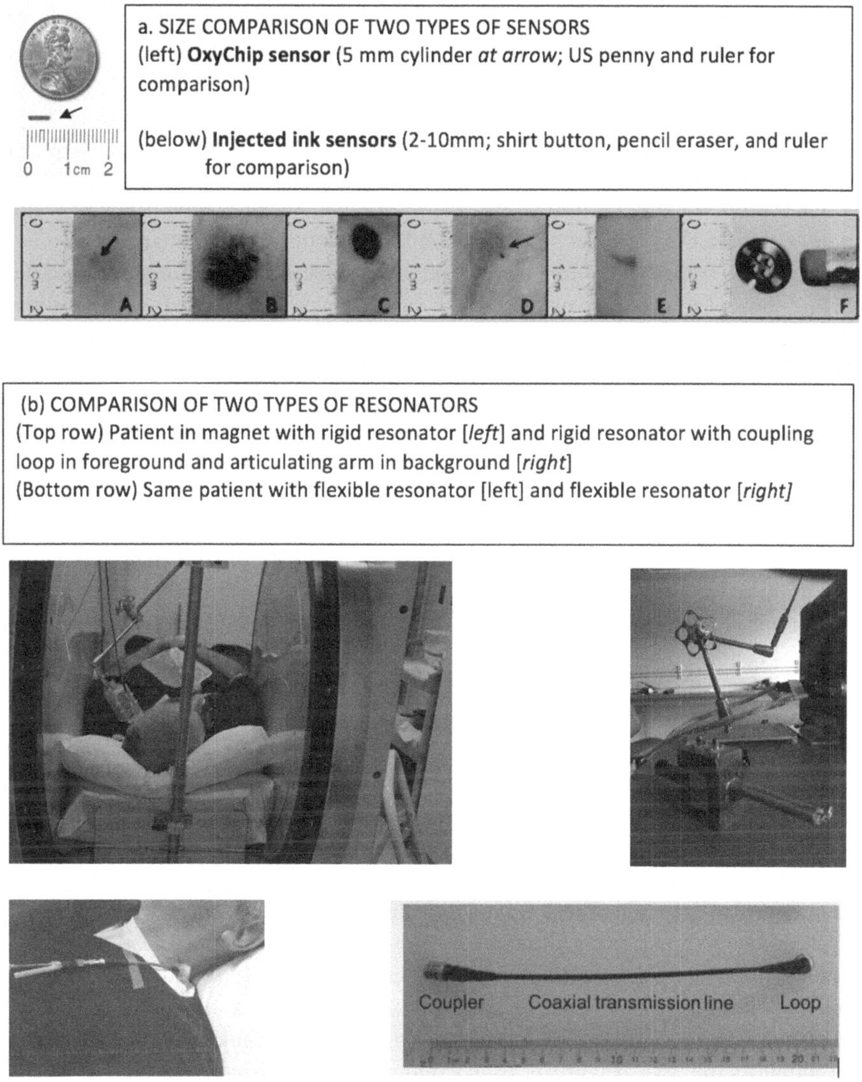

Fig. 1 Comparisons of oxygen sensors and resonators used in *in vivo* EPR oximetry

making the tumor volume queried considerably larger than the other types of sensors (an advantage), but variably so (a disadvantage). The carbon particles are typically permanently visible (analogous to India ink used in tattooing) but can be faint because they are injected deeper than a tattoo. (Figure 1a illustrates their typical variation in size and visual appearance.) Two inks have been used to date with different carbon particulates: Printex (carbon black) and Carlo Erba (charcoal). Both are restricted to tumor depths ≤5 mm due to the sensitivity limitations of EPR oximetry for this sensor.

The second sensor used in humans consists of lithium octa-n-butoxynaphthalocyanine (LiNc-BuO) crystals embedded in a silicon-based organic polymer (polydimethylsiloxane or PDMS) through which O_2 can move freely [33–35]. For humans, it is molded into a solid but flexible cylinder of specific diameter and length. Since the cylinder is impenetrable by cells, it detects tissue O_2 adjacent to its surface.

Basic properties of the third sensor, the implantable resonator (see [36]), are briefly compared to the other sensors in Table 1 but not otherwise detailed here.

Once these sensors are embedded in the tissue, measurements are made with the sensing loop of a resonator placed on the surface over the sensor. Figure 1b illustrates two configurations of sensing resonators, each with a small loop. The initial clinical measurements used the rigid resonator, which was held in place for 30 min by a mechanical arm. There were several clinical disadvantages of this technique. It is difficult for the operator to place (the rigid arm is difficult to control and needs to be placed with the patient located in the magnet). It is less comfortable for the patient. It increases the likelihood of introducing measurement artifacts due to pressure from the weight on the skin (potentially interfering with the O_2 dynamics in tissues adjacent to the loop) and to being inflexible in response to patient movement (including physiological processes such as breathing). The current flexible resonator eases placement (including being placed before the patient is inside the magnet), improves comfort, and moves with breathing, thereby improving the signal to noise ratio (SNR) and minimizing technical artifacts [37].

Collecting the data: Each EPR measurement 'session' in the ongoing studies consists of ~30 min of continuous data acquisition of EPR spectra, i.e., twelve 5-sec scans are taken per min and the 12 scans are used to create 1 median, call a 'set'. The ~30 min of a standard measurement session are divided into three ~equal segments, each differing by the gas the patient is breathing, i.e., room air (~21% O_2), 100% O_2 delivered via a non-rebreather mask at a constant flowrate, followed by breathing room air again. The software then fits the median spectra so that linewidth (LW) estimates can be extracted; the software will eventually convert LW estimates to pO_2 estimates, using a calibration curve derived separately for each type of sensor. (Only LWs are displayed here.) The software flags selected parameters that are outside of the expected settings (boundaries are currently somewhat arbitrarily set) and monitors the SNR. Figure 2c is an example of the software's initial tracking of SNR and ability to display data relative to the time when the patient is breathing different levels of O_2 (after dropping flagged scans).

Figures 1 and 2c illustrate some of the real-world complexities in acquiring 30 min of continuous scans. Patients sometimes also arrive late and have medical appointments after their measurement session, thereby not leaving enough time to complete all three phases. When the mask is placed over the nose and mouth, time may elapse before measurements can be restarted. Not infrequently, the patient moves enough during this action to require a retuning step before measurements can resume. While 100% O_2 is delivered at a constant rate during the hyperoxygenation treatment period, what is actually inspired is not the same across subjects. The fraction of inspired oxygen, with the type of mask and rate of delivery used, is typically

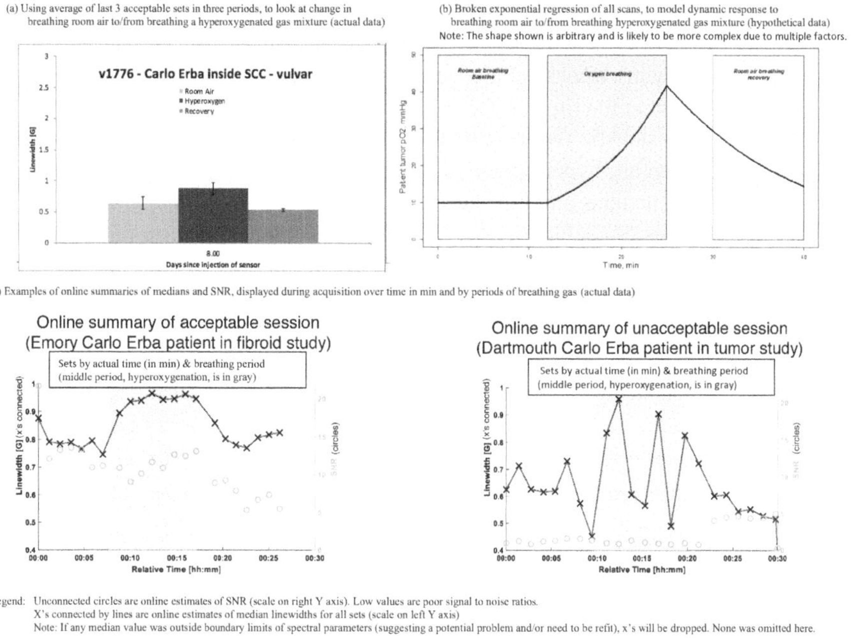

Fig 2 Analytic models of response to hyperoxygenation for EPR oximetry measurements taken in patients

listed as 60–90%, but may be less, especially when the resonator needs to be placed on the nose or face near the mask thereby preventing a tight connection to the face. Therefore, the amount of time that a patient is breathing the hyperoxygenated gas mixture and the fraction of O_2 in the gas mixture actually inspired may vary. So, in reality, the number of scans vary from patient to patient, their quality may vary, the amount of oxygen inspired varies, and the placement within the tumor and volume queried will vary from the 'intended ideal' of data about tissue O_2.

For all these reasons, the actual data that we use to characterize whether 'a tumor is hypoxic' and whether the tissue appears to be 'responsive to hyperoxygenation' still needs to be carefully considered. How should we measure these important variables and more importantly what do our measures mean - and not mean - in regard to addressing the fundamentally important clinical questions of interest?

Five patients and one healthy volunteer (out of 68 injected to date with carbon particulates) illustrate some ways to address these questions. Specifically, we report on 2 patients in a study with ink injected into the tumor; 1 healthy subject injected in the foot; 1 breast cancer patient injected in the foot who is enrolled in a study of chemotherapy-induced peripheral neuropathy; and 2 breast cancer patients injected in the irradiated postsurgical area who are in a study of radiation-induced fibrosis.

All spectra for these patients were re-analyzed for this study to ensure that rules of selection of sessions and scans were applied consistently. Sessions were excluded for two reasons: any measurement made on the day of the injection was assumed to be compromised by the injection/healing; any session with fewer than 6 scans per min during a breathing period was dropped as indicating an unresolved technical problem. Sets of scans were excluded if deemed ‘unacceptable’ by the operator of the EPR instrument at the time of the measurement.

As the primary statistic reported here, we characterize a period within a session (referred to as room air, hyperoxygenation, and recovery) by choosing the last three acceptable sets of medians and then averaging their LWs. This strategy assumes that the last few minutes of each period are a reasonable characterization of the steady-state of the actual dynamics of responding to breathing O_2-enriched gas and then responding dynamically to the return to breathing room air. Note, however, this rule may result in portraying quite different actual lengths of time since the patient started breathing O_2-enriched gas, due to delays already noted and also due to the potential occurrence of unacceptable sets at the end of the period, causing this rule to focus coincidentally on the early part of the period when the dynamic change may not be observable and therefore the response may appear to be ‘insignificant’.

We have proposed other ways to look at the dynamics of responding to hyper-oxygenation. One approach (a broken-exponential regression approach [38]) has the important advantage of using the full distribution of good scans across real time to examine the dynamics of the changes associated with breathing enriched oxygen and returning to room air. This model is an improvement over a continuous exponential approach for two reasons: (1) It is less impacted by practical issues that lead to real differences related to how long the patient has actually been breathing the gases. (2) It is less sensitive to whether the pO_2 has reached a steady-state plateau by the end of these dynamic periods. Figure 2b illustrates this with hypothetical data.

Another approach under consideration would have a different strength: it explicitly takes into account that a major driver of the clinical radio-sensitivity depends, not just on whether there is a significant response to breathing oxygen, but also on whether the tumor region being treated is initially hypoxic [39, 40].

Note, however, that none of these three measurement strategies fully addresses two important issues, and their consideration is important when deciding whether the assumptions underlying their applications are valid (or approximately so):

(1) [What is the ‘true’ pO_2?]: Tumors are well known to be heterogeneous and the distribution of pO_2 across the tumor is **not** normally distributed [41, 42]. Yet each EPR type of sensor only senses a specific subregion where it *happens* to be placed, i.e., we cannot identify a specific region within the tumor to place our sensor for maximum effect. Furthermore, if the subregion detected by the sensor happens itself to be heterogeneous, the EPR measure will still report only one value, which may or may not be weighted across time, space, and oxygen levels. The single value reported could really reflect an ‘average’ of the pO_2 sensed in the specific subregion, but for which there is no indication of the variation of O_2 sensed nor is the variation likely to be normally distributed (as is usually assumed when using an average). Of note for all three sensors, if there are differences in pO_2 in subregions within the volume being queried, there is a bias toward EPR’s sensing the LWs from the more

hypoxic sections of the subregion. This bias may be an advantage for the clinical meaningfulness of EPR estimates because an 'average' may overreport the hypoxia.

It is therefore important to understand how much of the tumor is represented by its subregion actually being sensed. To help quantify the volume our sensors can report relative to the mass of typical tumor, we used size estimates of breast carcinomas, based on several hundred US women with invasive breast cancer [43: p2016]; size was assessed by the largest diameter of the postsurgical specimen. Michaelson et al. [43] report that the median diameter for women never-screened before diagnosis was 15 mm and for those diagnosed after a first screening was 10 mm. Applying these sizes to a cylinder shape to approximate the total tumor volume (recall that the tumor subregion sensed by each sensor in Table 1 also used a cylinder), the median total tumor volume is ~785 mm^3 (for first-screened women) or ~2650 mm^3 (for never-screened women). Comparing these estimates to the estimated subregion sensed by carbon particles (Table 1), the subregion reported by our sensor is about 5x less than the total tumor volume (for first-screened tumors) and 16x less (for never-screened tumors). However, breast cancer patients in studies using ink are not intended to be injected in tumor tissue; suitable studies of hypoxia in breast cancer would need to be conducted using our other sensors. While the superficial tumors sensible by the carbon particulates are likely to be much smaller than breast carcinomas, these comparisons of subregion-volume to total-tumor-volume illustrate the concern that the subregion sensed is only a small fraction of the actual tumor. Note, however, that the clinically important interpretation of what our measures indicate in regard to 'true hypoxia' in tumors may be less of a problem if the main clinical indicator of interest is simply to find out if the tumor appears to be responsive to hyperoxygenation or to monitor for the presence of lower levels than typical or long-term changes in levels of pO_2 in non-tumor tissues. These issues are less likely to confound preclinical studies in rodents as well, due largely to the smaller size of the animal's tumor.

(2) [Uncertainties in the data/measures of pO_2]: There are many sources for uncertainties, e.g., instrumental factors such as data acquisition, modeling of the spectra, SNR or patient factors such as movement or having a tumor not easily placed in the best location within the magnet, or operator factors such as errors in settings or differences in judgments about which sets to drop. While none of these current measures takes these uncertainties fully into account, some do a better job than others, and it will be important to improve them to better address these issues.

3 Illustrative Results

Figures 2 and 3 illustrate these statistics used in five patients and one healthy subject. Figure 2 focuses on a patient whose sensor was placed in the tumor. Figure 2a presents the primary statistic, i.e., the average of the last 3 acceptable sets and the SD. There does appear to be a response to hyperoxygenation for all but one subject, but most subjects' responsiveness varies over time.

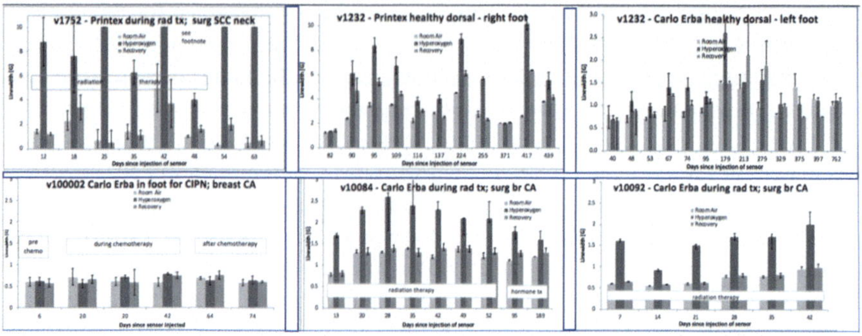

Fig. 3 Longitudinal oximetry of non-tumor tissues in healthy volunteer and cancer patients during radiation therapy or chemotherapy

Figure 2b presents an idealized model analyzing spectra over the 30 min of a measurement period, based on the broken-exponential regression technique to model the dynamics at a scan level. In preliminary analyses not presented here, this model portrays useful information about the distribution over time and its relationship to actual minutes breathing hyperoxygenated gas. Nonetheless, it identified the same sessions as showing a response to hyperoxygenation as the primary statistic.

The graphs in Fig. 2c are the online-generated portrayals of two *in vivo* measurement sessions for this patient. The individual dots portray the SNR, and the carets on the X-axis are automated 'warnings' that the spectral parameters of the scans may be out of bounds and should be investigated as to whether they warrant refitting or, in extreme cases, should be dropped from analyses. As expected, the session on the right with poorer data quality was excluded by our rules as well. While these warnings are currently based on somewhat arbitrary boundaries, they illustrate both the potential for automating the discarding or refitting on data and more importantly here, they are a reminder of the likelihood of experiencing uncertainties during measurements that, if overlooked, compromise the meaningfulness of the statistic.

Figure 3 presents data for a healthy subject and for patients for whom the sensor is deliberately *not* injected in the tumor; instead these patients are enrolled in studies of the potential for hypoxia to appear over time and during the course of therapy for their cancer, potentially predicting which patients develop debilitating side effects. Healthy subject v1232 had both types of ink injected and has been measured up to 762 days after injection, illustrating the potential for very long-term repetition of measurements. Many but far from all of v1232's sessions showed a response to hyperoxygenation and a lot of variability in the magnitude of the linewidth during the initial periods. The recovery period frequently does not return to the level of the initial period, suggesting perhaps that 10 min may not be sufficient to portray the full dynamics (at least in normal tissue in the foot). While not itself important for clinical decisions, these results suggest the dynamics of responses to breathing O_2-enriched gas bear more study if hyperoxygenation is to be used with actual therapy.

The responses of the patients in Fig. 3 are shown relative to whether they are undergoing cancer treatments. These results do not illustrate any major changes over the course of several weeks in the initial phase, nor are there obvious changes in relationship to their actively receiving treatment. Probably by coincidence, the patients receiving radiation therapy (v1752, v100084 and v100092) all showed a strong response to breathing a hyperoxygenated gas mixture while those receiving chemotherapy did not. While therapy per se may not have been related to these dynamics, the chemotherapy patient was measured in the periphery (foot), which may be slower to respond to hyperoxygenation than other regions of the body. Thus, it behooves us to remember the variability in O_2, even across types of normal tissues, and perhaps by peripheral locations. Note, however, that these remarks are not based on a systematic examination of patients, nor even all those currently enrolled.

4 Conclusions

There have been many promising developments in clinical applications of oximetry that are minimally invasive, potentially easily accomplished within usual clinical workflows and can be repeated over long periods of time. EPR sensors, particularly the carbon particulates injected as ink suspensions, have been successful in being able to assess O_2 in tissues in clinical studies and, perhaps more importantly, can assess changes in O_2 in response to hyperoxygenation. However, it is important to challenge our understandings of what our measures are actually able to tell us, in the context of what information is most needed to inform clinical decision making, whether it be to attempt to hyperoxygenate malignant tumors during radiation therapy or to monitor for indications of developing debilitating side effects. There are many important clinical studies remaining too, such as to determine whether a different method to try to increase pO_2 in the tumor would work better, at least in some patients, compared to the simple use of O_2-enriched gas mixtures. Questions such as the optimum timing of delivering hyperoxygenation or varying radiotherapy dose remain to be investigated, and, as suggested by these examples, may vary by anatomical location as well as by types of tumors or pathology being investigated [44].

This article has focused on some of the conundrums and how we are trying to improve our measures and overcome some difficulties in assessing heterogeneity in time and space with a specific sensor and EPR techniques. Despite the practical and statistical issues discussed here, it is important to keep in mind the potential advantages of EPR sensors to make repeated measurements of oxygen in the same patient from the same site. This information provides the potential to reach the long-sought goal of enhancing the effectiveness of radiation therapy by utilizing the radiation-sensitizing effects of oxygen. In order to reach this goal, it is important to continue to evaluate and improve upon both the techniques *and* the measures.

Acknowledgments Major funding is from the National Cancer Institute, PPG Grant P01CA190193 and Dept Neurol, Alexander Reeves Endowment Pilot Project 1 (CIPN). We gratefully acknowledge BW Pogue (Co- Principal investigator of the PPG), P Kuppusamy (PI of PPG's Project 2: Oximetry using the OxyChip), E Demidenko (Director of PPG's Biostatistics Core) and the study clinical coordinators (VA Wood and KA Hebert at Dartmouth and JJ Jeong and S Henry at Emory), as well as the engineers and clinicians who contributed to these studies at all participating institutions. All data reported here were gathered under IRB protocols at the respective institutions and all volunteers signed written informed consent. Disclaimer: ABF and HMS are owners of Clin-EPR, LLC which manufacturers clinical EPR instruments for investigational use only.

References

1. Höckel M, Schlenger K, Aral B et al (1996) Association between tumor hypoxia and malignant progression in advanced cancer of the uterine cervix. Cancer Res 56:4509–4515
2. Gray L, Conger A, Ebert M et al (1953) The concentration of oxygen dissolved in tissues at the time of irradiation as a factor in radiotherapy. Br J Radiol 26:638–648
3. Hall E, Giaccia A (2006) Radiobiology for the radiologist, 6th edn. Lippincott William and Wilkins, Philadelphia
4. Overgaard J (2007) Hypoxic radiosensitization: adored and ignored. J Clin Oncol 25(26):4066–4074. https://doi.org/10.1200/JCO.2007.12.7878
5. Vordermark D, Horsman MR (2016) Hypoxia as a biomarker and for personalized radiation oncology. Rec Res Cancer Res 198:123–142. https://doi.org/10.1007/978-3-662-49651-0_6
6. Horsman MR, Mortensen LS, Petersen JB et al (2012) Imaging hypoxia to improve radiotherapy outcome. Nat Rev Clin Oncol 9(12):674–687. https://doi.org/10.1038/nrclinonc.2012.171
7. Tatum JL, Kelloff GJ, Gillies RJ et al (2006) Hypoxia: importance in tumor biology, noninvasive measurement by imaging, and value of its measurement in the management of cancer therapy. Int J Radiat Biol 82(10):699–757. https://doi.org/10.1080/09553000601002324
8. Turaka A, Buyyounouski MK, Hanlon AL et al (2012) Hypoxic prostate/muscle pO_2 ratio predicts for outcome in patients with localized prostate cancer: long-term results. Int J Radiat Oncol Biol Phys 82(3):e433–e439. https://doi.org/10.1016/j.ijrobp.2011.05.037
9. Nordsmark M, Bentzen SM, Rudat V et al (2005) Prognostic value of tumor oxygenation in 397 head and neck tumors after primary radiation therapy. An international multi-center study. Radiother Oncol 77(1):18–24. https://doi.org/10.1016/j.radonc.2005.06.038
10. Nordsmark M, Loncaster J, Aquino-Parsons C et al (2006) The prognostic value of pimonidazole and tumour pO_2 in human cervix carcinomas after radiation therapy: a prospective international multi-center study. Radiother Oncol 80(2):123–131. https://doi.org/10.1016/j.radonc.2006.07.010
11. Janssens GO, Rademakers SE, Terhaard CH et al (2012) Accelerated radiotherapy with carbogen and nicotinamide for laryngeal cancer: results of a phase III randomized trial. J Clin Oncol 30(15):1777–1783
12. Vaupel P, Mayer A (2017) In: Schwab M (ed) Oxygenation of tumors Encyclopedia of Cancer, 4th edn. Springer, pp 3342–3346
13. Carreau A, El Hafny-Rahbi B, Matejuk A et al (2011) Why is the partial pressure of tissues a crucial parameter? J Cell Mol Med 15(6):1239–1253
14. Vaupel P, Höckel M, Mayer A (2007) Detection and characterization of tumor hypoxia using pO_2 histography. Antioxid Redox Signal 9:1221–1235
15. Epel B, Bowman MK, Mailer C et al (2014) Absolute oxygen R1e imaging in vivo with pulse electron paramagnetic resonance. Magn Reson Red 72(2):362–368. https://doi.org/10.1002/mrm.24926160
16. Krishna MC, English S, Yamada K et al (2002) Overhauser enhanced magnetic resonance imaging for tumor oximetry: Coregistration of tumor anatomy and tissue oxygen concentration. Proc Natl Acad Sci U S A 99(4):2216–2221. https://doi.org/10.1073/pnas.042671399162

17. Magat J, Jordan BF, Cron GO et al (2010) Noninvasive mapping of spontaneous fluctuations in tumor oxygenation using 19F MRI. Med Phys 37(10):5434–5441. https://doi.org/10.1118/1.3484056
18. Bayer C, Shi K, Astner ST et al (2011) Acute versus chronic hypoxia: why a simplified classification is simply not enough. Int J. Radiat Oncol Biol Phys 80:965–968
19. Vaupel P, Mayer A (2014) Hypoxia in tumors: pathogenesis- related classification, characterization and hypoxia subtypes, and associated biological and clinical implications. Adv Exp Med Biol 812:19–24
20. Vaupel P and Multhoff G (2019) Fatal alliance of hypoxia-/HIF-1α-driven microenvironmental traits promoting cancer progression. Adv Exp Med Bio (in press)
21. Yoshida EJ, Chen H, Torres MA et al (2011) Spectrophotometer and ultrasound evaluation of late toxicity following breast-cancer radiotherapy. Med Phys 38(10):5747–5755. 3203129
22. Yoshida EJ, Chen H, Torres MA et al (2012) Reliability of quantitative ultrasonic assessment of normal-tissue toxicity in breast cancer radiotherapy. Int J Radiat Oncol Biol Phys 82(2):724–731. 3156354
23. Fukuda Y, Li Y, Segal RA (2017) A mechanistic understanding of axon degeneration in chemotherapy-induced peripheral neuropathy. Front Neurosci 11:481. https://doi.org/10.3389/fnins.2017.00481
24. Park SB, Kwok JB, Asher R et al (2017) Clinical and genetic predictors of paclitaxel neurotoxicity based on patient- versus clinician-reported incidence and severity of neurotoxicity in the ICON7 trial. Ann Oncol 28(11):2733–2740. https://doi.org/10.1093/annonc/mdx491
25. Swartz HM, Vaupel P, Williams BB et al (2019) 'Oxygen level in a tissue' – What do available measurements really report? Adv Exp Med Bio (in press)
26. Swartz HM, Clarkson RB (1998) The measurement of oxygen in vivo using EPR techniques. Phys Med Biol 43(7):1957–1975
27. Swartz HM, Williams BB, Zaki BI et al (2014) Clinical EPR: unique opportunities and some challenges. Acad Rad 21(2):197–206
28. Swartz HM, Williams BB, Hou H et al (2016) Direct and repeated clinical measurements of pO_2 for enhancing cancer therapy and other applications. Adv Exp Med Biol 923:95–104
29. Gallez B, Baudelet C, Jordan BF (2004) Assessment of tumor oxygenation by electron paramagnetic resonance: principles and applications. NMR in Biomed 17:240–262
30. Charlier N, Beghein N, Gallez B (2004) Development and evaluation of biocompatible inks for the local measurement of oxygen using in vivo EPR. NMR in Biomed 17(5):303–310
31. Desmet CM, Binh L, An T et al (2018) Characterization of a clinically used charcoal suspension for in vivo EPR oximetry. MAGMA pub online at 32:205–212. https://doi.org/10.1007/s10334-018-0704-x
32. Flood AB, Wood VA, Swartz HM (2017) Using India ink as a sensor for oximetry: evidence of its safety as a medical device. Adv Exp Med and Biol 977:297–312. https://doi.org/10.1007/978-3-319-55231-6_40
33. Pandian RP, Parinandi NL, Ilangovan G et al (2003) Novel particulate spin probe for targeted determination of oxygen in cells and tissues. Free Radic Biol Med 35:1138–1148
34. Hou H, Khan N, Gohain S et al (2018) Pre-clinical evaluation of OxyChip for long-term EPR oximetry. Biomed microdev. 1 20(2):29
35. Jarvis LA, Williams BB, Schaner PE et al (2016) Phase 1 clinical trial of OxyChip, an implantable absolute pO_2 sensor for tumor oximetry. Int J Radiat Onc Biol Phys 96(2):S109–S110
36. Caston RM, Schreiber W, Hou H et al (2017) Development of the implantable resonator system for clinical EPR oximetry. Cell Biochem-Biophy 75(3–4):275–283
37. Flood AB, Wood VA, Schreiber W et al (2017) Guidance for academics to transfer 'bench-ready' medical technology into usual clinical practice. Case study: sensors and spectrometer used in EPR oximetry. Adv Exp med bio 1072:233–239. see suppl at 314496_1_En_37_MOESM1_ESM.docx
38. Demidenko E (2019) Advanced statistics with applications in R. Hoboken: Wiley (in press)
39. Churchill-Davidson I (1964) Oxygenation in radiotherapy of malignant disease of the upper air passages. The oxygen effect of radiotherapy. Proc R Soc med 57:635–638. 4

40. Brown JM (2007) Tumor hypoxia in cancer therapy. Methods Enzymol 435:297–321. https://doi.org/10.1016/S0076-6879(07)35015-5
41. Braun RD, Lanzen JL, Snyder SA et al (2001) Comparison of tumor and normal tissue oxygen tension measurements using OxyLite or microelectrodes in rodents. Am J Physiol Heart Circ Physiol 280: H2533–H2544, 2001
42. Vaupel P, Höckel M, Mayer A (2007) Detection and characterization of tumor hypoxia using pO_2 histography. Antioxid Redox Signal 9(8):1221–1235. https://doi.org/10.1089/ars.2007.1628
43. Michaelson JS, Satija S, Kopans D et al (2003) Gauging the impact of breast carcinoma screening in terms of tumor size and death rate. Cancer 98(10):2114–2124
44. Yang Y, Lei X (2006) Towards biologically conformal radiation therapy (BCRT): selective IMRT dose escalation under the guidance of spatial biology distribution. Med Phys 32(6):1473–1484

Fatal Alliance of Hypoxia-/HIF-1α-Driven Microenvironmental Traits Promoting Cancer Progression

Peter Vaupel and Gabriele Multhoff

Abstract Inhospitable conditions within the tumor microenvironment (TME) are a characteristic feature ('hallmark') of most solid malignancies. Regional tumor hypoxia is a primary deficiency since it plays a key role in malignant progression. Severe hypoxia is often associated with other detrimental conditions in the TME as a consequence of hypoxia-/HIF-1α-induced (with/without oncogene-direction and/or reciprocal interaction of cancer cells with TME cells) metabolic re-programming, exorbitant extracellular adenosine (ADO) generation and VEGF overexpression/VEGF-R activation. Re-programming of the tumor metabolism *inter alia* includes a 'selfish' upregulation of aerobic glycolysis/glycolytic flux ('Warburg effect'), a strongly enhanced glutaminolysis in tumor cells, ketogenesis in cancer-associated fibroblasts, and an acceleration of the tryptophan uptake/intensified catabolism yielding kynurenine, which can support the malignant phenotype. Aerobic glycolysis and glutaminolysis result in lactate accumulation (up to 40 mM), and together with the enhanced ketogenesis and CO_2/carbonic acid production lead to extracellular acidosis ($pH_e < 6.8$). These traits of the TME individually or collectively operate towards cancer progression via e.g. promotion of genetic instability and mutation, resistance to apoptosis, clonal selection, limitless cell survival and sustained proliferation, continuous angiogenesis and tumor growth, local invasion and distant metastasis, anti-tumor immunosuppression and resistance to therapy.

Keywords Tumor hypoxia · Metabolic re-programming · Aerobic glycolysis · Warburg effect · Glutaminolysis · Lactate · Tumor acidosis · Adenosine · Tumor progression · VEGF · HIF-1α

P. Vaupel (✉)
Department of Radiation Oncology, Klinikum rechts der Isar, Technical University Munich (TUM), Munich, Germany
e-mail: vaupel@uni-mainz.de

G. Multhoff
Center of Translational Cancer Research (TranslaTUM), Radiation Immuno-Oncology Group,Klinikum rechts der Isar, Technical University Munich (TUM), Munich, Germany

© Springer Nature Switzerland AG 2020
P.-D. Ryu et al. (eds.), *Oxygen Transport to Tissue XLI*, Advances in Experimental Medicine and Biology 1232, https://doi.org/10.1007/978-3-030-34461-0_21

1 Introduction

Adverse microenvironmental conditions are a 'hallmark' of most solid tumors. Scattered microregional and temporal heterogeneities in hypoxic areas are believed to be the most crucial deficiency since it has been well documented that hypoxia and/or upregulation of HIF-1α can play a critical role in (a) the multifaceted malignant progression, (b) inducing resistance to therapy [1–3], and (c) the suppression of anti-tumor immune responses [4–6]. Severe hypoxia is often associated with other detrimental conditions in the tumor microenvironment (TME). These traits individually or collectively operate towards cancer progression. Alternatively, upregulation of HIF-1α by oncogene activation, mutation of suppressor genes or epigenetics can likely provide a selective growth advantage of cancer cells with subsequent disease progression.

In this Chapter the following main features of the TME as key drivers for tumor progression are exemplarily discussed: role of hypoxia/HIF-1α pathway proteins, consequences of the phenotypic 'metabolic re-programming', generation and accumulation of lactate in anaerobic and aerobic glycolysis ('Warburg effect') and glutaminolysis, tumor acidosis, extracellular generation and accumulation of adenosine (ADO). These features of the hypoxic TME are key drivers for continuous malignant growth, sustained tumor angiogenesis, cell migration, local invasion, metastasis to distant sites, acquired treatment resistance and, finally, poor patient prognosis.

Hypoxia-/HIF-1α-driven features of the TME compromising anti-tumor immune responses are described in Multhoff and Vaupel [This Volume].

2 Microenvironmental Traits Promoting Cancer Progression

As described recently, the metabolic TME is characterized *inter alia* by critical O_2 depletion (moderate hypoxia: $pO_2 < 10$ mmHg, severe hypoxia: $pO_2 < 1$ mmHg), extracellular acidosis ($pH_e < 6.8$), high lactate levels (up to 40 mM) and extremely elevated ADO concentrations (10–100 μM) [4–6]. Hypoxia *per se* and hypoxia-dependent (and non-hypoxia-dependent) HIF-1α activation are pervasive stimuli and play a key role in orchestrating multifaceted activities in the development of these traits during tumor growth, especially in the metabolic re-programming of cancer cells ('metabolic adaptation') which supports the hypoxic, more aggressive and more resistant phenotype (Fig. 1).

2.1 Metabolic Re-Programming

Our current understanding of how HIF-1α can modulate the metabolism of hypoxic cancer cells (and immune cells), and how tumorigenesis-associated, altered metabolism upon phenotypic metabolic adaptation plays a role in cancer progression has

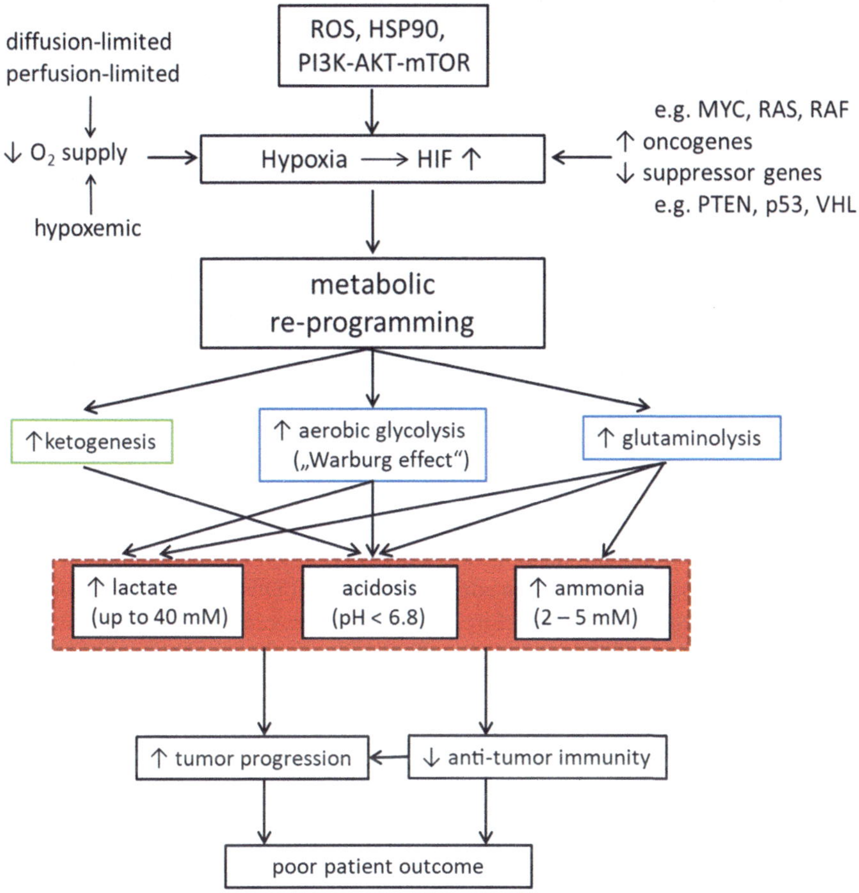

Fig. 1 Schematic representation of key metabolic alterations in cancer cells (blue boxes) and in cancer-associated fibroblasts (green box) in response to hypoxia-/HIF-1α–/oncogene-induced metabolic re-programming, evolving detrimental traits in the tumor microenvironment (TME, red box) and promoting tumor progression

been reviewed recently [7–10]. In these reviews, the alterations in the extracellular milieu elicited by cancer cells and their pleiotropic effects on stromal cells (and *vice versa*), and on the extracellular matrix are described. Reciprocally, the TME affects the metabolism and signaling response of cancer cells themselves [10]. Latest information suggests that HIF-1α-expressing tumor cells in hypoxic regions are likely to contribute to tumor progression by modifying the behaviour of tumor cells in normoxic regions of the local TME [11].

2.1.1 Upregulation of Aerobic Glycolysis

As a consequence of metabolic re-programming, cancer cells predominantly obtain their energy for cell growth and division through aerobic glycolysis, i.e., via glycolysis even in the presence of an adequate O_2 supply ('Warburg effect'). Cancer cells 'over-compensate' for the 16–18 times lower ATP production per mole glucose in cytosolic glycolysis, relative to mitochondrial ATP generation via Krebs cycle (TCA cycle) and oxidative phosphorylation (OXPHOS), by very rapid production of ATP since the speed of the cytosolic ATP generation is approximately 100-times faster than in OXPHOS, i.e., aerobic glycolysis is able to supply much more ATP *per unit time* than oxidative metabolism of glucose ('low-yield', but high-speed ATP production") [12, 13]. This is mainly accomplished by activation of the PI3K-AKT-mTOR pathway, as well as HIF-1α- and c-MYC-driven upregulation of the glucose transporter GLUT-1, substantially facilitating glucose transport into the cytosol, and in overexpressing key glycolytic enzymes. In addition to providing ATP, aerobic glycolysis generates antioxidant moieties and allows for the diversion of glycolytic intermediates ('carbon sources') into numerous biosynthetic pathways (e.g., generation of nucleosides, phospholipids and amino acids) thus supporting biosynthetic programs as long as an adequate glucose supply is maintained ('tumors act as glucose traps' [14]). Therefore, high glycolytic rates can lead to glucose depletion in the tumor TME (0–2 mM), which *per se* may exert detrimental effects that are not yet clearly understood. Furthermore, glycolysis can minimize the production of reactive oxygen species (ROS) which, at lower concentrations, can promote increased survival of cancer cells [15, 16].

2.1.2 Lactate, a Key Oncometabolite, Signaling Molecule and Fuel for Normoxic Cancer Cells

High lactate levels in the TME (up to 40 mM) primarily result from the upregulation of aerobic glycolysis. In addition, glutaminolysis, to a certain extent, contributes to lactate accumulation. Upon uptake into cancer cells through ASCT2-transporters and conversion to glutamate and α-ketoglutarate, the subsequent reaction steps in the Krebs cycle (TCA cycle) lead to malate. The conversion of malate to lactate is catalyzed by malic enzyme and lactate dehydrogenase A (LDH-A), both overexpressed in tumors.

Lactate is probably the only 'oncometabolite' involved and necessary in nearly all main sequelae for malignant progression. A series of these pathophysiological conditions results after binding of the ligand lactate to the GPR81-receptor and activation of the PI3K-AKT-mTOR pathway [17]. Sequelae *inter alia* include sustained angiogenesis, promotion of cell motility, local invasion (partly via hyaluronidase production by cancer-associated fibroblasts) and distant metastasis, resistance to apoptosis and promotion of a stem cell phenotype. In addition, lactate stabilizes HIF-1α through inhibition of prolyl-hydroxylase (PHD) [10, 18]

The export of lactate- anions and H^+ through hypoxia-driven MCT4 symporters into the extracellular space leads to a substantial TME acidification (see Sect. 2.1.5).

Upon accumulation in the extracellular space, lactate -by contrast- can be imported by normoxic cancer (and stromal) cells via MCT1 symporters and utilized to fuel oxidative phosphorylation (OXPHOS), thus sparing the uptake of glucose which is avidly consumed by hypoxic cells [19].

There is ample information that hypoxia, lactate- anions and H^+ (acidosis) are independent parameters (i.e., they can act independently) promoting malignant phenotypes in many instances [17, 20, 21].

The strong immunosuppressive actions of lactate are summarized in Multhoff and Vaupel [This Volume].

2.1.3 Role of upregulated glutaminolysis

The second principal growth supporting substrate for cancer cells is glutamine, providing the nitrogen required for the biosynthesis for purine and pyrimidine nucleotides and non-essential amino acids. In addition, glutamine serves as energy source in normoxic cancer cells as outlined above. Cancer cells are 'glutamine-addicted' (regulated by HIF-1α and c-MYC) and, thereby, act as 'perfect nitrogen traps' [14, 18, 22]. Glutaminolysis leads to strongly elevated levels of ammonia (up to 5 mM), which is highly immunosuppressive (see Multhoff and Vaupel [This Volume]). In addition, glutaminolysis contributes to extracellular acidification via lactate accumulation (see above).

2.1.4 Ketogenesis

Cancer-associated fibroblasts (CAFs) within the tumor stroma produce high-energy ketone bodies upon reciprocal interaction with cancer cells. These 'oncometabolites' can be used as mitochondrial fuels for OXPHOS by normoxic cancer cells. In addition, they contribute to tumor acidosis (see below). Ketone bodies can drive tumor growth, tumor recurrence and metastasis, and can increase cancer cell 'stemness' [22–25].

2.1.5 TME Acidification

Relevant pathomechanisms involved in and factors contributing to the acidification of the extracellular compartment ($pH_e < 6.8$) are as follows: anaerobic and aerobic glycolysis and glutaminolysis (through lactate accumulation), ketogenesis, ATP hydrolysis and CO_2-production by the TCA cycle and the pentose phosphate pathway. CO_2 is hydrated by hypoxia-activated extracellular, membrane-associated carbonic anhydrase CA IX and converted into bicarbonate (HCO_3^-) and H^+, the latter remaining extracellularly and contributing to TME acidification [20, 26]. In cancer (as well as in normal tissues) protons can also act as ligands, and the respective pH_e sensing and signaling are described in Multhoff and Vaupel [This Volume].

Acidosis is a detrimental trait since it drives *inter alia* genetic instability and mutagenesis, triggers resistance to apoptosis, promotes stem cell phenotypes, cancer cell motility, clonal selection of cells with high invasive capacity, upregulates MMP-2-, MMP-9- and cathepsin-activities, induces epithelial-to-mesenchymal transition (EMT) and promotes metastasis via enhanced ROS formation. Acidosis stabilizes HIF-1α, induces vigorous angiogenesis via VEGF-overexpression and triggers autophagy. Furthermore, it can lead to radio-resistance, impedes anti-tumor immune responses, diminishes the effectiveness of basic chemotherapeutic drugs and may contribute to drug resistance via mTOR-signaling [1, 10, 20].

Of note, the frequent (but not necessarily evolving) co-existence of hypoxia, lactate accumulation and acidosis in vivo often complicates the interpretation of their respective roles in tumor progression [1].

2.1.6 Accelerated Tryptophan Turnover and Kynurenine Accumulation

Besides glutamine, tryptophan is also fundamental for tumor progression [18, 27, 28]. Increased expression of indoleamine-2,3-dioxygenase (IDO) and tryptophan-2,3-dioxygenase (TDO) in cancer cells accelerates the catabolism of tryptophan into kynurenine. This 'oncometabolite' is known to favor tumor angiogenesis, degradation of the extracellular matrix and thus local invasion. Immunosuppressive effects of kynurenine are described in Multhoff and Vaupel [This Volume].

2.2 Extracellular Adenosine Generation

Hypoxia-/HIF-1α-driven adenosine (ADO) generation in tumors and adenosine-triggered effects on cancer cells have recently been summarized [3–5, 29]. Exorbitantly elevated ADO levels in tumors (10–100 μM) can lead to cell cycle activation, stimulation of cell proliferation and glycolytic fluxes. ADO can increase HIF-1α expression and the production of pro-angiogenic factors (e.g., VEGF). In addition, elevated extracellular ADO levels are highly immunosuppressive, as described in Multhoff and Vaupel [This Volume].

2.3 Overexpression of Vascular Endothelial Growth Factor (VEGF)

Hypoxia and/or HIF-1α directly or indirectly (in the latter case via ADO, lactate or acidosis) can drive the expression of VEGF and activation of VEGFR, thus promoting sustained tumor angiogenesis which supports tumor progression and metastasis [4, 6]. As recently shown, VEGF-A can exert diverse cellular effects via activation of the small G-proteins Rho and Rap. These effects include enhanced proliferation, migration and local invasion [30].

Overexpression of VEGF and activation of VEGF-R can promote tumor evasion from immune surveillance as described in Multhoff and Vaupel [This Volume] in more detail.

3 Conclusions

Detrimental traits of the TME as a consequence of hypoxia-/HIF-1α-driven, 'selfish' metabolic re-programming (e.g., upregulation of aerobic glycolysis, glutaminolysis, ketogenesis and accelerated tryptophan turnover), excessive ADO generation as well as VEGF-overexpression/VEGF-R-activation can individually or collectively operate towards cancer progression (via e.g. promotion of genetic instability and mutation, clonal selection, sustained proliferation, continuous angiogenesis and tumor growth, resistance to apoptosis, local invasion, distant metastasis), anti-cancer immunosuppression, resistance to therapy and ultimately lead to poor patient prognosis.

Acknowledgments The authors thank Anett Lange for her help in preparation of this manuscript.

References

1. Vaupel P, Mayer A, Höckel M (2004) Tumor hypoxia and malignant progression. Methods Enzymol 381:335–354
2. Vaupel P, Mayer A (2007) Hypoxia in cancer: significance and impact on clinical outcome. Cancer Metastasis Rev 26:225–239
3. Mayer A, Vaupel P (2013) Hypoxia, lactate accumulation, and acidosis: siblings or accomplices driving tumor progression and resistance to therapy? Adv Exp Med Biol 789:203–209
4. Vaupel P, Multhoff G (2016) Adenosine can thwart antitumor immune responses elicited by radiotherapy. Strahlenther Onkol 192:279–287
5. Vaupel P, Multhoff G (2018) Hypoxia-/HIF-1α-driven factors of the tumor microenvironment impeding antitumor immune responses and promoting malignant progression. Adv Exp Med Biol 1072:171–176
6. Vaupel P, Multhoff G (2017) Accomplices of the hypoxic tumor microenvironment compromising antitumor immunity: adenosine, lactate, acidosis vascular endothelial growth factor, potassium ions, and phosphatidylserine. Front Immunol 8:1887
7. Samanta D, Semenza GL (2018) Metabolic adaptation of cancer and immune cells mediated by hypoxia-inducible factors. Biochim Biophys Acta 1870:15–22. https://doi.org/10.1016/j.bbcan.2018.07.002
8. Sun L, Suo C, Li SF et al (2018) Metabolic reprogramming for cancer cells and their microenvironment. Beyond the Warburg effect. Biochim Biophys Acta 1870:51–66. https://doi.org/10.1016/j.bbcan.2018.06.005
9. Eales KL, Hollinshead KER, Tennant DA (2016) Hypoxia and metabolic adaptation of cancer cells. Oncogene 5:e190. https://doi.org/10.1038/oncosis.2015.50

10. Pavlova NN, Thompson CB (2016) The emerging hallmarks of cancer metabolism. Cell Metab 23:27–47
11. Harrison H, Pegg HJ, Thompson J et al (2018) HIF-1α expressing cells induce a hypoxic-like response in neighbouring cancer cells. BMC Cancer 18:674
12. Pfeiffer T, Schuster S, Bonhoeffer S (2001) Cooperation and competition in the evolution of ATP producing pathways. Science 292:504–507
13. Shestov AA, Liu X, Ser Z et al (2014) Quantitative determinants of aerobic glycolysis identifying flux through the enzyme GAPDH as a limiting step. elife 3. https://doi.org/10.7554/e/Life.03342
14. Shapot VS (1980) Biochemical aspects of tumour growth. MIR Publishers, Moscow
15. Sporn MB, Liby KT (2012) NRF2 and cancer: the good, the bad and the importance of context. Nat Rev Cancer 12:564–571
16. Lee M, Yoon JH (2015) Metabolic interplay between glycolysis and mitochondrial oxidation. The reverse Warburg effect and its therapeutic implication. World J Biol Chem 6:148–161
17. San-Millan I, Brooks GS (2017) Reexamining cancer metabolism: lactate production for carcinogenesis could be the purpose and explanation of the Warburg effect. Carcinogenesis 38:119–133
18. Sormendi S, Wielockx B (2018) Hypoxia pathway proteins as central mediators of metabolism in the tumor cells and their microenvironment. Front Immunol 9:40
19. Romero-Garcia S, Moreno-Altamirano MMB, Prado-Garcia H et al (2016) Lactate contribution to the tumor microenvironment: mechanisms, effects on immune cells and therapeutic relevance. Front Immunol 7:52
20. Corbet C, Feron O (2017) Tumour acidosis: from the passenger to the driver's seat. Nat Rev Cancer 17:577–593
21. Lacroix R, Rozeman EA, Kreutz M et al (2018) Targeting tumor-associated acidity in cancer immunotherapy. Cancer Immunol Immunother 67:1331–1348. https://doi.org/10.1007/s00262-018-2195-z
22. Kato Y, Maeda Z, Suzuki A et al (2018) Cancer metabolism: new insights into classic characteristics. Jap Dental Sci Rev 54:8–21
23. Bonuccelli G, Tsirigos A, Whitaker-Menezes D et al (2010) Ketones and lactate "fuel" tumor growth and metastasis: evidence that epithelial cancer cells use oxidative mitochondrial metabolism. Cell Cycle 9:3506–3514
24. Martinez-Outschoorn UE, Prisco M, Ertel A et al (2011) Ketones and lactate increase cancer cell "stemness", driving recurrence, metastasis and poor clinical outcome in breast cancer: achieving personalized medicine via Metabolo-genomics. Cell Cycle 10:1271–1286
25. Martinez-Outschoorn UE, Lin Z, Whitaker-Menezes D et al (2012) Ketone body utilization drives tumor growth and metastasis. Cell Cycle 11:3964–3971
26. Li Y, Patel SP, Roszik J et al (2018) Hypoxia-driven immunosuppressive metabolites in the tumor microenvironment: new approaches for combinational immunotherapy. Front Immunol 9:1591
27. Kouidhi S, Ayed FB, Elgaaied AB (2018) Targeting tumor metabolism: a new challenge to improve immunotherapy. Front Immunol 9:353
28. Wei L, Zhu S, Li M et al (2018) High indoleamine-2,3-dioxygenase is correlated with microvessel density and worse prognosis in breast cancer. Front Immunol 9:724
29. Vaupel P, Mayer A (2016) Hypoxia-driven adenosine accumulation: a crucial microenvironmental factor promoting tumor progression. Adv Exp Med Biol 876:177–183
30. Shimizu A, Zankov DP, Kurokawa M et al (2018) Vascular endothelial growth factor a exerts diverse cellular effects via small G proteins, rho and rap. Int J Mol Sci 19:1203

Quantification of Tumor Oxygenation Based on FMISO PET: Influence of Location and Oxygen Level of the Well-Oxygenated Reference Region

M. Lazzeroni, I. Toma-Dasu, A. Ureba, F. Schiavo, N. Wiedenmann, H. Bunea, B. Thomann, D. Baltas, M. Mix, C. Stoykow, A. Sörensen, and A. L. Grosu

Abstract Tumor hypoxia may play a fundamental role in determining the radiotherapy outcome for several cancer types. Functional imaging with hypoxia specific radiotracers offers a way to visualize and quantify regions of increased radioresistance, which may benefit from dose escalation strategies. Conversion of the uptake in positron emission tomography (PET) images into oxygenation maps offers a way to quantitatively characterize the microenvironment. However, normalization of the uptake with respect to a well-oxygenated reference volume (WOV), which should be properly selected, is necessary when using conversion functions. This study aims at assessing the sensitivity of quantifying tumor oxygenation based on ^{18}F-fluoromisonidazole (FMISO) PET with respect to the choice of the location and the oxygenation level of the WOV in head and neck cancer patients. WOVs varying not only in shape and location but also with respect to the assigned pO_2 level were considered. pO_2 values other than the standard 60 mmHg were selected according to the specific tissue type included in the volume. For comparison, the volume which would be considered as hypoxic based on a tissue-to-muscle ratio equal to 1.4 was also delineated, as conventionally done in clinical practice. Hypoxia mapping strategies are found highly sensitive to selection of the location of well-oxygenated region, but also on its assigned oxygenation level, which is crucial for hypoxia-guided adaptive dose escalation strategies.

M. Lazzeroni (✉) · I. Toma-Dasu · A. Ureba
Department of Physics, Stockholm University, Stockholm, Sweden
e-mail: marta.lazzeroni@fysik.su.se

F. Schiavo
Department of Information Engineering, University of Padova, Padova, Italy

N. Wiedenmann · H. Bunea · B. Thomann · D. Baltas · A. L. Grosu
Department of Radiation Oncology, Medical Center, Medical Faculty Freiburg, German Cancer Consortium (DKTK) Partner Site Freiburg, Freiburg, Germany

M. Mix · C. Stoykow · A. Sörensen
Department of Nuclear Medicine, University Medical Center, Freiburg, Germany

© Springer Nature Switzerland AG 2020

P.-D. Ryu et al. (eds.), *Oxygen Transport to Tissue XLI*, Advances in Experimental Medicine and Biology 1232, https://doi.org/10.1007/978-3-030-34461-0_22

Keywords Hypoxia · FMISO PET imaging · Treatment adaptation · Partial oxygen pressure · Head and neck cancer

1 Introduction

The role of functional imaging in radiotherapy is rapidly expanding from monitoring the status of the tumor before radiotherapy and its evolution during treatment to treatment outcome prediction [1]. Tumor microenvironment, in general, and tumor hypoxia, in particular, have been looked at as the main determinants of cell radioresistance and are investigated as leading causes of failure of tumor response to radiotherapy in several cancer types, including head and neck cancer [1, 2]. Positron emission tomography (PET) with hypoxia-specific agents, such as ^{18}F-fluoromisonidazole (FMISO), offers not only a way to visualize hypoxic areas, but also to quantitatively characterize the microenvironment by conversion of radiotracer uptake into oxygenation maps. Conversion functions necessarily make use of a well-oxygenated reference volume (WOV) for normalization purposes. The choice of the location of this region and its assigned oxygen level may play a crucial role in the determination of the hypoxic target volume (HTV) in a patient. It is, therefore, the aim of this study to investigate the influence of adopting different strategies for WOV determination in hypoxic volume definition.

2 Materials and Methods

2.1 *Patient Data, Treatment Protocol and PET/CT Acquisition*

Thirty patients with histologically confirmed T3/4, N0/N+, M0 squamous cell carcinomas of the oral cavity, oropharynx, hypopharynx, and larynx treated with concomitant chemoradiotherapy were included in the study. The protocol consisted of a total dose of 70 Gy in five fractions per week over 7 weeks, and three concomitant cycles of cisplatin of 100 mg/m^2 or carboplatin if indicated by renal insufficiency. Patients were imaged three times with ^{18}FMISO PET/CT in radiotherapy position: before the start of the treatment, in week 2, and in week 5. The image acquisition lasted 20 min after 167 ± 15 min from the injection of 302 ± 17 MBq of radiotracer.

2.2 *Hypoxic Sub-Volume Delineation Strategies*

To determine the HTV (with oxygen partial pressure threshold equal to 10 mmHg) from the distributions of FMISO uptake, a conversion function was applied following the method proposed by Toma-Dasu et al. [3, 4]. Equation 1 describes the sigmoid function applied at voxel level to the FMISO PET image in order to derive oxygen partial pressure, pO_2, distributions:

$$pO_2(\mathrm{r}) = \frac{c(a - Uptake(\mathrm{r}))}{b + Uptake(\mathrm{r}) - a} \tag{1}$$

with parameters a, b, and c equal to 10.9, 10.7, and 2.5 as described in more detail in [3–5]. The parameter denoted 'Uptake' in Eq. 1 is calculated in the following way: the voxel values in the FMISO PET images were divided to the average value in the WOV and the results were multiplied by the tracer uptake predicted by the conversion function for the assigned pO_2 in the WOV, which should be properly selected by the user.

For the purpose of studying the influence of the location of the reference region and its assigned oxygen level (i.e. oxygen partial pressure expressed in mmHg indicating well-oxygenation), three different methods for defining the WOV were considered:

I. A sphere located in the shoulder region (low density area in the CT) with pO_2 value equal to 60 mmHg;
II. Deep neck muscle volume with two alternative levels of assigned oxygenation:
   a. equal to 60 mmHg;
   b. equal to 29 mmHg, as from [6].

For comparison, the HTV was also delineated in the FMISO PET images following the clinical practice delineation, which often consists in considering all the voxels in the FMISO PET image having a value higher than 1.4 times the average in a reference region locate in the neck muscle (tissue-to-muscle ratio, TMR, equal to 1.4) [1, 7].

In order to quantify the similarity between HTV volumes delineated using the conversion function or the TMR (e.g. HTV1 and HTV2), the DICE coefficient was calculated as the ratio between the intersection of the volumes ($HTV1 \cap HTV2$) and their union ($HTV1 \cup HTV2$).

3 Results and Discussion

Figure 1 shows the gross tumor volume (GTV) and the HTV in one representative slice of the pO_2 maps generated by selecting different WOVs: a sphere in the shoulder region with 60 mmHg assigned oxygen level (**a**), a WOV corresponding to the neck muscle with 60 mmHg assigned oxygen level (**b**), or 29 mmHg, respectively (**c**). An HTV corresponding to the tissue to muscle ratio using the neck muscle as reference region, $HTV_{TMR = 1.4}$, is also shown in (**d**).

Figure 2 presents results of minimum (**a**) and mean (**b**) oxygen partial pressure values resulting from the conversion of FMISO PET uptake in one of the clinical target volumes (CTV) encompassing the HTV. The volumes defined based on a

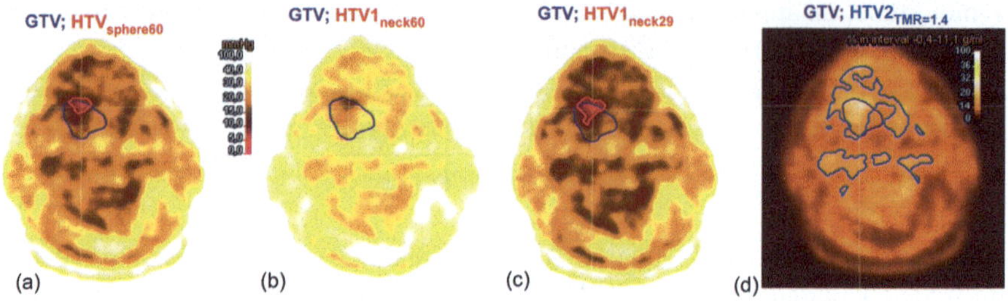

Fig. 1 Hypoxic target volumes (HTV) are delineated for a 10 mmHg threshold in one representative slice in oxygen partial pressure maps generated by considering as a well oxygenated region: a sphere in the shoulder region with 60 mmHg assigned oxygenation level, $HTV1_{sphere60}$, (**a**), a reference region corresponding to the deep neck muscle with 60 mmHg assigned oxygenation level, $HTV1_{neck60}$, (**b**), a reference region corresponding to the deep neck muscle with 29 mmHg assigned oxygenation level, $HTV1_{neck29}$, (**c**). An HTV corresponding to the tissue to muscle ratio using the neck muscle as reference region, $HTV2_{TMR=1.4}$, is also shown in (**d**)

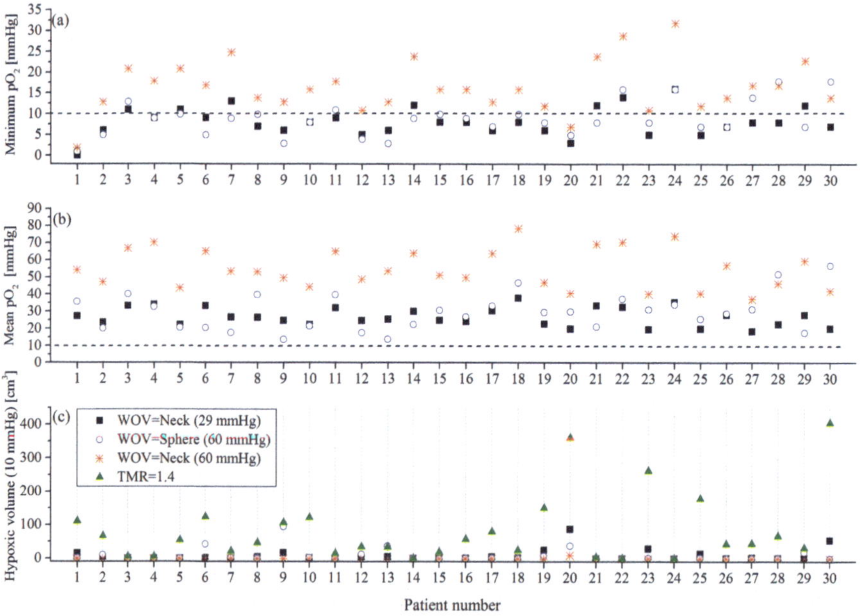

Fig. 2 Minimum (**a**) and mean (**b**) oxygen partial pressure values resulting from the conversion of FMISO PET uptake in one of the clinical target volumes encompassing the HTV are shown together with the volume of the HTV defined for a 10 mmHg threshold (**c**) for 30 head and neck cancer patients. Values are scored for different locations (neck, shoulder) and assigned pO_2 values of the well-oxygenated volume (WOV) (29 and 60 mmHg). The hypoxic tumor volume based on a tumor-to-muscle ratio (TMR) equal to 1.4 is also reported for comparison in (**c**)

10 mmHg threshold for different strategies of defining the WOV are reported and compared with the volume corresponding to a TMR of 1.4 (**c**).

In absence of precise information regarding the actual oxygenation of the tissue used as reference, the choice of the reference value of 60 mmHg in the assumed well-oxygenated reference volume was based on corroborating results of simulations and experimental observations. Thus, simulations of the oxygen partial pressure in tissue for a given distribution of capillaries expected to be characteristic to normal tissue [8], resulted in oxygen partial pressure distributions centred around 60 mmHg which was found to be in the same range of values experimentally measured [9]. This generic value should be, of course, replaced with specific ones when available [10, 11].

The classification of the patients as hypoxic/non-hypoxic (threshold 10 mmHg) shows about 70% agreement when a sphere with 60 mmHg and the neck with 29 mmHg are considered as WOVs. Considering as a WOV the neck region with an assigned pO_2 level equal to 60 mmHg does not appear to be a suitable option, since all patients result in being non-hypoxic, except for two cases (patients 1 and 20). On the other hand, the choice of a TMR level equal to 1.4 does not seem to be suitable for this patient dataset, since all patients show rather large hypoxic volumes.

Figure 3 shows the correlation between the hypoxic volume delineated for a TMR equal to 1.4 and the hypoxic volume contoured on oxygen partial pressure maps for a 10 mmHg threshold with a WOV located in the neck and an assigned pO_2 level of 29 mmHg. A linear trend (slope of about 5) is clearly shown in the figure.

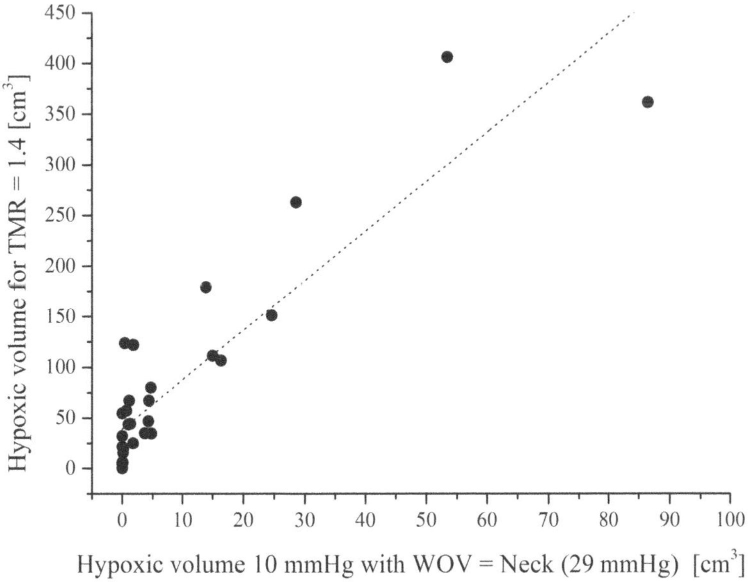

Fig. 3 Hypoxic volume contoured based on tissue to muscle ratio (TMR) equal to 1.4 as a function of the hypoxic volume contoured on oxygen partial pressure maps for a 10 mmHg threshold with a well-oxygenated volume (WOV) located in the neck with an assigned pO_2 level of 29 mmHg

Further investigation was conducted to study this aspect and, remarkably, the HTV corresponding to TMR equal to 1.4 was found to be similar to the volume which would be contoured in the pO_2 map corresponding to the WOV located in the neck region with 29 mmHg when the threshold for hypoxia is raised to 18 mmHg (18.0 ± 0.5 mmHg and median value equal to 18 mmHg for all patients in the study), instead of the standard hypoxia threshold of 10 mmHg. The DICE coefficient for the two volumes (i.e. $HTV_{TMR = 1.4}$ and $HTV_{neck29, threshold18}$) was 0.79 ± 0.17 and with median equal to 0.82 for this patient dataset.

4 Conclusions

The choice of the well-oxygenated reference region and its assigned oxygen partial pressure level is crucial when delineating the hypoxic target volume in PET images. Standardization of the method for delineation would be required when aiming for hypoxia driven treatment adaptation and dose-boosting strategies.

References

1. Wiedenmann NE, Bucher S, Hentschel M et al (2015) Serial [18F]-fluoromisonidazole PET during radiochemotherapy for locally advanced head and neck cancer and its correlation with outcome. Radiother Oncol 117:113–117
2. Sun A, Johansson S, Turesson I et al (2012) Imaging tumor perfusion and oxidative metabolism in patients with head-and-neck Cancer using 1- [^{11}C]-acetate PET during radiotherapy: preliminary results. Int J Radiat Oncol Biology Physics 82:554–560
3. Toma-Dasu I, D A, Brahme A (2009) Quantifying tumour hypoxia from PET - a theoretical analysis. Adv Exp Med Biol 645:267–227
4. Toma-Dasu I, Uhrdin J, Antonovic L et al (2012) Dose prescription and treatment planning based on FMISO-PET hypoxia. Acta Oncol 51:222–230
5. Toma-Dasu I, Uhrdin J, Dasu A, et al (2009) Therapy optimization based on non-linear uptake of PET tracers versus "linear dose painting". IFMBE Proceedings, 25/I:221–224
6. Carreau A, Hafny-Rahbi BE, Matejuk A et al (2011) Why is the partial oxygen pressure of human tissues a crucial parameter? Small molecules and hypoxia. J Cell Molec Med 15:1239–1253
7. Bittner MI, Wiedenmann N, Bucher S et al (2013) Exploratory geographical analysis of hypoxic subvolumes using 18F-MISO-PET imaging in patients with head and neck cancer in the course of primary chemoradiotherapy. Radiother Oncol 108(3):511–516
8. Konerding MA, Malkusch W, Klapthor B et al (1999) Evidence for characteristic vascular patterns in solid tumours: quantitative studies using corrosion casts. Br J Cancer 80:724–732
9. Dasu A, Toma-Dasu I, Karlsson M (2003) Theoretical simulation of tumour oxygenation and results from acute and chronic hypoxia. Phys Med Biol 48:2829–2842
10. Clavo B, Pérez JL, López L et al (2003) Influence of haemoglobin concentration and peripheral muscle pO_2 on tumour oxygenation in advanced head and neck tumours. Radiother Oncol 66(1):71–74
11. Vaupel P, Kallinowski F, Okunieff P (1989) Blood flow, oxygen and nutrient supply, and metabolic microenvironment of human tumors: a review. Cancer Res 49(23):6449–6465

Pathways of Oxygen Diffusion in Cells and Tissues

Hydrophobic Channeling *via* Networked Lipids

Sally C. Pias

Abstract Oxygen delivery to tissue mitochondria relies on simple diffusion in the target cells and tissues. As such, intracellular availability of O_2 in tissue depends on its solubility and diffusivity in complex and heterogeneous macromolecular environments. The path of oxygen diffusion is key to its rate of transfer, especially where pathways of differing favorability are present. Most commonly, aqueous media, such as interstitial fluid and cytoplasm, are assumed to provide the dominant diffusion path. Here, the 'hydrophobic channeling' hypothesis is revisited, and several lines of evidence pointing toward lipid-accelerated oxygen diffusion pathways are discussed. The implications of hydrophobic channeling are considered in light of extended membrane networks in cells and tissues.

Keywords Tumor hypoxia · Tissue engineering · Wound healing · Lung surfactant · Mitochondrial network · Oxygen flux

1 Oxygen Diffusion and Availability

The availability of oxygen (O_2) within cells and tissues has significant biomedical implications. Indeed, cellular oxygenation is a critical parameter in tumor radiotherapy [1, 2], anesthesia [3], wound healing [4], reperfusion injury [5], adipose tissue dysfunction [6], as well as brain function [7] and possibly neuronal hypometabolism [8]. Tissue-level hypoxia may select tumor cells resistant to apoptosis [9], and hypoxic cycling may favor tumor aggression and resistance to therapy [10]. Moreover, hypoxia is a major barrier to progress in tissue engineering, as 3D-printed cells toward the center of engineered constructs tend to languish and die because of poor diffusional oxygen delivery [11].

S. C. Pias (✉)
Department of Chemistry, New Mexico Institute of Mining and Technology (New Mexico Tech), Socorro, NM, USA
e-mail: sally.pias@nmt.edu

© Springer Nature Switzerland AG 2020
P.-D. Ryu et al. (eds.), *Oxygen Transport to Tissue XLI*, Advances in Experimental Medicine and Biology 1232, https://doi.org/10.1007/978-3-030-34461-0_23

While it is widely known that O_2 plays a crucial role in cellular energy metabolism, the mechanism of its delivery to tissue mitochondria is only partially understood. Existing physiological models provide reasonable estimates of the amount of O_2 leaving the lungs in the form of oxygenated hemoglobin within red blood cells, and hemoglobin O_2 release mechanisms are well studied. Physiological control of microvessel diameter in response to local oxygen demand is also fairly well understood. Yet, preceding uptake by red blood cells and following release in capillaries, O_2 transit occurs through simple diffusion [3].

With respect to oxygen diffusion rate, the inhomogeneity of cells and tissues has been largely neglected by the medical and scientific communities, although its importance was previously noted [12]. Tissues vary widely in macromolecular composition and physical properties. Such properties are well known to vary for diseased and aging tissues. For example, variations in lipid composition occur in breast tissues affected by cancer [13]. Moreover, tumor tissue commonly has a greater fraction of interstitium, compared with normal tissue of the same type [14]. Aging eye lens fiber cells have increased membrane cholesterol content [15], which is associated with increased rigidity and reduced oxygen permeability [16–18]. In patients with hypercholesterolemia, membrane cholesterol levels are elevated in red blood cells and possibly also in other cells [19], such as those forming the capillary endothelium. Consequent reduction in the rate of red blood cell O_2 unloading may decrease the amount of oxygen supplied to heart tissue under stress conditions [19]. These examples illustrate that tissues may be expected to have different levels of oxygen metabolic availability, depending on physical characteristics of the tissue and of the cells involved in oxygen diffusional delivery.

Metabolic availability is a dynamic parameter, reflecting a balance between metabolic demand and oxygen supply. Differences in tissue function and associated metabolic requirements give a wide range of 'normal' tissue oxygen levels [7]. Still, the supply to a particular tissue or portion of tissue depends not only on the amount of oxygen released in the capillaries (or culture media) but also on the rate of oxygen diffusion within the tissue, itself. As such, even tissue-specific O_2 measurements provide an incomplete picture of the amount of oxygen metabolically available to mitochondria. Accurate estimation of the *kinetics* of oxygen transit from air to red blood cells and from capillaries or media to tissue mitochondria will be key to understanding, predicting, and modulating tissue oxygenation.

Here, cellular- and tissue-level oxygen diffusional efficiency is addressed, with a focus on diffusion path and its impact on timely metabolic availability. Widely accepted theoretical aspects of oxygen diffusional flux are first discussed, followed by revisiting the 'hydrophobic channeling' hypothesis of lipid-mediated oxygen diffusion. Evidence in support of hydrophobic channeling is considered, especially in the context of interconnected membrane networks prevalent in cells and tissues.

2 Path of Least Resistance

The speed of a molecule's transit through complex surroundings depends on its path of travel. Where multiple paths are available, the molecule will move primarily along the path of least resistance. In energetic terms, the most favorable path will be that with the lowest free energy. Metabolite molecules such as O_2 are understood to diffuse *via* Brownian motion, exhibiting 'random walk' behavior. The overall direction of metabolite flux will be determined by the location of metabolic demand and the resulting concentration gradient.

The rate of metabolite transfer is affected both by the magnitude of the concentration gradient and by the permeability of the medium. Namely, the diffusional flux, J, is directly proportional to the permeability, P, and to the metabolite's concentration gradient, ΔC, as described by the equation $J = -P\Delta C$, derived from Fick's first law of diffusion [20]. Consistent with intuition, this equation predicts that higher-permeability environments will give rise to greater fluxes.

The solubility–diffusion model relates the permeability of a given environment to the solubility and diffusivity (diffusion coefficient) of a molecule traveling by Brownian motion. Most often used to characterize molecular diffusion across a cell membrane, the solubility–diffusion model can be expressed as $P = (K_P D)/h$ [20]. This relation is also known as Overton's rule. In it, K_P is the membrane/water partition coefficient, D is the diffusivity, and h is the thickness of the membrane. The partition coefficient describes the relative solubility of the molecule in the membrane, compared to adjacent bulk water.

Although quantitative application of Overton's rule may not be meaningful outside the context of membranes, the relation is conceptually valuable for predicting the preferred path of oxygen diffusion in the heterogeneous *milieu* of tissue. Where two regions of differing permeability are found next to one another, we can expect that oxygen will 'choose' a diffusion path through the higher permeability region because its relative solubility and/or diffusivity is greater there. That is, oxygen will diffuse preferentially within the portions of cells and tissues where it is most abundant and able to diffuse most readily. Further, because diffusional flux depends on permeability, we can expect the rate of oxygen transfer to be greatest along such preferential diffusion pathways.

3 Hydrophobic Channeling *via* Networked Lipids

Given the high water content of tissue, oxygen has been assumed to diffuse primarily *via* aqueous pathways. To the author's knowledge, this assumption is not supported by specific evidence but rather by the intuition that aqueous compartments would provide the most direct diffusional paths. It is especially easy to accept this view if one perceives cells as having a primarily aqueous interior and interstitial fluid as 'mostly water'. Yet, current knowledge of the complex and crowded macromolecular environment of cytoplasm [21] and interstitial fluid [22] poses a challenge. Several researchers have suggested that lipids may provide more favorable pathways and, thus, facilitate rapid oxygen delivery. The related hypothesis has sometimes been called 'hydrophobic channeling' [16, 23].

Given its nonpolar nature, O_2 is widely known to have substantially greater solubility in lipids *versus* water, by a factor of at least 3 or 4 [24, 25]. Further, the diffusivity of O_2 in lipids is comparable to that in water, although this finding was initially unexpected, given the much higher viscosity of lipids *versus* water [26, 27]. Taken together with Overton's rule, the higher solubility and comparable diffusivity in lipids point to enhanced O_2 permeability for lipids compared with water. The enhanced permeability would correspond with diffusional flux enhancement, encouraging rapid oxygen transfer within lipids and suggesting that cellular lipids may offer preferential diffusion pathways.

Consistent with these fundamental observations, Longmuir suggested in 1981 that oxygen transit from blood to mitochondria occurs *via* "channels of high solubility" comprised of lipids [28]. Skulachev later suggested that "extended membranous systems", especially mitochondrial membrane networks, may function as passageways for oxygen [27]. He proposed "lateral transfer" of oxygen by diffusion within the core of membranes, parallel to the membrane plane. He implied that lateral transfer may occur both within cells *via* mitochondrial networks and at longer range, within the muscle cell mitochondrial reticulum and through series of cells interconnected by gap junctions.

Skulachev additionally noted the presence of fat droplets in very close proximity to mitochondria, seeming to suggest that lipid droplets may also aid in oxygen diffusion [27]. This view was later supported by Sidell and colleagues, who found that fish adapted to cold water temperature (5 °C) develop high lipid droplet content in their skeletal muscle [29, 30]. The high lipid content is associated with enhanced oxygen solubility, predicting high oxygen permeability relative to aqueous cytoplasm, which is expected to be highly viscous at low temperature [30]. Skulachev's view of mitochondrial membranes as passageways for oxygen diffusion is supported by the finding by Sidell and colleagues that mitochondria, themselves, also proliferate in cold-adapted fish [30].

Dutta and Popel further developed the idea of hydrophobic channeling and reviewed a good deal of supportive experimental evidence [12]. Subczynski and colleagues also found support for such a model in their electron spin resonance (ESR) oximetry work, using spin-label probes placed at various depths within model lipid bilayers. The ESR measurements produce profiles of the 'oxygen transport parameter,' which reflects the product of O_2 solubility and diffusivity. This parameter varies according to the bilayer depth of the spin-label probes, and the resulting profiles indicate that O_2 solubility–diffusion is greater in the nonpolar center of the membrane versus the polar headgroup regions [16]. Oxygen concentration and diffusivity curves derived from nuclear magnetic resonance (NMR) experiments [31, 32] and molecular simulation studies [17, 31, 33, 34] support this observation. Simulation data additionally suggest that low molecular packing density promotes O_2 solubility and diffusion in the interleaflet region [17, 31].

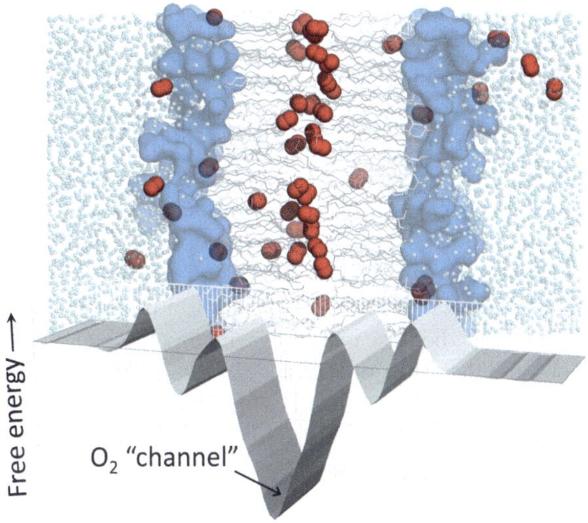

Fig. 1 Hydrophobic channeling is facilitated by high O_2 solubility and low free energy in the interleaflet region. Schematic representation showing a free energy curve juxtaposed with a molecular dynamics simulation image of a mixed phospholipid/cholesterol bilayer (1:1 ratio). O_2 shown as red spheres, phospholipids as gray lines and blue headgroup surface, cholesterol as white lines, and water molecules as cyan dots. H atoms omitted for clarity

Both ESR and simulations indicate that the membrane lipid composition substantially influences O_2 diffusion patterns [16–18, 35]. In particular, inclusion of membrane cholesterol modestly reduces oxygen permeability across a lipid bilayer but also enhances oxygen channeling toward the bilayer center [17]. Figure 1 provides a schematic illustration of the channeling effect, based on molecular dynamics simulation data for a bilayer incorporating cholesterol.

Molecular simulation studies by Ghysels and coworkers demonstrated that the *radial* diffusivity of O_2 parallel to the plane of phospholipid bilayers is greater than the transverse diffusivity perpendicular to the bilayer plane [34]. Moreover, O_2 molecules travel laterally in the interleaflet region across distances 3 to 10 times the bilayer thickness, prior to exiting into an adjacent aqueous layer and rapidly reentering a bilayer [36]. These findings indicate that oxygen diffuses more readily inside the core of a lipid bilayer, between the leaflets, than it does across a bilayer. Thus, travel within membranes is favored both by the enhanced concentration of oxygen in that region, compared with water, and by the enhanced radial diffusivity of oxygen in the membrane core.

Skulachev pointed out that high density of membrane proteins may attenuate lateral transport within membranous systems [27]. A recent simulation study partially addresses this issue [37]. A major finding of the study is that the apparent diffusivity of oxygen within a lipid bilayer is reduced by the presence of a potassium channel protein. This effect may stem from slow rotational dynamics of the protein side chains, relative to the lipid tail motions. Additionally, the presence of membrane proteins decreases the effective solubility of oxygen in the membrane because the portion of the membrane occupied by protein is not available to solvate O_2 [37]. With respect to oxygen permeability, the simulation study agrees with prior experimental work in bilayers incorporating bacteriorhodopsin protein [38]. Both methods indicate that the oxygen permeability is reduced, but the degree of change cannot be predicted solely by the physical presence of protein [17, 38]. Rather, the apparent permeability of the lipid surrounding the protein is also reduced [16, 37, 38], but this effect has not been satisfactorily explained.

It is important to note that the solubility of oxygen in the cytosol is expected to be lower than in pure water [27, 28]. First, the presence of salts can substantially reduce oxygen solubility [39]. Furthermore, water molecules surrounding other cytosolic solutes—proteins, cytoskeletal structures, and membrane polar groups—become tied up in solvent shells and are, thus, less available to solvate O_2 [27]. Macromolecular crowding in the cytosol is likely to reduce the effective diffusivity of $O_{2,}$ as well, because collisions with proteins and other macromolecules would tend to obscure the diffusional path.

Recent experimental work with lung surfactant has characterized the lung lipids as a network of interlinked lipid bilayers, thought to facilitate rapid O_2 uptake *via* diffusion from bilayer to bilayer along the network [40]. In that work, protein-mediated connection points among the bilayers are suggested to provide a roughly continuous hydrophobic conduit for oxygen diffusion. Absence of the lung surfactant protein fraction reduced the rate of oxygen movement by about 60% [40], suggesting that the protein contacts facilitate hydrophobic channeling.

In the *milieu* of cells and tissues, networked membranes are a common occurrence. Protein-mediated junctions such as gap junctions and organelle contact sites [41] place membranes in very close proximity. Relatively rapid exit from the membranes, due to low free energy barriers [17], should enable rapid supply of O_2 where needed, as well as diversion of O_2 to high-flux pathways affected by large O_2 concentration gradients.

4 Conclusion

The common assumption that oxygen diffuses primarily by way of aqueous pathways is challenged by contemporary understanding of cells and tissues as complex and crowded macromolecular environments. Rather, evidence to date supports a model of lipid-accelerated oxygen diffusion within membranes and lipid droplets held in close proximity by protein contacts. Further work is needed to account for the effects of macromolecules in cytoplasm/interstitium as well as in cellular membranes. Work is also needed to evaluate the potential role of lipid droplets as accelerants for oxygen diffusion, under various physiological and pathophysiological conditions. Clarifying the mechanism of oxygen diffusional delivery may reveal strategies for alleviating hypoxia in tumors, adipose tissue, chronic wounds, and engineered tissue constructs.

Acknowledgments Gary Angles provided simulation data for the figure, and PyMOL [42] was used to generate the image. This research is supported by the National Institute of General Medical Sciences of the National Institutes of Health under grant P20GM103451 and by a gift from the Glendorn Foundation.

References

1. Hou H, Dong R, Lariviere JP et al (2011) Synergistic combination of hyperoxygenation and radiotherapy by repeated assessments of tumor pO_2 with EPR oximetry. J Radiat Res 52:568–574
2. Multhoff G, Radons J, Vaupel P (2014) Critical role of aberrant angiogenesis in the development of tumor hypoxia and associated radioresistance. Cancers (Basel) 6:813–828. https://doi.org/10.3390/cancers6020813
3. Dunn JOC, Mythen MG, Grocott MP (2016) Physiology of oxygen transport. BJA Educ 16:341–348. https://doi.org/10.1093/bjaed/mkw012
4. Castilla DM, Liu Z-J, Velazquez OC (2012) Oxygen: implications for wound healing. Adv Wound Care 1:225–230. https://doi.org/10.1089/wound.2011.0319
5. Granger DN, Kvietys PR (2015) Reperfusion injury and reactive oxygen species: the evolution of a concept. Redox Biol 6:524–551. https://doi.org/10.1016/j.redox.2015.08.020
6. Netzer N, Gatterer H, Faulhaber M et al (2015) Hypoxia, oxidative stress and fat. Biomol Ther 5:1143–1150. https://doi.org/10.3390/biom5021143
7. Carreau A, El Hafny-Rahbi B, Matejuk A et al (2011) Why is the partial oxygen pressure of human tissues a crucial parameter? Small molecules and hypoxia. J Cell Mol Med 15:1239–1253. https://doi.org/10.1111/j.1582-4934.2011.01258.x
8. Rius-Pérez S, Tormos AM, Pérez S, Taléns-Visconti R (2017) Vascular pathology: cause or effect in Alzheimer disease? Neurol English Ed 33:112–120. https://doi.org/10.1016/j.nrleng.2015.07.008
9. Graeber TG, Osmanian C, Jacks T et al (1996) Hypoxia-mediated selection of cells with diminished apoptotic potential in solid tumours. Nature 379:88–91
10. Michiels C, Tellier C, Feron O (2016) Cycling hypoxia: a key feature of the tumor microenvironment. Biochim Biophys Acta – Rev Cancer 1866:76–86. https://doi.org/10.1016/j.bbcan.2016.06.004
11. Volkmer E, Drosse I, Otto S et al (2008) Hypoxia in static and dynamic 3D culture systems for tissue engineering of bone. Tissue Eng Part A 14:1331–1340. https://doi.org/10.1089/ten.tea.2007.0231
12. Dutta A, Popel AS (1995) A theoretical analysis of intracellular oxygen diffusion. J Theor Biol 176:433–445. https://doi.org/10.1006/jtbi.1995.0211
13. Hilvo M, Denkert C, Lehtinen L et al (2011) Novel theranostic opportunities offered by characterization of altered membrane lipid metabolism in breast cancer progression. Cancer Res 71:3236–3245. https://doi.org/10.1158/0008-5472.CAN-10-3894
14. Jain RK (1987) Transport of molecules in the tumor interstitium: a review. Cancer Res 47:3039–3051
15. Truscott RJ (2000) Age-related nuclear cataract: a lens transport problem. Ophthalmic Res 32:185–194. https://doi.org/10.1159/000055612
16. Widomska J, Raguz M, Subczynski WK (2007) Oxygen permeability of the lipid bilayer membrane made of calf lens lipids. Biochim Biophys Acta 1768:2635–2645. doi: S0005-2736(07)00233-7 [pii]. https://doi.org/10.1016/j.bbamem.2007.06.018
17. Dotson RJ, Smith CR, Bueche K et al (2017) Influence of cholesterol on the oxygen permeability of membranes: insight from atomistic simulations. Biophys J 112:2336–2347. https://doi.org/10.1016/j.bpj.2017.04.046
18. Plesnar E, Szczelina R, Subczynski WK, Pasenkiewicz-Gierula M (2018) Is the cholesterol bilayer domain a barrier to oxygen transport into the eye lens? Biochim Biophys Acta Biomembr 1860:434–441. https://doi.org/10.1016/j.bbamem.2017.10.020
19. Buchwald H, Menchaca HJ, Michalek VN et al (2000) Plasma cholesterol: an influencing factor in red blood cell oxygen release and cellular oxygen availability. J Am Coll Surg 191:490–497
20. Missner A, Pohl P (2009) 110 years of the Meyer-Overton rule: predicting membrane permeability of gases and other small compounds. Chem Phys Chem 10:1405–1414
21. Ellis RJ (2001) Macromolecular crowding: obvious but underappreciated. Trends Biochem Sci 26:597–604. https://doi.org/10.1016/S0968-0004(01)01938-7

22. Wiig H, Gyenge C, Iversen PO et al (2008) The role of the extracellular matrix in tissue distribution of macromolecules in normal and pathological tissues: potential therapeutic consequences. Microcirculation 15:283–296. https://doi.org/10.1080/10739680701671105
23. Subczynski WK, Wisniewska A, Yin JJ et al (1994) Hydrophobic barriers of lipid bilayer membranes formed by reduction of water penetration by alkyl chain unsaturation and cholesterol. Biochemistry 33:7670–7681. https://doi.org/10.1021/bi00190a022
24. Battino R, Evans FD, Danforth WF (1968) The solubilities of seven gases in olive oil with reference to theories of transport through the cell membrane. J Am Oil Chem Soc 45:830–833
25. Möller M, Botti H, Batthyany C et al (2005) Direct measurement of nitric oxide and oxygen partitioning into liposomes and low density lipoprotein. J Biol Chem 280:8850–8854. https://doi.org/10.1074/jbc.M413699200
26. Fischkoff S, Vanderkooi JM (1975) Oxygen diffusion in biological and artificial membranes determined by the fluorochrome pyrene. J Gen Physiol 65:663–676. https://doi.org/10.1085/jgp.65.5.663
27. Skulachev VP (1990) Power transmission along biological membranes. J Membr Biol 114:97–112
28. Longmuir IS (1981) Channels of oxygen transport from blood to mitochondria. Adv Physiol Sci 25:19–22. https://doi.org/10.1016/B978-0-08-027346-4.50007-3
29. Desaulniers N, Moerland TS, Sidell BD (1996) High lipid content enhances the rate of oxygen diffusion through fish skeletal muscle. Am J Phys 271:R42–R47
30. Sidell BD (1998) Intracellular oxygen diffusion: the roles of myoglobin and lipid at cold body temperature. J Exp Biol 201:1119–1128
31. Al-Abdul-Wahid MS, Yu CH, Batruch I et al (2006) A combined NMR and molecular dynamics study of the transmembrane solubility and diffusion rate profile of dioxygen in lipid bilayers. Biochemistry 45:10719–10728. https://doi.org/10.1021/bi060270f
32. Al-Abdul-Wahid MS, Evanics F, Prosser RS (2011) Dioxygen transmembrane distributions and partitioning thermodynamics in lipid bilayers and micelles. Biochemistry 50:3975–3983. https://doi.org/10.1021/bi200168n
33. Marrink SJ, Berendsen HJC (1996) Permeation process of small molecules across lipid membranes studied by molecular dynamics simulations. J Phys Chem 100:16729–16738. https://doi.org/10.1021/jp952956f
34. Ghysels A, Venable RM, Pastor RW, Hummer G (2017) Position-dependent diffusion tensors in anisotropic media from simulation: oxygen transport in and through membranes. J Chem Theory Comput 13:2962–2976. https://doi.org/10.1021/acs.jctc.7b00039
35. Subczynski WK, Hyde JS, Kusumi A (1991) Effect of alkyl chain unsaturation and cholesterol intercalation on oxygen transport in membranes: a pulse ESR spin labeling study. Biochemistry 30:8578–8590
36. De Vos O, Venable RM, Van Hecke T et al (2018) Membrane permeability: characteristic times and lengths for oxygen and a simulation-based test of the inhomogeneous solubility-diffusion model. J Chem Theory Comput 14:3811–3824. https://doi.org/10.1021/acs.jctc.8b00115
37. Dotson RJ, Pias SC (2018) Reduced oxygen permeability upon protein incorporation within phospholipid bilayers. Adv Exp Med Biol 1072:405–411. https://doi.org/10.1007/978-3-319-91287-5_65
38. Ashikawa I, Yin JJ, Subczynski WK et al (1994) Molecular organization and dynamics in bacteriorhodopsin-rich reconstituted membranes: discrimination of lipid environments by the oxygen transport parameter using a pulse ESR spin-labeling technique. Biochem 33:4947–4952
39. Battino R, Rettich TR, Tominaga T (1983) The solubility of oxygen and ozone in liquids. J Phys Chem Ref Data 12:163–178
40. Olmeda B, Villén L, Cruz A et al (2010) Pulmonary surfactant layers accelerate O_2 diffusion through the air-water interface. Biochim Biophys Acta Biomembr 1798:1281–1284. https://doi.org/10.1016/j.bbamem.2010.03.008
41. Helle SCJ, Kanfer G, Kolar K et al (2013) Organization and function of membrane contact sites. Biochim Biophys Acta, Mol Cell Res 1833:2526–2541. https://doi.org/10.1016/j.bbamcr.2013.01.028
42. The PyMOL Molecular Graphics System, Version 1.7.6.5 Schrödinger, LLC

Part III
Muscle Oxygenation and Sports Medicine

Effect of Exercise Duration on Post-Exercise Persistence of Oxyhemoglobin Changes in the Premotor Cortex: A Near-Infrared Spectroscopy Study in Moderate-Intensity Cycling Exercise

Atsuhiro Tsubaki, Shinichiro Morishita, Yuta Tokunaga, Daisuke Sato, Weixiang Qin, Sho Kojima, and Hideaki Onishi

Abstract Measurement of oxyhemoglobin (O_2Hb) changes in the cerebral cortex using near-infrared spectroscopy (NIRS) shows that its levels increase during moderate-intensity exercise and persists after exercise. However, the effects of exercise duration on O_2Hb persistence in the premotor cortex (PMC) are unknown. We aimed to determine the effects of exercise duration on the persistence of O_2Hb changes after moderate-intensity cycling as exercise. Healthy young volunteers were recruited to participate in this study. After a 3-min rest period, the exercise was initiated at a workload corresponding to 50% VO_2peak. The exercise continued for 10 min and 20 min, followed by 15 min of rest. The O_2Hb levels in the right (R-PMC) and left premotor cortices (L-PMC) were measured using an NIRS system. The O_2Hb values during the 15-min post-exercise rest period in the R-PMC were 0.010 ± 0.011 mM·cm after the 10-min exercise and 0.035 ± 0.010 mM·cm after the 20-min exercise, without significant differences ($p = 0.104$). The O_2Hb value in the L-PMC during post-exercise rest (0.055 ± 0.010 mM·cm) after the 20-min exercise was significantly higher than that after the 10-min exercise (0.023 ± 0.007 mM·cm; $p = 0.014$). Thus, the effects of exercise duration on O_2Hb persistence have laterality in the PMC.

Keywords Oxyhemoglobin · Post-exercise persistence · Premotor cortex · Moderate-intensity exercise · Near-infrared spectroscopy

A. Tsubaki (✉) · S. Morishita · Y. Tokunaga · D. Sato · W. Qin · S. Kojima · H. Onishi
Institute for Human Movement and Medical Sciences, Niigata University of Health and Welfare, Niigata, Japan
e-mail: tsubaki@nuhw.ac.jp

© Springer Nature Switzerland AG 2020
P.-D. Ryu et al. (eds.), *Oxygen Transport to Tissue XLI*, Advances in Experimental Medicine and Biology 1232, https://doi.org/10.1007/978-3-030-34461-0_24

1 Introduction

Moderate-intensity exercise (e.g. cycling) improves not only fitness but also brain function [1, 2]. Changes in oxyhemoglobin (O_2Hb) reflect changes in cortical activation [3, 4] as well as exercise intensity [5, 6]. O_2Hb increase is related to the improvement of the brain function [7, 8]. Moderate-intensity exercise induces increased cortical oxygenation, which persists even after the exercise in motor function-related areas using near-infrared spectroscopy (NIRS) [9, 10]. If the status of O_2Hb persistence were established, we might understand the effect of exercise on improvement of brain function. However, the effects of exercise duration on increased cortical oxygenation are unknown.

The premotor cortex (PMC) plays a role in the selection, planning, and performance of voluntary movements [11–13]. The PMC and the prefrontal cortex are involved in control of locomotion at different speeds [14]. However, few studies have investigated the acute effects of moderate-intensity exercise on PMC.

The aim of the present study was to compare the effects of exercise duration on the persistence of O_2Hb changes after moderate-intensity exercise (cycling) in the PMC bilaterally. We hypothesized that O_2Hb levels would be higher after the longer duration of exercise.

2 Methods

2.1 Participants

Fifteen healthy young volunteers participated in this study. None of the participants showed symptoms of neurological, medical, or cardiovascular disease, and all were free from medication use at the time of the study. Each participant provided a written informed consent after receiving information regarding the potential risks, study objectives, measurement techniques, and benefits associated with the study. This study was approved by the Ethics Committee of Niigata University of Health and Welfare and conformed to the standards outlined in the Declaration of Helsinki.

2.2 Experimental Procedure

Individual exercise workload was determined on the basis of maximal oxygen consumption (VO_2max) during an incremental cycling protocol (Aerobike 75XLII; Combi, Tokyo, Japan). Measurements of VO_2max were obtained before the main experiments based on published recommendations [15]. Exhaustion was defined as previously described [6].

In the main experiment, participants performed constant work-rate exercise corresponding to 50% of VO_2max on a cycle ergometer for 10 min and 20 min, following a 3-min pre-exercise rest period. A 15-min post-exercise rest period followed the main exercise period. NIRS signals, skin blood flow (SBF), and mean arterial pressure (MAP) were measured continuously during the experiment.

2.3 NIRS Measurements

A multichannel NIRS imaging system (OMM-3000; Shimadzu Co., Kyoto, Japan) with multiple continuous wavelengths (780, 805, and 830 nm) was used to detect changes in O_2Hb, deoxyhemoglobin (HHb), and total hemoglobin (THb) at a sampling rate of 130 ms, on the basis of the modified Beer-Lambert law [16]. NIRS optodes consisted of 12 light-source fibers and 12 detectors, which provided 24-channel simultaneous recording. The optodes were arranged in a 4 × 6 manner in a multichannel probe holder, and a 30-mm interoptode distance was utilized to measure cortical tissue oxygenation. The Cz position of the international 10–20 system was used to ensure consistent optode placement for all participants. Regions of interest (ROIs) included the right (R-PMC) and left premotor cortices (L-PMC) (Fig. 1).

2.4 Blood Pressure, and Skin Blood Flow Measurements

Beat-to-beat MAP was recorded via the volume clamping method at the left middle finger, using a finger photoplethysmograph (Finometer; Finapres Medical Systems, Amsterdam, the Netherlands). Changes in SBF were measured at the forehead using a laser Doppler blood flowmeter (Omegaflow FLO-CI; Omegawave Inc., Osaka, Japan). Analog data were converted to digital data using an A/D converter (PowerLab; AD Instruments, Australia) at a sampling rate of 1000 Hz.

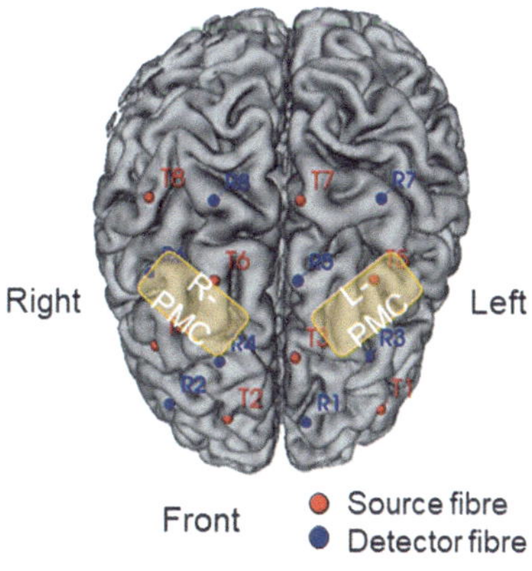

Fig. 1 NIRS optode placement and regions of interest. R-PMC, right premotor cortex; L-PMC, left premotor cortex

2.5 Statistical Analysis

SBF and MAP were down-sampled by adopting the sampling rate used for NIRS monitoring. To obtain temporal changes, the average O_2Hb, HHb, and THb levels for each ROI, SBF and MAP were expressed as changes from the average value obtained during the pre-exercise rest phase. O_2Hb, HHb, and THb levels, the delta value from the average value of the pre-exercise rest phase, were averaged during the 15 min post-exercise rest. The paired *t*-test was used to compare the exercise duration for each ROI. The level of statistical significance was set at $p < 0.05$.

3 Results

All 15 participants completed the incremental exercise test to measure the maximum oxygen consumption. Three participants from each group were excluded due to lack of data. In each group, out of 12 subjects, 9 who performed both the exercises were analyzed (Table 1). The temporal changes in O_2Hb, HHb, and THb are shown in Fig. 2 and those in SBF and MAP in Fig. 3. The elevated O_2Hb persisted throughout the 15-min post-exercise rest in both ROIs. SBF degraded over time, and MAP decreased immediately after the exercise. The O_2Hb values in the L-PMC during post-exercise rest after the 20-min exercise was significantly higher than that after the 10-min exercise. However, the O_2Hb value in the R-PMC after the 10-min exercise and after the 20-min exercise, have no significant difference during post-exercise rest. Values of HHb in both ROIs post-exercise did not show significant difference between the 10-min and 20-min exercise. The THb values in both ROIs during the post-exercise rest after the 20-min exercise were significantly higher than those after the 10-min exercise (Table 2).

Table 1 Characteristics of the participants

	Participants
Number	9
Age (years)	21.2 ± 0.8
Gender (female/ male)	6/3
Height (cm)	163.0 ± 8.6
Weight (kg)	55.0 ± 12.9
VO_2max (mL/kg/min)	31.6 ± 7.6

Values are presented as mean ± standard deviation.

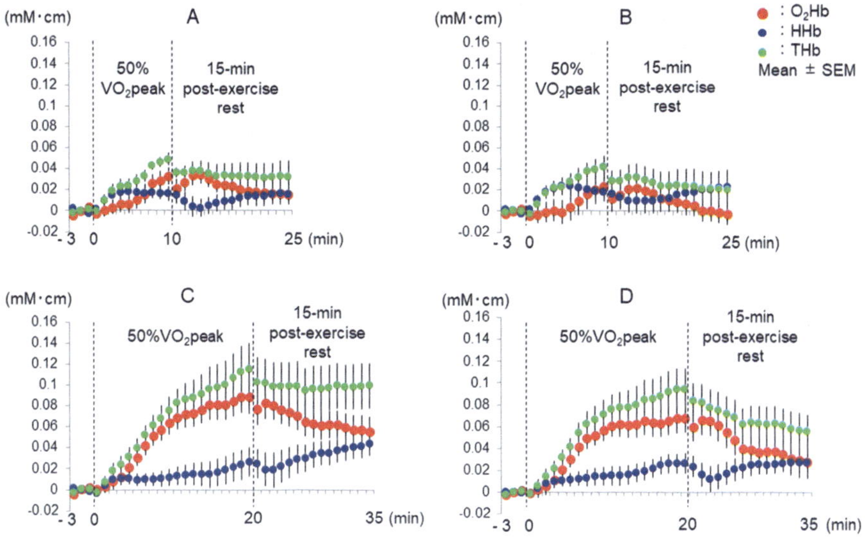

Fig. 2 Temporal changes in the average oxyhemoglobin (O_2Hb), deoxyhemoglobin (HHb) and total hemoglobin (THb) levels. Values are presented as the mean ± standard error of the mean (SEM). A: Left premotor cortex (L-PMC) 10-min exercise. B: Right premotor cortex (R-PMC) 10-min exercise. C: Left premotor cortex (L-PMC) 20-min exercise. D: Right premotor cortex (R-PMC) 20-min exercise

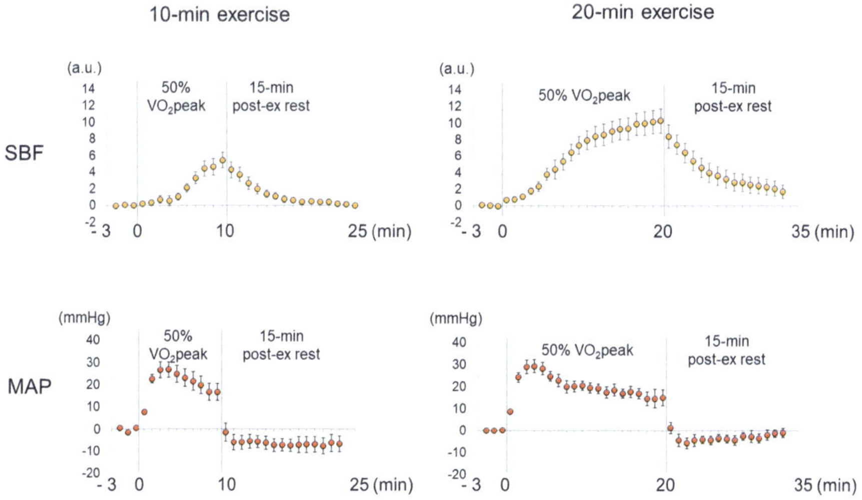

Fig. 3 Temporal changes in the average skin blood flow (SBF) and average mean arterial pressure (MAP). Values are presented as the mean ± standard error of the mean (SEM)

Table 2 Group comparison of O_2Hb, HHb and THb persisted throughout the 15-min post-exercise rest between exercise duration in both ROIs

		10-min exercise	20-min exercise	p value
O_2Hb (mM·cm)	R-PMC	0.008 ± 0.013	0.047 ± 0.010	0.075
	L-PMC	0.020 ± 0.007	0.063 ± 0.010	0.017
HHb (mM·cm)	R-PMC	0.013 ± 0.016	0.027 ± 0.011	0.517
	L-PMC	0.006 ± 0.011	0.015 ± 0.017	0.475
THb (mM·cm)	R-PMC	0.021 ± 0.014	0.073 ± 0.013	0.005
	L-PMC	0.026 ± 0.011	0.079 ± 0.020	0.012

O_2Hb, oxyhemoglobin; HHb, deoxyhemoglobin; THb, total hemoglobin; R-PMC, right premotor cortex; L-PMC, left premotor cortex. Values are presented as mean ± standard error of the mean (SEM)

4 Discussion

In the present study, we compared the effects of exercise duration on the persistence of O_2Hb levels in the PMC bilaterally after moderate-intensity cycling exercise. Our findings indicated that O_2Hb persistence was higher in the 20 min-exercise only in the L-PMC following cessation of exercise. As few studies have examined acute changes in cerebral oxygenation following exercise, our findings may provide insight into the mechanisms underlying exercise-induced neuroplasticity.

THb after the 20-min exercise was significantly higher than that after the 10-min exercise. However, O_2Hb after the 20-min exercise in L-PMC was higher than that after the 10-min exercise. These results suggested that cortical activation in L-PMC indicated by O_2Hb was higher after the 20-min exercise than that after the 10-min exercise although blood volume was higher after the 20-min exercise in both regions. Previous studies have reported that changes in O_2Hb reflect changes in cortical activation [3, 4]. The PMC plays a role in the preparation of movement for control and posture [17]. To maintain the sitting posture on the cycling ergometer, the PMC might maintain the activation after cessation of the exercise. This suggests that L-PMC may play an important role in posture control after the exercise depending on the exercise duration.

Our study had a limitation that the sites measuring SBF and O_2Hb were not close based on the methodological limitation. Although we could not measure the effect of SBF on O_2Hb changes, we estimated that the effect of SBF on O_2Hb might not be strong because we could observe asymmetrical O_2Hb changes during the 15-min post exercise rest.

This investigation found higher O_2Hb levels in the L-PMC after the 20-min exercise than that after the 10-min exercise. Some studies reported left-dominant O_2Hb elevation in the prefrontal cortex. Further studies are required to investigate the left-dominant oxygenation of the PMC.

Thus, the effects of exercise duration on O_2Hb persistence have laterality in the PMC, and this study may provide insight into the mechanism of neuroplasticity.

Acknowledgments This study was supported by a Grant-in-Aid for Scientific Research (C) from the Japan Society for the Promotion of Science (15 K01433) and a Grant-in-Aid for Exploratory Research from the Niigata University of Health and Welfare (H29C17).

References

1. Raichlen DA, Alexander GE (2017) Adaptive capacity: an evolutionary neuroscience model linking exercise, cognition, and brain health. Trends Neurosci 40(7):408–421. https://doi.org/10.1016/j.tins.2017.05.001
2. Hillman CH, Erickson KI, Kramer AF (2008) Be smart, exercise your heart: exercise effects on brain and cognition. Nat Rev Neurosci 9(1):58–65. https://doi.org/10.1038/nrn2298
3. Miyai I, Tanabe HC, Sase I et al (2001) Cortical mapping of gait in humans: a near-infrared spectroscopic topography study. NeuroImage 14(5):1186–1192. https://doi.org/10.1006/nimg.2001.0905
4. Obrig H, Wolf T, Doge C et al (1996) Cerebral oxygenation changes during motor and somatosensory stimulation in humans, as measured by near-infrared spectroscopy. Adv Exp Med Biol 388:219–224
5. Shibuya K, Kuboyama N, Tanaka J (2014) Changes in ipsilateral motor cortex activity during a unilateral isometric finger task are dependent on the muscle contraction force. Physiol Meas 35(3):417–428. https://doi.org/10.1088/0967-3334/35/3/417
6. Rupp T, Perrey S (2008) Prefrontal cortex oxygenation and neuromuscular responses to exhaustive exercise. Eur J Appl Physiol 102(2):153–163. https://doi.org/10.1007/s00421-007-0568-7
7. Yanagisawa H, Dan I, Tsuzuki D et al (2010) Acute moderate exercise elicits increased dorsolateral prefrontal activation and improves cognitive performance with Stroop test. NeuroImage 50(4):1702–1710. https://doi.org/10.1016/j.neuroimage.2009.12.023
8. Hyodo K, Dan I, Suwabe K et al (2012) Acute moderate exercise enhances compensatory brain activation in older adults. Neurobiol Aging 33(11):2621–2632. https://doi.org/10.1016/j.neurobiolaging.2011.12.022
9. Tsubaki A, Takehara N, Sato D et al (2017) Cortical oxyhemoglobin elevation persists after moderate-intensity cycling exercise: a near-infrared spectroscopy study. Adv Exp Med Biol 977:261–268. https://doi.org/10.1007/978-3-319-55231-6_36
10. Tsubaki A, Morishita S, Tokunaga Y (2018) Changes in cerebral oxyhaemoglobin levels during and after a single 20-minute bout of moderate-intensity cycling. Adv Exp Med Biol 1072:127–131. https://doi.org/10.1007/978-3-319-91287-5_20
11. Grafton ST, Fagg AH, Arbib MA (1998) Dorsal premotor cortex and conditional movement selection: a PET functional mapping study. J Neurophysiol 79:1092–1097. https://doi.org/10.1152/jn.1998.79.2.1092
12. Kubota K, Hamada I (1978) Visual tracking and neuron activity in the post-arcuate area in monkeys. J Physiol Paris 74:297–312
13. Weinrich M, Wise SP (1982) The premotor cortex of the monkey. J Neurosci 2:1329–1345
14. Suzuki M, Miyai I, Ono T et al (2004) Prefrontal and premotor cortices are involved in adapting walking and running speed on the treadmill: an optical imaging study. NeuroImage 23(3):1020–1026. https://doi.org/10.1016/j.neuroimage.2004.07.002
15. American Thoracic S, American College of Chest P (2003) ATS/ACCP statement on cardiopulmonary exercise testing. Am J Respir Crit Care Med 167(2):211–277. https://doi.org/10.1164/rccm.167.2.211
16. Boas DA, Gaudette T, Strangman G et al (2001) The accuracy of near infrared spectroscopy and imaging during focal changes in cerebral hemodynamics. NeuroImage 13(1):76–90. https://doi.org/10.1006/nimg.2000.0674
17. Leff DR, Orihuela-Espina F, Elwell CE et al (2011) Assessment of the cerebral cortex during motor task behaviours in adults: a systematic review of functional near infrared spectroscopy (fNIRS) studies. NeuroImage 54(4):2922–2936. https://doi.org/10.1016/j.neuroimage.2010.10.058

Relationship Between Muscle Oxygen Saturation and Exercise Load in Patients with Malignant Hematopoietic Disease

Tatsushi Wakasugi, Shinichiro Morishita, Katsuji Kaida, Yusuke Itani, Kazuhiro Ikegame, Norihiko Kodama, Hiroyasu Ogawa, Yoshihiro Fujimori, and Kazuhisa Domen

Abstract Our previous research confirmed that patients with malignant hematopoietic disease already had a low hemoglobin level before allogeneic hematopoietic stem cell transplantation (allo-HSCT). However, no study has determined whether a correlation exists between exercise load, hemoglobin level, and muscle oxygen saturation (SmO_2), during exercise. Therefore, the purpose of this study was to investigate whether near-infrared spectroscopy (NIRS)-derived SmO_2 is associated with exercise load, as determined by a dynamometer, before allo-HSCT. This study included 19 male patients who received allo-HSCT in Hyogo College of Medicine Hospital (Japan) between November 2009 and October 2012. Patients performed isometric repeated dorsiflexion at 50% maximum voluntary contraction for 180 s to determine exercise load, and SmO_2 was evaluated during exercise at the same time using NIRS (BOM-L1TRW, Omega Wave, Inc., Japan). The hemoglobin level was also evaluated before allo-HSCT. Patients with hematopoietic disease before allo-HSCT already had a low hemoglobin level. There was a significant correlation between exercise load and ΔSmO_2; however, the hemoglobin level was not correlated with exercise load. In these patients, exercise load might be affected by muscle oxygen consumption rather than by the hemoglobin level. This finding shows that NIRS can used to assess fatigue in patients with malignant hematopoietic disease.

T. Wakasugi (✉) · Y. Itani
Department of Physical Medicine and Rehabilitation, Hyogo Collage of Medicine Hospital, Nishinomiya, Hyogo, Japan

S. Morishita
Department of Rehabilitation Medicine, Hyogo College of Medicine, Nishinomiya, Japan

Institute for Human Movement and Medical Science, Niigata University of Health and Welfare, Niigata, Japan

K. Kaida · K. Ikegame · H. Ogawa · Y. Fujimori
Division of Hematology, Department of Internal Medicine, Hyogo College of Medicine, Nishinomiya, Japan

N. Kodama · K. Domen
Department of Rehabilitation Medicine, Hyogo College of Medicine, Nishinomiya, Japan

© Springer Nature Switzerland AG 2020
P.-D. Ryu et al. (eds.), *Oxygen Transport to Tissue XLI*, Advances in Experimental Medicine and Biology 1232, https://doi.org/10.1007/978-3-030-34461-0_25

Keywords Near-infrared spectroscopy · Malignant hematopoietic disease · Hemoglobin · Muscle · Exercise load

1 Introduction

Patients with malignant hematopoietic disease already have exercise intolerance before allogeneic hematopoietic stem cell transplantation (allo-HSCT) [1]. The exercise intolerance observed during allo-HSCT treatment in a sterile room affects patients' quality of life [2]. However, the mechanism of exercise intolerance in patients with malignant hematopoietic disease before allo-HSCT is unclear. Therefore, we investigated whether exercise intolerance is associated with the hemoglobin level or near-infrared spectroscopy (NIRS)-derived muscle oxygen consumption. Hemoglobin is responsible for the ability of the red blood cells to transport oxygen. In our previous study, patients with malignant hematopoietic disease already had a low hemoglobin level before allo-HSCT. The low hemoglobin level induced fatigue and exercise intolerance [3]. Furthermore, fatigue is associated with NIRS-derived muscle oxygen consumption [4]. Our previous study reported that there was a correlation between the hemoglobin level and exercise capacity according to the 6-min walking test [5]. However, no study has determined whether a correlation exists between exercise load, the hemoglobin level, and muscle oxygen saturation (SmO_2) during exercise. NIRS is used to non-invasively assess SmO_2 during exercise, and SmO_2 is a parameter that represents the dynamic balance between oxygen consumption and oxygen supply [6]. The purpose of this study was to investigate whether NIRS-derived SmO_2 during exercise is associated with exercise load, as determined by a dynamometer, in patients with malignant hematopoietic disease before all-HSCT.

2 Methods

2.1 Participants and Data Collection

In this observational study conducted between November 2009 and October 2012, we investigated the relationship between exercise load, the hemoglobin level, and SmO_2 during an exercise task by using NIRS in patients with malignant hematopoietic disease in Hyogo College of Medicine Hospital (Japan). The Hyogo College of Medicine Institutional Committee on Human Research approved the study, and written informed consent was obtained from each patient before study participation. The following information was collected from patients' medical records: age, sex, height, diagnosis, and hemoglobin level.

2.2 Exercise Load

A dynamometer (Biodex System 4, Biodex Medical Systems, Inc. USA) was used to measure exercise load on the ankle dorsiflexor (units = Nm/kg). The isometric measurement mode was used to assess exercise load. All patients were instructed to perform a repeated isometric contraction task at 50% maximum voluntary isometric contraction (MVIC) with their right leg. Exercise load was adjusted at 50% duty cycle (1 sof contraction/1 s of release) for 180 s (90 times) using pace sounds. A line representing the 50% MVIC target torque level was displayed on the computer screen with the actual torque output, which provided real-time feedback of torque to the patients. Exercise load was determined by the mean value of peak torque during the exercise task (units = Nm/kg × 100). The %MVIC (units = %) represented the ratio of the mean values of peak torque during the exercise task to peak torque during MVIC, and it was calculated by the following formula: [%MVIC (%) = peak torque mean (Nm/kg) during the exercise task / peak torque during MVIC (Nm/kg) × 100].

2.3 NIRS Measurements

A laser tissue blood oximeter (BOM-L1TRW, Omega Wave, Inc., Japan) was used to assess the decrease in SmO_2 values, which was determined by the relative change from the resting SmO_2 values (Fig. 1). The ΔSmO_2 values represent greater oxygen metabolic demand on the skeletal muscle [7]. The dorsiflexor muscle group was selected for this experiment because the skeletal muscles produce intramuscular pressures that lead to blood flow restriction during voluntary isometric contractions [8].

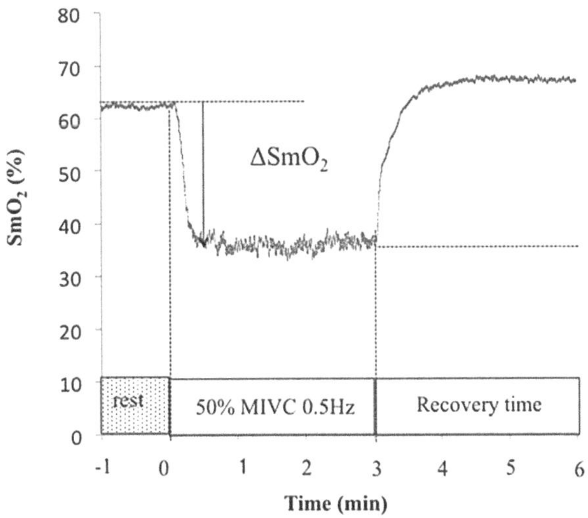

Fig. 1 Protocol of the experiment, an example of a tissue oxygen saturation trace, and example of dorsiflexor muscle oxygen saturation during 50% maximum voluntary isometric contraction in one patient

Patients were placed in a seated position with their foot fixed to the ankle attachment device. The optical probe was placed 100 mm from the lower edge of the patella on the tibialis anterior muscle of each patient [5].

2.4 Statistical Analysis

Pearson's correlation tests were used to evaluate the relationship between exercise load, the hemoglobin level, and ΔSmO_2. We also used Spearman's correlation test to evaluate the relationship between %MVIC and ΔSmO_2. Statistical analyses were performed using SPSS 21.0 (SPSS Japan, Inc., Tokyo, Japan) with statistical significance set at $p < 0.05$.

3 Results

This study included 19 male patients with malignant hematopoietic disease; their clinical characteristics at diagnosis are shown in Table 1. Exercise load had a significant correlation with ΔSmO_2 ($r = 0.537$, $R^2 = 0.286$, $p < 0.05$) (Fig. 2a); however, there was no correlation between exercise load and the serum hemoglobin level ($r = 0.05$, $p = 0.84$) (Fig. 3) Furthermore, %MVIC was correlated with ΔSmO_2 ($r = 0.484$, $p < 0.05$) (Fig. 2b).

Table 1 Characteristics of patients with malignant hematopoietic disease (n = 19)

Characteristic		Value
Age (in years)		42.6 ± 14.4
Sex	Male	19
Height (cm)		172.8 ± 6.01
Body weight (kg)		66.02 ± 10.4
Body fat (%)		19.64 ± 6.09
Body mass index		24.01 ± 9.11
Diagnosis	Acute lymphoblastic leukemia	3
	Acute myeloid leukemia	7
	Myelodysplastic syndrome	2
	Chronic myelogenous leukemia	2
	Hodgkin's lymphoma	1
	Non-Hodgkin's lymphoma	2
Hemoglobin level (g/dL)		11.1 ± 1.75
ΔSmO_2 (%)		22.03 ± 8.24
Exercise load (Nm/kg)		23.96 ± 8.04
%MVIC (%)		56.13 ± 5.86

Values are presented as a median ± standard deviation.

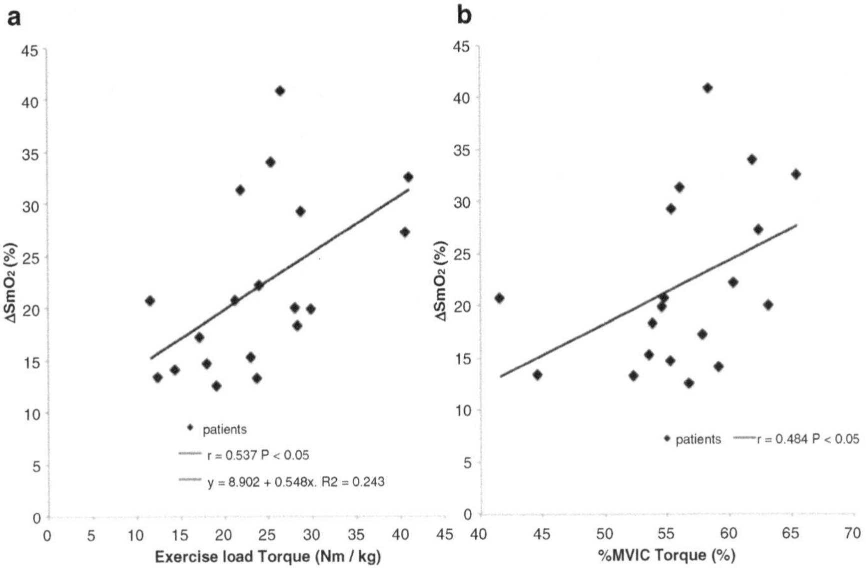

Fig. 2 Correlations between changes in muscle oxygen saturation and exercise load: (**a**) peak torque mean and (**b**) percent maximum voluntary isometric contraction

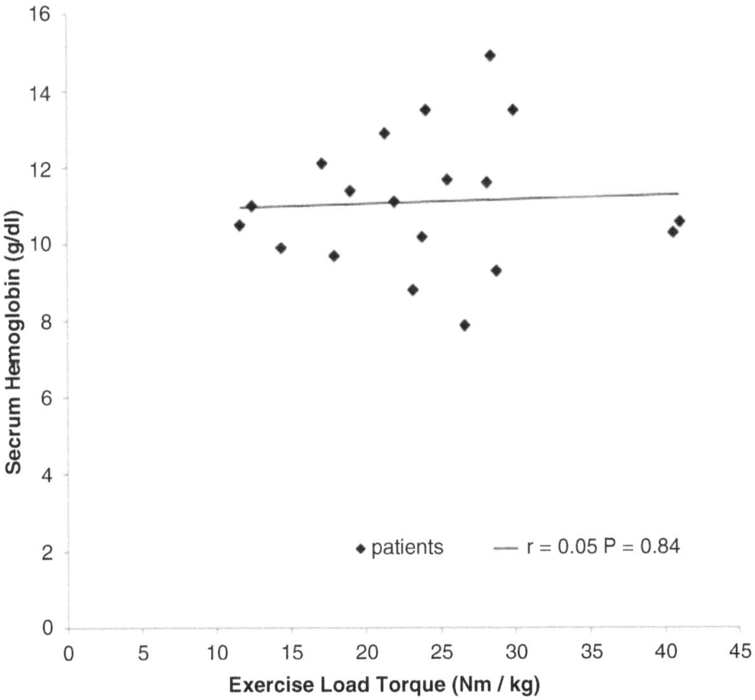

Fig. 3 Correlations between the serum hemoglobin level and dorsiflexor exercise load (in peak torque mean) for 3 min

4 Discussion

In the present study, patients with malignant hematopoietic disease before allo-HSCT already had a low hemoglobin level (Table 1). We found a significant correlation between exercise load and ΔSmO_2 in patients with malignant hematopoietic disease. However, the hemoglobin level was not correlated with exercise load. We think our findings suggest that in these patients, exercise load might be affected by muscle oxygen consumption rather than by the hemoglobin level. In this study, patients were instructed to perform an isometric contraction task at 50% MVC. A previous study reported that ΔSmO_2 values were different for each exercise load (i.e., low, moderate, and submaximal) [8]. In the present study, %MVIC was also correlated with ΔSmO2. These results suggest that oxygen consumption in skeletal muscle during moderate exercise might be affected by the amount of absolute workload or relative workload from MVIC that patients performed. SmO_2, as a parameter during exercise, might be useful to investigate patients' fatigue in the clinical setting. The present study has some limitations. First, the sample size of 19 subjects was small and it was a convenience sample. As a result of linear regression analysis between exercise load and ΔSmO_2 values, the regression equation was significant in variance analysis, and the regression coefficient was significant. However, the coefficient of determination was small ($R^2 = 0.286$), and predictive accuracy was low. In the future, we need to increase the sample size. Furthermore, our study did not have a control, so we will need to include an age-matched control. Additionally, longitudinal studies are required to evaluate this topic further and corroborate our findings.

5 Conclusions

The decrease in SmO_2 values during the isometric dorsiflexion exercise task (50% MVC) indicated that patients' exercise load was associated with muscle oxygen consumption rather than with the hemoglobin level. This indeed shows that NIRS can used to investigate fatigue in patients with malignant hematopoietic disease.

Acknowledgments This study was supported by the Japan Society for the Promotion of Science (KAKENHI grant number 18H00508.

References

1. Morishita S, Kaida K, Ikegame K et al (2012) Impaired physical function and health-related QOL in patients before hematopoietic stem-cell transplantation. Support Care Cancer 20:821–829
2. Morishita S, Kaida K, Tanaka T et al (2012) Prevalence of sarcopenia and relevance of body composition physiological function, fatigue, health related quality of life in patients before allogeneic hematopoietic stem cell transplantation. Support Care Cancer 20:3161–3168

3. Wiskemann J, Dreger P, Schwerdtfeger R et al (2011) Effects of a partly self-administered exercise program before, during, and after allogeneic stem cell transplantation. Blood 117:2604–2613
4. Morishita S, Wakasugi T, Kaida K et al (2018) Fatigue, muscle oxygen consumption and blood flow to the skeletal muscle after allogeneic hematopoietic stem cell transplantation. Adv Exp Med Biol
5. Wakasugi T, Morishita S, Kaida K et al (2018) Impaired skeletal muscle oxygenation following allogeneic hematopoietic stem cell transplantation is associated with exercise capacity. Support Care Cancer 26:2149–2160
6. Ferrari M, Muthalib M, Quaresima V (2011) The use of near-infrared spectroscopy in understanding skeletal muscle physiology: recent developments. Philos Trans A Math Phys Eng Sci 369:4577–4590
7. McNeil C, Murray B, Rice CL (2006) Differential changes in muscle oxygenation between voluntary and stimulated isometric fatigue of human dorsiflexors. J Appl Physiol 100:890–895
8. Paiziev A, Wolf M, Kerimov F (2017) Dorsiflexor muscle oxygenation during low, moderate and submaximal sustained isometric contraction. Adv Exp Med Biol 977:21–26

Comparison of the Effects of Continuous and Intermittent Exercise on Cerebral Oxygenation and Cognitive Function

Yuya Ichinose, Shinichiro Morishita, Rio Suzuki, Gaku Endo, and Atsuhiro Tsubaki

Abstract Cognitive function is reported to improve by moderate aerobic exercise. However, the effects of intermittent exercise with rest between the moderate-intensity exercise are unclear. Therefore, this study aimed to compare the effects of continuous and intermittent exercise on cerebral oxygenation and cognitive function. This study included 18 healthy adults. For the continuous exercise protocol, 5 min of rest was followed by 30 min of exercise; 5 min of rest was allowed after each exercise. For the intermittent exercise protocol, 3 sets of 10 min of exercise were completed, with 5 min of rest between the sets. Exercise intensity was 50% of maximum oxygen uptake. Oxyhemoglobin (O_2Hb) in the prefrontal cortex (PFC) was measured during each protocol, and cognitive tasks (Stroop test) were performed before and after exercise. O_2Hb levels for the left and right PFCs were significantly higher post-exercise than pre-exercise for both exercise protocols ($p < 0.01$). The average reaction time in the Stroop test was significantly shorter post-exercise than pre-exercise for both protocols ($p < 0.01$). There was no significant difference in the error rate pre- and post-exercise for both protocols (continuous $p = 0.22$; intermittent $p = 0.44$). There was no significant difference between both protocols in all measurement results (O_2Hb: $p = 0.67$; average reaction time $p = 0.50$; error rate $p = 0.24$). O_2Hb was higher and average reaction time was shorter after exercise than before exercise for both exercise protocols. Intermittent and continuous exercise may improve cognitive function to the same degree after exercise.

Keywords Intermittent exercise · Continuous exercise · Cognitive function · Oxygenated hemoglobin · NIRS

Y. Ichinose · R. Suzuki · G. Endo
Department of Physical Therapy, Niigata University of Health and Welfare, Niigata, Japan

S. Morishita · A. Tsubaki (✉)
Department of Physical Therapy, Niigata University of Health and Welfare, Niigata, Japan

Institute for Human Movement and Medical Sciences, Niigata University of Health and Welfare, Niigata, Japan
e-mail: tsubaki@nuhw.ac.jp

© Springer Nature Switzerland AG 2020

P.-D. Ryu et al. (eds.), *Oxygen Transport to Tissue XLI*, Advances in Experimental Medicine and Biology 1232, https://doi.org/10.1007/978-3-030-34461-0_26

1 Introduction

Studies have indicated that cognitive function can be improved by performing moderate-intensity exercise. Regarding the acute effects in young adults, 10 min of moderate-intensity exercise shortens the Stroop test reaction times and increases the oxyhemoglobin (O_2Hb) level in the prefrontal cortex (PFC) [1], while 15 min of exercise reduces the reaction time and increases neural activation in the PFC [2]. Further, the relationship between cognitive function and physical activity level has also been clarified, and it is reported that activities in the performance functional area were significantly higher in a high physical activity group than in a low physical activity group [3].

Moderate-intensity exercise of ≥30 min is recommended for increasing physical activity [4]. It is also recommended that rest intervals should be interposed between exercises to extend the exercise time for persons in whom exercise is difficult to continue [5]. However, to our knowledge, the effect of moderate-intensity intermittent exercise on brain function is unknown. Clarifying the effects of moderate-intensity exercise on brain function can inform clinicians and therapists about optimal exercise therapy strategies in the clinical setting.

Therefore, this study aimed to clarify the influence of moderate-intensity intermittent exercise and continuous exercise on PFC O_2Hb and cognitive function using near-infrared spectroscopy (NIRS).

2 Methods

2.1 *Participants*

Of the 18 healthy volunteers who participated in this study, none had symptoms of neurological, medical, or cardiovascular disease, and all were free of medication at the time of the study. Each participant provided written informed consent after receiving information regarding the potential risks, study objectives, measurement techniques, and benefits associated with the study. This study was approved by the Ethics Committee of Niigata University of Health and Welfare and conformed to the standards outlined in the Declaration of Helsinki.

2.2 *Experimental Procedure*

Individual exercise workload was determined based on maximal oxygen consumption (VO_2max) during an incremental cycling protocol (Aerobike 75XLII; Combi, Tokyo, Japan). Measurements of VO_2max were obtained prior to the main experiments using an automated metabolic analyzer (AE-310, Minato Medical Science, Osaka, Japan). Exhaustion was defined as previously described [6].

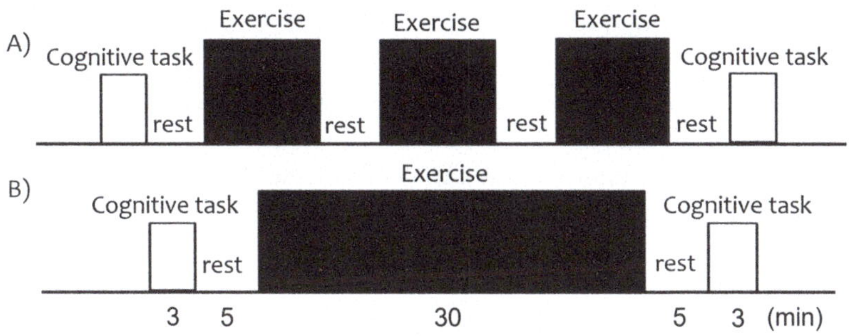

Fig. 1 Experimental protocol: (**A**) intermittent exercise and (**B**) continuous exercise

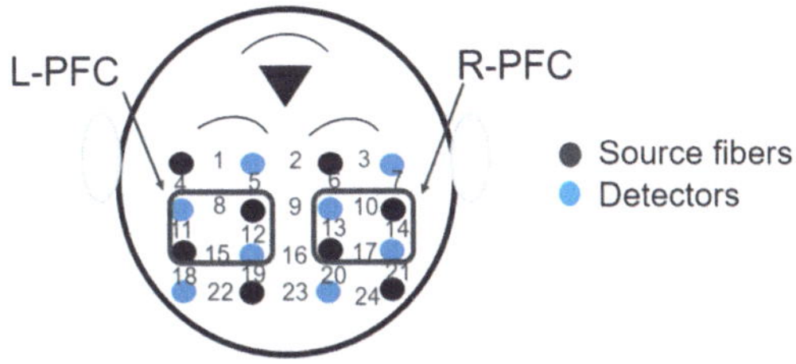

Fig. 2 Location of the 8 light-source fibers and 8 detectors, and regions of interest

Exercise intensity was considered as 50% of maximum oxygen intake (50% VO_2max). The intermittent exercise protocol comprised three sets of 10-min exercise with a rest period of 5 min between each set (Fig. 1a). For continuous exercise, the main exercise was performed continuously for 30 min (Fig. 1b). A cognitive task was performed for 3 min before and after exercise, with a rest period of 5 min before and after exercise. The NIRS signals were measured continuously during the experiment. Cognitive function was evaluated with a Stroop task (average reaction time [RT], error rate). Three difficulty levels were set for the Stroop task (neutral, congruent, and incongruent), with 30 problems and 10 difficulty levels for each problem.

A multichannel NIRS imaging system (OMM-3000; Shimadzu Co., Kyoto, Japan) with multiple continuous wavelengths (780, 805, and 830 nm) was utilized to detect changes in O_2Hb and deoxyhemoglobin (HHb) at a sampling rate of 130 ms. The NIRS optodes consisted of 12 light-source fibers and 12 detectors, which provided 24-channel simultaneous recording. The optodes were arranged in a 4 × 6 fashion in a multichannel probe holder, and a 30-mm interoptode distance was employed to measure cortical tissue oxygenation. The Fpz position of the international 10–20 system [7], which was originally developed for electroencephalography, was used to ensure consistent optode placement among all participants. Regions of interest included the right PFC (Chaps. 10, 13, 14 and 17; R-PFC) and left PFC (Chaps. 8, 11, 12 and 15; L-PFC) (Fig. 2).

L-PFC, left prefrontal cortex; R-PFC, right prefrontal cortex.

2.3 Statistical Analysis

O_2Hb was calculated with respect to the average value at rest and the average value was calculated every minute. O_2Hb values were averaged and compared before exercise for 5 min and following rest after 5 min of exercise. The average RT was the number of problems per RT, and the error rate was calculated as the number of incorrect answers per problem number. O_2Hb, average RT, and error rate were compared based on condition factors and time factors using two-way analysis of variance. Statistical significance was set at $p < 0.05$.

3 Results

Levels of O_2Hb of the left and right PFCs were significantly higher post-exercise than pre-exercise for both exercise protocols ($p < 0.01$). Levels of HHb of the left and right PFCs were also significantly higher post-exercise than pre-exercise for both protocols ($p < 0.01$). The average RT in the Stroop test was significantly shorter post-exercise than pre-exercise for both exercise protocols ($p < 0.01$). No significant difference was found in the error rate pre- and post-exercise for both protocols. Additionally, no significant difference was found between the exercise protocols for any of the measurement results (Table 1).

Table 1 Oxygenation kinetics in intermittent and continuous cycling exercise and changes in cognitive function

		Before exercise	After exercise	Time factor	Condition factor
Right PFC O_2Hb (mM·cm)	Intermittent	−0.000 ± 0.000	0.073 ± 0.084	p < 0.01	p = 0.79
	Continuous	−0.000 ± −0.000	0.079 ± 0.047		
Left PFC O_2Hb (mM·cm)	Intermittent	0.000 ± 0.002	0.092 ± 0.086	p < 0.01	p = 0.67
	Continuous	0.000 ± 0.004	0.081 ± 0.063		
Right PFC HHb (mM·cm)	Intermittent	0.000 ± 0.001	0.044 ± 0.075	p < 0.05	p = 0.44
	Continuous	−0.000 ± −0.000	0.027 ± 0.003		
Left PFC HHb (mM·cm)	Intermittent	−0.000 ± 0.000	0.012 ± 0.036	p < 0.05	p = 0.46
	Continuous	0.000 ± 0.002	0.022 ± 0.047		
Average RT (ms)	Intermittent	729.2 ± 106.9	689.7 ± 88.6	p < 0.01	p = 0.50
	Continuous	763.1 ± 149.0	711.2 ± 145.6		
Error rate (%)	Intermittent	2.57 ± 0.03	1.83 ± 0.02	p = 0.11	p = 0.24
	Continuous	3.86 ± 0.04	2.20 ± 0.02		

Values are presented as mean ± standard deviation.
PFC, prefrontal cortex; O_2Hb, oxyhemoglobin; HHb, deoxyhemoglobin; RT, reaction time

4 Discussion

This study compared the effects of intermittent and continuous cycling exercise at 50% peak VO_2 intensity on cerebral oxygenation kinetics and cognitive function. Levels of O_2Hb and HHb of the left and right PFCs showed a significant increase after exercise compared to before exercise. However, there was no significant difference between the kinetic modes of intermittent exercise and continuous exercise.

Changes in cerebral hemodynamics and metabolism can be evaluated with NIRS, and these factors can subsequently be used to evaluate changes in brain activity [8] based on neurovascular coupling [9]. Changes in O_2Hb are reported to reflect changes in cortical activation [10]. Studies showed that O_2Hb levels increased significantly even after short moderate-intensity exercise for 10 min [11]. Moreover, O_2Hb is maintained at a high level even after 5 min post-exercise [12]. These findings suggest that the level of O_2Hb of the left and right PFCs also increased significantly in intermittent exercise, which involves the repetition of moderate-intensity exercise over a short period, as in the present study. Further, it is reported that O_2Hb does not increase with exercise of 20% VO_2max [2]. From this report, it is considered that exercise intensity exerts an influence on the increase of the O_2Hb level. In this study, it is considered that the increase of O_2Hb did not show any difference from intermittent exercise or continuous exercise by setting exercise intensity to 50% VO_2max load for both exercise protocols.

In both intermittent and continuous exercise, the average RT was significantly shortened after exercise. However, there was no significant difference in the error rate between pre- and post-exercise. Moreover, there was no significant difference between the kinetic modes of intermittent exercise and continuous exercise. Studies also reported that exercise exerts acute effects on brain function. A similar study revealed that moderate-intensity exercise improved cognitive function, as indicated by a decreased post-exercise RT in the Stroop test [2]. Moreover, 10 min of moderate-intensity exercise improved cognitive performance in the Stroop test in both young and older adults, suggesting that exercise enhances prefrontal oxygenation during the cognitive task [1]. These results indicate that cognitive function improvement occurred due to the increased neural activation of the PFC as a result of exercise. An increase in O_2Hb and a decrease in HHb are considered indicators of an increase in neuron activation [13]. However, in another study, the increase in HHb reflected neuron activity [14]. It has been reported that HHb is related to the neurocoupling system [15]. In this study, both O_2Hb and HHb increased. This result is also thought to reflect neuron activity. However, NIRS response is reported to be affected by systemic physiological changes [13]. In this study, we have not measured the scalp blood flow and could not evaluate the extracranial blood flow state. As a result, it is difficult to identify whether improvement of cognitive function is due to neuron activity or increased blood flow, which is the limitation of this research. Future studies should conduct experiments by retreating the surface hemodynamics and capturing only neuron activity.

In conclusion, the results of this study suggest that cognitive function improves with both intermittent exercise with intervening rest periods, and with continuous exercise. However, there was no difference between exercise protocols.

Acknowledgments This study was supported by a Grant-in-Aid for Exploratory Research from the Niigata University of Health and Welfare (A. Tsubaki), Japan.

References

1. Yanagisawa H, Dan I, Tsuzuki D et al (2010) Acute moderate exercise elicits increased dorsolateral prefrontal activation and improves cognitive performance with Stroop test. NeuroImage 50:1702–1710. https://doi.org/10.1016/j.neuroimage.2009.12.023
2. Endo K, Matsukawa K, Liang N et al (2013) Dynamic exercise improves cognitive function in association with increased prefrontal oxygenation. J Physiol Sci 63:287–298. https://doi.org/10.1007/s12576-013-0267-6
3. Matsuda K, Ikeda S, Mitsutake T et al (2017) Factors influencing executive function by physical activity level among young adults: a near-infrared spectroscopy study. J Phys Ther Sci 29:470–475. https://doi.org/10.1589/jpts.29.470
4. Pate RR, Pratt M, Blair SN et al (1995) Physical activity and public health. A recommendation from the Centers for Disease Control and Prevention and the American college of sports medicine. JAMA 273:402–407. https://doi.org/10.1006/jama.1995.03520290054029
5. American Association of Cardiovascular and Pulmonary Rehabilitation (2004) Guideline for cardiac rehabilitation and secondary prevention, vol 4. Human Kinetics, Illinois, pp 135–175
6. Rupp T, Perrey S (2008) Prefrontal cortex oxygenation and neuromuscular responses to exhaustive exercise. Eur J Appl Physiol 102:153–163. https://doi.org/10.1007/s00421-007-0568-7
7. Jasper HH (1958) The ten–twenty electrode system of the international federation. Electroencephalogr Clin Neurophysiol 10:367–380
8. Tamura M, Hoshi Y, Okada F (1997) Localized near-infrared spectroscopy and functional optical imaging of brain activity. Philos Trans R Soc Lond Ser B Biol Sci 352:737–742. https://doi.org/10.1098/rstb.1997.0056
9. Phillips AA, Chan FH, Zheng MM et al (2016) Neurovascular coupling in humans: physiology, methodological advances and clinical implications. J Cereb Blood Flow Metab 36:647–664. https://doi.org/10.1177/0271678X15617954
10. Miyai I, Tanabe HC, Sase I et al (2001) Cortical mapping of gait in humans: a near-infrared spectroscopic topography study. NeuroImage 14:1186–1192. https://doi.org/10.1006/nimg.2001.0905
11. Tsubaki A, Takehara N, Sato D et al (2017) Cortical oxyhemoglobin elevation persists after moderate-intensity cycling exercise: a near-infrared spectroscopy study. Adv Exp Med Biol 977:261–268
12. Tsubaki A, Morishita S, Tokunaga Y et al (2018) Changes in cerebral oxyhaemoglobin levels during and after a single 20-minute bout of moderate-intensity cycling. Adv Exp Med Biol 1072:127–131
13. Tachtsidis I, Scholkmann F (2016) False positives and false negatives in functional near-infrared spectroscopy: issues, challenges, and the way forward. Neurophotonics 3:031405
14. Perrey S (2009) Decrease in cerebral oxygenation influences central motor output in humans. Acta Physiol 196:279–281
15. Magistretti PJ (2006) Neuron-glia metabolic coupling and plasticity. J Exper Biol 209: 2304–2311

Relationship Between Exercise Capacity and Muscle O_2Hb Saturation in Patients Before Hematopoietic Stem-Cell Transplantation

Shinichiro Morishita, Tatsushi Wakasugi, Katsuji Kaida, Yusuke Itani, Kazuhiro Ikegame, Hiroyasu Ogawa, Yoshihiro Fujimori, and Kazuhisa Domen

Abstract Patients with hematological malignancy might already have decreased muscle oxygen saturation at rest and exercise capacity before undergoing hematopoietic stem cell transplantation (HSCT). However, to date, no studies have investigated the relationship between exercise capacity and muscle oxygen saturation at rest in these patients. Therefore, purpose of this study was to investigate the relationship between exercise capacity and muscle oxygen–hemoglobin (O2Hb) saturation (SmO2) at rest and patients' hemoglobin level before undergoing HSCT. *Methods:* This study included 60 men with hematologic disease who underwent allo-HSCT. Patients performed a 6-minute walk test (6MWT) to determine exercise capacity, and muscle O2Hb saturation at rest was evaluatabed using near-infrared spectroscopy (BOM-L1TRW, Omegawave Inc., Japan); hemoglobin levels in hematological malignancy patients before undergoing HSCT were also evaluated. *Results:* There was a significant correlation between the 6MWT and muscle O2Hb saturation at rest in hematological malignancy patients ($p < 0.05$). Additionally, the 6MWT was significantly correlated to the hemoglobin level ($p < 0.05$). Furthermore,

---

S. Morishita (✉)
Institute for Human Movement and Medical Science, Niigata University of Health and Welfare, Niigata, Japan

Department of Physical Medicine and Rehabilitation, Hyogo College of Medicine, Nishinomiya, Japan
e-mail: morishita@nuhw.ac.jp

T. Wakasugi · Y. Itani
Department of Rehabilitation Medicine, Hyogo College of Medicine Hospital, Nishinomiya, Japan

K. Kaida · K. Ikegame · H. Ogawa · Y. Fujimori
Division of Hematology, Department of Internal Medicine, Hyogo College of Medicine, Nishinomiya, Japan

K. Domen
Department of Physical Medicine and Rehabilitation, Hyogo College of Medicine, Nishinomiya, Japan

© Springer Nature Switzerland AG 2020

P.-D. Ryu et al. (eds.), *Oxygen Transport to Tissue XLI*, Advances in Experimental Medicine and Biology 1232, https://doi.org/10.1007/978-3-030-34461-0_27

muscle O2Hb saturation at rest was significantly related to hemoglobin level ($p < 0.05$). *Conclusion*: In patients with hematological malignancy, a relationship exists between exercise capacity, muscle O2Hb saturation, and hemoglobin level before they undergo HSCT. Therefore, rehabilitation staff, nurses, and physicians should recognize these relationships in patients who undergo allo-HSCT. Moreover, physiotherapists may need to promote muscle oxidative metabolism through exercise to increase exercise capacity in these patients.

Keywords Hematopoietic stem cell transplantation · Muscle oxygen–hemoglobin · Near-infrared spectroscopy · Rehabilitation · Physical therapy

1 Introduction

Allogeneic hematopoietic stem cell transplantation (allo-HSCT) is a potentially curative treatment for patients with hematological malignancy [1, 2] and is being increasingly used to treat hematopoietic diseases worldwide [3, 4]. A patient with hematological malignancy who has undergone HSCT has decreased exercise capacity after transplantation compared to that before HSCT [5]. Furthermore, our previous research showed that a relationship exists between exercise capacity and hemoglobin levels in patients before HSCT [6]. Patients might already have decreased muscle oxygen saturation at rest and exercise capacity before undergoing HSCT. However, to date, no studies have investigated the relationship between exercise capacity and muscle oxygen saturation at rest in these patients. Near-infrared spectroscopy (NIRS) can be used for non-invasive assessment of muscle oxygenation and hemodynamic parameters during exercise [7]. The purpose of this study was to investigate the relationship between exercise capacity and muscle O_2Hb saturation (SmO_2) at rest and patients' hemoglobin level before undergoing HSCT.

2 Methods

2.1 Participants

In this prospective observational study, we investigated the relationship between hemoglobin, muscle O2Hb saturation (SmO_2) in skeletal muscles by using NIRS, and exercise capacity among patients who had undergone allo-HSCT at the Hyogo College of Medicine Hospital, Japan, between November 2009 and February 2016. Sixty patients met our inclusion criteria and were enrolled in the study. Ethical approval of the study was obtained from the Institutional Committee on Human Research of the Hyogo College of Medicine. The following information was collected from the medical records: age, sex, height, hemoglobin level, underlying hematological diagnosis, stem cell source, and conditioning. Patient evaluation was performed 3 weeks before transplantation. Consequently, 60 hematological malignancy patients were included in this study (Table 1).

Table 1 Demographic and clinical characteristics of HSCT in 60 patients

Characteristics		
		Median (range)
Age (in years)		38.5 (18-63)
Sex (number, n)	Male	60
		Mean (SD)
Height (cm)		170.9 (7.0)
Body weight (kg)		64.0 (11.1)
Diagnosis (n)	Acute leukemia	33
	Malignant lymphoma	13
	Myelodysplastic syndrome	10
	Chronic myelogenous leukemia	2
	Multiple myeloma	1
	Primary immunodeficiency	1
Donor (n)	HLA-matched/related	3
	HLA-matched/unrelated	2
	HLA-mismatched/related	47
	HLA-mismatched/unrelated	8
Stem cell source (n)	Peripheral blood stem cell	44
	Bone marrow	8
	Cord blood	8
Conditioning (n)	Myeloablative	16
	Reduced intensity	44
		Mean (SD)
Hemoglobin (g/dL)		10.2 (2.1)
SmO_2 rest (%)		59.8 (7.6)
6MWT (m)		520.4 (68.1)

HLA = human leukocyte antigen; HSCT = hematopoietic stem cell transplantation

2.2 NIRS Measurements

A laser tissue oximeter (BOM-L1TRW Omega Wave, Japan) was used to measure SmO_2. SmO_2 reflects the dynamic balance of O_2 supplied by the microcirculation and O_2 consumption by the muscle. The NIRS signals were continuously stored at 10 Hz using Power Lab (AD Instruments, Nagoya, Japan) on a personal computer and analyzed using Lab Chart software (AD Instruments, Nagoya, Japan). NIRS directly measures the oxygen-dependent absorption of hemoglobin (Hb) in microvessels (i.e., arterioles, capillaries, and venules) and myoglobin in the muscle cytoplasm. We evaluated SmO_2 rest during 60 s of rest. The resting values of SmO_2 were determined as the mean value for 60 s during rest. Using the tibialis anterior (TA) muscle, we monitored the muscle oxidative extraction and dynamics of hemoglobin. The dorsiflexor muscle group was selected for this experiment because the restrictive sheath of the anterior compartment induces high levels of intramuscular pressure during voluntary isometric contractions, and a proposed contraction intensity for complete occlusion has been identified in young males. The TA is suitable for clinical NIRS measurement because of its relatively small size and thin adipose layer, suggesting that the area beneath the probe is more representative of the whole muscle than it would be in a muscle like the quadriceps [8].

2.3 *Exercise Capacity (6MWT)*

The 6-minute walk test (6MWT) was used as a sub-maximal exercise capacity test and was conducted according to the American Thoracic Society guidelines [9]. Patients walked along a 20-m corridor at our department for 6 min at their own pace. Patients were encouraged to cover as much distance as possible but were permitted to rest as needed and to continue walking as soon as they felt able to, or to stop if they experienced symptoms of dyspnea or leg pain. The distance (in meters) traveled during the 6 min were measured.

2.4 *Statistical Analysis*

Pearson's product moment correlation coefficient was used to evaluate the relationship between the hemoglobin, SmO_2 rest, and 6MWT. Statistical analyses were performed using SPSS 21.0 (SPSS Japan Inc., Tokyo, Japan), with statistical significance set at $p < 0.05$.

3 Results

The median age of the patients in this study was 38.5 years; 100% were men. Patients' hematological diseases included acute leukemia, malignant lymphoma, myelodysplastic syndrome, chronic myelogenous leukemia, multiple myeloma, and primary immunodeficiency. Sixteen patients received myeloablative conditioning and 44 patients received reduced intensity conditioning. The mean hemoglobin value was 10.2 g/dL, SmO_2 at rest for the TA muscle was 59.8%, and the 6MWT was 520.4 m in patients with hematological malignancy (Table 1). The 6MWT showed a significant correlation with the hemoglobin level and was significantly correlated with SmO_2 at rest, and SmO_2 at rest was significantly correlated with the hemoglobin level ($p < 0.05$ for all) (Fig. 1a–c).

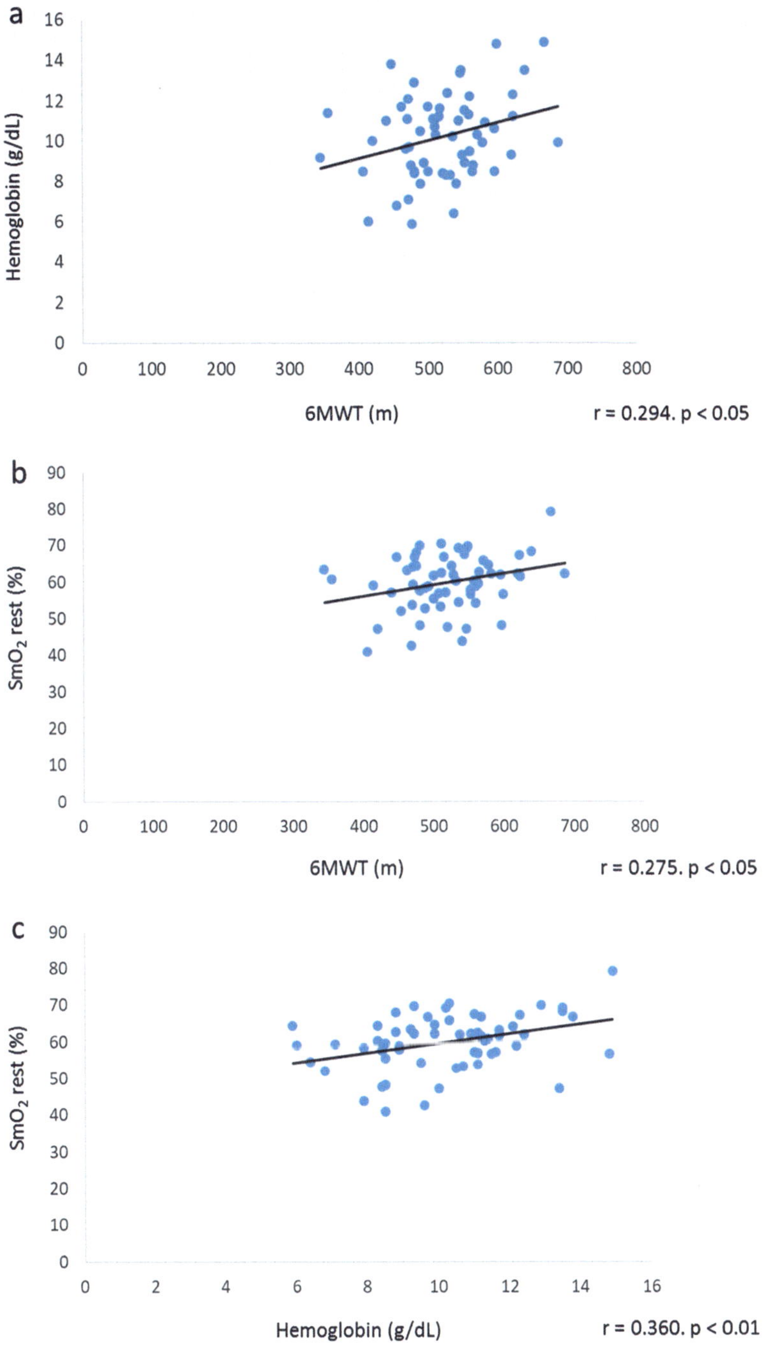

Fig. 1 Scatterplots illustrating the relationship between the 6MWT, SmO_2 at rest, and hemoglobin level. (**a**): the 6MWT and hemoglobin, (**b**): the 6MWT and SmO_2 at rest, c: SmO_2 at rest and hemoglobin

4 Discussion

In the present study, there was a significant correlation between the 6MWT and TA muscle O_2Hb saturation at rest in hematological malignancy patients. Additionally, the 6MWT was significantly correlated with hemoglobin levels. Furthermore, TA muscle O_2Hb saturation at rest was significantly related to the hemoglobin level. Our previous research showed that hematological malignancy in patients has a relationship with 6MWT findings and hemoglobin level [6]. Furthermore, our other research showed that SmO_2 during and after exercise was positively correlated with the distance of 6MWT [10]. The current study showed that SmO_2 is related to 6MWT not only during and after exercise, but also at rest. Furthermore, SmO_2 at rest has a relationship with hemoglobin levels in patients with hematological malignancy. In general, the 6MWT often has a relationship with blood oxygen saturation (SpO_2) in pulmonary disease patients [11]. On the basis of these findings, poor muscle saturation function may contribute to skeletal muscle oxygen consumption and blood flow during exercise; therefore, hematological malignancy patients may be at a risk of decreased oxygen carrying capacity.

This study has some limitations worth mentioning. We only measured hemoglobin levels, SmO_2 at rest, and exercise capacity in hematological malignancy patients before HSCT. Hemoglobin levels and SmO_2 may be related to muscle fatigue in patients with hematological malignancy. We have planned to investigate muscle fatigue with respect to hemoglobin levels and SmO_2 in patients with hematological malignancy in future studies. These findings may have helpful to develop specialized physical exercise programs for patients with hematological malignancy.

In conclusion, hematological malignancy in patients might have a relationship with exercise capacity, muscle O_2Hb saturation at rest, and hemoglobin level before HSCT in clinical measurements. Therefore, rehabilitation staff, nurses, and physicians should recognize these relationships in patients who undergo HSCT. Moreover, physiotherapists may need to promote muscle oxidative metabolism through exercise to increase exercise capacity in such patients.

Acknowledgments This study was supported by a Grant-in-Aid for Exploratory Research from the Niigata University of Health and Welfare, Japan.

References

1. Koreth J, Schlenk R, Kopecky KJ et al (2009) Allogeneic stem cell transplantation for acute myeloid leukemia in first complete remission: systematic review and meta-analysis of prospective clinical trials. JAMA 301:2349–2361
2. Pidala J, Djulbegovic B, Anasetti C, Kharfan-Dabaja M, Kumar A (2011) Allogeneic hematopoietic cell transplantation for adult acute lymphoblastic leukemia (ALL) in first complete remission. Cochrane Database Syst Rev:CD008818

3. Yoshimi A, Suzuki R, Atsuta Y et al (2010) Hematopoietic SCT activity in Asia: a report from the Asia-Pacific blood and marrow transplantation group. Bone Marrow Transplant 45:1682–1691
4. Passweg JR, Baldomero H, Gratwohl A et al (2012) The EBMT activity survey: 1990-2010. Bone Marrow Transplant 47:906–923
5. Morishita S, Kaida K, Yamauchi S et al (2013) Gender differences in health-related quality of life, physical function and psychological status among patients in the early phase following allogeneic haematopoietic stem cell transplantation. Psychooncology 22:1159–1166
6. Morishita S, Kaida K, Ikegame K et al (2012) Impaired physiological function and health-related QOL in patients before hematopoietic stem-cell transplantation. Support Care Cancer 20:821–829
7. Hamaoka T, McCully KK, Quaresima V, Yamamoto K, Chance B (2007) Near-infrared spectroscopy/imaging for monitoring muscle oxygenation and oxidative metabolism in healthy and diseased humans. J Biomed Opt 12:062105
8. McNeil CJ, Murray BJ, Rice CL (2006) Differential changes in muscle oxygenation between voluntary and stimulated isometric fatigue of human dorsiflexors. J Appl Physiol 100:890–895
9. ATS statement: guidelines for the six-minute walk test (2002) Am J Respir Crit Care Med 166:111–7
10. Wakasugi T, Morishita S, Kaida K et al (2018) Impaired skeletal muscle oxygenation following allogeneic hematopoietic stem cell transplantation is associated with exercise capacity. Support Care Cancer 26:2149–2160
11. Strickland SL, Hogan TM, Hogan RG, Sohal HS, McKenzie WN, Petroski GF (2009) A randomized multi-arm repeated-measures prospective study of several modalities of portable oxygen delivery during assessment of functional exercise capacity. Respir Care 54:344–349

Differences in Muscle O_2 Dynamics During Treadmill Exercise Between Aerobic Capacity-Matched Overweight and Normal-Weight Adults

Shun Takagi, Ryotaro Kime, Taishi Midorikawa, Masatsugu Niwayama, Shizuo Sakamoto, and Toshihito Katsumura

Abstract The aim of this study was to compare muscle O_2 dynamics during exercise between aerobic capacity-matched overweight and normal-weight adults. Overweight women (OW, n = 9) and normal-weight women (NW, n = 14) performed graded treadmill exercise until exhaustion. Muscle O_2 saturation (SmO_2) and relative changes from rest in deoxygenated hemoglobin concentration (Δdeoxy-Hb) and total hemoglobin concentration (Δtotal-Hb) were monitored continuously at gastrocnemius medialis muscle by near infrared spatial resolved spectroscopy. Significantly higher SmO_2 and lower Δdeoxy-Hb and Δtotal-Hb were observed in OW compared with NW. Pulmonary O_2 uptake (VO_2) normalized by fat-free mass was matched between groups. In both groups, peak VO_2 was significantly correlated with change in SmO_2 and Δdeoxy-Hb. Our findings suggest that both muscle blood volume and deoxygenation were lower in overweight adults, compared to aerobic capacity-matched normal-weight adults. Moreover, lowered muscle O_2 extraction was related to peak VO_2 in overweight adults, as well as in normal-weight adults.

Keywords Blood volume · Muscle O_2 extraction · Near infrared spectroscopy · Regional difference · Women

---

S. Takagi (✉)
Faculty of Health and Sports Science, Doshisha University, Kyoto, Japan
e-mail: shtakagi@mail.doshisha.ac.jp

R. Kime · T. Katsumura
Department of Sports Medicine for Health Promotion, Tokyo Medical University, Tokyo, Japan

T. Midorikawa
College of Health and Welfare, J. F. Oberlin University, Tokyo, Japan

M. Niwayama
Department of Electrical and Electronic Engineering, Shizuoka University, Shizuoka, Japan

S. Sakamoto
Faculty of Sport Sciences, Waseda University, Tokyo, Japan

© Springer Nature Switzerland AG 2020

P.-D. Ryu et al. (eds.), *Oxygen Transport to Tissue XLI*, Advances in Experimental Medicine and Biology 1232, https://doi.org/10.1007/978-3-030-34461-0_28

1 Introduction

Overweight is an important health issue worldwide, and severely obese people have been characterized by impaired vasodilation, muscle blood flow [1], or mitochondrial content and functions, especially with insulin resistance [2]. However, to date, the effects of overweight (i.e. mild degree/early stage obesity) on microcirculation and metabolism in skeletal muscle during exercise have not been established.

Previous studies have demonstrated that peak pulmonary O_2 uptake (VO_2) potentially affects hemodynamic and vascular responses [3]. Therefore, to evaluate the difference in muscle O_2 dynamics in overweight and normal-weight subjects, peak VO_2 should be matched between groups. The aim of this study was to compare muscle O_2 dynamics during treadmill exercise between aerobic capacity-matched overweight and normal-weight adults. Overweight adults may or may not have severe functional impairments, and muscle O_2 demand during treadmill exercise seems to be higher due to greater body weight. We hypothesized that muscle deoxygenation would be enhanced in overweight adults.

2 Methods

2.1 Subjects

Age- and aerobic capacity-matched overweight women (OW; n = 9) and normal-weight women (NW, n = 14) participated in the study (Table 1). In general, overweight is defined as a body mass index (BMI) value of ≥25. However, even if

Table 1 Physical and clinical characteristics of the study population

	Overweight (n = 9)	Normal weight (n = 14)	p-value
Age (years)	38 ± 5	39 ± 6	0.86
Height (cm)	162.6 ± 3.3	159.2 ± 5.6	0.19
Body weight (kg)	70.5 ± 8.0	52.7 ± 5.4	<0.01
BMI (kg/m^2)	26.7 ± 2.5	20.7 ± 1.1	<0.01
% body fat (%)	38.6 ± 2.5	29.1 ± 2.7	<0.01
FFM (kg)	43.1 ± 3.5	37.3 ± 3.4	<0.01
Fat layer thickness at gastrocnemius medialis muscle (mm)	7.2 ± 1.5	5.7 ± 1.4	<0.05
Fat layer thickness at vastus lateralis muscle (mm)	8.8 ± 1.4	7.3 ± 1.8	<0.05
Fasting glucose (mg/dL)	96 ± 9[a]	90 ± 5[b]	0.06
Fasting insulin (μU/mL)	7.4 ± 3.4[a]	5.4 ± 2.6[b]	0.13
Fasting HOMA-IR	1.7 ± 0.6[a]	1.2 ± 0.6[b]	0.08
Peak VO_2 per FFM (mL/kgFFM/min)	44.8 ± 4.1	44.0 ± 5.0	0.77

All data are given as mean ± SD. [a]: n = 8, [b]: n = 12.

subjects who have the same BMI are compared, there are relatively large inter-individual differences in percentage of body fat (%BF) [4]. Hence, in this study, overweight was defined as %BF corresponding to BMI value of ≥25, as reported in a previous study [4] (cutoff value for %BF depends on age, and the value was about 35.3 in this study). All subjects were untrained, and none had cardiovascular disease or diabetes mellitus (i.e. <126 mg/dL of fasting blood glucose [5]). This study was approved by the institutional ethics committee. All subjects were informed of the purpose of the study and written consent was given.

2.2 Experimental Design

The subjects performed graded ramp treadmill exercise (MAT-2700, Fukuda-Denshi, Japan) until exhaustion. The speed and grade of the treadmill were increased every 1 min by approximately 1 metabolic equivalent. VO_2 was measured continuously during the experiments to determine peak VO_2 (AE300S, Minato Medical Science, Japan). All subjects attained respiratory gas exchange ratio > 1.1 and heart rate > 90% of 220-age, at peak exercise. Fat-free mass (FFM) was determined by bio-impedance analysis (DC320, Tanita, Japan), and VO_2 was subsequently normalized by FFM. Muscle O_2 saturation (SmO_2) and relative changes from rest in oxygenated hemoglobin concentration (Δoxy-Hb), deoxygenated hemoglobin concentration (Δdeoxy-Hb), and total hemoglobin concentration (Δtotal-Hb) were measured at gastrocnemius medialis and vastus lateralis muscles in the left leg by near infrared spatial resolved spectroscopy (NIR_{SRS}). The NIR_{SRS} data were averaged over the last 10 s at rest, 20, 40, 60, 80, and 100% of peak VO_2. The NIR_{SRS} probe consisted of one light-emitting diode using two-wavelength (770 and 830 nm) and two photodiode detectors, and the optode distances were 20 and 30 mm (Hb12–4, Astem Co., Japan). Fat layer thickness at the measurement site was measured by using an ultrasound device (LogiQ3, GE-Yokokawa Medical Systems, Japan), and the light scattering effect of the fat layer on NIR_{SRS} data was corrected by normalizing measurement sensitivity [6].

2.3 Statistical Analysis

All data are given as means ± standard deviation (SD). To compare changes in muscle O_2 dynamics during exercise between groups, a 2-way repeated-measures analysis of variance (ANOVA) was used, with group and exercise intensity as factors. Where appropriate, the Bonferroni post hoc test was performed. Differences in physical and clinical variables and exercise time were compared by unpaired t-tests. For all statistical analyses, significance was accepted at $p < 0.05$.

3 Results

Body weight, FFM, and fat layer thickness at measurement sites were significantly higher in OW compared to NW (Table 1). Fasting blood glucose concentration and homeostasis model assessment-insulin resistance (HOMA-IR) tended to be higher in OW, while the difference in serum insulin concentration between groups did not reach significance. There was no significant difference in exercise time until exhaustion between groups.

In gastrocnemius medialis muscle, there was a significant interaction for SmO_2 ($p < 0.05$), Δdeoxy-Hb ($p < 0.01$) and Δtotal-Hb ($p < 0.05$) during exercise (Fig. 1). Consequently, significantly lower Δdeoxy-Hb and Δtotal-Hb and higher SmO_2 were observed in OW than NW. No significant interaction or main effects of group was observed in Δoxy-Hb. In contrast, in vastus lateralis muscle, there were no significant differences in muscle O_2 dynamics between groups.

At gastrocnemius medialis muscle, ΔSmO_2 (values at peak exercise minus values at resting) was significantly negatively related to peak VO_2 in OW ($r = -0.68$, $p < 0.05$, $R^2 = 0.48$) and in NW ($r = -0.84$, $p < 0.01$, $R^2 = 0.71$) (Fig. 2a). Similarly,

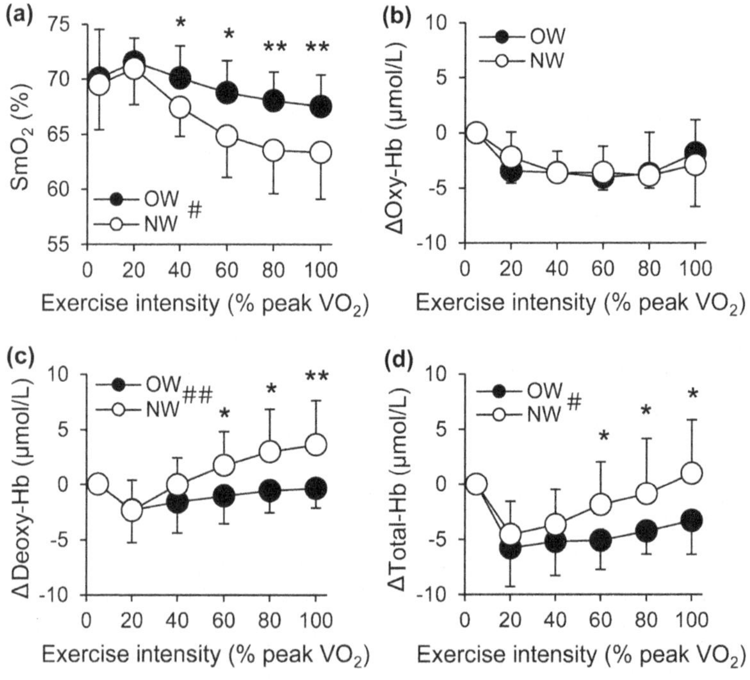

Fig. 1 Changes in muscle O_2 saturation (SmO_2: **a**), oxygenated hemoglobin (Δoxy-Hb: **b**), deoxygenated hemoglobin (Δdeoxy-Hb: **c**), and total hemoglobin (Δtotal-Hb: **d**) concentration at gastrocnemius medialis muscles during exercise in OW (closed circles) and NW (open circles). There were significant differences between groups (*: $p < 0.05$, **: $p < 0.01$). There was a significant group and exercise intensity interaction (#: $p < 0.05$, ##: $p < 0.01$). Symbols indicating a significant difference between exercise intensity have been omitted for the sake of clarity

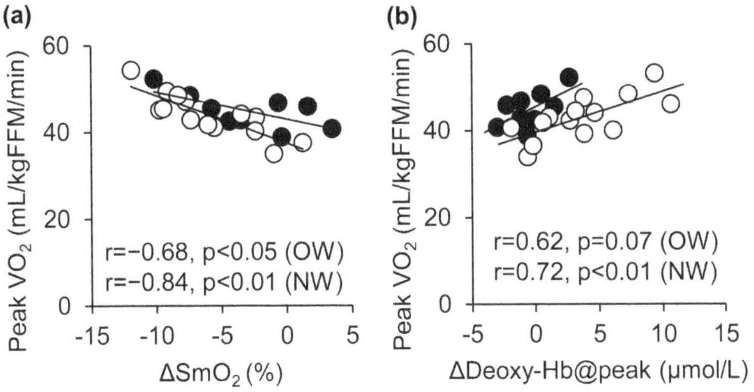

Fig. 2 Relationship between muscle deoxygenation at gastrocnemius medialis muscle and aerobic capacity in OW (closed circles) and NW (open circles). **a**, change in muscle O_2 saturation from rest to peak exercise (ΔSmO_2) and peak VO_2 normalized by FFM. **b**, change in deoxygenated hemoglobin from rest to peak exercise (Δdeoxy-Hb@peak) and peak VO_2 normalized by FFM

Δdeoxy-Hb at peak exercise tended to be positively correlated to peak VO_2 in OW ($r = 0.62$, $p = 0.07$, $R^2 = 0.39$), while a significant relationship was observed in NW ($r = 0.72$, $p < 0.01$, $R^2 = 0.52$) (Fig. 2b). In contrast, in vastus lateralis muscle, no significant relationship was observed between muscle O_2 dynamics and peak VO_2. Fat layer thickness at the measurement site was not significantly associated with any muscle O_2 dynamics.

4 Discussion

In gastrocnemius medialis muscle, significantly higher SmO_2 and lower Δdeoxy-Hb and Δtotal-Hb were found. These results indicate that deoxygenation and O_2 extraction in activating muscle were lowered in OW than NW, while blood volume was also diminished in OW. Severely obese subjects were not included in this study, and no one was clinically judged to have diabetes mellitus, evaluated by fasting glucose concentration. Moreover, all subjects represented less than 2.5 of HOMA-IR, even though >2.5 of HOMA-IR is generally assumed to be a high probability of insulin resistance [7]. However, HOMA-IR tended to be higher in OW than NW, and insulin resistance potentially impaired mitochondrial content and function [2]. Obese adults generally have lower capillary density, capillary-to-fiber area ratio [8], and vasodilation response [1] compared with normal-weight adults. Therefore, our findings lead us to speculate that O_2 diffusive transport and vasodilation response in exercising muscle may have already been blunted in overweight adults who were not severely obese with a mild degree of insulin resistance. Another possibility for lowered muscle O_2 extraction is higher muscle blood flow. Previous studies have demonstrated that obese adults have higher cardiac output normalized for body size, compared with aerobic capacity-matched normal-weight adults [9, 10]. Because NIR_{SRS} variables reflect very localized information, future studies are needed to measure muscle blood flow and/or cardiac output directly. However, in this study, because VO_2 was similar between groups, our findings using the NIR_{SRS} technique firstly demonstrate that muscle O_2 extraction, rather than convective O_2 transport may have been compromised in overweight adults. Notably, ΔSmO_2 and Δdeoxy-Hb at peak exercise are related to peak VO_2 in both groups. Hence, the lowered muscle O_2 extraction was related to peak VO_2 in overweight adults, as well as in normal-weight adults. Although the coefficient of determination was somewhat lower in OW than NW, 39–48% of variance in peak VO_2 can be explained by muscle O_2 extraction. Overweight and lowered peak VO_2 both potentially increase cardiovascular-related mortality, and maintaining peak VO_2 may be more important than preventing the development of obesity [11]. Therefore, there is a possibility that an enhancement of muscle O_2 extraction may be beneficial for overweight adults.

In the present study, no significant difference was observed in muscle O_2 dynamics at vastus lateralis muscle, in contrast to gastrocnemius medialis. Thigh muscles do not largely contribute during walking and running, compared to lower leg muscles. Hence, the regional differences in muscle deoxygenation and blood volume may be partly explained by the degree of muscle recruitment. Moreover, because sex-related differences in muscle O_2 dynamics have been observed in elderly men and women [12], only women were recruited for this study. Results in this study may be restricted to women.

In conclusion, both muscle blood volume and deoxygenation were reduced in overweight adults, compared to aerobic capacity-matched normal-weight adults. Because VO_2 was similar throughout exercise, muscle O_2 extraction, rather than convective O_2 transport, may have been compromised in overweight adults. Moreover, because lowered muscle O_2 extraction was related to peak VO_2 in overweight adults, an enhancement of muscle O_2 extraction may be beneficial for improvement of peak VO_2. However, alteration in muscle O_2 dynamics during exercise may be regional in overweight adults.

Acknowledgments The authors are grateful for revision of this manuscript by Andrea Hope. This work was supported in part by JSPS KAKENHI Grant Number 16 K16487 to Shun Takagi.

References

1. Hodnett BL, Hester RL (2007) Regulation of muscle blood flow in obesity. Microcirculation 14:273–288
2. Dumas JF, Simard G, Flamment M (2009) Is skeletal muscle mitochondrial dysfunction a cause or an indirect consequence of insulin resistance in humans? Diabetes Metab 35(3):159–167
3. Martin WH 3rd, Ogawa T, Kohrt WM et al (1991) Effects of aging, gender, and physical training on peripheral vascular function. Circulation 84:654–664
4. Gallagher D, Heymsfield SB, Heo M et al (2000) Healthy percentage body fat ranges: an approach for developing guidelines based on body mass index. Am J Clin Nutr 72(3):694–701

5. American Diabetes Association (2006) Diagnosis and classification of diabetes mellitus. Diabetes Care 29(Suppl 1):S43–S48
6. Niwayama M, Suzuki H, Yamashita T et al (2012) Error factors in oxygenation measurement using continuous wave and spatially resolved near-infrared spectroscopy. J Jpn Coll Angiol 52:211–215
7. Vogeser M, König D, Frey I et al (2007) Fasting serum insulin and the homeostasis model of insulin resistance (HOMA-IR) in the monitoring of lifestyle interventions in obese persons. Clin Biochem 40(13–14):964–968
8. Gavin TP, Stallings HW 3rd, Zwetsloot KA et al (2005) Lower capillary density but no difference in VEGF expression in obese vs. lean young skeletal muscle in humans. J Appl Physiol (1985) 98(1):315–321
9. Vella CA, Ontiveros D, Zubia RY (2011) Cardiac function and arteriovenous oxygen difference during exercise in obese adults. Eur J Appl Physiol 111(6):915–923
10. Vella CA, Paul DR, Bader J (2012) Cardiac response to exercise in normal-weight and obese, Hispanic men and women: implications for exercise prescription. Acta Physiol (Oxf) 205(1):113–123
11. Kennedy AB, Lavie CJ, Blair SN (2018) Fitness or fatness: which is more important? JAMA 319(3):231–232
12. Takagi S, Kime R, Niwayama M et al (2016) Sex-related difference in muscle deoxygenation responses between aerobic capacity-matched elderly men and women. Adv Exp Med Biol 876:55–61

Cerebral Oxygenation Dynamics of the Prefrontal Cortex and Motor-Related Area During Cardiopulmonary Exercise Test: A Near-Infrared Spectroscopy Study

Sho Kojima, Shinichiro Morishita, Weixiang Qin, and Atsuhiro Tsubaki

Abstract Near-infrared spectroscopy (NIRS) during cardiopulmonary exercise test (CPX) has shown a correlation between prefrontal cortex (PFC) oxygenated hemoglobin (O_2Hb) level and negative affective responses. We hypothesized that O2Hb changes differ between the PFC and motor-related areas. This study investigated changes in hemoglobin levels in the PFC and motor-related areas during CPX. Twelve young healthy adults participated in this study. They performed a CPX after 4 min of rest and 4 min of warming up. Cortical O2Hb, deoxygenated hemoglobin (HHb), and total hemoglobin (THb) levels were measured with NIRS during CPX. Regions of interest (ROI) were the PFC, premotor area (PMA), supplementary motor area (SMA), and primary motor cortex (M1). The anaerobic threshold (AT), respiratory compensation (RC), and peak oxygen uptake (Peak) points were determined. The rest, AT, RC and Peak points of O_2Hb, HHb, and THb were averaged over 5 s; hemoglobin slopes, from RC to the Peak points, were calculated to compare functional changes in cortical oxygenation. Average values of O_2Hb, HHb, and THb in each ROI were compared among the rest, AT, RC, and Peak points. Average values of hemoglobin slopes, from RC to Peak points, were compared among ROIs using Bonferroni multiple comparisons. The HHb of all ROIs significantly increased at Peak point, compared with at the AT point. THb of the PFC, PMA, and SMA significantly increased at the RC or Peak points, compared with at the rest point. Hemoglobin slopes, from RC to Peak, showed no significant differences among ROIs. Each ROI exhibited similar changes, regardless of cortical function.

Keywords Cardiopulmonary exercise test · Near-infrared spectroscopy · Motor-related area · Prefrontal cortex · Oxygenated hemoglobin

---

S. Kojima (✉) · S. Morishita · W. Qin · A. Tsubaki
Graduate School of Health and Welfare, Niigata University of Health and Welfare, Niigata, Japan

Institute for Human Movement and Medical Science, Niigata University of Health and Welfare, Niigata, Japan
e-mail: hpm18008@nuhw.ac.jp

© Springer Nature Switzerland AG 2020

P.-D. Ryu et al. (eds.), *Oxygen Transport to Tissue XLI*, Advances in Experimental Medicine and Biology 1232, https://doi.org/10.1007/978-3-030-34461-0_29

1 Introduction

Studies have shown that aerobic exercise increases cerebral oxygenation in the PFC and motor-related areas [1, 2]. Aerobic exercise intensity can be determined by cardiopulmonary exercise tests (CPX) [3]. Previous studies that used near-infrared spectroscopy (NIRS) during CPX have shown a correlation between prefrontal cortex (PFC) oxygenated hemoglobin (O_2Hb) level and negative affective responses [4]. Another study showed that correlations between regions were high, and that deoxygenated hemoglobin (HHb) was greater in prefrontal than premotor and motor regions [5]. PFC and motor-related areas have not been compared in terms of hemoglobin dynamics at the anaerobic threshold (AT) and respiratory compensation (RC) points. The purpose of this study was to investigate changes in the PFC and motor-related areas in terms of hemoglobin levels in the cerebral cortices during CPX.

2 Methods

2.1 *Participants*

Study participants comprised 12 healthy adult volunteers (8 females, mean age 21.6 ± 0.2 years, height 162.6 ± 2.0 cm, weight 57.3 ± 2.9 kg) recruited from among students enrolled at the Niigata University of Health and Welfare. Participants had no history of neurological disorder or orthopedic disorder. Each participant received oral and written descriptions of the objectives, measurement techniques, and risks and benefits of the investigation. All participants consented to inclusion in the study. The study was approved by the Ethics Committee of Niigata University of Health and Welfare, and was conducted in accordance with the Declaration of Helsinki.

2.2 *Procedures*

Participants were instructed to not consume alcohol and caffeine 24 h before the experiment. They were allowed to consume other food items until 3 h before the experiments. Moreover, food and drink intake were restricted altogether from 3 h prior to completion of the experiment. CPX was performed by pedaling with a cycle ergometer (Aerobike 75XLII; Combi, Tokyo, Japan). Participants performed incremental loading, corresponding to 20 watts/min, after 4 min of rest and 4 min of warming up. Pedaling speed was maintained at 50–60 rpm. CPX of all participants was completed upon dyspneic or leg fatigue. Electrocardiogram and blood pressure were measured to prevent sudden deterioration of the physical condition during CPX. In addition, respiratory metabolism parameters were measured using an exhaled gas analyzer (AE-310, Minato Medical Science, Osaka, Japan) during CPX. We subsequently determined the AT, RC, and peak oxygen uptake (Peak) points based on previously reported methods [6, 7].

2.3 NIRS and Skin Blood Flow Measurements

Cortical O_2Hb, HHb, and total hemoglobin (THb) were measured with a multi-channel NIRS imaging system (OMM-3000, Simadzu Co., Kyoto, Japan) during CPX. We instructed to participants to reduce head motion during the experiment. Measurements used 8 source probes and 8 detector probes (Fig. 1); a total of 24 channels were used. The 24 channels were placed parallel to the vertex (Cz) position of the international 10–20 system. The Cz position of the international 10–20 system was used to ensure consistent placement of optodes in all participants. The probe distance was set at 30 mm. Measurement was performed at a sampling interval of 130 ms. The regions of interest (ROI) were PFC, premotor area (PMA), supplementary motor area (SMA), and primary motor cortex (M1). The PFC used channels 1, 3, 4, 5, 6, and 7; PMA used channels 8, 10, 11, and 14; SMA used channels 12, 13, and 16; and M1 used channels 19, 20, and 23. Artifacts of head motion were filtered by bandpass filter. Afterward, O_2Hb, HHb, and THb were calculated as the differences from the average values of 4-min rest. O_2Hb, HHb, and THb were calculated by the average values over 5 s at the rest, AT, RC, and the Peak points. The slopes of each hemoglobin, from RC to the Peak points, were calculated to compare functional changes in cortical oxygenation. Changes in skin blood flow (SBF) were measured at the forehead using a laser tissue blood flow oxygen monitor (Omegaflow, FLO-Cl, Omega Wave Inc., Osaka, Japan). Analogue data were converted to digital data using an A/D converter (PowerLab, AD Instruments, Australia) at a 130-Hz sampling rate.

2.4 Statistical Analysis

Average values of O_2Hb, HHb, and THb in each ROI were compared among the rest, AT, RC, and Peak points using the Bonferroni multiple comparisons test. Average values of SBF were analyzed in a similar manner as the O_2Hb, HHb, and

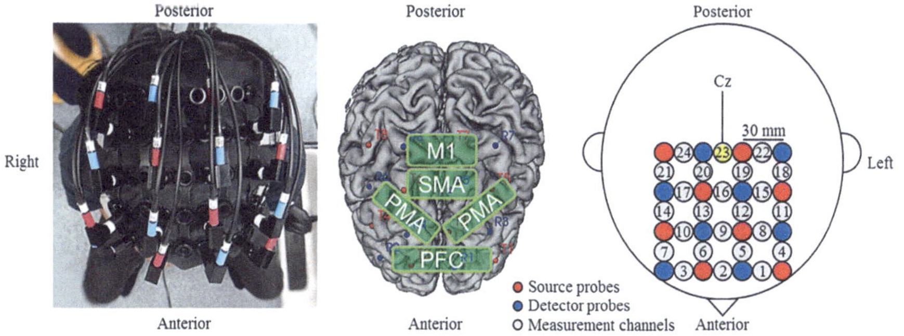

Fig. 1 Locations of the 8 source probes and 8 detector probes, as well as the region of interest Red dots are source probes; blue dots are detector probes. Source probes and detector probes are placed in an alternate manner. The probe distance was set at 30 mm

THb. Average values of the slopes for each hemoglobin, from RC to the Peak points, were compared between PFC, PMA, SMA, and M1 using the Bonferroni multiple comparisons test. Statistical analyses were performed using SPSS 21.0 (SPSS Japan Inc., Tokyo, Japan), with statistical significance set at $p < 0.05$.

3 Results

The O_2Hb of PFC showed a significant increase ($p < 0.05$) at the RC point, compared with at the rest point. The HHb of PFC and PMA showed a significant increase ($p < 0.05$) at the Peak point, compared with at the rest point. Also, the HHb of all ROIs showed a significant increase ($p < 0.05$) at the Peak point, compared with at the AT point. The THb of the PFC and PMA showed significant increases ($p < 0.05$) at the RC and Peak points, compared with at the rest and AT points. The SBF showed a significant increase ($p < 0.05$) at the AT, RC and Peak points, compared with at the rest point (Table 1). The slope of O_2Hb, HHb and THb, from RC to the Peak points, showed no significant difference among PFC, PMA, SMA, and M1 (Fig. 2).

Table 1 Change of the rest to the peak point (n = 12)

	Rest point	AT point	RC point	Peak point
PFC				
O_2Hb	0.00 ± 0.00	0.00 ± 0.00	0.01 ± 0.00[a]	0.00 ± 0.01
HHb	−0.00 ± 0.00	−0.00 ± 0.00	0.02 ± 0.00	0.04 ± 0.00[a, b]
THb	−0.00 ± 0.00	0.00 ± 0.00	0.04 ± 0.00[a, b]	0.05 ± 0.01[a, b]
PMA				
O_2Hb	0.00 ± 0.00	0.00 ± 0.00	0.01 ± 0.00	−0.00 ± 0.01
HHb	−0.00 ± 0.00	−0.00 ± 0.00	0.02 ± 0.00	0.03 ± 0.00[a, b]
THb	−0.00 ± 0.00	0.00 ± 0.00	0.03 ± 0.00[a, b]	0.03 ± 0.00[a]
SMA				
O_2Hb	0.00 ± 0.00	0.00 ± 0.00	0.02 ± 0.01	0.02 ± 0.01
HHb	−0.00 ± 0.00	−0.01 ± 0.00	0.00 ± 0.00	0.01 ± 0.00[b]
THb	−0.00 ± 0.00	−0.00 ± 0.01	0.02 ± 0.01	0.03 ± 0.01[b]
M1				
O_2Hb	−0.00 ± 0.00	0.01 ± 0.00	0.03 ± 0.01	0.02 ± 0.01
HHb	0.00 ± 0.00	−0.02 ± 0.00	−0.00 ± 0.00	0.01 ± 0.00[b]
THb	−0.00 ± 0.00	−0.00 ± 0.01	0.03 ± 0.01	0.03 ± 0.01
SBF	0.00 ± 0.00	3.13 ± 1.10[a]	5.67 ± 0.97[a]	6.93 ± 1.61[a]

Values are presented as mean ± standard error of the mean (SEM)
Bonferroni multiple comparison procedure was used to obtain p-values
[a]$p < 0.05$; significantly different from the rest point
[b]$p < 0.05$; significantly different from the AT point
AT: anaerobic threshold, RC: respiratory compensation, Peak: peak oxygen uptake

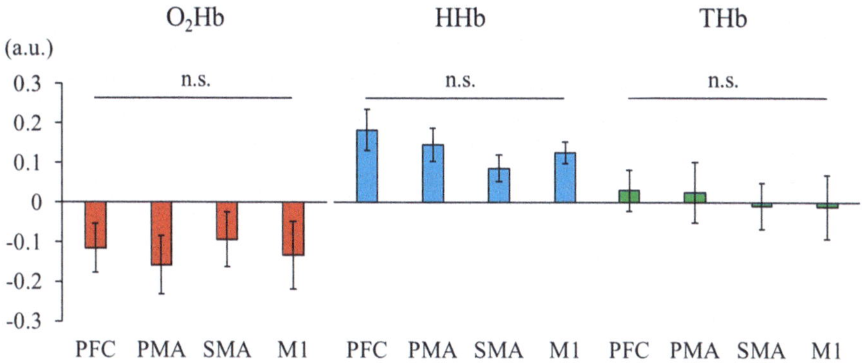

Fig. 2 Slopes of hemoglobin levels from the RC point to the peak point. Red bars are oxygenated hemoglobin (O_2Hb), blue bars are deoxygenated hemoglobin (HHb), green bars are total hemoglobin (THb). Values are presented as mean ± standard error of the mean (SEM)

4 Discussion

In this study, cortical O_2Hb, HHb, and THb in the PFC, PMA, SMA, and M1 were measured during CPX. We focused on changes in O_2Hb, HHb, and THb from the rest point to the AT, RC, and Peak points. The AT point involves ventilatory increase with an associated increase in lactate due to anaerobic metabolism [6, 7]. Lactate production is incrementally increased by exercise intensity. Increased lactate production results in metabolic acidosis, and respiratory compensation occurs to inhibit metabolic acidosis [6, 7]; this is the RC point.

The SBF showed a significant increase at the AT, RC, and Peak points, compared with at the rest point. The cortical O_2Hb, HHb, and THb did not show significant increases at the AT, RC, and Peak points, compared with at the rest point. Furthermore, the HHb and THb showed a significant increase at the RC or Peak points, compared with at the AT point. Therefore, we consider the influence of SBF to be small in relation to cortical hemoglobin.

The O_2Hb of PFC showed a significant increase at the RC point, compared with at the rest point. A previous study showed a correlation between increasing O_2Hb level in PFC and increasing negative affective responses [4]. Thus, O_2Hb of PFC might have been influenced by affective changes. The THb of the PFC and PMA showed significant increases at the RC point, compared with at the rest point; HHb did not show this increase. Furthermore, increasing O_2Hb is only PFC. Increased oxygen metabolism drives the conversion of O_2Hb to HHb [8]. Generally, the neuro-activation area exhibits reduced HHb and increased O_2Hb [9, 10]; this reduced HHb is produced by washout of HHb from the activation area. The present study considered that the increased exercise intensity drove the conversion of O_2Hb to HHb. Therefore, O_2Hb showed no significant increase, and HHb showed no significant decrease upon washout of HHb from the activation area. Consequently, THb increased at the RC point. The THb of PFC, PMA, and SMA showed a significant increase at the Peak point, compared with at the rest and AT points. The HHb of all ROIs showed a significant increase at the Peak point, compared with at the AT point. The Peak point of high intensity exercise drove the conversion of O_2Hb to HHb more strongly than the AT and the RC points. A previous study reported that only HHb greatly increased during incremental load exercise [11]. Conversely, another study reported increased O_2Hb and HHb during constant load exercise [12]. Therefore, O_2Hb and HHb changes may differ between CPX and steady load exercise.

The slopes of O_2Hb, HHb, and THb, from RC to the Peak points, showed no significant difference among the PFC, PMA, SMA, and M1. All ROIs showed a reduced slope of O2Hb from the RC point to the Peak point. Neural activity of cortical function is associated with oxygen metabolism [10]. In this study, all ROIs changed in a similar manner, regardless of cortical function, from the RC to the Peak points. Additionally, HHb of all ROIs increased at the Peak point, compared with at the AT point. Therefore, the wide range of cortex drove deoxygenation at the Peak point.

However, this study was limited in that it used extra-cerebral measurement. Here, the extra-cerebral parameter was skin blood flow, assessed using laser tissue blood flow oxygen monitoring. It may be insufficient to measure extra-cerebral tissue alone. In the future, we need to measure using short channel regression methods. In conclusion, the slopes of hemoglobin levels, from the RC to the Peak points, showed no significant differences among the PFC, PMA, SMA, and M1. However, the HHb of the PFC, PMA, SMA, and M1 at the Peak point showed significant increases, compared with at the AT point. Therefore, the wide range of cortex drove deoxygenation at the Peak point.

Acknowledgments This study was supported by a Grant-in-Aid for Scientific Research (C) from the Japan Society for the Promotion of Science (A. Tsubaki) and a Grant-in-Aid for Exploratory Research from Niigata University of Health and Welfare (A. Tsubaki).

References

1. Tsubaki A, Takai H, Kojima S et al (2016) Changes in cortical oxyhaemoglobin signal during low-intensity cycle ergometer activity: a near-infrared spectroscopy study. Adv Exp Med Biol 876:79–85
2. Takehara N, Tsubaki A, Yamazaki Y et al (2017) Changes in oxyhemoglobin concentration in the prefrontal cortex and primary motor cortex during low- and moderate-intensity exercise on a cycle ergometer. Adv Exp Med Biol 977:241–247
3. American Thoracic Society, American College of Chest Physicians (2003) ATS/ACCP statement on cardiopulmonary exercise testing. Am J Respir Crit Care Med 167:211–277
4. Tempest GD, Eston RG, Parfitt G (2014) Prefrontal cortex haemodynamics and affective responses during exercise: a multi-channel near infrared spectroscopy study. PLoS One 9:e95924
5. Subudhi AW, Miramon BR, Granger ME et al (2009) Frontal and motor cortex oxygenation during maximal exercise in normoxia and hypoxia. J Appl Physiol (1985) 106:1153–1158
6. Wasserman K, McIlroy MB (1964) Detecting the threshold of anaerobic metabolism in cardiac patients during exercise. Am J Cardiol 14:844–852

7. Wasserman K, Whipp BJ, Koyl SN et al (1973) Anaerobic threshold and respiratory gas exchange during exercise. J Appl Physiol 35:236–243
8. Lindauer U, Dirnagl U, Füchtemeier M et al (2010) Pathophysiological interference with neurovascular coupling - when imaging based on hemoglobin might go blind. Front Neuroenerg 2:25
9. Lindauer U, Royl G, Leithner C et al (2001) No evidence for early decrease in blood oxygenation in rat whisker cortex in response to functional activation. NeuroImage 13:988–1001
10. Fox PT, Raichle ME (1986) Focal physiological uncoupling of cerebral blood flow and oxidative metabolism during somatosensory stimulation in human subjects. Proc Natl Acad Sci U S A 83:1140–1144
11. Auger H, Bherer L, Boucher É et al (2016) Quantification of extra-cerebral and cerebral hemoglobin concentrations during physical exercise using time-domain near infrared spectroscopy. Biomed Opt Express 7:3826–3842
12. Giles GE, Brunyé TT, Eddy MD et al (2014) Acute exercise increases oxygenated and deoxygenated hemoglobin in the prefrontal cortex. Neuroreport 25:1320–1325

Reduced Optical Path Length in the Vastus Lateralis During Ramp Cycling Exercise

Tasuki Endo, Ryotaro Kime, Tsubasa Watanabe, Sayuri Fuse, Norio Murase, Yuko Kurosawa, and Takafumi Hamaoka

Abstract Near-infrared time-resolved spectroscopy (NIR_{TRS}) can quantitatively evaluate mean optical path length (MPL). Since an increase in optical absorbers in the NIR region (e.g. an increase in deoxygenated hemoglobin during exercise) would shorten the MPL, the NIRS measurement area may vary depending on physical and physiological characteristics of the measurement region and/or the exercise intensity. The aim of this study was to examine the changes in MPL measured by NIR_{TRS} during ramp cycling exercise between fat layer thickness-matched subjects with different aerobic capacities. Healthy control (CON, n = 8) and endurance-trained males (TR, n = 8) performed ramp cycling exercise until exhaustion. Deoxygenated hemoglobin concentration (Deoxy-Hb), total hemoglobin concentration (Total-Hb) and oxygenated hemoglobin concentration (Oxy-Hb) were evaluated by a three-wavelength NIR_{TRS} system. MPL in each wavelength (MPL_{760}, MPL_{800} and MPL_{830}) was monitored continuously. With increasing exercise intensity, Total- and Deoxy-Hb significantly increased and Oxy-Hb decreased in both groups. Total- and Oxy-Hb during exercise were significantly higher in TR than CON ($P < 0.05$, $P < 0.01$, respectively). Furthermore, Deoxy-Hb also tended to be higher in TR than CON ($P = 0.07$). In addition, MPL at all wavelengths significantly shortened with an increase in exercise intensity, with no differences between CON and TR. In particular, MPL_{760} at peak exercise shortened more than 10% compared to the start of exercise in both groups, even though MPL_{830} decreased only a few per cent. These findings suggest that the NIRS measurement area may be reduced during ramp cycling exercise due to shortened MPL. Additionally, the changes in MPL may be especially greater at 760 nm than at the other wavelengths due to greater changes in Deoxy-Hb during exercise. Furthermore, this study indicates that the measurements of muscle deoxygenation using continuous-wave NIRS can be less accurate since they are significantly affected by changes in the optical path length.

T. Endo · R. Kime (✉) · T. Watanabe · S. Fuse · N. Murase · Y. Kurosawa · T. Hamaoka
Department of Sports Medicine for Health Promotion, Tokyo Medical University, Shinjuku-ku, Tokyo, Japan
e-mail: zxc06104@nifty.com

© Springer Nature Switzerland AG 2020
P.-D. Ryu et al. (eds.), *Oxygen Transport to Tissue XLI*, Advances in Experimental Medicine and Biology 1232, https://doi.org/10.1007/978-3-030-34461-0_30

Keywords Optical path length · Ramp cycling exercise · Muscle deoxygenation · Near-infrared time-resolved spectroscopy · Endurance trained athlete

1 Introduction

Muscle deoxygenation can be monitored noninvasively by near-infrared spectroscopy (NIRS) [1]. It is evident that the changes in muscle deoxygenation during exercise are greater in subjects with higher peak pulmonary oxygen uptake [2]. However, an increase in optical absorbers in the NIR region (e.g. an increase in deoxygenated hemoglobin during exercise) would shorten the optical path length (PL). The NIRS measurement area may vary depending on the subject's aerobic capacity and/or the exercise intensity. If PL is varied during exercise, continuous-wave NIRS (NIR_{CWS}) based on the modified Beer-Lambert law, a widely used NIRS device, cannot correctly evaluate muscle deoxygenation because of the assumption that PL remains constant. NIR_{CWS} can measure only relative changes from rest with this assumption. Since time-resolved NIRS (NIR_{TRS}) can determine mean PL (MPL) by measuring the time of photon flight [3], NIR_{TRS} can evaluate the effects of each exercise intensity and aerobic capacity on the changes in MPL.

Studies have demonstrated that PL decreases during cuff occlusion or exercise [4–6]. However, factors affecting PL, such as muscle oxidative capacity or fat layer thickness (FLT) that lengthens PL, were not considered in these studies. Moreover, few studies have focused on the changes in PL in vastus lateralis muscle during cycling exercise: a frequently used NIRS measurement site and exercise protocol. Thus, the aim of this study was to examine the changes in MPL and muscle O_2 dynamics measured by NIR_{TRS} during ramp cycling exercise between FLT-matched subjects with different aerobic capacities.

2 Methods

Healthy control (CON, n = 8) and endurance-trained males (TR, n = 8) participated in this study. Physical characteristic data are shown in Table 1. All subjects were informed of the purpose of this study and gave their written informed consent before

Table 1 Healthy control (CON) and endurance-trained (TR) group physical characteristics. Values are expressed as mean ± SD

	CON (n = 8)	TR (n = 8)
Age (years)	21 ± 3	20 ± 1
Height (cm)	175.7 ± 6.8	173.6 ± 7.3
Weight (kg)	63.1 ± 6.0	62.8 ± 6.0
Fat free mass (kg)	56.3 ± 5.7	56.2 ± 5.4
VO_{2peak} (mL/kgFFM/min)	52.7 ± 5.8**	72.2 ± 3.8
Fat layer thickness (mm)	3.7 ± 0.6	3.7 ± 0.5

**Significant difference from TR ($P < 0.01$)

the experimental protocol. This study was approved by the local ethics committee of Tokyo Medical University.

The subjects were asked to avoid alcohol and intense exercise for 24 h before the test. After resting for at least 30 min after arrival in the laboratory, all subjects performed a ramp incremental exercise test on a cycle ergometer (Strength Ergo 8, FUKUDA DENSHI, Japan) in upright position until exhaustion to determine peak pulmonary oxygen uptake (VO_{2peak}). The exercise protocol consisted of 1-min rest, 1-min warm-up at 0 W followed by ramp incremental exercise at 20 W/min. The pedal frequency was maintained at 60 rpm. VO_2 was monitored by a breath-by-breath gas exchange measurement system (AE310S, Minato Medical Science, Japan). VO_{2peak} was normalized by fat-free mass (FFM) determined by bio-impedance analysis (InBody 720, InBody Japan, Japan).

Absolute oxygenated (Oxy-Hb), deoxygenated (Deoxy-Hb) and total hemoglobin concentration (Total-Hb) were measured continuously using a three wavelength (760 nm, 800 nm and 830 nm) NIR_{TRS} system (TRS-21, Hamamatsu Photonics K.K., Japan). MPL at each wavelength (MPL_{760}, MPL_{800} and MPL_{830}) was calculated continuously during the ramp incremental exercise. Details on the principle of the NIR_{TRS} system are already published [7]. The data sampling rate was 0.16 Hz (10 samples a minute). All NIR_{TRS} variables were resampled to values of every 10% relative intensity to peak workloads (100%W_{max}) for each subject. The NIR_{TRS} measurement site was the belly of the right vastus lateralis muscle, which is defined as 30% of the length between the patella and the greater trochanter. The NIR_{TRS} probe was firmly attached to the measurement site to reduce movement artifact and was protected against ambient light intrusion. The probe distance between the source and detector was 3 cm. FLT at the NIR_{TRS} measurement site was measured by an ultrasound device (Vscan Dual Probe, GE Healthcare, Japan).

An unpaired *t* test was used to compare the differences in physical characteristics between groups. Changes in NIR_{TRS} variables during exercise were analyzed by 2-way repeated-measures analysis of variance with group and exercise intensity as factors. The Bonferroni post-hoc test was performed to determine specific significant differences. All statistical analyses were performed using IBM SPSS Statistics (version 24, IBM Corporation, USA). For all statistical analyses, $P < 0.05$ was accepted as the level of significance. Data are expressed as mean ± standard deviation (SD).

3 Results

In physical characteristics, no significant differences were found between CON and TR, except for VO_{2peak} (Table 1).

After analysis of Deoxy- and Oxy-Hb, although there were no significant interactions, there were significant main effects of exercise intensity and group. Compared with 0%W_{max}, Oxy-Hb at peak exercise significantly decreased, while Deoxy-Hb significantly increased (Table 2). In addition, Oxy-Hb during exercise

Table 2 NIR_{TRS} variables at start ($0\%W_{max}$) and peak ($100\%W_{max}$) exercise in healthy control (CON) and endurance-trained (TR) group. MLP denotes mean optical path length at each wavelength. Values are expressed as mean ± SD. Significant difference from TR within intensity ($*P < 0.05$ and $** P < 0.01$). ††Significant difference from $0\%VO_{2peak}$ within group ($P < 0.01$)

	$0\%W_{max}$		$100\%W_{max}$	
	CON	TR	CON	TR
Deoxy-Hb (μM)	35.5 ± 7.2	42.6 ± 8.5	66.0 ± 18.1††	84.1 ± 20.9††
Total-Hb (μM)	128.3 ± 16.1**	154.2 ± 17.2	144.9 ± 23.2*††	176.1 ± 23.1††
Oxy-Hb (μM)	92.8 ± 10.1**	111.6 ± 11.2	78.9 ± 11.7**††	92.0 ± 7.1††
MPL_{760} (cm)	12.8 ± 1.1	12.3 ± 1.3	11.3 ± 1.5††	10.9 ± 1.4††
MPL_{800} (cm)	12.2 ± 1.4	11.9 ± 1.2	11.7 ± 1.3††	11.4 ± 1.2††
MPL_{830} (cm)	11.4 ± 1.4	11.3 ± 1.2	11.1 ± 1.3††	11.0 ± 1.1††

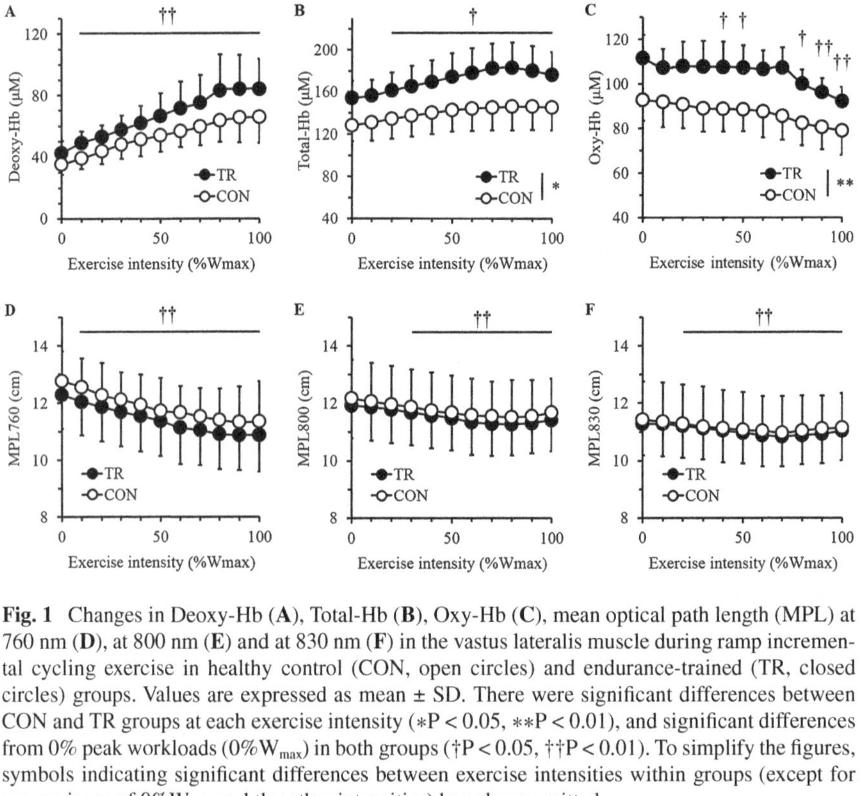

Fig. 1 Changes in Deoxy-Hb (**A**), Total-Hb (**B**), Oxy-Hb (**C**), mean optical path length (MPL) at 760 nm (**D**), at 800 nm (**E**) and at 830 nm (**F**) in the vastus lateralis muscle during ramp incremental cycling exercise in healthy control (CON, open circles) and endurance-trained (TR, closed circles) groups. Values are expressed as mean ± SD. There were significant differences between CON and TR groups at each exercise intensity ($*P < 0.05$, $**P < 0.01$), and significant differences from 0% peak workloads ($0\%W_{max}$) in both groups (†$P < 0.05$, ††$P < 0.01$). To simplify the figures, symbols indicating significant differences between exercise intensities within groups (except for comparisons of $0\%W_{max}$ and the other intensities) have been omitted

was significantly greater in TR than CON (Fig. 1C), and Deoxy-Hb tended to be greater ($P = 0.07$, Fig. 1A). In Total-Hb, there were significant exercise intensity × group interactions ($P < 0.05$). Compared with $0\%W_{max}$, Total-Hb at peak exercise significantly increased in both groups (Table 2). However, Total-Hb in TR significantly decreased from 90%W_{max} to 100%W_{max} ($P < 0.01$), in contrast to unchanged CON. Total-Hb in TR was significantly higher than CON throughout exercise (Fig. 1B).

In the analysis of MPL, there were no significant exercise intensity × group interactions for changes in MPL_{760}, MPL_{800} or MPL_{830}. A significant main effect of exercise intensity was observed in each MPL wavelength in both groups. Compared with 0%W_{max}, MPL at each wavelength was significantly decreased with increasing exercise intensity (MPL_{760}, Fig. 1D; MPL_{800}, Fig. 1E; MPL_{830}, Fig. 1F; Table 2).

4 Discussion

The present study is the first to compare the changes in MPL during ramp cycling exercise between FLT-matched subjects with different aerobic capacities. We found that MPL shortened during ramp incremental exercise, which was concordant with our original hypothesis. Although we hypothesized that MPL would show a greater decrease in endurance-trained subjects, there were no significant differences in changes in MPL at any wavelengths between groups. This result demonstrates that MPL changes during ramp cycling exercise regardless of whole body aerobic capacity.

This study reveals that MPL is reduced during exercise. Since NIR_{CWS} is based on the assumption that PL remains constant, muscle deoxygenation measurement using NIR_{CWS} may be underestimated. In addition, although Deoxy-Hb measured by NIR_{CWS} is widely used for evaluating O_2 unloading during exercise, the changes in MPL may be particularly large at 760 nm wavelength, which is well absorbed by Deoxy-Hb. These results imply that muscle deoxygenation measurements using NIR_{CWS} may be inaccurate since MPL during exercise is inconstant, especially at 760 nm wavelength. Thus, the measured values obtained from the NIR_{CWS} muscle measurements and their physiological implications should be interpreted with great care. Moreover, considering the depth direction using NIRS, there is a strong possibility that the NIRS measurement area may be reduced during exercise.

Unexpectedly, there were no significant differences in changes in MPL between CON and TR, which was not concordant with our hypothesis. We attempted to explain this as follows. In general, endurance-trained subjects have high capillary density [8]. This would mean that MPL in TR would become shorter than CON, as the higher Hb concentration has more optical absorbers in the NIR region. In contrast, Ferreira et al. demonstrated a positive correlation between Total-Hb and the reduced scattering coefficient (μ_s') [5]. The higher Hb concentration may also have more scatterers. Thus, in TR, high optical absorption and scattering in the NIR region may have offset the influence on MPL. Further studies on the changes in the absorption coefficient and μ_s' during exercise are needed.

Following the Beer-Lambert law, decreased Oxy-Hb during exercise can be interpreted as extended PL. Despite the decrease in Oxy-Hb during exercise, MPL_{830} also decreased. This may be explained by the optical absorption property in

Oxy- and Deoxy-Hb at 830 nm NIR light. A wavelength of 830 nm is a region where Oxy-Hb absorbs more than Deoxy-Hb. However, compared with NIR light at 760 nm, Deoxy-Hb also absorbs well at 830 nm. From the changes in Hb concentration during ramp exercise in this study, that is, the greater changes in Deoxy-Hb than Oxy-Hb (Table. 2), we suspect that MPL_{830} has become shortened due to the effects of absorption by Deoxy-Hb.

In summary, MPL measured by NIR_{TRS} was significantly shortened during ramp cycling exercise in both CON and TR groups. In particular, the change in MPL at 760 nm NIR light, primarily absorbed by Deoxy-Hb, was greater than at 800 and 830 nm light. These findings indicate that the NIRS measurement area may be reduced during ramp exercise due to shortened MPL derived from increased optical absorbers.

Acknowledgments The authors are grateful to Andrea Hope for revision of this manuscript. We also thank Mikiko Anjo and Ayaka Kime (Tokyo Medical University, Japan) for their helpful technical assistance. This study was supported by JSPS KAKENHI Grant Number 16 K01735.

References

1. Grassi B, Quaresima V (2016) Near-infrared spectroscopy and skeletal muscle oxidative function in vivo in health and disease: a review from an exercise physiology perspective. J Biomed Opt 21(9):091313
2. Takagi S (2016) Skeletal muscle oxygen dynamics and peak aerobic capacity. J Phys Fitness Sports Med 5(5):379–383
3. Delpy DT et al (1988) Estimation of optical pathlength through tissue from direct time of flight measurement. Phys Med Biol 33(12):1433–1442
4. Ferrari M et al (1992) Time-resolved spectroscopy of the human arm. J Photochem Photobiol B Biol 16:141–153
5. Ferreira LF et al (2007) Effects of assuming constant optical scattering on measurements of muscle oxygenation by near-infrared spectroscopy during exercise. J Appl Physiol 102:358–367
6. Duncan A et al (1995) Measurement of changes in optical pathlength through human muscle during cuff occlusion on the arm. Opt Laser Technol 27(4):269–274
7. Patterson MS et al (1989) Time resolved reflectance and transmittance for the noninvasive measurement of tissue optical properties. Appl Opt 28(12):2231–2236
8. Zoladz JA et al (2005) Capillary density and capillary-to-fibre ratio in vastus lateralis muscle of untrained and trained men. Folia Histochem Cyto 43(1):11–17

Improvements in Skeletal Muscle Can Be Detected Using Broadband NIRS in First-Time Marathon Runners

Siana Jones, Matthew Kinsella, Camilla Torlasco, Pardis Kaynezhad, Isabel de Roever, James C. Moon, Alun D. Hughes, and Gemma Bale

Abstract Skeletal muscle metabolic function is known to respond positively to endurance exercise interventions, such as marathon training. Studies investigating skeletal muscle have typically used muscle biopsy samples or magnetic resonance spectroscopy (MRS) to interrogate metabolic function. We aimed to non-invasively detect exercise-training-induced improvements in muscle function using broadband near-infrared spectroscopy (NIRS). We used NIRS to determine concentration changes in oxygenated haemoglobin (HbO_2) and the oxidation state of cytochrome-c-oxidase (oxCCO) in gastrocnemius during arterial occlusion in 14 volunteers. We also used a cardio-pulmonary exercise test (CPET) to assess peak total body oxygen uptake (peakVO_2; a measure of fitness). Measurements were made at baseline (BL) which was prior to a period of at least 16 weeks of training for the 2017 London Marathon, and then within 3 weeks after completion of the marathon, follow-up (FU). We observed an increase in locally measured muscle oxygen consumption and rate of oxCCO concentration change, but not in cardio-respiratory fitness measured as whole-body peak oxygen consumption (peakVO_2).

Keywords Near-infrared spectroscopy · Metabolism · Cytochrome-c-oxidase · Endurance exercise · Vascular

The original version of this chapter was revised. The correction to this chapter is available at https://doi.org/10.1007/978-3-030-34461-0_54

S. Jones · A. D. Hughes
MRC Unit for Lifelong Health & Ageing at UCL, Department of Population Science & Experimental Medicine, Institute for Cardiovascular Science, UCL, London, UK

M. Kinsella · P. Kaynezhad · I. de Roever · G. Bale (✉)
Medical Physics and Biomedical Engineering, University College London, London, UK
e-mail: g.bale@ucl.ac.uk

C. Torlasco · J. C. Moon
Barts Heart Centre, St Bartholomew's Hospital, London, UK

© Springer Nature Switzerland AG 2020
P.-D. Ryu et al. (eds.), *Oxygen Transport to Tissue XLI*, Advances in Experimental Medicine and Biology 1232, https://doi.org/10.1007/978-3-030-34461-0_31

1 Introduction

Skeletal muscle metabolic function is typically interrogated via muscle biopsy or magnetic resonance spectroscopy (MRS). While these techniques have the capacity to phenotype muscle in detail, they are not always appropriate, or available, in research and clinical environments. There is a need to develop skeletal muscle assessment tools which are non-invasive, widely available and sensitive enough to detect changes in function in response to intervention.

Continuous wave NIRS devices, applying 2–4 wavelengths of near-infrared light, have previously been used to measure local muscle oxygen consumption, which is represented by the rate of change in oxygenated haemoglobin/myoglobin (HbO_2) during an arterial occlusion [1]. Broadband NIRS can additionally monitor metabolism via the oxidation state of cytochrome-c-oxidase (oxCCO), from redox-dependent spectral changes in its copper A centre (Cu_A) [2]. Changes in oxCCO in skeletal muscle during arterial occlusions have not been fully examined previously.

Skeletal muscle metabolic function is known to respond positively to endurance exercise interventions. Evidence that has been gathered by measuring increases in the overall concentration of mitochondrial enzymes in biopsy samples, shows that exercise training stimulates mitochondrial growth, oxidative capacity, and capacity for syntheses of glycogen and lipid [3, 4].

In this study we use a miniature broadband NIRS system, called mini-CYRIL [5], to assess the effect of marathon training on muscle haemodynamic and metabolic functions at rest and after exercise.

2 Methods

Participants were healthy, non-athletic adults (>30 years old) enrolled in a study investigating cardiac adaptations to at least 16 weeks of endurance training for their first marathon. All procedures were in accordance with the Declaration of Helsinki; all participants gave written informed consent and the study was approved by the London Queen Square National Research Ethics Service Committee (15/LO/0086).

Before commencing training (baseline; BL), participants underwent measurements of HbO_2, deoxy-haemoglobin (HHb) and oxCCO concentration changes in the lateral gastrocnemius using an in-house built laboratory broadband NIRS device (mini-CYRIL) [5]. Two 3-minute arterial occlusions were applied proximal to the measurement site using a leg cuff inflated to supra-systolic pressure. The first occlusion was carried out at rest; the second, following a maximal exertion exercise test.

Height and weight were measured using a stadiometer and scales (BC-418, Tanita, USA), respectively. Adipose tissue thickness (ATT) was measured by ultrasound at the NIRS measurement site. Cardio-respiratory fitness was measured using a maximal cardio-pulmonary exercise test (CPET) carried out on a supine cycle ergometer (Ergoselect1200, Ergoline, Germany) to determine peak oxygen consumption (peakVO_2) by analysis of expired gases (Quark CPET, Cosmed, Italy).

All measurements were repeated within 3 weeks of participants completing the 2017 London marathon (follow-up; FU).

Data analysis was carried out in MATLAB 2015b (Mathworks, USA). NIRS spectral data were assessed for adequate signal to noise (SNR) and resolved concentration changes were assessed for cross-talk using residual analysis [2]. Data sets with poor signal to noise or evidence of cross-talk were excluded from further analysis. Concentration changes were determined from the mini-CYRIL spectral data using the modified Beer-Lambert law [2] with a differential pathlength factor of 5.51 [6] that was corrected for the wavelength dependency of the pathlength [7]. To check that the occlusion period did not induce changes in the optical pathlength, a dynamic measured pathlength was calculated for a sub-set of data sets using the second differential of water spectral peaks [8].

Linear fitting was applied to the HbO_2 and oxCCO signals during the occlusion periods to determine their rate of change. These represent local muscle oxygen consumption. While the HbO_2 signal captures changes in haemoglobin/myoglobin -bound oxygen in capillaries, small blood vessels and skeletal myocytes, oxCCO represents changes in mitochondrial oxygen availability. Statistical analysis was performed in STATA15 (StataCorp LLC, USA). Participant characteristics are presented as n (%) if data are categorical and mean ± standard deviation is normally distributed. NIRS data are presented as median (interquartile range; IQR). Differences in mean and median values were determined using a paired Student's t-test or signed-rank test, respectively. The level of significance was set at $p < 0.05$. The rate of change of each NIRS signal was compared before/after exercise and before/after marathon training.

3 Results

Complete data sets at both BL and FU were collected from 14 participants. An example NIRS trace is shown in Fig. 1. Participant characteristics and cardio-respiratory fitness at BL and FU are shown in Table 1. Overall, there were no discernable changes in weight or peakVO_2 after marathon training.

The group median for rate of change in HbO_2 during occlusions at rest was more negative (higher consumption) after marathon training (BL median (IQR): −0.027 (−0.025, −0.035) μM/s versus FU: −0.041 (−0.032, −0.046) μM/s, p = 0.004; Fig. 2, top left). This was also the case for rate of change measured directly after the CPET (post-exercise) (BL: −0.037 (−0.028, −0.040) μM/s versus FU: −0.047 (−0.061, −0.036) μM/s, p = 0.04; Fig. 2, bottom left).

The group median for rate of change in oxCCO during occlusions at rest was more negative (higher rate of concentration change) after marathon training (B: −0.0012 (−0.0025, 0.0032) μM/s versus FU: −0.0037 (−0.0050, −0.0022) μM/s, p = 0.02; Fig. 2, top right). This was also the case for rates of change measured directly after the CPET (post-exercise) (BL: −0.0014 (−0.0057, 0.0049) μM/s versus FU: −0.0060 (−0.014, −0.002) μM/s, p = 0.04; Fig. 2, bottom right).

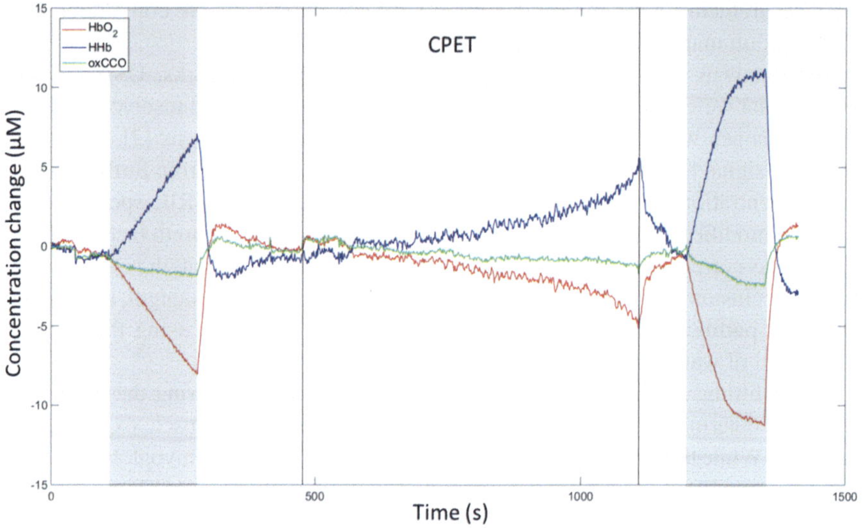

Fig. 1 Example NIRS data at FU during occlusions (grey) pre- and post-CPET (between black lines). Rate of change during occlusions- HbO_2: −0.04 and − 0.07 μM/s, oxCCO: −0.005 and − 0.014 μM/s

Table 1 Group characteristics of participants at baseline and follow-up. Data are mean ± standard deviation

	Baseline	Follow Up	p-value
Male n (%)	6 (43%)	–	–
Age (years)	43.4 ± .6	–	–
Height (cm)	175.4 ± 8.7	–	–
Weight (kg)	76.2 ± 16.7	75.2 ± 16.8	0.18
ATT (mm)	7.3 ± 1.9	6.6 ± 2.1	0.07
Peak VO_2 (ml/min/kg)	31.5 ± 5.7	31.0 ± 4.9	0.41

4 Discussion

We describe the novel application of broadband NIRS to measure changes in oxCCO and HbO_2 during arterial occlusions to estimate oxygen consumption in skeletal muscle. We found that, in middle-aged adults, endurance exercise training was associated with an increase in estimates of local muscle oxygen consumption in the absence of a detectable change in whole-body cardio-respiratory fitness (peakVO_2).

At rest, arterial occlusions induced a more rapid decline in HbO_2 after the period of endurance training (FU resting; Fig. 2, top left). A similar pattern was also seen during arterial occlusions made directly following a period of acute intense exercise (FU post-exercise; Fig. 2, bottom left), a finding that is in line with a previously described effect of marathon training on skeletal muscle oxygen consumption [9].

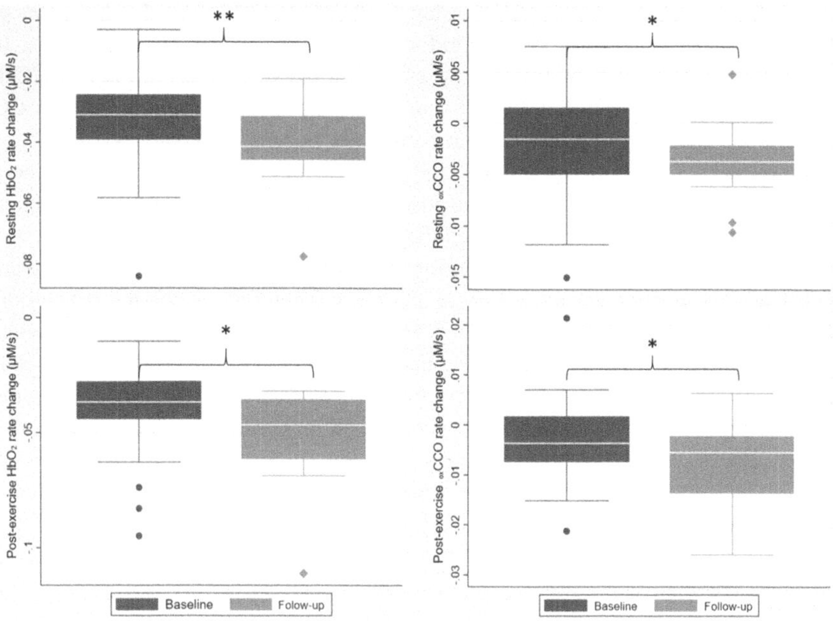

Fig. 2 Boxplots show median (IQR) rate of change of HbO_2 (left side) and oxCCO (right side) during occlusions before (BL, dark grey) and after (FU, light grey) marathon training. Top panels show resting (before CPET) and bottom panels show post-exercise (after CPET). * $p < 0.05$, ** $p < 0.01$

We interpret this as an improvement in extraction and/or consumption of oxygen by skeletal muscle. The general view is that oxygen delivery is the limiting factor for oxygen consumption in muscle, but evidence exists that mitochondrial capacity scales with O_2 delivery [10], so the situation is likely more complex.

oxCCO declined more rapidly during occlusions after a period of endurance training both at rest and post-exercise test (FU resting & post-exercise; Fig. 2, right panels). We interpret this as a greater oxidative capacity in the muscle due to training since more rapid reduction in oxCCO indicates a quicker depletion of oxygen, because an absence of oxygen prevents electron transfer leading to a reduced CuA [11]. Further, in brain tissue it has been observed that cytochrome c oxidase (CCO) reduction occurs only under extreme hypoxia and hence, our findings may be an indicator of oxygen depletion in the muscle.

Surprisingly, we observed an increase in oxCCO in several individuals during arterial occlusions at rest (BL: n = 6, FU: n = 3) and post-exercise (BL: n = 7, FU: n = 2). Note that this was observed in fewer individuals at FU, so could be associated with the effects of marathon training. It is possible that these increases are artefacts, or too small to be physiologically relevant. However, these increases are substantial (on the order of 0.1 to 1 μM), and were observed when both a fixed pathlength and an estimated pathlength were used to resolve them. Furthermore, the NIRS intensity data were scrutinized for high SNR, residual analysis was used to check for cross-talk, and there was no relationship between the ATT and the direction of oxCCO change. A possible explanation for this increase in oxCCO is an increase in nitric oxide (NO) due to ischaemia. NO competes with oxygen to bind to CCO, hence an increase in cellular NO will cause an apparent increase in oxidized CCO [12]. More studies are needed to confirm and understand this result.

There are several limitations to this study. First, while we inflated the cuff to more than 250 mmHg we cannot exclude the possibility of incomplete arterial occlusion in some individuals and, as we considered the change in HbO_2 only, we cannot be sure that volumetric shifts did not occur during the occlusion. Second, participants were not asked to complete a training diary in this study. Therefore, we do not have information about type or intensity of training. Finally, the sample size (n = 14) is small.

To conclude, in healthy middle-aged men and women preparing for a first marathon, training for a period of at least 16 weeks was associated with an increase in the ability of skeletal muscle to utilize oxygen, and an increase in the rate of mitochondrial oxygen depletion. Together these findings suggest an improvement in metabolic capacity with low-intensity endurance training. Metabolic adaptions can be identified non-invasively using broadband NIRS combined with arterial occlusions. However, further work in more subjects is warranted to investigate the changes in oxCCO observed.

Acknowledgments The authors would like to thank the volunteers who participated in this study. GB acknowledges support from The Wellcome Trust, grant 104580/Z/14/Z. SJ is supported by a grant from the British Heart Foundation (CS/13/1/30327). ADH receives support from the British Heart Foundation (PG/15/75/31748, CS/15/6/31468, CS/13/1/30327), the National Institute for Health Research University College London Hospitals Biomedical Research Centre, and the UK Medical Research Council (MC_UU_12019/1).

References

1. van Beekvelt MCP, van Engelen BGM, Wevers RA, Colier WNJM (2002) In vivo quantitative near-infrared spectroscopy in skeletal muscle during incremental isometric handgrip exercise. Clin Physiol Funct Imaging 22(3):210–217
2. Bale G, Elwell CE, Tachtsidis I (2016) From Jöbsis to the present day: a review of clinical near-infrared spectroscopy measurements of cerebral cytochrome-c-oxidase. J Biomed Opt 21(9):091307
3. Holloszy JO, Coyle EF (1984) Adaptations of skeletal muscle to endurance exercise and their metabolic consequences. J Appl Physiol 56:831–838
4. Morgan TE, Cobb LA, Short FA, Ross R, Gunn DR (1971) Effects of long-term exercise on human muscle mitochondria. In: Pernow B, Saltin B (eds) Muscle metabolism during exercise: proceedings of a Karolinska Institutet symposium held in Stockholm, Sweden, September 6–9, 1970 honorary guest: E Hohwü Christensen. Springer US, Boston, pp 87–95
5. Siddiqui MF, Lloyd-Fox S, Kaynezhad P, Tachtsidis I, Johnson MH, Elwell CE (Dec. 2017) Non-invasive measurement of a metabolic marker of infant brain function. Sci Rep 7(1):1330
6. Duncan A et al (1995) Optical pathlength measurements on adult head, calf and forearm and the head of the newborn infant using phase resolved optical spectroscopy. Phys Med Biol 40(2):295–304

7. Essenpreis M, Elwell CE, Cope M, van der Zee P, Arridge SR, Delpy DT (1993) Spectral dependence of temporal point spread functions in human tissues. Appl Opt 32(4):418–425
8. Matcher SJ, Cope M, Delpy DT (1994) Use of the water absorption spectrum to quantify tissue chromophore concentration changes in near-infrared spectroscopy. Phys Med Biol 39:177–196
9. Jones S et al (2017) Improved exercise-related skeletal muscle oxygen consumption following uptake of endurance training measured using near-infrared spectroscopy. Front Physiol 12(8):1018
10. van der Zwaard S et al (2016) Maximal oxygen uptake is proportional to muscle fiber oxidative capacity, from chronic heart failure patients to professional cyclists. J Appl Physiol
11. Cooper CE et al (Nov. 1994) Near-infrared spectroscopy of the brain: relevance to cytochrome oxidase bioenergetics. Biochem Soc Trans 22(4):974–980
12. Erusalimsky JD, Moncada S (2007) Nitric oxide and mitochondrial signaling: from physiology to pathophysiology. Arterioscler Thromb Vasc Biol 27(12):2524–2531

Comparison of Two NIRS Tissue Oximeters (Moxy and Nimo) for Non-Invasive Assessment of Muscle Oxygenation and Perfusion

Felix Scholkmann and Andrea Scherer-Vrana

Abstract Background: Near-infrared spectroscopy (NIRS) tissue oximeters enable non-invasive measurement of muscle oxygenation and perfusion. Several NIRS oximeters are currently available, particularly for muscle measurements. Aim: To evaluate the agreement of oxygenation and perfusion measurements obtained by two devices (Moxy, Fortiori Designs LLC, USA, and Nimo, Nirox, Italy) during an arterial occlusion test on the arm. Subject and Methods: Arterial occlusions were conducted at the arm of one individual for 10 min with 200 mmHg. Measurements were made twice a day on five different days. Both NIRS devices were fixed at the arm (covering the muscles extensor carpi ulnaris, extensor digitorum, and flexor carpi ulnaris). Results: The experiment revealed that i) both devices could detect changes in muscle oxygenation and perfusion during the occlusion, but ii) the magnitudes and dynamic changes differed between the two devices. Discussion and Conclusion: Both devices had different performances with regard to the measurement of tissue oxygenation and perfusion. This study shows that it might be worthwhile to compare all NIRS tissue oximeters currently available for muscle measurement in a large systematic study to increase the comparability of measurements obtained with different devices.

Keywords Near-infrared spectroscopy · NIRS · Muscle oxygenation and perfusion · Validation

---

F. Scholkmann (✉)
University Hospital Zurich, University of Zurich, Department of Neonatology, Biomedical Optics Research Laboratory, Zurich, Switzerland

Scholkmann Data Analysis Services, Scientific Consulting and Physical Engineering, Zurich, Switzerland
e-mail: Felix.Scholkmann@usz.ch

A. Scherer-Vrana
Interdisciplinary Spinal Research, Department of Chiropractic Medicine, Balgrist University Hospital, Zurich, Switzerland

© Springer Nature Switzerland AG 2020

P.-D. Ryu et al. (eds.), *Oxygen Transport to Tissue XLI*, Advances in Experimental Medicine and Biology 1232, https://doi.org/10.1007/978-3-030-34461-0_32

1 Introduction

One NIRS device relatively frequently used for muscle measurement is the Moxy (Fortiori Design LLC, Minnesota, USA). Another device currently used in studies on muscle physiology is the Nimo (Nirox srl, Borgosatello, Italy). Despite the extensive use of these devices in the exercise physiology community, only a few peer-reviewed papers have reported the application of the two devices (Moxy: [1, 2]; Nimo: [3–10]). Surprisingly, no study so far has compared these two devices with the respect to how the measured changes in muscle oxygenation and perfusion depend on the specific device used.

The aim of this study was to compare these two devices by performing an arm occlusion experiment. The main question was whether the devices measured similar changes in muscle oxygenation and perfusion (with respect to magnitude and dynamics) during the experiment.

2 Subject and Methods

NIRS Tissue Oximeters Two devices were quantitatively compared: the Moxy device (Fortiori Design LLC, Minnesota, USA) and the Nimo (Nirox srl, Borgosatollo, Italy). Table 1 shows the technical specifications and Fig. 1 additional details of the two devices. Both devices use different geometrical arrangements of the detectors and sources and employ different numbers, types and wavelengths.

Participant and Protocol One healthy male individual (aged 38 years; body mass index 25.7) was recruited for this study. Inclusion criteria were normotonia, the absence of any acute or chronic health problems, and no regular intake of any medication. The participant was orally informed about the experimental procedures and provided informed consent. The study was approved by the Swiss Ethical Committee (BASEC-Nr. Req-2017-00226). Ten arterial occlusions were conducted in this individual at the left biceps brachialis using a medical inflatable cuff for manual blood pressure measurement (Boso, Bosch & Sohn, Jungingen, Germany). The adipose tissue thickness at the measurement area was 3 mm and was assessed prior to the experiment using a caliper.

During the experiment, the subject was sitting in a comfortable position with both arms lying on a table in front of him beneath the level of the heart. The arterial occlusion lasted 10 min and was applied with a pressure of 200 mmHg by the inflatable cuff. Measurements were taken on five different days and twice per day, i.e. between 10:00 and 11:00 in the morning, and between 13:00 and 15:00 in the afternoon. Both NIRS devices were fixed at the arm (covering the muscles extensor carpi ulnaris, extensor digitorum, and flexor carpi ulnaris) with medical tape and a dark bandage to avoid potential influence from daylight. The position of the NIRS devices was randomly altered to guarantee that both devices measured at both loca-

Table 1 Technical specifications of the two devices

	Moxy	Nimo
Company	Fortiori Design LLC (Minnesota, USA)	Nirox (Borgosatollo, Italy)
	www.moxymonitor.com	www.nirox.it
NIRS operation mode	CW	CW
Sampling rate	0.5–2 Hz, depending on settings	40 Hz
Number of light sources	4	3
Number of light detectors	2	1
Wavelengths	680, 720, 760, 800 nm	685, 850, 980 nm
Type of light source	LEDs	Laser diodes
Source-detector distance	1.25 cm, 2.5 cm	3 cm
Number of light paths	2	3
Measurement of SmO_2 (absolute concentration)	Yes	Yes
Measurement of [tHbMb] (absolute concentration)	No	Yes
Fat-layer correction	Yes	Yes
Correction of temperature-dependent spectral changes of the light emitters	Yes	No
Water correction	Yes (water spectra with fixed water volume fraction included in the calibration model); however, no direct measurement of the water concentration	Yes (water absorption measured used to calculate the optical pathlength); however, no direct measurement of the water concentration
Weight	48 g	Probe: 100 g, device: 3 kg
Water resistant	Full	Splash-water proof
CE certified	Yes	Yes

CW: continuous wave, CE: European Conformity. Data were obtained from manuals provided by the manufacturers and by directly contacting the manufacturers. Manufacturers were asked to review the table and approve the correctness of the information

tions on both day times. The examination started with a baseline measurement of 2 min. After 2 min, the cuff was inflated within 5 s and maintained stable for the following 10 min. In case of a (minimal) decrease in pressure during the occlusion, the tester adjusted the pressure back to 200 mmHg by immediately pumping. Additionally, the tester auscultated the brachial artery at the elbow during the whole occlusion (by listening to the returning Korotkoff sound) to ensure the maintenance of arterial occlusion. Deflation was started after 10 min of occlusion and lasted approximately 3 s, followed by a 3-min recovery period.

Data Analysis The data (muscle oxygenation, SmO_2, and concentration of total hemoglobin plus the concentration of myoglobin, [tHbMb]) obtained from the two devices were analyzed as follows: first, the raw data were resampled to obtain signals with 0.2 Hz. Block averages of the data over all trials were calculated with the

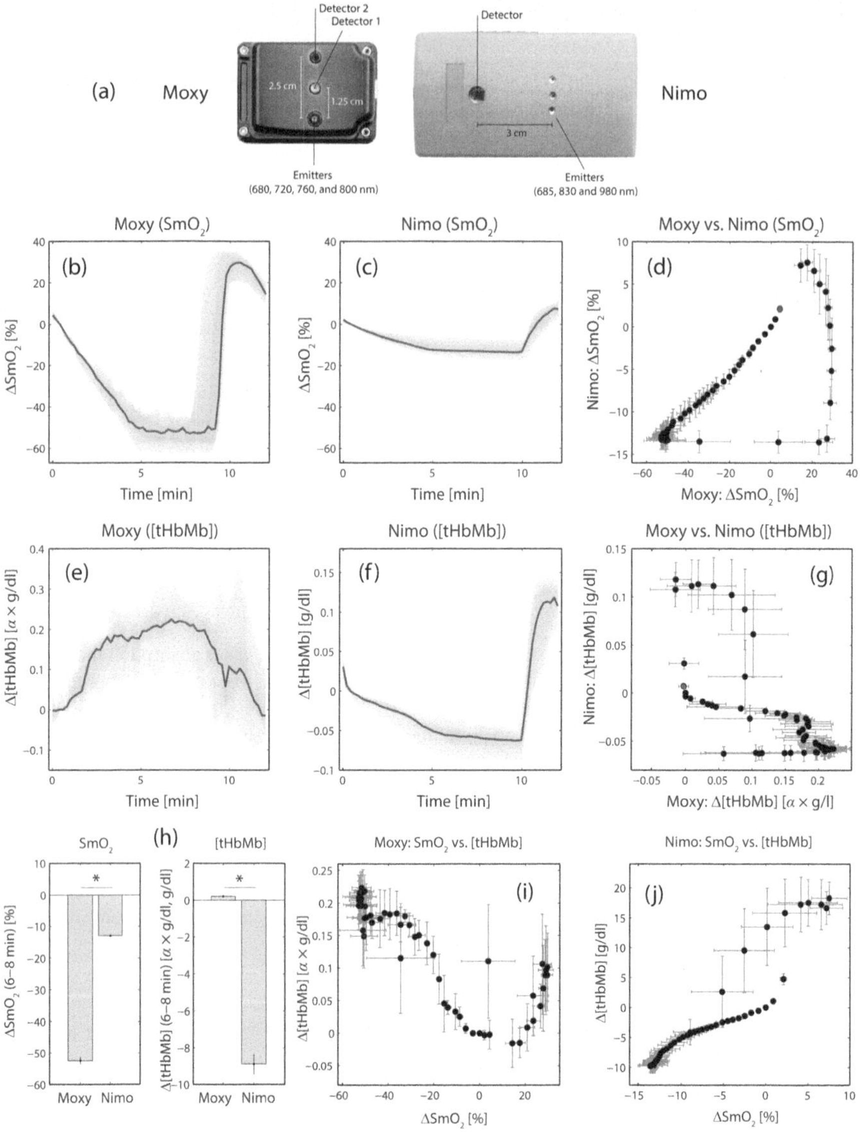

Fig. 1 (**a**) The devices tested. (**b**)–(**d**) Changes in SmO_2. (**e–g**) Changes in [tHbMb]. (**h**) Changes in SmO_2 and [tHbMb] during occlusion. (**i**, **j**) Scatter plots comparing the changes measured by both devices

resampled, or with the resampled and normalized data. Normalization was done by dividing the signals by the median value of the first 25 s. This set the individual baseline to a similar value, providing a better group-based analysis of the dynamic changes of SmO_2 and [tHbMb] due to occlusion. The normalized SmO_2 and [tHbMb] data are denoted as ΔSmO_2 and Δ[tHbMb], respectively.

Furthermore, the median and median absolute deviation (mad) values of SmO_2 and [tHbMb] (from both devices) were calculated for the interval 6–8 min to quantify the maximal change of SmO_2 and [tHbMb] measured by the devices during the occlusion.

Finally, correlation analyses were performed to compare the devices. Therefore, the following signal combinations were analyzed using the signals recorded during the occlusion: i) SmO_2 (Moxy) vs. SmO_2 (Nimo), ii) ΔSmO_2 (Moxy) vs. ΔSmO_2 (Nimo), iii) [tHbMb] (Moxy) vs. [tHbMb] (Nimo), iv) Δ[tHbMb] (Moxy) vs. Δ[tHbMb] (Nimo), v) Δ[tHbMb] (Moxy) vs. ΔStO_2 (Moxy), and vi) Δ[tHbMb] (Nimo) vs. ΔStO_2 (Nimo).

3 Results

Figure 1 shows that the magnitude and dynamics of the changes in SmO_2 and [tHbMb], as well as ΔSmO_2 and Δ[tHbMb], differed between the two devices.

Absolute Change in Muscle Oxygenation and Perfusion Both devices measured a decrease in SmO_2 during the occlusion; however, the decrease measured by the Moxy was much larger (decrease of SmO_2 of −52.50% (median), 95% confidence interval, CI 0.98%) compared with that obtained with the Nimo (−12.93%, 95% CI 0.24%). Also, both devices measured significantly different ($p < 0.0001$, Wilcoxon rank sum test) ΔSmO_2 values due to occlusion.

In parallel, [tHbMb] measured with the Moxy showed an increase (0.214 $\alpha \times$ g/dl, CI 0.013 $\alpha \times$ g/dl), while Nimo measured a decrease (−0.056 g/dl, CI 0.003 g/dl) (the α in the unit is a scaling factor of unknown numerical value, i.e. not given by the manufacturer). Both devices measured significantly different ($p < 0.0001$, Wilcoxon rank sum test) Δ[tHbMb] values due to occlusion.

Dynamics of Changes in Muscle Oxygenation and Perfusion Figure 1 shows that the *dynamics* of changes in muscle oxygenation and perfusion also differed between the devices. The Moxy showed a strong and fast decline of SmO_2 during occlusion with an overshoot after occlusion (reperfusion), whereas the Nimo's SmO_2 signal decreased moderately and slower, and the reperfusion increase was smaller and slower compared to that of the Moxy (Fig. 1(b) and (c)).

The [tHbMb] showed a completely different dynamic behavior depending on the device: during occlusion, the Moxy measured a rapid increase that stabilized and decreased to the baseline value after occlusion. In contrast, the Nimo measured a decrease that continued until the end of occlusion and reversed to an overshoot of [tHbMb] after release of the cuff (Fig. 1 (e) and (f).

Correlations The following correlations of the signals during the experiments were obtained (r: Spearman correlation coefficient, p: p-value for statistical significance of the correlation): i) SmO_2 (Moxy) vs. SmO_2 (Nimo): $r = 0.6437$, $p < 0.001$; ii) ΔSmO_2

(Moxy) vs. ΔSmO_2 (Nimo): $r = 0.6899$, $p < 0.001$; iii) [tHbMb] (Moxy) vs. [tHbMb] (Nimo): $r = -0.7395$, $p < 0.001$; iv) Δ[tHbMb] (Moxy) vs. Δ[tHbMb] (Nimo): $r = -0.6957$, $p < 0.001$; v) Δ[tHbMb] (Moxy) vs. ΔStO_2 (Moxy): $r = -0.8594$, $p < 0.001$; and vi) Δ[tHbMb] (Nimo) vs. ΔStO_2 (Nimo): $r = 0.9936$, $p < 0.001$.

Therefore, there is a good correlation between the signals measured by both devices. However, the scatter plots (Fig. 1(g), (i) and (j)) clearly indicate that the correlations are non-linear and show hysteresis. A quasi-linear hysteresis is present for the relationship between SmO_2 values, while a non-linear hysteresis is present for the [tHbMb] signals.

4 Discussion, Conclusion and Outlook

Our main finding that the magnitude and dynamics of the changes in SmO_2 and [tHbMb] were different for the two NIRS oximeters is generally in line with previous studies comparing the performance of NIRS oximeters [11–13].

Our study shows that the measured signals are correlated in a complex manner. SmO_2 values from both devices follow a relationship of linear hysteresis where the [tHbMb] signals are even more complex following a non-linear hysteresis. This finding is problematic since, in case of linear correlations, it would have been possible to create conversion (look-up) tables based on linear equations for the signals of the Nimo and the Moxy.

Why the NIRS devices tested delivered such different results? The main reason seems to be the differences how the devices measure the optical changes in the tissue and how they relate them to changes in oxygenation and perfusion. The selection of wavelengths, the mode of measurement (Nimo: single-distance mode, 3 cm; Moxy: multi-distance mode, 1.25 and 2.5 cm), the models for light-propagation used, and different methods to correct of the fat layer thickness (Moxy: assumed value from the literature; Nimo: direct measurement of the optical pathlength based on the water absorption peak) are obviously the causing differences in the final calculated values of tissue oxygenation and perfusion. To answer which device is closer to the "real" physiological changes in the muscle was not aim of the study since we solely wanted to investigate if the two devices deliver comparable signal, which they did not to a large extent.

The study shows that both NIRS-based muscle oximeters were able to detect changes in muscle oxygenation and perfusion during a vascular occlusion test on the arm. However, the magnitudes and the dynamic changes differed between the two devices. It might be worthwhile to compare all NIRS tissue oximeters for muscle measurement that are currently available in a large systematic study to increase the comparability of measurements obtained with different devices.

Acknowledgments The authors thank Prof. Dr. Martin Flück and Prof. Dr. Martin Wolf for support and technical advice. In addition, we thank the two companies (Maurizio Donini, Nirox; Roger Schmitz, Fortiori Design LLC) for technical advice and proofreading the sections describing the technical specifications of their devices.

References

1. Muller MD, Li Z, Sica CT et al (2016) Muscle oxygenation during dynamic plantar flexion exercise: combining BOLD MRI with traditional physiological measurements. Physiol Rep 4(20):e13004
2. Baláš J, Michailov M, Giles D et al (2015) Active recovery of the finger flexors enhances intermittent handgrip performance in rock climbers. Eur J Sport Sci 16(7):764–772
3. De Blasi RA, Palmisani S, Boezi M et al (2008) Effects of remifentanil-based general anaesthesia with propofol or sevoflurane on muscle microcirculation as assessed by near-infrared spectroscopy. Br J Anaesth 101(2):171–177
4. Lluch GL, Lanfranconi F, Pollastri L et al (2014) Near Infrared Spectroscopy (NIRS) as a new non-invasive tool to detect oxidative skeletal muscle impairment in children survived to acute lymphoblastic Leukaemia. PLoS One 9(6):e99282
5. De Blasi R, Luciani R, Punzo G et al (2009) Microcirculatory changes and skeletal muscle oxygenation measured at rest by non-infrared spectroscopy in patients with and without diabetes undergoing haemodialysis. Crit Care 13(Suppl 5):S9
6. Pipili C, Grapsa E, Ioannidou S et al (2015) Changes in skeletal muscle microcirculation after a hemodialysis session correlates with adequacy of dialysis. Int J Nephrol Renov Dis:59
7. Zerbini L, Brighenti A, Pellegrini B et al (2012) Effects of acute hypoxia on the oxygen uptake kinetics of older adults during cycling exercise. Appl Physiol Nutr Metab 37(4):744–752
8. De Blasi RA, Arcioni R (2014) Assessing skeletal muscle variations in microvascular pressure and unstressed blood volume at the bedside. Microcirculation 21(7):606–614
9. Macdonald JH, Fearn L, Jibani M et al (2012) Exertional fatigue in patients with CKD. Am J Kidney Dis 60(6):930–939
10. Casanova N, Reis JF, Vaz JR et al (2017) Effects of roller massager on muscle recovery after exercise-induced muscle damage. J Sports Sci:1–8
11. Fellahi J-L, Butin G, Fischer M-O et al (2013) Dynamic evaluation of near-infrared peripheral oximetry in healthy volunteers: a comparison between INVOS and EQUANOX. J Crit Care 28(5):881.e1–881.e6
12. Lee J-H, Park Y-H, Kim H-S et al (2014) Comparison of two devices using near-infrared spectroscopy for the measurement of tissue oxygenation during a vascular occlusion test in healthy volunteers (INVOS® vs. InSpectra™). J Clin Monit Comput 29(2):271–278
13. Nygren A, Rennerfelt K, Zhang Q (2013) Detection of changes in muscle oxygen saturation in the human leg: a comparison of two near-infrared spectroscopy devices. J Clin Monit Comput 28(1):57–62

Part IV
Cell Metabolism and Tissue Oxygenation

Effects of Pulsed Magnetic Field on the Hemolysis of Erythrocytes Exposed to Oxidative Stress

Hyoje Ahn, Kyunghun Shin, and Hyunsook Lee

Abstract Ahematological and morphological investigation was made of the effects of pulsed magnetic field (PMF) stimulus on oxidized erythrocyte membrane using the smear method and spectroscopic measurement. Tert-butyl hydroperoxide (tBHP) was used for oxidative stress, and verapamil was used as reduction agent on red blood cells (RBCs). Our PMF stimulator system was designed to generate a maximum intensity of 0.27 T at a transition time of 0.102 ms. The morphology of oxidized RBCs, and oxidative stressed RBCs after treatment with a reducing agent were observed before and after PMF. Light absorbance of hemoglobin (Hb) was measured in the membrane as well as plasma, through hemolysis of RBCs. Absorbance for a sample exposed to PMF before the oxidation treatment was lower than that for a sample not exposed to PMF in the plasma. This means that PMF plays a role in preventing hemolysis of erythrocyte membrane from oxidative stress. Our results were confirmed using an osmotic fragility test. Hemolysis in the case of PMF treatment is 28% lower than that of non-PMF treatment. As a result, PMF stimulus is proposed to achieve an improvement of RBCs aggregation and prevent RBCs from oxidative stress, and could be used in various clinical fields related to peripheral vascular diseases. For further clinical application, we need to optimize PMF intensity and stimulated duration.

Keywords Erythrocytes · Oxidative stress · Deformability · Hemoglobin · Spectrophotometer

---

H. Ahn · K. Shin · H. Lee (✉)
Department of Oriental Biomedical Engineering, College of Health Sciences, Sangji University, Wonju, South Korea
e-mail: hslee@sangji.ac.kr

© Springer Nature Switzerland AG 2020

P.-D. Ryu et al. (eds.), *Oxygen Transport to Tissue XLI*, Advances in Experimental Medicine and Biology 1232, https://doi.org/10.1007/978-3-030-34461-0_33

1 Introduction

Transportation of the respiratory gases of erythrocytes is not only a major contribution to blood circulation, but also an important factor in buffering the pH of the blood. Erythrocytes are naturally exposed to oxidative stress while circulating the blood vessels in the physiological state, but these circulatory cells are equipped with an effective anti-oxidative system that makes them mobile free radical scavengers, providing antioxidant protection to themselves as well as to other tissues and organs in the body [1, 2].

Under the hyper-oxidative stress, free radicals oxidize lipids, proteins and DNA, damaging cells and tissues, and ultimately leading to malignant diseases such as arteriosclerosis and cancer. Red blood cells (RBCs) are highly susceptible to oxidative damage due to the high cell concentration of oxygen and hemoglobin (Hb), a powerful promoter of the oxidative process [3]. Hb contained in RBCs can carry out vital gas transport functions smoothly, due to the deformability of RBCs. Accordingly, when RBCs are subjected to oxidative stress, it is useful to investigate the state of Hb and erythrocyte membrane changes.

The use of pulsed magnetic field (PMF) was proposed as an alternative non-invasive treatment to influence human physiology by inducing an electric current in deep tissue. Many studies have investigated the influence of a magnetic field on various biological phenomena both in vivo and in vitro [4–6].

This study elucidates both hematologically and morphologically the influence of PMF on oxidized RBCs and establishes whether PMF can prevent oxidative stress, through observation of morphological changes in erythrocyte membranes and light absorbance of Hb. In addition, the osmotic fragility test was performed to observe the effect of PMF on hemolysis of the erythrocyte membrane. Confirming that PMF relieves oxidative stress of erythrocytes, PMF system might apply to clinical treatment such as ischemic disease due to oxidized erythrocytes.

2 Experimental Materials and Methods

Oxidation and Reduction of Erythrocytes All blood samples were obtained by routine collection at the Sangji blood bank and preserved in vacuum tubes containing ethylenediaminetetraacetic acid (1.5 mg/ml) to prevent coagulation. Whole blood of 10 ml was centrifuged at 3000 g for 10 min at 4 °C. After careful removal of plasma and the buffy coat, RBCs were washed three times with phosphate buffered saline (PBS: pH 7.4). Finally, PBS and plasma were added to the washed RBCs for RBC suspension with a hematocrit (Ht) level of 25%.

Tert-butyl hydroperoxide (tBHP) was used to induce oxidative stress in RBCs, since the action mechanism of tBHP is very similar to that when RBCs are subjected to severe oxidative stress [7]; verapamil was used as a reducing agent. tBHP (0.8 mM) was added to the RBC suspension with ratio of one to one and kept for

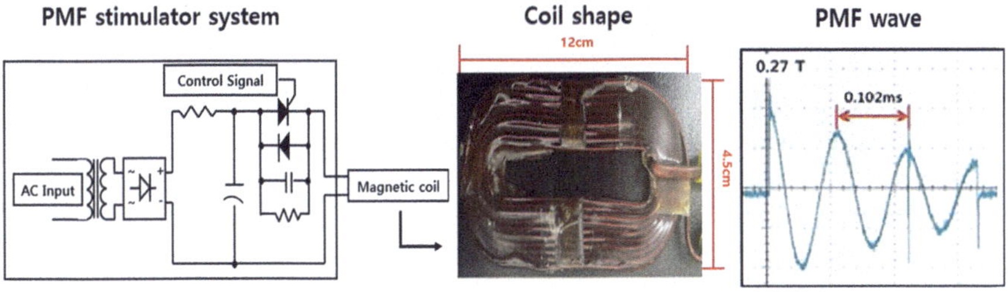

Fig. 1 Schematic diagram showing the experimental setup, the generated PMF waveform, and the shape of the coil

90 min at 37 °C. To determine how the reducing agent works on PMF alleviating oxidative stress, verapamil (0.1 μM) was first treated for 30 min before the oxidation treatment.

PMF Stimulus The schematic diagram for the experimental setup of PMF is shown in Fig. 1. The generating coil was turned to a single layer of 10 turns with an elliptical shape of 12 cm × 4.5 cm using a plat square-shaped single stranded wire of 1 mm in thickness and 3 mm in width. Our system generates time-varying PMF which has the peak magnetic field intensity of 0.27 T, 5 mm away from coil and magnetic field pulse of 0.102 ms in transition time. Pulse repetition rate was 1 Hz. Since the waveforms of generated PMF show rapidly decayed sinusoidal signal, averaging magnetic fields over a period were calculated as 0.63 Gauss. Collected blood samples of 0.5 mL were exposed to PMF for 3 min to compare the effect of PMF stimulus on RBCs. The smear method was used to observe morphological biochemical change in the erythrocyte membrane.

Spectroscopic Measurement For spectrophotometry the UV-VIS T60 U spectrophotometer (London, UK) was used: field wavelength 190~1100 nm; wavelength accuracy 1 nm. Using plastic spectrophotometry cuvettes with a 1-cm lightpath (Kartell, Italy), we measured the absorbance of 1 mL of sample diluted with 0.999 mL of buffer using the spectrum mode, with a diluent used as the blank.

To observe the state of Hb in deformed RBCs due to oxidation treatment, light absorbance was measured for the group treated with oxidation and the group applied with PMF stimulus before oxidation treatment, respectively. To observe the PMF effect on the hemolysis of the erythrocyte membrane, it is necessary to separate the inner and outer components of RBCs. To separate the inner and outer components of the erythrocyte membrane, two sample groups were centrifuged at 15,000 g for 10 min at 4 °C and then divided into RBCs and plasma layers. The plasma layer was only extracted, and the absorbance of Hb released from the membrane due to damage of the deformed erythrocyte was measured. The remaining RBCs were treated with triton-x100 to completely hemolyze and then centrifuged again to destroy the erythrocyte membrane; then, Hb absorbance in the membrane was measured.

3 Results and Discussion

In order to hematologically and morphologically elucidate the influence of PMF on oxidized RBCs, oxidation treatment with tBHP was performed before and after PMF treatment, respectively. RBCs were reduced with verapamil in order to confirm whether PMF could prevent oxidative stress, through observation of the morphological changes in the erythrocyte membrane.

Figure 2 shows the morphology of RBCs treated with tBHP and PMF. Under hyper- oxidative stress, Hb in RBCs is oxidized to MetHb, Heinz bodies are bound to the cell membrane, and continuously produce active oxygen, causing cell damage, degenerating the RBCs deformability [8]. In addition, tBHP causes cell membrane protein band 3 abnormality and cell expansion [9]. These phenomena can be observed in Fig. 2b, i.e. erythrocytes exposed to oxidative stress. Also deformed RBCs are aggregated together compared to RBCs suspended in the PBS solution (Fig. 2a). Morphology of RBCs oxidized after PMF stimulus, and RBCs exposed to PMF after oxidization, are shown in Figs. 2c and 2d, respectively. The extent of RBCs aggregation is much smaller in the oxidation after PMF treatment, compared to that in PMF stimulus after oxidation. It is thought that oxidation stress in RBCs might be alleviated by PMF stimulus. Therefore, the magnetic field might prevent the destruction of RBCs undergoing oxidative stress, thereby enhancing flow in the capillary blood vessels and, consequently, allowing supply of oxygen to the body.

Figure 3 show the morphology of RBCs treated with verapamil, tBHP and PMF stimulus. Figure 3a is the control image of reduced RBCs with reducing agents, verapamil. RBCs treated with tBHP after treatment of verapamil (Fig. 3b) were

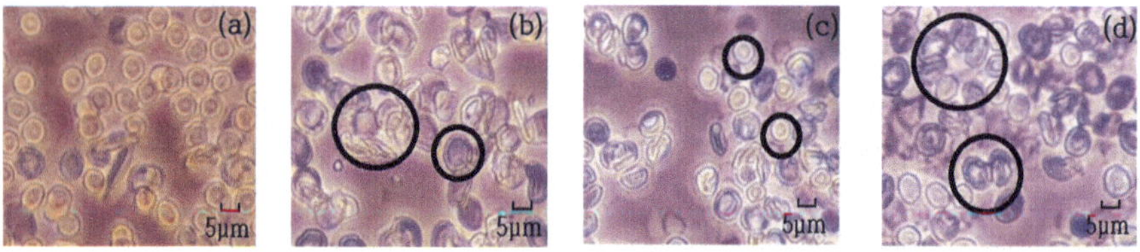

Fig. 2 Morphology of RBCs (**a**) suspended in PBS solution, (**b**) treated with tBHP, (**c**) treated with PMF-tBHP, and (**d**) treated with tBHP-PMF

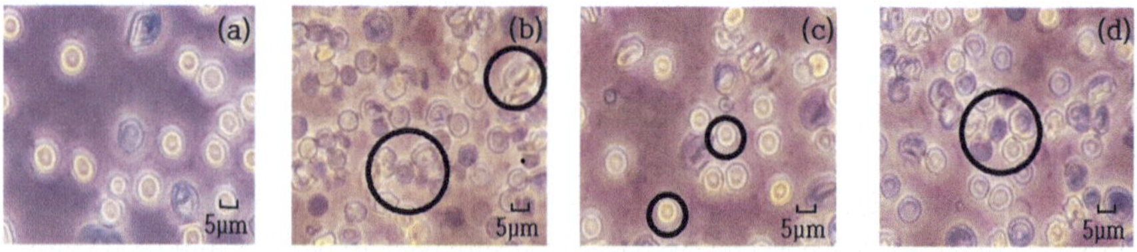

Fig. 3 Morphology of RBCs treated with (**a**) verapamil, (**b**) verapamil-tBHP, (**c**) verapamil-PMF-tBHP, and (**d**) verapamil-tBHP-PMF

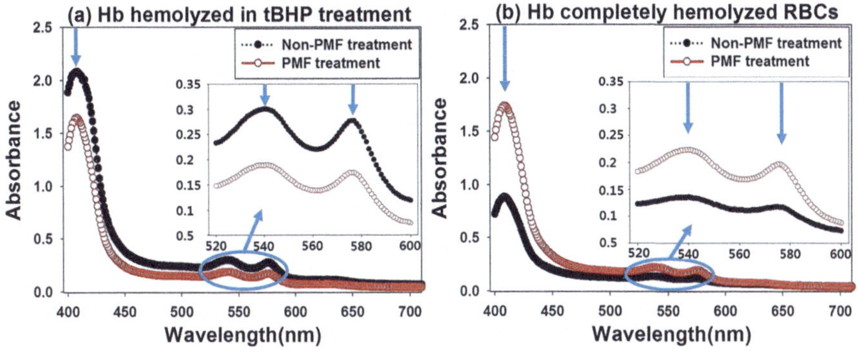

Fig. 4 Absorption spectra of hemoglobin (**a**) hemolyzed in tBHP treatment and (**b**) completely hemolyzed RBCs

aggregated, but less than in only oxidated RBCs (Fig. 2b); this is probably due to the reducing agents. When exposed to PMF stimulus in the sample of Fig. 3b, RBCs were disaggregated with recovery of the shape of a biconcave disk (Fig. 3c and 3d). For example, in Fig. 3c, for RBCs exposed to PMF after a reducing agent and then oxidative stress, aggregation occurred due to the oxidizing agents, but less than is shown in Fig. 3b. Therefore, PMF relieves oxidation stress and is effective for disaggregation of RBCs in addition to the reducing agent.

When RBCs become hemolyzed, Hb is released; with a greater release of Hb, the absorbance value increases overall. To confirm the state of Hb in RBCs deformed by oxidative stress, the blood sample was separated into two layers, i.e. RBCs and plasma, by centrifuging at 15,000 g. In the separated plasma layer, absorbance for the sample exposed to PMF before the oxidation treatment was lower than that for the sample not exposed to PMF. When PMF was not applied, the Hb outflow from the RBCs was relatively high and the absorbance was high (Fig. 4a).

On the other hand, Fig. 4b shows absorption spectra of hemoglobin released, after RBCs remained below the plasma layer were completely hemolyzed using TritonX-100. Hb absorbance after complete hemolysis is higher when PMF is applied. This means that before hemolysis, the number of normal RBCs exposed to PMF before the oxidation treatment was relatively larger than that for the RBCs not exposed to PMF. Therefore, the more oxyHb is leaked in the remaining RBCs exposed to PMF. These results might suggest that PMF plays a role in preventing RBCs hemolysis from oxidative stress.

The amount of hemolysis is determined by measuring the absorbance of the supernatants spectrophotometrically. As the saline concentration increases, the level of hemolysis gradually decreases. Figure 5 shows that hemolysis in the case of PMF treatment was maintained at 5% lower compared to that of non-PMF treatment at a saline concentration of 0.25~0.40%. However, at 0.40–0.45% in saline concentration, hemolysis in the case of PMF treatment is 28% lower than that of non-PMF treatment. These results demonstrate that PMF decreases osmotic lysis of RBCs. PMF might increase the deformability of erythrocyte membrane and prevent the hemolytic phenomenon that the erythrocyte membrane is destroyed due to osmotic pressure.

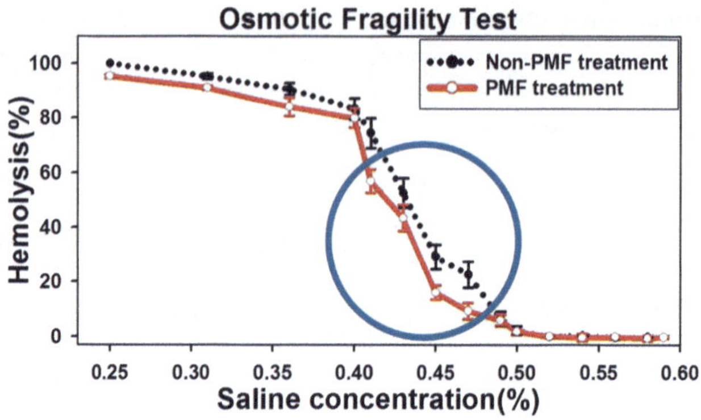

Fig. 5 Osmotic fragility test using sodium chloride to observe the effect of PMF on hemolysis of erythrocyte membrane

4 Conclusions

To investigate the effects of PMF on the hemolysis of erythrocytes exposed to oxygen stress, we observed the morphology of oxidized RBCs before and after PMF treatment. Also, for oxidative stressed RBCs after treatment with a reducing agent, morphology was observed before and after PMF. Our results demonstrate that PMF relieves oxidation stress and is effective for disaggregation of RBCs in addition to the reducing agent. In addition, to see hematologically the influence of PMF on RBCs deformed by oxidative stress, through hemolysis of RBCs, Hb absorbance was measured in membrane, as well as plasma, using spectroscopic measurement. These results might indicate that PMF plays a role in preventing RBCs hemolysis from oxidative stress. As a result of the osmotic fragility test, hemolysis in the case of PMF treatment is 28% lower than that of non-PMF treatment at 0.40–0.45% in saline concentration. PMF might increase the deformability of the erythrocyte membrane and prevent hemolytic phenomena. For further clinical application, we need to optimize the PMF intensity and stimulated duration.

Acknowledgments This research was supported by Basic Science Research Program through the National Research Foundation of Korea (NRF) funded by the Ministry of Education (2017R1D1A1B03034105).

References

1. Siems WG, Sommerburg O, Grune T (2000) Erythrocyte free radical and energy metabolism. Clin Nephrol 53:9–17
2. Arbos KA, Claro LM, Borges L et al (2008) Human erythrocytes as a system for evaluating the antioxidant capacity of vegetable extracts. Nutr Res 28:457–463

3. Bryszewska M, Zavodnik IB, Niekurzak A et al (1995) Oxidative processes in red blood cells from normal and diabetic individuals. Biochem Mol Biol Int 37:345–354
4. Kim YJ, Yoo JS, Hwang DG et al (2014) Comparative analysis of photoplethysmography under pulsed magnetic field and low level laser stimulus: motivation for blood flow increase using stimulus on acupoint LI4 (Hegu). J Magn 19:32–36
5. Tao R, Huang K (2011) Reducing blood viscosity with magnetic fields. Phys Rev E84:001900
6. Sun J, Kwan RL, Zheng Y et al (2016) Effects of pulsed electromagnetic fields on peripheral blood circulation in people with diabetes: a randomized controlled trial. Bioelectromagnetics 37:290–297
7. Deuticke B, Heller KB, Haest CW (1987) Progressive oxidative membrane damage in erythrocytes after pulse treatment with t-butyl hydroperoxide. Biochim Biophys Acta 899:113–124
8. Carrell R, Winterbourn C, Rachmilewitz E (1975) Annotation: activated oxygen and haemolysis. Br J Haematol 30:259–264
9. Arakawa T, Kobayashi-Yurugi T, Alguel Y et al (2015) Crystal structure of the anion exchanger domain of human erythrocyte band 3. Science 350:680–684

Role of Microtubule-Associated Factors in HIF1α Nuclear Translocation

Hyun Jik Lee and Ho Jae Han

Abstract Adaptation to hypoxia is essential for regulating the survival and functions of hypoxic cells; it is mainly mediated by the hypoxia-inducible factor 1 (HIF1). The alpha subunit of HIF1 (HIF1α) is a well-known regulatory component of HIF1, which is tightly controlled by various types of HIF1α-regulating processes. Previous research has shown that microtubule-regulated HIF1α nuclear translocation is a key factor for HIF1 activation under hypoxia. In this review, we summarize experimental reports on the role of microtubule-associated factors, such as microtubule, dynein, and dynein adaptor protein, in nuclear translocation of HIF1α. Based upon scientific evidence, we propose a bicaudal D homolog (BICD) as a novel HIF1α translocation regulating factor. A deeper understanding of the mechanism of the action of regulatory factors in controlling HIF1α nuclear translocation will provide novel insights into cell biology under hypoxia.

Keywords Hypoxia · Hypoxia-inducible factor 1 alpha (HIF1α) · Calcium · Prolyl hydroxylase (PHD) · Factor inhibiting HIF (FIH) · Microtubule · Bicaudal D homolog (BICD) · HIF1α co-activator · Stem cells

1 Introduction

Hypoxia-inducible factor (HIF) is a heterodimeric transcription factor, which comprises alpha (HIF1α) and beta (HIF1β) subunits [1, 2]. The alpha subunits of HIF in mammalian cells are encoded by *HIF1A*, *EPAS1/HIF2A*, and *HIF3A*. HIF1β is encoded by *ARNT1* and *ARNT2* [3–5]. HIF1 is considered a major target of HIF-mediated hypoxia adaptation response via the transcriptional stimulation of gene

H. J. Lee · H. J. Han (✉)
Department of Veterinary Physiology, College of Veterinary Medicine, Research Institute for Veterinary Science, and BK21 PLUS Program for Creative Veterinary Science Research, Seoul National University, Seoul, South Korea
e-mail: hjhan@snu.ac.kr

© Springer Nature Switzerland AG 2020

P.-D. Ryu et al. (eds.), *Oxygen Transport to Tissue XLI*, Advances in Experimental Medicine and Biology 1232, https://doi.org/10.1007/978-3-030-34461-0_34

expression involved in cell metabolism, proliferation, angiogenesis, and survival [6–8]. Under hypoxia, HIF1α is considered a key regulator subunit of HIF1, mainly controlled by oxygen-dependent mechanisms including transcription, translation, stabilization, and nuclear translocation. Among them, the mechanism of nuclear translocation of HIF1α remains poorly understood. However, understanding of the regulatory mechanism of HIF1α nuclear translocation will provide new insight into the regulation of HIF1α in hypoxic cells. Therefore, this review discusses previous evidence on the role of microtubule-associated factors, such as microtubule, dynein, and bicaudal D homolog (BICD) in HIF1α nuclear translocation.

2 HIF1α Nuclear Translocation

2.1 Role of Microtubule

The network of microtubules plays a crucial role in the regulation of cellular adaptation response to stress, including hypoxia conditions [9]. However, the effect of hypoxia on microtubule network has been widely debated. Chronic hypoxia incubation and hypoxic preconditioning disrupts this microtubule network in cardiomyocytes and cancer cells [10–12]. Conversely, hypoxia stabilizes the microtubule network by increasing chemoresistance to anticancer drugs in cancer cells [13, 14].

Previous research has demonstrated that the stabilization of microtubules is important for HIF1α nuclear translocation under hypoxia (Fig. 1). For example, Guo

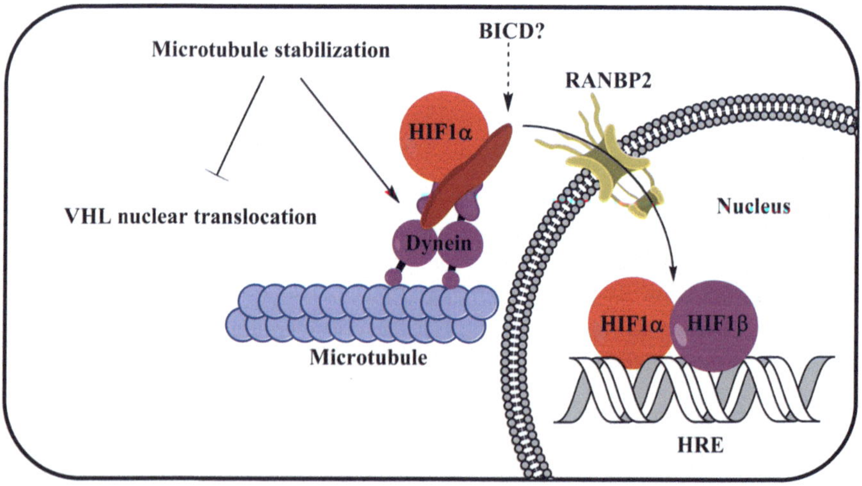

Fig. 1 Regulation of HIF1α nuclear translocation. Microtubule stabilization stimulates HIF1α nuclear translocation and inhibits VHL nuclear translocation, thus inducing HIF1α nuclear accumulation. Dynein activity is also important for HIF1α nuclear translocation. However, the identity of that dynein adaptor protein that mediates the binding of HIF1α to dynein remains unclear. The BICD family interacts with RANBP2 of NPC for nuclear translocation

et al. reported that chronic hypoxia stimulates microtubule depolymerization, leading to HIF1α clustering in the perinuclear region, and this effect is reversed by a microtubule stabilizer, paclitaxel, treatment [10]. Additionally, Teng et al. reported that the depolymerization of microtubules by colchicine abolished hypoxia-induced HIF1α nuclear translocation [15]. Microtubule stabilization by taxol further stimulated hypoxia-induced HIF1α nuclear translocation [15]. HIF1α ubiquitination in the nucleus is induced by Ran-mediated von Hippel-Lindau (VHL) nuclear import, and microtubule stabilization suppressed VHL-mediated HIF1α ubiquitination and accumulated nuclear HIF1α [16]. However, the role of microtubules in HIF1α translation is controversial. Carbonaro et al. showed that the regulation of microtubules using microtubule-targeting drugs, such as taxol, a microtubule stabilizer, and 2ME2, a microtubule depolymerizer, did not affect HIF1α translation [17]. Conversely, another study reported that treatment with taxol delayed *HIF1A* mRNA transport and released it from polysomes for the inactivation of HIF1α [18].

2.2 *Role of Dynein*

Dynein is a microtubule-associated motor protein that mediates minus end-directed cargo transport. A previous study reported that the cytoplasmic dynein mediates the interaction between HIF1α and microtubule for HIF1α nuclear translocation. Thus, dynein is emerging as a key motor protein that regulates HIF1α nuclear translocation (Fig. 1) [17]. However, the detailed mechanisms underlying the dynein-mediated nuclear translocation of HIF1 and dynein adaptor protein regulating the interaction between HIF1α and dynein remain unclear. Dynein adaptor proteins play an important role in various types of cargo protein transport [19, 20]. However, which adaptor protein interacts with HIF1α is not yet reported. Considering the low activity of von Hippel-Lindau protein (VHL) under hypoxia, the regulation of the interaction between dynein and HIF1α can be a potential strategy in enhancing HIF1α nuclear translocation.

2.3 *Role of BICD*

BICD is a motor adaptor protein that links cargo proteins to microtubule-associated motor proteins, including dynein and kinesin (Fig. 2). It has been reported that the BICD family contributes to Rab6-mediated intracellular cargo transport and to the central positioning of centrosomes during mitosis in mammalian cells [21]. Additionally, a recent study demonstrated that BICD2 stimulates the nuclear transport of the viral genome [22]. A structure-based study showed that coiled-coil domain 1 (CC1) in the N-terminal region plays a crucial role in the recruitment of microtubule motor proteins, including dynein and dynactin [23, 24]. CC2 interacts with the plus end-directed motor protein kinesin [20]. CC3 in the C-terminal region

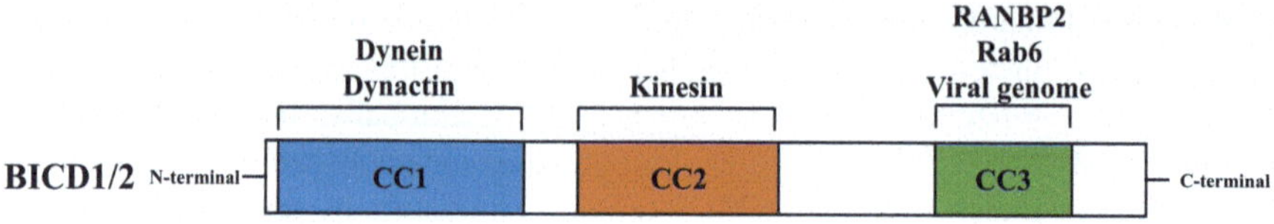

Fig. 2 Schematic domain structures of BICD1/2. The BICD family has three CC regions. The CC1 domain of N-terminal interacts with dynein and dynactin, whereas the middle CC2 domain binds to kinesin. The CC3 domain of the C-terminal of BICD recruits the Rab6-mediated vesicles RANBP2 and viral genome

of BICD interacts with various proteins, Rab6-mediated vesicles, and HIV-1 viral genome [22, 25, 26].

BICD upregulates the cargo-transporting efficacy of cytoplasmic dynein. Indeed, the addition of N-terminal fragment of BICD2 stabilizes the dynein-dynactin complex resulting in the enhancement of cytoplasmic dynein motility [19]. Also, full-length BICD1 overexpression enhances dynein-mediated cargo transport [25]. Splinter et al. showed that BICD2 binds to the nuclear pore complex (NPC) during the G2 phase [27]. Especially, the CC3 domain of BICD binds to an NPC component, RANBP2, involved in nuclear transport [20, 28]. RANBP2 is a SUMO E3 ligase, which contributes to the nuclear translocation of transcription factors [29]. The binding affinities of BICD1 and BICD2 for RANBP2 are controversial.

A previous structural study showed that BICD2, but not BICD1, binds to RANBP2 [27]. However, another investigator showed that the CC3 domain of BICD1 is capable of recruiting RANBP2 [30]. Additionally, we observed that both BICD1 and BICD2 interact with both HIF1α and RANBP2. BICD1 silencing suppressed hypoxia-induced HIF1α nuclear translocation in mesenchymal stem cells (unpublished data). Based on these findings, we suggest that the BICD family can function as a binding partner of HIF1α for its dynein-mediated nuclear translocation in stem cells. However, because the physiological role of BICDs in stem cell biology is poorly understood, further investigations using various stem cells are needed.

3 Conclusion

Microtubule-associated nuclear translocation of HIF1α is tightly controlled by various types of regulatory factors, including dynein and its adaptor proteins as well as microtubule stability. However, the regulatory mechanism of dynein-mediated HIF1α transport remains unclear. In addition, further investigation into the identification of the motor adaptor protein regulating dynein-associated HIF1α nuclear translocation is required to improve our understanding of the regulatory mechanism of HIF1α nuclear import. As discussed above, we suggest a BICD as a HIF1α nuclear translocation regulator. Identification of an interaction between BICD and HIF1α will provide novel insights into the regulation of cellular adaptation to hypoxia.

Acknowledgments This research was supported by National R&D Program through the National Research Foundation of Korea (NRF) funded by the Ministry of Science, ICT & Future Planning (NRF-2017R1A2B2008661) and BK21 PLUS Program for Creative Veterinary Science Research.

References

1. Wang GL, Jiang BH, Rue EA et al (1995) Hypoxia-inducible factor 1 is a basic-helix-loop-helix-PAS heterodimer regulated by cellular O_2 tension. Proc Natl Acad Sci U S A 92:5510–5514
2. Reyes H, Reisz-Porszasz S, Hankinson O (1992) Identification of the Ah receptor nuclear translocator protein (Arnt) as a component of the DNA binding form of the Ah receptor. Science 256:1193–1195
3. Ema M, Taya S, Yokotani N et al (1997) A novel bHLH-PAS factor with close sequence similarity to hypoxia-inducible factor 1α regulates the VEGF expression and is potentially involved in lung and vascular development. Proc Natl Acad Sci U S A 94:4273–4278
4. Iyer NV, Leung SW, Semenza GL (1998) The human hypoxia-inducible factor 1α gene: HIF1A structure and evolutionary conservation. Genomics 52:159–165
5. Gu YZ, Moran SM, Hogenesch JB et al (1998) Molecular characterization and chromosomal localization of a third α-class hypoxia inducible factor subunit, HIF3α. Gene Expr 7:205–213
6. Choudhry H, Harris AL (2018) Advances in hypoxia-inducible factor biology. Cell Metab 27:281–298
7. Semenza GL (2013) HIF-1 mediates metabolic responses to intratumoral hypoxia and oncogenic mutations. J Clin Invest 123:3664–3671
8. Man J, Yu X, Huang H et al (2018) Hypoxic induction of vasorin regulates notch1 turnover to maintain glioma stem-like cells. Cell Stem Cell 22(104–118):e106
9. Parker AL, Kavallaris M, McCarroll JA (2014) Microtubules and their role in cellular stress in cancer. Front Oncol 4:153
10. Guo H, Zheng H, Wu J et al (2017) The key role of microtubules in hypoxia preconditioning-induced nuclear translocation of HIF-1α in rat cardiomyocytes. PeerJ 5:e3662
11. Hu JY, Chu ZG, Han J et al (2010) The p38/MAPK pathway regulates microtubule polymerization through phosphorylation of MAP 4 and Op18 in hypoxic cells. Cell Mol Life Sci 67:321–333
12. Fang YD, Xu X, Dang YM et al (2011) MAP 4 mechanism that stabilizes mitochondrial permeability transition in hypoxia: microtubule enhancement and DYNLT1 interaction with VDAC1. PLoS One 6:e28052
13. Peng WX, Pan FY, Liu XJ et al (2010) Hypoxia stabilizes microtubule networks and decreases tumor cell chemosensitivity to anticancer drugs through Egr 1. Anat Rec (Hoboken) 293:414–420
14. Yoon SO, Shin S, Mercurio AM (2005) Hypoxia stimulates carcinoma invasion by stabilizing microtubules and promoting the Rab11 trafficking of the α6β4 integrin. Cancer Res 65:2761–2769
15. Teng M, Dang YM, Zhang JP et al (2010) Microtubular stability affects cardiomyocyte glycolysis by HIF-1α expression and endonuclear aggregation during early stages of hypoxia. Am J Physiol Heart Circ Physiol 298:H1919–H1931
16. Jiang X, Zhang D, Zhang H et al (2015) Role of Ran-regulated nuclear-cytoplasmic trafficking of pVHL in the regulation of microtubular stability-mediated HIF-1α in hypoxic cardiomyocytes. Sci Rep 5:9193
17. Carbonaro M, Escuin D, O'Brate A et al (2012) Microtubules regulate hypoxia-inducible factor-1α protein trafficking and activity: implications for taxane therapy. J Biol Chem 287:11859–11869
18. Carbonaro M, O'Brate A, Giannakakou P (2011) Microtubule disruption targets HIF-1α mRNA to cytoplasmic P-bodies for translational repression. J Cell Biol 192:83–99

19. Cianfrocco MA, Leschziner AE (2014) Traffic control: adaptor proteins guide dynein-cargo takeoff. EMBO J 33:1845–1846
20. Hoogenraad CC, Akhmanova A (2016) Bicaudal D family of motor adaptors: linking dynein motility to cargo binding. Trends Cell Biol 26:327–340
21. Budzinska M, Wicher KB, Terenzio M (2017) Neuronal roles of the bicaudal d family of motor adaptors. Vitamins & Hormones 104:133–152
22. Dharan A, Opp S, Abdel-Rahim O et al (2017) Bicaudal D2 facilitates the cytoplasmic trafficking and nuclear import of HIV-1 genomes during infection. Proc Natl Acad Sci U S A 114:E10707–E10716
23. Hoogenraad CC, Wulf P, Schiefermeier N et al (2003) Bicaudal D induces selective dynein-mediated microtubule minus end-directed transport. EMBO J 22:6004–6015
24. Hoogenraad CC, Akhmanova A, Howell SA et al (2001) Mammalian Golgi-associated Bicaudal-D2 functions in the dynein-dynactin pathway by interacting with these complexes. EMBO J 20:4041–4054
25. Matanis T, Akhmanova A, Wulf P et al (2002) Bicaudal-D regulates COPI-independent Golgi-ER transport by recruiting the dynein-dynactin motor complex. Nat Cell Biol 4:986–992
26. Liu Y, Salter HK, Holding AN et al (2013) Bicaudal-D uses a parallel, homodimeric coiled coil with heterotypic registry to coordinate recruitment of cargos to dynein. Genes Dev 27:1233–1246
27. Splinter D, Tanenbaum ME, Lindqvist A et al (2010) Bicaudal D2, dynein, and kinesin-1 associate with nuclear pore complexes and regulate centrosome and nuclear positioning during mitotic entry. PLoS Biol 8:e1000350
28. Terawaki S, Ootsuka H, Higuchi Y et al (2014) Crystallographic characterization of the C-terminal coiled-coil region of mouse Bicaudal-D1 (BICD1). Acta Crystallogr F Struct Biol Commun 70:1103–1106
29. Walde S, Thakar K, Hutten S et al (2012) The nucleoporin Nup358/RanBP2 promotes nuclear import in a cargo- and transport receptor-specific manner. Traffic 13:218–233
30. Terawaki S, Yoshikane A, Higuchi Y et al (2015) Structural basis for cargo binding and auto-inhibition of Bicaudal-D1 by a parallel coiled-coil with homotypic registry. Biochem Biophys Res Commun 460:451–456

Extracellular Acidosis Regulates the Expression of Inflammatory Mediators in Rat Epithelial Cells

A. Riemann, S. Reime, M. Gießelmann, and O. Thews

Abstract Acidification of the cellular microenvironment is found in different pathological states such as inflammation, ischemia and in solid tumors. It can affect cell function and phenotype, and by this aggravate the pathological process. Epithelial cells are a relevant functional part in several normal organs as well as in tumors and will thus be challenged by the acidic extracellular pH (acidosis). Therefore, the impact of acidosis on the expression of different inflammatory mediators (MCP-1, IL-6, osteopontin, iNOS, TNF-α, and COX-2), as well as the role of different signaling pathways regulating the expression, was studied in epithelial normal rat kidney cells (NRK-52E). Acidosis led to an increase in TNF-α expression but a down-regulation of MCP-1, iNOS and COX-2. Expression of IL-6 was only slightly modulated, while osteopontin was not regulated at all. Since acidosis activates ERK1/2 and p38 signaling in NRK-52E cells, the impact of MAP kinase signaling pathways on the expression of the inflammatory markers was analyzed. At normal pH, blocking ERK1/2 or p38 decreased the level of MCP-1, iNOS and partly TNF-α. However, the effect of acidosis on the expression of inflammatory mediators was not affected by inhibition of the MAP kinase pathways. In conclusion, our results show that an acidic microenvironment affects the transcriptional program of epithelial cells. Low pH mostly reduced the expression of pathological relevant genes and might thus repress inflammatory processes induced by epithelial cells.

Keywords Acidosis · MAP kinases · MCP-1 · iNOS · TNF-α

A. Riemann (✉) · S. Reime · M. Gießelmann · O. Thews
Julius-Bernstein-Institute of Physiology, University of Halle, Halle (Saale), Germany
e-mail: anne.riemann@medizin.uni-halle.de

© Springer Nature Switzerland AG 2020

P.-D. Ryu et al. (eds.), *Oxygen Transport to Tissue XLI*, Advances in Experimental Medicine and Biology 1232, https://doi.org/10.1007/978-3-030-34461-0_35

1 Introduction

Changes in the local cellular microenvironment are present in different pathological conditions and result in alterations of cell function which can in turn aggravate the pathophysiological state. In inflammation, ischemia and in solid tumors an acidification of the microenvironment is found within the range of pH 6.0–7.0 [1]. Amongst others, acidosis has an impact on cellular function by regulation of enzyme activity, ion transport and protein, as well as DNA synthesis. Former studies of our group described the impact of acidosis on immune cells, fibroblasts or tumor cells [2–4]. However, the response of normal epithelial cells, which are also part of the normal or malignant tissues, to an acidic microenvironment is not well understood. Thus, the aim of this study was to analyze changes in the inflammatory program of normal rat epithelial cells (NRK-52E) by acidosis. The expression of monocyte chemotactic protein 1 (MCP-1), interleukin-6 (IL-6), osteopontin (SPP1), inducible NO synthase (iNOS), tumor necrosis factor-α (TNF-α) and cyclooxygenase-2 (COX-2) were assessed. MCP-1 is involved in the recruitment of leukocytes and is linked to inflammation, ischemia and cancer [5]. IL-6 is produced in response to tissue injuries and has pro- or anti-inflammatory actions depending on the microenvironmental context [6]. Osteopontin regulates the recruitment as well as cytokine secretion of leukocytes, and it modulates tissue repair and inflammation [7]. TNF-α is one of the most important pro-inflammatory cytokines, while iNOS and COX-2 foster inflammation by producing reactive nitrogen species or prostaglandins [8–10].

2 Methods

2.1 Cell Line

Normal rat kidney epithelial cells (NRK-52E, ATCC CRL-1571, LGC Standards, Wesel, Germany) were grown in DMEM medium supplemented with 5% fetal calf serum (FCS), 4.5 g/l glucose and 1.5 g/l $NaHCO_3$. The cells were serum-starved for 24 h and afterwards were incubated for 3 or 6 h in bicarbonate-HEPES- (pH 7.4) or MES-(pH 6.6) buffered Ringer solutions at room air supplemented with 5% CO_2. For 24-h experiments, cells were incubated in HEPES- and MES-buffered medium lacking FCS at pH 7.4 (control) or pH 6.6 (acidosis) at 37 °C in a humidified atmosphere with 5% CO_2. Subsequently, the cells were harvested and total RNA was extracted using TRIzol reagent according to the manufacturer's protocol (Thermo Fisher Scientific, Waltham, MA, USA). MAP kinase function was studied by the use of 10 μM p38 inhibitor SB203580 or 10 μM ERK1/2 activation blocker U0126 (Merck, Darmstadt, Germany), which were added to the buffers during incubation at different pH.

2.2 Experimental Settings

By quantitative PCR, the expression of MCP-1, IL-6, osteopontin, iNOS, TNF-α and COX-2 was assessed after control or acidotic conditions as described in [9]. In brief, 1 μg RNA was subjected to reverse transcription with SuperScript II reverse transcriptase (Invitrogen, Carlsbad, CA, USA) and expression changes studied by qPCR using the Platinum SYBR Green qPCR Supermix (Invitrogen, Carlsbad, CA, USA). As housekeeping genes, 18S rRNA or hypoxanthine-guanine phosphoribosyltransferase (HPRT) were used. The qPCR data were normalized to the results at pH 7.4. All experiments were performed in triplicate with at least three passages, and results are presented as mean ± SEM.

3 Results

As shown in Fig. 1, acidification of the cellular microenvironment led to a strong reduction in the expression of MCP-1, iNOS and COX-2 in epithelial cells (NRK-52E) after an incubation period of 3 h, while after 6 h or 24 h these changes were diminished. Interestingly, TNF-α expression was strongly increased after 3 h and 6 h of acidosis, but downregulated after 24 h at pH 6.6. Regulation of IL-6

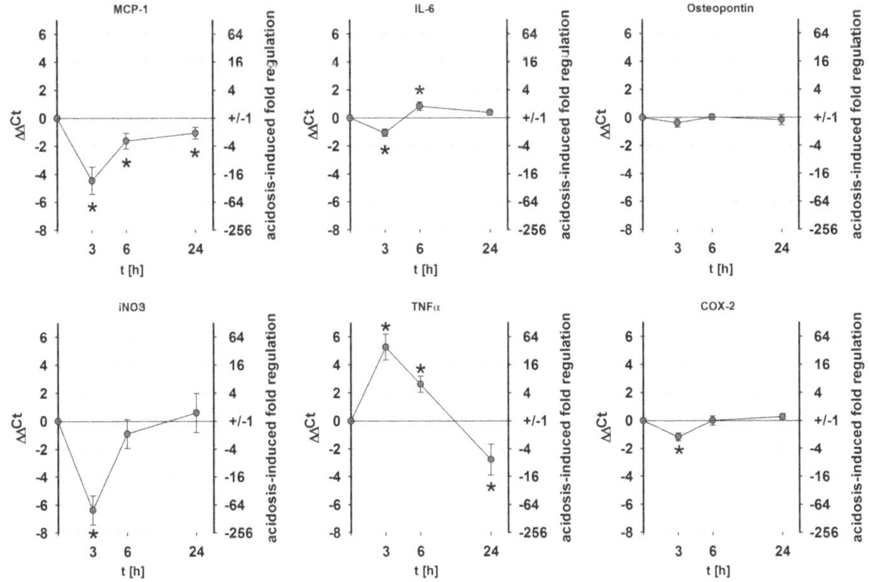

Fig. 1 Acidosis-induced modulation of the expression of inflammatory mediators in NRK-52E cells after different intervals at pH 6.6 (3–24 h). The values are normalized to control conditions at pH 7.4, n = 8–20. $*p < 0.05$

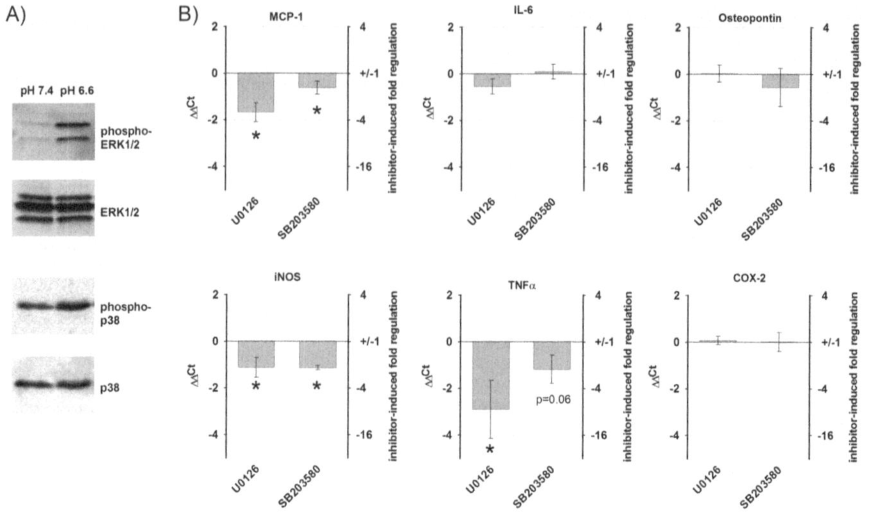

Fig. 2 (**A**) Representative western blot showing phosphorylated and overall ERK1/2 and p38 protein. (**B**) Effect of blocking ERK1/2 (U0126) or p38 (SB 203580) signaling on basal mRNA expression of inflammatory mediators under control conditions (pH 7.4). Fold changes after an incubation period of 3 h with the respective inhibitors in HEPES-Ringer solution pH 7.4 normalized to vehicle incubation (DMSO) are shown, n = 4–9. $*p < 0.05$

expression by acidosis was weak, displaying a minor reduction in IL-6 mRNA after 3 h and a small increase after 6 h at pH 6.6. The expression of osteopontin was almost not regulated by acidosis in epithelial cells. In former studies a strong activation of ERK1/2 and p38 MAP kinases in NRK-52E cells was detected [11] and (Fig. 2A). Hence, the impact of ERK1/2 and p38 in the regulation of inflammatory marker expression was studied. When ERK1/2 signaling was blocked by U0126 under control conditions (pH 7.4) the expression of MCP-1, iNOS and TNF-α was significantly reduced (Fig. 2B). Blocking of p38 activity with SB203580 weakly reduced basal expression of MCP-1 and iNOS at pH 7.4. However, the acidosis-induced modulation of MCP-1, iNOS and TNF-α expression was not prevented by ERK1/2 or p38 inhibition (Fig. 3). Compared to incubation with vehicle alone, inhibition of the MAPKs with U0126 or SB203580 had almost no impact on the acidosis-induced changes of inflammatory mediator expression.

4 Conclusion

Acidification of the cellular microenvironment, as found in inflammation, ischemia and in solid tumors, affects the transcriptional program of normal epithelial cells (NRK-52E). Acidosis downregulated the expression of MCP-1 which might lead to decreased immune cell recruitment, since MCP-1 is involved in chemotaxis of

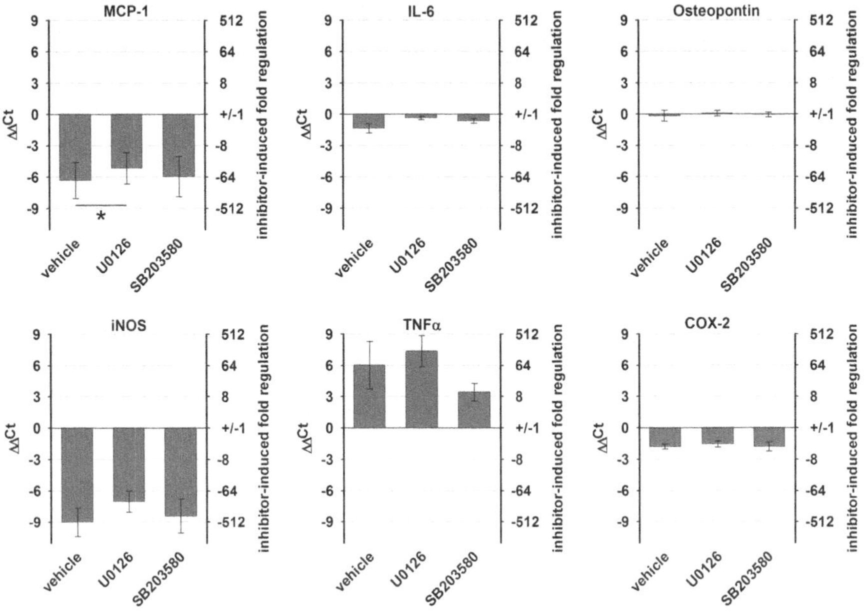

Fig. 3 Acidosis-induced changes in the expression of inflammatory markers in NRK-52E cells when ERK1/2 (U0126) or p38 (SB203580) signaling was blocked (at pH 6.6), vehicle = DMSO, n = 3–9. $*p < 0.05$

monocytes, NK and T cells [5]. Reduced expression of iNOS and COX-2 by acidosis might diminish the level of reactive nitrogen species or prostaglandins, respectively. Thus, acidosis possibly impairs macrophage cytotoxicity, leukocyte migration, proliferation and cytokine production by reduced NO production [12]. A decrease in the level of pro-inflammatory prostaglandins might impair inflammatory response as well as tumorigenesis (and tumor progression) [13]. Since the expression of MCP-1, iNOS and COX-2 was downregulated, acidosis might favor an anti-inflammatory response of epithelial cells restrict the recruitment of immune cells, and protect the tissue. However, acidosis also strongly increased the expression of TNF-α, at least after short-term incubation of 3 h and 6 h. TNF-α is involved in cell death and proliferation, migration, as well as differentiation (and tumorigenesis) [8]. Therefore, acidosis might create a para-inflammatory situation and lead to tissue remodeling. However, in the literature, an acidosis-induced decrease in TNF-α protein secretion has been described, although the TNF-α mRNA levels were increased [14]. In addition, long-term acidosis (24 h) rather reduced the expression of TNF-α. Thus, the results of acidosis-induced TNF-α regulation might not be opposing to a rather anti-inflammatory response of epithelial cells. Although, acidosis led to an activation of ERK1/2 and p38 signaling in NRK-52E cells [11], blocking of the MAP kinase activity had no effect on acidosis-induced modulation of the expression of inflammatory mediators. Thus, other signaling pathways must be involved in the impact of acidosis on MCP-1, iNOS, COX-2, IL-6 and TNF-α expression. Further studies are required to unravel the underlying signaling pathways and the mechanisms by which acidosis affects the inflammatory program in epithelial cells.

Acknowledgments This study was supported by the Deutsche Forschungsgemeinschaft DFG (grant TH482/6-1).

References

1. Rajamäki K, Nordström T, Nurmi K et al (2013) Extracellular acidosis is a novel danger signal alerting innate immunity via the NLRP3 inflammasome. J Biol Chem 288:13410–13419
2. Riemann A, Reime S, Thews O (2017) Tumor acidosis and hypoxia differently modulate the inflammatory program: measurements in vitro and in vivo. Neoplasia (United States) 19:1033–1042
3. Riemann A, Ihling A, Thomas J et al (2015) Acidic environment activates inflammatory programs in fibroblasts via a cAMP-MAPK pathway. Biochim Biophys Acta 1853:299–307
4. Riemann A, Wußling H, Loppnow H et al (2016) Acidosis differently modulates the inflammatory program in monocytes and macrophages. Biochim Biophys Acta Mol basis Dis 1862:72–81
5. Deshmane SL, Kremlev S, Amini S, Sawaya BE (2009) Monocyte chemoattractant protein-1 (MCP-1): an overview. J Interf Cytokine Res 29:313–326
6. Kamimura D, Ishihara K, Hirano T (2003) IL-6 signal transduction and its physiological roles: the signal orchestration model. Rev Physiol Biochem Pharmacol 149:1–38
7. Kahles F, Findeisen HM, Bruemmer D (2014) Osteopontin: a novel regulator at the cross roads of inflammation, obesity and diabetes. Mol Metab 3:384–393
8. Bradley JR (2008) TNF-mediated inflammatory disease. J Pathol 214:149–160
9. Simmons DL, Botting RM, Hla T (2004) Cyclooxygenase isozymes: the biology of prostaglandin synthesis and inhibition. Pharmacol Rev 56:387–437
10. Aktan F (2004) iNOS-mediated nitric oxide production and its regulation. Life Sci 75:639–653
11. Riemann A, Schneider B, Gündel D et al (2014) Acidic priming enhances metastatic potential of cancer cells. Pflügers Arch Eur J Physiol 466:2127–2138
12. Korhonen R, Lahti A, Kankaanranta H, Moilanen E (2005) Nitric oxide production and signaling in inflammation. Curr Drug Target -Inflammation Allergy 4:471–479
13. Morteau O (2000) Prostaglandins and inflammation: the cyclooxygenase controversy. Arch Immunol Ther Exp 48:473–480
14. Bidani A, Wang CZ, Saggi SJ, Heming TA (1998) Evidence for pH sensitivity of tumor necrosis factor-α release by alveolar macrophages. Lung 176:111–121

Part V
Methodology of O2 Measurements

Reducing False Alarm Rates in Neonatal Intensive Care: A New Machine Learning Approach

D. Ostojic, S. Guglielmini, V. Moser, J. C. Fauchère, H. U. Bucher, D. Bassler, M. Wolf, S. Kleiser, F. Scholkmann, and T. Karen

Abstract In neonatal intensive care units (NICUs), 87.5% of alarms by the monitoring system are false alarms, often caused by the movements of the neonates. Such false alarms are not only stressful for the neonates as well as for their parents and caregivers, but may also lead to longer response times in real critical situations. The aim of this project was to reduce the rates of false alarms by employing machine learning algorithms (MLA), which intelligently analyze data stemming from standard physiological monitoring in combination with cerebral oximetry data (in-house built, OxyPrem). *Materials & Methods:* Four popular MLAs were selected to categorize the alarms as false or real: (i) decision tree (DT), (ii) 5-nearest neighbors (5-NN), (iii) naïve Bayes (NB) and (iv) support vector machine (SVM). We acquired and processed monitoring data (median duration (SD): 54.6 (± 6.9) min) of 14 preterm infants (gestational age: 26 6/7 (± 2 5/7) weeks). A hybrid method of filter and wrapper feature selection generated the candidate subset for training these four MLAs. *Results:* A high specificity of >99% was achieved by all four approaches. DT showed the highest sensitivity (87%). The cerebral oximetry data improved the classification accuracy. *Discussion & Conclusion:* Despite a (as yet) low amount of data for training, the four MLAs achieved an excellent specificity and a promising sensitivity. Presently, the current sensitivity is insufficient since, in the NICU, it is

D. Ostojic and S. Guglielmini have contributed equally for this chapter.

D. Ostojic (✉) · S. Guglielmini · M. Wolf · S. Kleiser · F. Scholkmann · T. Karen
Biomedical Optics Research Laboratory (BORL), University of Zurich, Zurich, Switzerland

Department of Neonatology, University Hospital Zurich, University of Zurich, Zurich, Switzerland
e-mail: Daniel.Ostojic@usz.ch

J. C. Fauchère · H. U. Bucher · D. Bassler
Department of Neonatology, University Hospital Zurich, University of Zurich, Zurich, Switzerland

V. Moser
CSEM, Neuchâtel, Switzerland

© Springer Nature Switzerland AG 2020

P.-D. Ryu et al. (eds.), *Oxygen Transport to Tissue XLI*, Advances in Experimental Medicine and Biology 1232, https://doi.org/10.1007/978-3-030-34461-0_36

crucial that no real alarms are missed. This will most likely be improved by including more subjects and data in the training of the MLAs, which makes pursuing this approach worthwhile.

Keywords False alarms · Oxygen saturation · Neonatal intensive care · Machine learning · NICU

1 Introduction

Preterm infants are not able to regulate their oxygen levels reliably. Hypoxia or hyperoxia may lead to injury, in particular of the brain, which may lead to long-term disabilities. Therefore, oxygen saturation as the most commonly monitored proxy for oxygenation and vital parameters are continuously measured in neonatal intensive care units (NICUs). If the oxygen saturation is out of the set range, an alarm sounds and the staff reacts accordingly by adjusting the oxygen supply or stimulating the infant for breathing. However, 87.5% of the alarms have been shown to be false alarms, which are mostly caused by movements of the infants [1]. False alarms increase the stress for patients, parents, and staff. In particular, if an infant creates many false alarms and suddenly a real critical situation occurs, the response time of the caregivers may be increased. This is due to a phenomenon known as 'alarm fatigue' [2–4] or as the 'crying-wolf syndrome' [5]. Alarm fatigue is a real safety concern and may harm the patients [2–4]. One option to solve this problem is to harness technology to suppress false alarms, for example the Fuzzy-logic, a multi-valued logic for classification of mathematical objects with blurred boundaries. To caregivers, the vital signs are signals with fuzzy boundaries. For example, a value of SpO_2 slightly below its 87% threshold may mean the patient is still doing fine and the alarm can be dismissed as false. Using the Fuzzy-logic based system [1], a suppression of 99.4% of all false alarms was demonstrated. Unfortunately, neither Fuzzy logic nor machine learning algorithms (MLAs) have been implemented in monitoring devices in NICUs, due to insufficient accuracy and legal issues [6, 7]. MLAs are a promising modern approach that may solve the problem of false alarms in NICUs. The aim of our project, therefore, was to test how efficiently MLAs are able to reduce the rates of false alarms by intelligently analyzing data from standard physiological monitoring and from cerebral oximetry.

2 Methods

Data of 25 preterm infants were recorded in the NICU of the University Hospital Zurich (Switzerland) under a declaration of 'no objection' by the Ethics Committee of Zurich (KEK-ZH, Req-2016-00720). Parental consent was obtained prior to

Table 1 Information on the 14 participants whose monitoring data were included

	Median	Range
Gestational age (weeks)	26 6/7	24 6/7–32 5/7
Postmenstrual age (weeks)	32 4/7	29 1/7–38 6/7
Birth weight (g)	985	550–1870
Weight (g)	1585	980–2450

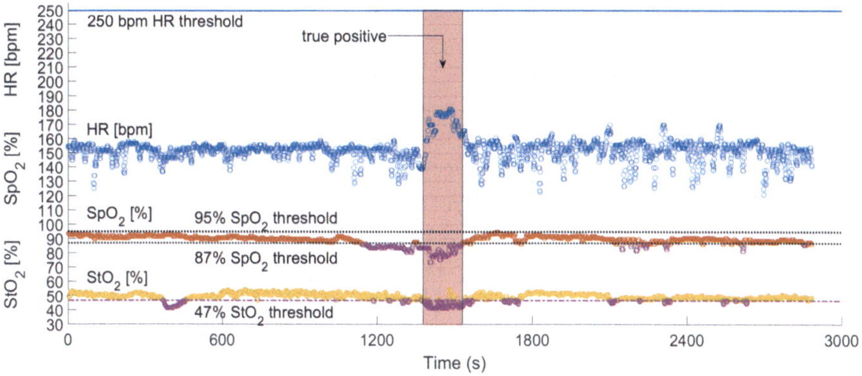

Fig. 1 Example of a recording showing one alarm labeled by the staff and logged (see Table 2)

enrolment. Data of 11 participants were excluded due to missing actionable alarms, or events labeled by the caregivers as real alarms, or due to poor signal quality. The demographic data of the remaining 14 subjects are shown in Table 1.

The standard monitoring device (SMD), the Infinity Delta XL (Dräger, Germany), provided arterial oxygen saturation (SpO_2) and the heart rate (HR). The data were streamed for (mean) 55 min via the serial port at a time resolution of 0.5 s. Simultaneously, our in-house built near-infrared spectroscopy (NIRS) oximeter (OxyPrem) [8] measured cerebral oxygen saturation (StO_2) from the parietal cortex.

An additional research SpO_2 sensor [9], on the opposite fronto-parietal side, measured HR and SpO_2. The alarm limits of the SMD were set to: $SpO_2 < 87\%$, $SpO_2 > 95\%$ (only for assisted ventilation or additional O_2 supply), HR < 80 bpm and HR > 250 bpm. These limits were frequently crossed and many alarms were created. The staff labeled these alarms as true (C_1) or false (C_0) according to their professional judgment (an example is shown in Fig. 1 and Table 2).

The pre-processing of the 14 datasets was performed in two steps: (i) the research SpO_2 sensor caused interferences on StO_2 (NIRS) and hence StO_2 was filtered to reduce this noise (Fig. 2), (ii) data were of different sampling rates and were resampled to the same rate of 2 Hz.

The HR and SpO_2 of the SMD and the StO_2, the oxy- and deoxy-hemoglobin concentration ([O_2Hb] and HHb]) of the OxyPrem were directly employed as MLA features. Three additional features that represent the area between the StO_2, SpO_2 and HR signals and their respective alarm limits were calculated. The rationale for this is that the severity of a deviation depends on both the time and the depth.

Table 2 Example of real-time transcriptions in the log-book (corresponding to Fig. 1)

Time [s]	Event
0–1383	Occasional SpO_2 drops <87%, triggering alarms deemed as false by physician in charge.
1383–1534	True positive. Drop of $StO_2 < 47\%$ and $SpO_2 < 87\%$. Onset of the true alarm treated by tactile stimulation to incite breathing.
1534–2884	End of true alarm. SpO_2 and StO_2 return to normal of 88% respectively 49–51%.

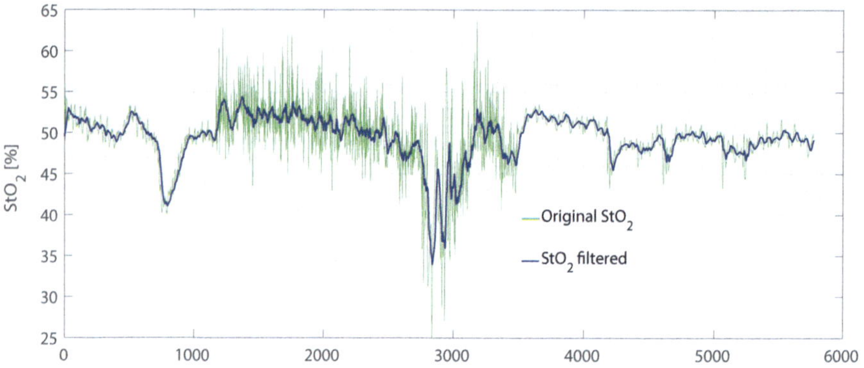

Fig. 2 Original StO_2, in green, affected by the interference coming from the research SpO_2 sensor. StO_2 signal in blue was filtered with 30 points (15 s) moving average filter

This also represents the concept of the caregivers. In addition, the last feature corresponds to the phase difference between the $[O_2Hb]$ and the [HHb].

To simplify the classifier's complexity and improve the accuracy of the classification, the most relevant features were automatically identified by a feature selection step. First, the Fisher's discriminant ratio [10] reduced the set from 10 to 6 features. The Sequential Backward Selection [11] decreased the set further to 4 features: Area SpO_2, HR, SpO_2 and StO_2. The feature selection was carried out on the individual subject level, and in two subjects solely HR and SpO_2 were selected. The resulting reduced feature sets were used to train and test the four supervised machine learning algorithms: (i) decision tree (DT), (ii) 5-nearest neighbors (5-NN), (iii) naïve Bayes (NB) and (iv) support vector machine (SVM). Each was implemented in the MATLAB Statistics and Machine Learning Toolbox. The learning phase was repeated 10 times. The classifier was tested each time on different data. To avoid overfitting [12], a ten-fold cross-validation procedure was employed, i.e. in a rotational manner, nine subsets were used as a training set and the remaining one as a test set.

3 Results

During a mean measurement time of 55 min in 14 subjects, 27 true and 578 false alarms occurred. The real alarms occurred at a rate of median 1.5 per measurement. The most important features to discriminate the type of alarm in the classification phase were the area below the SpO_2 threshold, HR, SpO_2 and StO_2, in this order. To evaluate the performance of classifications the *accuracy* (percentage of correctly classified instances over the total number of instances), *sensitivity* (percentage of situation classified as real alarms that actually were the real alarms), and *specificity* (percentage of situations reported as false alarms that actually were the false alarms) are shown in Fig. 3 and Table 3. These values are based on the average of the 10 iterations. It is noteworthy that the cerebral StO_2 improved the classification accuracy.

4 Discussion, Conclusions and Outlook

The achieved specificity of >99% and the sensitivity (87.52%) is comparable to the results reported in [13–15] for (N)ICUs, realized either with MLAs or with other approaches such as, e.g., the employment of multimodal descriptive statistics, Fourier and Hilbert transform to categorize the alarms. It has to be kept in mind that, generally, MLAs require a large amount of data to be trained effectively. In our case, the amount of data was certainly not optimal, because it was too few data with too few real alarms, due to the imbalance between true and false alarms. Taking this into consideration, impressive accuracy, specificity and sensitivity were, nevertheless, achieved. Of course, for a clinical application the highest sensitivity of 87.52% by

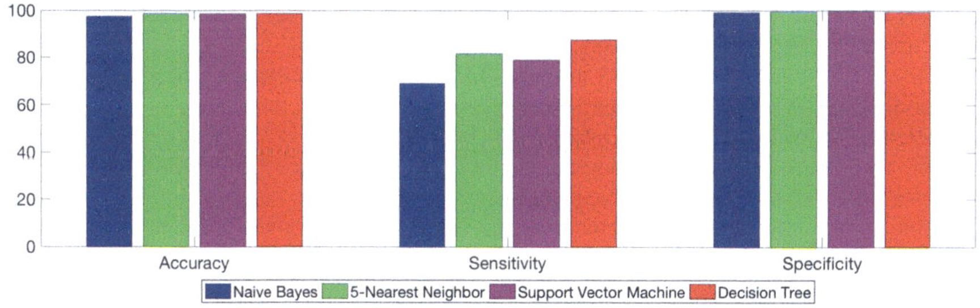

Fig. 3 Mean accuracy, mean sensitivity and mean specificity for NB, 5-NN, SVM and DT classifiers. DT has the highest accuracy and sensitivity of 98.67% and 87.52%, respectively

Table 3 Mean (standard deviation) performance of the four classifiers

	NB	5-NN	SVM	DT
Accuracy [%]	97.52 (0.030)	98.55 (0.020)	98.65 (0.020)	98.67 (0.020)
Sensitivity [%]	69.03 (0.260)	81.68 (0.140)	78.97 (0.150)	87.52 (0.100)
Specificity [%]	99.13 (0.010)	99.46 (0.010)	99.65 (0.005)	99.33 (0.010)

the DT MLA would not be sufficient. Since missing a real alarm could be detrimental for patients, 100% detection of the real alarms is needed. To obtain higher sensitivity in the future, we will include larger datasets and use strategies to handle the above-mentioned imbalance. We conclude that all four tested MLAs yield promising results and we are convinced that 100% sensitivity can be achieved by increased training. This study shows that indeed the false alarms can be eliminated with modern MLAs, and that once the legal problems are solved, MLAs can rapidly be implemented in the standard care of the NICU. This will lead to better working conditions for the staff and a higher quality of care, as well as less stress for the neonates and their parents. Ultimately, this will reduce brain injury and long-term disabilities.

Acknowledgments This work was supported by the Nano-Tera RTD project NewbornCare, the Clinical Research Priority Program (CRPP) Molecular Imaging Network Zürich (MINZ) of the University of Zurich and the Swiss National Science Foundation project 159490.

References

1. Wolf M, Keel M, von Siebenthal K et al (1996) Improved monitoring of preterm infants by Fuzzy logic. Technol Health Care 4:193–201
2. Sendelbach S, Funk M (2013) Alarm fatigue: a patient safety concern. AACN Adv Crit Care 24:378–386. quiz 87-8
3. Johnson KR, Hagadorn JI, Sink DW (2017) Alarm safety and alarm fatigue. Clin Perinatol 44:713–728
4. Li T, Matsushima M, Timpson W et al (2018) Epidemiology of patient monitoring alarms in the neonatal intensive care unit. J Perinatol
5. Lawless ST (1994) Crying wolf: false alarms in a pediatric intensive care unit. Crit Care Med 22:981–985
6. Johnson AEW, Ghassemi MM, Nemati S et al (2016) Machine learning and decision support in critical care. P Ieee 104:444–466
7. Cerka P, Grigiene J, Sirbikyte G (2015) Liability for damages caused by artificial intelligence. Comput Law Secur Rev 31:376–389
8. Kleiser S, Ostojic D, Nasseri N et al (2018) In vivo precision assessment of a near-infrared spectroscopy-based tissue oximeter (OxyPrem v1.3) in neonates considering systemic hemodynamic fluctuations. J Biomed Opt 23:1–10
9. Proença M, Grossenbacher O, Dasen S, et al. (2018) Performance assessment of a dedicated reflectance pulse oximeter in a neonatal intensive care unit. In: James patton UIaC, editor. 40th Annual International Conference of the IEEE Engineering in Medicine and Biology Society. Honolulu, HI
10. Webb AR (2002) Statistical pattern recognition, 2nd edn. Wiley, Chichester
11. Aha DW, Bankert RLA (1996) Comparative evaluation of sequential feature selection algorithms. Learning from data lecture notes in statistics, vol 112. Springer, New York
12. Chandrashekar G, Ferat S (2014) A survey on feature selection methods. Comput Electr Eng Elsevier 40:16–28
13. Eerikainen LM, Vanschoren J, Rooijakkers MJ et al (2016) Reduction of false arrhythmia alarms using signal selection and machine learning. Physiol Meas 37:1204–1216
14. Plesinger F, Klimes P, Halamek J et al (2016) Taming of the monitors: reducing false alarms in intensive care units. Physiol Meas 37:1313–1325
15. Monasterio V, Burgess F, Clifford GD (2012) Robust classification of neonatal apnoea-related desaturations. Physiol Meas 33:1503–1516

Development of an IoT-Based Monitoring System for Healthcare: A Preliminary Study

M. Ishida, S. Ushioda, Y. Nagasawa, Y. Komuroa, Z. Tang, L. Hu, T. Tamura, and K. Sakatani

Abstract We present an IoT-based monitoring system for healthcare that allows for long-term measurements of blood pressure (BP), heart rate (HR), and body weight (BW), as well as near-infrared spectroscopy (NIRS) for measurement of prefrontal cortex (PFC) activity. To verify the applicability of the system, it was set up in a local fitness gym for a preliminary study. A total of 39 subjects, selected from members of the gym, participated in the study. We analyzed the BP, HR, and BW data, collected from the subjects over one half-year. In addition, to assess the degree of mental stress of the subjects, we analysed left-right asymmetry of the PFC activity using the laterality index at rest (LIR) of the NIRS parameter. Results show that the subjects were able to measure their physiological data by themselves when they visited the gym, after being instructed how to perform the measurements. Furthermore, the results also indicate that ordinary people can continuously monitor physiological functions such as brain function in a non-medical facility, such as a fitness gym.

Keywords IoT · Health care · Prevention medicine · Big data · Near infrared spectroscopy

M. Ishida · S. Ushioda · Y. Nagasawa · Y. Komuroa · Z. Tang · L. Hu · T. Tamura
NEWCAT Research Institute, Department of Electrical and Electronic Engineering, College of Engineering, Koriyama, Japan

K. Sakatani (✉)
Department of Human and Engineered Environmental Studies, Universal Sports Health Science Laboratory, Graduate School of Frontier Sciences, The University of Tokyo, Kashiwanoha, Kashiwa-shi, Chiba, Japan
e-mail: k.sakatani@edu.k.u-tokyo.ac.jp

© Springer Nature Switzerland AG 2020

P.-D. Ryu et al. (eds.), *Oxygen Transport to Tissue XLI*, Advances in Experimental Medicine and Biology 1232, https://doi.org/10.1007/978-3-030-34461-0_37

1 Introduction

The rapidly aging global population has resulted in a significant increase in the prevalence of chronic diseases, such as diabetes, obesity and hypertension, and their related effects. Therefore, there is a rapidly increasing need for medical and welfare service resources. On the other hand, exceedingly low fertility rates of the populations of many countries, including Japan, and regions have resulted in a serious shortage of physicians, nurses, and home caregivers.

The remote health monitoring system (also known as telehealth or telemedicine) is one of the most modern forms of medical and healthcare services, and its purpose is to provide clinical healthcare from a distance by use of information and communication/telecommunication technology (ICT) [1]. It has been used to overcome obstacles such as distance, and to improve access to medical services that would often not be consistently available in distant rural communities. Such systems include not only remote clinical service delivery but also non-clinical elements of the healthcare system, such as continued medical education, long-term health monitoring and tracking for healthy older subjects. It actually refers to a broader spectrum of remote healthcare services. Therefore, the remote health monitoring system is considered to be one of the possible ways of solving the problems outlined above.

In the current study, in order to stablish a new medical and welfare service system corresponding to the declining birthrate and aging population, we developed an IoT-based monitoring system for healthcare, which allows for long-term measurement of blood pressure (BP), heart rate (HR), body weight (BW), and even mental stress measured from pre-frontal cortex (PFC) activity using a wearable near-infrared spectroscopy (NIRS) device. We observed that the subjects can continuously monitor physiological functions including brain function. Our results indicate the potential of the IoT-based healthcare monitoring system for improving the quality of life of older people as well as promoting their health.

2 Methods

2.1 Subjects and Study Protocol

Thirty-nine volunteers (7 males and 32 females, average age 62.0 ± 8.6 years) from a fitness gym called 'Sakura' (which belongs to Kasuga Rehabilitation Hospital, Fukushima) were recruited for this study. In general, the subjects visited the gym two to three times a week, and spent about one hour for aerobic exercise including walking and running. The subjects provided written informed consent as required by the Human Subjects Committee of the Rehabilitation Hospital.

The protocol is that, after instruction on the use of the IoT health monitoring system, the subjects were requested to monitor their physiological conditions by themselves when they visited the fitness gym. The participants were requested to sit in front of a tablet placed on a table where the on-screen instructions and measurement items are presented. Following the instructions displayed on the screen, the subjects were first requested to scan their membership card with the identification barcode, and then to measure PFC activity at rest using a NIRS device for 1 min, followed by measurements of their BP, HR, and BW. There were no limitations for the number of measurements that could be performed in a single day; it took about 5 mins for measurements of these physiological parameters. The experimental study was performed between July 2017 and March 2018.

2.2 System Design

We designed and developed an IoT-based healthcare monitoring system, which aims to take long-term measurements of BP, HR, and BW, as well as NIRS measurements of PFC activity. The system is composed of a tablet-based data receiver collecting physical and mental data using several kinds of medical instruments, and a remote control system used to store and analyse these collected data from the tablet. We developed an Android application for the receiver so that users can perform the daily health measurements through interaction operation by themselves. The objective health measurements include BP and HR using a sphygmomanometer (TM-2657, A&D Corp., Japan), and BW using an electronic scale (AD-6209PBT-C, A&D Corp., Japan). Note that the sphygmomanometer is a standard cuff-type sphygmomanometer.

In addition, we measured PFC activity using a wearable NIRS (HOT-1000, Hi-tachi High-Technologies Corporation, Japan). The HOT-1000 is a two-channel NIRS, which uses a single LED (800 nm) for measurement of total hemoglobin (t-Hb) concentration changes [2]. It is comprised of a light source and two light detectors, which are placed at distances of 1.0 cm and 3.0 cm from the source. It estimates the concentration changes of t-Hb using the modified Beer-Lambert law.

These devices have a Bluetooth communication function so that the measured data can be transported to the tablet receiver automatically. After being collected in the receiver, the data can be sent to the remote Amazon's AWS Cloud system at the end of each measurement session. The systemic diagram of the proposed system is presented in Fig. 1.

2.3 Data Processing

First, all the BP, BW and HR recordings of each subject are plotted in time series to analyse the changing trend with time. Next, we analyse the NIRS data. In order to analyse left/right asymmetry of PFC activity at rest, we calculated the laterality index at rest (LIR) as follows [3]:

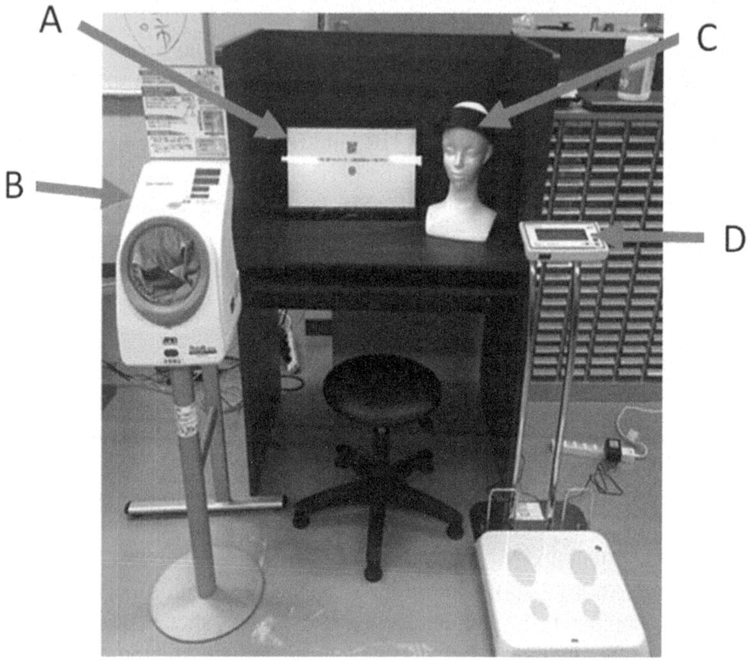

Fig. 1 The IoT-based monitoring system used for daily health measurements. (**A**) Control PC, (**B**) Sphygmomanometer (TM-2657; A&D), (**C**) NIRS device (HOT-1000; Hitachi), (**D**) Electronic scale (AD-6209PBT-C; A&D)

$$\mathrm{LIR} = \frac{\sum_{t \in analysis\ interval}\left[\left(\Delta totalR_t - \Delta totalR_{\min}\right) - \left(\Delta totalL_t - \Delta totalL_{\min}\right)\right]}{\sum_{t \in analysis\ interval}\left[\left(\Delta totalR_t - \Delta totalR_{\min}\right) + \left(\Delta totalL_t - \Delta totalL_{\min}\right)\right]}$$

In the above equation, $\Delta totalR_t$ and $\Delta totalL_t$ denote t-Hb concentration changes of the right and left PFC at rest, respectively. $\Delta totalR_{\min}$ and $\Delta totalL_{\min}$ denote the minimums of $\Delta totalR_t$ and $\Delta totalL_t$, respectively. Note that $\Delta totalR_t - \Delta totalR_{\min}$ and $\Delta totalL_t - \Delta totalL_{\min}$ are always non-negative. The index defined by the above equation provides values in the range of [−1, +1]. A positive LIR (0<) indicates right dominant PFC activity, which reflects negative emotion, while a negative LIR (<0) indicates left dominant PFC activity, which reflects positive emotion [4, 5].

3 Results

By the end of March 2018, over 3000 recordings were collected from the subjects. On average, each subject completed a measurement at a rate of once per day. When the subjects visited the gym, their systolic BP, diastolic BP, and HR were measured continuously. A typical example of the changing trends is shown in Fig. 2, which

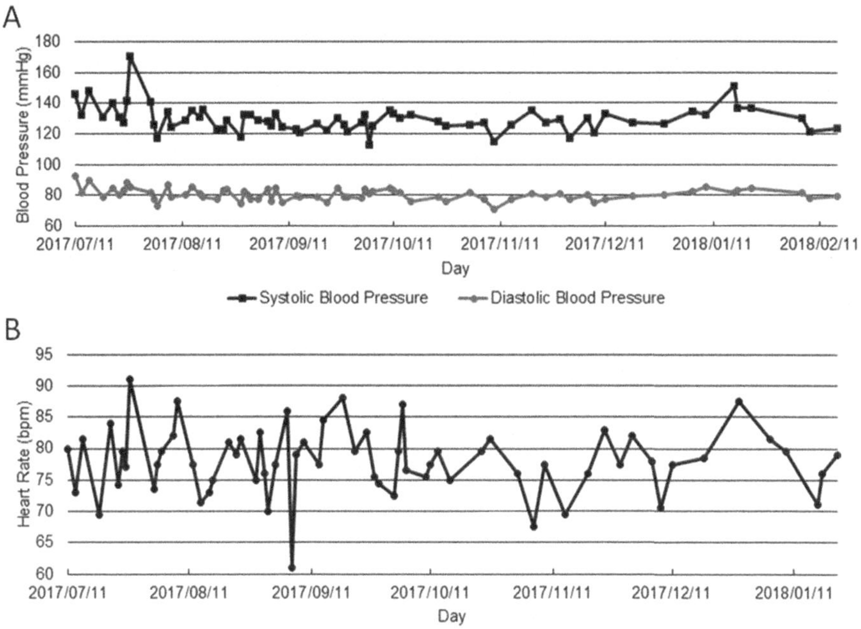

Fig. 2 Typical example of changing trends in systolic blood pressure (SBP), diastolic blood pressure (DBP) (**A**), and heart rate (HR) (**B**) in one subject over 6 months

depicts the systolic/diastolic BP and HR of a subject over one half-year. Correspondingly, a typical example of the changing trends in BW and calculated LIR index in the same subject is shown in Fig. 3. Through these plots, we can clearly evaluate the changes of the condition of the subjects.

We also analysed the average changes of BP, HR, BW, and NIRS (LIR) for all subjects during the experimental period to monitor their health condition; all data during the experimental period of the subjects were averaged (Fig. 4). Note that that the subjects had an overall healthy BP, BW and HR.

4 Discussions

The present study demonstrates that the developed IoT-based health monitoring system can easily make long-term and continuous measurements of the physical and mental condition. It should be emphasized that, after receiving instructions on the use of the system, ordinary people can monitor their physical and mental condition using the IoT health monitoring system by themselves. Analysis shows that there was a trend of a gradual decrease of BW and BP for many subjects, suggesting positive effects of fitness on the health condition. This suggests that the physical activities at the gym have a positive effect on reducing their BP and BW, and on

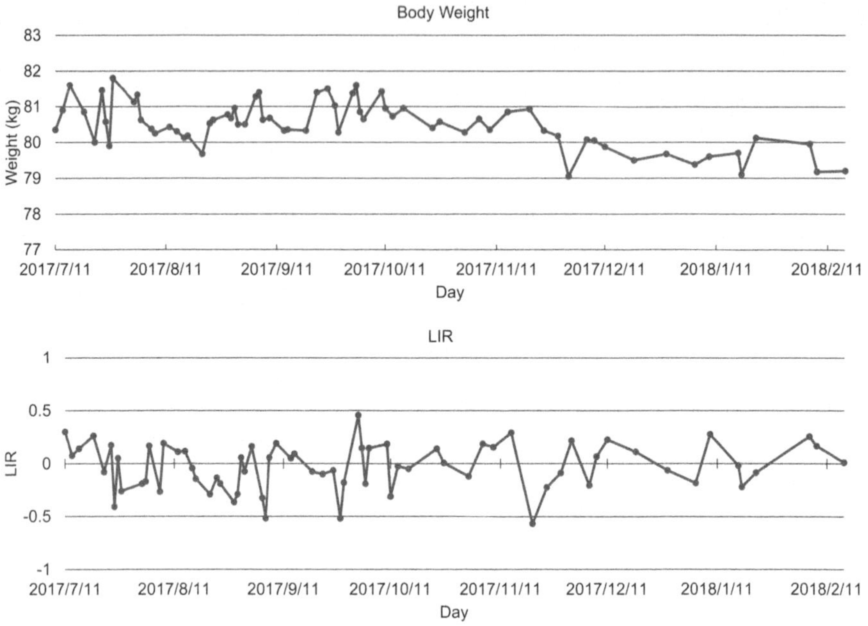

Fig. 3 Typical example of changing trends in body weight (BW) and laterality index at rest (LIR) of NIRS in one subject over 6 months

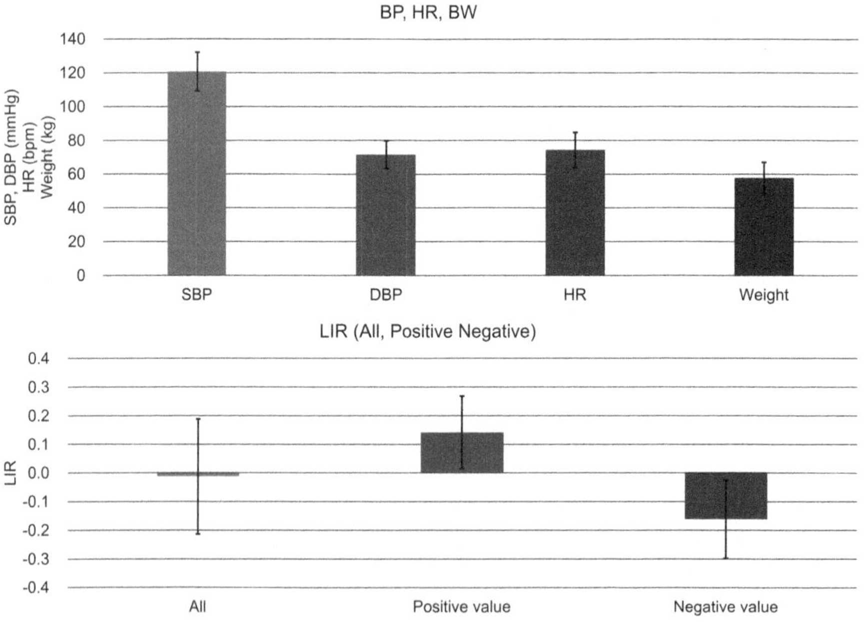

Fig. 4 Mean changes in blood pressure (BP), heart rate (HR), body weight (BW), and laterality index at rest (LIR) of NIRS for all subjects during the study period

promoting their health. This is consistent with another study on the effect of exercise on hypertension [6].

In addition, data on the LIR index shows small fluctuations between minus one and plus one for subjects during the experimental period, suggesting that the mental stress conditions were not stable in the subjects [3–5]. However, the average LIR of all subjects during the experimental period was about zero (Fig. 4). This suggests that the overall mental stress condition of the subjects was relatively low and stable since LIR below zero is associated with low anxiety levels [3].

In summary, we developed the IoT-based health monitoring system which allows ordinary people to monitor their physiological conditions such as BP, HR, BW, and mental stress by themselves. We believe that the IoT-based health monitoring system is useful for healthcare outside a medical facility, and can resolve the shortage of physicians, nurses, and home caregivers.

Acknowledgments This work was supported in part by Strategic Research Foundation Grant-aided Project for Private Universities (S1411017) from the MEXT, Groundwork Project for Creating Industrial Models Using IoT from the NEDO, and grants from Iing Co., Ltd. (Tokyo, Japan) and Southern Tohoku General Hospital (Fukushima, Japan).

References

1. Vollenbroek-Hutten M, Jansen-Kosterink S, Tabak M et al (2017) Possibilities of ICT-supported services in the clinical management of older adults. Aging Clin Exp Res 29:49–57
2. Nozawa T, Sasaki Y, Sasaki K et al (2016) Interpersonal frontopolar neural synchronization in group communication: an exploration toward fNIRS hyperscanning of natural interactions. NeuroImage 133:484–497
3. Ishikawa W, Sato M, Fukuda Y et al (2014) Correlation between asymmetry of spontaneous oscillation of hemodynamic changes in the prefrontal cortex and anxiety levels: a near-infrared spectroscopy study. J Biomed Optics 19(2):027005
4. Davidson RJ, Jackson DC, Kalin NH (2000) Emotion, plasticity, cortex, and regulation: perspectives from affective neuroscience. Psychol Bull 126:890–909
5. Fischer H, Andersson JL, Furmark T et al (2002) Right-sided human prefrontal brain activation during acquisition of conditioned fear. Emotion 2:233–241
6. Pagonas N, dimeo F, Bauer F et al (2014) The impact of aerobic exercise on blood pressure variability. J Hum Hypertens 28:367–371

Developing a Model to Simulate the Effect of Hypothermia on Cerebral Blood Flow and Metabolism

Joshua Russell-Buckland and Ilias Tachtsidis

Abstract Hypoxic ischemic encephalopathy (HIE) is a significant cause of death and neurological disability in newborns. Therapeutic hypothermia at 33.5 °C is one of the most common treatments in HIE and generally improves outcome; however 45–55% of injuries still result in death or severe neurodevelopmental disability. We have developed a systems biology model of cerebral oxygen transport and metabolism to model the impact of hypothermia on the piglet brain (the neonatal preclinical animal model) tissue physiology. This computational model is an extension of the BrainSignals model of the adult brain. The model predicts that during hypothermia there is a 5.1% decrease in cerebral metabolism, 1.1% decrease in blood flow and 2.3% increase in cerebral tissue oxygenation saturation. The model can be used to simulate effects of hypothermia on the brain and to help interpret bedside recordings.

Keywords Broadband NIRS · Hypothermia · Systems biology

1 Introduction

Hypoxic-ischaemic encephalopathy (HIE), often resulting from intrapartum hypoxic-ischemic (HI) injury, is a significant cause of death and morbidity. Somewhere between 700,000 deaths amongst neonates can be attributed to HIE alone [1]. Following neonatal HI injury or birth asphyxia, infants are treated with therapeutic hypothermia at a temperature of 33.5 °C, as well as a variety of medications such as morphine and atracurium [2]. However, 45–55% of cases treated with hypothermia end with death or moderate to severe neurodevelopmental disability [1, 3]. The brain of neonates undergoing hypothermia treatment is monitored through a variety of methods such as electro-encephalography (EEG) [4] and

J. Russell-Buckland (✉) · I. Tachtsidis
Biomedical Optics Research Laboratory, University College London, London, UK
e-mail: joshua.russell-buckland.15@ucl.ac.uk

© The Author(s) 2020

P.-D. Ryu et al. (eds.), *Oxygen Transport to Tissue XLI*, Advances in Experimental Medicine and Biology 1232, https://doi.org/10.1007/978-3-030-34461-0_38

near-infrared spectroscopy (NIRS) [2, 5]. Additionally, in the few hospitals with appropriate facilities, when the infant is stable enough (usually a week after birth) and following treatment they image the brain with magnetic resonance spectroscopy (MRS) [6]. The collected multimodal data can provide not only diagnostic and prognostic information but also insights on the mechanisms of the injury.

Our approach to analyse this multimodal data has been multifaceted and includes the development and application of (1) a physiology-informed 'mathematical model' of the cerebral circulation under a systems biology approach, which is specially designed for the interpretation of NIRS signals [7–12]; and (2) 'signal processing' methods quantifying the interrelationships between signals both in time- and frequency-domain to quantify indices of cerebral blood flow, oxygenation and metabolic regulation [2, 5].

The development of systems biology-based models begin with the 'BRAINCIRC' model in 2005 [7]. This built on an earlier circulatory model by Ursino and Lodi [13] and combined models for the biophysics of the circulatory system, the brain metabolic biochemistry and the function of vascular smooth muscle. This model was succeeded by the 'BrainSignals' model [8], which simplified the previous BRAINCIRC model and added a submodel of mitochondrial metabolism. Additional versions were then developed from this, such as the 'BrainPiglet' model [9] which was developed to interpret data collected from a piglet model. It involved modifying the default values for 11 of the 107 parameters used and was extended to include simulated measurements for magnetic resonance spectroscopy values, which are available for the piglet model. In 2015, Caldwell et al. modified the BrainSignals model to produce the 'BrainSignals Revisited' model [10]. This made various simplifications to the BrainSignals model to reduce complexity and decrease the time taken to run a simulation, whilst being able to reproduce the same results and behaviour of the original model. This reduced model was later extended in 2016 to simulate scalp haemodynamics to produce the 'BSX' model [11]. This could be used to investigate the potential for systemic haemodynamics to confound fNIRS haemoglobin signals. The BrainPiglet model was also extended to model cell death following HIE producing the 'BrainPigletHI' model [12]. This history is shown schematically in Fig. 1.

However, the existing mathematical models have been developed to model brain physiology under 'typical' conditions, particularly at normal body temperature. In order to properly interpret data collected during therapeutic hypothermia, the models need to be able to reflect these biological conditions. It has been observed that both cerebral metabolic rate of oxygen ($CMRO_2$) and cerebral blood flow (CBF) in piglets decrease with reduced body temperature [14]. For reliable inferences to be made through the use of systems biology models, they must be able to simulate this behaviour.

We present a new systems biology model of the piglet brain, a common animal model for the human neonatal brain, which incorporates temperature effects in the brain tissue physiology. This is an expansion of the BrainPigletHI model, as seen in [12]. The model is used to demonstrate how brain tissue temperature impacts brain physiology steady state behaviour for changing blood pressure, arterial oxygen saturation and partial pressure of CO_2. It is then shown how decreasing temperature impacts a variety of measurable signals.

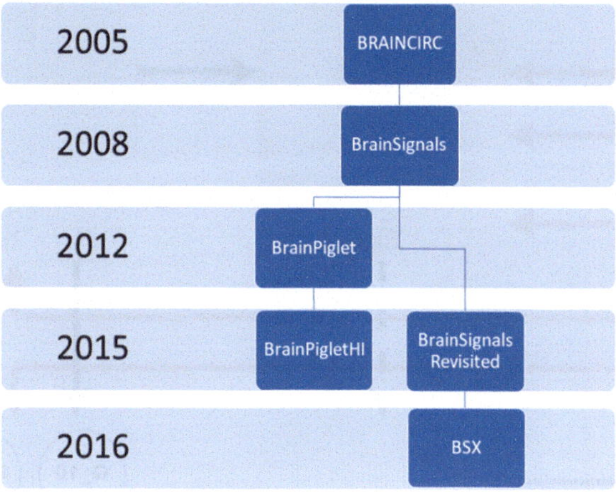

Fig. 1 History of the brainsignals family of models. A general overview of the brainsignals model history. The first model was the BRAINCIRC model in 2005, followed by the brainsignals model in 2008. This model was adapted for the physiology of piglets, a common neonatal preclinical animal model, in 2012 producing the brainpiglet model. The brainpiglet model was modified to include cell death in 2015, to produce the brainpigletHI model. Also in 2015, the brainsignal model was refactored for speed and clarity, producing the brainsignals revisited model. This was extended in 2016 to include scalp haemodynamics, producing the BSX model

2 Methods

Temperature is already incorporated into the BrainPiglet model as a constant value within the proportionality constant $Z = RT/F$, where R is the ideal gas constant, F is the Faraday constant and T is absolute body temperature. The constant Z is used within the model to determine the equilibrium constant for a variety of metabolic reactions, such as electron transfer within mitochondria. By making Z a function of temperature, temperature modulated electron transfer is incorporated into the metabolic submodel.

Temperature also impacts the rate of other reactions and processes, such as diffusion or Michaelis-Menten type behaviour. Orlowski et al. [15] expanded an existing model of cellular metabolism by incorporating temperature dependence into the rates of reaction and ion diffusion and a similar approach is taken here. Reaction rates, Michaelis-Menten rate constants and diffusion rates are modified by a quantity

$$k_{i,new} = k_{i,previous} \times Q_{10}^{\frac{T_{new} - T_{previous}}{10.}}$$

where $k_{i,\,new}$ is the new rate constant for reaction i at the new temperature T_{new}, $k_{i,\,previous}$ is the rate constant at temperature $T_{previous}$, and Q_{10} is the temperature

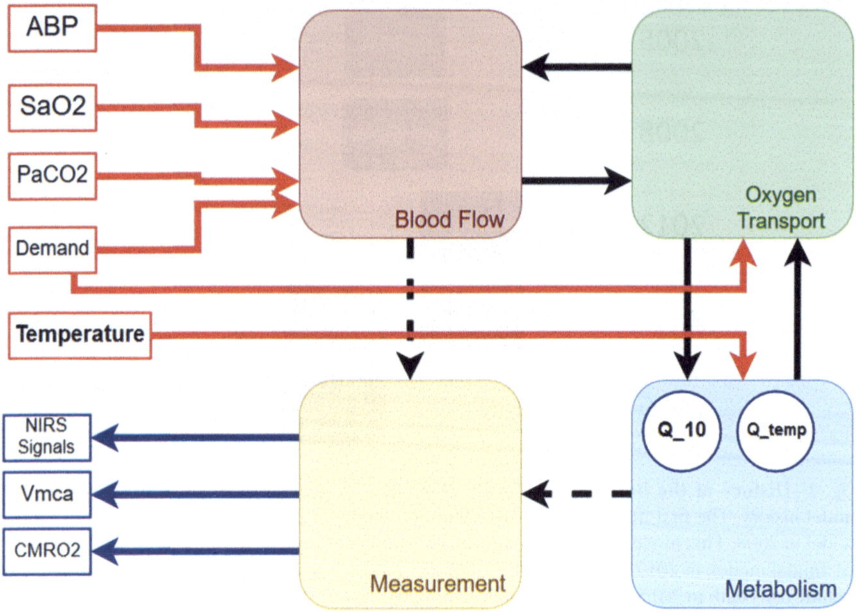

Fig. 2 General structure of the brainpiglet hypothermia model. Model inputs, arterial blood pressure (ABP, arterial oxygen saturation (SaO2), partial pressure of CO_2 (PaCO2) and demand, and outputs are shown, as well as each of the four sub-models and the general relations between each. New additions are shown in bold. Temperature is added as an input to the model. Q_10, a measure of the change in reaction rate when increasing temperature by 10 °C, is a new parameter. Q_temp, the factor by which a reaction rate is modified when changing temperature, is added as a new internal state variable local to the metabolism submodel

coefficient, defined as the ratio of reaction rates measured for the same reaction at two temperatures 10 °C apart, with an initial default value of 2.23, as per [15], but an expected final value within the range of approximately 2–3 as per most biological reactions [16]. Typically, $T_{previous}$ will be assumed to be normal body temperature of 37 °C, but this can be set as a model parameter. For simplification purposes, within the model

the temporary variable $Q_{temp} = Q_{10}^{\frac{T_{new} - T_{previous}}{10}}$ is defined. Figure 2 shows a simplified schematic of the model structure, with the new model additions of temperature, Q_{10} and Q_{temp} shown in bold.

Models were then tested and verified through steady state simulations, at 37 °C, 35 °C and 33.5 °C, varying arterial blood pressure, arterial oxygen saturation and partial pressure of CO_2. Following this, all model inputs except temperature were kept at their default values, whilst temperature was decreased between 37 °C and 33.5 °C for varying values of Q_{10}.

3 Results

Steady state simulations were carried out at three temperatures (33.5 °C, 35 °C and 37 °C) to investigate the effects of hypothermia on brain vascular autoregulation. The three main measured inputs of arterial blood pressure (P_a), arterial oxygen saturation (SaO_2) and partial pressure of CO_2 ($PaCO_2$) were both increased and decreased with CBF simulated at the end of 100 s at each step change. Figure 3 shows that cerebral autoregulation is preserved at all temperatures and for both increasing and decreasing changes in P_a, SaO_2 and $PaCO_2$.

Following this, the effect of decreasing temperature on physiology within the model was investigated through further use of steady state simulations. Temperature was decreased to 33.5 °C with all other inputs kept at baseline values for a range of Q_{10} values. Without a known value of Q_{10} it was important to investigate a range of values to ensure that the full range of model behaviour could be considered. As with the autoregulation simulations, output values were simulated after 100 s at each temperature step. Outputs considered are: (a) brain tissue oxygenation saturation (StO_2), (b) CBF, (c) brain tissue haemoglobin differences changes (ΔHbD = oxyhaemoglobin-deoxyhaemoglobin), (d) brain tissue changes in the concentration of the oxidation of cytochrome-*c*-oxidase (ΔoxCCO), and (e) cerebral metabolic rate of oxygen ($CMRO_2$). Figure 4 shows that, across all outputs except StO_2 and ΔHbD, the output decreases linearly, whilst for StO_2 and ΔHbD an increase in value is, instead, observed as temperature decreases. The rate of change increases with Q_{10}.

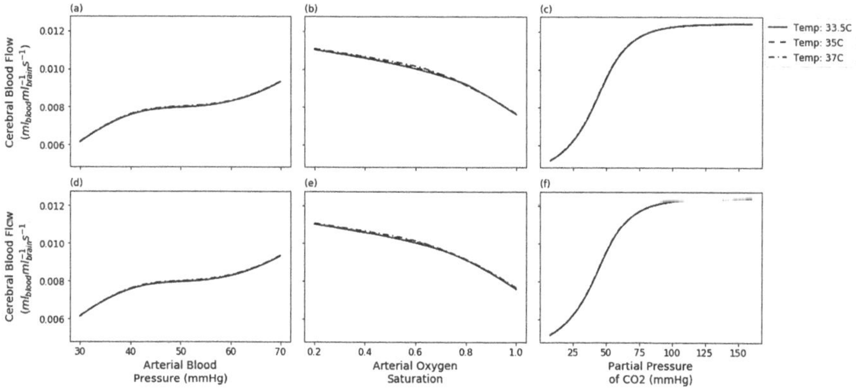

Fig. 3 Steady states curves showing cerebral blood flow against increasing (a) arterial blood pressure; (b) arterial oxygen saturation; (c) partial pressure of CO_2 and decreasing (d) arterial blood pressure; (e) arterial oxygen saturation; (f) partial pressure of CO_2 for temperatures of 33.5 °C, 35 °C and 37 °C. It can be seen in all figures that autoregulation is preserved across all three temperatures and there is little difference between increasing and decreasing values of input

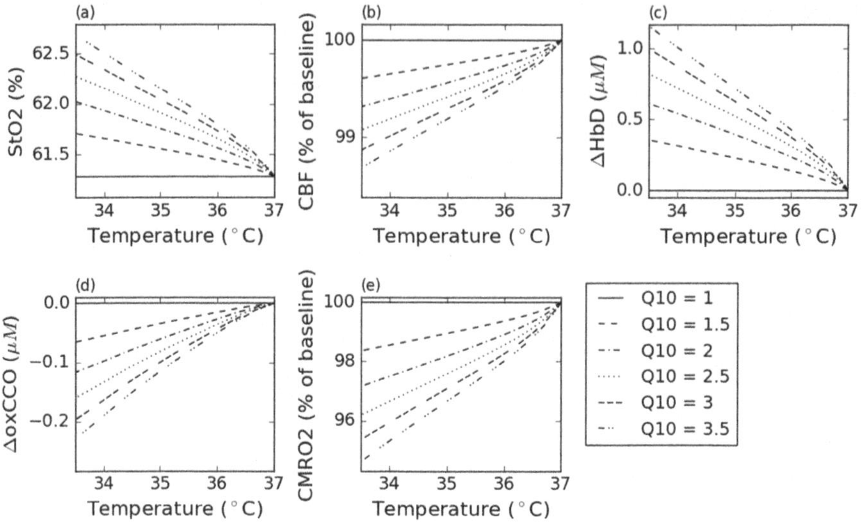

Fig. 4 Steady state curves showing the effect of decreasing temperature on (a) total oxygenation index; (b) cerebral blood flow; (c)velocity of the middle cerebral artery; (d) change in concentration of cytochrome-*c*-oxidase; (e) cerebral metabolic rate of oxygen for varying values of Q_{10}. Steady state simulations show expected behaviour across outputs, where information is available to confirm, such as the decrease cerebral blood flow and cerebral metabolic rate of oxygen with decreasing temperature down to 33.5 °C. The observed change is linear, with the rate of change increasing with the Q_{10} value

Considering Q_{10} values of 2.5, which is in the middle of the range given previously for most biological reactions, and 3.5, which is the largest value considered, CBF decreases by 1.1% and 1.6%, respectively whilst the $CMRO_2$ decrease by 5.1% and 7.1% respectively. StO_2 increases by 2.3% and 3.2% of normothermic values respectively.

4 Discussion

We have expanded an existing systems biology model of the piglet brain physiology to include the impact of hypothermia. This has been done by introducing a minimal number of new parameters and inputs and is able to produce qualitatively reasonable results. Simulations of cerebral autoregulation agree with the findings of Lee et al. who found that hypothermia did not change autoregulation within a piglet model for both hyper- and hypotensive changes [17] (Fig. 3).

When considering the effect of temperature on various measurable outcomes, we see that both CBF and $CMRO_2$ decrease with decreasing temperature, as found by Ehrlich et al. [9]. Whilst the model changes are smaller than those found by Ehrlich et al., the final cooled temperature is not as low and it is not the intention of the model to simulate below a temperature of 33.5 °C. We expect changes in brain physiology at this temperature to be subtle but important. Below this temperature damage to the brain may occur causing a change in brain physiology not captured by this model.

Systems biology models were previously used by our group to investigate the effect of HI in the piglet model [12]; however, they were not able to incorporate the impact of therapeutic hypothermia alongside this injury. In particular, it was found that the pre- and post-injury brain is sufficiently different to require refitting of the model and a number of measurable differences could be explained through the incorporation of a parameter representing cell death within the brain. By combining this previously developed approach with the new hypothermia model, it may be possible to further explain other behaviour. We aim to apply the model to broadband NIRS data, including cytochrome-*c*-oxidase measurements, collected within the group that show differing responses to hypothermia in piglets who received the same injury. We will apply the model to data collected from human neonates, where we expect the same model structure to apply but with different model parameters to reflect the difference in human and pig physiology.

Acknowledgments This research was funded by The Wellcome Trust, grant 104580/Z/14/Z

References

1. Hassell KJ, Ezzati M, Alonso-Alconada D et al (2015) New horizons for newborn brain protection: enhancing endogenous neuroprotection. Arch Di Child Fetal Neonatal Ed 100:F541F552
2. Bale G, Mitra S, de Roever I et al (2018) Oxygen dependency of mitochondrial metabolism indicates outcome of newborn brain injury. J Cerebral Blood Flow Metab 0(00):1–13
3. Gluckman P, Wyatt J, Azzopardinna D et al (2005) Selective head cooling with mild systemic hypothermia after neonatal encephalopathy: multicentre randomized trial. Lancet 365(9460):663–670
4. Murray D, Boylan GB, Ryan AC et al (2009) Early EEG findings in hypoxic-ischemic encephalopathy predict outcomes at 2 years. Pediatrics 124:e459–e467. https://doi.org/10.1542/peds.2008-2190
5. Bale G, Mitra S, Meek J et al (2014) A new broadband near-infrared spectroscopy system for in-vivo measurements of cerebral cytochrome-c-oxidase changes in neonatal brain injury. Biomed Opt Express 5:3450–3466. https://doi.org/10.1364/BOE.5.003450
6. Vries L, Groenendaal F (2010) Patterns of neonatal hypoxic-ischaemic brain injury. Neuroradiology 52:555–566. https://doi.org/10.1007/s00234-010-0674-9
7. Banaji M, Tachtsidis I, Delpy D, Baigent S (2005) A physiological model of cerebral blood flow control. Math Biosci 194(2):125–173. https://doi.org/10.1016/j.mbs.2004.10.005
8. Banaji M, Mallet A, Elwell CE, Nicholls P, Cooper CE (2008) A model of brain circulation and metabolism: NIRS signal changes during physiological challenges. PLoS Comput Biol 4(11):e1000212
9. Moroz T, Banaji M, Robertson NJ, Cooper CE, Tachtsidis I (2012) Computational modelling of the piglet brain to simulate near-infrared spectroscopy and magnetic resonance spectroscopy data collected during oxygen deprivation. J R Soc Interface 9(72):1499–1509
10. Caldwell M, Hapuarachchi T, Highton D et al (2015) BrainSignals revisited: simplifying a computational model of cerebral physiology. PLoS One 10:e0126695. https://doi.org/10.1371/journal.pone.0126695

11. Caldwell M, Scholkmann F, Wolf U, Wolf M, Elwell C, Tachtsidis I (2016) Modelling confounding effects from extracerebral contamination and systemic factors on functional near-infrared spectroscopy. NeuroImage 143:91–105. https://doi.org/10.1016/j.neuroimage.2016.08.058
12. Caldwell M, Moroz T, Hapuarachchi T et al (2015) Modelling blood flow and metabolism in the preclinical neonatal brain during and following hypoxic-Ischaemia. PLoS One 10:e0140171. https://doi.org/10.1371/journal.pone.0140171
13. Ursino M, Lodi CA (1997) A simple mathematical model of the interaction between intracranial pressure and cerebral hemodynamics. J Applied Physiology 82(4):1256–1269
14. Ehrlich MP, McCullough JN, Zhang N et al Effect of hypothermia on cerebral blood flow and metabolism in the pig. Ann Thoracic Surg 73:191–197
15. Orlowski P, McConnell FK, Payne S (2014 Feb) A mathematical model of cellular metabolism during ischemic stroke and hypothermia. IEEE Trans Biomed Eng 61(2):484–490
16. Reyes B, Pendergast J, Yamazaki S (2008) Mammalian peripheral circadian oscillators are temperature compensated. J Biol Rhythm 23:95–98. https://doi.org/10.1177/0748730407311855
17. Lee JK, Brady KM, Mytar JO et al (2011) Cerebral blood flow and cerebrovascular autoregulation in a swine model of pediatric cardiac arrest and hypothermia. Crit Care Med 39(10):2337–2345. https://doi.org/10.1097/ccm.0b013e318223b910

Open Access This chapter is licensed under the terms of the Creative Commons Attribution 4.0 International License (http://creativecommons.org/licenses/by/4.0/), which permits use, sharing, adaptation, distribution and reproduction in any medium or format, as long as you give appropriate credit to the original author(s) and the source, provide a link to the Creative Commons license and indicate if changes were made.

The images or other third party material in this chapter are included in the chapter's Creative Commons license, unless indicated otherwise in a credit line to the material. If material is not included in the chapter's Creative Commons license and your intended use is not permitted by statutory regulation or exceeds the permitted use, you will need to obtain permission directly from the copyright holder.

Validation and Comparison of Monte Carlo and Finite Element Method in Forward Modeling for Near Infrared Optical Tomography

Jingjing Jiang, Wuwei Ren, Helene Isler, Alexander Kalyanov, Scott Lindner, Di Costanzo Mata Aldo, Markus Rudin, and Martin Wolf

Abstract Near infrared optical tomography (NIROT) is a non-invasive imaging technique to provide physiological information e.g. the oxygenation of tissue. For image reconstruction in clinical and preclinical scenarios, models to accurately describe light propagation are needed. This work aims to assess the accuracy and efficiency of different models, which paves the way for an optimal design of model-based image reconstruction algorithms in NIROT for realistic tissue geometries and heterogeneities. Two popular simulators were evaluated: the Monte Carlo (MC) method based MCX and the finite element method (FEM) based Toast++. We compared simulated results with experimental data measured on a homogeneous silicone phantom with well-calibrated parameters. The laser light was focused on the center of the phantom surface and images were captured by a CCD camera in both reflection and transmission modes. For transmittance measurements, the two models showed good agreement. Both achieve a cosine similarity of ~99%. In contrast, for reflectance measurements, FEM results deviated more from the measured values than MC, yielding similarity values of 86% and 94%, respectively. This study recommends the use of MC for NIROT in reflection mode and both MC and FEM yield excellent results for transmission mode.

Keywords Near infrared optical tomography · Finite element method · Monte Carlo method · Experimental validation

Jingjing Jiang and Wuwei Ren have contributed equally for this chapter.

J. Jiang (✉) · H. Isler · A. Kalyanov · S. Lindner · D. C. M. Aldo · M. Wolf
Biomedical Optics Research Laboratory (BORL), Department of Neonatology, University Hospital Zurich (USZ), Zurich, Switzerland
e-mail: jingjing.jiang@usz.ch

W. Ren
Biomedical Optics Research Laboratory (BORL), Department of Neonatology, University Hospital Zurich (USZ), Zurich, Switzerland

Institute of Biomedical Engineering, ETH, Zurich, Zurich, Switzerland

M. Rudin
Institute of Biomedical Engineering, ETH, Zurich, Zurich, Switzerland

© Springer Nature Switzerland AG 2020

P.-D. Ryu et al. (eds.), *Oxygen Transport to Tissue XLI*, Advances in Experimental Medicine and Biology 1232, https://doi.org/10.1007/978-3-030-34461-0_39

1 Introduction

To image e.g. the oxygenation of tissue by high resolution near infrared optical tomography (NIROT), an accurate model for describing light propagation in tissue is critical irrespective of the actual algorithm used for the image reconstruction. The gold standard model for light propagation in tissue is the radiative transfer equation (RTE) [1]. However, the RTE is impractical because it cannot simply be solved analytically. The Monte Carlo (MC) method provides an accurate solution to the RTE by simulating the path of photons through the tissue. But MC is computationally expensive and hence time consuming. By using parallel computing techniques, the state-of-the-art MC-based toolkit, MCX, has improved this situation considerably [2]. Therefore, image reconstruction based on MC has become practical, in particular, when combined with high speed methods such as scaling methods, where the MC simulation is based on known reduced scattering coefficients μ_s', and the simulation results are scaled by absorption coefficients (μ_a) [3]. However, when the μ_s' values are also unknowns, the current hardware limits the use of MC particularly for a large number (e.g. >1000) of source-detector pairs and for time-domain data. An alternative method is to approximate the RTE by the diffusion theory. Simple analytical solutions exist for homogeneous infinite and semi-infinite geometries. For more complex geometries the diffusion equation can be solved numerically e.g. by finite element methods (FEM) [4]. The objective of this study was to model light propagation comparing the two currently popular simulators, a MC based model MCX [2] and a FEM based model Toast++ [4]. For model validation experiments have been carried out using silicone phantoms: the results of forward simulations by the two simulators were compared with the measured intensity distribution for both reflection and transmission mode.

2 Methods

2.1 Silicone Phantom Experiments

For the experiment, we fabricated a homogeneous slab silicone phantom with a dimension of $60 \times 30 \times 15\text{mm}^3$. The μ_a of the phantom was 0.007mm^{-1} and μ_s' was 0.87mm^{-1} according to published procedures [5]. The schematic of the experimental setup is illustrated in Fig. 1. Light was emitted from a solid-state laser (B&W Tek, Newark, USA) operated at 670 nm and collimated before entering an imaging chamber. The beam was then directed to the sample surface by a scan head (ScanLab, Puchheim, Germany), which contained two galvanometric driven mirrors. By deflecting the beam via mirrors, reflection and transmission mode operation can be implemented by illuminating the top or bottom surface, respectively. After interaction with tissue, backscattered light was captured with a 16-bit CCD camera (ANDOR Corporation, Northern Ireland) equipped with a macro lens (Nikkor, Tokyo, Japan).

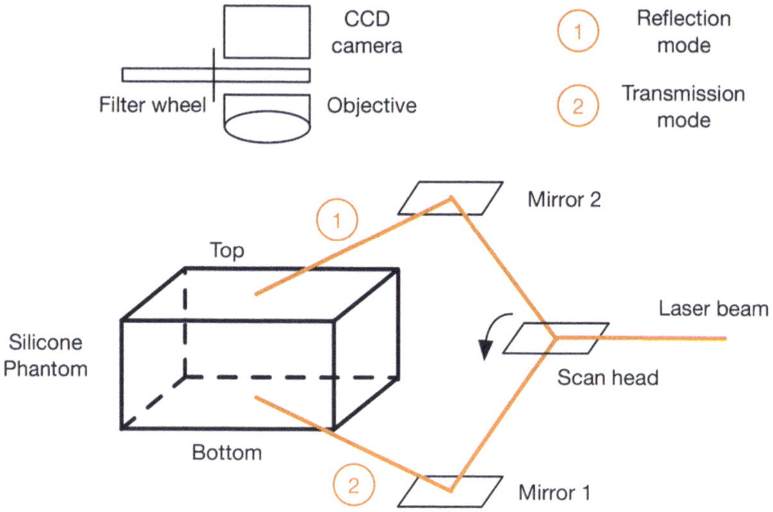

Fig. 1 Schematic of the experimental setup

2.2 *Simulation With MCXLAB*

We modeled the above measurement with MCXLAB, a MATLAB version of MCX with all core codes in C and CUDA C. We employed a discretized volume of 15 × 30 × 60 voxels with voxel size of 1 mm^3 for simulating the silicone phantom. The same optical properties were assigned to each voxel. Detectors of 2×2 mm^2 size covered the whole area of one side of the volume. A light source with Gaussian profile was placed on the center of the opposite side in transmission mode and on the same plane in reflection mode. To account for the continuous wave nature of the measurement, we utilized 5×10^7 photons to achieve smooth results. Traveling through the volume, the photons experienced multiple scattering and absorption events. The computation of their propagation was parallelized on a Geforce Titan xp GPU (Nvidia, USA) yielding an acceleration by a factor >1000 as compared to CPU based computation [2].

Once a photon escaped the boundary defined by detectors, the track was saved and tagged with the corresponding detector ID. The path length of the track s was used for calculating survival probability P of the photon given by $P = e^{-\mu_a s}$. After obtaining P for each detected photon, the energy for each detector can be calculated by accumulating P for photons detected by the same detector. This requires a loop over the list of photon tracks, which was facilitated by a MEX compilation of C code.

2.3 Simulation with Toast++

Tissue is highly scattering at the wavelength utilized in NIROT and, therefore, light propagation can be approximated as a diffusion process. FEM numerically solves diffusion equations for complex boundaries. We implemented FEM with Toast++ in MATLAB on a computer with an Intel Core i7@ 2.60 GHz and 8.00 GB RAM. First, we generated tetrahedral meshes for the slab phantom with an open-source meshing tool, iso2mesh [6]. To study the influence of the meshing configuration in FEM, we created a coarse mesh containing 7793 nodes and a refined mesh consisting of 107293 nodes. The illumination source was set to the center of the top and the bottom of the mesh for reflection and transmission mode, respectively. 30 × 15 virtual detector pixels were set to cover the top surface of the object, given that each pixel has a dimension of 2 × 2mm^2, and μ_s' and μ_a were assigned to the mesh. With all the setup information and presumed optical properties, a system matrix was generated. System matrix describes the linear relationship between the illumination source and light intensity within the simulated object [4].

3 Results

We generated transmittance and reflectance data with MCXLAB and FEM/TOAST++. It took 3.27 s on average to generate the forward results with MCXLAB. With Toast++, the procedure of calculating the system matrix took 1.07 s for the coarse mesh and 17.69 s for the refined mesh. The detected images were obtained by dividing the illumination profile with the system matrix. For the coarse and refined meshes, this last step took less than 0.5 s. FEM based Toast++ has the advantage of avoiding the time-consuming step of recalculating the system matrix for different source patterns, whereas MC has to be run for each new source pattern. MCXLAB was able to compete with Toast++ with respect to computational speed. The reason is the acceleration of the MC by the advanced GPUs. This result is true when combining a small number of sources with a large number of detectors, which is the case for many NIROT instruments based on continuous wave CCD cameras or time-resolved SPAD cameras.

To validate the models, we compared simulation and experimental data for both 2D images (Fig. 2) and two directional 1D plots (Fig. 3). The overall distributions appear similar in transmission mode whereas, in reflection mode, the values from FEM deviated more from the measured data, especially in the central area.

We calculated the cosine similarity between simulated I_s and measured results I_{m},

$$\text{cosine similarity} = \frac{I_{\mathrm{m}} \cdot I_{\mathrm{s}}}{\left\|I_{\mathrm{m}}\right\| \left\|I_{\mathrm{s}}\right\|} \tag{1}$$

to quantify the accuracy of the simulation results (Table 1).

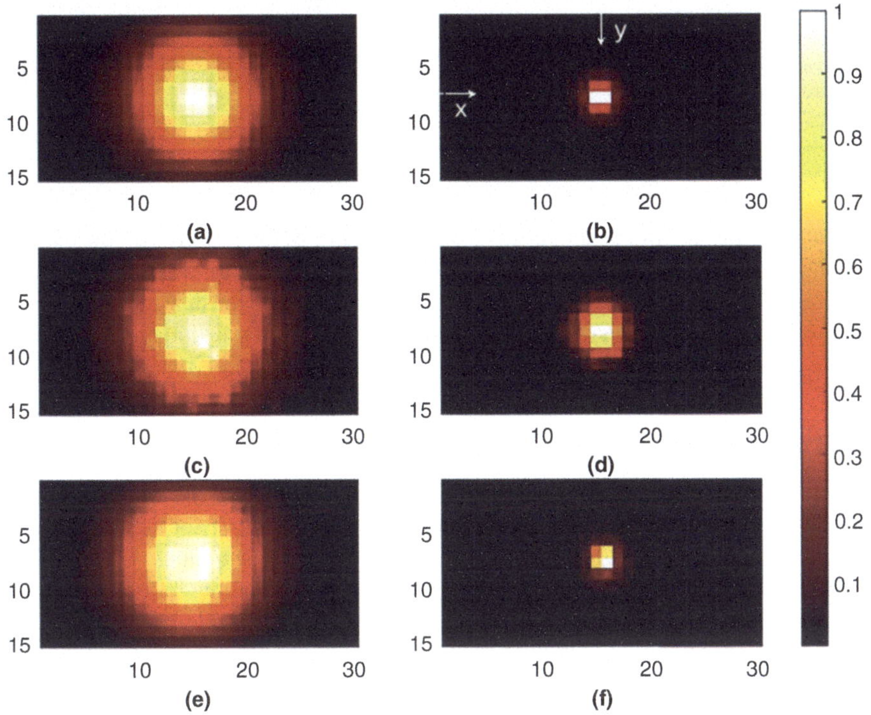

Fig. 2 Forward results of MC simulated (a, b), FEM simulated (c, d) and phantom experiments (e, f) in transmission mode (a, c, e) and reflection mode (b, d, f)

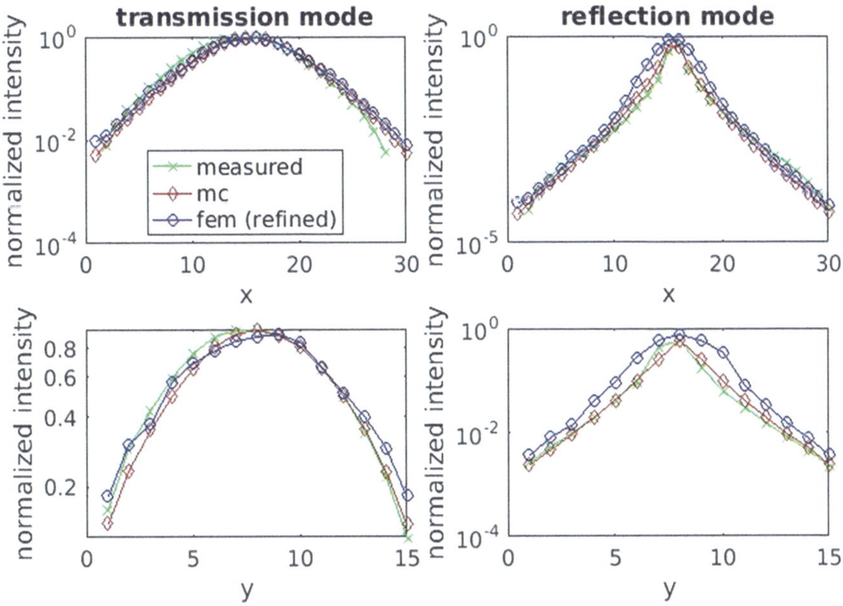

Fig. 3 Comparison between measured, MC and FEM simulated data along central lines

Table 1 Cosine similarity between simulated (MC, FEM) and experimental forward results

	Transmission mode	Reflection mode
MC	0.988	0.942
FEM with fine mesh	0.987	0.868
FEM with coarse mesh	0.983	0.865

For transmission mode, the results from MC and FEM agree well with the experiments. However, in reflection mode, MC outperformed FEM with 7.4% higher accuracy. In this study, FEM results obtained with the coarse mesh were not inferior to those obtained with the refined mesh in transmission and reflection mode.

4 Discussion, Conclusion and Outlook

We compared the MC-based MCX and the FEM based Toast++ for modeling light propagation in tissue with experimental results for the continuous wave mode. Based on these results, MCX is recommended for simulating the reflectance measurement. In most clinical applications, reflectance will be the relevant mode. FEM is not as accurate because, in typical NIROT setups, sources and detectors are placed too close together to apply FEM [7]. FEM relies on the diffusion approximation, which is not correct for short source-detector distances. When working in transmission mode, e.g. for breast cancer diagnosis, both MCX and Toast++ will yield appropriate modeling results.

In a next step, we will compare the two simulation approaches for time resolved measurements and compare the results with data acquired with our newly developed in-house TR NIROT system.

Acknowledgments This work was supported by the Clinical Research Priority Programs (CRPP) Tumor Oxygenation and Molecular Imaging Network Zürich (MINZ) of the University of Zurich, the Swiss Cancer Research grant KFS-3732-08-2015 and the Swiss National Science Foundation project 159490.

References

1. Welch AJ, Gemert MJC (2010) Optical-Thermal Response of Laser- Irradiated Tissue, 2nd edn. Springer
2. Fang Q, Boas DA (2009) Monte Carlo simulation of photon migration in 3D turbid media accelerated by graphics processing units. Opt Express 17:20178–20190
3. Zhu C, Liu Q (2013) Review of Monte Carlo modeling of light transport in tissues. J Biomed Opt 18:050902
4. Mand S, Arridge SR (2014) The Toast++ software suite for forward and inverse modeling in optical tomography. J Biomed Opt 19(4):040801

5. Ren W (2018) STIFT: a modular software platform for simulation, Optimization and reconstruction in fluorescence molecular tomography. (PhD thesis), ETH Zurich
6. Fang Q, Boas DA (2009) Tetrahedral mesh generation from volumetric binary and gray-scale images. IEEE international symposium on biomedical imaging: from nano to macro 1,2:1142–1145
7. Yoo M, Liu F, Alfano RR (1990) When does the diffusion- approximation fail to describe photon transport in random-media. Phys Rev Lett 64:2647–2650

Development of a Cuff-Less Blood Pressure Monitoring System and Its Application

S. Ushioda, Y. Nagasawa, M. Isida, Y. Komuro, Z. Tang, L. Hu, T. Tamura, and K. Sakatani

Abstract We present an unobtrusive cuff-less sphygmomanometer based on contact-type and optical pulse sensors for continuous and minimally invasive monitoring of blood pressure (BP). We developed a cuff-less sphygmomanometer that utilizes the pulse arrival time (PAT) to estimate continuous BP. To assess its accuracy, we recruited 10 healthy subjects in whom we carried out BP studies using the cuff-less sphygmomanometer compared with a standard cuff-type device in a stationary sitting patient. Preliminary results showed that the mean difference (MD) of estimated systolic blood pressure and diastolic blood pressure were 0.96 ± 9.6 (mean ± SD) mmHg and 1.14 ± 7.5 mmHg, respectively, compared to the control. The corresponding correlation between the estimated BP values and controls were 0.78 for systolic blood pressure ($p < 0.01$) and 0.69 for diastolic blood pressure ($p < 0.01$); thus, there were significant correlations. These results suggest that the developed cuff-less sphygmomanometer has the potential for continuous BP monitoring. Finally, we conducted a preliminary study of simultaneous monitoring of cuff-less BP and near-infrared spectroscopy to evaluate the potential for assessment of autonomic nervous system functions during mental stress tasks.

Keywords Blood pressure · Near infrared spectroscopy · Mental stress · Prefrontal cortex · Prevention medicine

S. Ushioda · Y. Nagasawa · M. Isida · Y. Komuro · Z. Tang · L. Hu · T. Tamura
NEWCAT Research Institute, Department of Electrical and Electronic Engineering, College of Engineering, Koriyama, Japan

K. Sakatani (✉)
Universal Sports Health Science Laboratory, Department of Human and Engineered Environmental Studies, Graduate School of Frontier Sciences, The University of Tokyo, Kashiwanoha, Chiba, Japan
e-mail: k.sakatani@edu.k.u-tokyo.ac.jp

© Springer Nature Switzerland AG 2020

P.-D. Ryu et al. (eds.), *Oxygen Transport to Tissue XLI*, Advances in Experimental Medicine and Biology 1232, https://doi.org/10.1007/978-3-030-34461-0_40

1 Introduction

Blood pressure (BP) is one of the important signs of the body's vital functions. High blood pressure (or hypertension) directly increases the risk of cardiovascular diseases (CVD), such as heart attack, heart failure, and stroke. Therefore, accurate and continuous (ambulatory) BP monitoring during daily life is imperative for improving hypertension detection in the general population, and may even help control hypertension by providing timely and continual feedback to hypertensive patients. Conventionally, for continuous blood pressure monitoring an invasive measurement method, such as inserting a catheter into an artery, is necessary. However, due to the invasiveness of such a method, it can be only performed in hospitals. Conventional standard cuff-based means of BP measurement, such as auscultation and oscillometry, are able to provide instantaneous information on BP status. However, these methods are not applicable for continuous BP measurements because of the population-averaged nature of the BP estimation algorithm and the limited frequency of measurement.

Studies have shown that BP estimation based on pulse arrival time (PAT), which is the time it takes for the cardiac wave to propagate through a length of the arterial tree or between the heart and a peripheral arterial site, has acceptable accuracy compared to the gold standard BP measurement method in some situations. Chen et al. [1] described a method of combining the high frequency information of the PAT method and low frequency information in an intermittently acquired systolic blood pressure (SBP) measurement. Poon and Zhang estimated SBP and diastolic blood pressure (DBP) using a weighted sum of log and squared PAT with reference BP, and acquired a mean error of 0.6 ± 9.8 mmHg and 0.9 ± 5.6 mmHg for the estimated SBP and DBP, respectively, compared to the reference measurement [2].

In the present study, we developed a cuff-less sphygmomanometer based on PAT measured using a contact-type sensor and an optical pulse sensor, i.e., electrocardiogram (ECG) and photoplethysmography (PPG), and further evaluated the accuracy of the developed cuff-less sphygmomanometer by comparison with a standard cuff-type device. We also conducted a preliminary study of simultaneous monitoring of cuff-less BP and near-infrared spectroscopy (NIRS) to evaluate the potential for assessment of autonomic nervous system functions during mental stress tasks.

2 Methods

2.1 Principle of Photoplethysmography (PPG)

PPG is a simple optical technique used to detect volumetric changes in blood in peripheral circulation. It is a low cost and non-invasive method that makes measurements at the surface of the skin, e.g. the fingers and earlobes. PPG uses low-intensity infrared (IR) light. When light travels through biological tissues, it is absorbed by bones, skin pigments and both venous and arterial blood. Since light is more strongly absorbed by blood than the surrounding tissues, the changes in blood flow can be detected using PPG sensors as changes in the intensity of light. The voltage signal from PPG is proportional to the quantity of blood flowing through the blood vessels. Even small changes in blood volume can be detected using this method, though it cannot be used to quantify the amount of blood. A PPG signal has several components, including volumetric changes in arterial blood, which are associated with cardiac activity, variations in venous blood volume that modulate the PPG signal, a Direct Current (DC) component showing the tissues' optical property, and subtle energy changes in the body.

This technique provides valuable information related to our cardiovascular system. Recent advances in technology have revived interest in the technique, which is widely used in clinical physiological measurement and monitoring, especially for ambulatory blood pressure monitoring.

2.2 Algorithm to Estimate Blood Pressure

There is increasing evidence [1, 2] that PAT can provide the basis for unconstrained and cuff-less BP measurement. PAT is defined as the time taken for an artery pulse to travel between two arterial sites, which is related to pulse wave velocity (PWV). Since PAT can be simplified as the time delay between the R-wave peak in ECG and the corresponding point in PPG signals, it is a potentially practical solution for ambulatory blood pressure monitoring. Here we refer to the method of estimating BP in [3]. Systolic BP can be estimated using the following equation:

$$SBP_e = SBP_0 - \frac{2}{\gamma T_0}(T - T_0)$$

where SBP_0 is the base SBP (also called the calibrated SBP), T_0 is the base pulse arrival time corresponding to SBP_0, and T is the measured PAT corresponding to SBP_e Note that γ is the interior radius of the vessel in the equation and it is viewed as a constant. The diastolic BP can be calculated as

$$DBP_e = SBP_0 - \frac{2}{\gamma T_0}(T - T_0) - (SBP_0 - DBP_0)\left(\frac{T_0}{T}\right)^2$$

where DBP_0 is the base DBP. Thus, BP estimations based on PAT can be conducted using the equation above, where the required parameters are only SBP_0, DBP_0, and T_0. These parameters can be obtained at the beginning of monitoring by a calibration using an additional cuff-type BP sphygmomanometer.

2.3 Structure of Cuff-Less Sphygmomanometer

The cuff-less sphygmomanometer was first developed to measure continuous ECG and PPG signals and then to further estimate BP. The prototype of the developed device is shown in Fig. 1. The device is mainly composed of an ECG with two movable electrodes (actually, three-lead ECG is adopted), a PPG sensor with a green LED (SML-M13MTT86, Rohm, Japan) and a photodetector (S11154-01CT, Hamamatsu, Japan), a control circuit with a Bluetooth module, and a high capacity battery. BP monitoring can be completed by pressing the two respective electrodes with the thumbs, while holding the device with two hands, or by placing both palms on the electrodes, while the subject is sitting and the device is mounted on a chair that has two armrests (Fig. 2). The measured ECG and PPG data were transmitted to a software terminal installed on a PC in order to calculate beat-by-beat PAT in real time. The PAT data were further used to estimate continuous BP values.

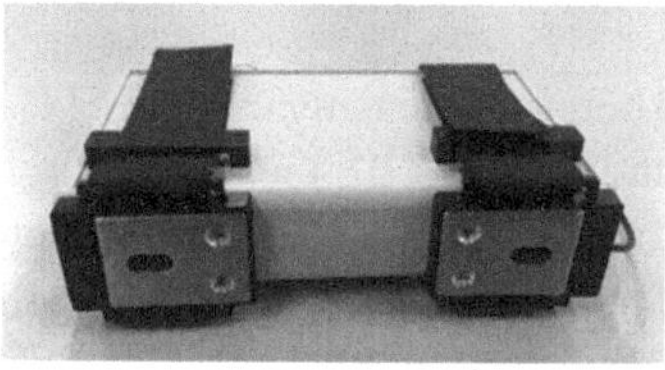

Fig. 1 Prototype of the developed cuff-less sphygmomanometer

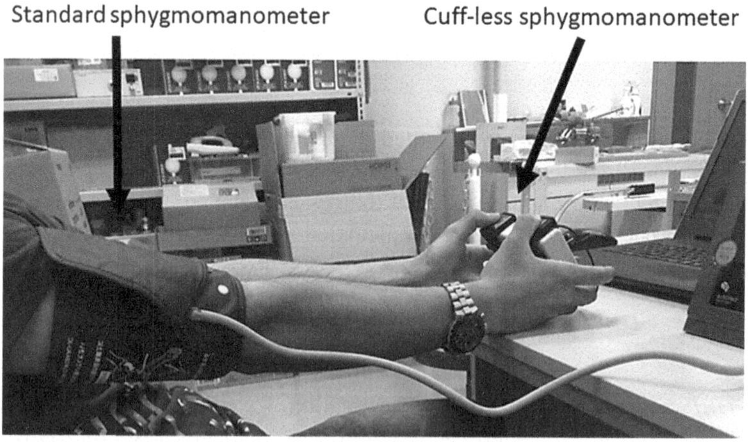

Fig. 2 Experimental setting

2.4 Subjects and Study Protocol

Ten healthy subjects (10 males, average age 21.2 ± 0.4 years) were recruited for this study. Following a detailed explanation of the investigation written informed consent was obtained from each subject. BP was measured to assess the health of all subjects prior to the measurement session.

The protocol consisted of two stages. The first stage was to take BP measurements five times, while the subject is sitting stationary, after making an initial calibration with a cuff BP sphygmomanometer (UA-851PBT, A&D Corp., Japan). All sessions were to be finished within 1 h after the initial calibration. In order to minimize changes of the autonomic nervous system during measurements, the subjects closed their eyes with seating in a comfortable chair, in an air-conditioned room. Our aim with this is to evaluate the accuracy of the estimated BP compared with a reference in a short time after calibration.

Then, we performed a preliminary study of simultaneous monitoring of cuff-less blood pressure and NIRS during stress tasks. The experimental protocol of this stage was firstly to calibrate the cuff-less sphygmomanometer with the subject's eyes closed. After 1 min, the subjects were asked to remain sitting stationary with their eyes closed for 1 min of rest. Next, the subjects were asked to perform mental arithmetic tasks for 2 min [4]. Finally, the subjects resumed their stationary sitting position with their eyes closed for 2 min. At this stage, we simultaneously monitored changes in systemic BP using the cuff-less sphygmomanometer and we monitored changes in cerebral blood oxygenation during the mental stress tasks using two- channel NIRS (PocketNIRS, Hamamatsu Photonics K.K, Japan) to evaluate the applicability of the proposed cuff-less sphygmomanometer in clinical physiological measurement and monitoring of stress responses.

The details of the NIRS equipment have been described previously [5–7]. Briefly, this system measures concentration changes of oxyhemoglobin (oxy-Hb), deoxy-Hb and total-Hb. The system is wireless (Bluetooth®), and equipped with two channels, where each uses LEDs with wavelengths 735, 810, and 850 nm as light sources (sampling rate = 61.3 Hz). The NIRS probes were set on Fp1 (left) and Fp2 (right) of the international electroencephalographic 10–20 system.

3 Results

In the present study, all BP readings taken prior to the measurement sessions were within the accepted 'normal' range (i.e. systolic blood pressure was 120~130 mmHg while diastolic pressure was 80~85 mmHg). In total, 50 pairs of BP recordings were collected. In our analysis, we found that the estimated BP values are mostly close to the corresponding reference BP values. Figure 3 presents a Bland-Altman plot comparing the performances of the estimated BP with the control BP for all recordings (n = 50). The mean differences (MD) of the estimated SBP and DBP were 0.96 ± 9.6 mmHg and 1.14 ± 7.5 mmHg, respectively. Figure 4 presents scatter plots

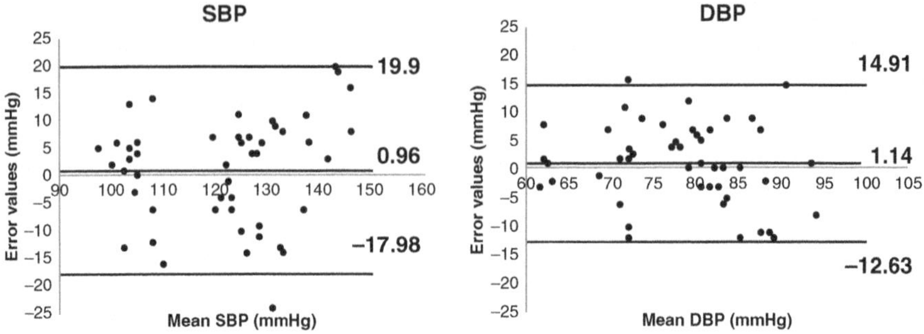

Fig. 3 Bland-Altman plot comparing the performance of the cuff-less sphygmomanometer with that of the reference sphygmomanometer

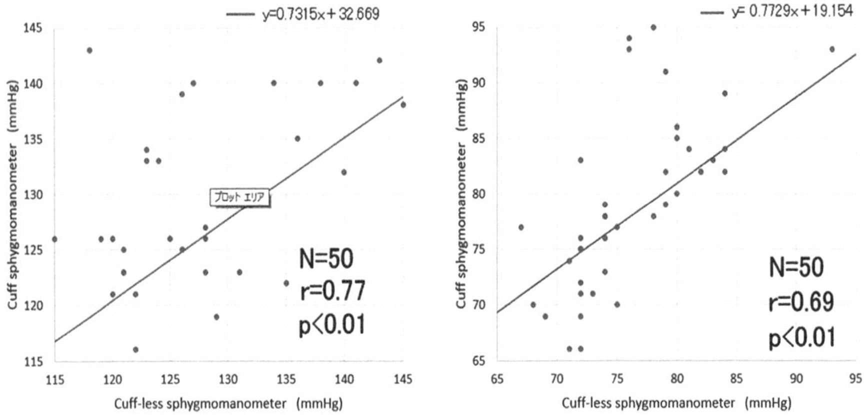

Fig. 4 Scatter plots of the reference BP and estimated BP for SBP (left) and DBP (right)

of the control BP and estimated BP method. The corresponding correlation coefficients between the control and estimated BP values were 0.78 for SBP ($p < 0.01$) and 0.69 for DBP ($p < 0.01$).

Figure 5 shows the preliminary results of simultaneous monitoring using the cuff-less sphygmomanometer and NIRS during the mental arithmetic tasks. NIRS demonstrated increases in oxy-Hb and total-Hb associated with a decrease of deoxy-Hb during the task. The cuff-less sphygmomanometer demonstrated increases in SBP, DBP and HR during the task

4 Discussion

We developed a cuff-less sphygmomanometer that can measure ECG and PPG signals to estimate BP in real-time, unlike the conventional cuff devices. Although some smart watches have a BP measurement function, the accuracy of BP monitoring

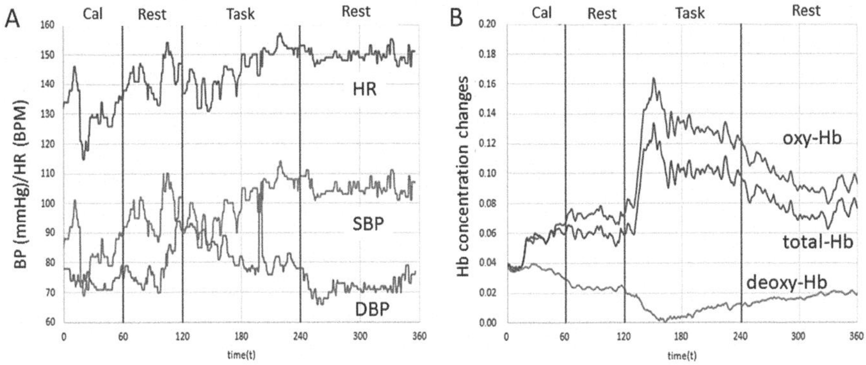

Fig. 5 A typical example of simultaneous monitoring of cuff-less BP (Left) and NIRS (Right) with mental stress tasks. (**A**): Changes in systolic blood pressure (SBP), diastolic blood pressure (DBP) and heart rate (HR) during mental stress tasks; (**B**): Cerebral blood oxygenation changes measured by NIRS simultaneously. The unit of NIRS parameters is expressed by arbitrary unit (a.u.)

is not yet clear. In the present study, by verifying the accuracy of the cuff-less sphygmomanometer compared to control measurements taken using a cuff-type sphygmomanometer, our sphygmomanometer obtained better performances. Of the measured values for SBP, 94% were within tolerance, and the mean square error was 9.6 mmHg. A significant correlation was obtained at 0.78 ($p < 0.01$). Of the measured values for DBP, 90% were within tolerance and the mean square error was 7.5 mmHg. A significant correlation was obtained at 0.69 ($p < 0.01$). These observations suggest that the cuff-less sphygmomanometer could monitor BP almost precisely.

In the preliminary study, the developed cuff-less sphygmomanometer demonstrated increases in SBP, DBP, and HR during the mental stress task. NIRS demonstrated increases in oxy-Hb and total-Hb associated with a decrease of deoxy-Hb during the task; these changes are consistent with the changes of NIRS parameters during activation [4]. However, interestingly, the peak HR changes were observed in the first half of the task period, whereas in the peaks of SBP and DBP changes were observed in the second half. In addition, the peak of oxy-Hb changes was observed in the first half of the task. In order to clarify the physiological mechanisms of the differences in changes of SBP, DBP, HR and oxy-Hb induced by mental stress tasks, further studies using simultaneous measurements of the cuff-less sphygmomanometer and NIRS are necessary. Finally, we should emphasize that further research is needed to clarify the accuracy of the cuff-less monitoring system.

Acknowledgments This research was supported in part by the Strategic Research Foundation Grant-aided Project for Private Universities (S1411017) and a Grant-in-Aid for Exploratory Research (25560356) from the Ministry of Education, Culture, Sports, Sciences, and Technology of Japan.

References

1. Chen W, Kobayashi T, Ichikawa S et al (2000) Continuous estimation of systolic blood pressure using the pulse arrival time and intermittent calibration. Med Biol Eng Comput 38(5):569–574
2. Poon C, Zhang Y (2005) Cuff-less and noninvasive measurements of arterial blood pressure by pulse transit time. Proc 27th Annu Int Conf IEEE Eng Med Biol Soc:5877–5880
3. Tang Z, Tamura T, Sekine M et al (2017) A chair–based unobtrusive Cuffless blood pressure monitoring system based on pulse arrival time. IEEE J Biomed Health Inform 21(5):1194–1205
4. Tanida M, Sakatani K, Takano R et al (2004) Relation between asymmetry of prefrontal cortex activities and the autonomic nervous system during a mental arithmetic task: near infrared spectroscopy study. Neurosci Lett 369:69–74
5. Matsumoto T, Fuchita Y, Ichikawa K et al (2016) Gender and age analysis of NIRS/STAI Pearson correlation coefficients at resting state. Adv Exp Med Biol 876:281–287
6. Fukuda Y, Ishikawa W, Kanayama R et al (2014) Bayesian prediction of anxiety level in aged people at rest using 2-channel NIRS data from prefrontal cortex. Adv Exp Med Biol 812:303–308
7. Ishikawa W, Sato M, Fukuda Y et al (2014) Correlation between asymmetry of spontaneous oscillation of hemodynamic changes in the prefrontal cortex and anxiety levels: a near-infrared spectroscopy study. J Biomed Opt 19:027005

Usefulness of a New Device to Monitor Cerebral Blood Oxygenation Using NIRS During Cardiopulmonary Resuscitation in Patients with Cardiac Arrest: A Pilot Study

Tsukasa Yagi, Tsuyoshi Kawamorita, Keiichiro Kuronuma, Eizo Tachibana, Kazuhiro Watanabe, Nobutaka Chiba, Tadashi Ashida, Wataru Atsumi, Satoshi Kunimoto, Shigemasa Tani, Naoya Matsumoto, Yasuo Okumura, Atsuo Yoshino, and Kaoru Sakatani

Abstract Recent guidelines on cardiopulmonary resuscitation (CPR) have stressed the necessity to improve the quality of CPR. Our previous studies demonstrated the usefulness of monitoring cerebral blood oxygenation (CBO) during CPR by near-infrared spectroscopy (NIRS). The present study evaluates whether the NIRO-CCR1, a new NIRS device, is as useful in the clinical setting as the NIRO-200NX. We monitored CBO in 20 patients with cardiac arrest by NIRS. On the arrival of patients at the emergency department, the attending physician immediately assessed whether the patient was eligible for this study after conventional advanced life support and, if eligible, measured CBO in the frontal lobe by NIRS. We found that in all patients,

T. Yagi (✉)
Department of Cardiology, Kawaguchi Municipal Medical Center, Kawaguchi, Japan

Department of Cardiology, Nihon University Hospital, Tokyo, Japan

T. Kawamorita · K. Kuronuma · E. Tachibana · W. Atsumi · S. Kunimoto
Department of Cardiology, Kawaguchi Municipal Medical Center, Kawaguchi, Japan

K. Watanabe
Department of Cardiology, Nihon University Hospital, Tokyo, Japan

Department of Emergency and Critical Care Medicine, Nihon University Hospital, Tokyo, Japan

N. Chiba
Department of Emergency and Critical Care Medicine, Nihon University Hospital, Tokyo, Japan

T. Ashida · S. Tani · N. Matsumoto
Department of Cardiology, Nihon University Hospital, Tokyo, Japan

Y. Okumura
Division of Cardiology, Department of Medicine, Nihon University School of Medicine, Tokyo, Japan

© Springer Nature Switzerland AG 2020
P.-D. Ryu et al. (eds.), *Oxygen Transport to Tissue XLI*, Advances in Experimental Medicine and Biology 1232, https://doi.org/10.1007/978-3-030-34461-0_41

the cerebral blood flow waveform was in synchrony with the chest compressions. Moreover, the tissue oxygenation index increased following cardiopulmonary bypass (CPB) in patients undergoing CPB, including one patient in whom CBO was monitored using the NIRO-CCR1. In addition, although the NIRO-CCR1 could display the pulse rate (Tempo) in real time, Tempo was not always detected, despite detection of the cerebral blood flow waveform. This suggested that chest compressions may not have been effective, indicating that the NIRO-CCR1 also seems useful to assess the quality of CPR. This study suggests that the NIRO-CCR1 can measure CBO during CPR in patients with cardiac arrest as effectively as the NIRO-200NX; in addition, the new NIRO-CCR1 may be even more useful, especially in prehospital fields (e.g. in an ambulance), since it is easy to carry.

Keywords Cardiopulmonary resuscitation · Near-infrared spectroscopy · Extracorporeal cardiopulmonary resuscitation · Quality of cardiopulmonary resuscitation · Veno-arterial extracorporeal membrane oxygenation

1 Introduction

Cardiac arrest is a major public health issue worldwide. Despite significant advances in the care of cardiac arrest victims, the survival rate of patients suffering from cardiac arrest remains low [1]. Recent guidelines on cardiopulmonary resuscitation (CPR) have stressed that high-quality CPR remains the key to improving the outcomes [2]. Chest compression with as few interruptions as possible is important for high-quality CPR. These guidelines indicated it may be reasonable to use physiologic parameters when feasible to monitor and optimize CPR quality, guide vasopressor therapy, and detect return of spontaneous circulation (ROSC) (Class IIb) [3]. However, these guidelines have not mentioned monitoring cerebral blood oxygenation (CBO) during CPR by near-infrared spectroscopy (NIRS) in order to improve the quality of CPR. In addition, studies have shown that extracorporeal CPR (ECPR) using emergency cardiopulmonary bypass (CPB) could improve neurologic outcome in cases of out-of-hospital cardiac arrest [4–6]. According to the guidelines, in settings where it can be immedi-

A. Yoshino
Division of Neurosurgery, Department of Neurological Surgery,
Nihon University School of Medicine, Tokyo, Japan

K. Sakatani
Division of Neurosurgery, Department of Neurological Surgery,
Nihon University School of Medicine, Tokyo, Japan

NEWCAT Research Institute, Department of Electrical and Electronic Engineering,
Nihon University College of Engineering, Koriyama, Japan

ately implemented, ECPR may be considered for selected patients in whom the suspected etiology of the cardiac arrest is potentially reversible during the limited period of CPB (Class IIb) [2].

We previously reported the usefulness of monitoring CBO during CPR and ECPR by NIRS (NIRO-200NX, Hamamatsu Photonics, Japan) [7, 8]. Moreover, Koyama et al. developed the NIRO-Pulse (Hamamatsu Photonics, Japan), a mode capable of depicting changes in hemoglobin concentrations as an indicator of cerebral blood flow, and simultaneously displaying the cerebral tissue oxygenation index (TOI) [9–11]. However, because the NIRO-200NX is heavy and big, it is difficult to use the NIRO-200NX in prehospital setting, such as inside an ambulance. Thus, the NIRO-CCR1 (Hamamatsu Photonics, Japan) which is smaller and lighter than the NIRO-200NX was developed. The NIRO-pulse can be used not only on the NIRO-200NX, but also on the NIRO-CCR1. However, it is unclear whether the NIRO-CCR1 can measure CBO during CPR and ECPR in patients with cardiac arrest as effectively as the NIRO-200NX in clinical setting. Therefore, this study evaluates whether the NIRO-CCR1 could be as useful in the clinical setting as the NIRO-200NX.

2 Methods

2.1 Patients

In this prospective observational study, NIRS (NIRO-200NX or NIRO-CCR1) was used to measure CBO in the frontal lobe in patients with cardiac arrest transported to the emergency department (ED) at Kawaguchi Municipal Medical Center or Surugadai Nihon University Hospital. The study was approved by the Kawaguchi Municipal Medical Center Ethics Committee. The informed consent was obtained from patients or their family for this study. Patients meeting the following criteria were enrolled in this study: persistent cardiac arrest on arrival at the ED, and successful ROSC after arrival at the ED with conventional advanced life support (ALS) and/or ECPR [4, 7, 8].

2.2 Procedures

The procedures used in the present study are described in detail elsewhere [7, 8]. Briefly, on arrival at the ED, the attending physicians rapidly assessed whether the patient was eligible for this study after conventional ALS, and employed NIRS to measure CBO in the frontal lobe. ECPR was initiated when ROSC could not be achieved within 10 min of arrival of the patient at the ED.

2.3 *Statistical Analysis*

Data are expressed as means ± standard deviation for continuous variables. Levels of the TOI and saturation of the waveform (SnO_2) were compared using the Mann-Whitney U test for continuous variables. *P*-values ≤0.05 were considered to be statistically significant. All analyses were performed using the SPSS software (version 25.0, J SPSS).

3 Results

Table 1 lists the characteristics of the NIRO-200NX and the NIRO-CCR1. Although the NIRO-CCR1 device is smaller and lighter than the NIRO-200NX, the internal data storage time of the NIRO-CCR1 is only 1 h. The blue, red and white waveforms obtained using the NIRO-Pulse mode on the NIRO-200NX and on the NIRO-CCR1 are displayed in real time. The blue, red and white waveforms show the delta-deoxyhemoglobin (Δ-Deoxy Hb), delta-oxyhemoglobin (Δ-Oxy Hb) and delta-total hemoglobin (Δ-total Hb) concentrations, respectively. Moreover, the

Table 1 Characteristics of the NIRO-200NX and NIRO-CCR1 devices

	NIRO-200NX	NIRO-CCR1
Size	264 (W) x 278 (H) x 190 (D) mm	230 (W) x 210 (H) x 80 (D) mm
Weight	6 kg	1.6 kg
Internal data storage	>400 h	1 h
Probe	2 channels	1 channel
Battery backup operation	30 min	2 h
Price	4,600,000 JPY	1,680,000 JPY
Display	1. TOI 2. nTHI 3. Oxy Hb 4. Deoxy Hb 5. Total Hb	1. TOI 2. Tempo 3. Δ-oxy Hb 4. Δ-deoxy Hb 5. Δ-total Hb
NIRO-pulse mode	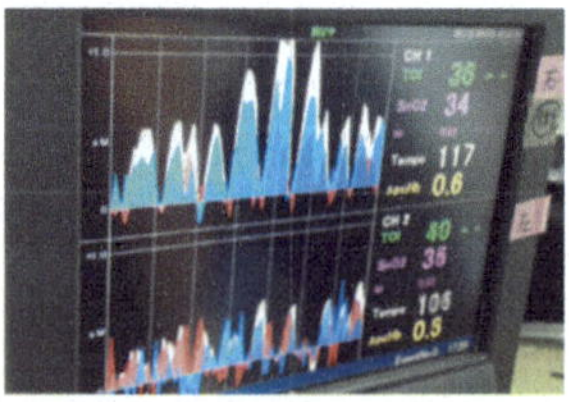 SnO_2 and tempo obtained using the NIRO-pulse mode.	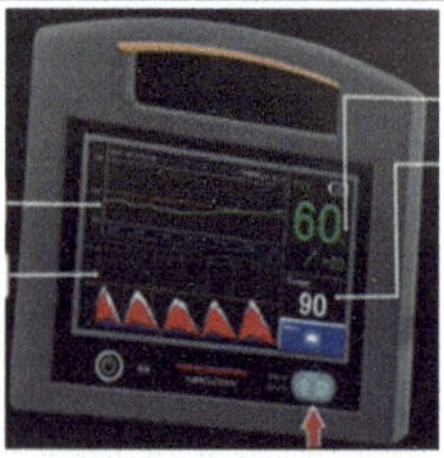 This can only be used with the NIRO-pulse mode.

TOI, Tissue oxygenation index; nTHI, normalized tissue hemoglobin index; Oxy Hb, Oxygenated hemoglobin change; Deoxy Hb, Deoxygenated hemoglobin change

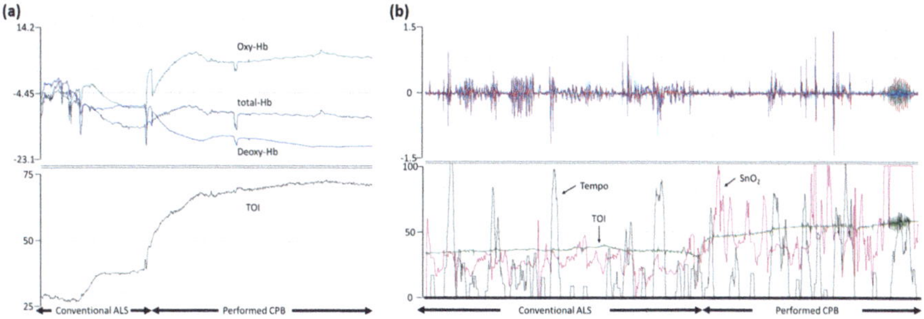

Fig. 1 (**a**) NIRO-200NX and (b) NIRO-CCR1 to measure cerebral blood oxygenation during cardiopulmonary resuscitation (CPR) and extracorporeal CPR. (**b**) The upper figure shows the total hemoglobin concentration, the oxidized hemoglobin and the deoxidized hemoglobin of the cerebral blood flow. Hb, hemoglobin; TOI, tissue oxygenation index; SnO_2, saturation of the waveform; Tempo, pulse/compression rate; ALS, advanced life support; CPB, cardiopulmonary bypass

TOI, SnO_2 and Tempo are also displayed on the NIRO-Pulse. The SnO_2 represents the ratio of Δ-Oxy Hb to Δ-total Hb (= Δ-Oxy Hb + Δ-Deoxy Hb), and Tempo represents the pulse rate.

We monitored CBO in 20 patients with cardiac arrest by NIRS (using the NIRO-200NX in 19 patients and the NIRO-CCR1 in one patient). Of these patients, after arrival at the ED, ROSC was achieved with conventional ALS in two patients and after ECPR in the remaining 18 patients. The mean age of the study population was 60.7 ± 14.2 years, and 95.0% was male.

Figure 1 shows typical profiles of patients in whom we employed the NIRO-200NX (Fig. 1a) or the NIRO-CCR1 (Fig. 1b) to measure CBO in the frontal lobe. In all patients, the cerebral blood flow waveform was in synchrony with the chest compressions. Moreover, the TOI increased following implementation of CPB in patients in whom CPB was performed, including the patient in whom CBO was monitored using the NIRO-CCR1. Figure 1b shows that the pulse rate (Tempo) was not always detected, despite detection of the cerebral blood flow waveform, and that the TOI and SnO_2 were significantly higher after implementation of CPB than before (TOI before implementation of CPB versus (vs.) after: 36.2 ± 1.61% vs. 52.9 ± 3.84%, $P < 0.001$; SnO_2 before implementation of CPB vs. after: 27.4 ± 8.29% vs. 54.6 ± 23.4%, $P < 0.001$).

4 Discussion

This study suggests that CBO during CPR and ECPR in patients with cardiac ar-rest might be measured as effectively with the NIRO-CCR1 as with the NIRO-200NX. That is, synchrony of the cerebral blood flow waveform with the chest compressions and a significant increase in the TOI after implementation of CPB were observed with both the NIRO-200NX and the NIRO-CCR1. When establishing CPB, emergency cannulation of a femoral vein and artery is usually performed under ultra-sonographic or fluoroscopic guidance. However, in EDs and prehospital setting [12], cannulation often has to be performed without ultrasonographic or fluoroscopic guidance. In these situations, it is often difficult to perform cannulation safely. Cannulation can be deemed as successful by confirming a significant increase in the TOI using NIRS after the establishment of CPB. In fact, in our patient in whom CBO was monitored using the NIRO-CCR1, CPB was established without ultrasonographic or fluoroscopic guidance (Fig. 1b).

In addition, the NIRO-Pulse could display the pulse rate (Tempo) in real time; however, we found that Tempo was not always detected, despite detection of the cerebral blood flow waveform. This suggests that some of the chest compressions may not have been effective; this implies that that the NIRO-Pulse may also be useful to assess the quality of CPR. Because recent guidelines recommend that, in adult victims of cardiac arrest, rescuers perform chest compressions at the rate of 100 to 120/min [2], it is important for rescuers to know the number of useful chest compressions per minute. Thus, it is important and necessary for rescuers to measure Tempo using the NIRO-Pulse during CPR in order to perform high-quality CPR. The NIRO-CCR1 can only be used together with the NIRO-Pulse.

The NIRO-CCR1 allows noninvasive, continuous monitoring of changes of CBO with high time resolution and is easy to carry. Therefore, the NIRO-CCR1 may be even more useful, especially in prehospital setting, such as inside an ambulance. On the other hand, the internal data storage time of the NIRO-CCR1 is only 1 h. Some studies suggest that it is important to observe TOI changes over several hours after the establishment of CPB [7, 10, 13]. Future improvements of the NIRO-CCR1 may help to resolve this issue.

There are several limitations to our study. First, this study was not a randomized controlled trial. Second, our findings should be considered preliminary because of the small sample size: there were only 20 patients in the present study and only one patient used NIRO-CCR1. Therefore, from now on, it is necessary to monitor CBO using the NIRO-CCR1 by more physicians and emergency medical responders in more cardiac arrest patients, especially in the prehospital setting.

5 Conclusions

On the basis of these findings, we conclude that the NIRO-CCR1 can measure CBO during CPR and ECPR in patients with cardiac arrest. Furthermore, the NIRO-CCR1 may be even more useful than the NIRO-200NX, especially in prehospital setting, as the device is easy to carry.

Disclosure The authors have no conflicts of interest to disclose.

References

1. Meaney PA, Bobrow BJ, Mancini ME et al (2013) Cardiopulmonary resuscitation quality: [corrected] improving cardiac resuscitation outcomes both inside and outside the hospital: a consensus statement from the American Heart Association. Circulation 128:417–435
2. Neumar RW, Shuster M, Callaway CW et al (2015) Part 1: executive summary: 2015 American Heart Association guidelines update for cardiopulmonary resuscitation and emergency cardiovascular care. Circulation 132:S315–S367
3. Link MS, Berkow LC, Kudenchuk PJ et al (2015) Part 7: adult advanced cardiovascular life support: 2015 American Heart Association guidelines update for cardiopulmonary resuscitation and emergency cardiovascular care. Circulation 132:S444–S464
4. Nagao K, Kikushima K, Watanabe K et al (2010) Early induction of hypothermia during cardiac arrest improves neurological outcomes in patients with out-of-hospital cardiac arrest who undergo emergency cardiopulmonary bypass and percutaneous coronary intervention. Circ J 74:77–85
5. Maekawa K, Tanno K, Hase M et al (2013) Extracorporeal cardiopulmonary resuscitation for patients with out-of-hospital cardiac arrest of cardiac origin: a propensity-matched study and predictor analysis. Crit Care Med 41:1186–1196
6. Sakamoto T, Morimura N, Nagao K et al (2014) Extracorporeal cardiopulmonary resuscitation versus conventional cardiopulmonary resuscitation in adults with out-of-hospital cardiac arrest: a prospective observational study. Resuscitation 85:762–768
7. Yagi T, Nagao K, Sakatani K et al (2013) Changes of cerebral oxygen metabolism and hemodynamics during ECPR with hypothermia measured by near-infrared spectroscopy: a pilot study. Adv Exp Med Biol 789:121–128
8. Yagi T, Nagao K, Kawamorita T et al (2016) Detection of ROSC in patients with cardiac arrest during chest compression using NIRS: a pilot study. Adv Exp Med Biol 876:151–157
9. Koyama Y, Wada T, Lohman BD et al (2013) A new method to detect cerebral blood flow waveform in synchrony with chest compression by near-infrared spectroscopy during CPR. Am J Emerg Med 31:1504–1508
10. Koyama Y, Mizutani T, Marushima A et al (2017) Cerebral tissue oxygenation index using near-infrared spectroscopy during extracorporeal cardio-pulmonary resuscitation predicted good neurological recovery in a patient with acute severe anemia. Intern Med 56:2451–2453
11. Koyama Y, Inoue Y, Hisago S et al (2018) Improving the neurological prognosis following OHCA using real-time evaluation of cerebral tissue oxygenation. Am J Emerg Med 36:344 e345–344 e347
12. Lamhaut L, Hutin A, Deutsch J et al (2017) Extracorporeal cardiopulmonary resuscitation (ECPR) in the prehospital setting: an illustrative case of ECPR performed in the louvre museum. Prehosp Emerg Care 21:386–389
13. Ehara N, Hirose T, Shiozaki T et al (2017) The relationship between cerebral regional oxygen saturation during extracorporeal cardiopulmonary resuscitation and the neurological outcome in a retrospective analysis of 16 cases. J Intensive Care 5:20

Application of Peripheral Near Infrared Spectroscopy to Assess Risk Factors in Patient with Coronary Artery Disease: Part 1

Tsuyoshi Kawamorita, Keiichiro Kuronuma, Tsukasa Yagi, Eizo Tachibana, Shonosuke Sugai, Satoshi Hayashida, Kazuki Iso, Korehito Iida, Wataru Atsumi, Satoshi Kunimoto, Yasuyuki Suzuki, Shigemasa Tani, Naoya Matsumoto, Yasuo Okumura, and Kaoru Sakatani

Abstract Obesity, a risk factor of coronary artery disease, is known to cause peripheral microcirculatory disturbances. This study evaluated the relationship between the degree of obesity and peripheral microcirculatory disturbances, using peripheral near infrared spectroscopy (NIRS) with a vascular occlusion test (VOT). We compared correlations between the NIRS parameter changes induced by VOT and body mass index (BMI) in patients with and without statin therapy. A NIRS probe was set on the right thenar eminence, brachial artery blood flow was blocked for 3 min, and then released. Although total hemoglobin (ΔcHb), deoxyhemoglobin (ΔHHb) and tissue oxygenation index (ΔTOI) were not correlated with BMI, a significant negative correlation was found between oxyhemoglobin (ΔO_2Hb) and BMI in the overall study population (r = −0.255, p-value 0.02). In addition, a significant negative correlation was found between ΔO_2Hb and BMI in patients without statin therapy (r = −0.353, p-value 0.02) but not in patients with statin therapy (r = −0.181, p-value 0.27). These findings suggest that ΔO_2Hb may be a useful indicator to assess peripheral microcirculation.

Keywords Coronary artery disease · Microcirculation · Near infrared spectroscopy · Obesity · Vascular occlusion test

T. Kawamorita · K. Kuronuma (✉) · E. Tachibana · S. Sugai · S. Hayashida · K. Iso · K. Iida
W. Atsumi · S. Kunimoto
Department of Cardiology, Kawaguchi Municipal Medical Center, Kawaguchi, Japan

T. Yagi · Y. Suzuki · S. Tani · N. Matsumoto
Department of Cardiology, Nihon University Hospital, Tokyo, Japan

Y. Okumura
Division of Cardiology, Department of Medicine, Nihon University Itabashi Hospital, Tokyo, Japan

K. Sakatani
NEWCAT Research Institute, Department of Electrical and Electronic Engineering, Nihon University College of Engineering, Koriyama, Tokyo, Japan

© Springer Nature Switzerland AG 2020

P.-D. Ryu et al. (eds.), *Oxygen Transport to Tissue XLI*, Advances in Experimental Medicine and Biology 1232, https://doi.org/10.1007/978-3-030-34461-0_42

1 Introduction

Obesity is a known cause of coronary artery disease, microcirculation disorder and endothelial dysfunction, typified by metabolic syndrome, as well as hypertension and insulin resistance [1].

Near infrared spectroscopy (NIRS) with a vascular occlusion test (VOT) is a noninvasive method used for evaluating oxidative metabolism and microcirculation. It is reported that NIRS with a VOT is useful for assessing peripheral microcirculation in sepsis [2] or post-cardiac surgical patients [3]; however, it has not yet been evaluated whether a correlation exists between body mass index (BMI) and microcirculation, as assessed using NIRS.

Statin therapy is widely used in patients with dyslipidemia and contributes to reducing coronary artery disease. A previous study showed that statin therapy could improve endothelial function and microcirculation [4]. The purpose of the present study was to clarify the relationship between BMI and changes of NIRS parameters with a VOT in patients with and without statin therapy.

2 Methods

2.1 Subjects

Patients with suspected coronary artery disease were prospectively enrolled between October 2017 and March 2018. The Ethical Committee of Kawaguchi Municipal Medical Center approved the study and its protocol. All subjects, or their family, provided written informed consent as required by the Ethical Committee.

2.2 BMI and NIRS Measurements

The body height and weight of all patients were measured before NIRS examination. BMI was derived using the following formula; body weight (kg)/body height $(m)^2$. All NIRS examinations were performed using a NIRO-200NX (Hamamatsu Photonics K.K., Japan), with the patient lying in the supine position. The NIRS probe was attached to the right thenar eminence with an adhesive sticker, and was shielded from external light. Then, a pneumatic pressure cuff was placed on the right upper arm. Two min after NIRS monitoring, brachial artery blood flow was blocked for 3 min at 50 mmHg above the resting systolic blood pressure. The cuff was deflated rapidly after the termination of VOT, to observe reperfusion. The measurements were taken after 3 min of reperfusion. All NIRS parameters were recorded every 0.2 s, continuously. Maximum and minimum values of after the vascular

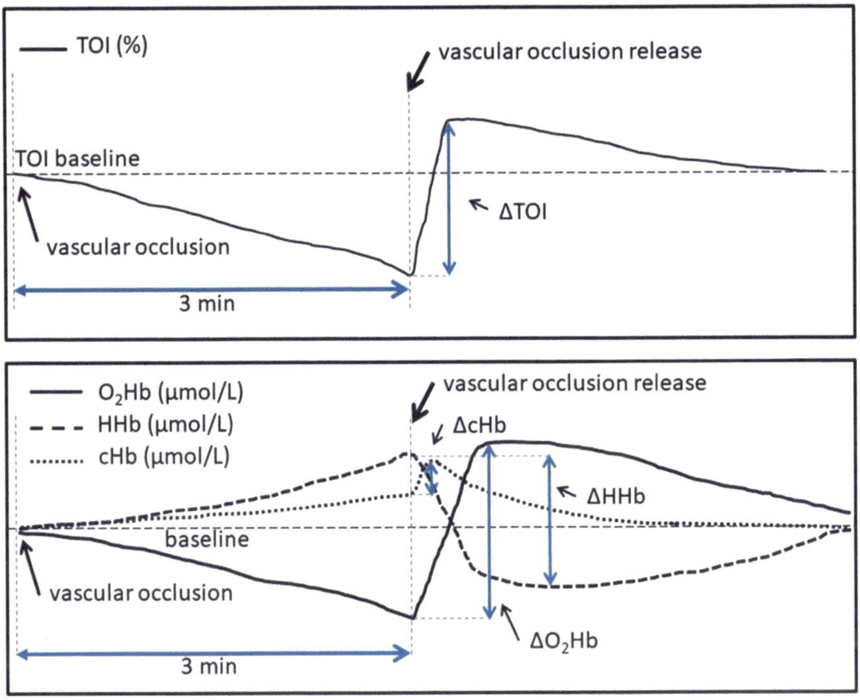

Fig. 1 Representative dynamic curve of near infrared spectroscopy parameters. cHb, total hemoglobin; HHb, deoxyhemoglobin; O_2Hb, oxyhemoglobin; TOI, tissue oxygen index; VOT, vascular occlusion test

occlusion were used to determine concentration changes for total hemoglobin (ΔcHb), oxyhemoglobin (ΔO_2Hb), deoxyhemoglobin (ΔHHb) and tissue oxygenation index (ΔTOI). The recovery curves of after the vascular occlusion was not linear and it is considered that the measurement of the gradient of the changes have variations, thus, we used the changes of NIRS parameters. These values were expressed semi-automatically using NIRO-200NX Display Software (U10898 Version 1.20, Hamamatsu Photonics K.K., Japan) (Fig. 1).

2.3 *Statistical Analysis*

Normality of the distribution of data was assessed using the Kolmogorov-Smirnov test. Numeric variables are expressed as mean ± standard deviation (SD) for normal distributions or median [interquartile range] for non-normal distributions. Categorical variables were compared using a Chi-squared test, and continuous variables were analyzed with Student's t-test or the Mann-Whitney U test. Correlations were assessed using Pearson's or Spearman's coefficient, as appropriate. A two-sided p-value of <0.05 was considered statistically significant. All statistical analyses were performed using EZR (Saitama Medical Center, Jichi Medical University, Saitama, Japan), which is a graphical user interface for R (The R Foundation for Statistical Computing, Vienna, Austria) [5].

3 Results

Of the 83 consecutive patients enrolled (52 males, median age 69.0 years, median BMI 23.9 kg/m^2), 39 were prescribed statins. Patient characteristics are presented in Table 1. The maximum and minimum values after the vascular occlusion were obtained within at least 1 min in all patients. All parameters derived from NIRS with VOT showed no significant difference between patients with and without statin therapy (Table 2). ΔTOI, ΔcHb and ΔHHb were not correlated with BMI

Table 1 Characteristics of the patient groups

	Total	Without statin	With statin	
	(n = 83)	(n = 44)	(n = 39)	p-value
Age (years)	69.0 [58.5, 77.5]	68.0 [52.8, 77.5]	71.0 [63.5, 77.5]	0.36
Male (%)	52 (62.7)	27 (61.4)	25 (64.1)	0.82
Height (cm)	160.7 ± 9.5	159.8 ± 10.0	161.7 ± 8.9	0.35
Body weight (kg)	63.0 [53.0, 71.0]	63.0 [51.0, 69.3]	66.0 [55.0, 72.5]	0.16
BMI (kg/m^2)	23.9 [22.0, 25.9]	23.6 [21.9, 25.7]	24.3 [22.1, 26.8]	0.37
Systolic BP (mmHg)	139.1 ± 17.3	139.3 ± 18.3	138.8 ± 16.3	0.90
Diastolic BP (mmHg)	74.3 ± 11.6	75.6 ± 11.0	72.8 ± 12.2	0.27
Heart rate (bpm)	69.3 ± 12.5	70.7 ± 11.8	67.7 ± 13.3	0.29
HTN (%)	55 (66.3)	25 (56.8)	30 (76.9)	0.06
DM (%)	26 (31.3)	9 (20.9)	17 (42.5)	0.06
DLP (%)	53 (63.9)	14 (31.8)	39 (100)	<0.001

BMI, body mass index; BP, blood pressure; DM, diabetes mellitus; DLP, dyslipidemia; HTN, hypertension

Table 2 Results of all parameters derived from near infrared spectroscopy with vascular occlusion test

	Total	Without statin	With statin	
	(n = 83)	(n = 44)	(n = 39)	p-value
baseTOI (%)	63.55 (7.54)	64.6 ± 7.1	62.4 ± 7.9	0.18
minTOI (%)	35.24 (13.18)	36.4 ± 12.6	33.9 ± 13.8	0.39
maxTOI (%)	79.30 [75.90, 82.60]	79.1 [75.7, 81.73]	79.4 [76.4, 82.8]	0.75
Δ TOI (%)	43.66 (12.84)	42.6 ± 12.8	44.8 ± 13.0	0.44
Δ cHb (μmol/L)	12.88 [9.71, 17.21]	13.0 [9.8, 17.2]	12.7 [9.8, 16.9]	0.93
Δ O_2Hb (μmol/L)	32.83 (8.20)	33.1 ± 8.72	32.5 ± 7.7	0.74
Δ HHb (μmol/L)	36.15 (6.55)	35.5 ± 7.3	36.9 ± 5.6	0.34

cHb, total hemoglobin; HHb, deoxyhemoglobin; O_2Hb, oxyhemoglobin; TOI, tissue oxygen index

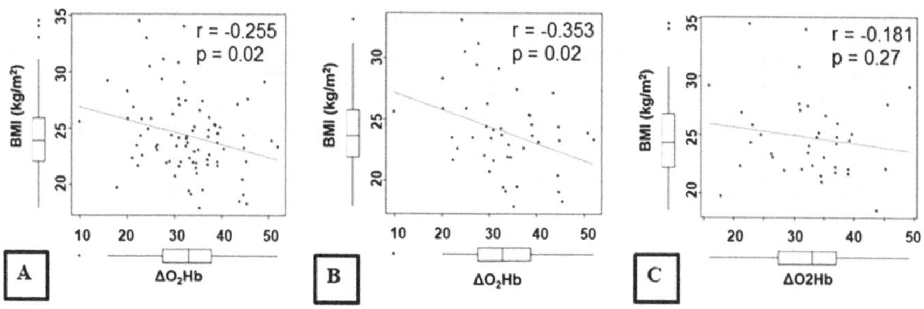

Fig. 2 Relationship between body mass index and changes of oxyhemoglobin in all patients (**A**), in patients without statin therapy (**B**), and in the patients with statin therapy (**C**). BMI, body mass index; O_2Hb, oxyhemoglobin

($r = -0.174$, $p = 0.12$; $r = -0.122$, $p = 0.27$; $r = 0.052$, $p = 0.64$, respectively). An inverse correlation was found between ΔO_2Hb and BMI ($r = -0.255$, $p = 0.02$) (Fig. 2A), and a stronger correlation was observed in patients without statin therapy ($r = -0.353$, $p = 0.02$) (Fig. 2B). Conversely, these correlations were absent in patients with statin therapy ($r = -0.181$, $p = 0.27$, Fig. 2C).

4 Discussion

The major findings from this study are that: 1) there was a significant inverse correlation between BMI and ΔO_2Hb, but not in the other parameters; 2) this correlation was stronger in patients *without* statin therapy.

NIRS can represent real-time tissue hemoglobin oxygen saturation using near infrared radiation, noninvasively and continuously. In the present study, we used a NIRO-200NX (which utilizes three lengths of near infrared light) and derived TOI, ΔcHb, ΔO_2Hb and ΔHHb. TOI was determined using spatially resolved methodology, and the other parameters were measured using the modified Beer-Lambert law. It is reported that the NIRS technique can evaluate peripheral microcirculation using the changes or area under the curve of StO_2, which is determined from the ratio $(O_2Hb) / (O_2Hb + HHb) \times 100\%$ [2, 3, 6].

In the present study, a negative correlation was only observed between BMI and ΔO_2Hb. ΔO_2Hb is the changes of oxyhemoglobin concentration during VOT, which becomes high value due to reactive hyperemia if the microcirculation is well maintained, thus, low ΔO_2Hb implies an impaired microcirculation. In addition, the negative correlation was particularly noticeable in the group without statin and, conversely, the correlation was absent in the group prescribed statin; this result may suggest that statin has an effect on the microcirculation. Our results suggest that ΔO_2Hb derived from NIRS with VOT may be useful to assess the microcirculation more effectively than other parameters. To the best of our knowledge, this is the first study to investigate the possibility to represent microcirculation using ΔO_2Hb.

Distinguishing between hemoglobin and myoglobin oxygenation is difficult using NIRS. Therefore, we placed the NIRS probe on the right thenar eminence, which has fewer muscles compared to other skeletal muscles, such as calf muscle. Additionally, the thenar has little fat and is steady enough to endure probe attachment; thus, there was little interference.

Brachial flow-mediated vasodilation (FMD) and reactive hyperemia-peripheral arterial tonometry (RH-PAT), which are widely used to examine endothelial function, are based on 5 min brachial artery occlusion to result in reactive hyperemia. However, because 5 min occlusion can lead to transient numbness, pain and redness, we set the occlusion time to 3 min and were able to observe correlations. This result might suggest that a 3 min VOT is sufficient to result in reactive hyperemia and assess microcirculation, especially for NIRS examination. Regarding monitoring period after the vascular occlusion, we fixed to 3 min. As a result, the maximum and minimum values could be obtained within at least 1 min after the vascular occlusion, thus, 3 min monitoring was enough to take those values. Furthermore, this simple protocol may contribute to the reduction of the total examination time to 8 min. In a previous study which performed StO_2-targeted VOT at 40%, the total time involved was reported to be approximately 60 min [7].

The present study has several limitations. First, we only used the right arm for assessment and did not examine the existence of peripheral artery disease. Second, the NIRS parameters were affected by the adipose tissue thickness under the site of the probe attached, however, we had not been investigated that in this study. Third, we did not collect data on vasoactive drugs and did not measure the duration of statin therapy. Fourth, the present study was conducted in a single center, which may limit the generalization of our findings to other institutions or the general population. Finally, The NIRS equipment (NIRO-200NX) was a continuous wave NIRS which does not allow measurements of optical pathlength. Therefore, the Hb concentration changes was semiquantitative data. A time-resolved NIRS is necessary to resolve this limitation [8].

The changes of O_2Hb derived from NIRS with VOT may better assess peripheral microcirculation than other NIRS parameters.

References

1. Karaca U, Schram MT, Houben AJ et al (2014) Microvascular dysfunction as a link between obesity, insulin resistance and hypertension. Diabetes Res Clin Pract 103:382–387
2. Soga T, Sakatani K, Yagi T et al (2014) The relationship between hyperlactatemia and microcirculation in the thenar eminence as measured using near-infrared spectroscopy in patients with sepsis. Emerg Med J 31:654–658
3. Butler E, Chin M, Aneman A (2017) Peripheral near-infrared spectroscopy: methodologic aspects and a systematic review in post-cardiac surgical patients. J Cardiothorac Vasc Anesth 31:1407–1416
4. Almuti K, Rimawi R, Spevack D et al (2006) Effects of statins beyond lipid lowering: potential for clinical benefits. Int J Cardiol 109:7–15

5. Kanda Y (2013) Investigation of the freely available easy-to-use software 'EZR' for medical statistics. Bone Marrow Transplant 48:452–458
6. Butler E, Nguyen J, Mahendran S et al (2018) Fluid responsiveness after CArdiac surgery (FRACAS): a prospective observational study using peripheral near-infrared spectroscopy. J Cardiothorac Vasc Anesth 32:197–204
7. Zamparini G, Butin G, Fischer MO et al (2015) Noninvasive assessment of peripheral microcirculation by near-infrared spectroscopy: a comparative study in healthy smoking and nonsmoking volunteers. J Clin Monit Comput 29:555–559
8. Lange F, Dunne L, Tachtsidis I (2017) Evaluation of Haemoglobin and cytochrome responses during forearm Ischaemia using multi-wavelength time domain NIRS. Adv Exp Med Biol 977:67–72

Broadband NIRS Cerebral Evaluation of the Hemodynamic and Oxidative State of Cytochrome-c-Oxidase Responses to +Gz Acceleration in Healthy Volunteers

F. Lange, G. Bale, P. Kaynezhad, R. D. Pollock, A. Stevenson, and I. Tachtsidis

Abstract We used a miniature broadband NIRS system to monitor concentration changes in brain oxygenation (oxy- and deoxy- haemoglobin [HbO_2], [HHb]) and oxidised cytochrome-c-oxidase ([oxCCO]) during a high +Gz acceleration, induced by a human centrifuge, on two healthy experienced volunteers (2 male, 34 and 37 years). We performed a sequence of several +Gz exposures that were terminated at the onset of visual symptoms (loss of peripheral vision). Systemic parameters were recorded (i.e. heart rate, blood pressure and arterial saturation), and brain tissue blood volume changes ([HbT] = [HbO_2] + [HHb]) and oxygen delivery ([HbDiff] = [HbO_2] - [HHb]) were calculated. Volunteer 1 demonstrated a decrease in [HbT] of -3.49 ± 0.02 μMol and [HbDiff] of -3.23 ± 0.44 μMol, and an increase of [oxCCO] of 0.42 ± 0.01μMol. Volunteer 2 demonstrated a decrease in [HbDiff] of -4.37 ± 0.23 μMol, and no significant change in [HbT] (0.53 ± 0.06 μMol) and [oxCCO] (0.09 ± 0.06 μMol). The variability of the brain metabolic response was related to the level of ischaemia, suggesting that suppression of metabolism was due to lack of glucose substrate delivery rather than oxygen availability.

Keywords NIRS · Broadband · Cytochrome-c-oxidase · Ischaemia · Human centrifuge

F. Lange (✉) · G. Bale · P. Kaynezhad · I. Tachtsidis
Department of Medical Physics and Biomedical Engineering, University College London, London, UK
e-mail: f.lange@ucl.ac.uk

R. D. Pollock
The Human Performance Group, QinetiQ PLC, Farnborough, UK

The Centre for Human and Applied Physiological Sciences, King's College London, London, UK

A. Stevenson
The Human Performance Group, QinetiQ PLC, Farnborough, UK

© The Author(s) 2020

P.-D. Ryu et al. (eds.), *Oxygen Transport to Tissue XLI*, Advances in Experimental Medicine and Biology 1232, https://doi.org/10.1007/978-3-030-34461-0_43

1 Introduction

Near-infrared spectroscopy (NIRS) is now a common tool for monitoring non-invasively the tissue in-vivo changes in oxy- and deoxy haemoglobin ([HbO_2] [HHb]) [1], and has been extensively used to monitor the function and physiology of the brain [2, 3].

Most NIRS systems use simple instrumentation and only measure the change in attenuation of 2 or 3 wavelengths, which is enough to calculate the changes in [HbO_2] and [HHb]. Recent developments in NIRS instrumentation enables measurement of the change in attenuation of more than a hundred wavelengths [4, 5]. This technique is called broadband NIRS and can be used to retrieve information of a third chromophore, cytochrome-c-oxidase (CCO). CCO is the terminal electron acceptor of the electron transport chain in the mitochondria. Broadband NIRS monitors the changes in the redox state of CCO using the difference between the oxidised and reduced CCO spectra ([oxCCO]), for further information on this topic see the review by Bale et al. [6]. CCO provides information about metabolism, and in particular mitochondrial oxygenation. For example, it has been demonstrated that broadband NIRS has the potential to provide a real-time assessment of brain metabolism during neonatal hypoxic-ischaemic encephalopathy (HIE), and that oxCCO could be a clinically relevant metabolic marker [7].

In recent years, NIRS has also been used to monitor cerebral cortical oxygenation during +Gz exposure [8]. The goal of the present study is to assess the feasibility of monitoring haemodynamic and CCO responses during +Gz exposure using a broadband NIRS system. This possibility could improve the understanding of +Gz-induced loss of consciousness (G-LOC) and also provide a framework to investigate the mechanisms of cerebral hypoxic-ischaemia (HI) in healthy volunteers.

2 Methods

Two healthy non-pilot male volunteers, one aged 34 years (height 1.79 m and mass 75 kg) and one aged 37 years (height 1.82 m and mass 95 kg), participated in this preliminary study. The study was conducted under an ethical approved centrifuge procedure (Approval number TI1501625).

Acceleration profiles were generated using a 9.4-m-radius human centrifuge (QinetiQ, Farnborough, UK).

Volunteer 1 performed 2 centrifuge exposures consisting of a gradual increase ($0.1G.s^{-1}$) in +Gz until the subject terminated the centrifuge run when peripheral light loss occurred. Each run was separated by 5 min of rest. Volunteer 2 performed 3 centrifuge exposures of these events.

Broadband NIRS measurements were made using an in-house developed miniature broadband system called miniCYRIL (CYtochrome Research Instrument and appLication) [9]. The system consists of a miniature Ocean Optics HL2000 white light source using a 20 W halogen-tungsten lamp and a customised Ocean Optics Ventana VIS-NIR miniature spectrometer. The miniCYRIL is a single channel system and the optodes were positioned over the left forehead with a source-detector separation of 3 cm, and secured with a headband and a custom 3D printed probe holder. It is worth mentioning that the probe holder was positioned with sufficient pressure to cause local blanching. Hence, we don't expect any response from the skin vasculature [13]. Light intensity spectra from 600-1100 nm were collected at 1 Hz. The changes in concentration in [HbO_2], [HHb] and [oxCCO] were calculated from the changes in attenuation from 780 to 900 nm using the UCLn algorithm [10]. Then, the change in concentration in total haemoglobin ([HbT]), which gives an indication of the blood volume changes, was calculated as [HbT] = [HbO_2] + [HHb]. Finally, the change in the oxygen delivery ([HbDiff]) was calculated as [HbDiff] = [HbO_2] - [HHb].

Systemic parameters were also recorded synchronously with the broadband NIRS data. Heart rate (HR) was recorded using a standard three-lead ECG from a proprietary system (locally manufactured) and beat-to-beat blood pressure (BP) from a Finapres device (Ohmeda). As we are interested in the brain's mean BP (BMBP), we computed an estimation of the BMBP based on the measurement at the heart level mean BP (HLMBP) as expressed in reference [11] (i.e. BMBP = HLMBP – 19 mmHg$*$Gz). Arterial saturation (SaO_2) was also recorded using a Masimo Rad-7 pulse oximeter with an ear probe (ear lobe). We observed a failure in the SaO_2 measurement on volunteer 2, therefore this parameter was excluded from the analysis. Data are presented as mean and standard deviation (std).

3 Results

Figures 1 and 2 present the response of the NIRS and systemic data for each event for volunteers 1 and 2, respectively.

Figure 1 shows that volunteer 1 had an increased in HR of 45.6 ± 5.7 bpm and a drop in BMBP of −65.1 ± 8.5 mmHg. Regarding the NIRS measurement, volunteer 1 had an increase in [oxCCO] of 0.42 ± 0.01 μM, a decrease in [HbO_2] of −3.36 ± 0.23 μM, [HbT] of −3.49 ± 0.02 μM and [HbDiff] of −3.23 ± 0.44 μM, and no meaningful change in [HHb] (−0.13 ± 0.21 μM). It is worth noting that volunteer 1 reported to be near G-LOC at the run termination time. Fig. 2 shows that volunteer 2 had an increased in HR of 40.7 ± 11.4 bpm and a drop in BMBP of −63.7 ± 6.4 mmHg. Regarding the NIRS measurement, volunteer 2 had no meaningful changes compared to volunteer 1 for [oxCCO] (0.09 ± 0.06 μM), an increase in [HHb] of 2.45 ± 0.14 μM, a decrease in [HbO_2] of −1.92 ± 0.09 μM, and [HbDiff] of −4.37 ± 0.23 μM, and no significant change in [HbT] (0.53 ± 0.06 μM)

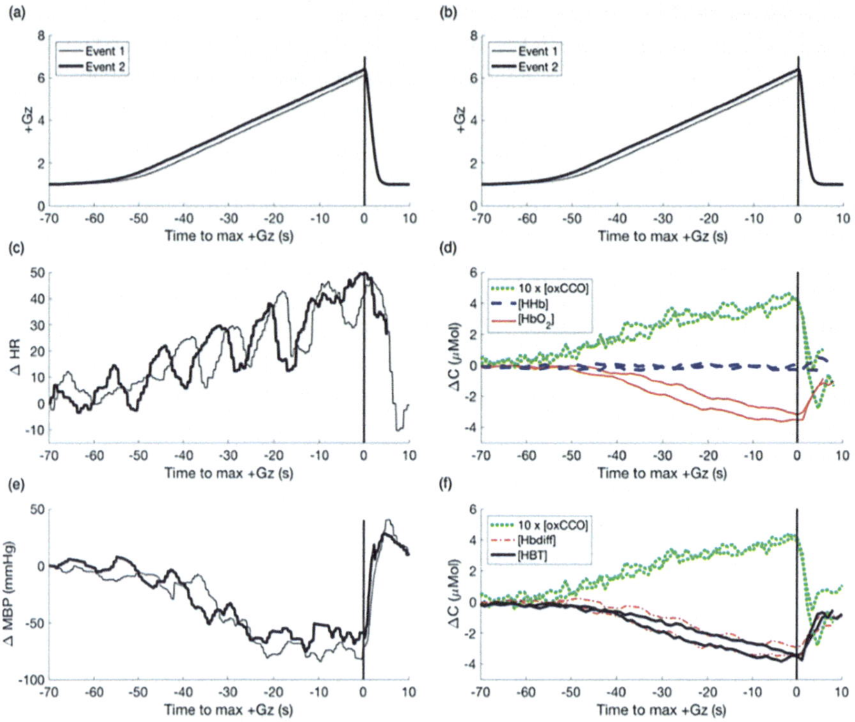

Fig. 1 NIRS and systemic responses to the +Gz events for volunteer 1. (**a**) and (**b**) present the +Gz events dynamic events and are repeated to help the visualisation of the systemic data (left panel) and NIRS data (right panel). (**c**) presents the changes in heart rate (HR). (**d**) presents the changes in [HbO_2] (solid red line) [HHb] (dashed blue lines), and [oxCCO] (scaled by a factor 10) (dotted green lines). (**e**) presents the changes of mean blood pressure (MBP) at head level. (**f**) presents the changes in [HbT] (solid black lines) and [HbDiff] together with the changes in [oxCCO] (scaled by a factor of 10) (dotted green lines). On all panels, the vertical black line presents the time of maximum +Gz

4 Discussion

A broadband NIRS system was used to evaluate the brain metabolic, oxygenation and haemodynamic responses during +Gz exposure. During these +Gz exposures, both volunteers experienced loss of vision (ischaemia of the retina), but volunteer 1 had a significant drop in [HbT] compared to volunteer 2. Also, both volunteers had similar reduction in brain oxygenation (drop in [HbDiff]) but volunteer 1 had a significant increase in [oxCCO] compared to volunteer 2.

Although some work investigating [oxCCO] in +Gz exposure was performed in the late 1980s [12–14], most NIRS studies focused only on the changes in brain oxygenation and haemodynamics to understand the mechanism of G-LOC. This is mainly due to the fact that the instrumentation required to be able to monitor this third chromophore is more complex and the interpretation of the [oxCCO] data can be difficult. However, the infor-

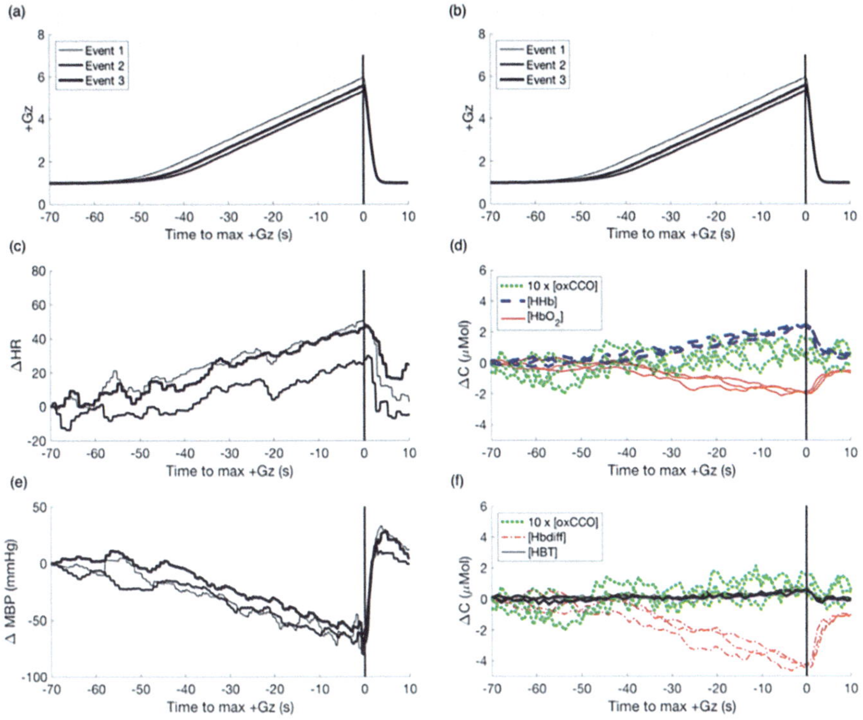

Fig. 2 NIRS and systemic responses to the +Gz events for volunteer 2. (**a**) and (**b**) present the +Gz events dynamic events and are repeated to help the visualisation of the systemic data (left panel) and NIRS data (right panel). (**c**) presents the changes in heart rate (HR). (**d**) presents the changes in $[HbO_2]$ (solid red line) [HHb] (dashed blue lines), and [oxCCO] (scaled by a factor 10) (dotted green lines). (**e**) presents the changes of mean blood pressure (MBP) at head level. (**f**) presents the changes in [HbT] (solid black lines) and [HbDiff] together with the changes in [oxCCO] (scaled by a factor of 10) (dotted green lines). On all panels, the vertical black line presents the time of maximum +Gz

mation provided from the current system can further elucidate the mechanism responsible for G-LOC. Thus, the development of a miniaturised system, such as used in the present study, provides new possibilities for the investigation of the interplay between brain oxygenation and metabolism in the high Gz environment.

The majority of the NIRS [oxCCO] contrast comes from the Copper A (CuA) centre in CCO. As CuA is a one-electron acceptor, changes in its redox state can be achieved by changing the rates of electron transfer to it or away from it. In HI, absence of oxygen prevents electron transfer from CuA, causing a reduction; additionally, a decrease of electrons to the chain will cause oxidation. Thus, changes in [oxCCO] reflect changes in (1) the supply of reducing equivalents to the respiratory chain; (2) the adenosine diphosphate (ADP) concentration, and (3) the cellular oxygen concentration [15].

It has been shown that HI produces a significant reduction in [oxCCO] in animal models [16, 17], due to oxygen depletion. However, it has also been shown in anaesthetised animals that only significant levels of hypoxia cause a reduction in oxCCO

[18]. Drury et al. showed that in asphyxia in foetal sheep (umbilical cord occlusion), an increase in [oxCCO] was observed that was dependent on gestational age, with the more mature foetuses demonstrating a later reduction in [oxCCO] [19].

In the present study, the increase in [oxCCO] observed in volunteer 1 is thus likely to reflect reduction in (1) the supply of reducing equivalents to the respiratory chain; and (2) the ADP concentration. This suggests that G-LOC may, in part, be driven by a lack of sufficient delivery of glucose substrate to the mitochondrial respiratory chain, rather than an absence of oxygen. It is worth mentioning that this hypothesis holds for an ischemic non-hypoxic volunteer and that further studies will be needed to investigate the effect of hypoxic-ischemic events.

In conclusion, we have demonstrated the feasibility of using a miniaturised broadband NIRS system in a centrifuge, which unlocks new possibilities for studying G-LOC and the effects of HI in healthy non-anaesthetised volunteers. In our two case studies, we found differences in the metabolic response related to the level of brain tissue ischaemia, which suggests that the delivery of glucose substrate affects metabolism more than it does oxygen. These preliminary findings also suggest that a human centrifuge could be used as a model to study HI in healthy volunteers in order to better understand the underlying physiology of the condition.

Acknowledgments The authors thank The Wellcome Trust (104580/Z/14/Z) for financial support of this work.

References

1. Ferrari M, Quaresima V (2012) A brief review on the history of human functional near-infrared spectroscopy (fNIRS) development and fields of application. NeuroImage 63:921–935
2. Wolf M, Ferrari M, Quaresima V (2007) Progress of near-infrared spectroscopy and topography for brain and muscle clinical applications. J Biomed Opt 12:62104
3. Scholkmann F, Kleiser S, Metz AJ et al (2014) A review on continuous wave functional near-infrared spectroscopy and imaging instrumentation and methodology. NeuroImage 85:6–27
4. Bale G, Mitra S, Meek J et al (2014) A new broadband near-infrared spectroscopy system for in-vivo measurements of cerebral cytochrome-c-oxidase changes in neonatal brain injury. Biomed Opt Express 5:3450–3466
5. Phan P, Highton D, Lai J et al (2016) Multi-channel multi-distance broadband near-infrared spectroscopy system to measure the spatial response of cellular oxygen metabolism and tissue oxygenation. Biomed Opt Express 7:4424–4440
6. Bale G, Elwell CE, Tachtsidis I (2016) From Jöbsis to the present day: a review of clinical near-infrared spectroscopy measurements of cerebral cytochrome-c-oxidase. J Biomed Opt 21:091307
7. Bale G, Mitra S, de Roever I, et al (2018) Oxygen dependency of mitochondrial metabolism indicates outcome of newborn brain injury. J Cereb Blood Flow Metab https://doi.org/10.1177/0271678X18777928
8. Glaister DH (1988) Current and emerging technology in G-LOC detection: noninvasive monitoring of cerebral microcirculation using near infrared. Aviat Sp Env Med 59:23–28
9. Siddiqui MF, Lloyd-Fox S, Kaynezhad P et al (2017) Non-invasive measurement of a metabolic marker of infant brain function. Sci Rep 7:1–6

10. Matcher SJ, Elwell CE, Cooper CE et al (1995) Performance comparison of several published tissue near-infrared spectroscopy algorithms. Anal Biochem 227:54–68
11. Ossard G, Clere JM, Kerguelen M et al (1994) Response of human cerebral blood flow to +Gz accelerations. J Appl Physiol 76:2114–2118
12. Glaister D (1988) Current and emerging technology in G-LOC detection: Noninvasive monitoring of cerebral microcirculation using near infrared. Aviat. Sp. Environ. Med. 59, 23–28.
13. Glaister DH, Jobsis-Vander Vliet FF (1988) A near-infrared spectrophotometric method for studying brain O2 sufficiency in man during +G(z) acceleration. Aviat Sp Environ Med
14. Glaister D, Miller N (1990) Cerebral tissue oxygen status and psychomotor performance during lower body negative pressure (LBNP). Aviat. Sp. Environ. Med. 61, 99–105.
15. Cooper CE, Wyatt JS, Cope M et al (1994) Near-infrared spectroscopy of the brain: relevance to cytochrome oxidase bioenergetics. Biochem. Soc. Trans 22:974–980
16. Rajaram A, Bale G, Kewin M et al Simultaneous monitoring of cerebral perfusion and cytochrome c oxidase by combining broadband near-infrared spectroscopy and diffuse correlation spectroscopy. Biomed. Opt. Express 9:2588–2603
17. Bainbridge A, Tachtsidis I, Faulkner SD et al (2014) Brain mitochondrial oxidative metabolism during and after cerebral hypoxia–ischemia studied by simultaneous phosphorus magnetic-resonance and broadband near-infrared spectroscopy. NeuroImage 102:173–183
18. Tsuji M, Naruse H, Volpe J, Holtzman D (1995) Reduction of cytochrome aa3 measured by near-infrared spectroscopy predicts cerebral energy loss in hypoxic piglets. Pediatr Res 37:253–259
19. Drury PP, Bennet L, Booth LC et al (2012) Maturation of the mitochondrial redox response to profound asphyxia in fetal sheep. PLoS One 7:1–8

Open Access This chapter is licensed under the terms of the Creative Commons Attribution 4.0 International License (http://creativecommons.org/licenses/by/4.0/), which permits use, sharing, adaptation, distribution and reproduction in any medium or format, as long as you give appropriate credit to the original author(s) and the source, provide a link to the Creative Commons license and indicate if changes were made.

The images or other third party material in this chapter are included in the chapter's Creative Commons license, unless indicated otherwise in a credit line to the material. If material is not included in the chapter's Creative Commons license and your intended use is not permitted by statutory regulation or exceeds the permitted use, you will need to obtain permission directly from the copyright holder.

Time-Resolved NIROT 'Pioneer' System for Imaging Oxygenation of the Preterm Brain: Preliminary Results

A. Di Costanzo-Mata, J. Jiang, S. Lindner, L. Ahnen, C. Zhang, S. Sánchez-Majos, M. Wolf, E. Charbon, and A. Kalyanov

Abstract In preterm infants, there is a risk of long-term cognitive, motor and behavioral impairments due to hemorrhagic and/or ischemic lesions. If detected early, lesions can be prevented. A bedside imaging modality, capable of early detection of both disorders, is necessary. We present the state of development of a tomographic imager (named Pioneer), that will be capable of determining the oxygenation of the preterm-infant brain with high spatial resolution. Pioneer is a time-resolved near-infrared optical tomography (TR NIROT) instrument. It employs multiple wavelength laser light in short pulses on 11 distinct locations and measures the re-emerging light in a contactless fashion by means of a time-correlated single-photon counting (TCSPC) camera (named Piccolo) covering ~4.9 cm^2 with 300 detectors. Timing response of the entire system is 116 ps. An in-house designed biocompatible source ring ensures fixed relative positions of sources and detectors and provides a secure interface between the patient and the probe. At the present state, the NIROT Pioneer system successfully detected a 6x6x50 mm^3 inclusion 3 cm deep inside a phantom. These results confirm that the Pioneer imager is working as expected and is on a solid path towards full 3D tissue oxygenation imaging.

A. Di Costanzo-Mata (✉) · J. Jiang · S. Lindner · S. Sánchez-Majos · A. Kalyanov
Biomedical Optics Research Laboratory (BORL), Department of Neonatology, University of Zurich, Zürich, Switzerland
e-mail: aldo.dicostanzomata@usz.ch

L. Ahnen · C. Zhang · E. Charbon
Advanced Quantum Architecture Laboratory (AQUA), School of Engineering, EPFL, Écublens, Switzerland

M. Wolf
Applied Quantum Architectures (AQUA), Delft University of Technology, Delft, The Netherlands

© Springer Nature Switzerland AG 2020

P.-D. Ryu et al. (eds.), *Oxygen Transport to Tissue XLI*, Advances in Experimental Medicine and Biology 1232, https://doi.org/10.1007/978-3-030-34461-0_44

1 Introduction

Despite the improved survival rate of extremely preterm infants within the last decades, long-term cognitive, motor and behavioral impairment remains a significant burden for preterm neonates and leads to substantial healthcare costs [1]. MRI is the best neuroimaging tool for detecting brain structural lesions, i.e. white matter injury (WMI) that causes neurodevelopmental impairments [2]. Nonetheless, MRI is unable to detect either hypoxia or ischemia, which causes the injury. Given that transporting of preterm infants is highly risky, the current diagnosis is based on bedside instrumentation only, such as ultrasound imaging. Ultrasound detects hemorrhagic brain lesions immediately, but ischemic brain lesions, which also lead to severe impairments, can only be detected after days and weeks, once the necrotic tissue has disintegrated. This causes considerable delay to therapeutic measures.

Near-infrared spectroscopy (NIRS) can be used to detect a lack of oxygen in a tissue, but it is not spatially specific. However, near-infrared optical tomography (NIROT) has the capability of detecting the oxygenation in high-spatial resolution (imaging) [3].

Image reconstruction in NIROT requires a solution of both a forward and an inverse problem. The diffusion equation is routinely used as the forward model to simulate the light propagation through tissue. The inverse problem corresponds to an iterative process to reconstruct the optical properties of the tissue. NIROT consists of a set of sources and detectors in different patterns, usually in transmission or reflection, depending on the anatomical shape under study. A light source emits light into the tissue, while several detectors measure the light re-emerging from the tissue. Setups with multiple light sources repeat the emission-detection process to acquire greater amounts of data [4]. NIROT is classified in three modes of illumination and acquisition: Time-resolved (TR), frequency-domain (FD) and continuous-wave (CW) NIROT. In TR NIROT, the source emits short pulses of light and the arrival times of the photons are measured at the detector. A histogram of the photon counts vs the arrival times is created in which photons that traveled deeply can be easily identified by their long arrival times and distinguished from superficial photons that arrived quickly. This timing data provides the most extensive set of information, compared to frequency domain or continuous wave NIROT modalities. In addition, this allows the determination of optical properties of relatively deep tissue, from which the absolute values for [HHb] and [HbO_2] can be calculated. Such characteristics make TR NIROT a promising technique for brain hypoxia detection. Here we introduce the Pioneer imager, a TR NIROT device that is based on a TR camera and ultrashort pulse laser light [5]. By imaging the oxygenation of brain tissue with high spatial resolution in preterm infants, it is hoped that ischemia, hemorrhage and hypoxia can be detected before an irreversible lesion has occurred, thereby preventing disabilities. The aim is to present the actual development state of the Pioneer tomographic imager and the results of the first laboratory tests on inhomogeneous phantoms.

2 The Pioneer System

The Pioneer instrument integrates state-of-the-art components into a system intended to measure 3D tissue oxygenation (Fig. 1). A supercontinuum (SC) laser (SuperK Extreme-15, NKT, Denmark) generates pulsed light in a broadband wavelengths range. The SC light is coupled to an acousto-optical tunable filter (AOTF) (SuperK-CROSS, NKT, Denmark), which selects a specific laser wavelength of 4 nm bandwidth. The AOTF wavelength selection-range on this setup ranges from 650 nm to 900 nm. For the current experiment we selected only one wavelength: 692 nm. This enables in principle multispectral measurements and wavelength normalization [6]. A fiber-splitter with a tap-channel power meter (PM100USB, Thorlabs, US) monitors the light intensity. This enables us to include the output light power in the reconstruction process. An optical fiber switch (Laser Components, Germany), with one input and 24 output channels (CH1, CH2 ...CHN), switches the light emission between several source locations on a subject. The light is guided by graded-index optical fibers to the tissue.

The actual setup consists of 11 sources arranged in a circular pattern. The optical fibers are hosted inside a biocompatible source ring (Fig. 2), with each fiber tip embedded in a transparent silicone window (SILPURAN, Wacker, Germany). The source ring stays in contact with the patient's skin [7]. The light is emitted at the

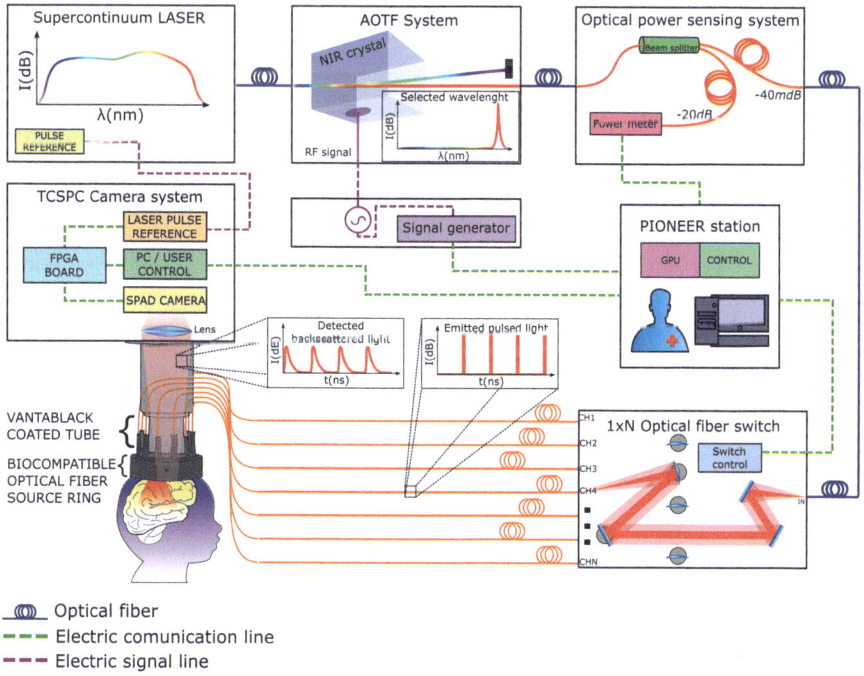

Fig. 1 Diagram of the pioneer system setup

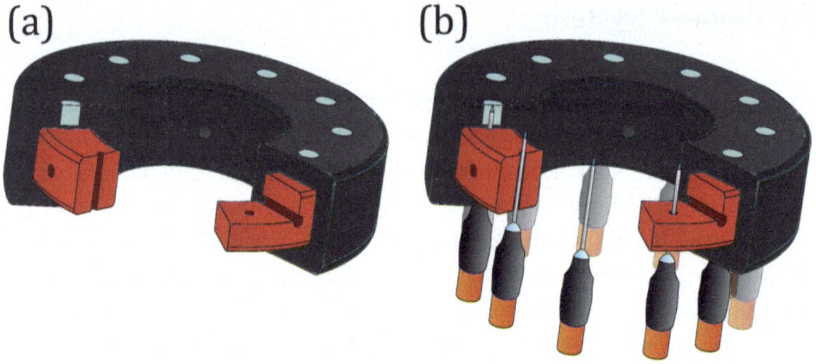

Fig. 2 Biocompatible source ring structural illustration (**a**) without fibers and (**b**) with fibers

optical windows with 1 ± 0.1 mW optical power. It penetrates the skin and interacts with the tissue.

The source ring has a circular field of view (FoV) of ~4.9 cm^2 in the middle, through which the backscattered reemerging light is detected in a contactless fashion. A time-correlated single-photon counting (TCSPC) camera chip (named Piccolo) was specifically designed for Pioneer [8]; it comprises an array of 32x32 single-photon avalanche diodes (SPADs) and with a timing jitter of 116 ps (FWHM). Currently, Pioneer employs 300 SPADs out of 1024 (due to the circular shape of the FoV) providing 3300 source-detector pairs. This high density of detectors provides a large amount of time-resolved data for image reconstruction. The space between Piccolo and the subject's skin is enclosed inside a tube, which shields the FoV from the ambient light. The lower section of the tube is inner-coated with a highly absorbing material (Vantablack, Surrey Nanosystems, UK) with an absorption rate of 99.965% [9]. This coating is needed to avoid internal reflections and enhance the SNR.

The acquisition sequence is controlled by an in-house C++ control software. Although we present only the preliminary test data here, we are currently working on embedded reconstruction algorithms. In the next stage of the project, all data will be processed by a reconstruction algorithm powered by a GPU, to produce the 3D reconstruction of the tissue oxygenation [10].

3 Testing and Results

We tested the effectiveness of Pioneer to detect a silicone inclusion with dimensions of 6x6x50 mm^3 at various depths and relative positions. Due to its length, which exceeds Pioneer's field-of-view (FoV), the inclusion was equivalent to an infinite square rod with 6x6 mm^2 section, which is commonly used to determine image resolution. To mimic hemorrhage, the inclusion had an absorption coefficient (μ_a) of 5.5 cm^{-1} and reduced scattering coefficient (μ_s') of 7.2 cm^{-1}. It was located inside a

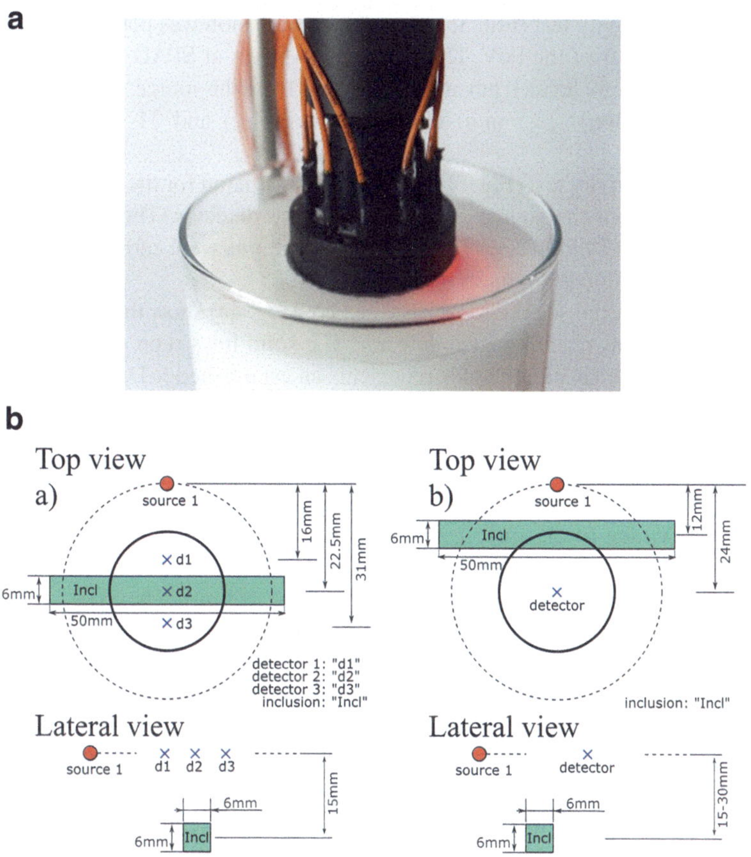

Fig. 3 Pioneer test setup on a liquid phantom (**a**) for axial selectivity and (**b**) for depth sensitivity

liquid phantom (water-Intralipid emulsion) with μ_a of 0.092 cm^{-1} and μ_s' of 5.5 cm^{-1}, such values are within the range of the head of a preterm infant [11]. The test consisted of comparing the signals acquired from the liquid phantom with no inclusion (homogeneous case, HC) against the liquid phantom with the inclusion (inhomogeneous case, IHC). The liquid phantom was in a glass container that had a cylindrical shape with 14 cm in diameter and 15 cm high. The sources were 4.7 cm away from the phantom's wall. The closest detector was 6.3 cm away. This long-distance warrants that the boundary has no influence on the measurements.

Pioneer was positioned over the liquid phantom (Fig. 3), and its location fixed using a mechanical arm (3arm, Spain). The source ring was manually immersed at a depth of ~1 mm in the liquid phantom to achieve a proper optical contact. The SC laser was set to 100% output power, the AOTF tuned at 692 nm with 100% throughput power, the fiber switch routed the light towards the channel 1 (CH1) of the biocompatible source ring.

For axial selectivity test (Fig. 3a), the silicone inclusion was placed at a depth of 15 mm in the center of the FoV. Three detectors (pixels at SPAD array) were used for the test. They were located at various distances from the source: 16 mm (between source and inclusion), 22.5 mm (above the inclusion) and 31 mm (behind the inclusion).

For depth sensitivity test (Fig. 3b), the silicone inclusion for the IHC was located ~12 mm away from the source (CH1) towards the detector. The source-detector distance (S-D) was 24 mm. The NIROT data acquisitions were carried out for inclusion depths of 15 mm, 20 mm, 25 mm and 30 mm.

The results for axial selectivity across the FoV (Fig. 4a) show the time histogram (TH) of the photons reaching each detector. The solid lines represent the IHC and the dashed lines the HC. Each color represents an established S-D pair. The 22 mm and 31 mm S-D show a considerable difference between the TH for HC vs IHC, an outcome of the inclusion being on the path of a larger number of photons. The 31 mm S-D shows a signal artifact, initially more photons for the IHC. This artifact is caused by reflected photons due to an irregular surface shape of the emulsion inside the FoV, due to the surface tension effect. For imaging inclusions, the late arriving photons are of higher interest. The 16 mm S-D shows a minor difference, since the inclusion is outside the effective detection volume. The axial selectivity, for a fixed depth inclusion, is enhanced by the high density of detectors provided by Pioneer. It is evident that detectors showing similar signals for the HC and ICH correspond to inclusion-free areas. Conversely, detectors showing increasing differences serve to resolve the inclusion location.

The results for depth sensitivity (Fig. 4b) show the ratio of I_{incl} (IHC TPSF) over I_{hom} (HC TPSF) vs time in ns. The colored lines show the attenuation (I_{incl}/I_{hom}) at different depths. For I_{incl}, when the inclusion is closer to the surface, the attenuation effect is greater due to the photons exposed to the higher absorption of the inclusion. A deeper inclusion has weaker attenuation due to more photons having the potential to backscatter in the Intralipid emulsion. Nevertheless, a 30 mm depth inclusion can be clearly observed.

4 Conclusion

It has been confirmed that the Pioneer imager system performs as expected. We have successfully integrated the optical components, the control software and the Piccolo camera together. The system has a high axial selectivity across the FoV due to the large array of detectors and has a penetration depth of at least 30 mm in reflection.

Having detected inclusions within a bulk, these axial selectivity and depth sensitivity results provide the first step towards detecting volumes inside the tissues that have different oxygenation levels than their surroundings, which is the case for hemorrhage, ischemia and hypoxia.

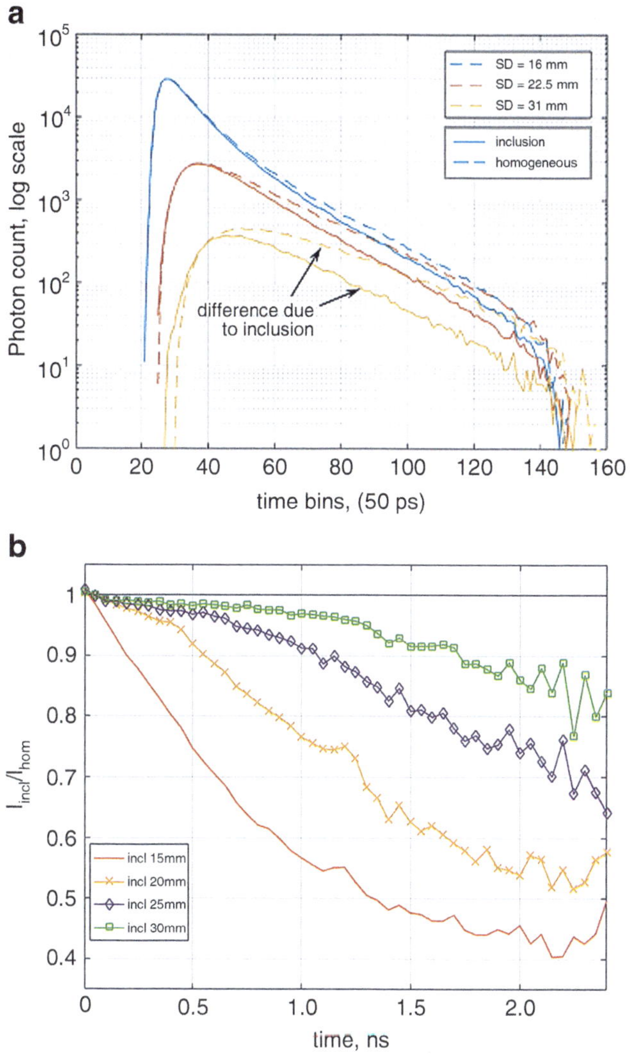

Fig. 4 (**a**) Results for the axial selectivity test across the field of view showing the time histogram of the photons arriving at the detectors. (**b**) Results for the depth sensitivity showing the ratio of the time histograms of the arriving photons for I_{incl} over I_{hom} (attenuation). The time scale is relative to the peak position of I_{incl} and I_{hom}

Acknowledgments This research was supported by Molecular Imaging Network Zurich MINZ and Tumor Oxygenation of the University of Zurich UZH, Swiss Cancer Research grant KFS-3732-08-2015, the Swiss National Science Foundation project 159490 and CONACyT by the CVU-627802.

References

1. Fanaroff AA et al (2007) Trends in neonatal morbidity and mortality for very low birthweight infants. American Journal of Obstetrics & Gynecology 196(2):147–1e1
2. Lee YA (2017) White matter injury of prematurity: its mechanisms and clinical features. Journal of pathology and translational medicine 51(5):449–455
3. Boas DA et al (2001) Imaging the body with diffuse optical tomography. IEEE Signal Process Mag 18(6):57–75
4. Wang LV et al (2012) Biomedical optics: principles and imaging. John Wiley & Sons
5. Pavia JM (2015) Near-infrared optical tomography with single-photon avalanche diode image sensors. Dissertation, EPFL
6. Kalyanov A et al (2018) Multispectral near-infrared optical tomography for Cancer hypoxia study in mice. In: Thews O, LaManna J, Harrison D (eds) Oxygen transport to tissue XL. Advances in experimental medicine and biology, vol 1072. Springer, Cham
7. Ahnen L et al (2017) Development and validation of a sensor prototype for near-infrared imaging of the newborn brain. In: Halpern H, LaManna J, Harrison D, Epel B (eds) Oxygen transport to tissue XXXIX. Advances in experimental medicine and biology, vol 977. Springer, Cham
8. Lindner S et al (2018). A Novel 32 x 32, 224 Mevents/s time resolved SPAD image sensor for near-infrared optical tomography. In Optics and the Brain (pp. JTh5A-6). Optical Society of America
9. Ball P (2016) Material witness: none more black. Nat Mater 15(5):500
10. Jiang J et al (2017) A new method based on graphics processing units for fast near-infrared optical tomography. In: Halpern H, LaManna J, Harrison D, Epel B (eds) Oxygen transport to tissue XXXIX. advances in experimental medicine and biology, vol 977. Springer, Cham
11. Arri SJ et al (2011) Precision of cerebral oxygenation and hemoglobin concentration measurements in neonates measured by near-infrared spectroscopy. J Biomed Opt 16(4):047005

Application of Peripheral Near Infrared Spectroscopy to Assess Risk Factors in Patient with Coronary Artery Disease: Part 2

Keiichiro Kuronuma, Tsuyoshi Kawamorita, Tsukasa Yagi, Eizo Tachibana, Shonosuke Sugai, Satoshi Hayashida, Kazuki Iso, Korehito Iida, Wataru Atsumi, Satoshi Kunimoto, Yasuyuki Suzuki, Shigemasa Tani, Naoya Matsumoto, Yasuo Okumura, and Kaoru Sakatani

Abstract Epicardial adipose tissue (EAT) is associated with visceral fat and various cardiac disorders, such as atrial fibrillation and adverse cardiovascular events. Therefore, it is important to develop a simple and non-invasive inspection method to assess EAT, to prevent unfavorable cardiac events. This study assessed correlations between near-infrared spectroscopy (NIRS) changes induced by a vascular occlusion test (VOT) and EAT volume measured by cardiac computed tomography (CCT) in patients with suspected coronary artery disease. We also assessed correlations between body mass index (BMI) and EAT volume in the same population. In addition, these correlations were compared in patients treated with statin therapy and in those without statin therapy. A NIRS probe was set on the right thenar eminence, and brachial artery blood flow was blocked for 3 min before being released. A negative correlation was found between oxyhemoglobin (ΔO_2Hb) and EAT volume in the overall study population ($r = -0.236$, $p = 0.03$). Interestingly, although a strong correlation was observed in patients *without* statin therapy ($r = -0.488$, $p < 0.001$), this correlation was not observed in patients *with* statin therapy ($r = 0.157$, $p = 0.34$). These findings suggest that NIRS measurements with VOT may be a useful method to identify patients with high EAT volume and high cardiovascular risks.

K. Kuronuma (✉) · T. Kawamorita · E. Tachibana · S. Sugai · S. Hayashida · K. Iso · K. Iida
W. Atsumi · S. Kunimoto
Department of Cardiology, Kawaguchi Municipal Medical Center, Kawaguchi, Japan

T. Yagi · Y. Suzuki · S. Tani · N. Matsumoto
Department of Cardiology, Nihon University Hospital, Tokyo, Japan

Y. Okumura
Division of Cardiology, Department of Medicine, Nihon University Itabashi Hospital, Tokyo, Japan

K. Sakatani
NEWCAT Research Institute, Department of Electrical and Electronic Engineering, Nihon University College of Engineering, Koriyama, Japan

© Springer Nature Switzerland AG 2020

P.-D. Ryu et al. (eds.), *Oxygen Transport to Tissue XLI*, Advances in Experimental Medicine and Biology 1232, https://doi.org/10.1007/978-3-030-34461-0_45

Keywords Cardiac computed tomography · Epicardial adipose tissue · Microcirculation · Near infrared spectroscopy · Vascular occlusion test

1 Introduction

Epicardial adipose tissue (EAT), which is located between the epicardium and visceral pericardium, is associated with visceral fat, atrial fibrillation [1] and major adverse cardiovascular events [2]. It is possible to measure EAT using transthoracic echocardiography (TTE), cardiac computed tomography (CCT) and cardiac magnetic resonance imaging. TTE can be used to assess EAT thickness readily and noninvasively. However, EAT measurement using TTE has disadvantages such as poor reproducibility and poor interobserver variability, whereas CCT can assess whole heart EAT more accurately and in detail.

Endothelial dysfunction leads impaired microcirculation and is the initial step of atherosclerosis. The relationship between EAT and endothelial function using flow-mediated dilatation (FMD) has been reported [3]; however, these correlations are not yet clear.

Near infrared spectroscopy (NIRS) is a noninvasive technique that allows to evaluate peripheral blood flow. A previous study demonstrated that NIRS with a vascular occlusion test (VOT) is useful in assessing peripheral microcirculation in post-cardiac surgical patients [4]. In the present study, we assessed the relationship between NIRS with VOT and EAT volume measured using CCT. Because EAT is also associated with visceral fat, we also assessed the relationship between EAT and body mass index (BMI). In addition, we evaluated the effect of statin therapy on those relationships; previous studies demonstrated that statin therapy affects EAT and microcirculation [5, 6].

2 Methods

2.1 Subjects

We studied patients with coronary artery disease who had undergone CCT between October 2017 and March 2018 in the Department of Cardiology at Kawaguchi Municipal Medical Center (Japan). The Ethical Committee of Kawaguchi Municipal Medical Center approved this study and protocol. All subjects (or their family) provided written informed consent, as required by the Ethical Committee.

2.2 NIRS, BMI Measurements and CCT Imaging

All patients had their body height and weight measured before NIRS examination. BMI was derived from the following formula; body weight (kg)/body height $(m)^2$. We employed NIRS (NIRO-200NX, Hamamatsu Photonics K.K., Japan) to evaluate peripheral blood flow during VOT before CCT scanning. The NIRS probe was set on the right thenar eminence and was then covered by a blanket to reduce light contamination. Next, a pneumatic pressure cuff was placed on the right upper arm. At 2 min after NIRS monitoring was started, brachial artery blood flow was blocked by the cuff for 3 min at 50 mmHg above the resting systolic pressure. The cuff was then deflated to observe reperfusion for a further 3 min. NIRS parameters included total hemoglobin (ΔcHb), oxyhemoglobin (ΔO_2Hb), deoxyhemoglobin (ΔHHb) and tissue oxygenation index (ΔTOI); these parameters were recorded every 0.2 s, continuously.

A Somatom Definition Flash (Siemens, Germany) was used to obtain CCT images. EAT volume was measured using non-contrast electrocardiography-gated CCT. CCT images were scanned at 120 keV and reconstructed with 3-mm thick slices. Pixels in the epicardium with densities of −230 to −30 Hounsfield units were considered EAT. The EAT volume was measured by manually tracing the pericardium from the level of the right pulmonary artery to the coronary sinus. All images were analyzed using a workstation (Ziostation2 Version 2.9.0.2, Ziosoft, Inc., Tokyo, Japan).

2.3 Statistical Analysis

Statistical analysis methods are the same as reported in Part 1 of this study.

3 Results

A total of 83 consecutive patients (52 male, median age 69.0 years, median BMI 23.9 kg/m^2) were enrolled, and 39 patients were prescribed statins. Histories of myocardial infarction and revascularization were significantly higher in the statin users (Table 1). No significant differences were observed between the parameters derived from NIRS with VOT and EAT in the patients with or without statin therapy (Table 2). ΔTOI, ΔcHb and ΔHHb were not correlated with EAT volume ($r = -0.08$, $p = 0.46$; $r = -0.098$, $p = 0.38$ and $r = 0.056$, $p = 0.62$, respectively). In the overall study population, an inverse correlation was found between ΔO_2Hb and EAT volume ($r = -0.236$; $p = 0.03$, Fig. 1A). A strong correlation was observed in the patients without statin therapy ($r = -0.488$; $p < 0.001$, Fig. 1B). Conversely, the correlation was absent in the patients with statin therapy ($r = 0.157$; $p = 0.34$, Fig. 1C).

Table 1 Characteristics of the patient groups

	Total	Without statin	With statin	
	(n = 83)	(n = 44)	(n = 39)	p-value
Age (years)	69.0 [58.5, 77.5]	68.0 [52.8, 77.5]	71.0 [63.5, 77.5]	0.36
Male (%)	52 (62.7)	27 (61.4)	25 (64.1)	0.82
Height (cm)	160.7 ± 9.5	159.8 ± 10.0	161.7 ± 8.9	0.35
Body weight (kg)	63.0 [53.0, 71.0]	63.0 [51.0, 69.3]	66.0 [55.0, 72.5]	0.16
BMI (kg/m^2)	23.9 [22.0, 25.9]	23.6 [21.9, 25.7]	24.3 [22.1, 26.8]	0.37
Systolic BP (mmHg)	139.1 ± 17.3	139.3 ± 18.3	138.8 ± 16.3	0.90
Diastolic BP (mmHg)	74.3 ± 11.6	75.6 ± 11.0	72.8 ± 12.2	0.27
Heart rate (bpm)	69.3 ± 12.5	70.7 ± 11.8	67.7 ± 13.3	0.29
HTN (%)	55 (66.3)	25 (56.8)	30 (76.9)	0.06
DM (%)	26 (31.3)	9 (20.9)	17 (42.5)	0.06
DLP (%)	53 (63.9)	14 (31.8)	39 (100)	<0.001
History of OMI (%)	10 (12.0)	1 (2.3)	9 (22.5)	0.006
Post CABG or PCI (%)	25 (30.1)	5 (11.4)	20 (51.3)	<0.001
eGFR (ml/min/l)	67.3 [57.8, 83.6]	70.2 [60.0, 84.1]	64.9 [53.2, 83.4]	0.31
Hemoglobin (g/dl)	13.5 ± 1.5	13.8 ± 1.4	13.2 ± 1.49	0.04
HbA1c (%)	5.8 [5.6, 6.5]	5.8 [5.6, 6.1]	6.1 [5.7, 7.0]	0.016
LDL (mg/dl)	105.0 ± 34.4	121.1 ± 32.5	87.8 ± 27.6	<0.001
HDL (mg/dl)	54.0 [44.0, 64.0]	54.6 [45.5, 66.8]	52.0 [44.0, 64.0]	0.72
TG (mg/dl)	106.0 [80.0, 166.0]	116.5 [86.3, 174.0]	98.0 [72.0, 159.5]	0.31

BMI, body mass index; BP, blood pressure; CABG, Coronary artery bypass graft; DM, diabetes mellitus; DLP, dyslipidemia; eGFR, estimated glomerular filtration rate; HDL; high density lipoprotein; HTN, hypertension; LDL, low density lipoprotein; OMI, old myocardial infarction; PCI, percutaneous coronary intervention; TG, triglyceride

Table 2 Results of all parameters derived from near infrared spectroscopy with vascular occlusion test and epicardial adipose tissue volume

	Total	Without statin	With statin	
	(n = 83)	(n = 44)	(n = 39)	p-value
baseTOI (%)	63.55 (7.54)	64.6 ± 7.1	62.4 ± 7.9	0.18
minTOI (%)	35.24 (13.18)	36.4 ± 12.6	33.9 ± 13.8	0.39
maxTOI (%)	79.30 [75.90, 82.60]	79.1 [75.7, 81.73]	79.4 [76.4, 82.8]	0.75
Δ TOI (%)	43.66 (12.84)	42.6 ± 12.8	44.8 ± 13.0	0.44
Δ cHb (μmol/L)	12.88 [9.71, 17.21]	13.0 [9.8, 17.2]	12.7 [9.8, 16.9]	0.93
Δ O_2Hb (μmol/L)	32.83 (8.20)	33.1 ± 8.72	32.5 ± 7.7	0.74
Δ HHb (μmol/L)	36.15 (6.55)	35.5 ± 7.3	36.9 ± 5.6	0.34
EAT volume (cm^3)	111.0 ± 43.0	105.4 ± 46.2	117.3 ± 41.1	0.21

cHb, total hemoglobin; EAT, epicardial adipose tissue; HHb, deoxyhemoglobin; O_2Hb, oxyhemoglobin; TOI, tissue oxygen index

In all cases, a positive correlation was observed between BMI and EAT volume ($r = 0.547$, $p < 0.001$) (Fig. 2A). A stronger correlation was observed in patients without statin therapy ($r = 0.722$, $p < 0.001$, Fig. 2B), while a significant but weak correlation was observed in patients with statin therapy ($r = 0.325$, $p = 0.044$, Fig. 2C).

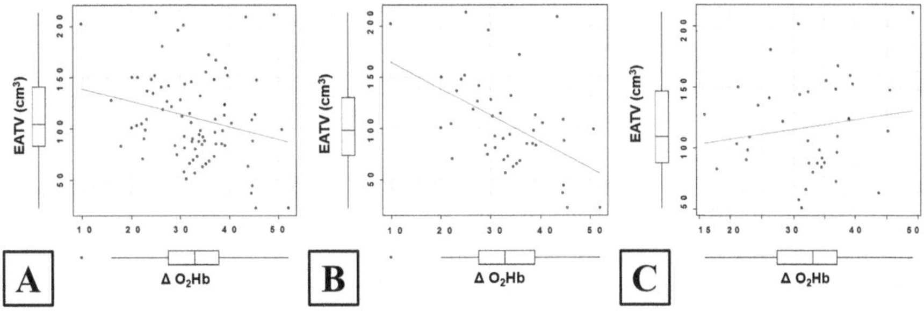

Fig. 1 Relationship between epicardial adipose tissue volume and changes of oxyhemoglobin in all patients (**A**), in patients without statin therapy (**B**) and in patients with statin therapy (**C**). EATV, epicardial adipose tissue volume; O_2Hb, oxyhemoglobin

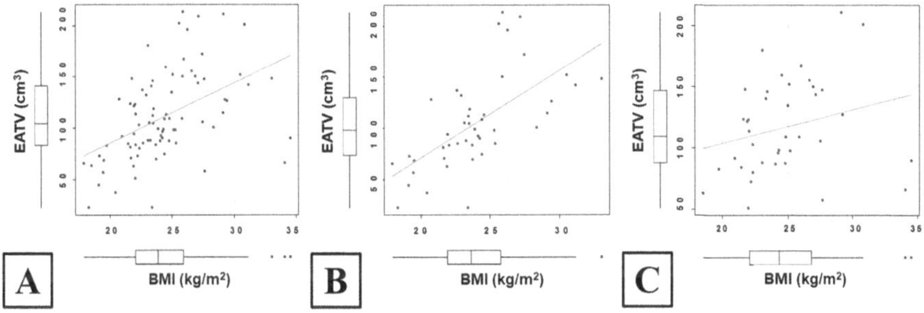

Fig. 2 Relationship between epicardial adipose tissue volume and body mass index in all patients (**A**), in patients without statin therapy (**B**) and in patients with statin therapy (**C**). EATV, epicardial adipose tissue volume; BMI, body mass index

4 Discussion

The major findings of this study are as follows: First, ΔO_2Hb, which was derived from NIRS with VOT, was associated with EAT volumes; however, no such association was observed in the other parameters. Second, BMI was also associated with EAT volumes. Third, stronger correlations were found in those relationships in patients without statin therapy.

EAT is the visceral fat depot of the heart and produces inflammatory adipokines [7]. Previous studies revealed that high EAT led to unfavorable events [1, 2]; therefore, EAT assessment has clinical implications regarding the prevention of such events. In the present study, a correlation was observed between ΔO_2Hb, BMI and EAT volume. Previous studies reported that statin can lower blood cholesterol and reduce cardiovascular events; however, caloric intake and BMI are reported to be increased among statin users [8]. Interestingly, in the present study, stronger correlations between ΔO_2Hb, BMI and EAT volume were observed in the non-statin group; these results may suggest that statin has an effect on EAT and peripheral microcirculations, beyond weight gain.

The findings of this study may be useful to identify patients with high EAT. In the clinical setting, physicians might consider additional intervention, such as statin therapy, for patients with low ΔO_2Hb to prevent future adverse events.

The present study has some limitations. First, we did not record other medications that can affect EAT and/or endothelial function, such as antidiabetic and antihypertensive drugs. Second, we had not investigated the dose or period of statin administration. Statin therapy have shown clinical benefit beyond lipid lowering which may be due to other actions such as anti-inflammatory effects, however, these mechanisms are still unclear. Further research would be needed.

The findings of this study may help to easily and noninvasively identify patients with high EAT volume and those at high cardiovascular risk.

Acknowledgement The authors cordially thank Mr. Yuichi Kusama and Tsuyoshi Ohtsuki for their assistance as radiological technologists.

References

1. Thanassoulis G, Massaro JM, O'Donnell CJ et al (2010) Pericardial fat is associated with prevalent atrial fibrillation: the Framingham heart study. Circ Arrhythm Electrophysiol 3:345–350
2. Cheng VY, Dey D, Tamarappoo B et al (2010) Pericardial fat burden on ECG-gated noncontrast CT in asymptomatic patients who subsequently experience adverse cardiovascular events. JACC Cardiovasc Imaging 3:352–360
3. Kocaman SA, Durakoglugil ME, Cetin M et al (2013) The independent relationship of epicardial adipose tissue with carotid intima-media thickness and endothelial functions: the association of pulse wave velocity with the active facilitated arterial conduction concept. Blood Press Monit 18:85–93
4. Butler E, Chin M, Aneman A (2017) Peripheral near-infrared spectroscopy: methodologic aspects and a systematic review in post-cardiac surgical patients. J Cardiothorac Vasc Anesth 31:1407–1416
5. Almuti K, Rimawi R, Spevack D et al (2006) Effects of statins beyond lipid lowering: potential for clinical benefits. Int J Cardiol 109:7–15
6. Alexopoulos N, Melek BH, Arepalli CD et al (2013) Effect of intensive versus moderate lipid-lowering therapy on Epicardial adipose tissue in Hyperlipidemic post-menopausal women: a substudy of the BELLES trial (beyond endorsed lipid lowering with EBT scanning). J Am Coll Cardiol 61:1956–1961
7. Mazurek T, Zhang L, Zalewski A et al (2003) Human epicardial adipose tissue is a source of inflammatory mediators. Circulation 108:2460–2466
8. Sugiyama T, Tsugawa Y, Tseng CH et al (2014) Different time trends of caloric and fat intake between statin users and nonusers among US adults: gluttony in the time of statins? JAMA Intern Med 174:1038–1045

Optimization of Band Selection in Multispectral and Narrow-Band Imaging: An Analytical Approach

Guennadi Saiko and Andrei Betlen

Abstract Hyperspectral imaging is a promising clinical imaging modality with multiple applications in wound care, dermatology, and ophthalmology. However, with current technologies, hyperspectral imagers are relatively large and expensive devices, mainly affordable only by hospitals. Multispectral imaging can be a cost-effective alternative for hyperspectral imaging and is capable of bringing diagnostics to primary health care. Multispectral imaging uses known features of tissue chromophores to simplify imaging device design. However, to maintain design simple and cost-effective the number of illumination bands should be minimal. Thus, proper band selection is very important. The goal of the current study is to develop an analytical model for the optimization of band selection for multispectral and narrow-band imaging techniques (e.g., narrow-band microscopy). *Methods*: The contrast ratio has been proposed for quantification of image quality of subsurface inhomogeneities in the skin. Based on the two-flux Kubelka-Munk model, we developed an analytical approach which links the contrast ratio with optical tissue parameters. *Results*: We obtained an explicit analytical solution for the dependence of maximal contrast ratio on optical tissue parameters. Then, we linked the minimally observable contrast ratio (c_{min}) with the bit depth of the camera, *d*: $c_{min} = 1/(2^d-1)$. Based on this analysis we were able to derive an explicit expression, which links camera properties with the minimally detectable changes in optical tissue parameters (both scattering and absorption). *Conclusions:* The proposed analytical model can be used for rapid assessment and optimization of multispectral and narrow band imaging techniques and for estimation of the accuracy of imaging techniques. The developed model confirms the utility of the contrast ratio for tissue imaging.

G. Saiko (✉)
Oxilight Inc, Toronto, Canada
e-mail: gennadi@oxilight.ca

A. Betlen
Oxilight Inc, Toronto, Canada

Department of Computer Science, Ryerson University, Toronto, Canada

© Springer Nature Switzerland AG 2020

P.-D. Ryu et al. (eds.), *Oxygen Transport to Tissue XLI*, Advances in Experimental Medicine and Biology 1232, https://doi.org/10.1007/978-3-030-34461-0_46

Keywords Biomedical imaging · Multispectral imaging · Blood vessels · Contrast ratio

1 Introduction

The inhomogeneous distribution of blood, chromophores and cellular structures in tissues produces variations in average optical properties. A number of tissue imaging modalities have been developed to visualize both absorption (diffuse imaging, tissue oximetry imaging, videocapillaroscopy) and scattering (OCT) tissue heterogeneities. The light scattering phenomena occur on boundaries with mismatched refractive indexes (e.g., collagen fibrils in the dermis). The light absorption phenomena in the visible and Near Infrared (NIR) range of the spectrum are linked primarily to hemoglobin, melanin, water, and lipids.

Imaging of light absorption heterogeneities in tissues is of particular importance because it is capable of visualizing tissue blood vessels, which is interesting for various medical fields. In particular, hyperspectral imaging is a promising clinical imaging modality with multiple applications in wound care, dermatology, and ophthalmology [1]. However, with current technologies, hyperspectral imagers are relatively large and expensive devices, mainly affordable only by hospitals. Multispectral imaging can be a cost-effective alternative for hyperspectral imaging and is capable of bringing diagnostics to primary health care. Multispectral imaging uses known features of tissue chromophores to simplify imaging device design. However, to maintain design simple and cost-effective the number of illumination bands should be minimal. Thus, proper band selection is very important.

Optimization and fine-tuning of imaging technology faces broader challenges: (a) various groups report different metrics; (b) there is no common approach to compare various imaging techniques, and (c) imaging optimization is generally performed on proprietary data or samples, and mostly empirically. To facilitate rapid technology development, there is a need for common metrics/approaches, which can be used for rapid comparison and assessment of various techniques. The contrast ratio has the potential to become such an approach. While introduced more than 150 years ago by Weber and Fechner [2], the contrast ratio is largely overlooked in the current tissue imaging literature. Instead, various alternatives (e.g., dynamic contrast ratio) have been proposed. In [3] we demonstrated the utility of the contrast ratio for biomedical imaging applications. However, further generalization is required before this approach can be useful for researchers.

The goal of the current study is to develop an approach for evaluation of the detection limits of the tissue imaging techniques and link them with the properties of an imaging device. In particular, this model can be helpful for optimization of band selection for multispectral and narrow-band imaging techniques (e.g., narrow-band microscopy).

2 Methods

2.1 *Tissue Model*

A tissue model which can be used for rapid assessment of tissue imaging techniques, is described in [3]. Briefly, the tissue is considered as a homogeneous medium and blood vessels (capillaries) are considered as perturbations. To assess an upper limit (theoretical maximum) of the sensitivity, the model can be reduced to a single layer.

In realistic settings, the tissue absorption is a result of the contribution of several pigments and chromophores. In particular, the relative contribution of melanin absorption can be high for dark-pigmented skin in the visible spectrum. Human skin is characterized by variable concentrations of melanin, ranging from very low in fair-skinned individuals (skin type I) to very high in dark skinned individuals (skin type VI) [4]. Jacques [5] reported that the volume fraction of melanin in the epidermis is 1–3% for light-skinned Caucasians, 11–16% for Mediterranean types, and 18–43% for dark pigmented Africans.

Blood normally occupies around 0.2–0.6% of the physical volume of the dermis [6]. In some conditions (e.g., hyperemia) the blood content can be higher.

2.2 *Contrast Ratio*

We start with the standard definition of the contrast ratio $c = (I - I_d)/I$, where I and I_d are the light intensities of the background and feature (defect), respectively. Considering that reflected light is the product of external illumination (which can be assumed constant within a small area) and the reflectance of the tissue, we can move from the intensity of reflected light (I) to the reflectance of the tissue (R). If we consider the tissue heterogeneity (e.g. capillary) as absorption (or scattering) perturbation $\Delta\mu$, then in the first order approximation we can write

$$c = \frac{I - I_d}{I} = \frac{R - R_d}{R} = \frac{-\Delta R}{R} = \frac{-1}{R}\frac{\partial R}{\partial \mu}\Delta\mu \tag{1}$$

Here μ denotes a coefficient of absorption (for an absorption defect) or a coefficient of scattering (for a scattering defect).

2.3 Tissue Light Propagation Model

Further, we need to specify the model of light propagation in the tissue. The two-flux Kubelka-Munk model (see e.g. [7]) is a well-known approach in tissue optics, which provides reasonable estimations in wide a range of conditions. For the semi-infinite slab the solution for the tissue reflectance R is well known:

$$R = x + 1 - \sqrt{(x+1)^2 - 1} \tag{2}$$

Here $x = k/s$, where k and s are the tissue absorption and scattering per unit length, respectively. For diffuse illumination, $k = 2\mu_a$ and $s = 2\mu_s$, (where μ_a and μ_s are tissue absorption and scattering coefficients). Taking into account that $\frac{\partial R}{\partial \mu_a} = \frac{\partial R}{\partial x}\frac{\partial x}{\partial \mu_a}$ and $\frac{\partial x}{\partial \mu_a} = \frac{1}{\mu_s}$ one can write $c_a = \frac{-1}{R}\frac{\partial R}{\partial \mu_a}\Delta\mu_a = \frac{x}{\sqrt{(x+1)^2 - 1}}\frac{\Delta\mu_a}{\mu_a}$ for the contrast ratio of an absorption defect. Expressing x as a function of R from Eq.2: $x = (1-R)^2 / 2R$ and substituting it into the last equation gives us

$$c_a = \frac{(1-R)}{(1+R)}\frac{\Delta\mu_a}{\mu_a} \tag{3a}$$

Similarly for the scattering defect:

$$c_s = -\frac{(1-R)}{(1+R)}\frac{\Delta\mu_s}{\mu_s} \tag{3b}$$

Eqs.3a–b are explicit relationships between the relative changes in absorption (scattering) coefficient and the contrast ratio. Tissue reflectance R can be measured experimentally.

2.4 Camera Model

Now, we try to link the properties of the camera with the limits of its imaging capabilities. In particular, if we consider illumination by a narrow band light source, then the signal will most likely be detected by a single channel (when it is an RGB or monochrome camera). Thus, the relevant parameter is the bit depth of the camera, d. Typically, it is 8 bits for a consumer-grade camera, and 12 bits for a scientific grade camera. The minimal contrast, which can be captured by a camera with bit depth d, can be found by taking into account the smallest detectable change in channel intensity (one) and the maximal background intensity (2^d-1):

$$c_{\min} = \frac{1}{2^d - 1} \tag{4}$$

In particular, the minimal contrast ratio is close to 0.4% for consumer grade cameras ($d = 8$). From Eq.3–4 we can get an explicit expression for the minimal relative change in the absorption (scattering) coefficient, which can be detected by a particular type of camera

$$\frac{\Delta\mu}{\mu} = \frac{(1+R)}{(1-R)} \frac{1}{2^d - 1} \tag{5}$$

3 Results

We can consider a multiplier $(1-R)/(1+R)$ in Eq.3 as an 'amplification factor', which shows how the relative change in absorption (scattering) translates into the contrast ratio. Figure 1a shows the dependence of the amplification factor on the tissue reflectance. In the practically important NIR and blue-green ranges of the visible spectrum (tissue reflectance R is 30–40% and 20–30%, correspondingly) the amplification factor is around 0.5–0.6 and 0.6–0.7, respectively. Figure 1b shows the results of emulation of spectral dependence of visualization of an absorption defect (background: 3% fully oxygenated blood; defect: 3.3% fully oxygenated blood, which corresponds to 10% increase in the blood content) for various skin types [3]: light skin tone (4% melanin content), medium skin tone (12% melanin content) and dark skin (30% melanin content). It was assumed that the epidermis thickness is 1/3 of the probing depth, which is approximately 0.5 mm in the visible spectrum [8]. It can be seen that the contrast is maximal at the absorption peaks.

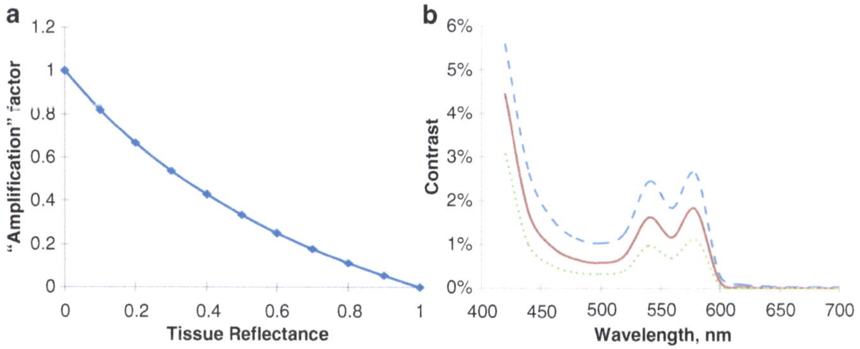

Fig. 1 (**A**) Dependence of amplification factor on tissue reflectance R. (**B**): spectral dependence of the contrast ratio of an absorption defect for various skin types i.e. light (dashed line, blue), medium (solid line, red), and dark (dotted line, green)

4 Discussion

In the proposed analytical model, the contrast ratio is the product of the amplification factor and the relative change in the absorption (scattering) coefficient. Thus, to increase the contrast we can either (a) increase the relative change in the absorption (scattering) coefficient, and/or (b) increase the amplification factor.

Just as the tissue absorption is a result of the contribution of several pigments and chromophores, the relative change in absorption coefficient can be increased either by increasing the contribution of the primary component (e.g., absorption peak) or decreasing the contribution of the undesirable components (melanin). In particular, even though absorption of melanin drops significantly with the wavelength λ as $\lambda^{-3.33}$ [9], the relative contribution of hemoglobin is higher in the 400-600 nm range than for absorption peaks in the 700-1000 nm range (e.g., deoxyhemoglobin at 760 nm).

Narrow-band techniques at absorption maximums may have better (2x-3x) sensitivity than broadband ones. This is a result of the contribution of both factors: increased relative change in the absorption coefficient and increased amplification factor (due to increased absorption). Wavelength selection is very important: the increase in absorption leads to a decrease in reflectance, and to an increase in sensitivity, consequently.

A trivial consequence of Eqs. 3a, b is that absorption and scattering defects have the opposite impact on brightness. Increased absorption leads to reduced intensity (positive contrast). Increased scattering leads to increased intensity (negative contrast). A less trivial consequence is that for defects with high absorption and high scattering, these effects can cancel each other out.

It should be noted that the contrast ratio provided by Eq.4 is probably not attainable in practice. Practically, the dynamic imaging range is 30–50% of the maximum value. Thus, 2–3 times larger values of contrast ratio (0.8–1.2% for a consumer grade camera) are more realistic. Thus, in the NIR range, where melanin impact is minimal, and tissue reflectance R is 50–60%, the 2.5–3.5% relative changes in absorption and scattering could be detectable.

5 Conclusions

The proposed analytical model provides specific relationships between the relative changes in absorption (scattering) coefficient and the contrast ratio. This can be used for rapid assessment and optimization of multispectral and narrow band imaging techniques. Also, it can be used for estimation of the accuracy and limitations of imaging techniques. The developed model confirms the utility of the contrast ratio as a versatile metric for tissue imaging, which can be used in various analytical and numerical models.

References

1. Lu G, Fei B (2014) Medical hyperspectral imaging: a review. JBO 19(1). https://doi.org/10.1117/1.JBO.19.1.010901
2. Fechner GT (1860) Elemente der Psychophysik. band 2. Breitkopf und Härtel, Leipzig
3. Saiko G, Douplik A (2018) Contrast Ratio Quantification During Visualization of Microvasculature. Adv Exp Med Biol 1072:369–373. https://doi.org/10.1007/978-3-319-91287-5_59
4. Fitzpatrick TB (1975) Soleil et peau. J Med Esthet. 2:33–34
5. Jacques SL (1996) Origins of tissue optical properties in the UVA, visible and NIR regions" in Advances in Optical Imaging and Photon Migration, R. R. Alfano, J. G. Fujimoto (eds.), pp. 364–371, OSATOPS: Optical Society of America, Vol. 2,Washington, DC
6. Lister T, Wright PA, Chappell PH (2012) Optical properties of human skin. JBO 17(9). https://doi.org/10.1117/1.JBO.17.9.090901
7. Saiko G, Douplik A (2014) Reflectance of Biological Turbid Tissues under Wide Area Illumination: Single Backward Scattering Approach. Int. J.Photoenergy 241364. https://doi.org/10.1155/2014/241364
8. Douplik A, Saiko G, Schelkanova I, Tuchin VV (2013) The response of tissue to laser light. In: Jelinkova H (ed) Lasers for Medical Applications. Diagnostics, Therapy and Surgery. Woodhead Publishing, pp 47–109. https://doi.org/10.1533/9780857097545.1.47
9. Meglinski IV, Matcher SJ (2002) Quantitative assessment of skin layers absorption and skin reflectance spectra simulation in the visible and near-infrared spectral regions. Physiol. Meas. 23:741–753

Fabrication and Optical Characterization of Gelatin-Based Phantoms for Tissue Oximetry

G. Saiko, X. Zheng, A. Betlen, and A. Douplik

Abstract Multispectral/hyperspectral imaging is one of the imaging modalities to visualize and quantify blood supply in surface tissues such as skin or mucosa. The results of visualization can be potentially affected by various factors, for instance by elevated methemoglobin (MetHb) content (e.g., methemoglobinemia). The scope of the current study is to develop a robust approach for fabrication and validation of tissue-mimicking phantoms, which can be used to assess and improve tissue oximetry. *Methods*: The realistic tissue mimicking gelatin-based phantoms with intralipid (4% v/v) and/or hemoglobins (oxy-, deoxyhemoglobins, and MetHb) were molded between two coverslips separated by 2-mm wires. The hemoglobin solutions were prepared by dissolving the lyophilized human hemoglobin powder (H7379, Sigma-Aldrich) in the deionized water. Sodium dithionite (85% purity, 157,953, Sigma-Aldrich) was used to reduce MetHb solution. The phantoms were imaged using a multispectral imaging device (Oxilight, Canada).To demonstrate the utility, the developed approach is applied to emulate elevated systemic MetHb content. *Results*: Initial results show that elevated systemic MetHb (2.0–6.7% of total blood) does not impact the accuracy of tissue oximetry imaging. *Discussion*: A robust method for fabrication and optical validation of biocompatible tissue-mimicking phantoms has been developed.The proposed phantom design allows combining different phantoms into multilayer (sandwich) structures, which can be used to emulate a wide range of topical and systemic conditions.

Keywords Biomedical imaging · Multispectral imaging · Tissue oximetry · Hemoglobin · Tissue phantom

---

G. Saiko (✉)
Oxilight Inc, Toronto, Canada
e-mail: gennadi@oxilight.ca

X. Zheng · A. Douplik
Department of Physics, Ryerson University, Toronto, Canada

iBEST, Keenan Research Centre of the LKS Knowledge Institute, Toronto, Canada

A. Betlen
Oxilight Inc, Toronto, Canada

Department of Computer Science, Ryerson University, Toronto, Canada

© Springer Nature Switzerland AG 2020

P.-D. Ryu et al. (eds.), *Oxygen Transport to Tissue XLI*, Advances in Experimental Medicine and Biology 1232, https://doi.org/10.1007/978-3-030-34461-0_47

1 Introduction

Multispectral/hyperspectral imaging is one of the imaging modalities to visualize and quantify blood supply in surface tissues, such as skin or mucosa. It allows to obtain information about concentrations of chromophores including oxy- and deoxyhemoglobins in biotissue noninvasively and (quasi)real-time, which makes it a useful tool adjuvant to diagnostics of peripheral vascular disease.

The principles of measuring the concentration of tissue chromophores, including oxyhemoglobin (HbO2) and deoxyhemoglobin (RHb), with multispectral or hyperspectral imaging are well understood. Briefly, the tissue is illuminated with narrowband (multispectral imaging) or broadband (hyperspectral imaging) illumination. Photons penetrate into the tissue and experience absorption and scattering events. Components of the blood (HbO2 and RHb) are major tissue chromophores in visible and NIR ranges. They have distinct absorption spectra, which allow to quantitatively assess their relative concentrations and, consequently, hemoglobin oxygen saturation. In addition to HbO2 and RHb, several other hemoglobins absorb visible and NIR light, e.g., methemoglobin (MetHb). However, the concentration of MetHb in the blood generally does not exceed 1% [1], and its absorption maximum (630 nm) is far from oxy/deoxy absorption peaks. Melanin is another skin chromophore relevant to the visible spectrum. The light penetration (sampling) depth is dependent on an illumination wavelength. Shortwave visible light (below 600 nm) penetrates typical tissues to a depth of 0.5–2.5 mm [2].

The results of tissue oximetry imaging can be potentially affected by various endogenous (e.g. elevated MetHb content or methemoglobinemia [1]) and exogenous (e.g., blood clots, tattoos, ointments) factors. Extensive validations are required to make it a valuable clinical methodology.

While the exogenous factors are relatively easy to control, the endogenous factors (e.g., epidermis thickness, systemic MetHb content) are more difficult to assess or measure in vivo. For example, it is well known that elevated MetHb content can decrease pulse oximeter reading to 85% [3]. Thus, skin phantoms can be invaluable tools for technology development, testing, and calibration. With a broad range of matrix, absorption, and scattering media proposed[4], the selection of a proper methodology is of great importance. In our previous work [5] we developed gelatin-based phantoms to demonstrate the feasibility of multispectral MetHb visualization in the tissue; however, there was a necessity to prepare and cure various solutions to emulate each set of conditions thereby adding a significant amount of time and complexity. A modular approach, where several solid parts can be combined sticking as a 'sandwich' to simulate a number of scenarios, would be of considerable use.

The aim of the current study is to develop a robust approach for fabrication and validation of skin-mimicking phantoms, which can be used to assess and improve tissue oximetry. As a particular example of potential applications, we have used developed phantoms to determine whether elevated systemic MetHb levels may impact the accuracy of tissue oximetry imaging.

2 Methods

Realistic gelatin-based phantoms, which mimic light propagation in the skin, have been developed and imaged using a multispectral imaging system.

2.1 *Materials*

The phantoms were based on the type A gelatin derived from porcine skin, with 300 g gel strength (G2500, Sigma-Aldrich, Canada), which does not have significant optical absorption and scattering in the visible range. The intralipid (20%, Sigma-Aldrich, Canada) was used to mimic the scattering property of the skin. HbO2, RHb, and MetHb were used to provide spectroscopy contrast.

Each phantom contained 10% (w/w) of type A gelatin. The hemoglobin solutions were prepared by dissolved the lyophilized human hemoglobin powder (H7379, Sigma-Aldrich, USA) in the deionized water. The resulted solution contained approximately 98% of MetHb molecules. The solution used sodium dithionite ($Na_2S_2O_4$ or NaDi) (85% purity, 157,953, Sigma-Aldrich) to reduce into RHb. A 2:1 solution Hb/NaDi was used to prepare RHb. M:1 solutions (where M is a number, $1 < M < 2$) were used to prepare partially oxygenated hemoglobin.

2.2 *Phantom Fabrication*

The realistic tissue simulating phantoms were prepared using coverslips separated by wires with various thicknesses. We have designed and prepared several types of phantoms: (a) phantoms mimicking the normal skin (dermis and epidermis), (b) phantoms mimicking the thick epidermis, and (c) phantoms mimicking the elevated systemic level of chromophores (e.g., MetHb). In a typical scenario, two 2-mm wires were used to obtain phantoms with homogeneous thickness. The phantoms can be stacked onto each other, like a 'sandwich' thus simulating various skin conditions.

Skin phantoms were prepared with intralipid (IL) and HbO2/RHb. Blood normally occupies 0.2–0.6% of the dermis volume [6]. However, in some conditions (e.g., hyperemia) the blood content can be higher. Hemoglobin concentrations: 1, 2, 5, and 10% (w/w) and 4% of IL were used to emulate skin tissue.

Epidermis layer thickness varies depending on anatomical locations. While it is generally only 50 μm thick, it can be up to 2-5 mm thick on soles or palms. To emulate the effect of the thick epidermis, the 2-mm thick *epidermis phantoms* were prepared. *Epidermis phantoms* were prepared using 4% of IL (v/v). Since epidermis does not contain blood components, no absorption contrast was added to the phantom.

Table 1 Parameters of phantoms

Parameter	Skin	Skin Phantom	Epidermis Phantom	MetHb Phantom
Thickness	1.5-2 mm[7]	2 mm	2 mm, 0-2 mm	2 mm
Scattering		4% intralipid (v/v)	4% intralipid (v/v)	
Blood	0.2–0.6%(v/v)[6]	1,2,5,10% Hb (w/w)		
MetHb	1% of blood [1]			0.1 and 0.2%(v/v)

Chromophore phantoms are phantoms which contain chromophore(s), but do not contain scatterer. The phantom can be placed on top of the skin or skin phantom and adds 2 mm to the optical path each way. As an example, we prepared 0.1 and 0.2%MetHb (v/v) phantoms. In a healthy individual, the systemic level of MetHb does not exceed 1% of total hemoglobin, Thus, even if we assumed that the blood content in the skin is in the 3–10% range (e.g., hyperaemia), then the normal MetHb content in the skin should not exceed 0.03–0.1% (v/v). Consequently, 0.1 and 0.2% MetHb phantoms with 2-mm thickness placed on top of the skin should emulate 1%–3.3% and 2%–6.7% systemic MetHb increase, respectively. Parameters of phantoms are summarized in Table 1.

The phantom fabrication steps were discussed in [5]. The final phantom was poured between the two coverslips separated by wires to solidify.

To validate phantom compositions, the phantoms transmission spectra were measured using a spectrometer (Shimadzu, UV3600 with Integrating sphere, Japan).

2.3 Imaging

The OxiLight (Oxilight Inc., Toronto, Canada) is a multispectral imaging system for visualization of blood oxygenation in surface tissues. It provides 2D false-color maps of blood oxygenation with a 6.5x12.5 cm field of view. The OxiLight system consists of a small illumination device (OxiLight device) and a smartphone with an app. The illumination device produces a sequence of light flashes, each flash at a particular wavelength. It consists of a ring of LEDs, the hardware,and software to run multispectral flash and synchronize it with the smartphone. Upon positioning at a certain distance from a target area (10 cm) the smartphone automatically captures the sequence of images (each illuminated at a particular wavelength); the app creates a reflectance hypercube (i, j, λ) and performs least square fitting for each pixel (i, j) to find concentrations of known chromophores (HbO2, RHb, and melanin). Concentrations of HbO2 and RHb are used to produce a blood oxygenation (SO_2 = HbO2/(HbO2 + RHb)) map, which is presented to a user on the smartphone screen. The user can interpret point data on a false-color oxygenation map using a color bar or use an averaging tool, which provides average oxygenation for a small circular area (1.5 cm diameter).

To mimic the intended use by healthcare professionals, the averaging tool for data collection and analysiswas used. The user could click on any point of the image to get average blood oxygenation for a small circular area.

Various phantoms were stacked on top of each other or the skin and imaged by the OxiLight system: MetHb phantom on skin phantom, epidermis phantom on skin phantom, MetHb phantom on the skin, and epidermis phantom on the skin. The volar side of the forearm of one of the investigators was used for *in vivo* experimentation. The study on volunteers was approved by the Research Ethics Board at Ryerson University. The imaging distance was 10 cm. Here we present only the results of MetHb phantoms on skin experiments.

3 Results

The imaging showed good homogeneity of the prepared samples. The heterogeneity (defined as a standard deviation) measured by oxygenation averaging tool did not exceed 3% (excluding edges and areas with specular reflection). To test the utility of the phantoms we performed *in vivo* imaging to simulate elevated MetHb levels. A volar forearm was covered with MetHb phantoms. Figure 1 shows false-color oxygenation maps of the volar forearm covered with 0.1% (A) and 0.2% (B) MetHb phantoms. It can be seen that the presence of the MetHb does not change calculated oxygenation by more than 2–3%.

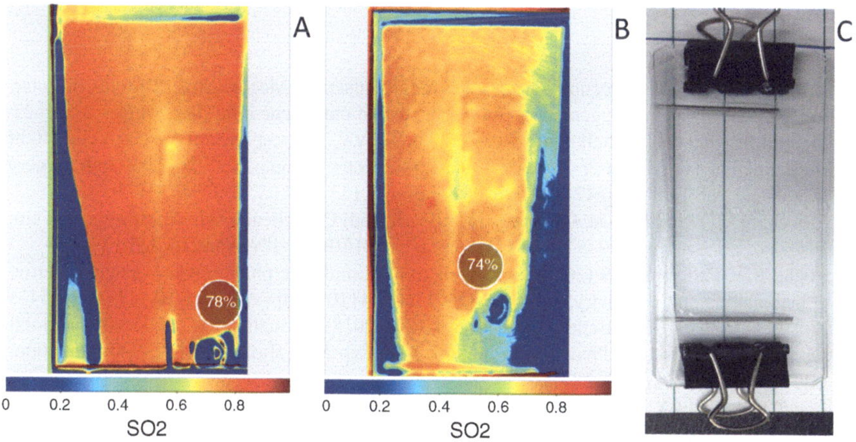

Fig. 1 False-color oxygenation maps of a volar forearm covered with 0.1%MetHb phantom (panel A) and 0.2% MetHb phantom (panel B). The averaging tool is seen as a grey circle. Panel C: the mould for phantoms (coverslips and wires)

4 Conclusions

The initial experiments show that the developed phantoms can be used to emulate a broad range of topical and systemic conditions. Gelatin phantoms are biocompatible [4] and can be used on the human skin. In addition to their standalone use, they can be easily combined in multilayer structures. They are versatile and can be used in bench and *in vivo* experiments.

In particular, using the developed phantoms, we found that elevated MetHb levels do not affect retrieved skin blood oxygenation by more than 2–3%.

The present study was designed to prove the concept. In future work, we plan to conduct more rigorous validation on volunteers. We also plan to investigate the influence of carboxyhemoglobin on oximetry imaging. Also, we plan to consider polyacrylamide as a more stable substrate, which can prevent rapid oxygenation.

In summary, a robust method for fabrication and optical validation of biocompatible tissue-mimicking phantoms has been developed. *Skin phantoms* can be used to emulate the optical properties of skin tissues. *Epidermis phantoms* can be used to emulate the epidermis layer of various thicknesses. *Chromophore phantoms* can be used to emulate elevated systemic chromospheres (e.g., MetHb or carboxyhemoglobin). *Epidermis* and *chromophore phantoms* can be used in combination with *skin phantoms* or placed on the skin for in vivo measurements.

Acknowledgments Guennadi Saiko thanks NRC-IRAP for their support as well as NSERC Individual Discovery of Prof. Alexandre Douplik.

References

1. Bradberry SM (2003) Occupational methaemoglobinaemia. Mechanisms of production, features, diagnosis and management including the use of methylene blue. Toxicol Rev 22:13–27
2. Douplik A, Saiko G, Schelkanova I (2013) Tuchin VV The response of tissue to laser light. In: Jelinkova H (ed) Lasers for Medical Applications. Diagnostics, Therapy and Surgery, Woodhead Publishing, pp 47–109. https://doi.org/10.1533/9780857097545.1.47
3. Stoneham MD (2007) Pulse Oximetry. In: Atlee JL (ed) Complications in Anesthesia, 2nd edn. Elsevier/Saunders, pp 570–573. https://doi.org/10.1016/B978-1-4160-2215-2.50145-9
4. Pogue BW, Patterson MS (2006) Review of tissue simulating phantoms for optical spectroscopy, imaging and dosimetry. J Biomed Opt 11(4):041102. https://doi.org/10.1117/1.2335429
5. Saiko G, Zheng X, Betlen A, Douplik A (2018) Visualization of Methemoglobin Distribution in Tissues: Phantom Validation. Adv Exp Med Biol 1072:387–390. https://doi.org/10.1007/978-3-319-91287-5_62
6. Lister T, Wright PA, Chappell PH (2012) Optical properties of human skin. JBO 17(9). https://doi.org/10.1117/1.JBO.17.9.090901
7. Meglinski IV, Matcher SJ (2002) Quantitative assessment of skin layers absorption and skin reflectance spectra simulation in the visible and near-infrared spectral regions. Physiol. Meas. 23:741–753

Two-Photon Autofluorescence Imaging of Fixed Tissues: Feasibility and Potential Values for Biomedical Applications

Lin Z. Li, Marissa Masek, Ting Wang, He N. Xu, Shoko Nioka, Joseph A. Baur, and Timothy M. Ragan

Abstract The value of optical redox imaging (ORI) of cells/tissues based on the intrinsic fluorescences of NADH (nicotinamide adenine dinucleotide) and oxidized flavoproteins (containing flavin adenine dinucleotide, i.e., FAD) has been demonstrated for potential biomedical applications including diagnosis, prognosis, and determining treatment response. However, the Chance redox scanner (a 3D cryogenic tissue imager) is limited by spatial resolution (~50 μm), and tissue ORI using fluorescence microscopy (single or multi-photon) is limited by the light penetration depth. Furthermore, viable or snap-frozen tissues are usually required. In this project, we aimed to study whether ORI may be achieved for unstained fixed tissue using a state-of-the-art modern Serial Two-Photon (STP) Tomography scanner that can rapidly acquire multi-plane images at micron resolution. Tissue specimens of mouse muscle, liver, and tumor xenografts were harvested and fixed in 4% paraformaldehyde (PFA) for 24 h. Tissue blocks were scanned by STP Tomography under room temperature to acquire the autofluorescence signals (NADH channel:

L. Z. Li (✉)
Department of Radiology & Britton Chance Laboratory of Redox Imaging, Johnson Research Foundation, Perelman School of Medicine, University of Pennsylvania, Philadelphia, PA, USA

Abramson Cancer Center, University of Pennsylvania, Philadelphia, PA, USA

Institute of Translational Medicine and Therapeutics, Perelman School of Medicine, University of Pennsylvania, Philadelphia, PA, USA
e-mail: linli@pennmedicine.upenn.edu

M. Masek · T. M. Ragan (✉)
TissueVision, Inc, Somerville, MA, USA
e-mail: tragan@tissuevision.com

T. Wang · H. N. Xu · S. Nioka
Department of Radiology & Britton Chance Laboratory of Redox Imaging, Johnson Research Foundation, Perelman School of Medicine, University of Pennsylvania, Philadelphia, PA, USA

J. A. Baur
Department of Physiology, Institute for Diabetes, Obesity and Metabolism, University of Pennsylvania, Philadelphia, PA, USA

© Springer Nature Switzerland AG 2020

P.-D. Ryu et al. (eds.), *Oxygen Transport to Tissue XLI*, Advances in Experimental Medicine and Biology 1232, https://doi.org/10.1007/978-3-030-34461-0_48

excitation 750 nm, blue emission filter; FAD channel: excitation 860 nm, green emission filter). We observed remarkable signals with significant intra-tissue heterogeneity in images of NADH, FAD and redox ratio (FAD/(NADH+FAD)), which are worthy of further investigation for extracting biological information.

Keywords Autofluorescence · NADH · FAD · Two photon imaging · Fixed tissue

1 Introduction

Optical redox imaging (ORI) or optical metabolic imaging (OMI) based on endogenous fluorescence signal sources including NADH and oxidized flavoproteins containing FAD have been increasingly employed for probing the metabolic/redox status of tissues and cells in order to understand disease pathology and develop tools for diagnosis and monitoring and predicting treatment response [1–6]. Optical redox ratio FAD/(NADH+FAD) is commonly used as an index sensitive to metabolic and redox status, and has been shown to correlate linearly with NAD^+/(NAD^++NADH) measured biochemically [7]. However, ORI is limited by the light penetration depth for tissue imaging with conventional fluorescence, confocal, or two-photon microscopes.

The 3D metabolic/redox indices (FAD, NADH, and redox ratio FAD/(NADH+FAD)) of deep tissues can be imaged by a cryogenic fluorescence imager (e.g. the Chance redox scanner [8, 9]) that is coupled to a cryostat or microtome with alternating tissue sectioning and imaging. Since NADH and FAD signals are labile with time in resected fresh tissue, tissue snap-freezing and imaging under cryogenic condition are used as necessary means to preserve or minimize the change of metabolism in tissue during sample harvesting, post-processing and imaging. Nevertheless, these procedures pose technical or operational challenges to applying ORI to clinical specimens.

In the clinic, paraffin embedded fixed tissue blocks and slides are widely available to provide pathophysiological evaluation. The long-term goal of this study is to evaluate whether ORI can be applicable to unstained fixed tissues so as to obtain metabolic/redox information that may potentially be clinically useful. We have reported some preliminary ORI results of formalin-fixed-paraffin-embedded unstained tissue slides using a conventional fluorescence microscope [10]. Here we present some ORI results for tissue blocks using two-photon microscopy.

2 Methods

Various fresh or frozen tissue blocks (size ~4 mm or less) including mouse organs and xenograft tumors were fixed in PFA (4%) for 24 h and then imaged on a STP Tomography scanner (TissueCyte® 1000, TissueVision Inc., Somerville, MA,

USA) [11–13]. Specifically, the formalin-fixed tissues were embedded in a 4.5% oxidized agarose block and was subsequently placed in a solution of 0.5% sodium borohydride in a 0.5 M sodium borate buffer to covalently link the tissue to the agarose. Tissue blocks were sectioned by a microtome to expose a surface plane for imaging. 2D or 3D imaging was achieved with the TissueCyte® 1000 coupled to a titanium sapphire laser (Spectra Physics InSight DeepSee™, Santa Clara, CA, USA) operating at 750 nm and 860 nm. A Nikon 16× 0.8 NA objective (Nikon, Melville, NY, USA) was used and the sampling resolution was 1.2 μm in the XY plane. The emitted fluorescent light was separated into three spectral channels: red (≥560 nm), green (500–560 nm), and blue (≤500 nm). Images generated from 750 nm excitation and blue emission corresponded to the NADH channel, whereas images with 860 nm excitation and green emission corresponded to the FAD channel. These images were post-processed with a customized Matlab® program to generate pseudocolor images of NADH, FAD and redox ratio FAD/(FAD+NADH).

3 Results and Discussion

Figure 1 shows the white light photo and 2D ORI images of a typical mouse muscle sample obtained by STP imaging. The muscle fiber structures are clearly seen. The ORI images of NADH and FAD demonstrate significant signal heterogeneities within the whole muscle. This is even clearer in the blown-up images such as a field of interest shown in Fig. 1d–f, indicating fibers with either high or low redox indices (FAD, NADH and redox ratio). Similar phenomena are observed in the ORI images of three additional muscle samples.

It is known that muscle fibers exhibit two major metabolic subtypes, i.e., glycolytic and oxidative with different mitochondrial functional phenotypes [14]. Since redox indices correlate with the metabolic state and oxygen consumption rate [1, 7, 15], it would be interesting to investigate whether and how the redox subtypes of the fixed muscle relate to the known metabolic subtypes.

Figure 2 shows the white light photo and ORI images of a liver sample from a mouse of 19 weeks old. In addition to the general intra-tissue heterogeneity across the whole sample, a new but very interesting phenomenon was observed as shown in the blown-up images of FOVs (Fig. 2 d–f). Both the FAD and NADH images exhibit scattered patterns indicating localized areas of high signals surrounded by areas of low signals. The size of these localized high-signal areas range from ~5–20 microns in NADH images and relatively less in FAD images. The distribution of these high-signal areas in FAD and NADH channels appears to be highly correlated but not fully matched in locations. This can be shown more clearly by the redox ratio image in Fig. 2e, in which a number of blue areas correlate spatially with the high intensity areas in FAD and NADH images. For such blue areas in the redox ratio image, we observed the dark blue regions indicating low FAD and high NADH and the light blue regions indicating high FAD and high NADH. Thus, there is a spatial mismatch between the high signal areas of FAD and NADH images.

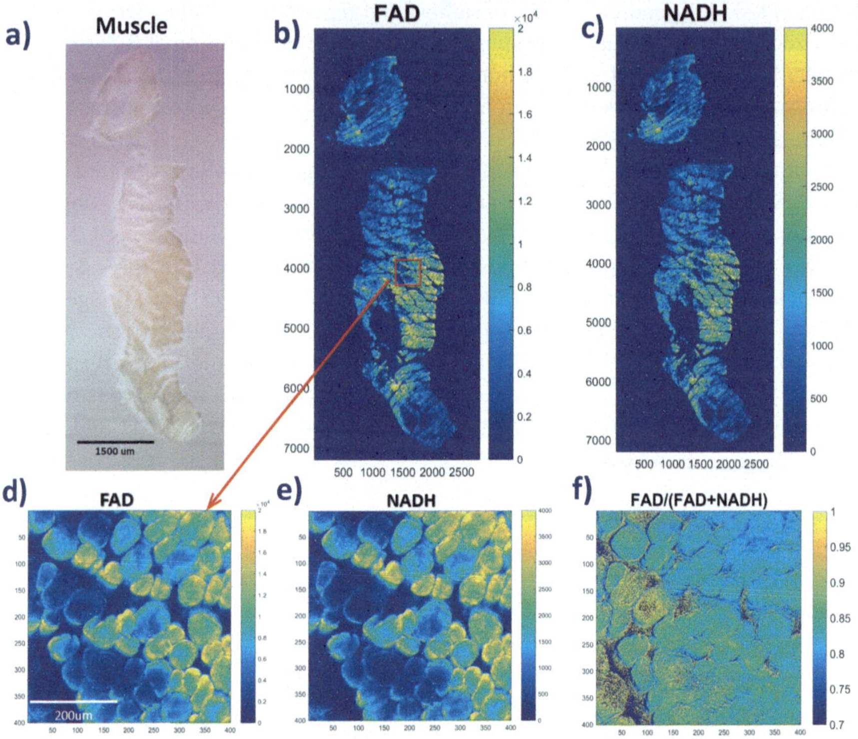

Fig. 1 ORI of a typical fixed mouse muscle block. (**a**) White light photo of the sample; (**b**) FAD and (**c**) NADH images for the sample; (**d–f**) FAD, NADH and redox ratios images, respectively, for a FOV blown-up from (**b**). The numbers below and on the left sides of individual images represent x and y coordinates of the image matrices. The color bars on the right sides of images indicate the ranges of displayed parameters

The ORI images from a mouse xenograft of human breast cancer MDA-MB-231 cell line are shown in Fig. 3. Again we can see significant intratumor heterogeneity for all three indices, i.e., FAD, NADH and redox ratio.

In summary, we have obtained high resolution autofluorescence images of fixed unstained tissue blocks and observed significant intra-tissue signal variations. It is known that mitochondria in cytosol account for the most of autofluorescence signals in the NADH and FAD channels [16], whereas nuclei should be relatively dark. The intratissue spatial heterogeneity of NADH and FAD signals have been reported in normal and cancer tissues imaged by cryogenic redox scanner [16, 17]. However, the interpretation of these spatial heterogeneity remains open. Other biological sources may contribute to these autofluorescence signals including NADPH, keratin, elastin, collagen, and lipofuscin [7, 18, 19]. More sophisticated imaging and data analysis approaches can be used to resolve specifically the NADH and FAD signals and exclude contributions from other sources [7, 18, 20]. Co-registration of autofluorescence imaging of tissue slides with H&E staining may also help to understand the histological basis of autofluorescence [21].

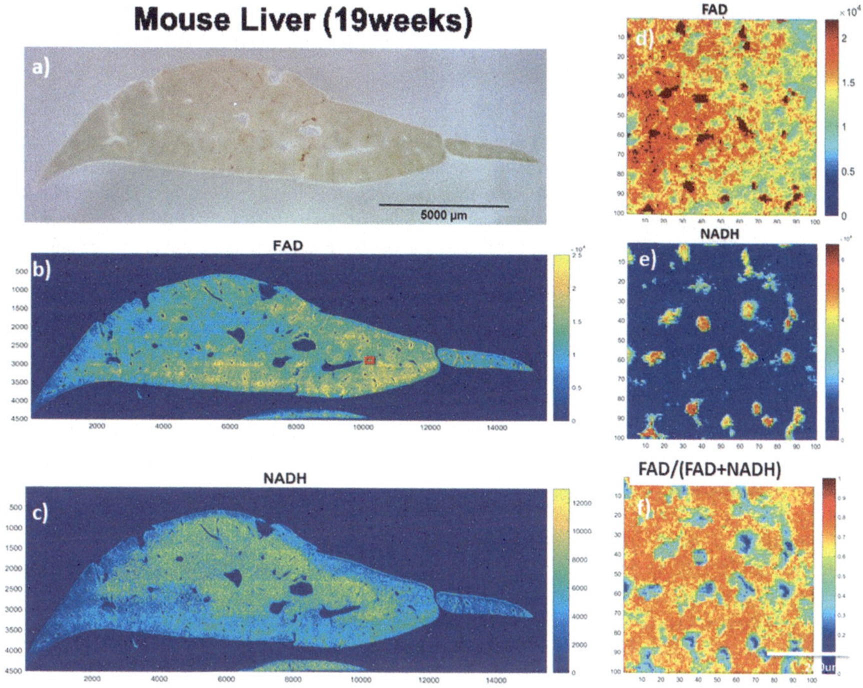

Fig. 2 Optical redox images of a fixed mouse liver sample from the two-photon scanner. (**a**) White light photo of the liver sample (19 weeks); (**b, c**) FAD and NADH images, respectively; (**d–f**) Blown-up FAD, NADH and redox ratios images, respectively, for an area of interest (100 × 100 pixel) marked as a red square in (**b**)

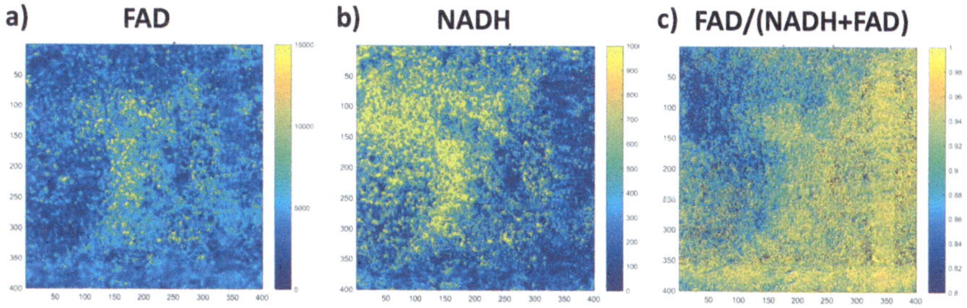

Fig. 3 FAD, NADH, and redox ratio images of a region of interest in a fixed mouse xenograft of human breast cancer MDA-MB-231 cells

Moreover, tissue NADH and FAD signals are expected to change due to the deprivation of oxygen during the period after death and before fixation. Fixation may further change the tissue micro- and ultra-structure, and autofluorescence intensity may depend on the tissue penetration speed and depth of fixatives. More studies are needed to understand the effects of tissue processing and PFA fixation on tissue autofluorescence [10], and to investigate whether these signals from fixed tissues may contain any biological or pathological information that could be useful for the clinic.

Acknowledgments We would like to thank Ms. Lily Moon, Ms. Min Feng and Dr. Karthikeyani Chellappa for preparation and handling of tissue samples. If there are any competing interest statements that are needed, I want like to note that Tim Ragan is an employee and shareholder of TissueVision Inc and Marissa Masek was an employee of TissueVision. TissueVision manufactures and sells the TissueCyte system on which some of the data taken in the paper was taken.

References

1. Chance B, Schoener B, Oshino R et al (1979) Oxidation-reduction ratio studies of mitochondria in freeze-trapped samples. NADH and flavoprotein fluorescence signals. Journal of Biological Chemistry 254:4764–4771
2. Li LZ, Zhou R, Xu HN et al (2009) Quantitative magnetic resonance and optical imaging biomarkers of melanoma metastatic potential. Proc Natl Acad Sci U S A 106:6608–6613
3. Li LZ, Xu HN, Ranji M et al (2009) Mitochondrial redox imaging for cancer diagnostic and therapeutic studies. J Innov Opt Health Sci 2:325–341
4. Georgakoudi I, Quinn KP (2012) Optical imaging using endogenous contrast to assess metabolic state. Annu Rev Biomed Eng 14:351–367
5. Walsh AJ, Cook RS, Sanders ME et al (2014) Quantitative optical imaging of primary tumor organoid metabolism predicts drug response in breast cancer. Cancer Res 74:5184–5194
6. Xu HN, Tchou J, Feng M et al (2016) Optical redox imaging indices discriminate human breast cancer from normal tissues. J Biomed Opt 21:114003
7. Varone A, Xylas J, Quinn KP et al (2014) Endogenous two-photon fluorescence imaging elucidates metabolic changes related to enhanced glycolysis and glutamine consumption in precancerous epithelial tissues. Cancer Res 74:3067–3075
8. Quistorff B, Haselgrove JC, Chance B (1985) High spatial resolution readout of 3-D metabolic organ structure: an automated, low-temperature redox ratio-scanning instrument. Anal Biochem 148:389–400
9. Gu Y, Qian Z, Chen J et al (2002) High-resolution three-dimensional scanning optical image system for intrinsic and extrinsic contrast agents in tissue. Rev Sci Instrum 73:172–178
10. Xu HN, Tchou J, Li Y et al (2018) Optical redox imaging of fixed unstained tissue slides to identify biomarkers for breast cancer diagnosis/prognosis: feasibility study. Proc SPIE 10472:104720U1–6
11. Ragan T, Kadiri LR, Venkataraju KU et al (2012) Serial two-photon tomography for automated ex vivo mouse brain imaging. Nat Methods 9:255–258
12. Amato SP, Pan F, Schwartz J et al (2016) Whole brain imaging with serial two-photon tomography. Front Neuroanat 10:31
13. Ragan T, Sylvan JD, Kim KH et al (2007) High-resolution whole organ imaging using two-photon tissue cytometry. J Biomed Opt 12:014015
14. Picard M, Hepple RT, Burelle Y (2012) Mitochondrial functional specialization in glycolytic and oxidative muscle fibers: tailoring the organelle for optimal function. Am J Physiol Cell Physiol 302:26
15. Hou J, Wright HJ, Chan N et al (2016) Correlating two-photon excited fluorescence imaging of breast cancer cellular redox state with seahorse flux analysis of normalized cellular oxygen consumption. J Biomed Opt 21:060503–060503
16. Xu HN, Li LZ (2014) Quantitative redox imaging biomarkers for studying tissue metabolic state and its heterogeneity. Journal of Innovative Optical Health Sciences 7:1430002

17. Xu HN, Zhou R, Moon L et al (2014) 3D imaging of the mitochondrial redox state of rat hearts under normal and fasting conditions. Journal of Innovative Optical Health Sciences 7:1350045
18. Xu Z, Reilley M, Li R et al (2017) Mapping absolute tissue endogenous fluorophore concentrations with chemometric wide-field fluorescence microscopy. J Biomed Opt 22:66009
19. Alzbeta C, Dusan C (2014) Tissue fluorophores and their spectroscopic characteristics. In: Fluorescence lifetime spectroscopy and imaging. CRC Press, pp 47–84
20. Blacker TS, Duchen MR (2016) Investigating mitochondrial redox state using NADH and NADPH autofluorescence. Free Radic Biol Med 100:53–65
21. Xu HN, Zhou R, Nioka S et al (2009) Histological basis of MR/optical imaging of human melanoma mouse xenografts spanning a range of metastatic potentials. Adv Exp Med Biol 645:247–253

Part VI
Special Topics

Acute Anemia Induces Erythropoiesis in Rat Organ Surface Primo-Vascular Tissue

Yiming Shen, Chae Jeong Lim, So Yeong Lee, and Pan-Dong Ryu

Abstract The primo-vascular system (PVS) is a newly identified vascular tissue composed of primo-nodes (PNs) and primo-vessels (PVs). Previously, we reported erythropoietic activity in the organ-surface PVS (osPVS) tissue of rats with heart failure. In this study, we further investigated whether acute anemia could induce erythropoiesis in the PVS of rats, based on the hypothesis that erythropoiesis in osPVS tissue is due to anemia accompanying heart failure. Acute anemia was induced by an intraperitoneal injection of phenylhydrazine (PHZ). Circulating red blood cells (RBCs) and hematocrit decreased by 31.6%, whereas reticulocytes and white blood cells increased at day 3 and day 6 after PHZ treatment. All these parameters recovered to control levels at day 10. At days 3 and 6, we observed an increase in the size of the PNs ($P < 0.05$), the number of the osPVS tissue samples per rat ($P < 0.01$), and the proportion of osPVS tissue samples with red chromophore ($P < 0.001$), which was from the RBCs in the PVS tissue. The number of RBCs, estimated from the PN sections stained with hematoxylin and eosin, increased at day 6 in the rats with anemia ($P < 0.01$). All these anemia-induced changes in the osPVS tissue recovered to the control levels by day 10. Taken together, the results showed that the morphological and cytological changes in the osPVS tissue appear to be related to the erythropoietic activity induced by acute anemia in rats. This study confirmed the previous findings that the osPVS can exert erythropoietic activity in disease states accompanied by anemia, such as heart failure.

Keywords Primo-node · Phenylhydrazine · Red blood cells · Hemolytic anemia · Hematopoiesis

Yiming Shen and Chae Jeong Lim contributed equally to this work.

Y. Shen · C. J. Lim · S. Y. Lee
Department of Veterinary Pharmacology, College of Veterinary Medicine and Research Institute for Veterinary Science, Seoul National University, Seoul, Republic of Korea

P.-D. Ryu (✉)
Department of Veterinary Pharmacology, College of Veterinary Medicine, Seoul National University, Seoul, Republic of Korea
e-mail: pdryu@snu.ac.kr

© Springer Nature Switzerland AG 2020

P.-D. Ryu et al. (eds.), *Oxygen Transport to Tissue XLI*, Advances in Experimental Medicine and Biology 1232, https://doi.org/10.1007/978-3-030-34461-0_49

1 Introduction

The primo-vascular system (PVS), which consists of primo-nodes (PNs) and primo-vessels (PV), is a novel circulatory system identified in various parts of the body, such as the abdominal organs, blood and lymphatic vessels, heart, brain, and subcutaneous layer [1, 2]. PNs are tightly filled with small round cells, including various white blood cells (WBCs), red blood cells (RBCs), mast cells and hematopoietic progenitor cells [3–5]. Currently, its structure and function is largely unknown. Previously, we reported morphological changes supporting erythropoietic activity in the organ-system PVS (osPVS) of rats with heart failure [10]. The number of RBCs and reticulocytes in the PNs of the osPVS of rats with heart failure was larger than that in the control rats. However, underlying mechanisms for such extramedullary erythropoiesis is not yet known.

Anemia frequently accompanies heart failure [6, 7]. Therefore, we hypothesized that anemia caused the erythropoiesis in the osPVS of the rats with heart failure. To test this hypothesis, we induced acute anemia in rats and then examined the morphological and cytological changes of the osPVS tissue in the rats with anemia. Acute hemolytic anemia was induced using phenylhydrazine (PHZ) [13]. PHZ induces the anemia through the oxidative stress causing the precipitation of hemoglobin, the lipid peroxidation, the damage of cell structure and membrane deformability reduction [14].

2 Material and Methods

Sprague-Dawley rats weighing 120–130 g (male, 5 weeks old; Orient Bio, Gyeonggi-do, Korea) were used in this study. The experiments were conducted in accordance with the Guide for the Laboratory Animal Care Advisory Committee of Seoul National University, and approved by the Institute of Laboratory Animal Resources of Seoul National University (SNU-180727-4).

The rats were randomly divided into a hemolytic anemia and a control group. PHZ was injected intraperitoneally to the rats in the hemolytic anemia group for 2 consecutive days at 40 mg/kg and the same volume of saline was injected to the control group rats.

For hematological tests, all rats were anesthetized with isoflurane. Blood samples (0.25–0.5 mL) were collected from the retro-orbital sinus in tubes with K_2EDTA (BD microtainer, USA) on the day before PHZ administration (or saline administration in the Control group), and on days 3, 6, and 10 after the first PHZ injection (Day 3, Day 6 and Day 10 group). Hematological parameters such as the RBC count, WBC count, hematocrit, and mean cell volume (MCV) were determined using a high-volume hematology analyzer (ADVIA 2120). The remaining blood samples were stained with new methylene blue for counting reticulocytes (%).

Organ surface PVS tissue samples were obtained from the control and anemic rats (at day 3, day 6, and day 10 after PHZ injection). Areas of milky-colored osPVS tissues were collected from the surface of abdominal organs of the rats under a stereomicroscope with ×10 magnification. The one unit of osPVS tissue was defined as a PVS tissue consisting of 1 or more PNs connected by a PV.

The PN size was estimated from the area of the tissue image using Image J software (NIH). Three PVS tissue samples from each group were sectioned from the paraffin block, and stained using hematoxylin and eosin (H&E) according to conventional protocols. All data are expressed as mean ± standard error. Student's t-test or the Fisher test were used to analyze the data. One-way analysis of variance with the Bonferroni post-test was used to determine the significance of the differences in hematological parameters among the 4 groups. The threshold for statistical significance was set at $P < 0.05$.

3 Results

The results were based on 143 osPVS tissue samples (control, 21; day 3, 52; day 6, 37; day 10, 33) from 5 rats in each group. The changes in hematological parameters are summarized in Fig. 1. There was a significant reduction in the number of RBCs

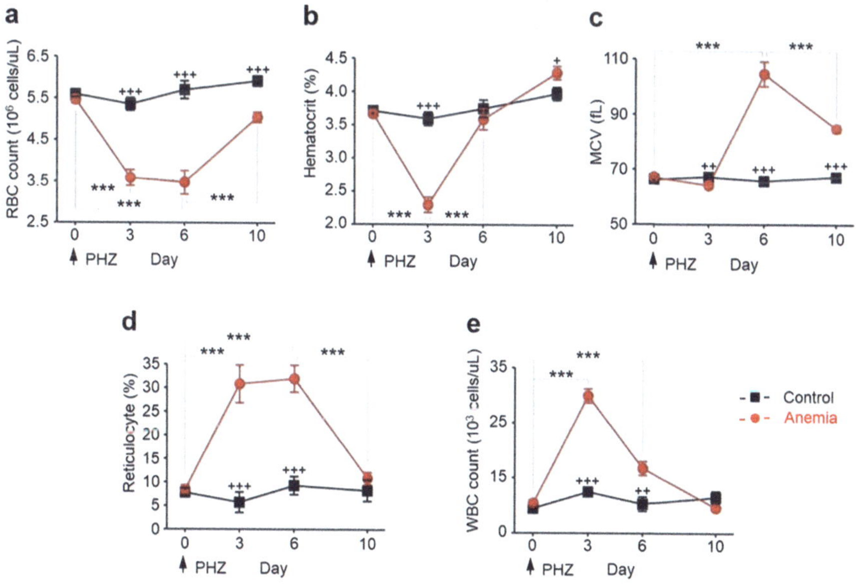

Fig. 1 Time course of RBC, hematocrit, MCV, reticulocyte (%), and WBC in saline-injected (n = 20, 5, 5, 6) and PHZ-injected (n = 21, 7, 6, 8) rats at day 0, day 3, day 6 and day 10 (a–e). The arrow was the PHZ injecting time. RBC (**a**) and hematocrit (**b**) were significantly decreased at day 3, the reticulocyte (**d**) and WBC (**e**) were significantly increased, and the MCV (**c**) increased at 6th day. All the parameters (a–e) were trend to be normal level at 10th day. The results are mean ± standard error. *** P<0.001 in PHZ-injected group. +P<0.05, ++ P<0.01 and +++ P<0.001 between saline-injected and PHZ-injected rats at same time point by Student's t-test

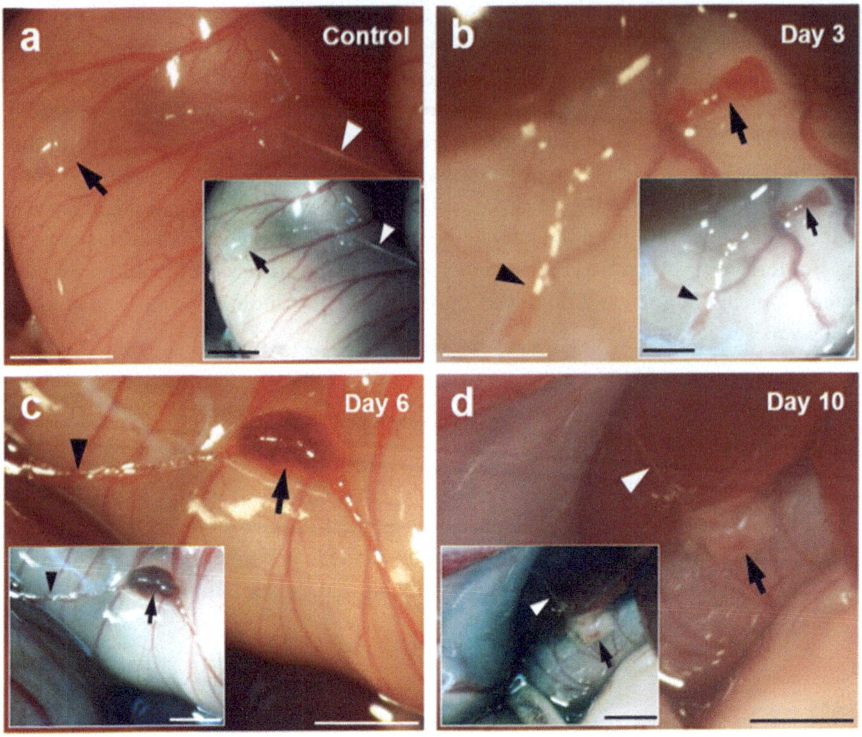

Fig. 2 Identification of osPVS tissue on the surface of the abdominal organs from control and anemic rats. **(a–d)** Representative examples of osPVS areas composed of a PN (arrowhead) and PV (arrow) on the surface of the small intestine from the control (**a**) and anemic rats at day 3 (**b**), day 6 (**c**), and day 10 (**d**). The insets in a-d were color-phase homogenized in GIMP version 2.10. The PNs were red at day 3 and day 6 after PHZ injection. In the control and PHZ injection groups, the size of the PNs was 1.057 (**a**), 1.462 (**b**), 2.146 (**c**), and 1.422 mm^2 (**d**). Scale bars: 2 mm

and hematocrit, and a significant increase in reticulocytes and WBCs at day 3 after PHZ injection. In contrast, the MCV was significantly increased at day 6 after PHZ injection. All these parameters ameliorated by day 10 after PHZ injection.

Figure 2 shows representative areas of osPVS identified on the surface of the small intestine from the control and anemia group rats. The PNs were enlarged and red at day 3 (Fig. 2b, arrow) and day 6 (Fig. 2c, arrow) after PHZ injection. Fig. 3 (a-d) shows isolated osPVS samples in phosphate-buffered saline solution from control and anemic rats. Cross-sectioned PN slices (4 μm) stained with H&E showed disseminated red chromophore from inside the osPVS at day 3 (Fig. 3f) and day 6 (Fig. 3 g). The total number of osPVS samples per rat was higher at day 3 ($n = 52$) than at day 6 ($n = 37$), at day 10 ($n = 33$), or in the control group ($n = 21$) (Fig. 3i). The proportion of osPVS tissue samples containing red chromophore reversibly increased at day 3, peaked at day 6, and then decreased at day 10 (control, 13.3% vs.

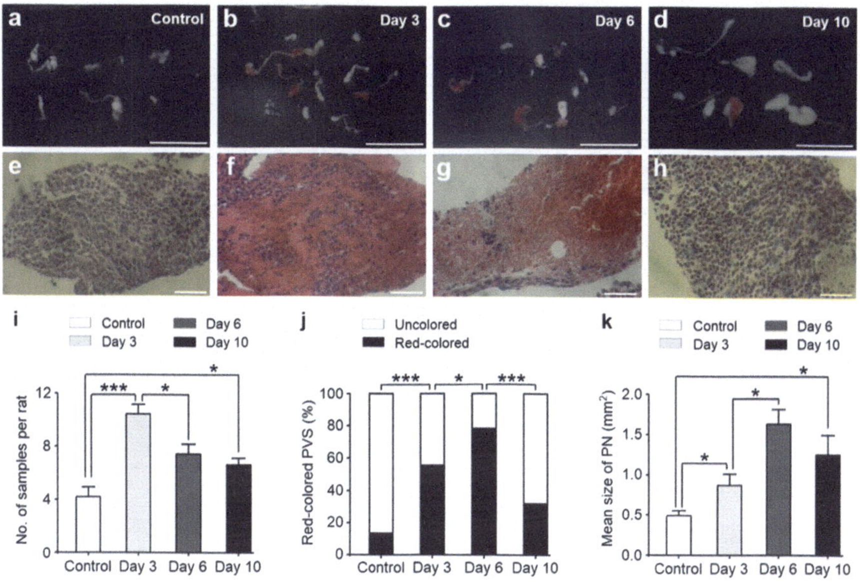

Fig. 3 Comparison of the morphological properties of osPVS tissue samples from control and anemic rats. **(a–d)** Collection of isolated intact PVS tissue samples in PBS solution from the control (a) and anemic rats at day 3 (**b**), day 6 (**c**), and day 10 (**d**) after PHZ injection. Scale bars: 5 mm. **(e–h)** Representative images (×200) of cross-sectioned PN slices (4 μm) stained using H&E from the control (**e**) and anemic rats at day 3 (**f**), day 6 (**g**) and day 10 (**h**) after PHZ injection. Scale bars: 50 μm. Note that the intensity of disseminated red chromophore is more strongly revealed in the PN from rats at day 3, 6, and 9 after PHZ injection. **(i–k)** Summary bar graphs showing the number of osPVS samples (**i**), the proportion of osPVS samples containing red chromophore (**j**), and the size of the PN (**k**) in control rats ($n = 21$ from 5 rats) and at day 3 ($n = 52$ from 5 rats), day 6 ($n = 37$ from 5 rats) and day 10 ($n = 33$ from 5 rats) after PHZ injection. Values are mean ± standard error. $*P < 0.05$, $***P < 0.001$, by Student's t-test or the Fisher test

day 10, 32.0%, $P > 0.05$) (Fig. 3j). In addition, the size of the PNs increased at day 3 and peaked at day 6, but decreased at day 10 (Fig. 3k) (control, 0.50 ± 0.06 vs. day 10, 1.25 ± 0.24, $P < 0.05$).

To further confirm the changes at the cytological level, we examined the cells in the osPVS tissue sections after H&E staining. Fig. 4 (a–d) illustrates the H&E stains of representative PN sections (4 μm) from rats in the control (Fig. 4a) and anemia (Figs. 4b–4d) groups. The level of red chromophore inside the osPVS tissue samples was remarkable at day 3 (Fig. 4b) and day 6 (Fig. 4c). The RBCs within the osPVS were spread throughout the tissue (Fig. 3f) or locally clustered (Fig. 4c). Single RBCs were identified at day 6, but not at day 3, in which dense overlapping of numerous RBCs made it difficult to distinguish their boundaries. Fig. 4e illustrates the 3 major cell groups identified in the osPVS tissue sections after H&E staining: RBCs, WBCs, and mast cells. The cells in the WBC category may include neutrophils, lymphocytes, eosinophils, and nucleated RBCs. RBCs and mast cells were

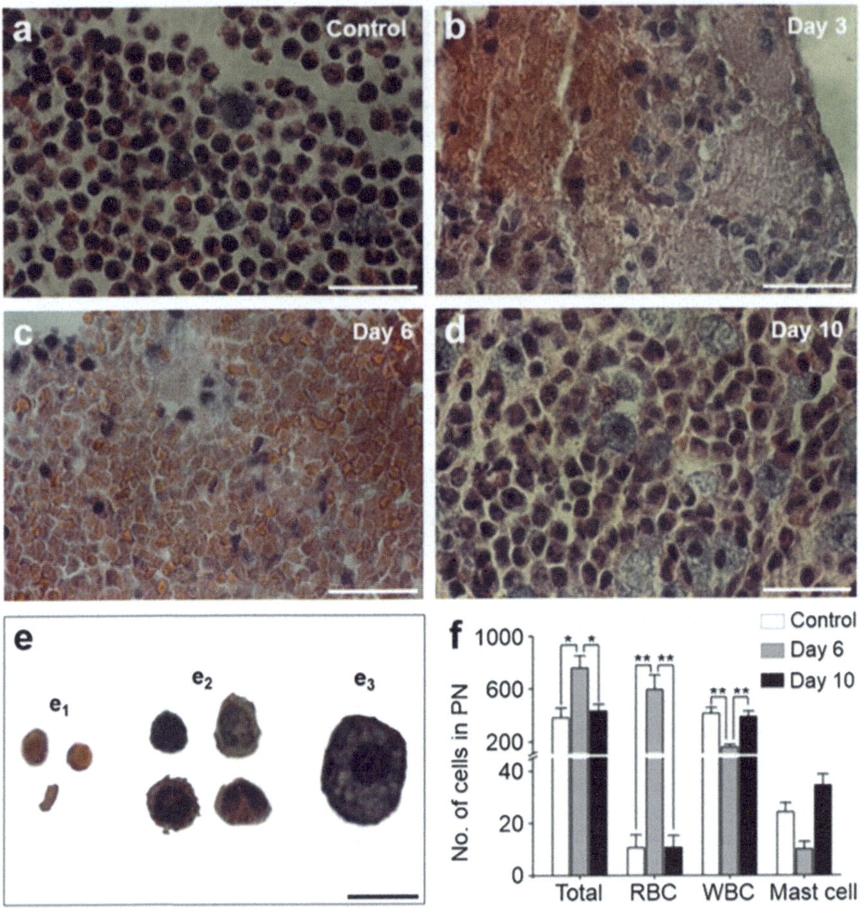

Fig. 4 Comparison of the cytological properties of the osPVS from control and anemic rats. **(a–d)** Representative images (×1000) of cross-sectioned PN slices (4 μm) stained using H&E from control rats (a) and anemic rats at day 3 (b), day 6 (c), and day 10 (d) after PHZ injection. Scale bars: 20 μm. **(e)** Three major groups of cells in the osPVS. Typical examples of RBCs (e_1), WBCs (e_2) and mast cells (e_3). Scale bar: 10 μm. **(f)** Summary bar graphs showing the number of cells in the osPVS in the control rats and at days 6 and 10 after PHZ injection. The number of cells was obtained from 3 rats. In each rat, a representative tissue section was selected and the cell numbers were counted in 3 rectangular fields (134 × 89 μm). Values are mean ± standard error. ***$P < 0.001$, by Student's t-test or the Fisher test

easily recognized by red chromophore without a nucleus and by their large size with typical granules, respectively [8]. The number of RBCs significantly increased, whereas the number of WBCs decreased at day 6 compared with the control group (Fig. 4f). The cell numbers had returned to the control level by day 10. There was no significant change in mast cells.

4 Discussion

In the present study, we found that erythropoietic morphological and cytological changes in the osPVS occurred in parallel with the progress of acute hemolytic anemia in the rats. In the acute anemia model used in this study, the hematological parameters showed an anemic state at days 3 and 6 after PHZ injection, followed by recovery to the control state at day 10. The osPVS in the rats with anemia showed a 2.5-fold increase in the number of samples taken from each rat, a 3.2-fold increase in the size of the PNs, a 5-fold increase in the proportion of the PNs with red chromophore, and a 55-fold increase in RBCs. All these morphological and cytological changes in the osPVS were recovered to control levels by day 10 after PHZ injection. Taken together, these findings indicate that the erythropoietic changes occurred in the osPVS tissue are likely due to the hemolytic anemia induced by PHZ.

In this study, the hematological parameters were recovered to control levels at day 10, and this observation is consistent with the previous report in mice [15]. In the present study, the number of RBC at day 6 was not restored, but the hematocrit is recovered to the control level. This result is considered due to the larger size of new RBCs since the MCV at day 6 is larger by 61% than those at day 0 and day 3 (Fig. 1a). This observation is also consistent with the findings of Higgins JM et.al [16].

Our observations further confirm previous reports in that the PVS can function as an erythopoietic tissue [5, 9]. In particular, known hematopoietic progenitors were identified in the osPVS [5]. Our findings may also provide the underlying mechanisms of the extra marrow erythropoiesis observed in the osPVS of heart failure rats [10]. It is of note that at day 3 it was difficult to count the number of RBCs in the PN sections stained with H&E, which indicates that the cytology of the PNs of osPVS tissue at day 3 is different from that at day 6. This could be due to the hemolysis of newborn RBCs in the osPVS, but further study is needed to fully understand the peculiar cytology at day 3 after PHZ injection (Fig. 4).

The results from previous studies showing an erythopoietic activity in the PVS of the heart failure rats [10] and the present study strongly indicate that the PVS may produce RBCs, like the bone marrow, when the number of circulating RBCs is reduced. In the bone marrow, reticulocytes increased at day 3 and returned to the control level at day 14 after PHZ treatment (50 mg/kg for 3 days) in rats [11], indicating that similar changes occur in both tissues.in hemolytic anemia. In addition to the erythropoiesis, the increase in the number of RBC and red chromophore could be also due to a translocation of the plasma RBC or the PHZ-induced cell-free haemoglobin, in particular at day 3. Further study is needed to determine whether the RBCs and the red chromophore observed in the osPVS of the PHZ-treated rats are locally originated, or translocated from the blood vessels.

In conclusion, we identified morphological and cytological changes supporting possible extra-marrow erythropoiesis in the osPVS in rats with PHZ-induced hemolytic anemia. These findings suggest that the PVS might be a site of extra-marrow hematopoiesis in certain disease states accompanied by anemia such as heart failure [12]. The physiological significance of the erythropoiesis in the PVS is remained to be studied further.

Acknowledgments This study was supported by the National Research Foundation of Korea funded by the Ministry of Education (2015R 1D 1A 1A02061732).

References

1. Soh KS (2009) Bonghan circulatory system as an extension of acupuncture meridians. J Acupunct Meridian Stud 2:93–106
2. Lim CJ, Lee SY, Ryu PD (2015) Identification of primo-vascular system in abdominal subcutaneous tissue layer of rats. Evid Based Complement Alternat Med 2015:13. https://doi.org/10.1155/2015/751937
3. Lee BC, Yoo JS, Ogay V et al (2007) Electron microscopic study of novel threadlike structures on the surfaces of mammalian organs. Microsc Res Tech 70:34–43
4. Lim CJ, Yoo JH, Kim Y et al (2013) Gross morphological features of the organ surface primovascular system revealed by hemacolor staining. Evid based complement Alternat med 2013:12. https://doi.org/10.1155/2013/350815
5. Hwang S, Lee SJ, Park SH et al (2014) Nonmarrow hematopoiesis occurs in a hyaluronic-acid-rich node and duct system in mice. Stem Cells Dev 1:2661–2671
6. Ruifrok WP, Qian C, Sillje HH et al (2011) Heart failure-associated anemia: bone marrow dysfunction and response to erythropoietin. J Mol Med (Berl) 9:377–387
7. Anand IS (2008) Anemia and chronic heart failure implications and treatment options. J Am Coll Cardiol 52:501–511
8. Eroschenko VP (2008) DiFiore's Atlas of Histology With Functional Correlations, 11th edn. Lippincott Williams & Wilkins
9. Kim BH (1965) Sanal and hematopoiesis. J Jo Sun Med 108:1–6
10. Lim CJ, Shen Y, Lee SY et al (2017) Potential erythropoiesis in the primo-vascular system in heart failure. Adv Exp Med Biol 977:409–415
11. Criswell KA, Sulkanen AP, Hochbaum AF et al (2000) Effects of phenylhydrazine or phlebotomy on peripheral blood, bone marrow and erythropoietin in Wistar rats. J Appl Toxicol 20(1):25–34
12. Orphanidou-Vlachou E, Tziakouri-Shiakalli C, Georgiades CS (2014) Extramedullary Hemopoiesis. Semin Ultrasound CT MR 35:255–262
13. Diallo A, Gbeassor M, Vovor A et al (2008) Effect of Tectona grandis on phenylhydrazine-induced anaemia in rats. Fitoterapia 79(5):332–336
14. Pandey K, Meena AK, Jain A (2014) Molecular mechanism of Phenylhydrazine induced Haematotoxicity: a review. Am J Phytomed Clin The 2(3):390–394
15. Angulo O, Gandrillon O, Crauste F (2018) Investigating the role of the experimental protocol in phenylhydrazine-induced anemia on mice recovery. J Theor Biol 437:286–298
16. Higgins JM (2015) Red blood cell population dynamics. Clin Lab Med 35(1):43–57

Analysis and Differential Expression of Primo Genes Using RNA-Seq and qRT-PCR Experiments

Jun-Young Shin, Jong-Ok Ji, Sang-Heon Choi, Da-Woon Choi, Ye-Jin An, Jae-Hyeok Seo, Jong-Gu Choi, Min-Suk Rho, Ji Yoon Lee, Sujung Yeo, and Sang-Suk Lee

Abstract Although the existence of the primo vasculature system has been shown in many species, including mice, rats, rabbits and humans, the biological role of this system, including expression of genes and proteins, has not yet been investigated. Especially the transcriptional action by mRNA, which is required for biological action, needs to be studied in primo vasculature biology. Differentially expressed genes in both isolated primo vessels and lymphatic vessels of rabbits were analyzed by RNA sequencing experiments. Primer efficiency and RNA purity of the primo vessels under lipopolysaccharides were confirmed prior to performing real-time qRT-PCR analysis following RNA extraction. We demonstrated that FLT4 was enriched in primo vessels and that several genes, including HSPH1 and EPHB2, were highly expressed in primo vessels compared with lymphatic vessels. Our data show that almost all genes, except HSPA4, were increased or sustained in isolated primo vessels compared with lymphatic vessels (FLT4 2.58 fold, HSPH1 1.83 fold, EPHB2 1.52 fold; whereas HSPA4 decreased 0.50 fold), suggesting primo vessels as a central regulator in diverse physiology. This implies that FLT4, HSPH1, and

J.-Y. Shin · S.-H. Choi · D.-W. Choi · Y.-J. An · J.-H. Seo · J.-G. Choi · M.-S. Rho
Department of Oriental Biomedical Engineering, College of Health Sciences, Sangji University, Wonju, Republic of Korea

J.-O. Ji
Goodpl Co., Ltd, Wonju, Republic of Korea

J. Y. Lee
Department of Biomedical Science, CHA Stem Cell Institute, CHA University, Pocheon, Gyeonggi-do, Republic of Korea

S. Yeo
Department of Meridian and Acupuncture, College of Korean Medicine, Sangji University, Wonju, Republic of Korea

S.-S. Lee (✉)
Department of Oriental Biomedical Engineering, Sangji University, Wonju, Republic of Korea
e-mail: sslee@sangji.ac.kr

© Springer Nature Switzerland AG 2020
P.-D. Ryu et al. (eds.), *Oxygen Transport to Tissue XLI*, Advances in Experimental Medicine and Biology 1232, https://doi.org/10.1007/978-3-030-34461-0_50

EPHB2 in high amounts may be involved in the functional activity of primo vessels. Our experimental data show that several genes are highly enriched in primo vessels in the lymphatic vessels of the rabbit.

Keywords FLT4 · RNA Seq · qRT-PCR · Primo vessel · Differentially expressed gene (DEG)

1 Introduction

The primo vascular system (also known as the Bong-Han circulatory system) is comprised of corpuscles and ducts, and is found in many species including mice, rats, rabbits and humans [1]. A primo vessel is considered to be a part of the vascular network within the human body that refers to meridians in oriental medicine. It has been shown that the primo vascular system (which consists of the anatomical vessel) exists in the form of a fine tube floating within lymphatic vessels [2]. However, since it is unknown whether very small primo vessels are more common in the lymphatic system, it is important to study the biological identification to enable improved understanding of the role of the primo vessel.

Previously, based on continuous dissection experiments in rabbits, we demonstrated that alcian blue (AB) staining visualizes the presence of smaller primo vessels in the lymphatic vessel [3], as also identified by others [1, 2]. Lymphatic vessels absorb lymphocytes and fats, maintain body fluid homeostasis, and play an essential role in immune function. An aim of the current study is to identify genes expressed by small primo vessels in the lymphatic system [4]. We investigated differentially expressed genes, including the lymphatic marker FLT4 gene, in the primo sample using RNA sequencing (Seq) followed by real-time reverse transcription polymerase chain reaction (RT-PCR) analysis of changes in the expression pattern of target genes due to inflammation induced by lipopolysaccharides (LPS).

2 Preparation of Sample and RNA-Seq Analysis

Protocols using New Zealand female rabbits were approved by the Institution of Animal Care and Use Committees of Sangji University. The rabbits used in the anatomical experiment were sacrificed by injecting 3.0 mL of a mixture Zoletil (2.5 ml) and Rumpun (0.5 ml) on the leg muscle. Especially, because the Zoletil reagent is classified controlled substance, we approved from Ministry of Food and Drug Safety, R.O.K. In this study, 200 μg/kg of LPS was injected into the lymphatic node near the abdominal vein of the rabbit. Immediately following injection of AB concentration and staining, the primo vessel was observed and extracted from inside the lymphatic vessel of the rabbit. The passed samples of two experimental groups on RNA-QC proceeded to the library construction stage automatically. For differential expression gene (DEG) analysis, gene level count data were generated using the HTSeq-count v0.5.4p3 tool, with the option '-m intersection-nonempty' and –r option considering paired-end sequence. Based on the calculated read count data, DEGs were identified using the R package, called TCC [5]. The TCC package applies robust normalization strategies to compare tag count data. Normalization factors were calculated using the iterative DEG elimination strategy/edgeR method. The Q-value was calculated based on the p-value using the p.adjust function of the R package with default parameter settings. DEGs were identified based on the q-value threshold of ≤0.05.

3 DEG Analysis in Primo and Lymphatic Vessels

Figure 1 shows the DEG analyses for the five genes obtained from the RNA-Seq data for: (i) lymphatic vessels including primo vessels, and (ii) the pure primo vessels of ten rabbits. Fragments per kilobase of exon per million (FPKM) as expression level is the average of duplicated experiments (at least two per experiment). FPKMs of FLT4, EPHB2, HSPH1, and HSPA4 were increased or decreased when compared with lymphatic vessels including primo vessels, and with pure primo vessels (Fig. 1). Similar to FLT4 and EPHB2, FPKM slightly decreased in pure primo vessels compared to lymphatic vessels including primo vessels. On the other hand, FPKMs of HSPH1 and HSPA4 were slightly and markedly increased in pure primo vessels, respectively.

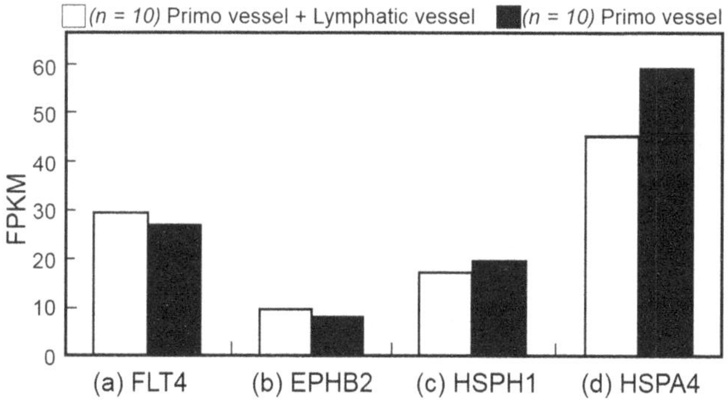

Fig. 1 DEG analysis of four genes of FLT4, EPHB2, HSPH1, and HSPA4. Expression level (FPKM) of gene markers in (□) lymphatic vessels including primo vessels and in (■) pure primo vessels. Samples were harvested and subjected to RNA-Seq. Each value is the average of duplicated experiments (at least two per experiment). The p-value for each gene is <0.05. FPKM, fragments per kilobase of exon per million

4 RNA Purity and Stability of Primo Vessels

Experimental procedures after RNA-Seq analysis were performed in the order of LPS injection: disease induction for 15 min, AB staining, primo vessel extraction, structural image acquisition, and real-time quantitative reverse transcription polymerase chain reaction (qRT-PCR) analysis. The primo circulatory system was successfully isolated from the lymphatic endothelium by AB staining of lymphatic nodes: Fig. 2(a), (b), and (c). We examined the expression of several lymphatic genes, including FLT4, in rabbit. On the basis of RNA-Seq analysis, several gene markers were selected to analyze qRT-PCR for the expression of genes in the pure primo and lymphatic vessels. Determination of the RNA extraction yield and purity of a small primo vessel was performed with measurement of candidate gene expression using qRT-PCR. The work described in this study was performed over a period of 14 days in three steps, i.e. rabbit preparation, dissection, and PCR analysis (Fig. 2). Images of (i) lymphatic vessels after LPS and AB injection in the vena cava lymphatic node of a rabbit, (ii) a floating primo vessel inside a lymphatic vessel, and (iii) an isolated primo vessel extracted from the lymphatic vessel are shown in Fig. 2(a), (b), and (c), respectively.

Because the primo vessel may be contaminated during separation from the lymphatic vessel, all manipulations were carefully performed using micro-forceps and scissors. The ratio of pure primo vessel to non-pure was 90%; 6 primo and lymphatic

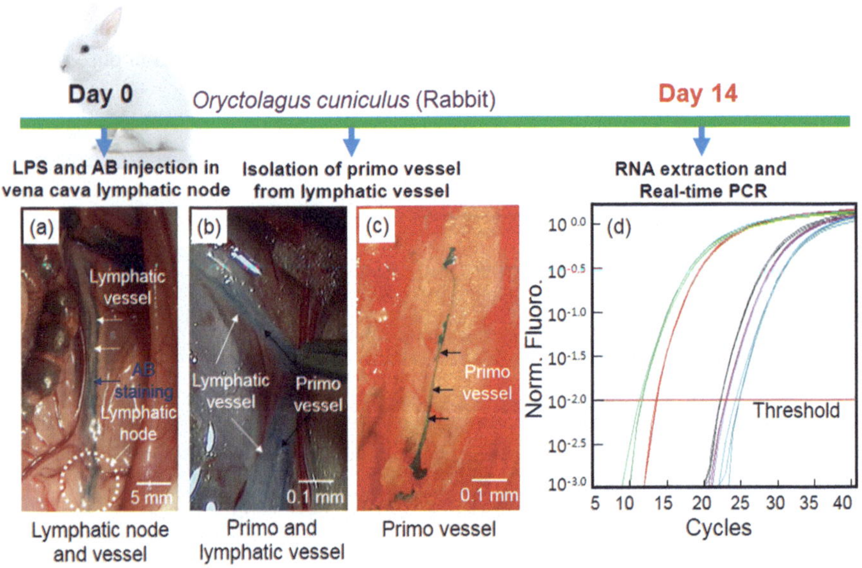

Fig. 2 Design of gene expression study of primo vessels in rabbit. (**a**) Image of lymphatic vessels after LPS and AB injection in a vena cava lymphatic node. (**b**) Image of a floating primo vessel inside a lymphatic vessel and (**c**) image of an isolated primo vessel extracted from a lymphatic vessel. (**d**) Amplification plots of normalized fluorescence versus number of cycles

Table 1 Data on RNA purity and stability from samples of (i) lymphatic vessels including primo vessels (n = 6) and (ii) pure primo vessels (n = 4)

Sample #	260/280*	Concentration (ng/μL)	GAPDH Curve	Sample type
1-1	2.00	276.661	21.85	Primo vessel + lymphatic vessel
1-2	1.99	62.200	20.40	
1-3	2.00	681.090	24.64	
1-4	2.01	539.064	22.58	
1-5	2.01	214.842	24.76	
1-6	2.03	134.769	23.20	
Mean			22.905	
2-1	1.99	859.765	26.18	Primo vessel
2-2	2.00	454.840	22.87	
2-3	2.02	681.759	20.63	
2-4	2.00	207.783	22.70	
Mean			23.095	

*The ratio of absorbance at 260 nm and 280 nm

vessels and 4 pure primo vessels were obtained from anatomical experiments using 10 rabbits for gene expression experiments. Data on RNA purity and stability from small primo vessels with a diameter ≤ 30 μm are presented in Table 1. The ratio of absorbance at 260 nm and 280 nm measured using a spectrophotometer was used to assess RNA purity, with a ratio of ~2.0 considered 'pure' RNA. Further, because the R^2 value of the primers used for gene expression analysis is 0.998, which is greater than a threshold of 0.98, the effectiveness of the primers is considered excellent. In this study, we used qRT-PCR to evaluate expression of marker genes in lymphatic and primo vessels following total RNA isolation and reverse transcription using samples from rabbit. Relative mRNA expression of the target gene was calculated using the comparative CT method, and two independent reactions were performed. Expression of all target genes was normalized to that of GAPDH expression. The difference in CT values for each target mRNA was calculated by subtracting the mean value of GAPDH expression (relative expression = $e^{-\triangle CT}$).

5 Gene Expression of Primo Vasculature in Lymphatic Vessels of Rabbits Stressed by LPS

FLT4, HSPH1, EPHB2, and HSPA4 are known well as markers for lymphatic endothelial cells (LECs). Fms related tyrosine kinase 4 (FLT4), heat shock protein H (HSPH1), EPH receptor B2 (EPHB2), and heat shock protein family A (Hsp70) member 4 (HSPA4), which are known to be expressed in the LV of rabbit, were investigated. The house keeping gene is Glyceraldehyde-3-phosphate dehydrogenase (GAPDH). The following three genes expressed in primo vessels were upregulated compared with primo and lymphatic vessels: FLT4, HPSH1, and EPHB2.

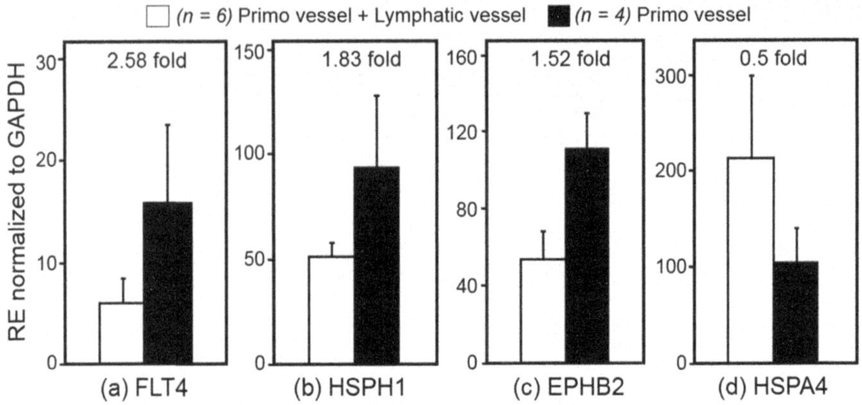

Fig. 3 Plots of target gene expression normalized to GAPDH showing upregulation of the genes, (**a**) FLT4, (**b**) HSPH1, and (**c**) EPHB2, and downregulation of the gene (**d**) HSPA4 in primo vessels versus lymphatic vessels including primo vessels. RE, relative expression. P-value is <0.05

Comparative expression of target genes, normalized to GAPDH as housekeeper gene, between the sample types is shown in Fig. 3(a), (b) and (c), and includes significantly increased expression in FLT4 (2.58 fold), HPSH1(1.83 fold), and EPHB2 (1.52 fold). In contrast, the decreased expression of HSPA4 (−0.5 fold) was found in primo vessels compared to lymphatic vessels including primo vessels.

The greatest expression change was found in FLT4 (also known as VEGFR-3), which was 2.58 times higher in primo vessels compared to lymphatic vessels including primo vessels. Based on this finding, the molecular function of FLT4 (which can be instigated by inflammation) may be greater in primo vessels than in lymphatic vessels, and indirectly suggests that, although FLT4 is a typical gene of the lymphatic vessels, it may play a greater role in primo vessels.

FLT4 (VEGFR-3) limits expression of the pseudotyrosine kinase 4 gene in the lymphatic endothelium [6]. These genes, such as FLT4, HSPH1, EPHB2 and HSPA4, are representative of those in rabbits that provide basic marker information for LECs [4, 6]. Genes expressed in stem cells and other related genes providing information on the lymphatic system in rabbits have been divided into three categories: (i) emerging marker genes for LECs, (ii) stem cell marker genes, and (iii) preliminary candidate genes for primo vessels. Although we will continue our evaluation of the function of major genes known in rabbit lymphatic nodes after this study, we investigated the background of FLT4 (VEGFR-3) which showed the greatest upregulation in the present study.

6 Conclusions

Primo vasculatures could be successfully isolated from floating lymphatic endothelium via LPS injection and AB staining of the lymphatic node in the vena cava of rabbit. Several gene markers were selected on the basis of RNA-Seq analysis for the pure primo vessels and the lymphatic vessels. RT-PCR following RNA extraction was performed using tiny primo vessels and lymphatic vessels. Primer efficiency and RNA purity were confirmed prior to qRT-PCR in 10 samples, consisting of 6 samples of lymphatic vessels containing primo vessels and 4 samples of pure primo vessels. Stable RNA extraction from tiny primo tissues was accomplished while maintaining a high level of purity. The FLT4 gene was enriched in primo vessels, and HPSH1 and EPHB2 genes were highly expressed in primo vessels compared with lymphatic vessels. Three target genes, with the exception of HSPA4, were increased in isolated primo vessels compared with those found in the lymphatic vessels. In addition, a classic marker for lymphatic endothelial cells, FLT4, showed the highest relative expression change in primo vessels under LPS conditions compared with lymphatic endothelium, suggesting an essential role of primo vessels in inflammation.

Acknowledgments This work was supported by the National Research Foundation of Korea (NRF) funded by the Korea government (Ministry of Science and ICT) under Grant No. 2016R1E1A2A01953467.

References

1. Soh KS (2009) Bonghan circulatory system as an extension of acupuncture meridians. J Acup Meridian Stud 2:93–106
2. Noh YI, Rho M, Yoo YM, Jung SJ, Lee SS (2012) Isolation and morphological features of primo vessels in rabbit lymph vessels. J Acupunct Meridian Stud 5:201–205
3. Lee HR, Rho M, Hong HJ, Ha YE, Kim JY, Noh YI, Park DY, Kim CK, Kim EJ, Jang IH, Kang SY, Lee SS (2015) Primo vessel stressed by lipopolysaccharide in rabbits. J Acupunct Meridian Stud 8:301–306
4. Shin JY, Ji JO, Choi DW, Choi SH, Choi JG, Rho M, Lee JY, Lee SS (2018) Expression of genes in primo vasculature floating in lymphatic endothelium under lipopolysaccharide and acupuncture electric stimulation. J Acupunct Meridian Stud 11. Online Published
5. Sun J, Nishiyama T, Shimizu K, Kadota K (2013) TCC: an R package for comparing tag count data with robust normalization strategies. BMC Bioinformatics 14:219–232
6. Lee JY, Kim HJ (2014) Lymph angiogenic influences on hematopoietic cells in acute myeloid leukemia. Exp Mole Med 46:122–132

Acupuncture Inhibits the Increase in Alpha-Synuclein in Substantia Nigra in an MPTP- Induced Parkinsonism Mouse Model

Sujung Yeo, Jongbeom Song, and Sabina Lim

Abstract Parkinson's disease, a progressive neurodegenerative disease, is caused by the loss of dopaminergic neurons in the substantia nigra (SN). It is characterized by the formation of intracytoplasmic Lewy bodies that are primarily composed of the protein alpha-synuclein (α-syn), along with dystrophic neurites. Acupuncture stimulation results in an enhanced survival of dopaminergic neurons in the SN in Parkinsonism animal models. We investigated the role of acupuncture in inhibiting the increase in α-syn expression that is related to dopaminergic cell loss in the SN in a chronic 1-methyl-4-phenyl-1,2,3,6-tetrahydropyridine (MPTP) Parkinsonism mouse model. In this model, acupuncture stimulation at GB34 and LR3 attenuated the decrease in tyrosine hydroxylase in the SN. Moreover, acupuncture stimulation attenuated the increase in α-syn in SN. Acupuncture stimulation also maintained the phosphorylated α-syn on serine 129 at levels similar to the control group. Our findings indicate that the MPTP-mediated increase in α-syn, and the acupuncture-mediated inhibition of the increase in α-syn, may be responsible for the neuroprotective effects of acupuncture in the SN following damage induced by MPTP.

Keywords Acupuncture · Alpha-synuclein · Parkinson's disease · GB34 · LR3

1 Introduction

Parkinson's disease (PD) is a progressive neurodegenerative disease that is caused by the loss of dopaminergic neurons in the substantia sigra (SN) [1]. It is characterized by the formation of intracytoplasmic Lewy bodies and dystrophic neurites

S. Yeo (✉) · J. Song
College of Korean Medicine, Sang Ji University, Wonju, Republic of Korea

S. Lim
Department of Meridian & Acupoint, College of Korean Medicine, Kyung Hee University, Seoul, Republic of Korea
e-mail: lims@khu.ac.kr

© Springer Nature Switzerland AG 2020

P.-D. Ryu et al. (eds.), *Oxygen Transport to Tissue XLI*, Advances in Experimental Medicine and Biology 1232, https://doi.org/10.1007/978-3-030-34461-0_51

[2, 3]. The Lewy bodies are primarily composed of the protein alpha-synuclein (α-syn) [4].

Animal models of Parkinsonism have been produced by using neurotoxic compounds such as 1-methyl-4-phenyl-1,2,3,6-tetrahydropyridine (MPTP) [5]. In the process, after MPTP is transformed into 1-methyl-4-phenylpyridinium ion (MPP+) by the monoamine oxidase B (MAO-B) in glial cells, toxic MPP+ is released and transported into dopaminergic neurons through the dopamine transporters [6]. The uptake and accumulation of MPP+ in the dopaminergic neurons results in the impairment of mitochondrial function and ATP synthesis, and the aggregation of α-syn, which is widely recognized as the most prominent element of the Lewy body [4, 7].

A previous study found that acupuncture stimulation at acupoints GB34 and LR3 results in the enhanced survival of dopaminergic neurons in the SN and an approximately 87.7% improvement in motor dysfunction in a 6-OHDA-induced Parkinsonism model [8]. Similar observations were made following MPTP administration, where the acupuncture-induced enhancement of synaptic dopamine availability may play a critical role in the observed motor function improvement [9]. Based on the literature, we hypothesized that acupuncture stimulation causes inhibition of the increase in α-syn expression, which is an important event associated with PD, and dopaminergic cell loss in the SN.

2 Methods

2.1 Animal and MPTP Model

Six-week-old male inbred C57BL/6 mice (Samtaco, Korea) were divided into the following four groups: (i) control (CTL); (ii) MPTP-treatment only (MPTP); (iii) MPTP and acupuncture treatment at GB34 and LR3 (MPTP-A); (iv) and MPTP and acupuncture treatment at non-acupoints (MPTP-NA, $n = 6$ in each group). The mice in the control group were intraperitoneally injected with saline 0.9% (100 μl) once daily for 28 days. The mice in the MPTP group were intraperitoneally injected with MPTP-HCl (20 mg/kg of free base) dissolved in saline 0.9% (100 μl) at 24 h intervals for 28 days.

2.2 Acupuncture Administration

Acupuncture was performed manually 2 h after the first MPTP injection and at 48-h intervals thereafter for a total of 14 sessions. The acupuncture needles were inserted bilaterally to depths of 1 mm at LR3 and 3 mm at GB34 before being turned at a rate of two spins per second for 15 s. In the non-acupoints group, the needles were inserted to a depth of 3 mm on both sides of the hips.

2.3 Western Blot

The striatum (ST) and substantia nigra (SN) regions were homogenized in 20-mM radioimmunoprecipitation assay buffer (RIPA). After centrifugation at 12,000 rpm at 4 °C for 20 min, the supernatant soluble samples of equal protein concentration were separated by a 12% sodium dodecyl sulfate-polyacrylamide gel electrophoresis (SDS-PAGE), and then transferred to the nitrocellulose membranes (Pharmacia Biotech, USA). The membranes were blocked and then incubated with the specific antibodies, anti-TH (1:2000; Santa Cruz Biotechnology, USA), phosphorylated-α-syn (p-α-syn, 1:1000) or anti-α-syn antibody (1:500; Abcam, Cambridge, UK). The band intensity of the detected proteins was measured by densitometry. β-actin was used as an internal control.

2.4 Immunohistochemistry

After 28 days, the brains were immediately removed, postfixed in a 0.05 M sodium phosphate buffer containing 4% paraformaldehyde for 12 h at 4 °C, rinsed with a 0.05 M sodium phosphate buffer, dehydrated with sucrose for 24 h at 4 °C, and then cryosected. The sections that encompassed the entire ST or SN regions were incubated with 3% H_2O_2 in PBS (pH 7.4), exposed to 3% BSA and 0.3% Triton X-100 in PBS for 1 h for blocking, and then treated with an avidin/biotin blocking kit (Vector Laboratories, CA) to block the endogenous avidin and biotin. When using the monoclonal IgG, the sections were treated with an M.O.M mouse Ig blocking reagent (Vector Laboratories, CA) at room temperature prior to the incubation with the primary antibodies. Thereafter, each section was stained at 4 °C.

2.5 Immunofluorescence

After having been incubated with the primary antibodies and then a biotinylated anti-mouse IgG, each section was treated with a Fluorescein Avidin DCS (Vector Laboratories, CA). The sections were then additionally treated with an avidin/biotin blocking kit and an M.O.M mouse Ig blocking reagent (Vector Laboratories, CA), after which they were stained with anti-α-syn or anti-p-α-syn IgG at 4 °C overnight. Each section was treated with a biotinylated antimouse IgG, followed by incubation with Rhodamine Avidin D (Vector Laboratories, CA).

2.6 Statistical Analysis

Statistical analysis was performed by a student t-test or ANOVA. All values are expressed as a percentage of the mean ± standard error.

3 Results

3.1 *Parkinsonism Mouse Model and the Ameliorative Effects of Acupuncture*

To verify the establishment of a chronic MPTP-induced Parkinsonism mouse model, we first evaluated the change in the expression of tyrosine hydroxylase (TH) because its expression has been found to be significantly reduced in the brains of Parkinsonism animals [10, 11]. TH is the enzyme responsible for catalyzing the conversion of the amino acid L-tyrosine to L-3,4-dihydroxyphenylalanine [12, 13]. TH was noticeably lower in the striatal (ST) and SN pars compacta (SNpc) regions in the MPTP group (Figs. 1b and f) than in the control group (Figs. 1a and e). Acupuncture stimulation at GB34 and LR3 (MPTP-A) attenuated the decrease in TH in both areas (Figs. 1c and g), but acupuncture at non-acupoints (MPTP-NA) did not similarly influence TH (Fig. 1d and h). In concordance with the immunohistochemical observations, immunoblot analyses also showed that the significant decrease in TH (p-value <0.05) in the ST and SNpc regions in the brains of MPTP mice (Fig. 1b) was significantly inhibited by acupuncture at acupoints (MPTP-A, Fig. 1c) but not at non-acupoints (MPTP-NA; Fig. 1d). These results confirm that acupuncture stimulation suppresses the pathological change in TH levels in the ST and SNpc regions that is induced by MPTP. Immunoblot analyses showed that the reversal of the MPTP-mediated decrease in TH expression was maintained in MPTP-A (Fig. 1I, $p < 0.05$), and this effect was significant compared to the MPTP condition.

3.2 *Changes of α-Syn Expression and the Ameliorative Effects of Acupuncture*

As in the immunohistochemical observations, immunoblot analyses showed that the significant increase in α-syn in the ST ($p < 0.005$) and SN ($p < 0.0005$) regions of mice treated with MPTP (Figs. 2b, f and j) was significantly inhibited by acu-

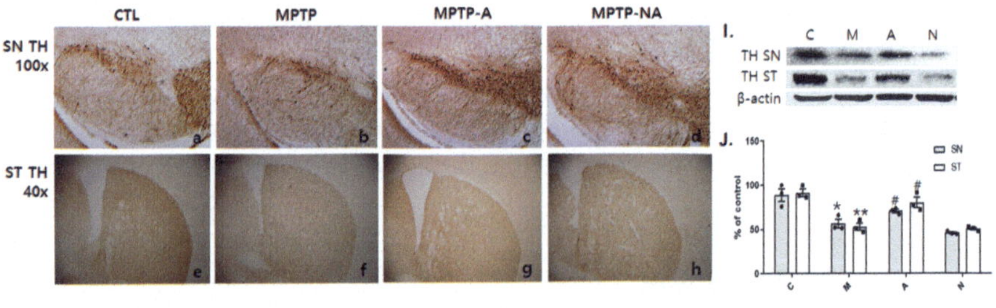

Fig. 1 Dopaminergic cell expression is maintained by acupuncture in a chronic MPTP-induced Parkinsonism model. The substantia nigra (SN, a–d) and striatum (ST, e–l) were immunostained using an anti-tyrosine hydroxylase (TH; a–d, 100×; e–h, 40×) antibody. Immunoblot analyses (I) showed that TH expression decreases of MPTP was maintained in MPTP-A; these were statistically significant compared to the MPTP that was normalized to 100% of control (J)

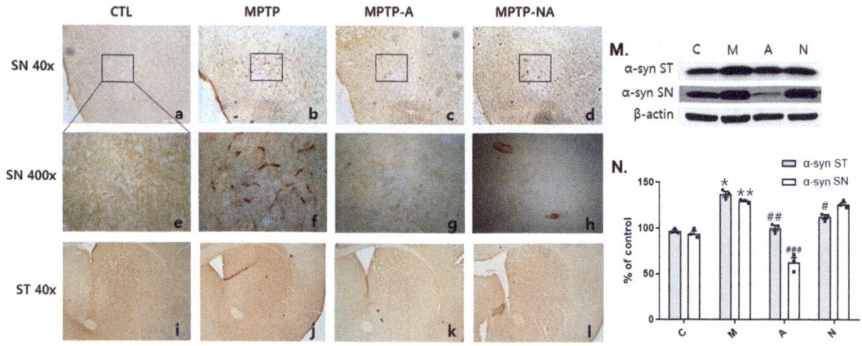

Fig. 2 Alpha synuclein (α-syn) expression and fibrillation are suppressed by acupuncture in a chronic MPTP-induced Parkinsonism model. The substantia nigra (SN, a–h) and striatum (ST, i–l) were immunostained using an anti-alpha synuclein (a–d, i–l, 40×; e–h, 400×) antibody. Immunoblot analyses (M) showed that α-syn expression increases of MPTP was inhibited in MPTP-A; these were statistically significant compared to the MPTP that was normalized to 100% of control (N). A $* p < 0.005$ compared to control, a $** p < 0.0005$ compared to control, a # $p < 0.005$ compared to MPTP, a ## $p < 0.001$ compared to MPTP and a ### $p < 0.0005$ compared to MPTP were considered significant

puncture at acupoints (ST, $p < 0.001$ and SN, $p < 0.0005$; Figs. 2c, g and k) but not when acupuncture was performed at non-acupoints (MPTP-NA; Figs. 2d, h and l). These results confirm that acupuncture stimulation suppresses the pathological change in α-syn levels induced by MPTP in the ST and SN.

3.3 Changes in Phospholylated Alpha Synuclein Expression and the Attenuative Effects of Acupuncture

Phosphorylated-α-syn (p-α-syn) expression was maintained by acupuncture. The SN (a-d) was immunofluorescently labeled with NF-1G anti-p-α-syn antibody. Western immunoblot analyses (I) showed that p-α-syn expression changes of MPTP was maintained in MPTP-A. Acupuncture stimulation inhibited the decrease in p-α-syn 32 (dimer, 32 kDa, $p < 0.001$) that was induced by MPTP ($p < 0.05$). Moreover, acupuncture stimulation inhibited an increase in p-α-syn 16 (monomer, 16 kDa, $p < 0.05$) at a level similar to the control. Thus, acupuncture stimulation attenuated the phosphorylation of α-syn. Previous research has shown that patients with PD have abnormal p-α-syn levels [14, 15]. Moreover, it is reported that p-α–syn increased α-syn fibrillization [16] and correlated with α-syn inclusion formation [17]. Stimulation with acupuncture maintained p-α-syn at levels comparable to control, suggesting that acupuncture stimulation confers neuroprotective effects (Fig. 3).

The p-α-syn 32 values devided by total α-syn values were maintained by acupuncture at the similar level to control (Fig. 4). It is thought that acupuncture stimulation might control the p-α-syn 32 values so as to have neuroprotective effects.

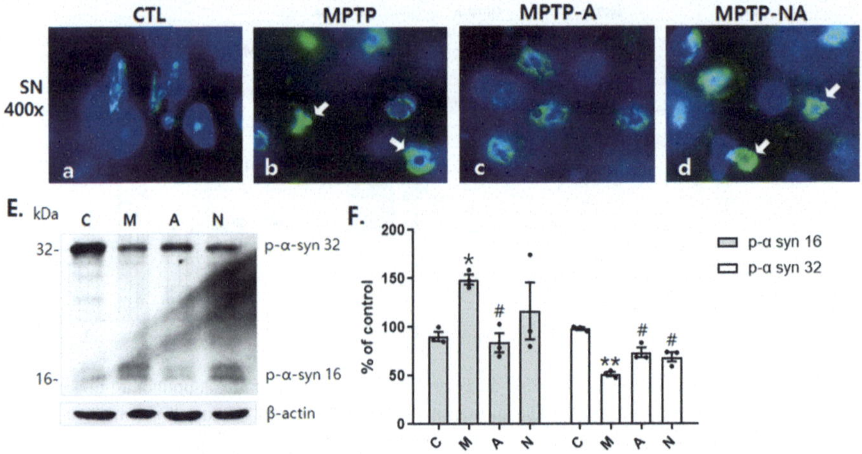

Fig. 3 Phospholylated alpha-synuclein (p-α-syn) expression is maintained by acupuncture in a chronic MPTP-induced Parkinsonism model. The substantia nigra (a–d) was immunofluorescently labeled with NF-1G anti-p-α-syn (a–d, 400×, blue is DAPI nuclear counter-stain). Immunoblot analyses (E) showed that p-α-syn expression changes of MPTP was maintained in MPTP-A; these were statistically significant compared to the MPTP that as normalized to 100% of control (F). A ∗ $p < 0.05$ compared to control, a ∗∗ $p < 0.001$ compared to control and a # $p < 0.05$ compared to MPTP were considered significant

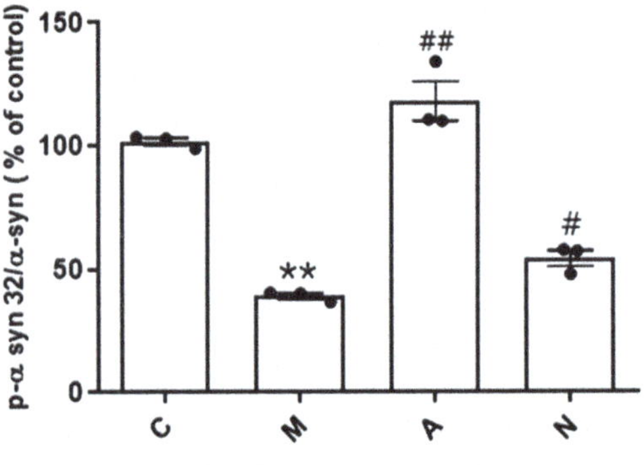

Fig. 4 Phospholylated alpha-synuclein dimer (p-α-syn 32) values devided by total α-syn values were maintained by acupuncture at the similar level to control in a chronic MPTP-induced Parkinsonism model. A ∗∗ $p < 0.0005$ compared to control, a # $p < 0.05$ compared to MPTP and ## $p < 0.001$ compared to MPTP were considered significant

4 Conclusions

Patients with Parkinson's disease are treated with levodopa medication [18] or brain surgery [19, 20]. However, medicine and surgery are only for symptom relief, but it is not the fundamental treatment. Up to 50% of PD patients experience dyskinesia or motor fluctuations within 5 years from the onset of levodopa medication [18]. Acupuncture stimulation controlled α-syn and phosphorylated α-syn in a manner that promoted neuroprotection. Our study suggests a role of acupuncture in the control of α-syn expression in the chronic MPTP-induced Parkinsonism mouse model. Acupuncture stimulation has been reported to have a therapeutic value for other neurodegenerative diseases, including PD, and our results suggest a mechanism for this effect. Our research provides support for the observation that acupuncture stimulation may be an important therapeutic avenue that could be explored in patients with PD and other α-syn-related diseases.

Acknowledgments This research was supported by Sangji University Research Fund, 2016.

References

1. Barzilai A, Melamed E (2003) Molecular mechanisms of selective dopaminergic neuronal death in Parkinson's disease. Trends Mol Med 9:126–132
2. Jellinger KA (1991) Pathology of Parkinson's disease. Changes other than the nigrostriatal pathway. Mol Chem Neuropathol 14:153–197
3. Kalia LV, Lang AE (2015) Parkinson's disease. Lancet 386:896–912
4. Shults CW (2006) Lewy bodies. Proc Natl Acad Sci U S A 103:1661–1668
5. Emborg ME (2007) Nonhuman primate models of Parkinson's disease. ILAR J 48:339–355
6. Schmidt N, Ferger B (2001) Neurochemical findings in the MPTP model of Parkinson's disease. J Neural Transm (Vienna) 108:1263–1282
7. Choi YG, Lim S (2010) N(varepsilon)-(carboxymethyl)lysine linkage to alpha-synuclein and involvement of advanced glycation end products in alpha-synuclein deposits in an MPTP-intoxicated mouse model. Biochimie 92:1379–1386
8. Park HJ, Lim S, Joo WS et al (2003) Acupuncture prevents 6-hydroxydopamine-induced neuronal death in the nigrostriatal dopaminergic system in the rat Parkinson's disease model. Exp Neurol 180:93–98
9. Kim SN, Doo AR, Park JY et al (2011) Acupuncture enhances the synaptic dopamine availability to improve motor function in a mouse model of Parkinson's disease. PLoS One 6:e27566
10. Kang JM, Park HJ, Choi YG et al (2007) Acupuncture inhibits microglial activation and inflammatory events in the MPTP-induced mouse model. Brain Res 1131:211–219
11. Yeo S, An KS, Hong YM et al (2015) Neuroprotective changes in degeneration-related gene expression in the substantia nigra following acupuncture in an MPTP mouse model of parkinsonism: microarray analysis. Genet Mol Biol 38:115–127
12. Kaufman S (1995) Tyrosine hydroxylase. Adv Enzymol Relat Areas Mol Biol 70:103–220
13. Nagatsu T (1995) Tyrosine hydroxylase: human isoforms, structure and regulation in physiology and pathology. Essays Biochem 30:15–35
14. Foulds PG, Diggle P, Mitchell JD et al (2013) A longitudinal study on alpha-synuclein in blood plasma as a biomarker for Parkinson's disease. Sci Rep 3:2540
15. Tenreiro S, Eckermann K, Outeiro TF (2014) Protein phosphorylation in neurodegeneration: friend or foe? Front Mol Neurosci 7:42
16. Fujiwara H, Hasegawa M, Dohmae N et al (2002) Alpha-Synuclein is phosphorylated in synucleinopathy lesions. Nat Cell Biol 4:160–164
17. Zabrocki P, Bastiaens I, Delay C et al (2008) Phosphorylation, lipid raft interaction and traffic of alpha-synuclein in a yeast model for Parkinson. Biochim Biophys Acta 1783:1767–1780

18. Lewitt PA (2008) Levodopa for the treatment of Parkinson's disease. N Engl J Med 359:2468–2476
19. Lang AE, Widner H (2002) Deep brain stimulation for Parkinson's disease: patient selection and evaluation. Mov Disord 17(Suppl 3):94–101
20. Obeso JA, Olanow CW, Rodriguez-Oroz MC et al (2001) Deep-brain stimulation of the subthalamic nucleus or the pars interna of the globus pallidus in Parkinson's disease. N Engl J Med 345:956–963

On the Biomarkers of Alzheimer's Disease

Timon Cheng-Yi Liu, Tao Zheng, Rui Duan, Ling Zhu, and Quan-Guang Zhang

Abstract Nakamura et al. examined the evidence, using a discovery and a validation database, that amyloid-β precursor protein $(APP)_{669-711}$/amyloid-β $(A\beta)_{1-42}$ and $A\beta_{1-40}/A\beta_{1-42}$ ratios, and composites based on traditional statistics; they concluded that these may be useful as biomarkers of Alzheimer's Disease (AD). We reexamined the same datasets, each of which included cognitively normal individuals (CN), individuals with mild cognitive impairment (MCI) and individuals with AD. We used fractal self-similar analyses and reexamined their data from (1) the Japanese National Center for Geriatrics and Gerontology (NCGG) (discovery database) and (2) the Australian Imaging, Biomarker and Lifestyle Study of Ageing (AIBL) cohort (validation database). Results: Using our methods, the three groups of individuals were found to be self-similar, i.e., they could not be differentiated quantitatively, in contrast to the findings of Nakamura et al. Conclusion: Appropriate biomarkers need further study. Our results suggest that $APP_{669-711}/A\beta_{1-42}$ and $A\beta_{1-40}/A\beta_{1-42}$ ratios and their composites may not be valid biomarkers of AD, when reexamined using fractal methods for comparing biomarkers across populations.

Keywords Alzheimer's disease · Biomarker · Self-similarity · Topology · Homeostasis

1 Introduction

The potential contribution of impaired oxygen delivery to the brain causing neuronal dysfunction associated with Alzheimer's disease (AD) has been considered an important factor in AD [6], but supportive biomarker information is needed.

Timon Cheng-Yi Liu, Tao Zheng, Rui Duan contributed equally to this work.

T. C.-Y. Liu (✉) · T. Zheng · R. Duan · L. Zhu · Q.-G. Zhang
Laboratory of Laser Sports Medicine, South China Normal University, Guangzhou, Guangdong, China
e-mail: liutcy@scnu.edu.cn

© Springer Nature Switzerland AG 2020

P.-D. Ryu et al. (eds.), *Oxygen Transport to Tissue XLI*, Advances in Experimental Medicine and Biology 1232, https://doi.org/10.1007/978-3-030-34461-0_52

Nakamura et al. found that the biomarkers of AD may be amyloid-β precursor protein $(APP)_{669-711}$/amyloid-β $(A\beta)_{1-42}$ and $A\beta_{1-40}/A\beta_{1-42}$ ratios, and their composites by using two independent datasets: a discovery dataset from the Japanese National Center for Geriatrics and Gerontology (NCGG) and a validation dataset derived from the Australian Imaging, Biomarker and Lifestyle Study of Ageing (AIBL) cohort, each of which included cognitively normal individuals (CN), individuals with mild cognitive impairment (MCI) and individuals with AD (AD) [7]. However, although the BACE inhibitors successfully blocked the accumulation of amyloid protein in mice, they seemed to worsen cognitive decline and brain shrinkage in people in three recent large, late-stage clinical trials. Their data analysis was based on p-values, the 'gold standard' of statistical validation; however, p-values are not always as reliable as many scientists have assumed [5]. Here, we re-analyze their data in terms of fractal self-similarity and quantitative difference (QD), a novel algorithm recently developed by us [4, 5]. However, our analysis did not support their conclusions.

2 Self-Similarity

Self-similarity was studied in the fractal literature: a pattern is self-similar if it does not vary with spatial or temporal scale. A self-similarity condition leads to the power law between two parameters [1, 8] x and y, $y = ax^{SSE}$, in which the exponent was called the self-similar exponent (SSE) between x and y. For the first-order self-similarity, SSE = 1. We have.

$$y / x = a \tag{1}$$

The power law and (Eq. 1) hold exactly true in physics [1, 8], but could be approximately true in biology in terms of QD [4, 5]. For a process of function x from x_1 to x_2, the process logarithm, $l_x(1,2)$ and its QD, $|l_x(1,2)|$, were introduced to represent the process [4, 5], where lt is the logarithm to base τ:

$$l_x(1,2) = \mathrm{lt}(x_2 / x_1) = \log_\tau(x_2 / x_1), \tau = \left(\sqrt{5}-1\right)/2 \approx 0.618 \tag{2}$$

There is QD threshold $(\alpha_x, \beta_x, \gamma_x)$ of a function x. It is $(0.268, 0.805, 1.221)$ for the molecular data sets AIBL and NCGG in Table 1. The function x is kept to be constant if $|l_x(1,2)| < \alpha_x$. In a biological system, negative feedback response can maintain a biological function that can be performed perfectly under certain condition. We have defined such a condition as function-specific homeostasis (FSH). A function in/far from its FSH is called a normal/dysfunctional function. A normal function can resist a disturbance under its threshold so that $|l_x(1,2)| < \beta_x$. A dysfunctional function is defined as the QD is significant if $\beta_x \le |l_x(1,2)| < \gamma_x$ and

Table 1 Group averages of seven parameters from AIBL and NCGG

	AIBL CN	AIBL MCI	AIBL AD	NCGG CN	NCGG MCI	NCGG AD
$A\beta_{40}$	8.0559	8.0857	8.2649	9.2150	8.8744	6.9785
$A\beta_{42}$	0.31890	0.30354	0.28082	0.41891	0.31880	0.24865
APP_{669}	0.27461	0.27116	0.27160	0.27066	0.29146	0.25200
$A\beta_{40}/A\beta_{40}$	2.5947	2.7162	2.9611	2.2470	2.7202	2.6981
Composite	1.7717	2.3047	2.2604	1.7316	3.0062	2.9535
PiB SUVR Be	1.3952	2.3177	2.3700	1.2104	2.1960	2.1627
$APP_{669}/A\beta_{42}$	0.87455	0.90409	0.97370	0.67861	0.90254	0.92051

extraordinarily significant if $|l_x(1,2)| \geq \gamma_x$. The function x is kept to be conserved if $|l_x(1,2)| < \beta_x$.

Equation 1 holds approximately true in biology. For two sets of N-dimension dimensionless data, A and B, we have the ratio, $a_i = x_i(A)/x_i(B)$, and the QD, $QD_i = |l_i(a_i, \bar{a})|$, in which $\bar{a} = \sum_i a_i / N$. The ratios were homogenized so that all of them are not smaller than 1. Biologically, the first-order self-similarity holds true if $QD_i < \beta_{\max}$ and $\overline{QD} < \beta_{\min}$ according to (Eq. 1):

$$\beta_{\max} = \max\{\beta_i\}, \ \beta_{\min} = \min\{\beta_i\} \tag{3}$$

The power law holds approximately true in biology. Topology is the mathematical study of shapes and their arrangement in space. It can be also used to discuss the topological differences between two sets of N-dimension dimensionless and homogenized data A and B [4]. In general, Data A were chosen as reference data for Data B. It was then normalized so that

$$\{x_i(A) : x_{i+1}(A) \geq x_i(A), i = 1,2,\ldots,N\} QD\left(\text{ltx}_1(A), \overline{\text{ltx}(A)}\right) \approx QD\left(\text{ltx}_N(A), \overline{\text{ltx}(A)}\right) \tag{4}$$

Here, the QD of two logarithms was modified from (Eq. 2).

$$QD(\text{ltx}, \text{lty}) = |\ln(\text{ltx}/\text{lty})(\text{ltx} + \text{lty})/2| \tag{5}$$

The process logarithm of two parameters of Data A or B was used to represent the topological relationship between the two parameters, and its SSE between Data A and B was used to represent the topological difference of Data A and B:

$$SSE_i(1,A,B) = l_x(1,i)(A)/l_x(1,i)(B), i = 2,3,\ldots,N \tag{6a}$$

$$SSE_i(A,B,N) = l_x(i,N)(A)/l_x(i,N)(B), i = 2,\ldots,N-1 \tag{6b}$$

We do not calculate the SSE when the absolute value of one of the process logarithm is smaller than the related α. However, the number of SSEs of significant Weber (NSW) needs to be recorded according to the following condition.

$$NSW = 1, if \left|l_x(1,i)\right| < \alpha_x, and \left|l_y(1,i)\right| \geq \beta_y, \\ x, y = A, B, A \neq B, i = 2,3,\ldots, or\, N \tag{7a}$$

$$NSW = 1, if \left|l_x(i,N)\right| < \alpha_x, and \left|l_y(i,N)\right| \geq \beta_y, \\ x, y = A, B, A \neq B, i = 2,3,\ldots, or\, N-1 \tag{7b}$$

The average of all the SSEs except NSW in (Eqs. 6) was denoted as $\overline{SSE(A,B)}$. The QD between each SSE and $\overline{SSE}$, $QD_{\overline{SSE}}(i)$, and the one between subsequent SSEs, $QD(i,i+1)$, were calculated according to (Eq. 5). In addition, the number of SSEs of significance (NSS) also needs to be recorded,

$$NSS = 1, if\, QD(i,i+1) \geq \beta_{i\max}, \beta_{i\max} = \max\{\beta_i, \beta_{i+1}\}, i = 2,3,\ldots, N-1; \\ QD_{\overline{SSE}}(i) \geq \beta_{\max}, i = 2,3,\ldots, N, \beta_{\max} = \max\{\beta_i\}; \text{or} \\ \overline{QD_{\overline{SSE}}} \geq \beta_{\min}, \beta_{\min} = \min\{\beta_i\} \tag{8}$$

We do not calculate the $\overline{SSE(A,B)}$ when $QD(i,i+1) \geq \beta_{i\max}$, $QD_{\overline{SSE}}(i) \geq \beta_{\max}$ or $\overline{QD_{\overline{SSE}}} \geq \beta_{\min}$ until NSS is zero. It is noteworthy that there are different forms of $\overline{SSE}$, $\overline{SSE(A,B)}$ and $\overline{SSE(B,A)}$, we choose $\overline{SSE} = \max\left\{\overline{SSE(A,B)}, \overline{SSE(B,A)}\right\}$. All the SSEs except NSW and NSS are consered,so that $NSS + NSW$ was defined as the topological number of the topological relationship. $NSS + NSW = 0$ indicates that the topological relationship between Data *A* and *B* was self-similar, and the larger the sum $NSS + NSW$ is, the more significant the irrelevance between Data *A* and *B* is. Those parameters that contribute to $NSS + NSW \neq 0$ were the biomarkers.

3 Data Topology of NCGG and AIBL

The group averages of group CN, MCI or AD from dataset AIBL or NCGG are listed in Table 1. We do not calculate the parameter group average of group CN, MCI or AD from dataset AIBL or NCGG when the QD between the parameter and its group average is not smaller than the QD threshold β, 0.805. With regards to the first-order self-similarity from two datasets of 7-dimension data in Table 1, any two groups among groups CN, MCI and AD in either dataset AIBL or NCGG or between them are self-similar between data sets AIBL and NCGG, respectively.

4 Discussion

Nakamura et al. (2018) found the biomarkers of AD are $APP_{669-711}/A\beta_{1-42}$ and $A\beta_{1-40}/A\beta_{1-42}$ ratios, and their composites by using two independent datasets, NCGG and AIBL, each of which included groups CN, MCI and AD [7]. However, the QD of $APP_{669-711}/A\beta_{1-42}$ or $A\beta_{1-40}/A\beta_{1-42}$ ratio between groups CN and MCI or AD was smaller than the QD significant threshold β, 0.805, in the dataset of AIBL or NCGG. The QD of the composite between CN and MCI or AD was larger than the QD significant threshold β, 0.805, in the dataset AIBL, but it was not in dataset NCGG. Moreover, any two groups among Groups AD, CN and MCI were self-similar in both datasets AIBL and NCGG. In other words, the $APP_{669-711}/A\beta_{1-42}$ and $A\beta_{1-40}/A\beta_{1-42}$ ratios and their composites may not be the biomarkers of AD. It was supported by three recent large, late-stage clinical trials. Although the BACE inhibitors successfully blocked the accumulation of amyloid protein in mice, they seemed to worsen cognitive decline and brain shrinkage in people.

Any two groups among Groups AD, CN and MCI were self-similar in dataset AIBL or NCGG. It was further supported by the clinic studies of AD treatment. Honig *et al.* conducted a double-blind, placebo-controlled, phase 3 trial involving patients with mild dementia due to AD [2]. Patients were randomly assigned to receive solanezumab at a dose of 400 mg or placebo intravenously every 4 weeks for 76 weeks. They found the solanezumab did not significantly affect cognitive decline. The first-order self-similarity of 7-dimension data holds true between baseline and 80 weeks for placebo or solanezumab group, and the one of 7-dimension ratio data between baseline and 80 weeks also holds true between placebo and solanezumab groups. Lamb *et al.* conducted a randomized controlled trial of moderate to high intensity exercise training for people with AD for 12 months [3]. They found that a moderate to high intensity aerobic and strength exercise training program did not slow cognitive impairment in people with mild to moderate dementia. The first-order self-similarity of 14-dimension data holds true between 6 and 12 months for the usual care or exercise group, and the one of 14-dimension ratio data between 6 and 12 months also holds true between the usual care and exercise group.

There should be biomarkers of AD. Wu *et al.* examined the effects of swimming exercise pretreatment on a streptozotocin (STZ)-induced sporadic AD rat model [9]. Male 2.5-month-old SD rats were divided into the following four groups: control (Cont), swim + vehicle (SW), STZ without swim (STZ) and swim + STZ (SS). The Barnes maze task and novel object recognition test were used to measure hippocampus-dependent spatial learning and working memory, respectively. Immunofluorescence staining, Western blot analysis, enzyme-linked immunosorbent assay (ELISA) analysis, and related assay kits were used to assess synaptic proteins, inflammatory cytokines, total antioxidant capacity, antioxidant enzymes, Aβ production, and tau hyperphosphorylation. The 28-dimension dataset consisted of all the 28 assessed parameters. The first-order self-similarity of the 28-dimension dataset held true between Cont and SW groups. The topological algorithm of the other groups suggested three AD biomarkers, protein carbonyl, granules density of presynaptic synaptophysin in the hippocampal CA1, and malondialdehyde (MDA) intensity. The three biomarkers of STZ-induced AD were completely reversed by exercise pretreatment. The MDA intensity may be partly contributed by impaired oxygen delivery due to red blood cell oxidative stress [1], but it need to be further verified.

5 Conclusion

Appropriate biomarkers need further study. Our results suggest that $APP_{669-711}/A\beta_{1-42}$ and $A\beta_{1-40}/A\beta_{1-42}$ ratios and their composites may not be valid biomarkers of AD, when reexamined using fractal methods for comparing biomarkers across populations.

Acknowledgments This work was supported by The National Key Research and Development Program of China (2017YFB0403800).

References

1. Harte J, Kinzig A, Green J (1999) Self-similarity in the distribution and abundance of species. Science 284(5412):334–336
2. Honig LS, Vellas B, Woodward M et al (2018) Trial of Solanezumab for mild dementia due to Alzheimer's disease. N Engl J Med 378(4):321–330
3. Lamb SE, Sheehan B, Atherton N, Nichols V, Collins H, Mistry D, Dosanjh S, Slowther AM, Khan I, Petrou S, Lall R et al (2018) Dementia And Physical Activity (DAPA) trial of moderate to high intensity exercise training for people with dementia: randomised controlled trial. BMJ 361:k1675
4. Liu TC, Liu G, Hu SJ et al (2017) Quantitative biology of exercise-induced signal transduction pathways. Adv Exp Med Biol 977:419–424
5. Liu TCY, Tang XM, Duan R et al (2018) The mitochondrial Na^+/Ca^{2+} exchanger is necessary but not sufficient for Ca^{2+} homeostasis and viability. Adv Exp Med Biol 1072:281–285
6. Mohanty JG, Eckley DM, Williamson JD et al (2008) Do red blood cell-beta-amyloid interactions alter oxygen delivery in Alzheimer's disease? Adv Exp Med Biol 614:29–35
7. Nakamura A, Kaneko N, Villemagne VL et al (2018) High performance plasma amyloid-Beta biomarkers for Alzheimer's disease. Nature 554(7691):249–254
8. West G (2017) Scale: the universal Laws of growth, innovation, sustainability, and the pace of life in organisms, cities, economies, and companies. Penguin Press, New York
9. Wu C, Yang L, Tucker D et al (2018) Beneficial effects of exercise pretreatment in a sporadic Alzheimer's rat model. Med Sci Sports Exerc 50(5):945–956

Effective Murine Model Induction for Niche Study in Immune Cells Against Leukemia

Dae Yong Kim, Sarah Lee, Dong Yu Kim, and Ji Yoon Lee

Abstract Murine models have become powerful tools in leukemia research for investigating interactions between blast cells niche factors. In the tumor microenvironment, immune cells are one of the most important niche factors, capable of mounting dynamic innate or adoptive responses against leukemic cells. Acute myeloid leukemia (AML) is a systemic cancer accompanied by immune disruption. In order to exploit the enhanced activity of immune cells in AML treatment, the use of syngeneic mouse models is necessary. Studies of crosstalk between cancer blast cells and immune cells in syngeneic mouse models are beneficial, as the absence of immune functions in syngeneic models enables focus on cancer-associated immune reactions. Once AML is induced, innate and adoptive immune cells respond differently, ultimately resulting in suppression of the immune cells. Murine AML models are commonly induced by intravenous or subcutaneous injection of C1498 cells. Despite the popularity of murine models, they have not yet resulted in the elucidation of distinct differences in immune cells by the injection

Dae Yong Kim and Ji Yoon Lee, the corresponding authors contributed equally to this work.

D. Y. Kim (✉)
Department of Pharmaceutical Science & Engineering, Seowon University, Chungbuk, Cheongju, South Korea
e-mail: dykim@seowon.ac.kr

S. Lee
Department of Biomedical Laboratory Science, College of Health Sciences, Sangji University, Gangwon, Wonju, Republic of Korea

D. Y. Kim
Yonsei University Wonju College of Medicine, Gangwon, Wonju, Republic of Korea

J. Y. Lee (✉)
Department of Biomedical Science, CHA Stem Cell Institute, CHA University, Gyeonggi-do, Seongnam, Republic of Korea

Department of Biomedical Laboratory Science, College of Health Sciences, Sangji University, Gangwon, Wonju, Republic of Korea
e-mail: leejiyoon@cha.ac.kr

© Springer Nature Switzerland AG 2020

P.-D. Ryu et al. (eds.), *Oxygen Transport to Tissue XLI*, Advances in Experimental Medicine and Biology 1232, https://doi.org/10.1007/978-3-030-34461-0_53

method. Here, we investigated the frequency of immune cells and survival rate of mice with AML induced using both injection methods.

Keywords Leukemia · Murine model · Immune cells · Intravenous injection · Subcutaneous injection

1 Introduction

Acute myeloid leukemia (AML) is characterized by systemic proliferation of undifferentiated myeloid cells [1]. The disease causes dysfunction in the immune system, resulting in hematopoietic insufficiency [2]. Most types of leukemia, including AML, affect immune cell function, which in turn influences the survival of leukemic cells in the tumor microenvironment. Since the pivotal role of the tumour microenvironment was revealed by Mercier et al. [3], the concept of the microenvironment as a therapeutic indicator of the recapitulated *in vivo* condition has gained acceptance. The tumor microenvironment can be readily studied using syngeneic mouse models, which enable investigation of both cellular and molecular events [2]. Syngeneic mouse models have been used in leukemia research to investigate the pathophysiologic activation of immune cells and red blood cells. A deeper understanding of immune reactions and risk of oxygen transport in leukemic mice is crucial to developing adequate treatments for the disease [4, 5]. Although the importance of using proper models in cancer biology is often highlighted, there are no data regarding how differences in injection methods affect the disease course in animal models.

In the present study, we compared several leukemic properties in mice models in which the disease was induced using i.v. and s.c. methods, including induction speed, the frequency of various immune cells arising from blast cells, and survival rate. Ultimately, these data may provide benefits for researchers planning to study interactions between immune cells and blast cells.

2 Materials and Methods

2.1 Murine Cell Lines C1498 Cell Culture

The murine AML cell line, C1498 cells (a murine myelogenous leukemia cell line, TIB-49™;ATCC), were cultured in Dulbecco's Modified Eagle's Medium (DMEM; Gibco, Grand Island, NY, USA) supplemented with 10% fetal bovine serum (FBS; RMBIO) and antibiotics (Invitrogen, Carlsbad, CA, USA) in a humidified atmosphere of 5% CO_2 at 37 °C.

2.2 Syngeneic Leukemic Mouse Model

C57Bl/6 J mice were purchased from the Jackson Laboratory (Bar Harbor, ME, USA). For the syngeneic model, two million C1498 cells were suspended in 200 μl phosphate-buffered saline (PBS) and were intravenously or subcutaneously injected; then, samples were obtained from the sacrificed mice until day 26 post-injection.

2.3 Gross Examination, Histology and Survival Monitoring

Tissues were fixed in 4% paraformaldehyde, then embedded in paraffin blocks and sectioned. The sections were stained with hematoxylin and eosin (H&E) for detection of leukemic blasts. Survival was monitored up to 40 days.

2.4 Flow Cytometry

PB cells were isolated, prepared and FACS analysis was performed. The following antibodies were used: CD115 (ASF98; Biolegend), CD3 (555,274; BD Biosciences), CD8a (45–0081-80; eBioscience), NK1.1 (553,165; BD Biosciences), and B220 (45–0452-82; eBioscience). Flow cytometric data were analyzed using appropriate controls with proper isotype-matched IgG and unstained controls.

2.5 Statistical Analysis

The results are presented as the mean ± standard error (SE). Values of $p < 0.05$ were considered statistically significant.

3 Results

3.1 Injected C1498 Cells Found in Peripheral Blood: Mice Injected with C1498 Cells Exhibit Leukemic Properties

To induce leukemia, C1498 cells were cultured *in vitro* and injected using two different injection methods, i.v. ands.c.C1498 cells were found in PB at 1-day post-injection, suggesting successful inoculation (Fig. 1A). Compared with wild-type leukocytes, C1498 cells were larger in size and higher in frequency (Fig. 1B). Leukemic mice exhibited enlarged ovaries, spleen, and aberrant-pigmented lungs, confirming the infiltration of leukemic cells (Fig. 1C). The tissues were examined

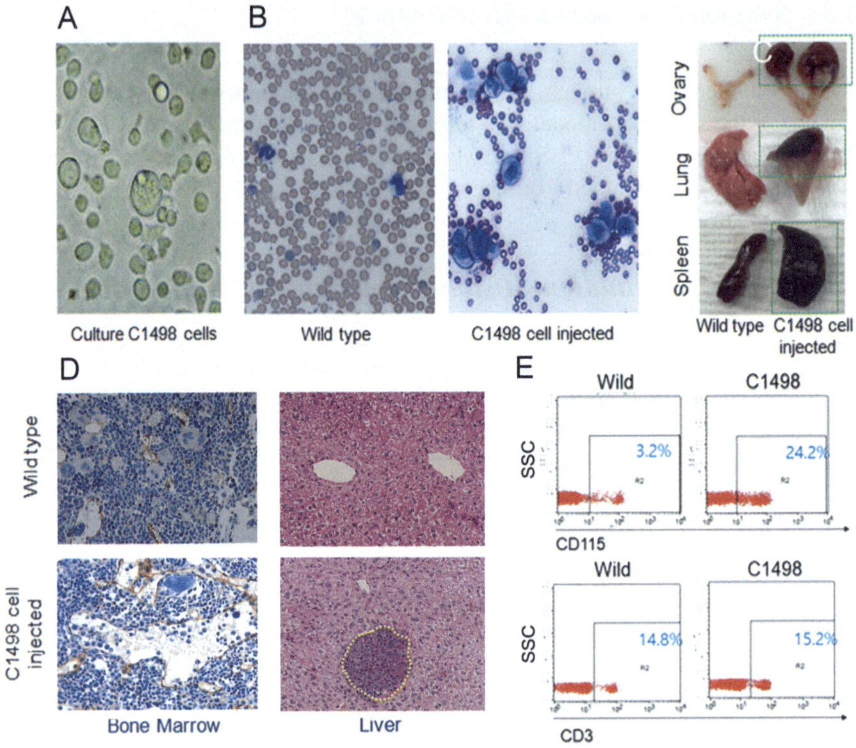

Fig. 1 Successful establishment of a leukemic murine model by i.v. and s.c. injection. (**A**) Cultured C1498 cells rapidly proliferated. (**B**) Blood films showing injected C1498 cells in peripheral blood (PB) of leukemic mice. (**C**) Gross examination of ovaries, lung, and spleen of leukemic mice. (**D**) Leukemic mice showed an engraftment of blasts in bone marrow and liver, brown sinusoidal vessels and yellow line, respectively. (**E**) FACS analysis revealed that expression of CD115, a myeloid marker, was increased in the PB of C1498-injected mice, but expression of CD3, a lymphoid marker, was not increased, suggesting successful induction of the myeloid lineage leukemic mouse model

with H&E staining, and tumor clusters in the liver and atypical morphology of hematopoietic cells in BM were found in leukemic mice, confirming successful establishment of disease. Next, we directly examined the BM for expression of vascular endothelial growth factor receptor 3 (VEGFR-3), which is a known marker of sinusoidal vessels. The sinusoidal vessels in the leukemic BM were larger than those of normal mice. Additionally, irregular and uncharacteristic shapes were common (Fig. 1D).To confirm whether myeloid lineage leukemic cells proliferated in the PB, FACS analysis was performed and data showed that e 1E, C1498-injected mice exhibited a marked increase (7.5-fold) in the frequency of monocytic CD115+ cells but not lymphocytic CD3+ cells (no difference), suggesting myeloid lineage leukemia induction by C1498 cells (Fig. 1E).

3.2 *High Frequency of Blast Cells Sustained by I.V. Injection: Frequency of Immune Cells and Survival Rate Differ with Injection Method*

Next, to confirm the generation of leukemia cells, we counted the number of blast cells in both models. It was found that the number of blasts in PB was significantly increased (3.9-fold) with i.v. injection compared with s.c. injection (Fig. 2A). FACS analysis was then performed using antibodies against B220, CD8, and NK1.1. The numbers of adaptive immune cells, such as cytotoxic T cells, were significantly higher with s.c. injection compared with i.v. injection in both the BM and PB (BM i.v. 3.7 ± 0.6%, s.c. 5.9 ± 0.6%; PB i.v. 14.6 ± 1.7%, s.c. 20.1 ± 1.7%). In contrast, the number of natural killer (NK) cells in the i.v.-injected group was significantly higher than in the s.c.-injected group (BM i.v. 1.9 ± 0.1%, s.c. 3.5 ± 0.4%; PB i.v. 2.0 ± 0.4%, s.c. 3.1 ± 1.2%). No significant difference in the number of B cells was detected (Fig. 2B). These data clearly show a marked difference in immune cells with the different injection methods. Finally, we examined the survival rate in both models. As shown in Fig. 2C, s.c.-injected leukemic mice demonstrated a significantly higher survival rate compared to i.v.-injected leukemic mice (Fig. 2C).

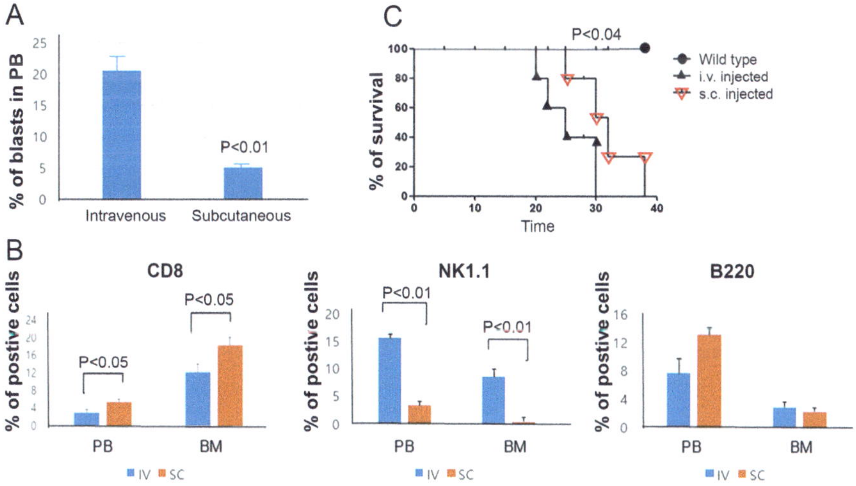

Fig. 2 Comparison of the frequency of immune cells with i.v. versus s.c. injection methods. (**A**) Induction by i.v. injection resulted in a significant increase in leukemic blasts in peripheral blood (PB) compared with s.c. injection. (**B**) FACS analysis showed that the frequency of immune cells in both bone marrow and PB depends on the induction method. Higher frequencies of CD8 T cells and NK cells were observed with the i.v. and s.c. methods, respectively. No significant difference in the number of B cells with the two induction methods were observed

4 Conclusion

In the present study, we demonstrated that both i.v. and s.c. injection methods can be used to induce a stable leukemic mouse model to study the interactions between leukemic and immune cells. The syngeneic leukemia model described here is thus useful for cancer research. NK cells can kill cancer cells, which lack MHC-I antigens [6]. NK cells also play a particularly important role in the maintenance of immune surveillance in the tumor microenvironment post-hematopoietic stem cell transplantation [7]. A proper leukemia model would thus provide a basic platform for niche studies. In future research, we will examine the activity of immune cells and oxygen transport using disease model. Collectively, our data demonstrate that model mice generated by i.v. and s.c. injection exhibit differences in subsets of immune cells. These data also provide technical information for future studies of the relationship between immune cells and cancer cells.

Acknowledgments This work was supported by National Research Foundation of Korea (NRF) funded by the Ministry of Education (2017R1D1A1B03031406).

References

1. Ferrar F, Schiffer CA (2013) Acute myeloid leukaemia in adults. Lancet 381:484–495
2. Lee JY, Park S, Kim DC et al (2013) A VEGFR-3 antagonist increases IFN-γ expression onlow functioning NK cells in acute myeloid leukemia. J Clin Immunol 33(4):826–837
3. Mercier FE, Ragu C, Scadden DT (2011) The bone marrow at the crossroads of blood and immunity. Nat Rev Immunol 23(12):49–60
4. Couzin-Frankel J (2013) Breakthrough of the year 2013. Cancer immunotherapy. Science 342:1432–1433
5. Velez J, Pan R, Lee JT et al (2016) Biquanides sensitize leukemia cells to BT-737-induced apoptosis by inhibiting mitochondrial electron transport. Oncotarget 7(32):51435–51449. https://doi.org/10.18632/oncotarget.9843
6. Ljunggren HG, Karre K (1990) In search of the `missing self': MHC molecules and NK cell recognition. Immunol Today 11(7):237–244
7. Parham P, McQeen KL (2003) Alloreactive killer cells: hindrance and help for haematopoietic transplants. Nat Rev Immunol 3:108–122

Correction to: Improvements in Skeletal Muscle Can Be Detected Using Broadband NIRS in First-Time Marathon Runners

Siana Jones, Matthew Kinsella, Camilla Torlasco, Pardis Kaynezhad, Isabel de Roever, James C. Moon, Alun D. Hughes, and Gemma Bale

Correction to:
Chapter 31 in: P.-D. Ryu et al. (eds.), *Oxygen Transport to Tissue XLI*, Advances in Experimental Medicine and Biology 1232, https://doi.org/10.1007/978-3-030-34461-0_31

This chapter was inadvertently published as an open access chapter. However, the open access for this chapter has now been reverted.

The updated online version of this chapter can be found at
https://doi.org/10.1007/978-3-030-34461-0_31

© Springer Nature Switzerland AG 2020

P.-D. Ryu et al. (eds.), *Oxygen Transport to Tissue XLI*, Advances in Experimental Medicine and Biology 1232, https://doi.org/10.1007/978-3-030-34461-0_54

Index

© Springer Nature Switzerland AG 2020

P.-D. Ryu et al. (eds.), *Oxygen Transport to Tissue XLI*, Advances in Experimental Medicine and Biology 1232, https://doi.org/10.1007/978-3-030-34461-0

I

The manufacturer's authorised representative in the EU is Springer Nature Customer Service Centre GmbH, Europaplatz 3, 69115 Heidelberg, Germany. If you have any concerns regarding our products, please contact ProductSafety@springernature.com

Printed and bound by CPI Group (UK) Ltd, Croydon, CR0 4YY
30/09/2026
02225458-0018

Women Accused of Sexual Harassment

Leslie Margolin

Women Accused of Sexual Harassment

palgrave
macmillan

Leslie Margolin
University of Iowa
Iowa City, IA, USA

ISBN 978-3-031-79020-1 ISBN 978-3-031-79021-8 (eBook)
https://doi.org/10.1007/978-3-031-79021-8

© The Editor(s) (if applicable) and The Author(s), under exclusive license to Springer Nature Switzerland AG 2024

This work is subject to copyright. All rights are solely and exclusively licensed by the Publisher, whether the whole or part of the material is concerned, specifically the rights of translation, reprinting, reuse of illustrations, recitation, broadcasting, reproduction on microfilms or in any other physical way, and transmission or information storage and retrieval, electronic adaptation, computer software, or by similar or dissimilar methodology now known or hereafter developed.
The use of general descriptive names, registered names, trademarks, service marks, etc. in this publication does not imply, even in the absence of a specific statement, that such names are exempt from the relevant protective laws and regulations and therefore free for general use.
The publisher, the authors and the editors are safe to assume that the advice and information in this book are believed to be true and accurate at the date of publication. Neither the publisher nor the authors or the editors give a warranty, expressed or implied, with respect to the material contained herein or for any errors or omissions that may have been made. The publisher remains neutral with regard to jurisdictional claims in published maps and institutional affiliations.

Cover illustration: Maram_shutterstock

This Palgrave Macmillan imprint is published by the registered company Springer Nature Switzerland AG.
The registered company address is: Gewerbestrasse 11, 6330 Cham, Switzerland

If disposing of this product, please recycle the paper.

For Mary Trachsel, with love

Preface

In Western society, false, extravagant constructions of women's sexuality have a long and well-known history. Consider the Christian belief that women succumb more readily to sexual temptation than men, as exemplified by the original sinner, Eve, the prototype of the pleasure seeking, sexually unmanageable woman. As Tertullian, an early Christian theologian, put it, "And do you not know you are Eve? … Woman, you are the gate to hell and her gaping genitals the mouth to hell" (quoted in Ukockis, 2019, p. 80).

Consider also that the criminal justice system has historically treated female offenders differently than male offenders: more leniently when they conformed to traditional feminine gender roles—when seen as submissive and chaste, good mothers, wives, and daughters—but more harshly when their behaviors seemed to fall outside gender norms (Belknap, 2001; Franklin, 2008, p. 345; Heidensohn, 1985; Nagel et al., 1981; Rafter, 1990). We know, for example, that during the seventeenth century, in Puritan New England, men were as likely as women to practice witchcraft. The difference was in indictments, convictions, and punishments: women who were not mothers, caretakers, or homemakers—"masculine" women—were seen as more vulnerable to the devil's influence and were often identified as "Satan's servants" (Godbeer, 2011, p. 11). Thus, the custom of imposing severe penalties on gender-norm-defying women, especially those accused of committing so-called "masculine" offenses (Albonetti, 1988; Koons-Witt, 2002). This research explores the possibility that the same bias applies to women accused of sexual harassment: they are judged and punished for two possible offenses simultaneously, the formal charge of sexual harassment and the informal charge of defying female gender norms. In this research, I examine what happens to women who defy conventional versions of feminine virtue and delicacy: how several successful, albeit gender-norm-defying, female faculty and administrators (e.g., Jane Gallop, Avital Ronell, Anna Stubblefield, and Marybeth Gasman) came to be accused of sexual harassment despite the weakness (even absurdity) of the charges and evidence brought against them.

I wish to thank Carol Harrington and Rebecca Longtin for reading drafts and making incredibly sharp suggestions. The anonymous reviewers were also exceptionally helpful. Mary Trachsel helped shape the book and provided countless theoretical and editorial suggestions. I could not have written this book without her. Finally, I wish to thank Jane Gallop for inspiring me.

Iowa City, IA, USA Leslie Margolin

References

Albonetti, C. (1988). The role of gender and departures in the sentencing of defendants convicted of a white-collar offense under the federal sentencing guidelines. *Sociology of Crime, Law, and Deviance, 1*, 3–48.

Belknap, J. (2001). *The invisible woman: Gender, crime, and justice.* Wadsworth.

Franklin, C. A. (2008). Women offenders, disparate treatment, and criminal justice: A theoretical, historical, and contemporary overview. *Criminal Justice Studies, 21*(4), 341–360. https://doi.org/10.1080/14786010802554238. http://www.informaworld.com

Godbeer, R. (2011). *The Salem witch hunt: A brief history with documents.* St. Martin's Press.

Heidensohn, F. (1985). *Women and crime.* Macmillan.

Koons-Witt, B. (2002). The effect of gender on the decision to incarcerate before and after the introduction of sentencing guidelines. *Criminology, 40*, 297–327.

Nagel, I., Cardascia, J., & Ross, C. E. (1981). Sex differences in the processing of criminal defendants. In D. K. Weisberg (Ed.), *Women and the law: The socio-historical perspective* (Vol. 1, pp. 259–282). Schenkman. https://www.nsvrc.org/resource/facts-behind-metoo-movement-national-study-sexual-harassment-and-assault

Rafter, N. H. (1990). *Partial justice: Women, prisons, and social control.* Transaction Books.

Ukockis, G. (2019). *Misogyny: The new activism.* Oxford University Press.

Contents

CHAPTER 1

Introduction

"The Brazen Kiss"

In 1992, Jane Gallop, a professor of English and comparative literature from the University of Wisconsin-Milwaukee, was accused of sexual harassment. Two of her female graduate students pinpointed the precise location and time they reached the conclusion that Gallop had been harassing them: it was at a gay and lesbian studies conference, when Gallop stood up and announced: "Graduate students are my sexual preference" (Gallop, 1997, p. 86). That statement, Gallop said, was intended as a joke; it was her first gay and lesbian conference, she was excited, and she wanted to appear clever and sassy, like the other participants. Also, as a Freudian, she believes that people's professional and artistic impulses are sublimated sexual drives: "The pleasure I get from working with graduate students, the intensity of my wish that certain promising graduate students will choose to work with me, and the satisfaction I get from seeing the imprint of my teaching in their work all strongly suggest a sexual analogy" (p. 87). But at the time no one got the joke, and no one saw the Freudian connection. Although Gallop had a reputation as a sex-gender provocateur—a sort of academic Mae West—people thought she was serious, especially the graduate students who filed the sexual harassment complaint against her. They concluded that all the time that Gallop had been talking to them about sex, she was not trying to teach them about sex as an academic topic; it was to talk them into *having sex*—with her. And because they did

© The Author(s), under exclusive license to Springer Nature Switzerland AG 2024

L. Margolin, *Women Accused of Sexual Harassment*,
https://doi.org/10.1007/978-3-031-79021-8_1

not give Gallop a green light, because they did not encourage Gallop's sexual advances, they claimed Gallop retaliated by making one of them rewrite her papers and by refusing to write letters of recommendation for the other.

Unfortunately, Gallop had no idea her students were jumping to these kinds of conclusions. So, hours after she made her "graduate students are my sexual preference" joke-flop, she accompanied a group of graduate students, including Dana Beckelman, one of the harassment complainants, to a local bar, unaware that some had taken her joke seriously. At the bar, Gallop and Beckelman got into an intense conversation about sex, power, and the erotic dynamics of their own relationship: "We were not discussing sex, power, and pedagogy in the abstract," Gallop said, "we were inevitably thinking of our own highly charged relationship" (p. 89).

When Beckelman got up to leave, she and Gallop hugged and kissed, as was their custom. But this time, perhaps because they were in a crowded bar and had an audience, the kiss was different. "The kiss was brazen and public," Gallop said, "and thus particularly appropriate for a conference distinguished by its intellectual and sexual daring. This was a performance tailor-made for the First Annual Graduate Student Gay and Lesbian Conference, whose title, after all, was 'Flaunting It'" (Gallop, p. 92). In her sexual harassment complaint, Beckelman described the kiss as distinctly upsetting, even though she said she was an active participant: "So I kissed her until she responded, more as a vindictive act than as a reciprocally sexual one. I was angry and hurt, and saw kissing as a form of revenge, a way to manipulate her desire, knowing I would never go any further" (Talbot, 1994, p. 15). Beckelman said Gallop "mashed her lips against mine" and "shoved her tongue in my mouth" (Talbot, p. 15). Gallop offered her own description of the kiss: "Somehow the usual goodbye peck became a real kiss. I don't actually know who started it. I know it surprised me and seemed to occur simultaneously to both of us, as if spontaneously generated out of the moment" (Gallop, p. 91),

Beckelman and another student, whose name was not disclosed, went on to file harassment complaints. The latter claimed that Gallop had tried to seduce her when she visited Gallop's home to drop off a paper. During the visit, she said that Gallop paused in a sexually suggestive way in front of her downstairs bedroom, and at another point, Gallop placed her bare foot on the rocker of the chair she was sitting on, again suggestively, causing the chair to rock. The student claimed that because she thwarted these apparent advances, Gallop refused to write letters of recommendation for her to Brown and Johns Hopkins, though she acknowledged that Gallop did agree to write a letter of recommendation to the University of California at Santa Cruz. The graduate student told harassment investigators that "it is at the level of the institutionally enforced power differential (which Gallop knowingly exploited) that I wish to locate the harassment" (Talbot, p. 19).

When investigations into Gallop's conduct commenced, the graduate student complainants led campus demonstrations against Gallop and started an organization called "Students Against Sexual Harassment" (SASH), to protest a conference Gallop was organizing. At the conference entrance, they sold bumper stickers which read, "Distinguished Professors Do It Pedagogically" (Gallop is a distinguished professor), and informed conference participants that Gallop was under investigation for sexual harassment, though the investigation was supposed to be confidential. One of their handouts even revealed Gallop's salary. Another read: "You have in your power today, the ability to take a stand on sexual harassment in a concrete and meaningful way. Do not allow yourselves to be co-opted into Jane's deluded world. Make a statement: Boycott!" (Gallop, p. 68)

As for the investigation's outcome, investigators could not find evidence that Gallop had coerced or sexually harassed Beckelman: "[The student] was a willing participant in sexual banter; Professor Gallop did not condition [her] grades or participation in an academic program on [her] submission to sexual advances or sexual acts; [the student] was not and did not feel physically threatened, psychologically harmed or humiliated by any of Professor Gallop's conduct or words" (Talbot, p. 3). Despite these findings, the University concluded that Gallop had violated University policy prohibiting "amorous consensual relations between students and faculty," albeit without specifying the nature of the so-called "amorous consensual relations" or the ways a close pedagogical relationship can veer off course and become "amorous." The University concluded that Gallop should have a letter of reprimand placed in her file. So, even though the investigators found nothing to suggest that Gallop's conversations with Beckelman on the topic of sex were coercive or that Gallop had in any way threatened or harmed her, they ruled that Gallop, "as the person in the more powerful position," did wrong by failing to report her relationship with Beckelman to a dean and failing to excuse herself from evaluating Beckelman's academic performances (Talbot, p. 3).

A year later, in 1993, another graduate student from the same University of Wisconsin-Milwaukee, Christine Ruh, filed a complaint in federal court against an associate professor of art, Stephen Samerjan, for sexually harassing her. Ruh sued the UW-Systems Board of Regents and the University of Wisconsin-Milwaukee for failing to properly investigate Samerjan and for dismissing her claim that she had been sexually harassed. Ruh alleged that Samerjan began a sexual relationship with her in 1983, when she was his student in the School of Fine Arts at UMW. Two years later, when she complained to him about their relationship, she said he retaliated by demeaning her, failing to show-up for scheduled academic appointments, and by giving her lower grades than she believed she deserved. She described Samerjan as a serial harasser who treated other female students in an exploitive and damaging manner: "What he did is … took you out for a date, got you in bed, made you think he would be your boyfriend or whatever, and then he dumped you.... And so I just dropped out of school" (Shelbourne, 2017, p. 15).

In 1986, when Ruh first tried to file charges against Samerjan with the UMW affirmative action office, the charges were dismissed; she was told that "everything has been taken care of." The next year, when she filed a second complaint, she was told that her "allegations did not meet the time requirements for an individual case." Then, in 1991, when she complained about Samerjan for a third time, the UMW Chancellor's office informed her that Samerjan did not violate Ruh's rights since "UWM policy did not prohibit consensual relationships between instructors and students." Finally, after hearing the evidence in Ruh's civil suit against Samerjan, a federal court ruled that he had not committed sexual harassment for the reason that "The alleged misconduct of Professor Samerjan ('inappropriate,' 'unprofessional,' failure to attend appointments, giving her lower grades, demeaning her) are all personal matters and not gender related. The professor's conduct, assuming it took place, did not stem from his discriminatory action against 'women' but, rather, is the way he ended their love affair" (Shelbourne, p. 17).

We have, then, a charge of female-to-female sexual harassment with Jane Gallop as the accused and a charge of male-to-female sexual harassment with Stephen Samerjan as the accused. These two charges/cases occurred at the same school, during the same time-period, and both involved professors as presumptive harassers and female students as presumptive victims. But these cases also have several critical differences. In the male-to-female case, both parties publicly confirmed their sexual relationship, while in the female-to-female case, both parties merely confirmed conversations of about sex, gender, and sexuality—and one public performance of a kiss. In the female-to-female case, the alleged perpetrator had no history of having had sexual relationships or having made sexual advances toward other UWM students. But in the male-to-female case, the man had allegedly been sexually involved with several other female students. In the female-to-female case, Beckelman, the central complainant, went on to earn her Ph.D., but in the male-to-female case, the complainant dropped out: "Because of what he did to me, because I came forward … I lost a $40,000 doctoral scholarship and my access to my education and eventually my stuff and my house" (Shelbourne, p. 15).

Among so many differences, the University community's response stands out: only in the female-to-female case did the University of Wisconsin-Milwaukee immediately launch an investigation into the harassment charges; only in the female-to-female case did students organize public demonstrations against the alleged harasser; only in the female-to-female case did members of the University of Wisconsin-Milwaukee community, long after the alleged harasser's offenses, continue to publicly proclaim her guilt. Consider that on April 19, 1993, two years after Gallop kissed her student in a bar, the student newspaper ran the front-page headline, "Professor Accused of Kissing Students," and one journalist, while photocopying articles about Gallop, was interrupted by a student, "O yeah, Jane Gallop," said the student, "Didn't she attack somebody or something?" (Talbot, p. 2).

This book explores these differences. My plan is to examine whether sexual harassment allegations against women in colleges and universities are different from harassment allegations levelled against men. I am also interested in exploring whether responses to allegations are different, whether they are taken more seriously when a woman is charged and, if so, whether that enforces women's subordination and men's dominance. Through a thematic/narrative analysis of publicly available sexual harassment records, I consider the possibility that harassment allegations wrongfully discriminate against women.

Materials and Procedures

This book addresses these questions through an exploration of public records of individuals listed on the "Academic Sexual Misconduct Database," https://academic-sexual-misconduct-database.org/, an ongoing archive of university and college employees who have been accused of sexual harassment. The archive began in February 2016 and has been continuously updated by voluntary submissions from colleges and universities across the United States. Though most of the cases on the archive are from the last 20 years, a few reach back much further: the earliest is from the first decades of the twentieth century when the president of Colorado College was accused of sexually harassing women on his staff.

The archive lists the names of male and female faculty, administrators, coaches, researchers, and support staff accused of sexual harassment (N = 1291 as of Aug. 2024) and includes links to publicly available reports documenting the harassment allegations against them. To find additional information on these individuals—in pursuit of civil lawsuits by individuals alleging harassment, lawsuits by individuals accused of harassment, federal civil rights investigations, college and university inquiries, victim and perpetrator interviews, diaries, and journalistic investigations and reports—I surveyed the entire media landscape through *LexisNexis* and other archival sources such as the *New York Times*, the *Chronicle of Higher Education*, the *Washington Post*, as well as college/university newspapers, social media posts, blogs, and videos.

The fact that information on a sexual harassment case is publicly available doesn't, of course, make the information representative or typical. And it doesn't ensure that the information is complete or clear. To address these limitations, I excluded cases that appeared fragmentary, equivocal, and/or obscure. Thus, for instance, I excluded the case of a female faculty member accused of sexually harassing a female student "by subjecting student to inappropriate comments of a sexual nature," because the publicly available data provided no information on the nature or context of the "inappropriate comments"; in another excluded case, the university shared that a female faculty committed a "violation of the consensual relationship policy under EO 1097," but nothing more. In a third excluded case, a senior administrator with the University of California-Berkeley was found guilty of arranging exorbitant raises for another UC-Berkeley employee who happened to be her lover. Although the case was listed on the Academic Sexual Misconduct Database, it was excluded from the study because there were no allegations of hostile/harmful behavior or unwelcome/prohibited sexual advances: the object of the alleged harassment, in this instance—the lover who saw his salary go from $70,000 to $110,000—appeared to welcome and benefit from his interactions with the senior administrator. As a result of this winnowing, the final research population came to 29 women listed on the Academic Sexual Misconduct Database.

Among the 29 women identified on the Database as harassment suspects, only three were indicted and found guilty. And while some eventually acknowledged the validity of all or most of the harassment charges, most did not: they consistently maintained their innocence. Technically speaking, then, this research is less about sexual harassment committed by women, than it is about sexual harassment *allegations* against women: their content, how they are constructed, what they represent, and the responses they elicited.

Since hardly anybody admits to committing harassment, even when offered anonymity, most harassment research has relied on standardized, quantitative surveys of victims' perceptions and experiences (Fitzgerald et al., 1988; McLauglin et al., 2012; Reinicke, 2022; Uggen & Blackstone, 2004). The advantage of standardized quantitative surveys is that they allow researchers to reach generalizable conclusions about sexual harassment and its impact on harassment victims. The primary advantage of research based on public records is that, instead of relying on victims' responses to close-ended prompts, they provide access to multiple stories and points of view. Given the variety and complexity of public records' data, it becomes possible to develop a fuller, richer understanding of the people and situations involved in sexual harassment than research exclusively reliant on survey data. This study, for example, contains first-person accounts of individuals charged with harassment, along with documentary evidence of their harassment, including email and text messages, witness testimony, and accounts by attorneys, investigators, and journalists, and thus has the potential to provide a deeper, more comprehensive understanding of how harassment behaviors unfold, the contexts in which they occur, and how harassers and their targets interact.

While public records are not optimal for detecting general population distributions, they are useful for examining stereotypical assumptions about sexual harassment (see Gillespie & Leffler, 1987; Leffler, 1982). And in sexual harassment, stereotypes abound, the most common being that sexual harassment is committed only by men and that only women are victims. Public records show that women harass too and that the victims can be either men or women. A second advantage is that, because the Academic Sexual Misconduct Database contains data on both men and women accused of harassment, it becomes possible to match the subsample of women accused of harassment to a randomly selected subsample of men so accused. The data on women's harassment can then serve as reference points, "negative cases" (Emigh, 1997), to delineate the characteristics of men's harassment, and vice versa. Such comparisons make it possible to specify the features of sexual harassment characteristic of each gender. In other words, the study of the minority population, women accused of sexual harassment, has the potential to enlighten us on the majority population, men accused of sexual harassment.

I make these comparisons in two ways. In the first (Part I), I examine exceptional cases of women accused of sexual harassment—exceptional either because of the weakness of the evidence or the idiosyncratic nature of the harassment charges. I then compare these exceptional cases to the cases of men accused of sexual harassment from the same or similar institutions and disciplines. In the second type of gender comparison (Part II), I compare women's cases which appear exceptional *and* nonexceptional (cases which appear to follow normal investigative procedures with allegations based on noncontroversial factual evidence), to cases of men randomly selected from the Academic Sexual Misconduct Database. To develop the latter sample, I generated a series of random numbers between 1 and the final number on the Database (1291 as of Aug. 2024) and selected the first 29 cases which attributed harassment to a man. Table 1 in the Appendix provides a list of the 29 cases of women charged with sexual harassment and the 29 men identified in the random sample.

Sexual Harassment on Campus

Sexual harassment on college campuses is a ubiquitous and deeply rooted problem, with nearly 50% of female college students reporting some form of sexual harassment (Cortina et al., 1998; Ivy & Hamlet, 1996; Thakur & Paul, 2017; Witze, 2018). Studies suggest that as many as one in five women have encountered serious harassment such as sexual coercion (e.g., Vohlídalová, 1999, p. 1130), with female victims consistently and substantially outpacing male victims (Berdahl, 2007; Buchanan et al., 2009; Campbell et al., 2017; Cantor et al., 2015; Hill & Silva, 2005; Kalof et al., 2001; Krebs et al., 2016; McGinley et al., 2016; Rosenthal et al., 2016; Rospenda et al., 2000). Studies also show that graduate students are at far greater risk of being sexually harassed by male faculty and staff than by their male or female peers, while undergraduates are at greater risk of being harassed by male peers (Klein & Martin, 2021). This is despite the fact that most institutions of higher education within the United States cannot be described as bastions of male power: in 2021, women made up 58% of total undergraduate enrollment compared to 42% for men (National Center for Educational Statistics, 2021) and the percentage of female professors, 49.8%, is now almost equal to that of male professors, 50.2% (National Center for Educational Statistics, 2021). Other studies show that female students belonging to marginalized groups, such as gay and bisexual women, younger women, students with disabilities, and racial minorities, are more exposed to sexual harassment than other women in academia (Bondestam & Lundqvist, 2020; D'augelli, 1992; Fedina et al., 2018; Ong, 2005; Vladutinu et al., 2011).

Incidence levels of sexual harassment vary from campus to campus, partly because harassment reports depend on the type of assessment and investigative procedures each campus utilizes. A second explanation for this unevenness is underreporting (Fisher, 2000; Ilies et al., 2003; Vohlídalová, 1999). In many instances victims do not come forward because they blame themselves (Fitzgerald et al., 1995; Woodzicka & LaFrance, 2001); they also anticipate being blamed by others (McDonald, 2012; Pina & Gannon, 2012). Harassment victims often express doubt that their institution will support them (McLaughlin et al., 2012), and, in general, see sexual harassment as a stigmatizing experience, one which marks victims as weak, as failing to properly assert themselves, and thus, as being partially responsible for their own victimization (Vohlídalová, 1999, p. 1141).

At least eight studies have assessed victimization rates for specific kinds of sexual harassment on campus (see Klein & Martin, 2021, p. 785), with inappropriate comments, such as jokes or remarks about bodies, appearance, or sexual behavior, representing the most common type of harassment (Cantor et al., 2015; Huerta, et al., 2006; Krebs et al., 2016; Yoon et al., 2010). However, inappropriate comments and jokes are also the harassment behaviors least likely to be recognized by students as harassment. By contrast, the types of behavior most likely to be seen as harassment are, in descending order, attempts at physical contact which are unwelcome and resisted, rape attempts, repeated verbal attempts at obtaining an intimate relationship, unwelcome conversation about intimate topics, light touches, private invitations for a date from a teacher, comments on appearance, lewd teaching materials, sex-based workplace advantages, and sex-based workplace disadvantages (Vohlidalova, 1999, p. 1137).

How the Book Is Organized

The book's main organizational principle is to tell the stories of women accused of sexual harassment in detail when the detail is available in public records (as in the case of Jane Gallop), and to offer thematic sketches when the detail is limited, always organizing the stories and sketches around comparisons with the stories and sketches of men accused of harassment.

The book begins with a review of controversies surrounding sexual harassment research—the topic of Chap. 2—why workplace sexual harassment occurs, the motivations behind it, whether harassment attributed to women is different than harassment attributed to men, whether some women are more likely to be accused of harassment than others, and how gender role performance influences judgments and penalties against women accused of harassment.

Chapter 3, "A Real Monster," and Chap. 4, "A Predator Preying on Their Prey," tell the stories of two successful female professors listed on the Academic Sexual Misconduct Database, Avital Ronell and Anna Stubblefield, who, like Jane Gallop, were treated as pariahs for sexual offenses which appear far less severe than offenses attributed to male professors from their own and comparable institutions. These chapters also show that Ronell and Stubblefield were subjected to an unusual form of gaslighting. While gaslighting is typically understood as an effort to make targets think of themselves as cognitively or morally defective (the type of gaslighting popularized in the 1944 movie, *Gaslight*, in which a husband knowingly and consistently attempts to make his wife think she is losing her mind), in the harassment cases involving Ronell and Stubblefield, as well as in the Gallop case, the gaslighting did not represent efforts to make them doubt themselves. Rather, the goal was to convince others—university administrators, faculty, alumni, students, as well as members of the judicial system and general public—to doubt them. Gaslighters' goal was to show that Gallop, Ronnell, and Stubblefield belong, in essence, to a lower species (Garfinkel, 1956). This was accomplished by projecting new, inferior identities onto them—a process that Weinstein and Deutschberger (1963) dubbed "altercasting." Because the sexual harassment attributed to Gallop, Ronell, and Stubblefield may have lacked the "normality" of harassment attributed to men—because these women appeared to behave in ways that deviated from traditional female gender roles—altercasters were able to attribute meanings and motivations to them that had little or nothing to do with the ways they saw themselves. In short, these chapters should illustrate, not only the weakness of the evidence used to convict Ronell and Stubblefield of sexual harassment, but also how the weak evidence used against them came to be seen as strong and compelling.

Chapter 5, "Lock Her Up!", examines the harassment charges levelled against several other women listed on the Academic Sexual Misconduct Database who, like Gallop, Ronell, and Stubblefield, were subject to false and exaggerated harassment charges. The allegations against them and the institutional responses to the allegations were characterized by hostility, ambiguity, inconsistency, and/or minimal evidence of harm to their putative victims. The chapter shows that women accused of sexual harassment not only faced different and harsher rules and judgements than men accused of harassment from comparable institutions and disciplines, but that their presumptive offenses were also less offensive, less frequent, and, overall, more ambiguous.

Chapter 6, "Disconnected Cases," focuses on another kind of gender issue. Instead of attending to procedural irregularities which occur when women are charged with sexual harassment—instead of questioning whether the sexual harassment attributed to women is fair or not, or whether it occurred or not, as in the earlier chapters—this chapter examines how the harassment attributed to women fails to conform to men's patterns and, indeed, fails to conform to any pattern. This chapter examines the idiosyncrasies—the heterogeneity—of allegations levelled against women.

Chapters 7 through 12 compare the cases of women listed on the Academic Sexual Misconduct Database to a sample of men's cases randomly selected from the Database. To facilitate these comparisons, sexual harassment allegations against women and men were divided into the same five categories. The first category, the topic of Chap. 7, is defined as harassment among consenting adults. In this type of harassment allegation, the wrong-doing is based on the presumptive harasser's institutional position—the fact that he or she occupies a higher status and has greater power than the presumptive victim. While individuals accused of this kind of harassment and their presumptive victims may claim that they began a sexual relationship freely and willingly, without coercion, investigators sometimes argue that a relationship with a substantial power imbalance—for example, involving a professor and student—is inherently coercive since it takes place under the cloak of the professor's greater power and authority.

Chapter 8 centers on the second harassment category, quid pro quo harassment, defined as allegations which assume that the presumptive harasser offered the victim workplace/career bribes or threats to gain sexual favors: sleep with me and I'll make sure you are hired, sleep with me and I'll support your promotion, deny me and you can forget about the favorable letter of recommendation, deny me and you're fired.

Chapter 9 centers on the third harassment category, "offensive fun and games," defined as allegations of joking or play which feel aggressive and exploitive, and which make the victim's work environment intimidating, hostile, and oppressive.

Chapter 10 concerns the fourth harassment category, "overtly hostile verbal harassment," defined as undisguised attempts to harm the target. These can take the form of a single hostile comment or persistent hounding/hectoring; they can occur over electronic media (online harassment), through face-to-face interactions, or in combinations of both.

Finally, Chaps. 11 and 12 concern the fifth harassment category, physical sexual intrusions, the most common allegation levelled against men, representing 45% of the men's random sample. Physical sexual intrusions, like other forms of harassment, can represent a single incident or a series of incidents, and can range from the relatively mild, such as unwelcome touching, kissing, and groping, to extremes such as stalking, sexual assault, and attempted murder. Physical sexual intrusions may be reported immediately after they occur, or they may be reported decades later. Hence, Chap. 12 on delayed physical sexual intrusions.

To sum up, Chaps. 7 through 12, each of which compares harassment allegations against women to allegations against a sample of men randomly selected from the Academic Sexual Misconduct Database, have three central goals: first, to determine how sexual harassment allegations against women and men are different, both in terms of the behaviors attributed to the presumptive harassers and their underlying motivations, second, to determine how women's and men's harassment appears to overlap—to identify similarities in women's and men's harassment behaviors and motivations—and third, to assess whether women accused of sexual harassment are subject to reactions, judgments, and penalties which are different and more severe than those experienced by men.

In Chap. 13, "conclusions and recommendations," the final chapter, I discuss the research's limitations, the research findings, the knowns and unknowns, and the implications for theory, prevention, and further research.

References

Berdahl, J. L. (2007). The sexual harassment of uppity women. *Journal of Applied Psychology, 92*(2), 425–437. https://doi.org/10.1037/0021-9010.92.2.425

Bondestam, F., & Lundqvist, M. (2020). Sexual harassment in higher education—A systematic review. *European Journal of Higher Education, 10*(4), 397–419. https://doi.org/10.1080/21568235.2020.1729833

Buchanan, N. T., Bergman, M. E., Bruce, T. A., Woods, K. C., & Lichty, L. L. (2009). Unique and joint effects of sexual and racial harassment on college students' well-being. *Basic and Applied Social Psychology, 31*, 267–285. https://doi.org/10.1080/01973530903058532

Campbell, J. C., Sabri, B., Budhathoki, C., Kaufman, M. R., Alhusen, J., & Decker, M. R. (2017). Unwanted sexual acts among university students: Correlates of victimization and perpetration. *Journal of Interpersonal Violence, 36*(1–2), NP504–NP526. https://doi.org/10.1177/0886260517734221

Cantor, D., Fisher, B., Chibnall, S., Townsend, R., Lee, H., Bruce, C., & Thomas, G. (2015). *Report on the AAU campus climate survey on sexual assault and sexual misconduct.* Westat.

Cortina, L. M., Swan, S., Fitzgerald, L. F., & Waldo, C. (1998). Sexual harassment and assault: Chilling the climate for women in academia. *Psychology of Women Quarterly, 22*, 419–441.

D'augelli, A. (1992). Lesbian and gay male undergraduates experiences of harassment and fear. *Journal of Interpersonal Violence, 7*(3), 383–396. https://doi.org/10.1177/088626092007003007

Emigh, R. (1997). The power of negative thinking: The use of negative case methodology in the development of sociological theory. *Theory and Society, 26*, 649–684.

Fedina, L., Holmes, J. L., & Backes, B. L. (2018). Campus sexual assault: A systematic review of prevalence research from 2000 to 2015. *Trauma, Violence & Abuse, 19*(1), 76–93. https://doi.org/10.1177/1524838016631129

Fisher, B. (2000). *The sexual victimization of college women.* US Department of Justice, Office of Justice Programs, National Institute of Justice.

Fitzgerald, L. F., Gelfand, M. J., & Drasgow, F. (1995). Measuring sexual harassment: Theoretical and psychometric advances. *Basic and Applied Social Psychology, 17*(4), 425–445. https://doi.org/10.1207/s15324834basp1704_2

Fitzgerald, L. F., Shullman, S. L., Bailey, N., Richards, M., Swecker, J., Gold, Y., et al. (1988). The incidence and dimensions of sexual harassment in academia and the workplace. *Journal of Vocational Behavior, 32*(2), 152–175. https://doi.org/10.1016/0001-8791(88)90012-7

Gallop, J. (1997). *Feminist accused of sexual harassment.* Duke University Press.

Garfinkel, H. (1956). Conditions of successful degradation ceremonies. *American Journal of Sociology, 61*(5), 420–424.

Gillespie, D. L., & Leffler, A. (1987). The politics of research methodology in claims-making activities: Social science and sexual harassment. *Social Problems, 34*(5), 490–501. https://doi.org/10.2307/800543

Hill, C., & Silva, E. (2005). *Drawing the line: Sexual harassment on campus.* American Association of University Women Educational Foundation.

Huerta, M., Cortina, L. M., Pang, J. S., Torges, C. M., & Magley, V. J. (2006). Sex and power in the academy: Modeling sexual harassment in the lives of college women. *Personality and Social Psychology Bulletin, 32*, 616–628. https://doi.org/10.1177/0146167205284281

Ilies, R., Hauserman, N., Schwochau, S., & Stibal, J. (2003). Reported incidence rates of work-related sexual harassment in the United States: Using meta-analysis to explain reported rate disparities. *Personnel Psychology, 56*(3), 607–631.

Ivy, D. K., & Hamlet, S. (1996). College students and sexual dynamics: Two studies of peer sexual harassment. *Communication Education, 45*, 149–166.

Kalof, L., Eby, K. K., Matheson, J. L., & Kroska, R. J. (2001). The influence of race and gender on student self-reports on sexual harassment by college professors. *Gender & Society, 15*, 282–302. https://doi.org/10.1177/089124301015002007

Klein, L. B., & Martin, S. L. (2021). Sexual harassment of college and university students: A systematic review. *Trauma, Violence & Abuse, 22*(4), 777–792. https://doi.org/10.1177/1524838019881731

Krebs, C., Lindquist, C., Berzofsky, M., Shook-Sa, B., & Peterson, K. (2016). *Campus climate survey validation study final technical support.* Bureau of Justice Statistics Research and Development Series.

Leffler, A. (1982). Review of woman battering: Victims and their experiences. *Sex Roles, 8*, 1160–1164.

McDonald, P. (2012). Workplace sexual harassment 30 years on: A review of the literature. *International Journal of Management Reviews, 14*(1), 1–17. https://doi.org/10.1111/j.1468-2370.2011.00300.x

McGinley, M., Wolff, J. M., Rospenda, K. M., Liu, L., & Richman, J. A. (2016). Risk factors and outcomes of chronic sexual harassment during the transition to college: Examination of a two-part growth mixture model. *Social Science Research, 60*, 297–310.

McLaughlin, H., Uggen, C., & Blackstone, A. (2012). Sexual harassment, workplace authority, and the paradox of power. *American Sociological Review, 77*(4), 625–647. https://doi.org/10.1177/0003122412451728

National Center for Educational Statistics. (2021). https://nces.ed.gov/fastFacts/display.asp?id=98

Ong, M. (2005). Body projects of young women of color in physics: Intersections of Gender, Race, and Science. *Social Problems, 52*(4), 593–617. https://doi.org/10.1525/sp.2005.52.4.593

Pina, A., & Gannon, T. A. (2012). An overview of the literature on antecedents, perceptions and behavioural consequences of sexual harassment. *Journal of*

Sexual Aggression, 18(2), 209–232. https://doi.org/10.1080/13552600.2010.501909

Reinicke, K. (2022). *Men after #MeToo: Being an ally in the fight against sexual harassment*. Springer Nature.

Rosenthal, M. N., Smidt, A. M., & Freyd, J. J. (2016). Still second class: Sexual harassment of graduate students. *Psychology of Women Quarterly, 40*(3), 364–377. https://doi.org/10.1177/0361684316644838

Rospenda, K. M., Richman, J. A., Wislar, J. S., & Flaherty, J. A. (2000). Chronicity of sexual harassment and generalized workplace abuse: Effects on drinking outcomes. *Addiction, 95*, 1805–1820. https://doi.org/10.1080/09652140020011117

Shelbourne, T. (2017, December 31). Professors accused of sexual harassment speak out. *Media Milwaukee*, 1–26. https://mediamilwaukee.com/news/jane-gallop-uwm-feminist-accused-of-sexual-harassment-uw-milwaukee/

Talbot, M. (1994, January/February). A most dangerous method: The pedagogical problem of Jane Gallop. *Lingua Franca*, 1–25. http://linguafranca.mirror.theinfo.org/Archive/method.html

Thakur, M. B., & Paul, P. (2017). Sexual harassment in academic institutions: A conceptual review. *Journal of Psychosocial Research, 12*(1), 33–40.

Uggen, C., & Blackstone, A. (2004). Sexual harassment as a gendered expression of power. *American Sociological Review, 69*(1), 64–92. https://doi.org/10.1177/000312240406900105

Vladutinu, C. J., Martin, S. L., & Macy, R. J. (2011). College- or university-based sexual assault prevention programs: A review of program outcomes: Characteristics and recommendations. *Trauma, Violence & Abuse, 12*(2), 67–86.

Vohlídalová, M. (1999). The perception and construction of sexual harassment by Czech university students. *Sociologický časopis/Czech Sociological Review, 47*(6), 1119–1147. https://www.jstor.org/stable/23535017

Weinstein, E. A., & Deutschberger, P. (1963). Some dimensions of altercasting. *Sociometry, 26*(4), 454–466.

Witze, A. (2018). Sexual harassment is rife in US science. *Nature, 558*(7710), 352–353.

Woodzicka, J. A., & LaFrance, M. (2001). Real versus imagined gender harassment. *Journal of Social Issues, 57*(1), 15–30. https://doi.org/10.1111/0022-4537.00199

Yoon, E., Funk, R. S., & Kropf, N. P. (2010). Sexual harassment experiences and their psychological correlates among a diverse sample of college women. *Affilia: Journal of Women & Social Work, 25*, 8–18. https://doi.org/10.1177/0886109909354979

CHAPTER 2

Controversies

"Power Is Neither Male nor Female"

Since the 1970s, most researchers viewed sexual harassment as a manifestation of men's workplace dominance. They examined sexual harassment through the male perpetrator/female victim lens according to which sexual harassment is a manifestation of men's interest in keeping women from obtaining desirable jobs—the kind of jobs men have—coupled with men's power to keep women from obtaining the desirable jobs they already have or aspire to (Barak et al., 1995; Farley, 1978; Gutek, 1985; MacKinnon, 1979; Schultz, 1997).

Which raises the question: what about harassment in workplaces dominated by women? In female-dominated workplaces, such as veterinary medicine and social welfare, do we find higher levels of sexual harassment committed by women? When women's power in the workplace exceeds men's, does their level of sexual harassment also exceed men's? Michael Crichton, in the epigraph to his novel, *Disclosure*, answered affirmatively: "Power is neither male nor female." As the seductive female boss explained to her male victim in the novel, "Because the fact is, harassment is a power issue. And power is neither male nor female. Whoever is behind the desk has the opportunity to abuse power."

So far, research on Crichton's hypothesis has been unclear. Women in workplaces dominated by men appear to be at greater risk of sexual harassment (Chamberlain et al., 2008; De Coster et al., 1999; Fitzgerald et al.,

© The Author(s), under exclusive license to Springer Nature Switzerland AG 2024

L. Margolin, *Women Accused of Sexual Harassment*,
https://doi.org/10.1007/978-3-031-79021-8_2

1997; Jackson & Newman, 2004; Uggen & Blackstone, 2004), and women in workplaces not dominated by men appear to experience less harassment (Raj et al., 2020; Riddle & Heaton, 2023). But little evidence supports the hypothesis that sexual harassment *committed by women* increases when women are the ones "behind the desk"—when women are in power. We know that in some male-dominated occupations such as the armed forces, sexual harassment committed by women represents a significant percentage of all harassment: a survey of sexual harassment allegations among active-duty members of the US Armed Services found that 24% of allegations were attributed to both men and women, with 4% of allegations attributed to women alone (Breslin et al., 2019). But what do these statistics mean? What kinds of harassment are women and men in the military accused of? And how do men and women collaborate to commit sexual harassment? How do they work together? When survey respondents checked the box indicating that they observed sexual harassment involving both men and women as perpetrators, were they thinking of men and women teaming up to harass a specific individual? Or were they thinking of men and women indirectly supporting a "hostile work environment" but no specific target? A survey of federal employees found that men who experienced some form of "unwanted sexual attention" at work (19% of all respondents) were more likely to say they received this unwanted sexual attention from women than from men (Newman et al., 2003). But, again, these statistics—these quantitative surveys—tell us nothing about the women responsible for harassment, their motivations, the circumstances surrounding their alleged harassment, and the types of harassment they are accused of committing.

After more than four decades of research on sexual harassment, no qualitative (or quantitative) studies of sexual harassment have been conducted with the aim of specifying the nature of sexual harassment attributed to women: how the harassment they allegedly commit and the penalties they experience compare to the allegations and penalties associated with men's harassment. While that neglect might be due to the small—perhaps even microscopic—portion of sexual harassment attributed to women, Jane Gallop suggests a reason why this topic should be studied: sexual harassment allegations against women might be a locus of sexism; they might function, like witchcraft, as a type of denunciation that unfairly targets women.

Why Do Men Harass?

Popular explanations for men's higher rates of sexual aggression often reference their higher levels of testosterone (e.g., Hsu et al., 2021), alongside cortisol and serotonin (Montoya et al., 2012). Social learning theory posits that the more men are exposed to other men's sexual aggression, the more behaviors they might otherwise see as deviant and unacceptable appear to them as normal and acceptable, and perhaps even required (Bandura, 1977). Sexually harassing behaviors such as "girl watching" are learned by men from observing other men's social behavior and by seeing this behavior valorized in popular media (Quinn, 2002). Several studies report that men who endorse traditional masculine norms are more sexually aggressive (Flood & Pease, 2009; Murnen et al., 2002), perpetrate more violence against women (Moore & Stuart, 2005), and display more physical aggression, in general (Mahalik et al., 2007; Mahalik et al., 2006). Studies also show that male aggression functions to establish and maintain men's power over women (Lawson, 2012; Taft et al., 2009), a perspective supported by research on precarious manhood (Bosson & Vandello, 2011; Bosson et al., 2009; Dagirmanjian et al., 2017; Vandello & Bosson, 2013; Vandello et al., 2008), the idea that achieving patriarchal dominance, and being perceived by others as a "real man," is something that men have to earn (Bosson & Vandello, 2011).

The earliest studies of sexual harassment argued that it is primarily motivated by sexual desire (cf. Franke, 1996; Gutek, 1985; Schultz, 1997). But over time, scholars have come to view sexual harassment differently: they see it as motivated less by sexual desire than by the pursuit of power, arguing that men who harass women tend to be motivated by ideologies of male dominance (Pryor, 1987), and select as their victims women they see as challenging or threatening male dominance (Berdahl, 2007b; Dall'Ara & Maass, 1999; Maass et al., 2003). Sexual harassment, in other words, is men's way of putting "uppity" women down, getting them out of the way, and eliminating them as potential and actual threats. In the words of Cortina and Areguin (2021, p. 286):

> People commonly think that sexual harassment is mostly about sex or romance gone awry, although nothing could be farther from the truth. More often than not, sexual harassment is a put-down not a come-on. It typically has contempt at its core, not sexual conquest (and certainly not romance).

Contemporary research argues that harassment is part of men's efforts to pursue their social, economic, and personal goals (Berdahl & Bhattacharyya, 2021; O'Leary-Kelly et al., 2000; Maass et al., 2013), and as such, belongs to the executive branch of the patriarchal order, the part concerned with policing and enforcing men's interests, privileges, and positions. From this perspective, harassment is a manifestation of Nietzschean *ressentiment*: men's awareness of their vulnerable or declining social status prompts them to lash-out at women to keep them "out of, or down in, male-dominated jobs, roles and spaces" (Berdahl & Bhattacharyya, 2021, p. 478; Manne, 2018); it is also a manifestation of men's power to lash-out (Barak et al., 1995; Connell, 2013, 2020; Farley, 1978; Gutek, 1985; MacKinnon, 1979; Schultz, 1997). Given men's higher socio-economic status—given that upper management has historically been male-dominated—they are well-positioned to protect their privileges by sexually demeaning and humiliating potential female competitors (Barak et al., 1995; Tangri et al., 1982). The sexual harassment of women, thus, not only reinforces men's entitlement and privilege; it's an effect of their entitlement and privilege (Anderson, 2006; MacKinnon, 1979).

According to this line of thinking, if earlier scholars were correct in assuming that men's sexual desire, not their social status and power, is the primary incentive for their harassment of women, then we would have found that male harassers target women who are especially "feminine" and sexually attractive. But we haven't, not according to studies utilizing the Sexual Experience Questionnaire (Fitzgerald et al., 1988, 1995; McLaughlin et al., 2012), a 17-item measure designed to assess the frequency of sexual harassment. Subjects' responses to that instrument—for instance, to the question of whether they have had harassment-like experiences (e.g., whether a supervisor or coworker may have "made sexist comments or jokes … never, rarely, sometimes, always, often")—consistently support the "not-for-sex" harassment model. They show that women with stereotypically "masculine" personalities, as measured by the Bem Sex Role Inventory (Bem, 1978)—women who would presumably be more threatening to men—report more sexual harassment than women with "feminine" personalities (Berdahl, 2007a, b; Maass et al., 2013), prompting researchers to conclude that sexual harassment "aims to put people down and push them out, not pull them into sexual activity" (Cortina & Areguin, 2021, p. 285).

Does this mean the matter is settled? Can we now speak definitively about sexual harassment aims based on the findings of randomly circulated survey instruments? Berdahl and Bhattacharyya (2021, p. 479) suggest that we can: the core motivation driving sexual harassment is "dominance," they argue, while conceding that "it is easy to get confused by the 'sexual' part of some forms of harassment."

Yes, it is easy to get confused. Confusion and uncertainty come with the territory, raising yet another question: is it possible that we sometimes get confused by the "dominance" part of some forms of sexual harassment and lose sight of the "sexual" component? The harassment case, Ellerth v. Burlington Industries (United States District Court, N. D. Illinois, Jan. 19, 1996), illustrates. In this case, a vice president of sales and marketing, Theodore Slowik, was accused of sexually harassing a woman during a preemployment interview. The woman, Kimberly Ellerth, claimed that while Slowik was discussing a sales representative position with her, he was staring at her breasts and legs. "Ellerth contends the stares were constant throughout the entire interview and she felt 'humiliated' during the interview." She also testified that in subsequent meetings, the vice president rubbed her knee and commented, "You have great legs, Kim" (Ellerth v. Burlington Industries, p. 3). Ellerth said she had no doubt that Slowik was disrespecting her: he was putting her down, humiliating her, and thus, making it difficult for her to succeed in the corporation. The court agreed, but also concluded that Slowik's behavior revealed that Ellerth's value to him was as a sex object and that her position in the company depended, to a large degree, on her sexual availability to him.

Apart from the range and variety of harassment motivations that can be attributed to Slowik—how, for example, his "putting down" motivation may have combined with a "coming on" motivation—it is, nonetheless, hard to imagine how a company vice president felt a need to "put down" someone interviewing for an entry-level job. In what ways could he have felt threatened by her?

He might, of course, have felt threatened by someone—a woman—who represented a threat to his "masculinity" rather than to his career or his workplace status. He might have believed that to earn and maintain his status as a "real man," he had to behave in sexist, sexually aggressive ways (DiMuccio & Knowles, 2020; O'Connor et al., 2017). As Lucero et al. (2003) have argued, the impulse to sexually harass is not a monolithic construct: so, Slowik might have believed that to affirm his masculinity he had to put this prospective employee down *and* attempt to pull her into sexual activity—because she is a woman. And he may have believed that putting her down could best be accomplished by pulling her into sexual activity. Another possibility is that Slowik harassed Ellerth, not only because she represented a threat to his masculinity, but also because, as someone who might become an entry-level employee—and was thus someone he had the power to hire or dismiss—she was vulnerable; she was relatively defenseless, an interpretation corroborated by studies showing that women who belong to marginalized groups—lesbians, people of color, younger women, women with insecure employment, women with functional disabilities, and those who have a history of victimization—are at greater risk of harassment (D'augelli, 1992; Fedina et al., 2018; Ong, 2005; Vladutinu et al., 2011).

Historical records tell the same story: victims of workplace sexual violence from earlier times were often female domestic servants assaulted by their male employers (Baker, 2008; Clark, 1987), suggesting that their inability to defend themselves—their vulnerability—acted as a catalyst or precondition for sexual exploitation. As an enslaved woman recalled how she came to have five children by her master: "I didn't want him, but I couldn't do nothin'" (Jennings, 1990, p. 65). If human behavior is guided by the pursuit of rewards and the avoidance of costs (Homans, 1967), a perpetrator, like the slave master who fathered multiple children with an enslaved woman, may have been encouraged by the belief that the costs of sexual aggression are relatively insignificant. Likewise, Slowik may have believed that he could harass a woman who was seeking a job, not because he was threatened by her, but rather because he felt safe—because he understood that he already had power over her. He may have harassed her because he felt he could without risk of penalty.

To be sure, there is no way to fully decipher Slowik's motivations, or the motivations of other perpetrators, not only because motivations are covert and intangible, existing only in people's minds, but also because people often hold multiple motivations, simultaneously, reflecting the possibility that expressions of contempt (put-downs), misogyny (woman-hatred), and expressions of sexual desire (come-ons) can coexist as mutually reinforcing actions and states of mind (Gilmore, 2001; Ukockis, 2019). We see this in BDSM sex, where performing activities and making comments expressing contempt for women can be experienced, by men as well as by women, as sexually exciting and desirable (Airaksinen, 2018; Turley et al., 2018; Williams, 2006). We also see multiple motivations behind the sexual objectification of women, whereby men see and interact with women, not as autonomous subjects, but as vehicles for satisfying their sexual appetites (Jütten, 2016; MacKinnon, 1989, p. 140; Nussbaum,

1995). In sexual objectification, put-downs, misogyny, and come-ons can work together, synergistically (Roberts et al., 2018).

To compound the difficulty of deciphering harassment motivations, people are often unaware of their own motivations. Motivations are inherently elusive. Imagine, then, the challenge of determining harassers' motivations from the checkmarks of randomly selected SEQ survey respondents, especially considering that the statistical association between the dependent variable (the reported occurrence of harassment experiences, such as a supervisor of coworker making "sexist comments or jokes") and the independent variable (the victim's possession of a "masculine" or "feminine" personality) may be a statistical artefact: individuals with a "masculine" personality may be more likely than others to *perceive and recall* "sexist comments and jokes" (Berdahl, 2007b; Gutek et al., 2004; McLaughlin et al., 2012). These issues may explain why a federal judge, in a 2002 sexual harassment trial, refused to admit SEQ survey data into evidence on the grounds that the SEQ "survey materials are too flawed to be useful in assisting the fact finder in this case" (quoted in Gutek et al., 2004, p. 458). These issues may also explain why it might be premature to say we understand the motivations underlying men's decisions to commit sexual harassment.

Why Do Women Harass?

The title of Gallop's book, *Feminist Accused of Sexual Harassment*, comes across as sensational/paradoxical because, as Gallop explains, "Feminist sexual harasser seems like a contradiction in terms" (p. 7). Feminists don't harass women; they support and protect them. Sexual harassment is something men do, and the victims are generally, and sometimes almost exclusively, women. Sexual harassment is about men's sexually demeaning conduct toward women in the workplace. When viewed through this lens—when sexual harassment is examined through the male perpetrator/female victim paradigm (Stemple & Meyer, 2014)—the possibility that a woman could sexually harass a man or another woman seems remote, anomalous, even absurd. That point of view may explain why scholars have paid little attention to sexual harassment attributed to women; it may also explain why scholars sometimes conflate men's and women's harassment motivations. In the words of one scholar, "the primary motive underlying *all harassment* is a desire to protect one's social status when it becomes threatened, *a desire held by men and women alike*" (Berdahl, 2007a, p. 641, italics added).

Which raises the question: if women's sexual harassment motivations are the same as men's—if both men and women harass out of a desire to protect their threatened social status—then how do we explain why observers (including researchers and scholars) attribute such a small share of harassment to women? Another, perhaps even more important question comes to mind: what informs researchers and scholars that women's motivations for harassment are the same as men's? Why assume the absence of gender differences?

The few qualitative studies which describe sexual harassment attributed to women, while very limited in scope and detail, suggest that women's sexual interest and desire play a significant role in motivating their harassment—a role that might be more significant than their interest in protecting their social status. Consider the earliest of these, a single case study (Clair, 1994) which examined the experience of a man who claimed that, shortly after he had been hired by a medical facility as a nursing assistant, he was sexually harassed by his female co-workers. His description of the harassment suggests that these coworkers made him uncomfortable, less because they were threatened by him and wanted to cut him down to size, but rather because, as the only man in their crew, he could contribute sexual information that, till his arrival, was unavailable for coffee-break conversation: he could provide new and interesting tidbits about a man's sexual proclivities:

> I was sitting at a table with my fellow nursing assistants, all female, when I suddenly became the object of an inquisition. They demanded to know if I was a virgin, if I had ever had oral sex, if I had ever been with a black woman, and so on.... (p. 259).

Two qualitative studies on sexual harassment by women which appeared in 2008 and 2010 (Scarduzio & Geist-Martin, 2008, 2010) also emphasized the sexual motivation behind women's harassment. The studies' authors sent out flyers seeking men who had experienced "unwanted sexual attention" at their university, leading to interviews with 41 respondents, four of whom were full professors who claimed that they received unwanted sexual attention from female subordinates. While it may be a stretch to claim that receiving "unwanted sexual attention," alone, is sufficient to warrant the status of "sexual harassment victim," in these studies, that is how the concept was operationalized. Among the so-called "victims," two attributed their harassment to subordinates with whom they had prior consensual sexual relationships. That each of the so-called "harassers"—three students and a staff member—occupied positions of little power relative to their so-called "victims," raises the question of how the female perpetrators managed to take advantage of the professors. It also raises the question: how do we know that the reverse was not true—that the male professors who claimed victimization by their female subordinates had not, in fact, victimized them?

The most recent qualitative study (Adikaram & Weerakotuwa, 2022) on sexual harassment attributed to women comes from interviews with heterosexual men occupying executive-level positions. Seven of the 19 respondents interviewed for the study claimed they had been victimized by women. But as in the other qualitative studies, the data is limited and imprecise. In one case, for example, an executive simply claimed a female subordinate tried to kiss him. A second executive claimed that a female subordinate with whom he once had a sexual relationship,had recorded their telephone conversations, including those in which he complained about work, and had used them to extort his sexual/romantic cooperation: she threatened to release them to management if he attempted to end their relationship. A third complained that a woman who was applying for a job at his company obtained his phone number and started calling him, oversharing about personal and sexual matters. A fourth said that a female subordinate "came on to him" once, and tried to kiss his cheeks and lips and "other sensitive parts," sometimes forcibly. A fifth stated that a female subordinate pursued him "relentlessly" even after he tried to discourage her. A sixth said his victimization consisted of female colleagues sending him unwanted text messages and inviting him on dates, even though he is married. And a seventh reported that, upon entering his cabin, he discovered a woman touching women's underwear in a sexually provocative manner, with the goal, he imagined, of arousing him. "Actually, she did not try anything physical or didn't say anything. But I think what she did was harassing" (p. 556). Perhaps because these reports provide only few and vague details on the sexual harassment attributed to women, the authors drew no conclusions on the characteristics of their alleged harassment—whether they might be similar or different from the characteristics of harassment attributed to men.

Are Women as Bad as—or Different Than—Men Who Harass?

If we compare attributions of sexual harassment by perpetrator gender, we may find that men and women harass in similar ways and are driven by similar motivations. But we may also find that those similar behaviors and motivations have radically different effects. Gender stereotypes predict that when a woman touches a man's body in a sexual way without first obtaining his consent, he won't feel particularly threatened, surely not to the same degree a woman would feel threatened when a man touches her body without first obtaining her consent, a difference confirmed by several studies (Berdahl et al., 1996; Fiske & Stevens, 1993; Gutek, 1985). Unwanted sexual attention from a woman may not traumatize a man or make him feel inferior in the ways unwanted sexual attention from a man can traumatize her or make her feel inferior because, given the way society is structured, he is not inferior, at least not in terms of his cultural and economic power (Superson, 1993, p. 55).

A woman who calls her male co-worker a "prick" or "player" may seem to be engaging in the same kind of behavior as a man who calls his female co-worker a "cunt" or "slut." But the effects are very different. The words "cunt" and "slut" have been and are used by men to dehumanize women, to reduce them to sexual acts and body parts, while the same cannot be said of "prick" and "player." That isn't to say that men cannot be sexually harassed by these kinds of smears. They can be and are (Holland et al., 2016). But the fact remains that these terms are not reinforcing a history of men's gender inferiority the way "cunt" and "slut" reinforce a history of women's gender inferiority. As MacKinnon (1979) observed, "references to sexuality have a pejorative connotation for women as a gender that is not comparable for men" (p. 182), an observation supported by the finding that men tend to rate sexually aggressive behavior from women as less threatening than similar behavior from men (Kessler et al., 2020). In general, men are less likely than women to identify either the heterosexual or homosexual encounters they've experienced as harassment (Dardis et al., 2018; Weziak-Bialowolska et al., 2020).

When it comes to gender antilocutions, it is possible that women are not only more limited in the repertoire of slurs they can use against men, but the ones they have—like "prick," "dick," "stud," "player," and "scumbag"—often sound more comical than threatening. Such a finding would be consistent with what Gutek (1985) showed four decades ago: men tend to experience sexual harassment by women as trivial, benign, and sometimes even welcome.

A "Dear Abby" letter (Van Buren, 2020) from a woman married to a Scotsman who wears kilts illustrates how sexist language and gestures work differently on men than on women. In the letter, she describes her outrage over the fact that when she and her husband go out, women frequently approach and lift his kilt, screaming with glee, yet the police respond as if it is insignificant. The last time this happened, she said, the police "kind of laughed it off." They didn't do anything. The letter concluded: "Why is there a double standard that women feel they can lift a man's kilt to expose him and call it fun, yet the same women would scream sexual assault if a man lifted their skirt?"

To be sure, under most circumstances, anyone who lifts or rips off a man's kilt in public is behaving inappropriately and offensively. But the same offense, when committed against a woman by a man, appears more serious. The double standard comes from the fact that while ripping off a man's kilt may embarrass him personally, it is not powered by the kind of stereotyping that underlies the sexual harassment of women, and it does not have the power to affect a man's social/economic/political privileges. It does not have the power to frighten, provoke, intimidate, and humiliate him in the way analogous gestures and comments can frighten, provoke, intimidate, and humiliate women, an interpretation supported by several studies (e.g., Katz et al., 1996; LaRocca & Kromrey, 1999; Smirles, 2004) which show that when a man is harassed by a woman, observers don't feel a strong reaction is required. They feel it's enough for the man (the victim) to simply "ask her (the perpetrator) to leave him alone" (Smirles, 2004, p. 358). By contrast, when a woman is harassed by a man—when he behaves offensively—observers feel he should be reported; his harassment should be taken very seriously.

I can suggest three reasons for these differences: first, men have much more cultural and economic power than women, and thus have greater capacity to inflict cultural and economic damage. They can hurt their targets in ways that go far beyond the immediate acts of harassment. Second, men are not taught to fear women's sexual predation in the ways women are, and for good reason: the victims of sexual violence are overwhelmingly women, and the victimizers are overwhelmingly men (Uggen & Blackstone, 2004). A third, paradoxical reason why male-to-female sexual harassment might be more impactful: it is relatively common, and hence, more likely to be seen as a normal part of social interaction (Quinn, 2002;

Schrock & Schwalbe, 2009). As a result, it is often excused with palliatives such as "boys will be boys" and "it's only locker room talk," language which makes it possible for men to sexually harass women with minimal risk of being called out—with minimal risk of anyone noticing or caring. As Shulamith Firestone (1970, p. 100) explained, "A man is allowed to blaspheme the world because it belongs to him … but the same curse out of the mouth of a woman or a minor, i. e., an incomplete 'man' to whom the world does not yet belong, is considered presumptuous, and thus an impropriety or worse …." Simply put, what may separate sexual harassment committed by men from sexual harassment by women, what may make the former seem more biting and more dangerous, is its likelihood of being taken for granted, going unheeded, coupled with its enormous capacity to change the lives of its victims.

The question of whether victims react differently to harassment by women than to harassment by men raises a related question: Do observers such as employers, co-workers, and investigators also react differently? Are employers and co-workers more dismissive of sexual harassment attributed to women because women have less power to harm their targets? Alternatively, since sexual harassment by women is less common, more abnormal, and thus, like "man bites dog," more noteworthy, perhaps employers and co-workers are more likely to have stronger, more negative reactions.

MacKinnon (1979, p. 6) argues that the harm of sexual harassment consists not only of disadvantaging women as individuals, but also of disadvantaging women as a gender ("sexual harassment is sex discrimination *per se* because the practice differentially injures one gender-defined group in a sphere—sexuality in employment—in which the treatment of women and men can be compared"). By implication, sexual harassment allegations when directed against women, as well as people's responses to those allegations, might represent another way of impugning and subjugating (harassing) women. Punishing a woman for sexual harassment might be another way of "putting her in her place"; it might be another way of informing her that she is not wanted, that she is too assertive, too loud, too masculine, and too overtly sexual. That is how Jane Gallop represented the sexual harassment charges levelled against her: because she, as a woman, was not expected to have power in the way men do, when she seemed to exercise power in that way—when she seemed to be acting like a man—she was seen as worse than a man. Thus, Gallop noted that a student whom she had never met, a self-styled "activist against sexual harassment," was quite willing to comment on her case to a reporter: "Jane Gallop is as bad as—no, worse than—the men who do this kind of thing" (Gallop, 1997, pp. 22–23).

Following Gallop's and MacKinnon's lead, one of my main goals is to understand the institutional processes involved in formulating sexual harassment allegations against women—to learn whether women's workplace sexual expressions and gender antilocutions are judged differently. Does perpetrator gender matter? Does the discriminatory treatment that Jane Gallop described apply to women in general? Do women accused of sexual harassment receive less social support and more condemnation than men accused of sexual harassment? Or, as illustrated in the Dear Abby letter, is the opposite true: do women accused of sexual harassment receive more social support and less condemnation?

What Is Sexual Harassment?

Richard Nixon, in signing the Higher Education Amendments of 1972, created a section, "Title IX," which states that "No person in the United States shall, on the basis of sex, be excluded from participation in, be denied the benefits of, or be subjected to discrimination under any education or activity receiving Federal financial assistance." Under Title IX, institutions of higher learning define sexual harassment as a form of discrimination. As such, the U.S. Department of Education's Office for Civil Rights (OCR) requires educational institutions that receive federal financial assistance to have policies in place for preventing and responding to sexual harassment in a timely manner. Each institution must designate a Title IX coordinator to oversee complaints and must promptly adopt and publish equitable complaint procedures.

Still, considerable uncertainty remains regarding what constitutes sexual harassment. While this offense is generally understood as any behavior that degrades, demeans, humiliates, or violates an individual in the workplace based on their sex or gender (Berdahl, 2007a; Lopez et al., 2009), the term has no single, universally accepted definition, and as a result, is often used and applied in different ways.

In the United States, one of the most widely quoted and accepted definitions of sexual harassment is that of the Equal Employment Opportunity Commission (Code of Federal Regulations, Title 29, 1604.11):

> Unwelcome sexual advances, requests for sexual favors, and other verbal or physical conduct of a sexual nature constitutes sexual harassment when: (1) submission to such conduct is made either explicitly or implicitly a term or condition of an individual's employment, (2) submission to or rejection of such conduct by an individual is used as the basis for employment decisions affecting such an individual, or (3) such conduct has the purpose or effect of unreasonably interfering with an individual's work performance, or creating an intimidating, hostile or offensive working environment (EEOC, 2016).

That this definition does not assume that the harasser is a man or the victim is a woman may be its most positive feature. It recognizes the reality that women can be harassers and men can be victims. Another positive feature of this definition is that it does not limit sexual harassment to the supervisor/supervisee relationship. Again, it recognizes the reality that sexual harassment is not restricted to any group or status: peers and subordinates—co-workers of any rank—can engage in sexual harassment.

On the negative side, the definition relies on loaded, ambiguous terms. For example, the term "unwelcome sexual advances" raises several questions. Unwelcome to whom? Unwelcome in what way? Sexual according to what measure? These uncertainties can cause confusion in harassment investigations since they highlight the potential gap between the victims' and perpetrators' interpretations of the kinds of harassment that may or may not have taken place. A look, a smile, a touch, or a hug can be interpreted in any number of ways: as innocuous, friendly, supportive, or as an "unwelcome sexual advance," which suggests that sexual harassment is often a matter of perspective, something that exists differently in the eyes of different beholders (Craig & Cossette, 2022). An additional source of confusion is that the EEOC definition, while based on the occurrence of so-called unwanted sexual advances, does not distinguish among types of unwanted advances, thus creating a technical equivalency between a look or smile and a sexual assault, a conflation that is both mystifying and impractical.

Other issues include the fact that the EEOC definition does not specify contingencies such as social context or the actors' intentions (either the accused's good intentions or the accuser's bad intentions), nor does it allow investigators to emphasize (or deemphasize) any ameliorating or aggravating conditions, such as the putative harasser's belief that a victim may have invited the sexual advance, the victim may have enjoyed the unwanted kisses, and that the victim may have even signaled an interest in receiving aggressive sexual attention.

The terms "sexual favors" and "sexual nature" are similarly ambiguous. Again, the EEOC definition disregards the question of how gestures, facial expressions, verbal allusions or innuendoes, jokes, or written communication should be defined as "sexual"—what makes a gesture or facial expression sufficiently sexual to warrant the label *sexual* harassment. It also disregards the question, not only of how to distinguish unwanted sexual gestures from unwanted sexual *advances*—how exactly are we to define a sexual advance?—but also why such distinctions matter.

Then there is the issue of hostile actions and motivations—where they fit into the EEOC definition of sexual harassment. Consider, for example, the term "intimidating, hostile or offensive working environment." While it may be possible to identify offensive behaviors or activities that interfere with an individual's work performance, it remains to be seen how an *environment* can be assessed as either "intimidating" or "nonintimidating," "hostile" or "nonhostile," "offensive" or "inoffensive." Can any unwelcome behavior or comment that somehow connects to sex or gender suffice to make a working environment "intimidating," "hostile," or "offensive"? If not, what behaviors or comments (and how many) should be treated as capable of imposing such conditions on an entire working environment? Because the concept lacks specificity, it can be applied in widely different ways, depending on investigators' biases and priorities. It can expand or contract indefinitely, making it what Patai (1998) calls an "accordion concept." As a result of this indefiniteness, exaggerated or false allegations of sexual harassment may be treated as true and allegations of harassment that are true may be dismissed as false or exaggerated.

A final question that the EEOC definition leaves unanswered is how to distinguish *sexual* harassment from general workplace harassment, defined as "interpersonal interaction that affects the terms, conditions, or employment decisions related to an individual's job, or creates an intimidating, hostile or oppressive work environment, but is not based on any legally protected characteristic" such as sex or gender (Rospenda & Richman, 2004, pp. 221–222). If general workplace harassment is driven mainly by hostility, but a portion of this hostility can be related to sex or gender, how are we to disentangle sexual harassment from general workplace harassment? How are we to disentangle them when, in practice, in peoples' perceptions and decision-making, sexual harassment and other forms of harassment often overlap? For example, many kinds of sexual harassment can be interpreted as hostile—as intended to hurt or to harm: pinching, grabbing, biting, groping, bra-flicking, teasing, ridiculing, name-calling, forcibly pulling a person's underpants upwards from the back, not to mention rape and attempted rape—but these behaviors can also be interpreted as driven, to some degree, by sexual desire and gender performance, leaving open the question of whether the offensive behaviors in question should be identified as sexual harassment or general workplace harassment.

There is, of course, no objective answer to any of these questions. That Title IX investigators, universities, colleges, and courts lack clear guidelines on how to identify sexual harassment, much less differentiate it from other workplace offenses, means that some individuals accused of serious offenses will walk away—they'll be excused—while others who are accused of lesser offenses will face significant penalties. The system, in short, lacks coherence.

Hypotheses

This research anticipates differences in the ways men and women perform (or are accused of performing) sexual harassment because there are so many well-established gender differences in other areas: in men's and women's physical and mental health (Kawachi et al., 1999; Otten et al., 2021; Rosenfield & Mouzon, 2013), in their psychosocial, cultural, and personality patterns (Codorow, 1978; Ezzedeen et al., 2015; Tavris, 1993; Tannen, 1994), and in their moral decision making (Gilligan, 1982). When these differences in men's and women's functioning are coupled with the evidence that women commit far less sexual harassment than men, it makes sense to expect differences in the ways that men and women perform and interpret sexual harassment.

A second expected gender difference in sexual harassment is how investigators and public opinion assess harassment attributed to women and men—measurable in part by how women and men are treated after the allegations have occurred. Studies of female and male sentencing in courts consistently show that women are treated differently than men, receiving significantly lighter sentences than their male counterparts (Doerner & Demuth, 2014; Kim et al., 2019), even in cases involving sexual offenses (Beeby et al., 2021; Shields & Cochran, 2020). Those findings suggest that sexual harassment attributed to women is judged more tolerantly, with more forgiveness, than sexual harassment attributed to men, a hypothesis consistent with the relatively small number of women listed on the Academic Sexual Misconduct Database. What these studies do not explain, however, is why the sexual harassment allegations against Jane Gallop and several other women appear inflated, and the penalties they endured appear extraordinary, so much harsher than those endured by male faculty and administrators from the same or similar institutions accused of more serious offenses—offenses representing elevated levels of hostility and aggression. Given these discrepancies, this research explores the possibility that Jane Gallop and other women are subject to stiffer penalties and greater condemnation because they occupy high-status, masculine-coded positions, an explanation consistent with psychologist L. A. Rudman's (Rudman et al., 2012) belief that people often unknowingly punish women who compete for, or otherwise seek advancement to, high-status positions. They are punished, according to Rudman, because they are seen as threats to existing gender hierarchies and because they possess agentic qualities (i.e., confidence, competence, independence) deemed undesirable in women. Rudman calls this the "status incongruity hypothesis," a hypothesis which extends to both men and women who stray from traditional gender roles and norms (see Leskinen et al., 2015; McLaughlin et al., 2012).

Research consistently shows that women accused of criminal offenses are treated more leniently than men accused of comparable offenses, but there is little data on whether women's membership (or apparent membership) in the LGBTQ community may influence judgments against them (Buist & Lenning, 2022; Woods, 2014). However, following the status incongruity hypothesis, this research predicts that women who identify as lesbian or who are accused of targeting other women are more likely to be identified as sexual harassers.

Finally, consistent with research showing that sexual harassment victims' perceived vulnerability—their youth, economic insecurity, membership in minority groups, and history of victimization—is associated with future victimization (D'augelli, 1992; Klein & Martin, 2021; Vladutinu et al., 2011; Zijlstra et al., 2017), this research predicts that victims of sexual harassment occupy lower, more vulnerable positions than their presumptive harassers, whether the harassers are men or women. While many individuals who are relatively powerless do not experience harassment, and many who are relatively powerful do, a person's perceived inability to defend themselves—their vulnerability—can act as an impetus for exploitation. Because people are more likely to engage in behavior that maximizes their rewards and minimizes their costs (Homans, 1967), individuals who are inclined to sexually harass will be more likely to follow that inclination when they believe the costs are insignificant—when they believe they won't experience resistance or punishment. Like slave masters who raped and exploited enslaved women and girls, probably men and boys too, they will be encouraged by the belief that they can transgress with impunity. Burn (2019) calls this the "vulnerable victim hypothesis."

References

Adikaram, A., & Weerakotuwa, S. (2022). Scorned by men and pursued by women: Sexual harassment of heterosexual working men. *Gender in Management: An International Journal, 37*(4), 549–565. https://doi.org/10.1108/GM-08-2021-0242

Airaksinen, T. (2018). The language of pain: A philosophical study of BDSM. *Sexualities, 8*(2), 1–9. https://doi.org/10.1177/2158244018771730

Anderson, E. (2006). Recent thinking about sexual harassment: A review essay. *Philosophy & Public Affairs, 34*(3), 284–311. https://www.jstor.org/stable/3876394

Baker, C. N. (2008). *The women's movement against sexual harassment*. Cambridge University Press.

Bandura, A. (1977). *Social learning theory*. Prentice-Hall.

Barak, A., Pitterman, Y., & Yitzhaki, R. (1995). An empirical test of the role of power differential in originating sexual harassment. *Basic and Applied Social Psychology, 17*(4), 497–517. https://doi.org/10.1207/s15324834basp1704_5

Beeby, A., Hobbs, L., Gross, J., Hayne, H., & Patterson, T. (2021). Gender disparities in sentencing outcomes for sexual offenders. *Journal of Sexual Aggression, 27*(3), 319–337. https://doi.org/10.1080/13552600.2020.1784476

Bem, S. L. (1978). *The Bem sex role inventory*. Consulting Psychologists Press.

Berdahl, J. L. (2007a). Harassment based on sex: Protecting social status in the context of gender hierarchy. *Academy of Management Review, 32*(2), 641–658. https://www.jstor.org/stable/20159319

Berdahl, J. L. (2007b). The sexual harassment of uppity women. *Journal of Applied Psychology, 92*(2), 425–437. https://doi.org/10.1037/0021-9010.92.2.425

Berdahl, J., & Bhattacharyya, B. (2021). Four ways forward in studying sex-based harassment. *Equality, Diversity and Inclusion: An International Journal, 40*(4), 477–492. https://www.emerald.com/insight/2040-7149.htm

Berdahl, J., Magley, V. J., & Waldo, C. R. (1996). The sexual harassment of men? *Psychology of Women Quarterly, 20*, 527–547.

Bosson, J. K., & Vandello, J. A. (2011). Precarious manhood and its links to action and aggression. *Current Directions in Psychological Science, 20*, 82–86. https://doi.org/10.1177/0963721411402669

Bosson, J. K., Vandello, J. A., Burnaford, R. M., Weaver, J. R., & Wasti, S. A. (2009). Precarious manhood and displays of physical aggression. *Personality and Social Psychology Bulletin, 35*, 625–634. https://doi.org/10.1177/0146167208331161

Breslin, R. A., Davis, E., Hylton, K., Hill, A., Klauberg, W., Petusky, M., & Klahr, A. (2019). *2018 workplace and gender relations survey of active duty members: Overview report (Report no. 2019–027)*. Office of People Analytics.

Buist, C. L., & Lenning, E. (2022). *Queer Criminology*. Routledge.

Burn, S. M. (2019). The psychology of sexual harassment. *Teaching of Psychology, 46*(1), 96–103. https://doi.org/10.1177/0098628318816183

Chamberlain, L. J., Crowley, M., Tope, M., & Hodson, R. (2008). Sexual harassment in organizational context. *Work and Occupations, 35*(3), 262–295. https://doi.org/10.1177/0730888408322008

Clair, R. P. (1994). Resistance and oppression as a self-contained opposite: An organizational communication analysis of one man's story of sexual harassment. *Western Journal of Communication, 58*, 235–262.

Clark, A. (1987). *Women's silence, men's violence. Sexual assault in England 1770–1845*. Pandora Press.

Codorow, N. (1978). *The Reproduction of Mothering: Psychoanalysis and the Sociology of Gender*. Berkeley.

Connell, R. (2013). *Gender and power: Society, the person and sexual politics*. John Wiley & Sons.

Connell, R. W. (2020). *Masculinities*. Routledge.

Cortina, L. M., & Areguin, M. A. (2021). Putting people down and pushing them out: Sexual harassment in the workplace. *Annual Review of Organizational Psychology and Organizational Behavior, 8*, 285–309. https://doi.org/10.1146/annurev-orgpsych-012420-055606

Craig, S. C., & Cossette, P. S. (2022). Eye of the beholder: Partisanship, identity, and the politics of sexual harassment. *Political Behavior, 44*, 749–777.

D'augelli, A. (1992). Lesbian and gay male undergraduates experiences of harassment and fear. *Journal of Interpersonal Violence, 7*(3), 383–396. https://doi.org/10.1177/088626092007003007

Dagirmanjian, F. B., Mahalik, J. R., Boland, J., Colbow, A., Dunn, J., Pomarico, A., & Rappaport, D. (2017). How do men construct and explain men's violence? *Journal of Interpersonal Violence, 32*(15), 2275–2297. https://doi.org/10.1177/0886260515625511

Dall'Ara, E., & Maass, A. (1999). Studying sexual harassment in the laboratory: Are egalitarian women at higher risk? *Sex Roles, 41*(9), 681–704.

Dardis, C. M., Vento, S. A., Gradus, J. L., & Street, A. E. (2018). Labeling of deployment sexual harassment experiences among male and female veterans. *Psychological Trauma Theory Research Practice and Policy, 10*(4), 452–455. https://doi.org/10.1037/tra0000330

De Coster, S., Estes, S. B., & Mueller, W. C. (1999). Routine activities and sexual harassment in the workplace. *Work and Occupations, 26*, 21–49.

DiMuccio, E. D., & Knowles, E. D. (2020). The political significance of fragile masculinity. *Current Opinion in Behavioral Sciences, 34*, 25–28.

Doerner, J. K., & Demuth, S. (2014). Gender and sentencing in the federal courts: Are women treated more leniently? *Criminal Justice Policy Review, 25*(2), 242–269.

Equal Employment Opportunity Commission (EEOC). (2016). https://www.eeoc.gov/select-task-force-study-harassment-workplace

Ezzedeen, S. R., Budworth, M.-H., & Baker, S. D. (2015). The Glass ceiling and executive careers: Still an issue for pre-career women. *Journal of Career Development, 42*, 355–369. https://doi.org/10.1177/0894845314566943

Farley, L. (1978). *Sexual shakedown: The sexual harassment of women on the job.* McGraw-Hill.

Fedina, L., Holmes, J. L., & Backes, B. L. (2018). Campus sexual assault: A systematic review of prevalence research from 2000 to 2015. *Trauma, Violence & Abuse, 19*(1), 76–93. https://doi.org/10.1177/1524838016631129

Firestone, S. (1970). *The dialectic of sex.* William Morrow.

Fiske, S. T., & Stevens, L. E. (1993). What's so special about sex? Gender stereotyping and discrimination. In S. Oskamp & M. Costanzo (Eds.), *Gender issues in contemporary society* (pp. 173–196). Sage.

Fitzgerald, L., Drasgow, F., Hulin, C. L., Gefland, M. J., & Magley, V. J. (1997). Antecedents and consequences of sexual harassment in organizations: A test of an integrated model. *Journal of Applied Psychology, 82*, 578–589.

Fitzgerald, L. F., Gelfand, M. J., & Drasgow, F. (1995). Measuring sexual harassment: Theoretical and psychometric advances. *Basic and Applied Social Psychology, 17*(4), 425–445. https://doi.org/10.1207/s15324834basp1704_2

Fitzgerald, L. F., Shullman, S. L., Bailey, N., Richards, M., Swecker, J., Gold, Y., et al. (1988). The incidence and dimensions of sexual harassment in academia and the workplace. *Journal of Vocational Behavior, 32*(2), 152–175. https://doi.org/10.1016/0001-8791(88)90012-7

Flood, M., & Pease, B. (2009). Factors influencing attitudes to violence against women. *Trauma Violence Abuse, 10*, 125–142. https://doi.org/10.1177/1524838009334131

Franke, K. M. (1996). What's wrong with sexual harassment. *Stanford Law Review, 49*, 691–772.

Gallop, J. (1997). *Feminist accused of sexual harassment.* Duke University Press.

Gilligan, C. (1982). In a different voice: Women's conception of the self and of morality. *Harvard Educational Review, 49*, 481–517.

Gilmore, D. D. (2001). *Misogyny: The male malady*. University of Pennsylvania Press.

Gutek, B. (1985). *Sex and the workplace: The impact of sexual behavior and harassment on women, men, and organizations*. Jossey-Bass.

Gutek, B. A., Murphy, R. O., & Douma, B. (2004). A review and critique of the Sexual Experiences Questionnaire (SEQ). *Law and Human Behavior, 28*(4), 457–482.

Holland, K. J., Rabelo, V. C., Gustafson, A. M., Seabrook, R. C., & Cortina, L. M. (2016). Sexual harassment against men: Examining the roles of feminist activism, sexuality, and organizational context. *Psychology of Men & Masculinity, 17*(1), 17–29.

Homans, G. C. (1967). Fundamental social processes. In N. Smelser (Ed.), *Sociology* (pp. 549–594). Wiley.

Hsu, N., Badura, K. L., Newman, D. A., & Speach, M. E. P. (2021). Gender, "masculinity," and "femininity": A meta-analytic review of gender differences in agency and communion. *Psychological Bulletin, 147*(10), 987–1011. https://doi.org/10.1037/bul0000343

Jackson, R. A., & Newman, M. A. (2004). Sexual harassment in the federal workplace revisited: Influences on sexual harassment by gender. *Public Administration Review, 64*(6), 705–717.

Jennings, T. (1990). "Us colored women had to go through a plenty": Sexual exploitation of African-American slave women. *Journal of Women's History, 1*(3), 45–74. https://doi.org/10.1353/jowh.2010.0050

Jütten, T. (2016). Sexual objectification. *Ethics, 127*(1), 27–49. https://doi.org/10.1086/687331open

Katz, R. C., Hannon, R., & Whitten, L. (1996). Effects of gender and situation on the perception of sexual harassment. *Sex Roles, 34*, 35–42.

Kawachi, I., Kennedy, B. P., Gupta, V., & Prothrow-Stith, D. (1999). Women's status and the health of women and men: A view from the States. *Social Science & Medicine, 48*(1), 21–32.

Kessler, A. M., Kennair, L. E. O., Grøntvedt, T. V., Bjørkheim, I., Drejer, I., & Bendixen, M. (2020). The effect of prototypical# MeToo features on the perception of social-sexual behavior as sexual harassment. *Sexuality and Culture, 24*(5), 1271–1291.

Kim, B., Wang, X., & Cheon, H. (2019). Examining the impact of contexts on gender disparity in federal sentencing. *Justice Quarterly, 36*(3), 466–502.

Klein, L. B., & Martin, S. L. (2021). Sexual harassment of college and university students: A systematic review. *Trauma, Violence & Abuse, 22*(4), 777–792. https://doi.org/10.1177/1524838019881731

LaRocca, M. A., & Kromrey, J. D. (1999). The perception of sexual harassment in higher education: Impact of gender and attractiveness. *Sex Roles, 40*, 921–936.

Lawson, J. (2012). Sociological theories of intimate partner violence. *Journal of Human Behavior in the Social Environment, 22*, 572–590. https://doi.org/10.1080/10911359.2011.598748

Leskinen, E. A., Rabelo, V. C., & Cortina, L. M. (2015). Gender stereotyping and harassment: A 'Catch-22' for women in the workplace. *Psychology, Public Policy, and Law, 21*(2), 192–204.

Lopez, S. H., Hodson, R., & Roscigno, V. J. (2009). Power, status, and abuse at work: General and sexual harassment compared. *The Sociological Quarterly, 50*(1), 3–27.

Lucero, M. A., Middleton, K. L., Finch, W. A., & Valentine, S. R. (2003). An empirical investigation of sexual harassers: Toward a perpetrator typology. *Human Relations, 56*, 1461–1483.

Maass, A., Cadinu, M., & Galdi, S. (2013). Sexual harassment: Motivations and consequences. In M. K. Ryan & N. R. Branscombe (Eds.), *The Sage handbook of gender and psychology* (pp. 341–358). Sage.

Maass, A., Cadinu, M., Guarnieri, G., & Guarnieri, A. (2003). Sexual harassment under social identity threat: The computer harassment paradigm. *Journal of Personality and Social Psychology, 85*(5), 853–870. https://doi.org/10.1037/0022-3514.85.5.853

MacKinnon, C. A. (1979). *Sexual harassment of working women: A case of sex discrimination.* Yale University Press.

MacKinnon, C. A. (1989). *Toward a feminist theory of the state.* Harvard University Press.

Mahalik, J. R., Burns, S. M., & Syzdek, M. (2007). Masculinity and perceived normative health behaviors as predictors of men's health behaviors. *Social Science & Medicine, 64*, 2201–2209. https://doi.org/10.1016/j.socscimed.2007.02.035

Mahalik, J. R., Lagan, H. D., & Morrison, J. A. (2006). Health behaviors and masculinity in Kenyan and U.S. male college students. *Psychology of Men & Masculinity, 7*, 191–202. https://doi.org/10.1037/1524-9220.7.4.191

Manne, K. (2018). *Down girl: The logic of misogyny.* Oxford University Press.

McLaughlin, H., Uggen, C., & Blackstone, A. (2012). Sexual harassment, workplace authority, and the paradox of power. *American Sociological Review, 77*(4), 625–647. https://doi.org/10.1177/0003122412451728

Montoya, E. R., Terburg, D., Bos, P. A., & van Honk, J. (2012). Testosterone, cortisol, and serotonin as key regulators of social aggression: A review and theoretical perspective. *Motivation and Emotion, 36*, 65–73. https://doi.org/10.1007/s11031-011-9264-3

Moore, T. M., & Stuart, G. L. (2005). A review of the literature on masculinity and partner violence. *Psychology of Men & Masculinity, 6*, 46–61. https://doi.org/10.1037/1524-9220.6.1.46

Murnen, S. K., Wright, C., & Kaluzny, G. (2002). If "boys will be boys," Then girls will be victims? A metaanalytic review of the research that relates masculine ideology to sexual aggression. *Sex Roles, 46*, 359–375.

Newman, M. A., Jackson, R. A., & Baker, D. D. (2003). Sexual harassment in the federal workforce. *Public Administration Review, 63*(4), 472–483. https://doi.org/10.1111/1540-6210.00309

Nussbaum, M. C. (1995). Objectification. *Philosophy & Public Affairs, 24*(4), 249–291. https://doi.org/10.1111/j.1088-4963.1995.tb00032.x

O'Connor, E. C., Ford, T. E., & Bamos, N. C. (2017). Restoring threatened masculinity: The appeal of sexist and anti-gay humor. *Sex Roles, 77*, 567–580.

O'Leary-Kelly, A. M., Paetzold, R. L., & Griffin, R. W. (2000). Sexual harassment as aggressive behavior: An actor-based perspective. *Academy of Management Review, 25*(2), 372–388. https://doi.org/10.5465/amr.2000.3312924

Ong, M. (2005). Body projects of young women of color in physics: Intersections of Gender, Race, and Science. *Social Problems, 52*(4), 593–617. https://doi.org/10.1525/sp.2005.52.4.593

Otten, D., Tibubos, A. N., Schomerus, G., Brähler, E., Binder, H., Kruse, J., et al. (2021). Similarities and differences of mental health in women and men: A systematic review of findings in three large German cohorts. *Frontiers in Public Health, 9*, 553071. https://doi.org/10.3389/fpubh.2021.553071

Patai, D. (1998). *Heterophobia*. Rowman and Littlefield.

Pryor, J. B. (1987). Sexual harassment proclivities in men. *Sex Roles, 17*, 269–290.

Quinn, B. A. (2002). Sexual harassment and masculinity: The power and meaning of "girl watching". *Gender & Society, 16*, 386–402.

Raj, A., Johns, N. E., & Jose, R. (2020). Gender parity at work and its association with workplace sexual harassment. *Workplace Health & Safety, 68*(6), 279–292.

Riddle, K., & Heaton, K. (2023). Antecedents to sexual harassment of women in selected male-dominated occupations: A systematic review. *Workplace Health & Safety, 71*(8), 356–365.

Roberts, T., Calogero, R. M., & Gervais, S. J. (2018). Objectification theory: Continuing contributions to feminist psychology. In C. B. Travis, J. W. White, A. Rutherford, W. S. Williams, S. L. Cook, & K. F. Wyche (Eds.), *APA handbook of the psychology of women: History, theory, and battlegrounds* (pp. 249–271). American Psychological Association.

Rosenfield, S., & Mouzon, D. (2013). Gender and mental health. In C. Aneshensel, J. Phelan, & A. Bierman (Eds.), *Handbook of the sociology of mental health* (2nd ed., pp. 277–296). Springer.

Rospenda, K. M., & Richman, J. A. (2004). The factor structure of generalized workplace harassment. *Violence and Victims, 19*, 221–238.

Rudman, L. A., Moss-Racusin, C., Phelan, J. E., & Nauts, S. (2012). Status incongruity and backlash effects: Defending the gender hierarchy motivates prejudice against female leaders. *Journal of Experimental Social Psychology, 48*, 165–179. https://doi.org/10.1016/j.jesp.2011.10.008

Scarduzio, J. A., & Geist-Martin, P. (2008). Making sense of fractured identities: Male professors' narratives of sexual harassment. *Communication Monographs, 75*, 369–395.

Scarduzio, J. A., & Geist-Martin, P. (2010). Accounting for victimization: Male professors' ideological positioning in stories of sexual harassment. *Management Communication Quarterly, 24*(3), 419–445. https://doi.org/10.1177/0893318909358746

Schrock, D., & Schwalbe, M. (2009). Men, masculinity, and manhood acts. *Annual Review of Sociology, 35*, 277–295.

Schultz, V. (1997). Reconceptualizing sexual harassment. *The Yale Law Journal, 107*, 1683.

Shields, R. T., & Cochran, J. C. (2020). The gender gap in sex offender punishment. *Journal of Quantitative Criminology, 36*(1), 95–118. https://doi.org/10.1007/s10940-019-09416-x

Smirles, K. E. (2004). Attributions of responsibility in cases of sexual harassment: The person and the situation. *Journal of Applied Social Psychology, 34*(2), 342–365.

Stemple, L., & Meyer, I. H. (2014). The sexual victimization of men in America: New data Challenge old assumptions. *American Journal of Public Health, 104*(6), 19–26.

Superson, A. (1993). A feminist definition of sexual harassment. *Journal of Social Philosophy, 24*(1), 46–64.

Taft, C., Bryant-Davis, T., Woodward, H., Tillman, S., & Torres, S. (2009). Intimate partner violence against African American women: An examination of the sociocultural context. *Aggression and Violent Behavior, 14*, 50–58. https://doi.org/10.1016/j.avb.2008.10.001

Tangri, S., Burt, M. R., & Johnson, L. B. (1982). Sexual harassment at work: Three explanatory models. *Journal of Social Issues, 38*(4), 33–54. https://doi.org/10.1111/j.1540-4560.1982.tb01909.x

Tannen, D. (1994). *Gender and discourse*. Oxford University Press.

Tavris, C. (1993). The mismeasure of woman. *Feminism & Psychology, 3*(2), 149–168.

Turley, E. L., King, N., & Monro, S. (2018). 'You want to be swept up in it all': Illuminating the erotic in BDSM. *Psychology & Sexuality, 9*(2), 148–160. https://doi.org/10.1080/19419899.2018.1448297

Uggen, C., & Blackstone, A. (2004). Sexual harassment as a gendered expression of power. *American Sociological Review, 69*(1), 64–92. https://doi.org/10.1177/000312240406900105

Ukockis, G. (2019). *Misogyny: The new activism*. Oxford University Press.

Van Buren, A. (2020, October 13). Dear Abby: When women lift man's kilt, it isn't funny, it's a Crime. *Chicago Sun-Times*. https://chicago.suntimes.com/2021/10/13/22722959/dear-abby-when-women-lift-mans-kilt-it-isnt-funny-its-a-crime

Vandello, J. A., & Bosson, J. K. (2013). Hard won and easily lost: A review and synthesis of theory and research on precarious manhood. *Psychology of Men & Masculinity, 14*, 101–113. https://doi.org/10.1037/a0029826

Vandello, J. A., Bosson, J. K., Cohen, D., Burnaford, R. M., & Weaver, J. R. (2008). Precarious manhood. *Journal of Personality and Social Psychology, 95*(60), 1325–1339.

Vladutinu, C. J., Martin, S. L., & Macy, R. J. (2011). College- or university-based sexual assault prevention programs: A review of program outcomes: Characteristics and recommendations. *Trauma, Violence & Abuse, 12*(2), 67–86.

Węziak-Białowolska, D., Białowolski, P., Mordukhovich, I., & McNeely, E. (2020). Work, gender and sexual harassment on the frontlines of commercial travel: A cross-sectional study of flight crew well-being. *The International Journal of Aerospace Psychology, 30*(3/4), 171–189.

Williams, D. J. (2006). Different (painful¡) strokes for different folks: A general overview of sexual sadomasochism (SM) and its diversity. *Sexual Addiction & Compulsivity, 13*(4), 333–346. https://doi.org/10.1080/10720160601011240

Woods, J. B. (2014). Queering criminology: Overview of the state of the field. In D. Peterson & V. R. Panfil (Eds.), *Handbook of LGBT communities, crime and justice* (pp. 15–41). Springer.

Zijlstra, E., Esselink, G., Moors, M. L., LoFoWong, S., Hutschemaekers, G., & Lagro-Janssen, A. (2017). Vulnerability and revictimization: Victim characteristics in a Dutch assault center. *Journal of Forensic and Legal Medicine, 52*, 199–207.

PART I

CHAPTER 3

"A Real Monster"

On August 13, 2018, in a front-page story, the *New York Times* reported that Avital Ronell, "one of the very few philosopher-stars of the world" had been suspended from New York University for a year without pay for sexually harassing her graduate student, Nimrod Reitman. The harassment began, according to Reitman's deposition (see Nimrod Reitman v Avital Ronell and New York University, Supreme Court of the State of New York, 8/16/2018), in the spring of 2012, before he had officially launched his doctoral studies, when Ronell invited him to visit her in Paris. Reitman claimed that although Ronell assured him that he would have his own bedroom and full privacy in her apartment, on his first night there, she asked him to read to her in her bedroom. Soon after, she insisted he get on the bed beside her, and he did so, he said, because he did not want to anger or alienate his future dissertation advisor. She then began kissing him, he said, several times attempting open-mouth kisses, then started groping him both over and under his clothing, and at one point, pushed her buttocks into his groin and put his hands on her breasts, behaviors which made him profoundly uncomfortable, and which continued, he claimed, during the entirety of the time she served as his advisor.

The first question raised by this narrative is, why did Reitman appear to encourage Ronell's expressions of attraction and affection? Why did he appear to lead her to believe that he reciprocated much, if not all, of what she felt for him? Why did he send her email messages such as:

© The Author(s), under exclusive license to Springer Nature Switzerland AG 2024

L. Margolin, *Women Accused of Sexual Harassment*,
https://doi.org/10.1007/978-3-031-79021-8_3

> Sweet Beloved, I was so happy to see you tonight, and spend time together. It was so magical and important, crucial on [sic] so many ways. Our shared intimacy was a glorious cadence to our time in Berlin. Thank you for these moments of togetherness and utter pure love!...Infinitely, - n. (Avital Ronell's press release, 2018, p. 3)

> My beloved Avital, Just sending you infinite kisses and love. Thank you for your being my most precious blessing. Loving, you – n. (p. 3)

> Beloved...Missing you and loving you ! – n. (p. 3)

> Baby. It was so wonderful seeing you today. You looked wonderful...I miss you terribly and await seeing you already.... (p. 3)

Reitman acknowledged that he often communicated with Ronell in extravagant, romantic language, but claimed he did so only because Ronell pressured him. She "demands that I voice certain phrases that I do not want to say..." (see Reitman v Ronell, p. 12). And he attempted to prove that Ronell abused her power over him by sharing several email and voicemail messages with the court in which she describes the urgency of her need for him. But instead of illustrating her domination, as he claimed, these messages may also be read as evidence that Ronell, as one who was in love with someone who did not fully reciprocate, experienced devastating powerlessness. They may be read as evidence of Reitman's domination over her:

> I am struggling but you address me as though I were another. ...You occupy an immense place in my life, in my heart, and I need to hear from yours... (Reitman v Ronell, p. 10)

> ... Maybe we can find a way for this not to happen, for me not to feel unnecessarily abandoned... (Reitman v Ronell, p. 10)

> Hi Sweetie. I'm checking in on you. I was wondering when you were planning to tell me how great our session was and how elated you are, over the moon, and so on... (Reitman v Ronell, p. 16)

Reitman testified that Ronell required him to always be available, to always be on call, day or night—as if her life and her needs should be his singular priorities. As evidence of her power over him (and of his victimization), he cited a series of messages from her, which, again, can be interpreted in an alternative way, as evidence of Reitman's power over her: "are you awake?"

she messaged one night, "I really do need to talk to you as promised!" "is it too late to hear yr beautiful voice?" "I guess it's too late for you at this point—I sought solace by imagining some more talk, wanting to hear your voice..." (p. 12).

To understand how these emails and voicemails were submitted to the court as evidence of Ronell's power over Reitman, we should turn to the concept of gaslighting, but not only to the kind of personal gaslighting which Reitman appears to have been using on Ronell—when he knowingly and consistently led her to believe things about their relationship which were untrue and thus undermined her capacity to assess the nature of their relationship (see Abramson, 2014)—but to the kind that Berenstain (2020) identifies as *structural gaslighting*. In the latter, gaslighting occurs when rhetors attempt to "obscure the nonaccidental connections between structures of oppression and the patterns of harm they produce and license"—when they invoke epistemologies and ideologies of oppression that tend to obscure the actual causes, mechanisms, and effects of oppression (p. 734). In the Reitman/Ronell case, for example, structural gaslighting occurred when Reitman and his supporters appeared to dismiss the existence of men's systematic violence against women, as in these comments that appeared on page one of the *New York Times* on August 17, 2018:

> Nimrod Reitman's very credible accusations against Avital Ronell point to what many women and men know firsthand: Women, too, can be abusers, and can inflict as much pain, humiliation, and shame as any man .... Women are not angels, and men are not sadists; predator and prey are not gendered roles. (Macaux, 2018).

By citing Ronell's emails and voicemails as evidence of her power to control his behavior, Reitman and his supporters appealed to the well-accepted dynamics of sexual harassment, only in those dynamics, the genders are reversed. So, instead of "dastardly men ... bend[ing] passive damsels to their wills" as Kipnis (2017, p. 53) described the conventional understanding of sexual harassment on campus, we have "dastardly women ... bending passive young men to their wills." By equating women's violence to men's—by representing sexual harassment as fundamentally, even pragmatically, genderless (women "can inflict as much pain, humiliation, and shame as any man")—the ongoing reality in which women are disproportionately harassed, raped, physically attacked, and killed by men becomes obfuscated. That obfuscation not only normalizes men's violence against women, but, on a micro-level, characterizes a man, Reitman, as a victim, and a woman, Ronell, as violent as "any man" (cf. Davis & Ernst, 2019; Berenstain, 2020).

One of the ways Ronell succeeded in forcing herself into Reitman's life, Reitman said, was to portray herself as extraordinarily fragile, needy, and infantile. She playacted fragility as a ruse to control him, he argued. However, the email messages which Reitman shared as evidence of Ronell's manipulativeness can also be read as evidence of her authenticity. Ronell may have been as profoundly needy and vulnerable as she claimed, especially since, to all appearances, she never deviated from these positions. It is possible that the following messages from Ronell, which Reitman cited as evidence of the power she wielded over him, came from a self-identified lesbian who—defying all cultural expectations—was emotionally dependent on a gay man who was not only 30 years younger than she, but who was also her student.

> I was crying when I did not hear back from you. It was a hard night, but I'm pulling back together. (p. 12)
>
> Hi my darling Nimrod, I am a bit weepy and confused, a normal aftermath I suppose, and also a response to the separation from you …But I will try to gain some ground with a visit to shrinky-winky and see if I can't develop another kind of report for you! …So many kisses for my guardian angel… (p. 13)
>
> I am having a hard time letting you go and want, if possible, to retrieve the idea of a 'date' …Please be kind to me as only you know how… (p. 13)
>
> My dearest Nimrod, …I am deeply sorry when I fail at distance, at least sometimes (but not always) and that I suffer your absence with such inelegance. I hope you can continue to have and hold compassion and not feel a downturn in our tremendous closeness at all times, …I simply wanted to talk to you. You told me that we would do so quite a lot: I didn't realize this was something very hard for me to calibrate and assimilate:… (p. 13)

In the press release Ronell (2017) distributed in her defense, she claimed she had no idea that she was making Reitman uncomfortable until she read the NYU investigators' report two years after he secured his degree. That's also when she realized that he had been using her. He had pretended to care for her, professed boundless affection to her face, but when she was not there, he berated her. So, while Reitman alleged that Ronell "created a false romantic relationship" between them, "by threat of, among other things, not allowing him to advance his Ph.D., [and] asserted complete domination and control over his life," Ronell contended that Reitman "created a false romantic relationship" by intentionally misrepresenting his feelings, leading her to believe that he loved her, as she loved him. To illustrate, Ronell cited the following email, sent to her on June 29, 2013: "Mon Avital, beloved and special one, I only now relieved (sic) your beautiful and exquisite message…I thank you for your infinite understanding and sensitivities which are always beyond measure, all of which I reciprocate with tenderness and love. I thank you so much for walking me through this catabasis [descent]. I don't know how I would have survived without you. You are the best!!! I love you so much. You are the best, my joy, my miracle. Kisses and devotion always. Yours – n." Yet, three weeks later, Reitman sent an email to a friend in which he acknowledged his true feelings for Ronell: "Tomorrow, I see the monster." To Reitman's friends, he referred to her as "monster," "witch," "evil," "psychotic," "bitter old lady," and on April 2013, he told a friend via email that, far from feeling that Ronell is his "beloved and special one … my joy, my miracle," when he is with her, "I want to throw up from disgust …."

In his civil suit against Ronell, Reitman made the case that, in her effort to retaliate against him—to injure him for rejecting her—she attempted to undermine his career prospects. He cited as an example that, when the time came for him to apply for faculty positions, she made no attempt to reach out to potential employers on his behalf, nor did she write letters of recommendation for him specifically crafted toward each school. Instead, he claimed she sent the same pro-forma letter to each school and called faculty members from other universities to poison their minds against him, with the result that Reitman, notwithstanding his excellent qualifications, which included a Ph.D. from NYU with Ronell as his advisor, was not offered a single interview for a full-time academic appointment. Reitman's only academic positions, following graduation, consisted of three post-doc fellowships at prestigious institutions, including Harvard.

Ronell (2017) denied Reitman's claim that she had attempted to kneecap his academic prospects, pointing to NYU investigators' finding that the letters of recommendation she sent out to support his job search were "comparable to those of other former students." She also claimed that she lacked motivation to harm Reitman's job search because, in her mind, she had nothing to retaliate against: she did not know about Reitman's harassment complaint until long after she had written letters of recommendation for him. Indeed, Reitman did not make a formal complaint against Ronell to NYU's Office of Equal Opportunity until 2017, two years after he graduated.

Nonetheless, Ronell's defense was widely discredited and condemned, and she was subjected to extraordinary personal attacks. Much of this hostility may have been stimulated by a letter sent to NYU's president and provost in support of Ronell (see Nell Gluckman, 2018). More than four dozen well-known scholars, including Judith Butler, author of *Gender Trouble* and president-elect of the Modern Language Association, delivered a letter on May 11, 2018, arguing, in effect, that Ronell's academic and intellectual stature should be factored into any possible judgments against her. Expressing their concern that Ronell might lose her job as a result of exaggerated harassment allegations, they requested that she receive a "fair hearing," and listed her many accomplishments in philosophy and literature as a kind of defense. The letter also stated that although the signatories had no access to the formal complaints against Ronell, "we have all seen her relationship with students, and some of us know the individual who has waged this malicious campaign against her."

The letter drew almost immediate condemnation from academic bloggers for victim-blaming and as evidence that feminist scholars expected special treatment for one of their own. For example, shortly after the letter was sent, Brian Leiter (2018), a law professor at the University of Chicago and author of a widely read blog, accused the signatories of hypocrisy and elitism: "Blaming the victim is apparently OK when the accused in a Title IX proceeding is a feminist literary theorist." Lili Loofbourow, writing for *Slate*, described the letter-in-support-of-Ronell as a retrograde effort to torpedo a complainant's case: "It [the letter] reproduces, with eerie exactitude, the reductive patterns of strategic victim-blaming … blindly parroting the playbook that has during the #MeToo almost exclusively been used by men." Loofbourow concluded: "Perhaps we can agree, at minimum, that people who claim they've been abused deserve to be spared drive-by character assassinations by their alleged assailants' more famous and powerful colleagues." James J. Marino, an associate professor of English at Cleveland State University, who started an online petition to remove Judith Butler as the President-Elect of the Modern Language Association because she signed the letter, described it as "a page from the old school boy's playbook. … It's uncannily like the letters used to defend male harassers." And Amy Elizabeth Robinson, in an article titled "On

Power and Aporia in the Academy," mocked the letter-writers as cultish genius worshippers: "Ronell possesses 'singular brilliance,' holds (in case you missed it the first time) an 'international reputation,' has created an 'illuminated world,' (She also sent a graduate student emails calling him her 'baby love' and 'cocker-er spaniel,' among other things, and asked him to touch her breasts.) 'She deserves a fair hearing, one that expresses respect, dignity, and human solicitude in addition to our enduring admiration.' It makes me nauseous."

Following publication of the letter, the attacks against Ronell became extravagant and personal. Among the most egregious, one critic described Ronell as "attractive as a rotten prune (indeed, she even looks like one)" (DeGroot, 2018). Another opined on Twitter, "NYU professor Avital Ronell is a straight up rapist" (pangmeli, 2018). Yet another likened Ronell to a pedophile (Park, 2018): "...there are in fact significant similarities between the Catholic pedophile priest scandal and the Ronell case.... Most significantly, just as with the Catholic Church and its ideology of canonical authority, so Ronell uses ideology to obscure her crimes and divert attention from them.... The Real is known: the Real is what Ronell is; a Real thing, a Real monster." Several critics tore into her personality: "At the very least, it seems the poor old cougar [Ronell] needs 24/7 narcissistic supply, and encircles herself with those who—for whatever personal reasons—are willing to comply" (Sewall, 2018). The theme of Ronell's "malignant" and "boundless" narcissism came up again and again: "...why are we even surprised that malignant narcissists make their way into these star positions then make others miserable, which is exactly what it sounds like Ronell did" (Schweitzer, 2018). "She pursued one goal: The work of Avital Ronell and Jacques Derrida must be at the center of all teaching and research. Instead of an academic program, we were left with boundless narcissism" (Huppauf, 2018). A former student of Ronell's added this: "It is simply no secret to anyone within a mile of the German or comp-lit departments at NYU that Avital is abusive. This is boring and socially agreed upon, like the weather" (Chu, 2018). Among the more curious and extreme attacks against Ronell was a movement to remove her books from academic syllabi, as well as the books of those, like Judith Butler, who offered her their support (Ciccota, 2018).

After Ronell returned from her year-long suspension, a student protest movement, much like the one organized against Jane Gallop, greeted her with a petition signed by more than 800 students, faculty, staff, and alumni. "NYU's decision to continue Ronell's employment constitutes an attack on survivors of sexual abuse and contributes to a hostile learning and working environment...," the petition read. "Moreover, Ronell's behavior is not isolated to this particular instance, but is part of a long-standing pattern of intimidation and misconduct, as testified by other students and faculty.... We therefore call on NYU to enforce its policy 'to maintain a safe learning, living, and working environment,' and immediately terminate Avital Ronell's employment" (see DiLillo, 2019). Among the protests which targeted Ronell after her return to NYU, one of the most dramatic consisted of students following her through the University's halls, chanting "No to abusers! Justice for survivors!" One such protest, filmed and published on Twitter, revealed a woman of advanced age and diminutive stature entering her classroom with five or six students trailing behind her, shouting: "You are a sex abuser and have no right to be on campus!" (NYUtoo).

According to public documents, three other NYU faculty were charged with sexual harassment. One was a male assistant professor of music, Cliff Eisen, who, in 1993, was found responsible for propositioning a trans-female student during a tutorial session, also of attempting to force a kiss, touch her breasts, buttocks, and crotch, and of sexually harassing three other students in similar fashion (see Miles v. New York University, United States District Court, S. D. New York, Oct. 7, 1997). NYU's response was to place a letter of reprimand in Eisen's file, while allowing him to continue teaching without interruption. The second male NYU faculty charged with harassment is Arnold Baskin, an associate professor of film, who, in 2013, was accused of exposing himself to a non-tenured female instructor, of forcibly kissing and touching her, threatening to sabotage her career if she didn't play along, and of calling her crude, gender-demeaning names such as "big mouth, big rack," "tiny Jew with the big tits," all in front of witnesses. According to the presumptive victim, when she reported the abuse to NYU, authorities conducted a "sham investigation," characterized Baskin's behavior as "collegial banter" and blamed her for the problem. NYU authorities, on the other hand, claimed they took the harassment allegations seriously and launched an investigation, although, to date, the investigation has been inconclusive. Baskin did not receive an official reprimand and, like Eisen, was allowed to continue teaching at NYU without interruption (Kazlowsky, 2020; Levine, 2020). The third NYU male faculty charged with sexual harassment is Robert Benevides, assistant professor in the Tisch film and television department. He was accused of asking a student to come to his office where he told her about his sexual fantasies, including his interest in pornography and having sex with students. That led to his disclosure that he would "totally do" her as well. The student responded by freezing in place: "I couldn't move," she said. "I was just so dissociated." A week later, she reported the incident to Title IX. An investigation ensued which concluded, in the summer of 2023, that Benevides violated the University's non-discrimination and anti-harassment policy. However, despite that ruling, and multiple current and former NYU students coming forward with similar harassment complaints against Benevides, his appointment in the NYU, Tisch School of Arts, was uninterrupted. His penalty, if indeed NYU penalized him, was not publicly disclosed. As one student described her frustration, "The fact that Tisch is offering classes taught by him with no disclosure of his past actions to new, unaware, vulnerable students—it is just so upsetting. We didn't know how that could happen..." (Moniz, 2024).

Obviously, Ronell was treated more harshly than Eisen, Baskin, and Benevides, but the reasons are unclear. Ronell's gender and the fiercely criticized letter written on her behalf may have made a difference. Another possibility is that, unlike Ronell, Eisen, Baskin, and Benevides were not "academic stars." Ronell's academic fame (like Jane Gallop's) may have inspired her academic critics to cut her down to size. To test this possibility, we should consider the treatment of two men listed on the Academic Sexual Misconduct Database, who, like Ronell, were renowned philosophy professors, Thomas Pogge of Yale University and John R. Searle of the University of California-Berkeley, both of whom have long records of sexually harassing female students, as well as long records of highly acclaimed teaching and scholarship.

In 2010, a 21-year-old woman who had taken a job as Pogge's translator for a conference in Chile claimed that one night, as she sat at her desk translating documents for him, he slid up behind her, pressed his erection against her, then fondled her breast and thigh. She said she rejected his advances, fled, and shortly thereafter, in what she alleged was an act of retaliation, Pogge fired her. When she filed a formal complaint against him the following year, investigators concluded that Pogge had engaged in "unprofessional conduct" but cleared him of charges of sexual harassment. As part of the fall-out from the harassment allegation, however, several similar allegations against Pogge came to light, dating back to the early 1990s. In response, more than 200 philosophy professors in 2016 signed an open letter condemning Pogge's alleged misconduct. The signatories expressed their belief that "Pogge engaged in behavior that violates the norms of appropriate conduct .... Based on the information that has been made public, we strongly condemn his harmful actions toward women, most notably women of color, and the entire academic community" (Rodrigues et al., 2016). What should be noted about this letter is that, unlike the petition against Ronell, the signatories condemned Pogge's behavior but did not condemn *him*. Also unlike the petition against Ronell, the Pogge petition did not call for firing or even suspension. Nor was Pogge portrayed as a threat to the academic community, despite his long history of allegedly forcing himself—*physically* forcing himself—on young women. Pogge has continued to teach at Yale without interruption and without reports of the kinds of personal attacks, protests, and demonstrations that followed the sexual harassment allegations against Ronell and Gallop.

John Searle's story is much the same. According to the civil suit launched by the 24-year-old complainant, in 2016, a week after she began working for Searle as a research assistant, he attacked her in his office. First, he asked the other research assistant to leave, then he locked the door behind him, approached, and began sliding his hands down her spine to her buttocks; he told the research assistant that she was going to become his lover (Asimov, 2017). She reported the assault to the director of the John Searle Center for Social Ontology, where she worked, and was told that Searle did this kind of thing: he had sexual relationships with his students in exchange for academic, monetary, and other benefits. As in the Pogge case, shortly thereafter, in what was allegedly an act of retaliation, the research assistant was fired, and as in the Pogge case, additional allegations surfaced which were similar in nature and decades old (Baker, 2017). Although graduate students had long expressed concerns about Searle, it was not until 2019, after Searle, then 86, had voluntarily retired, that UC-Berkeley stripped him of his teaching privileges.

Why was Ronell treated more harshly than these male professors? Her status as a woman, an academic star, and feminist may have played a role. It is also likely that the poorly conceived letter of support authored by dozens of feminist scholars added oxygen to the fire, not to mention the possibility that the image of a lesbian in her sixties forcing a virile gay man in his thirties to engage in baby talk—billing and cooing together on a daily basis for years—may have struck people as uniquely unwholesome. Consistent with Rudman's "status incongruity hypothesis," the fact that this clever and powerful woman had the aura of one who defies all the delicate and noble instincts of femininity may have made her appear, in the eyes of many, more corrupt and threatening than any man.

References

Abramson, K. (2014). Turning up the lights on gaslighting. *Philosophical Perspectives, 28*, 1–30. https://www.jstor.org/stable/26614542

Asimov, N. (2017, March 23). UC Berkeley worker says professor sexually assaulted her, Then fired her. *SFGate*. https://www.sfgate.com/education/article/UC-Berkeley-worker-says-prominent-professor-11023471.php

Baker, K. J. M. (2017, April 17). UC Berkeley Was Warned about Its Star Professor Years Before Sexual Harassment Lawsuit. *BuzzFeedNews*. https://www.buzzfeednews.com/article/katiejmbaker/john-searle-complaints-uc-berkeley

Berenstain, N. (2020). White feminist gaslighting. *Hypatia, 20*, 733–758. https://doi.org/10.1017/hyp.2020.31

Chu, A. L. (2018, August 30). I worked for Avital Ronell. I believe her accuser. *Chronicle of Higher Education*. https://www.chronicle.com/article/i-worked-with-avital-ronell-i-believe-her-accuser/

Ciccota, T. (2018, September 18). NYU professor accused of underage affair has her works removed From classes. *Breitbart*. https://www.breitbart.com/tech/2018/09/12/nyu-professor-accused-of-underage-affair-has-her-works-removed-from-classes/

Davis, A. M., & Ernst, R. (2019). Racial gaslighting. *Politics, Groups and Identities, 7*(4), 761–774. https://doi.org/10.1080/21565503.2017.1403934

DeGroot, C. (2018, August 24). The sorrows of young Rimrod the toady. *Taki's Magazine*. https://www.takimag.com/article/the-sorrows-of-young-nimrod-the-toady/

DiLillo, J. (2019, September 5). Graduate student union circulates petition to terminate professor found responsible for sexual harassment. *NYU Local*. https://nyulocal.com/graduate-student-union-petitions-to-terminate-avital-ronell-professor-accused-of-sexual-misconduct-1b4de4761458

Gluckman, N. (2018, June 12). How a letter defending Avital Ronell sparked confusion and condemnation. *Chronicle of Higher Education*. https://www.chronicle.com/article/how-a-letter-defending-avital-ronell-sparked-confusion-and-condemnation/

Huppauf, B. (2018, September 8). A witch hunt or a quest for justice: An insider's perspective on Disgraced academic Avital Ronell. *Salon*. https://www.salon.com/2018/09/08/a-witch-hunt-or-a-quest-for-justice-an-insiders-perspective-on-disgraced-academic-avital-ronell/

Kazlowsky, T. (2020, June 24). NYU film school prof claims deceased colleague sexually abused her. *The Jewish Voice*. https://thejewishvoice.com/2020/06/nyu-film-school-prof-claims-deceased-colleague-sexually-abused-her/

Kipnis, L. (2017). *Unwanted advances: Sexual paranoia comes to campus*. HarperCollins.

Leiter, Brian. (2018, June 10). Blaming the victim is apparently OK when the accused in a Title IX proceeding is a feminist literary theorist. *Leiter Reports: A Philosophy Blog*. https://leiterreports.typepad.com/blog/2018/06/blaming-the-victim-is-apparently-ok-when-the-accused-is-a-feminist-literary-theorist.html

Levine, J. (2020, June 20). NYU film school lecturer accuses acclaimed professor of flashing her. *New York Post*. nypost.com/2020/06/20/nyu-facing-sexual-harassment-lawsuit-against-dead-professor/

Macaux, E. J. (2018, August 17). A female professor, her male student and the limits of "MeToo." *New York Times*. https://www.nytimes.com/2018/08/17/opinion/letters/women-sexual-harassment.html

Moniz, C. (2024, May 3). A Tisch professor disappeared during a misconduct investigation. Two semesters later, he's scheduled to teach again. *Washington Square News*. https://nyunews.com/news/2024/05/03/tisch-professor-misconduct-investigation/

pangmeli. (2018, August 19). https://twitter.com/pangmeli/status/1032026245461094400

Park, P, (2018, September 20). *Avital Ronell & Judith Butler: A cautionary tale of power & accountability in Academia*. https://paulinepark.com/2018/09/19/avital-ronell-judith-butler-a-cautionary-tale-of-power-accountability-in-academia/

Rodrigues, A., Wang, M., & Wang, V. (2016, June 20). Philosophy community signs open letter in striking rebuke of Pogge. *Yale Daily Press*. https://yaledailynews.com/blog/2016/06/20/philosophy-community-signs-open-letter-in-striking-rebuke-of-pogge/

Ronell, A. (2017, August 16). *Press release on behalf of Professor Avital Ronell*. https://docplayer.net/88214318-Press-release-on-behalf-of-professor-avital-ronell-professor-avital-ronell-an-nyu-tenured-professor-has-been-the-subject-of-title-ix.html

Schweitzer, L. (2018, September 17). *Avital Ronell and a bunch of dudes*. https://lisaschweitzer.com/2018/09/17/avital-ronell-and-a-bunch-of-dudes/

Sewall, G. T. (2018, August 28). Bonfire of the humanities. *The American Conservative*. https://www.theamericanconservative.com/bonfire-of-the-humanities/

CHAPTER 4

"A Predator Preying on Their Prey"

Anna Stubblefield, a philosophy professor from Rutgers University, was accused of violating the sexual consent of a 30-year-old man who had severe motor disabilities, could not speak, and never has. D.J., as he is called, cannot use the toilet, walk, or dress without assistance, has trouble making eye contact and focusing on objects, and is prone to muscle spasms in his face, neck, torso, arms, and hands (Baron, 2017; Engber, 2015). Although he had been diagnosed with the intellectual ability of a three-year-old, his family had doubts. So, in 2019, they asked Stubblefield if she would be willing to assess his intellectual functioning without financial compensation—as a favor—and she agreed.

D.J.'s brother, Wesley, had taken a course with her at Rutgers, where he learned about a method of teaching communication skills to nonverbal persons with seemingly implacable disabilities. The method is known as "facilitated communication" or FC, and relies on a facilitator holding the disabled person's elbow, wrist, or hand as they point to pictures, and then letters, and eventually at a keyboard with a built-in screen. Proponents of FC claim that this kind of support provides people who can neither speak nor control their movements—those with the severest physical disabilities—the hope of one day expressing themselves. But the scientific community strongly disagrees (Mostert, 2012; Hemsley et al., 2018). Disability scholars and researchers argue that FC resembles ventriloquism: the words that FC facilitators claim come from the person with the speech disorder

© The Author(s), under exclusive license to Springer Nature Switzerland AG 2024
L. Margolin, *Women Accused of Sexual Harassment*,
https://doi.org/10.1007/978-3-031-79021-8_4

are, in fact, the words of the facilitator. The main difference between ventriloquism and facilitated communication, scientists claim, is that in ventriloquism, the ventriloquist knows where the words originate, but in FC, the facilitator incorrectly attributes the origin of the words to the person with the speech disorder (Boyton, 2012).

In Anna Stubblefield's case, she appeared to fully believe that the words she spelled out with D.J. were D.J.'s words. And after two years of instruction based on the principles of facilitated communication, D.J.'s family appeared to believe it too. He seemed to be making miraculous progress: a man whom many had thought had the cognitive capacity of a toddler, whose chief pleasures, prior to Stubblefield's involvement, were eating and playing with plastic coat hangers, was now sharing opinions, reading books, attending college classes, and, with Stubblefield's help, presenting papers at conferences, one of which was on the effects of facilitated communication: "The right to communication is the right to hope," the essay read. "I am jumping for joy knowing I can talk, but don't minimize how humiliating it can be to know people jump to the conclusion I am mentally disabled" (Engber, 2015, p. 5).

Those who knew D.J. best—his mother and brother—believed that facilitated communication had unlocked the prison of D.J.'s intellect. They believed that the words Stubblefield attributed to him were his own. However, that assessment went into reverse on Memorial Day 2011, during Stubblefield's visit to D.J.'s home, when she announced to his mother and Wesley, "We have something to tell you.... We're in love" (Engber, 2015, p. 1).

"What do you mean, *in love*?" D.J.'s mother asked, stunned. A moment later, after Wesley suggested that Stubblefield may have taken advantage of his brother, Stubblefield helped D.J. type out this message: "No one's been taken advantage of. I've been trying to seduce Anna for years, and she resisted valiantly." Then he typed another message intended for Stubblefield: "Kiss me." It was at this point that Wesley walked out (Engber, 2015, p. 1).

What made D.J.'s family profoundly uncomfortable with the romantic revelation was not only that it represented a betrayal of Stubblefield's professional responsibility to D.J. and to them. It was the incompatibility—what D.J.'s family saw as the fundamental absurdity—of their relationship: Stubblefield was 11 years older than D.J., a married, tenured professor, with a teenage daughter, and, perhaps most importantly to D.J.'s family, she is white and D.J. is Black. Wesley invoked critical race theory to suggest that Stubblefield, in taking charge of D.J.'s voice, had, in effect, colonized his racial identity, replacing "a life steeped in the history and culture of his God-fearing, Southern-rooted, African-American family. She tried to supplant that with some version of life she thought was better" (Randall, 2021, p. 386).

In August 2011, D.J.'s family accused Stubblefield of sexually assaulting D.J., a decision that unfolded after she resisted their demand to stop seeing him. First, the family contacted Rutgers University to express their concerns about Stubblefield; then Rutgers referred the case to the police, and then, as part of the investigation, the police recorded a call between Stubblefield and D.J.'s mother—a sting operation—in which Stubblefield, without knowing about the police involvement, was led to acknowledge her sexual relationship with D.J.: "Yes, [D.J.] wanted to be physically involved with me," she said over the phone, "and I wanted to be physically involved with him. But our relationship is not just about or primarily about the sex part. We love each other very, very, very much, and I wouldn't have sex with somebody that I didn't love" (Engber, 2015, p. 11).

According to Stubblefield, the idea of having sex originated with D.J.: "Okay, I believe you really love me," he typed with Stubblefield's assistance, but then he questioned whether she could be physically attracted to him. "That broke my heart all over again," she later testified. "'I'm in love with you the whole way.' Then he said, 'Kiss me,' and I did. He said, 'Kiss me again,' I kissed him again." With Stubblefield's hand guiding D.J.'s, she claimed he next typed, "Do you think it's even possible with my cerebral palsy for us to make love?" And the following Sunday, seeking to answer D.J.'s question, she met him at his home, while his family was away. Stubblefield claimed that, at D.J.'s request, she pulled his pants down, loosened his diaper, and performed oral sex for him. A week later, she said they attempted penis-vagina intercourse, but without success. The following week they tried again and succeeded, and when they were finished, Stubblefield testified that D.J. typed "I feel alive for the first time in my life" (Engber, 2015, p. 7).

Stubblefield was charged with two counts of first-degree aggravated sexual assault—or, to put it simply, two counts of rape—for performing sex acts on the body of an individual so cognitively impaired that he was incapable of understanding the meaning of those acts. The case for her defense depended on persuading jurors that D.J. was capable of understanding and consenting to sex. But while the judge allowed the prosecution to call experts to testify that facilitated communication is a sham and could not possibly represent D.J.'s sexual wishes, the judge refused to allow Stubblefield's defense to call experts who were prepared to testify to the opposite, that through FC, it might have been possible for D.J. to give and understand sexual consent. The judge also refused to allow D.J. to testify in the only way he might have been capable—through facilitated communication. Because the judge ruled that FC failed the test for scientific evidence, D.J.'s only appearance in court was not as a witness, but at the behest of the prosecution, as a "demonstrative exhibit." His mother led him to the jury, holding him up by his armpits. "This is my son," she said. Then she turned him to the judge, "Your honor, this is my son." What the jurors and judge saw was a diminutive man whose head lolled back and forth, and whose eyes focused on the ceiling—a man seemingly incapable of consenting to sex (Engber, 2015, p. 11).

After the jury deliberated for less than three hours, the verdict came in: Stubblefield was guilty of violating D.J.'s sexual consent. She raped him. The former professor of philosophy, who had devoted her academic career to social-justice activism and to championing the rights of people with disabilities, was sentenced to two concurrent 12-year prison terms. What is more, the judge felt called upon to denounce Stubblefield from the bench as "The perfect example of a predator preying on their prey" (McMahan & Singer, 2017, p. 3).

Philosophers Jeff McMahon and Peter Singer, in their article, "Who Is the Victim in the Anna Stubblefield Case?" expressed astonishment over the conduct of Stubblefield's trial—especially over the fact that the judge, while admitting expert testimony discrediting facilitated communication, refused to allow expert testimony affirming its credibility. McMahon and Singer were also astonished by the sentence: even supposing that Stubblefield was guilty of having sex with a man who could not give consent, the decision to sentence her to 12 years in prison was absurd. That kind of sentence might have been reasonable for a repeat offender—a hardened criminal—but Stubblefield had no criminal record. Until her involvement with D.J., she had lived the life of a model citizen. There was also no evidence from D.J., or from any other source, that sexual activity with her had harmed him. This is not to say he may not have been harmed in some way; it is simply to assert that no effort was made to establish D.J.'s injury or discomfort from the sexual activity; nor, indeed, was any effort made to establish Stubblefield's malicious motivation. On the contrary, all the evidence confirmed Stubblefield's claim that her principal motivation in working with him was altruistic. Even allowing the prosecution's argument that the words she helped D.J. type out were hers rather than his—even allowing that D.J. never consented to sex—attorney Marcia Baron (2017) argues that it is plausible that Stubblefield *believed* he had consented to sex, in which case the sexual activity which ensued would have been nothing more than a simple, well-intentioned misunderstanding. Stubblefield's guilt would then consist of acting out a benevolent fantasy without any awareness that it was a fantasy—the fantasy of rescuing D.J. from a life of total silence. The judge may have called Stubblefield a "predator preying on their prey," but this so-called predator had never pursued D.J. Rather, D.J.'s family pursued her. They saw Stubblefield as someone who might be able to help him communicate with the world around him. They asked for her help without offering, and without Stubblefield seeking, a fee. In addition, Stubblefield never tried to hide her feelings for D.J. or their sexual relationship: no one would have known that she and D.J. were sexually involved had Stubblefield not volunteered to share this information with his family.

Two years later, an appellate court tossed Stubblefield's conviction based on the judge's refusal to allow her to call experts willing to testify to the validity of facilitated communication. However, rather than go to trial again, Stubblefield chose to change her plea from innocent to guilty, and on that basis, the prosecutor's office agreed to release her with time served. But in Stubblefield's new plea, she did not concede that D.J. lacked the cognitive power of a normal adult nor that she had unwittingly put her words in his mouth. Her account of their relationship did not change. Her concession was only that she "should have known that the victim had been determined to be 'mentally defective' to the point of being incapable of providing consent" (Engber, 2017).

Contrary to legal precedent, the original judge, in sentencing Stubblefield to 12 years in prison, disregarded her exemplary record and good intentions. Instead, the judge treated Stubblefield's exemplary record and good intentions as evidence of her debased moral character, seeming to believe that, because Stubblefield was educated, successful, and smart, she should have known better. She should have concluded that D.J. lacked moral agency and intellectual understanding of his own sexuality. As Daniel Engber, who covered the case for the *New York Times*, noted, "several times, the judge cited Anna's intelligence—her 'high intellect'—as a point against her" (Engber, 2016, p. 4). However, in comparing her sentence to the punishments and penalties exacted against men charged with sexual misconduct who were also on the Rutgers faculty—also highly successful, educated individuals of "high intellect"—the harshness of Stubblefield's punishment appears exceptional. Consider, for example, the case of former Rutgers professor of bioscience, Douglas Fugman, who was accused in civil court of raping a subordinate repeatedly over the course of a decade. Rutgers eventually fired him but he was never charged with a crime (Bichao, 2018). The only sexual harassment case from Rutgers, apart from that of Anna Stubblefield, that ended in criminal court, involved James Goydos, a former professor of medicine. In early 2018, Goydos was accused of filming as many as 30 women in a bathroom. He was indicted on charges of violating these women's privacy and acknowledged that he had set-up cameras in the bathroom for the purpose of spying on women. But those charges were dropped as part of his agreement to plead guilty to a series of other, non-sex-related crimes such as burglary, computer theft, and illegal possession of an assault weapon. For those crimes, he was sentenced to 300 days in jail (Panico, 2020).

To understand why Stubblefield was punished more severely than male faculty who committed more serious offenses, we should consider people's difficulty seeing someone with disabilities as severe as D.J.'s as anything other than abject or pitiable—and as anything other than nonsexual (Loeser et al., 2018). Thus, the prosecution's decision to bring D.J. into the courtroom, not as a witness, but as an "exhibit," to convey the magnitude and breadth of his disabilities, and as a way of conveying the magnitude and breadth of Stubblefield's guilt (Mintz, 2017).

We should also consider how the concept of "structural gaslighting" (Berenstain, 2020) was mobilized to emphasize Stubblefield's culpability—how prosecutors and observers repeatedly invoked racial, gender, and disability ideologies to demonize her. For example, one scholar, impressed by the racial dimensions of Stubblefield's relationship with D.J., wrote, "To believe that she could interpret D.J.'s body, movements, and desires through FC alone … required that Anna contain a violent arrogance that cannot be disentangled from histories of racial violence" (Randall, 2021, p. 386). Another scholar, Mark Sherry (2016, p. 979) who focused on the racial and disability dimensions of the case, condemned Stubblefield's elitist privilege and arrogance: "I saw [disability] scholars advocate on behalf of Stubblefield, who is a white, non-disabled woman, but I never saw anything to support the black disabled man who was the victim of this sexual assault.… In my view, this response to rape is not only misdirected, it is unethical and shameful. The lack of concern for the victim and his family was chilling, disturbing, and unethical." Sherry affirmed Stubblefield's guilt in the strongest possible terms based on the racial and social differences between her and D.J., without mentioning the fact that romantic relationships often develop between disability professionals and their clients (Mintz, 2017), "Stubblefield was a well-paid white academic; the victim is a person of color. These dynamics cannot be ignored—imbalances of power underlie most cases of sexual abuse, rape, and other forms of sexual violence" (p. 979).

Wesley, D.J.'s brother, argued that Stubblefield's offense was being treated lightly because she is a woman, and asked the court to imagine how they would judge the perpetrator if the genders were reversed: if Anna were a man and D.J. were a woman. "This was rape," he said. "She did godawful things to him, and I believe the punishment is woefully inadequate." Wesley concluded by invoking the survivor-led movement against sexual violence, "On behalf of my brother, who is nonverbal, I want to say, 'Me, too'" (Engber, 2016, 2018).

Stubblefields's case, as well as Ronell's and Gallop's, shows that the ritual denunciation of norm-breaking women, a tradition that reaches as far back as the Ancient Greeks and Old Testament and is reflected, not only in ecclesiastical literature, but also in biological, gynecological, medical, and philosophical discourse (Bloch, 1987, p. 1), continues to this day. It continues, in part, through a kind of epistemic reversal according to which those who have been fighting oppression for themselves and others are portrayed as agents of oppression (Berenstain, 2020; Fricker, 1999). Anna Stubblefield's case shows how an anti-racist scholar and activist, the first and only white person to serve as chair of the American Philosophical Association's Committee on the status of Black Philosophers (Engber, 2015), could be cast as a racist for trying—pro bono—to help a Black man with profound disabilities, an example of what Davis and Ernst (2019) call racial gaslighting: the process "that perpetuates and normalizes a white supremacist reality through pathologizing those who resist" (p. 761).

References

Baron, M. (2017). Sexual consent, reasonable mistakes, and the case of Anna Stubblefield. *Ohio State Journal of Criminal Law, 15*, 429–449.

Berenstain, N. (2020). White feminist gaslighting. *Hypatia, 20*, 733–758. https://doi.org/10.1017/hyp.2020.31

Bichao, S. (2018, June 18). Rutgers official accused of raping, harassing employee for 10 years. *My Central Jersey*. https://www.mycentraljersey.com/story/

news/local/middlesex-county/2015/06/18/rutgers-sued-employee-rape-claim/28947849/

Bloch, R. H. (1987). Medieval misogyny. *Representations, 20*, 1–24. https://doi.org/10.2307/2928500

Boyton, J. (2012). Facilitated communication—What harm can it do: Confessions of a former facilitator. *Evidence-Based Communication Assessment and Intervention, 6*, 3–13. http://www.psypress.com/EBCAI. https://doi.org/10.1080/17489539.2012.674680

Davis, A. M., & Ernst, R. (2019). Racial gaslighting. *Politics, Groups and Identities, 7*(4), 761–774. https://doi.org/10.1080/21565503.2017.1403934

Engber, D. (2015, October 20). The strange case of Anna Stubblefield. *The New York Times Magazine*. https://www.nytimes.com/2015/10/25/magazine/the-strange-case-of-anna-stubblefield.html

Engber, D. (2016, February 3). What Anna Stubblefield believed she was doing. *New York Times*. nytimes.com/2016/02/03/magazine/what-anna-stubblefield-believed-she-was-doing.html#:~:text=The%20defendant%20believes%20she%20was,never%20meant%20to%20hurt%20anyone.

Engber, D. (2017, June 4). A second chance for Anna Stubblefield. *Slate*. https://slate.com/technology/2017/06/the-conviction-in-the-anna-stubblefield-facilitated-communication-case-has-been-overturned.html

Engber, D. (2018, April 5). The strange case of Anna Stubblefield, revisited. *New York Times Magazine*. https://www.nytimes.com/2018/04/05/magazine/the-strange-case-of-anna-stubblefield-revisited.html

Fricker, M. (1999). Epistemic oppression and epistemic privilege. *Canadian Journal of Philosophy, 29*(Suppl. 1), 191–210.

Hemsley, B., Bryant, L., Schlosser, R. W., Shane, H. C., Lang, R., Paul, D., Banajee, M., & Ireland, M. (2018). Systematic review of facilitated communication 2014–2018 finds no new evidence that messages delivered using facilitated communication are authored by the person with disability. *Autism & Developmental Language Impairments, 3*, 2396941518821570.

Loeser, C., Pini, B., & Crowley, V. (2018). Disability and sexuality: Desires and pleasures. *Sexualities, 21*(3), 255–270. https://doi.org/10.1177/1363460716688682

McMahan, J., & Singer, P. (2017, April 3). Who is the victim in the Anna Stubblefied case? *New York Times*. https://www.nytimes.com/2017/04/03/opinion/who-is-the-victim-in-the-anna-stubblefield-case.html

Mintz, K. (2017). Ableism, ambiguity, and the Anna Stubblefield case. *Disability & Society, 32*, 1–5.

Mostert, M. P. (2012). Facilitated communication: The empirical imperative to prevent further professional malpractice. *Evidence-Based Communication Assessment and Intervention, 6*(1), 18–27.

Panico, R. (2020, July 16). Ex-Rutgers cancer doc admits theft, gets 300 days in jail. *Middlesex*, 16. https://www.nj.com/middlesex/2020/07/ex-rutgers-cancer-doc-admits-theft-gets-300-days-in-jail.html

Randall, L. C. (2021). Consent as rhetorical ability in "The strange case of Anna Stubblefield". *Rhetoric Society Quarterly, 51*(5), 377–391.

Sherry, M. (2016). Facilitated communication, Anna Stubblefield and disability studies. *Disability & Society, 31*(7), 974–982.

CHAPTER 5

"Lock Her Up!"

"Lock her up!" Clinton's detractors chanted with delight during the months leading up to and following the 2016 election, though it is safe to say they had no idea what Clinton's incriminating conduct might have been. This chapter shows that the same "Lock her up!" mentality often comes into play when women are charged with sexual harassment. It shows that, regardless of a woman's good record and good intentions, if she is accused of sexual harassment but also appears to have behaved in ways that defy the norms traditionally associated with femininity, people will find things to dislike, doubt, and revile about her—things they would excuse or dismiss in a man.

When a Conversation About Sexual Feelings = Sexual Coercion

In 2015, Macalester College concluded that the relationship between Kristin Naca, a female professor of English, and her student, Jane Doe, the pseudonym for Naca's presumptive victim, involved sexual harassment. Jane Doe had studied English under Naca for three years. During her last semester at Macalester, she worked as Naca's assistant and took a workshop with her. Then, 11 days before Doe graduated, on May 6, 2014, Naca invited her to her home, presumably to grade papers. Naca later

© The Author(s), under exclusive license to Springer Nature Switzerland AG 2024

L. Margolin, *Women Accused of Sexual Harassment*,
https://doi.org/10.1007/978-3-031-79021-8_5

acknowledged that during the visit she initiated a conversation with Doe about what she perceived as the sexual tension between them. Naca said she began the conversation by saying she sensed that Doe had been flirting with her and that there seemed to be an intensity or attraction between them that might be physical or might just be creative. “Either way,” she continued, recalling how she introduced the topic to her student, “I wanted to have a conversation because I don’t want us to be working together and for me, or you, to be put in an awkward position.” Naca further recalled saying:

> I’m going to be frank. I need to know, first, if you noticed the intensity? And if you do, do you want me to make a pass at you? If you don’t want or intend that, we need to get whatever it is out in the open and clear the air (Naca v. Macalester College, No 18-3264 [8th Cir. 2020]).

A year later, Macalester College terminated Naca for asking these questions and making these comments to her student. And in the civil suit which followed, in which Naca contested her termination, the court found in favor of Macalester, a decision based on the assumption that Naca forced herself on Jane Doe, not physically, and not by cutting a quid pro quo deal with her to engage in sex at a future time. Rather, the court assumed that Naca’s sexual coercion came from her status as professor and Doe’s status as student, a relationship that, the judge claimed, always involves disparities in power and authority, and that, “as a result of these disparities, a student cannot give authentic consent to sex with a professor.” The judge went on to write that, “In continually emphasizing that she did not have sex with the student until three days after she graduated, Naca ignores that the student testified (and Macalester found) that Naca solicited sex from the student *while she was still a student*” (italics in the original, p. 13).

According to Doe, during the May 6th meeting at Naca’s home, she felt “pressured” into having a sexual relationship with Naca. However, Doe did not describe what that pressure consisted of; she did not say how Naca inspired her subjective sense of coercion (Naca v. Macalester College). Nor did the Macalester representatives or the court ask Jane Doe why, on May 20th, three days after she graduated from Macalester, when Naca no longer had an institutional relationship with her, she chose (or felt compelled) to enter into a sexual relationship with Naca which lasted several weeks, evolving into an emotionally intimate friendship/romance which ended in September 2014 at Naca's request.

Regarding the weeks-long sexual relationship between Naca and Jane Doe "who propositioned whom?" is, of course, a crucial question. Did Naca come on to Doe, or did Doe come on to Naca? But the question, according to court records, was not asked. Additional unasked questions include the following: Did Doe at some point want to be in a relationship with Naca? If yes, why complain about coercion? If not, why did she remain in the relationship for an extended period? And how did Doe feel about ending the relationship at Naca's request? Was she resentful, hurt? These questions were unasked because Jane Doe's passivity seemed an implicit element in the case against Naca. Naca came on to Doe with bad intentions. Naca was the actor, the predator, and Doe the acted upon, the prey.

What Macalester and the court appeared to assume is Naca's nefarious state of mind in meeting with Doe on May 6th when Doe was still enrolled in course work with Naca. The Macalester provost argued that, by inviting Doe to her home, Naca "intended to set the stage for a sexual relationship" and "initiated the relationship by offering to make a pass at the student." However, the provost did not attempt to square that interpretation with Naca's description of that meeting, which all parties appeared to accept as factual, and which provides a radically different picture of what took place. It reveals that, instead of Naca intending "to set the stage for a sexual relationship" with Jane Doe, she was asking Doe how she *felt* about having such a relationship (e.g., "do you want me to make a pass at you? If you don't want or intend that, we need to get whatever it is out in the open and clear the air"). Curiously, the provost further argued that "if Naca had truly intended to clear the air rather than invite a sexual relationship, she should have conducted the discussion in an office space or a public place" (p. 10), suggesting that if Naca and Jane Doe had had the same conversation in a different location, there would not have been a problem. By implication, Kristin Naca, the only faculty member from Macalester College listed on the Academic Sexual Misconduct Database, was terminated from Macalester, not for having sex with an active student—no one claims she had sex with Doe until after she graduated—and not for having a conversation with the Doe about their sexual feelings, but rather for the offense of having that kind of conversation in her home.

A Homonegative Spectacle

In July 2021, University of Mississippi assistant softball coach, Katie Rietkovich Browder, was accused of having a sexual relationship with a student-athlete on her team. The complainant, a member of the softball team, taped a copy of a text message to her head coach's computer which pointed to a possible relationship between her teammate and their assistant coach. The complaint was forwarded to the University of Mississippi athletic director, an investigation was launched, and one week after these accusations were made public, the presumptive victim denied the allegation and the assistant coach was exonerated. The school's Title IX office concluded that the allegation of inappropriate behavior was without substance (Axon, 2021; Kinsey, 2021). Nonetheless, in the brief interval between the time the allegations were first disclosed, in late August, and the finding that they were baseless, in early September, journalists and bloggers across the United States and Great Britain plunged in with a series of articles so homonegative and overblown, that you would have had to laugh out loud at the authors' cluelessness—unless you were Katie Rietkovich Browder and had to cope with the fear of losing your job and your reputation. This is from the *Barstool Sports*: "Katie Rietkovich is an assistant coach at Ole Miss and she's in some deep shit for fooling around with one of the girls.... Finding anything out via text message sucks, much less that your girlfriend's going to the dildo factory with the outfield coach" (Carl, 2021). One blogger wrote about the allegations against Rietkovich Browder under the title, "College Softball Lesbian Scandal!"

> This is not a scandal. Everybody in college sports knows that "varsity softball" is a synonym for lesbian. The lesbian coach who molested one of her players hates Trump? I'm shocked, but what's even more shocking is the suggestion that there could be ... heterosexuals on a Division I varsity softball team (McCain & Smitty, 2021).

Another blog was titled, "Ole Miss under Investigation for Incident Involving Scissors" (Secreant.com, 2021). And another ran with the title, "Ole Miss Softball Coach Caught Fucking One of her Players." The blogger, Mailman Dave, expressed inside knowledge of Rietkovich Browder's infractions: "Not only was the coach fucking one of her players, but that same player had a girlfriend on the team. How awkward was that? Here you are fielding ground balls, you go to Ole Miss, one of the best party schools, you're a D1 athlete, and you have no idea that the coach hitting you ground balls is also grinding clams against your girlfriend. What an absolute shit show." This is from the *New York Post*: "The Ole Miss softball coach at the center of a steamy love triangle involving a student … is married" (Byrne, 2021). The article went on to describe the "curve-hugging" dress Rietkovich Browder wore at her same-sex wedding, and how the current "sex scandal that threatens to break up their marriage may also consume the entire Ole Miss sports program." Even after Rietkovich Browder was cleared through the Title IX investigation, this was not the end of the homonegative rubbish. *Barstool Sports*, for example, decided against apologizing for its inflammatory and inaccurate commentary, but chose, instead, to construct a pornographic fantasy: "as much as we all enjoy a nice, juicy scandal about two consenting adults (allegedly) scissoring one another behind the backs of their significant others, when it turns out to be untrue, we've just got to take that L and move on to the next scandal" (Thorton, 2021).

Are Women Held to a Different Standard?

To dig more deeply into the question of whether women charged with sexual harassment are treated differently, we should consider the case of Jacqueline Hoffarth, a social work instructor from the University of North Dakota who was accused of having a sexual relationship with a student. However, the allegation had a problem: uncertainty as to when the relationship began. Was it before or after the student graduated (Port, 2020)? The uncertainty arose from the fact that the University of North Dakota only got wind of this relationship when Hoffarth announced over Facebook that she was "in a relationship" with the student, a few days after he had already graduated, in August 2019. A second problem with the allegation is that there was no inquiry into how the student might have been harmed by the relationship or how the relationship might have been coercive. Nonetheless, almost as soon as the chair of the social work department heard about the Facebook announcement, in August 2019, Hoffarth was fired. This is from Hoffarth's termination letter:

> Your relationship with an individual while they were enrolled in the Social Work undergraduate program and accepted (now enrolled) in the graduate program… is a violation of Department and University policies.… This is adequate cause for termination (Port, 2020).

Hoffarth appealed on the grounds that she did not teach in the graduate program, and thus would not be involved in the student's education. But the general counsel for UND rejected her appeal, arguing that, even if Hoffarth had no direct role in the graduate program, she would still be in an unequal and potentially coercive relationship since "her position as a faculty member in the department means she has a position of authority, especially as it relates to students" (Port, 2020).

Regarding the question of whether women are held to a different standard, it is important to note that the harassment allegation against Hoffarth was handled very differently than the much more serious, multiple allegations levelled against another UND instructor, Andrew Quinn, who was teaching in Hoffarth's social work department at the same time as Hoffarth. In December 2018, a UND student accused Quinn of seeking sexual favors in return for a positive letter of recommendation. She also accused him of oral rape, of posting Craigslist ads that solicited other men to have sexual encounters with her, and of making almost daily requests for personal information about her (Houle v. University of North Dakota, District Court of North Dakota, Sept. 27, 2021). However, the student claimed that when she reported the harassment to UND officials, they did nothing for more than a year, until January 2019, when Quinn was finally placed on paid administrative leave and forbidden to have contact with her. He resigned shortly thereafter, but two years later, in March 2021, the student sued UND for failing to protect her from Quinn and for fostering "a culture of silence" around reports of sexual misconduct, a charge that seems ironic considering how swiftly UND responded to the allegation against Hoffarth (Mook, 2021).

In summary, North Dakota treated Hoffarth's possible sexual harassment with urgency and harshness—she was fired immediately—even though she openly acknowledged the relationship, the relationship was consensual, and the presumptive victim had just graduated. By comparison, North Dakota treated Quinn, a male faculty from Hoffarth's department, in a relatively laid back, easygoing manner, though he was accused of multiple sexual offenses, including assaulting an active student.

"You Can Get Fired for Saying That?"

To illustrate how the Hoffarth case is not an isolated instance of gender discrimination, I turn now to the sexual harassment actions and policies of Louisiana State University where two women and several men were identified as possible harassers at about the same time but were treated in radically different ways. One of those cases involves a former tenured associate professor of early childhood education, Teresa Buchanan, one of two women from LSU listed on the Academic Sexual Misconduct Database. In December 2013, she was accused of saying something offensive to one of her female students. As the student was describing how her fiancé had helped with her service project—a coat drive for needy children—Buchanan allegedly interjected, "Well, he might support you now when the sex is good, but trust me, he won't support you in five years when it's not so good." The comment, according to Buchanan, was just a joke. She didn't intend to hurt her student. However, the student claimed she was "mortified." The idea that Buchanan, a professor, would make assumptions about her sex life was so upsetting that she said she considered changing majors or transferring out of LSU (Goldman, 2017).

After the student reported the incident to LSU administrators, Buchanan's 18-year career as a professor at LSU came to an end. She was never again allowed to teach a class. What makes this sexual harassment case extraordinary is the punishment Buchanan received. Did her poorly conceived joke deserve termination? A second, related issue is whether Buchanan's offensive joke amounted to sexual harassment. Did it conform to the EEOC definition of sexual harassment? Was it framed for "the purpose or effect of unreasonably interfering with an individual's work performance, or creating an intimidating, hostile or offensive working environment" (EEOC, 2016)? Or was it framed, perhaps, for the purpose of delivering a message about women's oppression—a warning about how men often use women for sex? If the latter possibility reflected Buchanan's intention, then LSU's decision to label Buchanan's comment "harassment," and fire her based on that assessment, can be interpreted, not only as a strike against Buchanan, but as a strike against women's license to voice feminist issues (see Faludi, 2009; Van Wormer, 2008). Thus, the title of Andrew Goldman's (2017) essay on LSU's decision to fire Buchanan: "You Can Get Fired for Saying That?"

The ensuing investigation included interviews with Buchanan's colleagues and students, as well as a close examination of Buchanan's teaching evaluations to see if former students made negative comments about her. What the investigators discovered is that Buchanan had a history of using profanity and making references to sex in the presence of students: they found that she used the word "*pussy*" three times during a meeting with student-teachers, she sometimes said "*fuck no*" in the presence of students; she once allegedly declared that only a dyke would wear brown pants, and allegedly opined that female students who became pregnant should not expect to graduate, a comment which was followed by an offer to buy condoms for her students to prevent that possible outcome. She also allegedly told a student who was expecting her third child that her education program was not designed for "mommies and wives," adding that the special accommodations granted her because of her disability were "bullshit," a comment that Buchanan forcefully denied. She said she would "never in a million years" refer to someone's disability as "bullshit." Finally, one of Buchanan's colleagues who sat in on one of Buchanan's classes claimed she was shocked to hear Buchanan remark that all men cared about was sex, which she allegedly followed by turning to a female student and asking, "Isn't that right, Amanda?" These discoveries convinced the LSU president and administration that Buchanan should be terminated (Goldman, 2017), even though terminating her violated LSU standard operating procedures. Under LSU rules, firing a tenured professor requires at least two unsatisfactory reviews in a row, coupled with evidence that the professor failed to remedy their transgressions. But there was nothing in Buchanan's record to indicate that she had in fact received negative reviews (Goldman, 2017).

Firing Buchanan seemed massively irregular when compared to the way LSU handled the cases of two male faculty also listed on the Academic Sexual Misconduct Database. In one of these cases, Niranjan Baisakh, an associate professor in the LSU school of plant, environmental, and soil sciences—the AgCenter—was accused, in 2014, of sexually assaulting one of his female graduate students. According to the police report, the student said that Baisakh entered her office, locked the door behind him and told her that "everyone in the department was having immoral relationships." She said that he then exposed his penis, restrained her when she tried to leave, and pushed her down, causing her to fall. The only way she could get him to back off, she said, was to threaten to hurt herself with a knife she took from her desk. But that isn't all. She also accused him of taking unwanted photos of her, hugging her, touching her breast, kissing her, and begging her to "please love me, please be mine." She said that on other occasions he showed up at her apartment uninvited, stalked her as she walked around campus, even following her when she went shopping and to her gym. After she rejected him, she said he threatened to kill himself if she were to report him, and told her that if he did kill himself, she would be responsible. In other words, the student reported an extraordinarily wide range of physical and psychological assaults to the police and to LSU investigators who corroborated her story. But Baisakh's punishment, unlike Buchanan's, did not involve termination. Instead, his tenure was suspended for three years. Although LSU did not allow Baisakh to resume working with graduate students, he was allowed to retain his position as professor at the University. Then, after three years, his tenure was reinstated. Finally, in 2020, six years after he was first accused of assaulting a student, LSU gave him permission to resume working with graduate students (Lim, 2021).

A second male professor from the LSU AgCenter to appear in the Academic Sexual Misconduct Database, Magdi Selim, was also investigated for threatening and sexually assaulting a female staff member between 2017 and 2019. According to the investigation report, he grabbed the staff member's buttocks, asked if her breasts were fake, offered to pay $1,000 to see her breasts, and asked about her genital grooming. He also repeatedly threatened to kill her if she were to tell anyone about his comments or threats. The charges against Selim, in short, like those levelled against Baisakh, were of the most serious nature, but unlike the Teresa Buchanan case, the investigation did not result in any disciplinary action. Instead, Selim, who was in his 70s, was allowed to voluntarily retire (Riegel, 2021).

In summary, LSU's response to two male professors charged with sexually threatening and assaultive behavior consisted of suspending one man's tenure for three years; the other received no disciplinary action at all. They managed to keep their jobs even though the allegations against them amounted to criminal assault. Teresa Buchanan, by contrast, was terminated, though the allegations against her were strictly verbal. She was fired for talking to her students in a blunt, "unladylike" style.

A Different Standard for Lesbians?

A second woman from LSU listed on the Academic Sexual Misconduct Database, Pokey Chatman, the former coach of LSU's women's basketball team, did not seem to live up to LSU's standards of female conduct. Chatman had a 90-14 winning record since taking the coach position in 2004, winning numerous awards such as Black Coaches Association Coach of the Year, SEC Coach of the Year, and Louisiana Coach of the Year. But, in March 2007, with her team ranked the 10th best in the country, someone, whose name was not disclosed, informed LSU that Chatman had an intimate relationship with one of her basketball players. Chatman acknowledged the relationship, describing it as noncoercive, but LSU administrators were profoundly unhappy. Though LSU had no policy forbidding consensual intimate relationships between faculty and students, Chatman was told that if she did not resign in two hours, she would be fired. Chatman's lawyer argued that LSU lacked the authority to fire someone for breaking a nonexistent rule. But the University's general counsel responded, "Does anybody believe you can do this kind of stuff and not have sanctions?" Chatman did resign in March 2007, and though she sought the remaining $900,000 on her contract, she settled for $160,000 (Gallo, 2021). She was then replaced by an interim coach, a man. The following year, LSU appointed a permanent coach to the women's basketball team, also a man (Longman, 2007a, b).

The main questions surrounding Chatman's forced resignation are, first, why the two-hour deadline? And second, like the main question surrounding the termination of Teresa Buchanan, what about discrepancies in the ways LSU responded to sexual harassment allegations against men? Consider, for example, how LSU managed the harassment charges against head football coach Les Miles. While LSU began investigating Miles in 2013, following charges that he demanded that the football program prioritize hiring "pretty girls with big breasts" and that he made unwelcome sexual advances to numerous female students, rather than publicly and immediately reporting Miles' harassment charges, as LSU did in Chatman's case, the University kept his investigation secret (Gallo, 2021). Miles was eventually terminated, but unlike Chatman's termination, it was not for sexual harassment. In 2016, the LSU football team got off to a disappointing, 2-2, start; his termination was about his failure to win football games (Kirk, 2016).

To further assess whether LSU may have handled harassment allegations against men differently than allegations against women, we should consider how LSU fielded sexual assault complaints against their star running back, Derrius Guice, who, in the spring 2016, was charged with raping a student after she passed out drunk at a party. As reported in *USA Today*, Guice was also charged with taking a nude photo of a student and sharing it with several others, including the team equipment manager. Then, in April 2017, another student claimed that Guice raped her. While federal laws and LSU's own policies require University officials to report such allegations to the Title IX office as well as to campus police, LSU did neither (Jacoby et al., 2020). The University did not investigate, did not call the police, and appeared to doubt the women's stories. *USA Today* further reported three cases where LSU allowed male students who allegedly committed sexual assault of female students to remain on campus, their only penalty consisting of a probationary period called "deferred suspension" which required the students "to stay out of trouble" for an indeterminate "period of time." *USA Today* reported that, in a fourth case involving a male student sexually assaulting two women, even after investigators found the student guilty of the assaults, the University refused to transfer him out of classes that he and his alleged victims were set to share. Instead, one of the victims was told she was the one who would have to transfer since her alleged assailant was not complaining; only she was (Jacoby et al., 2020).

The obvious question: Why did LSU allow male students charged with heterosexual assault to remain on campus but forced Pokey Chatman to leave campus and resign her position for engaging in a consensual same-sex relationship? To venture a guess: LSU was less concerned about the risk of a woman being sexually assaulted by a man than the risk that its athletics programs could be seen as tolerating and harboring lesbian sexual activity; LSU was concerned that retaining Chatman would make it possible for rival coaches to tell prospective players and their parents: "You don't want to go to LSU because the coach is a lesbian…." (Longman, 2007a, b).

The Academic Sexual Misconduct Database identified another basketball coach, a man accused of sexually assaulting a student, who may have been treated with greater tolerance and leniency than Chatman. Walter McCarty coached men's basketball at the University of Evansville until December 2019 when he was placed on leave while being investigated for violating a student's sexual consent. The student alleged that McCarty sent her inappropriate messages on Instagram, Snapchat, and text, which escalated to his finally pressuring her to visit his home, which she did on December 9, 2019. Once inside his home, the student claimed McCarty grabbed her, touched her breasts and buttocks, and digitally penetrated her. She reported the incident to campus police three days later, at which time she also began seeing a counselor who diagnosed her with PTSD (*TMZ Sports News*, 2021). The investigation which followed uncovered a series of sexual harassment reports against McCarty at the University of Evansville. Since he was hired in March 2018, he had been accused of sending persistent and unwanted messages to university employees, inviting them to bars, restaurants, and to his home. In one instance, he requested to see a swimsuit photo of an athletic department employee; in another he initiated unwanted physical contact with a female student who was working in a university café. When McCarty's complainant learned about the earlier allegations against him, she initiated a civil suit against the University for failing to protect her. She said, "I am heartbroken that my school knew about Coach McCarty's misconduct before what happened to me, and looked the other way." While Pokey Chatman, a gay woman, was given two hours to resign at LSU for having a consensual relationship with a female student, more than a year passed before McCarty, a heterosexual man, was finally fired in January 2020 for sexually assaulting a female student (Lindskog, 2021). The victim's attorney found that delay stunning and inexplicable: "If the university had just paid attention to what a long line of women were trying to tell them, it could have stopped a woman from being raped … but they sat on their hands and did nothing" (Lindskog, 2021).

A Frame-up?

Joanna Warmington was a nationally recognized collegiate cross country and track and field coach for the University of Minnesota-Duluth from 2009 to 2018 with many successes, including four NSIC (Northern Sun Intercollegiate Conference) championships, 38 all-Americans, three individual national champions, and three NSIC coach of the year awards. But in March 2018, the University placed her on leave and subsequently fired her, following complaints about her "sexualized" coaching behavior. That prompted a lawsuit from Warmington, who, when she told her side of the story in court, described a frame-up based on sex discrimination.

She said the University "was coordinating an effort through my supervisor, the men's head coach for cross country and track and field, and our shared assistant coaches (all males) to remove me from my position as head coach." She argued that University investigators had grossly and purposefully misinterpreted her actions, so that almost anything she did or said, in their eyes, was seen as "sexual in nature, even if it was innocent," as in her comment to an athlete that she had beautiful legs (St. George, 2018). Warmington acknowledged telling a student-athlete that she had "beautiful legs" but clarified that the comment had nothing to do with the student's sexual attractiveness; rather, it was to tell her that her legs "were toned and powerful and would serve her well as we discussed what kind of events were best for her physique and training." Warmington also noted that she was accused of having had "inappropriate discussions with athletes about their eating habits and weight," (Warmington v Bd of Regents of University of Minnesota, 455 F. Supp. 3d 871, April 21, 2020, p. 3), an allegation which, she contended, made no sense since a female track coach is expected to talk to her athletes about their eating habits and weight. She said that "[o]ver the years, several male members of the track and field coaching staff ... would make comments about certain female athletes gaining weight and ask that [she] talk to the athlete because she was a woman" (Warmington vs Bd of Regents, p. 7). Warmington gave one more example of how her actions were misinterpreted: after going on a run during the summer, she sent an inspirational text message to her athletes with a picture of herself in running gear, wearing a running bra. "This picture was cited as an example of a 'sexual picture' just because I was wearing my running bra," Warmington said. "My student-athletes always run in their running bras in the summer and there is no difference between me doing so and them—this is normal summer running attire for women" (St. George, 2018).

She pleaded in court that unlike herself, male coaches were not terminated for disciplining athletes and giving them personal advice on their mental health and sexuality, nor were they terminated for making sexual comments (Warmington v. Bd of Regents, p. 6). She also argued that the University had no problem when other coaches and athletes practiced in revealing shorts or running bras, and no one had ever complained about male coaches discussing nutrition and body weight with their athletes, the third alleged reason for her termination (Joanna Warmington v. Bd of Regents, p. 6).

Still, Warmington was fired, an outcome that other University of Minnesota-Duluth employees who were accused of sexual harassment and who appear on the Academic Sexual Misconduct Database, managed to avoid. Unlike Warmington, they kept their jobs. Also, unlike Warmington, they are men. One is a former fitness trainer, Rod Raymond, who, in 2009, allegedly tickled a female student's stomach during a fitness test. Other women accused him of nuzzling their necks, hugging them, and making unwelcome sexual advances. In response, UMD ordered Raymond to take a series of classes on sexual harassment. Shortly thereafter, the harassment allegations against Raymond seemed forgiven, as he was promoted to the position of fitness and wellness coordinator for the University (Busch, 2012). The other UMD faculty listed on the Academic Sexual Misconduct Database is psychology professor Randall Gordon, who, in

1996, gave one of his students a letter soliciting a personal relationship. After the student indicated she was not interested, he continued calling her. Then, in 1997, he gave another student a similar letter, again soliciting a personal relationship. After the student claimed he touched her without obtaining consent, she reported him to the University, and an internal investigation corroborated her story. His punishment consisted of suspension without pay or benefits for the fall quarter, 1997. He was also forbidden to have any further contact with the student (Ann Yochum at al. v. University of Minnesota, Duluth, Minnesota Court of Appeals, June 15, 1999, c4-98-2255).

Two other former track coaches, both men, appear on the Academic Sexual Misconduct Database, their cases distinguished by the seriousness of the allegations against them and the absence of any sense of urgency in the ensuing Title IX investigation. One, Sesar Figueroa, coached at Houston Christian University, where, according to court documents, he "physically assaulted and degraded" his female student-athletes for several years. One student recalled how Figueroa got her drunk, forced her to engage in unprotected intercourse, and then forced her to take Plan B emergency contraception to prevent pregnancy. HCU terminated Figueroa, but so slowly, without any sense of urgency, that several students claimed that the University "turned a blind eye" to his abusive behavior, doing nothing even after they reported his misconduct to University administrators (Vasquez, 2024).

The second male track coach listed on the Academic Sexual Misconduct Database is onetime Olympian, Conrad Mainwaring, who coached at Syracuse University, Colgate, UCLA, and a summer sports camp in Massachusetts. He also coached at the California Institute of Technology but was fired in less than a year following a student's complaint. The nature of that complaint is not publicly available, but an ESPN "Outside the Lines" investigation uncovered a pattern of sexual misconduct allegations against Mainwaring dating as far back as the mid-1970s, which continued until 2016, with one of his victims reportedly as young as 14-years-old. Mainwaring allegedly used his Olympic credentials and relationships with well-known athletes to persuade boys and young men that his training methods—which included genital manipulation—were legitimate and successful (Kessler & Fainaru-Wada, 2019). Mainwaring allegedly referred to genital manipulation as "physiotherapy," and one of the men who accused Mainwaring recalled asking him, "When is this going to stop?" with Mainwaring answering, "It's going to stop when you realize what's necessary in your training, and your training isn't there. If you stop, I won't coach you." In 2024, after Mainwaring's arrest on charges of sexual assault, he pleaded guilty to assaulting nine boys ages 13 to 19, and was sentenced to up to 11 years in prison (Lenthang, 2024).

Another Frame-up?

Why would a college or university or any other organization contrive sexual harassment allegations against a woman? What is to be gained? A possible answer is that, like the sexual harassment of women, in general, falsely accusing a woman of sexual harassment, particularly one who is high-ranking and successful, improves men's chances of obtaining promotions and retaining desirable positions. Because women wrongly accused of sexual harassment are likely to suffer anxiety and lowered self-esteem, not to mention damaged reputations, their male competitors, by comparison, are likely to feel more confident and secure. Broadcasting the message that women are sexually loose and predatory can make women doubt themselves and stifle their ambition. Bringing women down with false or exaggerated accusations can increase the likelihood that men who occupy lower positions can move up; they can then apply for the positions vacated by women driven out by contrived harassment accusations.

Consider the case of Rosalyn Templeton, the former provost of Montana State University-Northern, a school with 1,300 students, located in the high plains of north central Montana. In 2013, one of the University deans, Randy Bachmeier, accused Templeton, his direct supervisor, of sexually harassing him. According to Bachmeier, Templeton touched him—"slow and lingering" sexual touches—without his consent, and did so continuously from 2010 to 2013. The first time this occurred, he said, was during a meeting in Templeton's office, when she began rubbing his upper leg with the palm of her hand. He said he was so shocked he abruptly rose to his feet, causing Templeton's hand to fall from his leg. Then, on April 30, 2013, two and a half years after the alleged harassment began, Bachmeier claimed he finally told Templeton to stop touching him, a claim which Templeton disputed: she insisted that Bachmeier never said anything like this. When asked why he waited so long before telling her to stop, Bachmeier did not cite a quid pro quo bargain or any other kind of coercion. Rather, he said, "I have a hard time talking about things like this ... it's very hard to talk about being sexually harassed by a woman and have people believe you" (Schmidt, 2014).

As reported by Bachmeier, the final straw—what made him decide to charge Templeton with harassment—occurred on May 6, 2013, at a dinner party in the home of the University chancellor, Templeton's supervisor: Bachmeier and Templeton were standing on the buffet-line with Bachmeier in front and Templeton directly behind, when, according to Bachmeier, Templeton began stroking his shoulders and back in a sexual manner. The next day, Bachmeier notified Montana State University-Northern's human service department that Templeton had been sexually harassing him (Schmidt, 2014).

The key questions in Bachmeier's harassment allegation are how Templeton's touches were sexual and how were they coercive. If her touching made him uncomfortable, what prevented him from moving away or asking Templeton to stop? Templeton admitted to patting Bachmeier on the back at the chancellor's dinner party, but she denied *stroking* his back and shoulders, as Bachmeier asserted. She said her pats had nothing to do with sexual desire; rather, she briefly patted him as a way to encourage him to take the ice cream. "Take two scoops," she said, "it's really good." She explained that she sometimes uses "touching as a means of communicating with others in the workplace.... The touching is a means of providing a sense of reassurance or comfort," but she denied sexual intent (Schmidt, 2014).

In attempting to resolve the disparity between Bachmeier's and Templeton's accounts, it might help to think through a few hypotheticals: first, the matter of where the last alleged harassment took place—a dinner party buffet-line, a place where one could be observed by many others, including one's boss, the chancellor of the University. On the face of it, initiating an unwelcome sexual advance on a buffet-line at the boss's party does not make much sense, particularly since such advances are prohibited, not only by the University, but by Bachmeier himself who claimed he told Templeton point blank to never touch him again. We also need to consider that Bachmeier claimed that the day after he told Templeton to never touch him again, she berated him and as retaliation excluded him from meetings with other deans, raising the question, not only why Templeton would want to touch someone sexually with whom she recently fought, but also why, if their relationship was as rocky as Bachmeier claimed, she would choose such a moment—the boss's dinner party—to act out sexually with him. Then there is the issue of whether Bachmeier might have had something to gain by falsely accusing Templeton of sexually harassing him, given that Bachmeier had applied for Templeton's position—the provost position—before Templeton was hired, and that the day after Templeton resigned MSU-Northern, largely because of the negative fall-out from Bachmeier's allegations, Bachmeier again put himself forward as a candidate for the provost position. While he did not gain this promotion—the provost position called for a candidate who held the rank of associate or full professor, and Bachmeier, though one of the University's deans, was only an assistant professor—it is a position he coveted, as evidenced by the fact that he lobbied for a change in the qualifications for the provost position, so that an assistant professor could apply. Bachmeier proposed changing the qualifications "to include experience that merits the title of associate or full professor because the original language establishes a requirement based on a title rather than necessary skills and abilities to perform the duties of the position." However, Montana State University-Northern's chancellor reportedly shot Bachmeier's proposal down, saying, "It wouldn't look good for someone who had filed a complaint to get the position" (Associated Press, 2014).

To Bachmeier, this smacked of retaliation. In his mind, he had reported an instance of sexual harassment in good faith and now, because he had made that report, was being denied an opportunity to apply for a position for which he believed himself qualified. He therefore sued Montana State University-Northern and the chancellor for unfairly penalizing him for reporting his supervisor's sexual harassment, a claim that was upheld by the Montana State Supreme Court in a ruling which awarded Bachmeier more than $460,000 in damages and legal fees (Vigliotti, 2021).

Although MSU-Northern's internal investigation and the Montana Supreme Court concluded that Templeton had not sexually harassed Bachmeier, the investigation did unearth a long list of other, nonsexual complaints against Templeton. The complaints included comments such as: Templeton "doesn't let me come to meetings," "She doesn't communicate," "She's trying to get into the curriculum," "She comes to work late," "She has a humidifier going." So, even though, following a Title IX investigation, Templeton was not held responsible for violating the University's sexual harassment policies, the allegations Bachmeier levelled against her and the ensuing investigation created a volume of negative fallout sufficient to force her to vacate her position. On the one hand, she reported how "incredibly hard" it had been for her and her daughter to continue living in this closely knit Montana community following the harassment investigation. On the other hand, Bachmeier's allegations triggered the chancellor's decision to request Templeton's resignation. In the chancellor's words, "I made the decision that she needed to leave immediately, so we could begin, as I say, the process of healing" (Rivard, 2014).

Rosalyn Templeton is the only individual listed on the Academic Sexual Misconduct Database from Montana State University-Northern.

When Bawdy Jokes = Sexual Harassment

Marybeth Gasman was the Judy and Howard Berkowitz Professor of Higher Education at the University of Pennsylvania and Director of the Penn Center for Minority Serving Institutions when, in 2017, she was accused of sexual harassment, specifically, of creating a "culture of sexual harassment" at the Penn Center by repeatedly making comments to staff which contained sexual references. For example, she was accused of texting a male and female staff member, "Please get a room, you two," and, in response to a staff member's joke about her sexual prowess, she was accused of texting, "Damn! I want a man that I can cling to! All night long!" To another staff member, she allegedly wrote on the GroupMe app, "You can visit my penthouse anytime," a comment which came with a photo of an apartment interior, presumably her own, and included this: "I'm going to need some lovin' or this is a view you'll never see in the morning." She was also accused of sharing her breast size with staff, of commenting on whether she was wearing a bra, and of discussing how she lost her virginity. During a birthday party for a staff member, guests played "Pin the Penis on the Naked White Man," and Gasman once reportedly wore an apron that bore the message "I keep the best snacks under my apron." Gasman, who is white, was also accused of "fetishizing" some of her Latinx and Black staff and students, and of making more jokes about people of color than about whites. Although no complaints surfaced from individuals whom Gasman may have touched inappropriately, a former graduate assistant accused her of rubbing men's arms and chests and claimed she once asked two staff members to compare butt sizes (Flaherty, 2019a, b).

Because Gasman's comments were documented in text messages and performed in public, they were not contested. What could have been contested, however, is whether any of her comments were demeaning, reflected hostile intent, and were enough to qualify as "sexual harassment." Did they meet the EEOC standard of "unreasonably interfering with an individual's work performance, or creating an intimidating, hostile, or offensive working environment"?

One of the complainants—a former graduate assistant of Gasman's—said that Gasman's bawdy jokes and comments were "inappropriate" for a professor of her power and stature, an administrator who "gatekeeps access to a lot of academic resources not otherwise available to marginalized students." Which, of course, raises the question: Can comments be deemed sexual harassment simply because they are seen as undignified—when they appear too crude for someone who occupies a high-ranking position? A former Center employee claimed that Gasman's wisecracks were divisive: those who joined in were "seen as the 'in crowd'" and those who didn't, didn't get "the benefits of being invited to outings or professional development events" (Flaherty, 2019a, b). Which, again, raises the question: Can comments or wisecracks be deemed sexual harassment simply because they appeal to some but not to others—when they seem divisive? Another former staff member accused Gasman of intimidation—of demeaning other faculty members and administrators as weak. But when asked how, precisely, she intimidated faculty and administrators, the complainant only cited a text message that Gasman sent to her staff: "most students don't know how academic power works as we don't tell them. Faculty have the power at Penn. Admin don't" (Flaherty, 2019a, b).

The major problem in assessing whether any of these allegations qualify as sexual harassment is their lack of specificity. How did Gasman's sexualized jokes and comments, her so-called "inappropriate" behavior and divisive wisecracks, and her remarks on how academic power works, interfere with people's work performance or create an intimidating work environment? Because Gasman's alleged sexual harassment appeared to have no identified or identifiable victims—because no one came forward to claim they had been injured by Gasman's language or behavior—those questions could not, and perhaps, cannot be answered. That Gasman's staff at the Center for Minority Serving Institutions had been required to sign a blanket nondisclosure agreement, stating that anyone who worked in the Center could not discuss publicly anything that occurred in the Center, may have been raised as a sexual harassment issue—as a potential cover for sexual harassment ((Nguyen, 2019). However, no one at the Center claimed they had been harmed by signing the nondisclosure agreement. And while some of Gasman's staff insinuated that her sexual banter was harmful and racist *in general*, no one testified that her jokes and comments disrupted *their* workplace performance. No one provided evidence that Gasman's sexualized banter was intended to harm them.

Nonetheless, Penn took these complaints seriously, launched an investigation, and though the results were not shared with the public or with the complainants, Penn decided, based upon the findings, to move Gasman's graduate students away from her administrative hub, the Center for Minority Serving Institutions, to another location on campus. Graduate students and staff members from another campus location, in turn, were moved to the Center to surveil Gasman—"to provide oversight." Penn also promised to offer "relevant training" to Center employees. And the following year, Gasman resigned after having served on the Penn faculty for 16 years (Flaherty, 2019a, b).

To address the question of whether Gasman's alleged sexual harassment was treated differently than harassment allegations against men, we should consider, first, that the three former male professors and rowing coach from Penn who are listed on the Database, unlike Gasman, were not singled out for their sexually suggestive jokes and comments. Rather, they were accused of sexual assault and/or for having sex with their own students. One was convicted in court of sexually assaulting a student he was showing around campus and was sentenced to 3½ to seven years in prison (Garrett & McBride, 2008). A second was accused of several sexual offenses, including rape, but the latter charge did not come to light until after he had resigned from Penn (Tan, 2017). A third and fourth were accused of having sex with their undergraduate students. They also resigned (Berry, 1994; Mondon, 2018).

Several men listed on the Academic Sexual Misconduct Database but affiliated with institutions other than Penn had been accused sexual harassment for their racy, sexualized humor, among them, Robert Wiseman, a physiology professor from Michigan State University; Buck Ryan, a journalism professor from the University of Kentucky; Charles D. Hays, former president of Century College, a community college near Minneapolis-St. Paul; and Gilbert Rodman, a communications professor from the University of Minnesota. The first of these, Wiseman, allegedly had a decades-long history of making MSU women uncomfortable with his sexualized comments and jokes (e.g., after a woman mentioned that her knees were sore from playing volleyball over the weekend, he allegedly responded, "Oh, I'm sure that's not the only reason why you were on your knees this weekend") (Berg, 2019). Ryan, from Kentucky, was criticized for singing a version of the Beach Boys song, "California Girls," at a Chinese educational ceremony (e.g., "Well, Shanghai girls are hip; I really dig those styles they wear") (Thomason, 2018). Hays, from Century

College, was criticized for vulgar, sexist humor (e.g., his comment, "The color I like is titty pink.") (Bassinger, 2000). And Rodman, from Minnesota, was criticized for his vulgarity and sexism (e.g., during dinner with a University of Minnesota student he joked about her dog: "maybe his wang smells like bacon" and "I don't know, maybe you fellated [the dog]" (Hewitt & Marisam, 2013). The problem with comparing these professors' alleged offenses to Gasman's, apart from differences in the kinds of humor they employed, is that the allegations against Wiseman, Ryan, Hays, and Rodman went beyond sexual jokes and comments. Wiseman was also accused of making unwelcome sexual and romantic advances to MSU women. He was punished with a six-week suspension without pay. In Ryan's case, a University of Kentucky spokesperson reported that "a preponderance of evidence concluded that he engaged in 'inappropriate touching,'" the details of which were redacted to protect the "privacy and confidentiality of the victim." As punishment, he was banned from receiving international travel funds and was stripped of a teaching award worth thousands of dollars. In Hays' case, an internal investigation found that he "transgressed a state policy that prohibits employees from receiving, keeping, or sending obscenity or pornography." As punishment, he was asked to resign. And in Rodman's case, University of Minnesota investigators found him responsible for repeatedly touching subordinate women without their consent and for pressuring them to have a personal relationship with him after they made it clear that they did not want such a relationship. His penalty: a formal reprimand was placed in his file, and he was required to take sexual harassment training.

When Bawdy Jokes = Sexual Harassment (Part II)

The harassment case listed on the Academic Sexual Misconduct Database that bears the closest connection to Gasman's is that of another woman, Donna Laird, former director of the radiography program at St. Philip's College, a historically Black community college in San Antonio, Texas. In 2011, a male instructor accused her of harassing him via email repartee. As evidence, he turned over hundreds of emails containing links to jokes and satirical skits that Laird sent to him and other radiography staff over a six-year period. Many of these links included sexually explicit images and racial stereotypes: a musical slideshow starring scantily clad vaginas, young Black men dressed for prom in "ghetto" attire, a woman simulating fellatio on a car's stick shift, a young man lighting fireworks stuck in his anus, a satirical exercise program in which white women run from Black men posing as muggers.

Laird, like Gasman, disclaimed malicious intent. She said her goal in sharing what many might have been construed as outrageous humor was to "alleviate stress at work." Nonetheless, Philips College investigators opined that sending such a high volume of emails of a sexual nature was inconsistent with the school's policies and "certainly raises the potential for claims of a sexually hostile environment." Shortly after this finding was shared with the College administration, Laird was asked to resign, as was her supervisor, who knew about the raunchy emails but did nothing to stop them.

What makes the harassment allegations against Laird similar to the allegations against Gasman is that her controversial emails, the ones containing links to satirical sketches, did not have an individual target. Rather, she sent these emails to her radiography staff en masse. Furthermore, none of the email recipients claimed they suffered injury; the goal of the emails was to divert and entertain. The faculty member whose complaint launched the harassment investigation—the self-identified victim—far from suffering harm from Laird's emails, sometimes used the links from them as "icebreakers" for his own classes and business seminars. Moreover, the fact that he waited years before speaking out raised the question, why is he speaking out now? According to Melissa Ludwig (2011), author of "Bawdy Emails Cost Administrator Her Job" a possible answer is that he "believed that his tenure bid was in jeopardy" and that charging Laird with sexual harassment while he was going up for tenure could have been used to distract from, and possibly even to excuse, his weak portfolio. In short, the sexual harassment charge in this instance may have been manufactured as a means of buoying a man's career. Ultimately, he was denied tenure and lost his job, but Donna Laird and her supervisor, another woman, also lost theirs.

To compare Laird's case with that of men listed on the Academic Sexual Misconduct Database, we need to go outside St. Philip's College, since Laird is the only individual from St. Philip's on the Database. The closest male comparisons appear to be Eric Rasmusen, a business professor at the University of Indiana, and Rob Smith, a computer science professor from the University of Montana. Like Laird, they did not target any individual, but rather sent out messages en masse that were construed as sexist, racist, and homophobic. However, unlike Laird, Rasmusen and Smith sent their messages through social media platforms, and not in the workplace, and their goal, they said, was not to amuse or entertain. Rather, for Rasmusen, the goal was to share his controversial opinions and values. Rasmusen's Tweets, for example, included the messages, "Women do not belong in the workplace," "black students ... are generally inferior academically to white students," and "Women and gay men do not belong in academia" (Herron & Reschke, 2019). Smith's goal, much like Rasmusen's, was to share his sexist cultural beliefs: on his blog he urged men to date young women because they peak at 16 and then quickly "lose value." Thus, he advised women to recognize that their physical attractiveness is their "most valuable asset in finding a husband" and that their "pool of potential husbands shrinks significantly with every year past 18" (Assuncao, Oct. 23, 2021). Also, both Rasumsen and Smith, unlike Laird, managed to keep their jobs long after their objectionable messages became an issue. In 2019, a spokesperson for the University of Indiana stated that, although the University condemned Rasmusen's Tweets, his First Amendment rights preclude the possibility of firing him. Smith's blog began in 2013, but he did not resign his position until 2021, in response to a student-organized protest movement which had a website titled "Fire Rob Smith."

When Facts Don't Matter

In 2007, Karen Lopez Austen was hired as chair of the kinesiology department at Weatherford College, a community college in Weatherford, Texas. Shortly after she was hired, a secretary in the department complained that Austen had "inappropriately" invited the secretary's daughter to her office, showed her "inappropriate" photos, and asked to measure her with a measuring tape. In a second harassment complaint, the assistant men's basketball coach claimed that Austen made "improper" comments to him about his physique; he also accused her of taking "secret" photographs of him as he was working out. However, the circumstances and details surrounding these episodes and comments—what made them "inappropriate," "improper," and "secret"—were never publicly disclosed (Greenwald, 2014).

After Austen tried to defend herself by claiming that the sexual harassment charges initiated by the assistant men's basketball coach and the departmental secretary were discriminatory and unfair, she was replaced as chair of her department by a man with less experience and inferior credentials. Then Austen filed a complaint with the Equal Employment

Opportunity Commission (EEOC) claiming that the sexual misconduct allegations levelled against her amounted to sexual discrimination and harassment and had been used as justifications to demote her. Weatherford College, in response, proposed a settlement, promising to remove all the disciplinary warnings from Austen's file if she would agree to drop her discrimination and harassment charges against Weatherford, an agreement which Austen accepted, and which suggests that her complaints against Weatherford had merit (Austen v. Weatherford Coll, United States District Court Norther District of Texas, Aug. 8, 2012).

The next year, however, the conflict between Austen and Weatherford continued as a long list of new complaints surfaced, most of which appeared to have only a loose or meager connection to sexual misconduct: (1) a coach complained that Austen forced his students off of treadmills during class time; (2) a faculty member asserted that Austen had yelled at her, shut the door in her face, and made her feel harassed when signing payroll notifications; (3) a department secretary said that Austen had forced her to do a task that would require her to leave her desk even though her boss had instructed her to remain at her desk to answer an important phone call; (4) a student complained that Austen had made an inappropriate sexual comment to her when she was using an abductor machine: "Let's see if she is loose," Austen reportedly said. "Let's see if she is a virgin"; (5) other students complained that Austin had threatened to count them absent and fail them if they did not stay after class; (6) several witnesses described a series of inappropriate behaviors in the college bookstore which included Austen telling an African-American student, "You'll have to go to another register because she [the cashier] doesn't wait on Black people," telling a Hispanic student, "They [the bookstore staff] charge Hispanics 20 percent more," and telling an overweight student, "I can tell you where the lo-cal snacks are." Finally, (7) Austen reportedly answered the bookstore phone and responded to a student's question by saying, "First you have to tell me if you are Black or white because it is different times for different people" (Cmaadmin, 2014).

Although Austen and her attorney claimed they had an abundance of evidence which directly refuted these allegations—they had witnesses who could prove that the so-called incriminating incidents had been distorted and taken out of context—the president of Weatherford and the College's board of trustees decided against giving Austen a hearing: they refused to interview any of the parties who had filed reports about her or who had any first-hand knowledge of the allegations. Then, without examining actual evidence associated with the allegations—relying solely on hearsay—the Weatherford president and board of trustees decided against renewing Austen's contract (see letter by Mark W. Robinett, attorney, July 6, 2015).

Austen countered by filing suit in the U. S. District Court in Fort Worth, alleging sexual and racial discrimination, but the Court granted Weatherford's motion for summary judgment, again dismissing Austen's case by denying her an opportunity to present evidence. She then appealed to the Fifth Circuit Court of Appeals which is required to remand a case for trial if the plaintiff can present enough evidence to raise doubts about the allegations. However, the Court's panel of three judges held, like the U.S. District Court and the Weatherford president and board of trustees, that evidence was not needed, and went so far as to say,

> What matters is *not the truth* of the underlying complaints and reports, however, but rather whether the college could legitimately have relied on them in deciding to terminate Austen (italics added).

The Appeals Court panel decided that there was no need to weigh evidence before a fair and impartial tribunal. Instead, the judges elected to determine the legitimacy of Austen's termination without hearing Austen's side of the story and without checking to see if the allegations against her were true or false, decisions which sabotaged any attempt to assess the seriousness of the allegations against her. They also sabotaged any attempt to compare Austen's case to that of others, with perhaps one exception: the case of Catherine Woytowicz, another woman listed on the Academic Sexual Misconduct Database who was also fired for sexual harassment despite the absence of evidence. In the official version of events, as decided by her university and the courts, evidence was unnecessary.

When Investigating Sexual Harassment = Sexual Harassment

Woytowicz was an adjunct professor at the George Washington University from 2000 to 2017. She taught in both the department of chemistry and school of international affairs, and was accused, in January 2016, of threatening her former student, a 19-year-old male undergraduate, with dire consequences if he did not comply with her sexual demands. What makes this case comparable to Austen's is the disregard for facts, so that, when

George Washington investigators initially found scant evidence to support the student's harassment charge against Woytowicz, instead of dropping the case, they changed the rules: they expanded "the coverage of their prohibitions so that they mean anything and everything" (Larimer, 2018). Investigators appeared to launch a fishing expedition to find some kind of sexual misconduct with which to charge Woytowicz, a pursuit which she described as harassment. To illustrate how she was harassed, she described her first meeting with the Title IX investigator in charge of the case, on March 2016, during which he "peppered [her] with invasive questions about her personal life and sexual relationships," including questions about her relationship with an adult who had never been a student at GWU. She said the investigator even asked if she had ever had, or wanted to have, a "three-way" with this person. She also alleged that after she asked the investigator if she could look at the notebook containing the allegations against her, he held it over her head, toying with her, seeming "to delight in this, as if playing a child's game of keep away" (Brown, 2018; Larimer, 2018).

The University finally decided to charge Woytowicz with the offense of having a *consensual* sexual relationship with her former student. What made the ensuing investigation appear almost fact-free was, first, that investigators failed to give credence to the 19-year-old student's roommate's testimony that he had never seen or heard anything to indicate that Woyhowicz and the complainant had been sexually involved, and second, that the University failed to give credence to the possibility that the 19-year-old complainant might have had disingenuous motives for making the harassment allegations against Woytowwicz given "his admitted interest in 'mindfucking' her the same way Iago did to Othello, a technique he learned from a book titled *Mindfucking: A Critique of Mental Manipulation*" (Brown, 2018).

In the absence of evidence supporting the charge that Woytowicz and her student had been engaged in a *physical* sexual relationship, the University redefined "sexual relationship" in a highly original way: by claiming that a consensual sexual relationship exists when two individuals exchange text messages which "could be interpreted as [containing] sexual innuendo" (see Woytowicz vs, George Washington University, p. 3). Such messages, the University argued, violated the University's prohibition against "faculty member[s] … hav[ing] a sexual relationship with a student who is currently in his/her course or is subject to his/her supervision." In other words, George Washington University did not maintain that the text messages exchanged between Woytowicz and the complainant revealed that they had ever been, or desired to be, in a physical sexual relationship, but rather that these text messages constituted, in themselves, a type of sexual relationship, an allegation which the University supported by providing snippets of text messages which were purported to include inappropriate phrases, paraphrases, and quotations exchanged between Woytowicz and her student. Those snippets did not appear in court documents and never became publicly available, but the University attempted to support its claim that these texts were sexually inappropriate by pointing to the "frequency of communication, late hours of communication, meetings, multiple requests to see [the student complainant] or talk to [him], restaurants and drinks," in addition to talk about "emotional feelings" (Brown, Jan. 9, 2018).

In Woytowicz's suit against George Washington University, she reported that some of these text quotations were manufactured—they were either made up or framed in false contexts—while others consisted of "cherry-picked words or phrases to suggest something was meant sexually, and ignored the context showing they either had no such meaning or were ambiguous" (Brown, 2018). Woytowicz also argued that the so-called "improper" exchanges she had with the complainant were not any different from the kind of exchanges she had with other students at George Washington: as an adjunct professor who held another full-time position, she claimed she routinely arranged one-on-one meetings with students during weekends and evenings in coffee shops and other non-academic locales, which included inviting them to cultural and educational events, and helping them with their studies and academic applications.

Still, the University insisted that Woytowicz had violated its policies, and in September 2016, offered her a chance to continue at George Washington if she agreed to enter into an "informal resolution" in which she acknowledged guilt. According to this "informal resolution" she would need to accept a written reprimand for her inappropriate sexual relationship with the complainant and agree to undergo anti-sexual harassment training. She rejected the proposal, however, on the grounds that it "would require her to submit to a written reprimand for conduct of which she knows she is innocent" (Brown, 2018). As a result of her unwillingness to acknowledge something she believed was untrue, in 2017, George Washington University severed ties with her. She was terminated. As for Woytowicz's suit against the University for sex discrimination, sexual harassment, and wrongful termination, that too ended painfully for her:

the court ruled that George Washington University, as a private institution, had broad discretion to carry out its business as it saw fit.

Woytowicz is the only individual listed on the Academic Sexual Misconduct Database from George Washington University, but one case from the Database, in addition to Austen's, resembles hers: the case of Jeffrey Menaker, the former Hofstra University tennis coach was accused of having "a strange obsession with [a student's] menstrual cycle" and of making "quid pro quo threats [to a student that] were severe, pervasive, hostile, and disgusting." Menaker denied all the allegations, provided exculpatory documents, and the names of witnesses who could support his denials, but two months later, Hofstra University fired him. Like Weatherford College's decision to fire Karen Lopez Austen and George Washington University's decision to fire Catherine Woytowicz, Hofstra arrived at the decision fire Jeffrey Menaker without interviewing witnesses who Menaker claimed could have testified in his behalf and despite the absence of evidence supporting the complainant's allegations. Hofstra's grounds for termination, like those used against Austen and Woytowicz, were also vague in the extreme: he was fired for "unprofessional conduct" and "the totality of circumstances." The main difference between Menaker's case and Austen's and Woytowicz's is that after Menaker sued Hofstra, alleging discrimination, the court decided in his favor, ruling that Hofstra deviated from its own investigative procedures, failing, in particular, to interview possible exculpatory witnesses (see Menaker v. Hofstra University, on appeal from United District Court for the Eastern District of New York, Aug. 15, 2019).

References

Associated Press. (2014, June 12). MSU-Norther sexual harassment complaint to be heard. *Havre Daily News*. https://www.greatfallstribune.com/story/news/local/2014/06/12/msu-northern-sexual-harassment-complaint-heard/10369301/

Axon, S. (2021, September 8). Ole Miss coach cleared after Title IX allegations over improper relationship. *USA Today*. https://www.usatoday.com/story/sports/2021/09/08/ole-miss-softball-coaches-cleared-title-ix-improper-relationship/5778004001/

Bassinger, J. (2000, March 17). College president resigns after being accused of making offensive jokes. *The Chronicle of Higher Education*. https://www.chronicle.com/article/college-president-resigns-after-being-accused-of-making-offensive-jokes/

Berg, K. (2019, June 25). Report: MSU physiology professor sexually harassed at least 6 women over 17-year period. *Lansing State Journal*. https://www.lansingstatejournal.com/story/news/2019/06/25/michigan-state-sexual-harassment-msu-professor-sex-oie-osteopathic-wiseman/1511348001/

Berry, M. (1994, June 30). English prof resigns amidst sex scandal. *The Daily Pennsylvanian*.. https://www.thedp.com/article/1994/06/english-prof-resigns-amidst-sex-scandal

Brown, E. N. (2018, January 9). Exchanging dirty jokes is now a “sexual relationship” at George Washington University. *Reason*. https://reason.com/2018/01/09/woytowicz-sues-gwu-over-title-ix-farce/

Busch, M. (2012, November 5). UMD fitness and wellness coordinator faces more complaints. *The Statesman*. https://www.theumdstatesman.com/blog/2012/11/05/umd-fitness-and-wellness-coordinator-faces-more-allegations-of-sexual-harassment

Byrne, K. J. (2021, September 4). Ole Miss softball coach accused of tryst with student recently married. *New York Post*: https://nypost.com/2021/09/04/ole-miss-softball-coach-katie-browder-recently-married/

Carl. (2021, September 2). Sex scandal in the sec: Ole Miss softball coach is in hot water for Secretly hooking up with one of her players. *Bar Stool Sports*. https://www.barstoolsports.com/blog/3381748/sex-scandal-in-the-sec-ole-miss-softball-coach-is-in-hot-water-for-secretly-hooking-up-with-one-of-her-players

Cmaadmin. (2014, April 30). Diverse docket: Weatherford College prevails in discrimination suit. *Diverse*. https://www.diverseeducation.com/sports/article/15094694/diverse-docket-weatherford-college-prevails-in-discrimination-suit

Equal Employment Opportunity Commission (EEOC). (2016). https://www.eeoc.gov/select-task-force-study-harassment-workplace

Faludi, S. (2009). *Backlash: The undeclared war against American women*. Crown.

Flaherty, C. (2019a, January 30). U of Michigan music professor arrested for assault. *Inside Higher Ed*. https://www.insidehighered.com/quicktakes/2019/01/31/u-michigan-music-professor-arrested-assault

Flaherty, C. (2019b, August 26). A culture of sexual harassment. *Inside Higher Ed*. https://www.insidehighered.com/news/2019/08/27/star-scholar-minority-serving-institutions-was-accused-fostering-hypersexualized-and

Gallo, A. (2021, May 7). How Pokey Chatman’s 2-hour deadline to retire compares with how LSU Handles Les Miles. *The Advocate*. https://www.theadvocate.com/baton_rouge/sports/lsu/how-pokey-chatmans-2-hour-deadline-to-resign-compares-with-how-lsu-handled-les-miles/article_eb450386-add7-11eb-b27e-237b0ae912e0.html

Garrett, E., & McBride, M. A. (2008, February 14). Ex-prof gets prison sentence for sex assault. *The Daily Pennsylvanian*. https://www.thedp.com/article/2008/02/exprof_gets_prison_sentence_for_sex_assault_w_interactive_

feature#:~:text=Former%20Neurosurgery%20professor%20Tracy%20McIntosh,of%20his%20college%20roommate's%20niece.
Goldman, A. (2017, July 17). You can get fired for saying that? *Elle*. https://www.elle.com/culture/career-politics/a45922/louisiana-state-university-sexual-harassment-investigation/
Greenwald, J. (2014, April 21). Dismissal of lawsuit by teacher fired for inappropriate sexual comments upheld. *Business Insurance*. https://www.businessinsurance.com/article/20140421/NEWS07/140429975
Herron, A., & Reschke, M. (2019, November 20). IU won't fire professor for Tweets provost called 'racist, sexist, and homophobic.' *Indy Star*. https://www.indystar.com/story/news/education/2019/11/20/indiana-university-iu-professor-tweets-women-gay-men-academia/4255142002/
Hewitt, K., & Marisam, D. (2013, July 3). *Investigative findings*. University of Minnesota. https://csminnesota.wordpress.com/wp-content/uploads/2013/11/g-rodman.pdf
Jacoby, K., Armour, N., & Luther, J. (2020, November 16). LSU mishandled sexual misconduct complaints against students, including top athletes. *USA Today*. https://www.usatoday.com/in-depth/sports/ncaaf/2020/11/16/lsu-ignored-campus-sexual-assault-allegations-against-derrius-guice-drake-davis-other-students/6056388002/
Kessler, M., & Fainaru-Wada. (2019, August 1). 44 years. 41 allegations. Now the past is catching up. *ESPN*. https://www.espn.com/espn/feature/story/_/id/27244072/44-years-41-allegations-how-caught-former-olympian
Kinsey, John. (2021, September 10). The Ole Miss coach-player sex scandal is over. *Outkick*. https://www.outkick.com/mlb/the-ole-miss-coach-player-sex-scandal-is-over
Kirk, J. (2016, September). LSU fired Les Miles. Here's everything to know about that in a 5-minute read. *SBNation*. https://www.sbnation.com/college-football/2016/9/26/13055108/les-miles-fired-lsu-coaching-search-replacements-candidates
Larimer, S. (2018, July 4). Woman files suit over handling of George Washington University sexual harassment case. *Washington Post*. https://www.washingtonpost.com/local/education/woman-files-suit-over-handling-of-george-washington-university-sexual-harassment-case/2018/01/04/b53d4fea-f175-11e7-b390-a36dc3fa2842_story.html
Lenthang, M. (2024, February 14). Ex-Olympian pleads guilty to sexually assaulting 9 boys—But the true number of victims is unknown. *NBC News*. https://www.espn.com/espn/feature/story/_/id/27244072/44-years-41-allegations-how-caught-former-olympian
Lim, C. (2021, July 11). LSU AgCenter researcher to return from paid leave after review of Title IX case against him. *Reveille*. https://www.lsureveille.com/news/lsu-agcenter-researcher-to-return-from-paid-leave-after-review-of-title-ix-case-against/article_bd331006-d9c8-11eb-85d0-932041fe2fa1.html

Lindskog, C. (2021, April 12). Student sues University of Evansville, accuses ex-coach Walter McCarty of rape. *Courier & Press*. https://www.courierpress.com/story/sports/college/evansville/2021/04/12/student-sues-university-evansville-accuses-nba-walter-mccarty-rape/7197840002/

Longman, J. (2007a, May 5). Negative recruiting fears follow Chatman incident at LSU. *The Virginian-Pilot*. https://www.pilotonline.com/2007/05/05/negative-recruiting-fears-follow-chatman-incident-at-lsu/

Longman, J. (2007b, November 25). After a coach's scandal, the L.S.U. women rebound. *New York Times*. https://www.nytimes.com/2007/11/25/sports/ncaabasketball/25lsu.html

Ludwig, M. (2011, June 9). Bawdy emails cost administrator her job. *MYSA*. https://www.mysanantonio.com/news/local_news/article/Bawdy-emails-cost-administrator-her-job-1416298.php

McCain, R. S., & Smitty, B. S. (2021, August 28). College softball sex scandal! *The Other McCain*. https://theothermccain.com/2021/08/28/college-softball-lesbian-sex-scandal/

Mondon, M. (2018, July 25). Penn professor resigns following allegations of inappropriate relationships with students. *Philly Voice*. https://www.phillyvoice.com/penn-professor-kurzban-resigns-sexual-misconduct-allegations-relationships-students/

Mook, S. (2021, March 4). Lawsuit alleges UND "fostered a culture of silence" around sexual Misconduct reports. *INFORUM*. https://www.inforum.com/news/lawsuit-alleges-und-fostered-a-culture-of-silence-around-sexual-misconduct-reports

Nguyen, C. (2019, September 10). U Penn professor previously accused of sexual harassment starts Job at Rutgers. *Daily Targun*. https://dailytargum.com/article/2019/09/upenn-professor-previously-accused-of-sexual-harassment-starts-job-at-rutgers

Port, R. (2020, August 28). Public records show democratic legislative candidate was dismissed from UND for having a romantic relationship with a student. *Say Anything*. https://www.sayanythingblog.com/entry/public-records-show-democratic-legislative-candidate-was-dismissed-from-und-for-having-romantic-relationship-with-a-student/

Riegel, S. (2021, May 3). Second LSU AgCenter researcher shown leniency amid sexual misconduct findings. *Greater Baton Rouge Business Report*. https://www.businessreport.com/business/second-lsu-agcenter-researcher-shown-leniency-amid-sexual-misconduct-findings

Rivard, R. (2014, June 12). Unwelcome touch. *Inside Higher Ed*. https://www.insidehighered.com/news/2014/06/13/female-provost-accused-repeatedly-touching-her-male-colleagues

Schmidt, J. P. (2014, June 6). Sexual harassment claim against ex-provost surfaces. *Havre Daily News*. https://www.havredailynews.com/story/2014/06/06/local/sexual-harassment-claim-against-ex-provost-surfaces/301072.html

Secreant.com. (2021, August 28). *Ole Miss under investigation for incident involving scissors.* https://www.secrant.com/rant/sec-football/ole-miss-under-investigation-for-incident-involving-scissors/98006778/page-2/

St. George, L. (2018, August 21). Report alleges sexual misconduct by UMD Coack. *MPR News.* https://www.mprnews.org/story/2018/08/21/report-alleges-sexual-misconduct-umd-coach-warmington

Tan, R. (2017, December 26). A former Penn women's rowing coach faces multiple allegations of Sexual misconduct. *The Daily Pennsylvanian.* https://www.thedp.com/article/2017/12/larry-wittig-sexual-harassment-upenn-pa-education-crewrowing#:~:text=Larry%20Wittig%2C%20a%20longtime%20rowing,he%20worked%20as%20a%20coach

Thomason, A. (2018, May 25). U. of Kentucky moves to fire tenured professor for telling students to buy his book. *The Chronicle of Higher Education.* https://www.chronicle.com/article/u-of-kentucky-moves-to-fire-tenured-professor-for-telling-students-to-buy-his-book/

Thorton, J. (2021, September 9). The Ole Miss softball coaches accused of a sex scandal have been cleared of all charges. *Barstool Sports.* https://www.barstoolsports.com/blog/3382857/the-ole-miss-softball-coaches-accused-of-a-sex-scandal-have-been-cleared-of-all-charges

TMZ Sports. (2021, April 13). *Ex NBA player Walter McCarty denies raping college student. "I've never assaulted anyone".* https://www.tmz.com/2021/04/13/walter-mccarty-sexual-assault-lawsuit-rape-evansville-denial/

Van Wormer, K. (2008). Anti-feminist backlash and violence against women worldwide. *Social Work and Society, 6*, 324–337.

Vasquez, L. (2024, March 19). Former track coach accused of sexual misconduct against students at Houston Christian University, new lawsuit says. *Houston Public Media.* https://www.houstonpublicmedia.org/articles/news/criminal-justice/2024/03/19/480983/former-track-coach-accused-of-sexual-misconduct-against-students-at-houston-christian-university-new-lawsuit-says/

Vigliotti, T. (2021, February 4). Montana Supreme Court rules MSU-Northern faculty was harassed, Retaliated against. *Hi-Line Today.* https://hilinetoday.com/montana-supreme-court-rules-msu-northern-faculty-member-was-harassed-retaliated-against/

CHAPTER 6

Disconnected Cases

The previous chapters showcased how investigators, in pursuing sexual harassment allegations against women, made little or no effort to find evidence that women's so-called "victims" had been coerced or harmed. Investigators appeared to operate as if the matter of coercion or harm was irrelevant, representing a dramatic break in how sexual harassment allegations are managed when the accused are men. This chapter is about a second kind of break with tradition and a second way that sexual harassment allegations against women stand out. This chapter examines how allegations against women in colleges and universities are different from harassment allegations levelled against men, not only in terms of the investigative goals and procedures, but in terms of the kinds of harassment—the specific offenses—women commit or are alleged to have committed. In this chapter, I examine how the harassment behaviors attributed to six additional women listed on the Academic Sexual Misconduct Database are unique—how different they appear—when compared to the sexual harassment attributed to men but also how different they appear when compared to each other. These cases illustrate the disconnect between women's and men's harassment cases, and also the disconnect between women's cases—how women's cases are often strikingly dissimilar to each other.

© The Author(s), under exclusive license to Springer Nature Switzerland AG 2024
L. Margolin, *Women Accused of Sexual Harassment*,
https://doi.org/10.1007/978-3-031-79021-8_6

Drunk Woman Kisses "Anybody Who Would Stand Still"

Nicole Rovig, a former Michigan State University registrar, was accused of committing a series of sexually intrusive acts one night in October 2016, during a Big Ten Alliance Conference in Ann Arbor, Michigan. She was charged with touching, kissing, and groping several of her staff who were patronizing a bar. According to one of the observers, Rovig was "ridiculously drunk," so drunk she needed help getting to the bar's bathroom. When she came out of the bathroom, her clothing was askew, her belt unbuckled, and her shirt and pants unbuttoned. She asked one of her staff for help, but the staff member refused, at least initially: "I made her buckle her own belt and button [her] pants." However, when the top button of her pants proved too challenging for Rovig, she again asked for help, and the staff member acquiesced. But as she leaned in to help with the button, she claimed Rovig grabbed her head, "pulled it in [and] gave me a big kiss." The staff member said she pushed Rovig away, told her to behave herself, but Rovig did not behave herself; she continued drinking and as the night wore on, she "had her hands down people's pants…. [She] played with several people's hair, kissed people on the lips, tried to stick her tongue in people's mouths, and rubbed people's legs." Another member of Rovig's staff said that Rovig was kissing and touching "anybody who would stand still. She kissed me on my lips. She asked if she could kiss me. I guess I said yes. It was weird. It was everybody. My boss said, 'kiss me'" (*WLNS.com*, June 15, 2017).

Rovig, in her defense, admitted to kissing someone at the bar. She claimed that that person had given consent, but she denied the other accusations. To support her denials, she gave Title IX investigators a doctor's note which said that she has "an unusually short lingual frenulum"—she was "tongue tied"—which, she said, would make it prohibitively difficult to extend her tongue into anyone's mouth while kissing, one of the offenses attributed to her. The investigators, notwithstanding the doctor's note, concluded that Rovig had indeed violated the University's sexual harassment policy and she was forced to resign (*WLNS.com,* June 15, 2017).

In three other cases listed on the Academic Sexual Misconduct Database which involve sexual harassment at an off-campus bar or party by an intoxicated faculty member or administrator, the alleged perpetrator was a man. In one case, a former associate dean at the University of Buffalo, Jude A. Fabiano, was accused of making unwelcome sexual advances to a woman who worked as a clerk at the School of Dental Medicine; he was also accused of pressuring her to kiss another clerk at an office party. He allegedly put his arms around their necks and pulled them together. "You could tell he had too much to drink," an observer said. About two months after the party, Fabiano was suspended without pay, lost his dean appointment, and had to pay $255,00 (with the University chipping in $215,000) to settle the lawsuit brought by one of the clerks (Lakamp, 2013). In a second case, Harry Whitaker, a former psychology professor from Northern Michigan University, was accused of asking a student for sex while intoxicated at a party, and then telling her, several days later, "the offer still stands." He explained that he "had been drinking excessively that evening and would never have remembered the alleged incident except for the fact that the woman showed up in my office a few weeks later, to ask me if I remembered what happened at the party." When he said he did not, the woman reminded him that he had invited her to his hotel room. "I interpreted this as light banter," he said, which is why he replied that the offer still stands. The University suspended him without pay, and soon after, he retired (Keefer, 2018). In a third case, a Grand Rapids Community College professor, Harold Lee, was accused of repeatedly kissing a student against her will at a bar. He said that he had been drinking—three or four beers—and would not have behaved like this had he not been intoxicated. He later resigned under pressure (Tucker, 2016).

In comparing the men's cases to Rovig's, what stands out is her level of intoxication: she was so drunk she could not button her pants without assistance. And her sexual acting out—in which she "had her hand down people's pants ... played with several people's hair, kissed people on the lips, tried to stick her tongue in people's mouths...."—unlike that of the three men with comparable offenses—appeared random. The men charged with sexual harassment after drinking excessively at parties or bars appeared to have selected their targets, while Rovig appeared to have targeted people without first selecting them. Instead, she touched, groped, and kissed "anybody who would stand still." Her alleged harassment was so disorganized, arbitrary, and incoherent, she appeared unaware of what she was doing or whom she was harassing.

When a Woman Is Charged with Attempted Murder

On December 12, 2019, at 8 p.m., Rie Hachiyanagi, a Mt. Holyoke art professor, showed up unannounced at the home of her friend and fellow Holyoke professor, Lauret Savoy. Hachiyanagi said she needed to talk to Savoy "about feelings" because her boyfriend had just broken up with her. However, as soon as Hachiyanagi stepped inside, she hit Savoy on the head with something hard, and continued to rain blows down on her with anything she could find, including a rock, a fire poker, and garden shears, proclaiming for the next four hours—the duration of the attack—her intention to blind, disfigure, and finally murder Savoy. During the attack, Savoy asked why she was doing this to her. Hachiyanagi replied that it was because she had been in love with Savoy for years and was bitter that Savoy did not return her love. Although Savoy and Hachiyanagi had been friends for over a decade, they had never been involved romantically; and, at the time of the assault, Savoy was in a long-term relationship with a man (Frisch, 2021). In a ploy to end the attack, Savoy tried to convince Hachiyanagi that she did in fact return her love and pleaded with her to call for help, but Hachiyanagi hesitated. She said she could not handle going to jail. "If I go to jail," Hachiyanagi told Savoy, "I'll kill myself" (Frisch, 2021).

Savoy continued proclaiming her love for Hachiyanagi, promising not to tell anyone what happened, in the hope of making Hachiyanagi quit her attack. This seemed effective as Hachiyanagi finally relented and called 911. When the police arrived, they found Hachiyanagi on the floor, holding Savoy in her arms, both covered in blood. The story Hachiyanagi told investigators is that she went to her friend's house shortly before midnight for a visit, but when she opened the door, she discovered Savoy was semiconscious, barely breathing, with severe injuries to her face and head, the victim, she imagined, of some unknown intruder. Savoy, for her part, did not tell the police what really happened. At first, she said she had no idea who the attacker was. But once in the hospital, safely away from the crime scene, Savoy, who suffered significant blood loss, many stab and puncture wounds with multiple broken bones near her nose and eyes, identified her assailant (Flynn, 2020).

Hachiyanagi was arrested and charged with nine felonies, including three counts of armed assault with intent to murder. She pleaded guilty and at the sentence hearing, Savoy shared her struggle to find a word that could capture her experience of the attack. She finally settled on the word "torture" which she defined as the infliction of "severe or excruciating pain or suffering of mind and body; anguish, agony, torment." She went on to say that "for four hours I experienced literal torture of body and mind, not knowing if I would survive the next minute—yet needing to find some way to save my life.... The emotional, physical, financial, and professional impacts of this crime have been huge and they continue. Now the defendant's violation of me is becoming part of a public persona that I did not choose. She had invaded my persona, my career, my life" (Monastesse, 2021). The judge, who described Hachiyanagi's crime as "the most horrific set of facts I've ever heard," sentenced her to 10–12 years in prison, coincidentally, a slightly weaker sentence than Anna Stubblefield received for having sex with a man who may have been too cognitively impaired to give sexual consent. Nonetheless, few harassment allegations on the Academic Sexual Misconduct Database compare to this one in terms of their brutality, the victim's trauma, and the absence of reason—the senselessness of every feature of the attack. To add to the uniqueness of Hachiyanagi's assault, she claimed that she was not in love with Savoy. That was a lie, Hachiyanagi said. She described her state of mind at the time of the attack on Savoy as despair after learning that her live-in boyfriend had left the state, and that their relationship was over. She said she needed to do something to break out of her despair—something that "made her feel alive" again—and the attack on Savoy was the method she chose (Frisch, 2021).

How to Increase Spanish Class Enrollments

In 2013, an Amherst College teaching assistant in the Spanish department complained that one of the instructors in her department became angry with her upon learning that she was dating a student from the University of Massachusetts. According to the teaching assistant, the instructor who became angry, Victoria Maillo, said that she wanted her and the other teaching assistants to go on dates and sleep with Amherst men, exclusively. When the teaching assistant, bemused, asked Maillo if she wanted her to sleep with a different Amherst man every night, Maillo allegedly responded in the affirmative, saying "that is what I brought you here for." The teaching assistant said that she felt degraded and objectified, as if the Spanish department saw her as nothing more than a prostitute, which prompted her to share her complaint with another Spanish instructor, Dimaris Barrios-Beltran, who recalled that Maillo had once told her that when she looked up potential teaching assistants online, she liked to pick the ones with "pretty faces" to help attract more students to their Spanish classes. After Barrios-Beltran checked with the other Spanish teaching assistants to see if they had also been asked to date and become sexually intimate with Amherst men, she discovered that they had, and that, in addition, Maillo had tried to arrange dates between them and Amherst men, a strategy allegedly designed to counter flagging enrollments in Spanish classes (Barry, 2016; Svluga, 2015).

The next day, Barrios-Beltran met with the chair of the Spanish department to complain that Maillo had been instructing teaching assistants to become sexually involved with Amherst students. When Maillo learned that Barrios-Beltran had complained about her, she reportedly became angry and retaliatory: Barrios-Beltran claimed that Maillo began telling other Spanish department faculty that her Puerto Rican dialect was not sophisticated, referring to Barrios-Beltran's Spanish as "ghetto," and characterized her not only as lower class and poorly educated, but also as an ineffective instructor who could not control her students or command their respect. Barrios-Beltran then complained to Title IX about the hurtful and discriminatory messages Maillo had been giving the Spanish department teaching assistants. However, these complaints appeared to generate little or no interest among Amherst officials. According to public records, no disciplinary action was taken against Maillo, although when Maillo's contract expired, it was not renewed, a decision attributed to Maillo's newness in the department, her untenured status, and falling Spanish enrollments, the same reasons cited for the nonrenewal of Barrios-Beltran's own contract (Siemaszko, 2015). Maillo is the only individual from Amherst College listed on the Academic Sexual Misconduct Database and the only individual listed on the Database accused of requiring teaching assistants to have sexual encounters with students.

Stalking in Pursuit of Emotional Intimacy

Stalking is typically defined as a pattern of repeated unwanted attention that causes the targeted person(s) to feel inferior and fearful (Spitzberg & Cupach, 2014). But stalking is not always an expression of hostility (James & MacKenzie, 2018). Stalking can sometimes consist of nothing more than the repetition of seemingly routine, harmless behaviors, such as declarations of affection and personal interest (Sheridan & Davies, 2001; Sheridan et al., 2003). Taken in isolation, these behaviors might seem "normal." But when they continue over an extended period, the cumulative effects can be highly distressing (Quinn-Evans et al., 2021). If these kinds of intrusions occur over electronic media, such as email, they are often referred to as cyberstalking. That is the type of harassment attributed to Roxana Recio, a professor of Spanish from Creighton University.

What Recio wanted from her target, someone she barely knew, wasn't sex; it was affection and friendship—emotional intimacy—a type of stalking rarely found among male stalkers (Mullen et al., 1999; Purcell et al., 2001). The email messages she sent to her target, when examined individually, were almost always warm and positive. She did not seek to harass. She did not intend to make her target uncomfortable. The problem—what made Recio's messages pernicious, according to the complainant—was their cumulative and progressive impact: how they not only expressed too much positive feeling, with each email more effusive than the last, but how the expressions of unbridled affection appeared increasingly detached from reality. Like a celebrity-obsessed fan who only knows the celebrity from movies and TV, yet whose adoration knows no limits, Recio barely knew the object of her affection, a newly hired professor from Creighton University who had not yet assumed her position when Recio began sending her immoderate messages.

Recio was an associate professor of Spanish in the department of modern languages and literatures when Michelle Evers applied for a position as an assistant professor of Spanish. From January 2001, one month before Creighton hired Evers, through April 2001, about three months before Evers was scheduled to actively begin her position, Recio and Evers engaged in an email correspondence which formed the basis of Evers' harassment complaint. While this correspondence took place online, and was profoundly disturbing to Evers, Recio did not transmit threatening, hateful, or obscene messages. On the contrary, her singular goal appeared to be that of forming a positive relationship with Evers, a type of harassment which had no counterpart in the entire Academic Sexual Misconduct Database.

The first email message at issue, dated April 16, 2001, concerned Recio's sharing her summer travel plans with Evers. Recio wrote, "I'll write you from everywhere and you don't have to answer my postcards, of course, what I would like though would be to receive a letter from you sometime, short, but at least send me one" (Recio v. Evers, Supreme Court of Nebraska, Aug. 28, 2009, p. 408). Recio went on to write about how important Evers was to her in language that is surprisingly intense, considering that they had a professional relationship, with Recio in the senior position, and that they had only known each other for a few months:

> I want to be your friend, do you understand? I hope so, because if you don't understand, you will end up hating me and I will have an attack. If I don't see you in August as we were saying this morning ... UFFF!... I think I would shoot myself in the head (think that I'm bad off in the head if you want, I don't care, but I *will* shoot myself (Recio v. Evers, p. 408).

The following day, Recio sent another email to Evers in which she continued to discuss how important Evers was to her, again with over-the-top intensity.

> The truth is, I really feel like talking to you and I don't know if I'll have time and if I'll be able to tell you all that I want.... The most important thing is to communicate and I am happy with your e-mails in any case. Of course, I haven't erased your voice from my answering machine. It makes me happy and I love it. I'll leave it there a few days. I just feel like it. I'm trying hard not to call you ... but I won't do it because I don't want to take advantage of you. I was thrilled to talk to you yesterday. You already know that I don't have to tell you what I feel because you know quite well and I am always repeating to you like a parrot (Recio v. Evers, p. 408).

Recio went on to say how happy she was that she and Evers were reading and enjoying the same poet's work: "How great, I figured out what you like! Could you keep telling me what you like to read? I want to share with you." Recio then implored Evers to write to her, while promising to write continuously.

That same day, she sent Evers another email message which began by asking her if she was a Castro supporter, and if she believed all the pro-Castro propaganda:

> It would hurt me but I would still have the same caring feelings for you. The truth is, I already care so much for you that I don't know what I would say. It would be terribly hard to discuss with you. I'll tell you seriously, you are in charge. I am at your feet, I am not a man ... (that last part is a joke) (p. 409).

In the same email, Recio wrote that she imagined that Evers saw her as "some nice person who tortures you with e-mails and who you will work with," but for her, their relationship is deeper and more significant:

"Michelle, I feel so much for you, don't you notice? Don't you see that I talk to you not just to pass the time, but rather because it makes me happy? ...Let's see if some day you have half of the affection that I feel for you. Let's see. I doubt it but oh well. Today people are just plain savage (that's a joke)[.]" Recio concluded by attempting to reassure Evers that although she is obsessive, she is far from sinister or threatening: "don't freak out, I'm not like Jeffrey Dohmer, is that how you write his name? It's just that when I really like someone I'm like that..." (p. 411).

The next day, Recio sent this message: "Where are you? The truth is, I've been going on all day without any news from you and it's making me crazy. Have you heard of a drug called 'Michelle,' I have an addiction to it now" (Recio v. Evers, p. 412). And the following day, Recio sent two new messages. This passage from the second message is particularly significant because it reveals a shift in Recio's attitude toward Evers: she is beginning to feel the sting of rejection:

> I answered your message and you didn't answer me, especially knowing what I said to you yesterday.... Your hard attitude has insulted me. You know, it's better just to be colleagues in our work and that's it. Don't give me any lessons and I'm sorry for having been so sincere and sentimental with you. But I don't want to deal with a person so tough who forgets all my good traits for one little error. Thanks for the punch. We'll see each other (what choice do we have?) in August (Recio v. Evers, pp. 412–413).

In Recio's final email message to Evers, sent several days later, she tries to explain her extravagant language in what appears as an attempt to restore their relationship to a more professional footing:

> We'll see each other in August and with peace, and pardon me if I reacted like that but it's just that it hurt me like a pair of swords in my side.... You can blame my emotional immaturity or whatever you like. But everything's alright, eh? Nothing happened. August is just around the corner (Recio v. Evers, p. 413).

The email messages which Michelle Evers cited as evidence of sexual harassment were all sent during April 2001. However, Evers did not file a formal harassment complaint against Recio until two and a half years later, on February 12, 2004. What prompted the filing was Recio's apparent effort to retaliate.

Online stalking, initially based on strong positive feeling, often devolves over time (Quinn-Evans et al., 2021). Those who believe they have been ignored, unappreciated, or forsaken may try to exact revenge: they can be tempted to engage in some form of retaliation (Keatley, 2022). This kind of devolution may explain how the relationship between Recio and Evers ended: on February 10, 2004, the Creighton University Spanish faculty held a contentious meeting attended by both Recio and Evers, and two days later, Recio, perhaps still festering over Evers' personal rejection, complained in writing to administrators that Evers had behaved inappropriately during the meeting. The specifics of Recio's complaint are not publicly available; however, six days later, Evers filed her own complaint against Recio, citing her "inappropriate and offensive" email messages from April 2001. Creighton investigators, after examining those emails, concluded that they were "inappropriate, shocking, and of a sexual nature." They also concluded that the letter Recio wrote complaining about Evers' behavior during a faculty meeting appeared retaliatory, a likely effect of Evers' personal rejection of her (Recio v. Evers, p. 415). Although investigators recommended Recio's termination, the Creighton president felt that a year's probation would be more appropriate if coupled with the directive that Recio have no further contact or communication with Evers and that Recio enroll in "a program of psychological counseling and educational programs on communication, appropriate interactions with others, teamwork, etc." (Recio v. Evers, p. 415). Recio later challenged these recommendations in civil court on the grounds that Evers' complaints against her were "false, inflated and fabricated." The court, however, concluded that Evers' harassment complaint had been justified (Recio v. Evers, p. 427).

Stalking an Entire Firefighter Team

Most stalking complaints represent the unwanted pursuit of another with the goal of forming a relationship. But in some cases, the stalker's goal is not to form a relationship per se, but rather to injure or destroy the object of pursuit (Spitzberg & Cupach, 2003). Melissa Ann Santana, a former professor of interior design from Northern Arizona University, had the latter goal. Her stalking represented an attempt to intimidate and terrorize, and her target was very specific: an elite group of firefighters known as "hot shots" deployed by the Forest Service and National Park Service to battle wildland forest fires. Santana is the only individual on the Academic Sexual Misconduct Database accused of stalking an entire community. She was arrested in October 2017, fired the following month, and then indicted on two counts of stalking and one count of making false statements. A possible explanation of why she targeted "hot shot" firefighters is that she matched with one on Tinder in 2015 under the pretext of "looking for friends for daytime fun," but reacted badly when he ended the relationship. This is what she wrote to him after the break-up:

> You are a worthless piece of shit. You do a job that requires no brains what so ever. You are just a tree cutter and hole digger. The government finds you as a disposable front line against fire. You can easily be replaced by a younger dumber version. You are [so] worthless that they don't really care if a whole crew [of] the granite mountain guys die. Because you guys don't provide a unique service.... Be a success like the granite guys and die at your next fire (Gabbert, 2017).

Santana's attacks against the firefighters were both systematic and wide-ranging, as evidenced by her efforts to surveil and terrorize the firefighters' families and associates. For example, she posted this message on the Facebook page of the fiancée of one of the firefighters, below their engagement photo:

> Look at these lovebirds, Too bad I fucked her fiancé over and over while he was out fighting a fire. He even wanted to keep the relationship going. Said he regretted proposing (Gabbert, 2017).

Two weeks later, Santana sent a text message to the firefighter's fiancée proclaiming that she and the firefighter were in love. That was followed by a text message, saying, "You'll regret not talking to me," and by another that threatened, "I will show up at your work to address this." Later that day, the fiancée went to a restaurant, near her work. Soon after arriving, she received another text from Santana in which she identified the restaurant where she was eating, thus informing the fiancée that she was being followed. In Santana's next message, she referenced the place of the planned wedding, "I guess I will see you [there]. I will probably be fucking in the coat check before you walk down the aisle, unless he dumps your ass before then."

In Sept. 2016, she sent an email message to the superintendent of the Flagstaff Interagency Hotshot Crew, informing him that her (nonexistent) teenaged daughter had been sexually assaulted by his firefighters.

> I am disgusted by the behavior of your hotshot crew when they passed through my town. Several weeks ago your guys were on the way to a fire in Wyoming. I intercepted messages between your crew members and my UNDERAGE 15 year old daughter. She won't tell me which website they met on but I did read that they invited her back to their hotel, gave her alcohol and had sex with her. This is statutory rape and I want these men charged (Swenson, 2017).

She listed the names of three firefighters who she claimed assaulted her fictional daughter and threatened to "contact your local newspapers if I don't hear back" (Swenson, 2017). She was also accused of spray painting and stealing the license plate of one firefighter's vehicle and of puncturing his tires and scratching the word "shit" into the paint of another firefighter's vehicle.

Stalker Claims She's the Victim

Ivonne del Valle, a professor at the University of California-Berkeley, became preoccupied with Joshua Clover, a professor at the University of California-Davis, after a meeting with him in 2018. The pretext of the meeting was innocuous: she asked Clover to join her for drinks to discuss his participation in a forthcoming conference, but Clover later told investigators that the meeting went badly. First, he said del Valle acted as though they were on a date; then he said she became "visibly flustered" when he mentioned his partner (Mangan, 2023a, b). From there, things rapidly deteriorated, with del Valle attempting to intimidate and terrorize Clover by leaving threatening messages for him (e.g., "I can do whatever the fuck I want piece of shit" and "You need to still call me and apologize or you'll see what I'm going to do"). Her harassment of Clover included spray painting insults outside his door and dumping chunks of oily pineapple at his mother's doorstep, posting a message that proclaimed she "raised a psychopath." Why did del Valle do this? She claimed that Clover was stalking her: he was supposedly tweeting a series of deeply personal, yet coded, messages for the purpose of insulting and taunting her. She would message someone, she said, and then, within hours, a post would pop up on Clover's Twitter feed that indirectly referenced her original message. To illustrate, after she messaged a friend about a particular restaurant, she claimed she saw a tweet about the same restaurant posted by Clover. The same thing happened, she said, after she had searched the internet for a place to study French; shortly afterward, he tweeted something in French, "Moving on to daily vous, daily ils elles." And then, after a phone conversation about a song called "Humble," she found that the word "humble" appeared on two Twitter feeds traceable to Clover. In perhaps the most preposterous and delusional complaint about Clover's Twitter activity, del Valle said that a few hours after she took her phone to the shower to play music, a message appeared over Twitter ("Are those your two? They're huge!"), which she claimed was an oblique reference of her breasts, convincing her that Clover had access to her phone camera (Mangen, 2023a, b).

Del Valle acknowledged much of her offensive behavior. "I did write outside his door, 'Here lies a pervert.' I did that," and added that she's not proud of doing these things, but she also said she had to do them to bring attention to her plight: she had to find a way to show the world what she, an ethnic minority woman, has been forced to endure at the hands of a white male, senior professor. "I never received help from anyone" (McDede, 2023). This kind of explanation—her insistence on her victimization as an ethnic minority woman—may explain why her stalking was largely forgiven. Not only were no criminal charges pressed against her, but she retained her faculty position at Berkeley until January 2022, when the University placed her on involuntary medical leave, almost four years after her harassment of Clover had begun. Unlike other women listed on the Academic Sexual Misconduct Database for sexual harassment, del Valle continued to be respected and well-liked on campus long after Title IX investigators found her responsible for sexual harassment. Perhaps because Clover did not publicize his victimization, and perhaps because del Valle, unlike other women accused of sexual harassment, was quite successful at portraying herself as a victim, students and faculty did not launch protests seeking to ban her from campus, one of the most common responses to someone suspected of harassment. Indeed, students and faculty, and other members of the UC-Berkeley community, went in the opposite direction: they protested to retain del Valle as a faculty member; they also sought punishment for the man she identified as her harasser, going so far as to stage a sit-in on her behalf at the beginning of a University of California football game that ended in the arrest of several students wearing "Justice for Ivonne" T-shirts. Protesters cast both Clover and the University of California-Berkeley as the real harassers, he for sadistically taunting del Valle and the University for taking his side. Consider, for example, this open letter to the UC-Berkeley provost circulated by del Valle's supporters:

> We have witnessed the harsh and unfair treatment that our most beloved Latina professor, Dr. Ivonne del Valle, has received at the hands of the administration. We are here to say "Ya Basta!", meaning 'enough already'! If UC Berkeley really wants to become a Hispanic Serving Institution (HSIs), it needs to start treating our Latinx professors with respect. Professor del Valle was the one being harassed, yet your administration engaged in victim-blaming, retaliatory behavior.... We are supporting Professor Ivonne publicly because she deserves justice and dignity. We need Dr. del Valle back on campus....

Del Valle's insistence that Clover was sexually harassing her, despite Title IX investigators' failure, after multiple inquiries, to find any evidence of Clover's misconduct, suggests that her harassment of him was motivated by a delusion, what is known as "false victimization syndrome," a rare disorder based on an individual's false belief that they are being stalked (Mohandie et al., 1998; Mullen et al., 2000; Sheridan & Blaauw, 2004). No other sexual harassment allegations in the entire Academic Sexual Misconduct Database match-up with those levelled against del Valle. Indeed, no other harassment allegations match-up with the stalking attributed to Roxanna Recio and Melissa Ann Santana. Consider that the men listed on the Academic Sexual Misconduct Database for stalking limited their stalking to two behavioral categories. In one, the stalker is accused of relentlessly pursuing a former partner with the goal of resuming their sexual/romantic relationship, as in the case of a former adjunct professor at Harrison Areas Community College, Daniel Shafer, who was arrested and charged with stalking a former student with whom he had three-month sexual relationship. The student told him to stop sending her messages, but he persisted, even after she transferred to another school, which led her to believe that he was going to harm her (Crable, 2009). In a second type, the man pursues someone he became acquainted with—someone he may have worked or shared a class with—but not someone with whom he had a prior sexual or romantic involvement. In this variation, the stalker's goal is to initiate an intimate relationship, a type of stalking illustrated in

Chap. 5, in the discussion of Niranjan Baisakh's harassment of one of his female grad students—harassment which included following her around campus, showing up at her apartment uninvited, begging her to love him, and, finally, assaulting her (Lim, 2021).

* * *

The sexual harassment of women by men is commonly understood as the way harassment operates. Women are victims and men are perpetrators. But based on the cases examined here, women are accused of sexual harassment too, albeit, with far less frequency and in far different ways. Women's harassment also seems driven by different motivations, for example, Recio's stalking as an effort attain emotional intimacy with her same-sex target, Maillo's efforts to increase Spanish class enrollments, and del Valle's efforts to fend off the imagined intrusions of a man she believed was after her. Santana's stalking was different too: she went after a whole team of firefighters, sending all sorts of threatening and slanderous messages to them and their families, even though almost all were complete strangers to her. While the Academic Sexual Misconduct Database lists several men who attributed their sexual harassment to alcohol intoxication—they claimed they behaved improperly with a specific target because they were drunk—the one woman, Nicole Rovig, listed on the Database who attributed her sexual harassment to alcohol intoxication was unable to identify her targets. Her sexual acting out appeared random. And Rie Hachiyanagi's assault on a fellow faculty member—what amounted to hours of torture—while motivated, she said, by the feeling that her target had rejected her, was like nothing else in the entire Academic Sexual Misconduct Database in its brutality and senselessness.

But when it comes to gender differences, there are reasons to be cautious. For while women's sexual harassment frequently appears exceptional both in the ways it is performed and the ways it is assessed, there are times when women's and men's harassment represent similar behaviors, motivations, and outcomes. The book's second part seeks to clarify differences *and* similarities between women's and men's sexual harassment by comparing the sexual harassment charges levelled against the 29 women listed on the Academic Sexual Misconduct Database and 29 men randomly selected from the Database.

References

Barry, S. (2016, May 11). Lawyers for former Amherst College professor accused in federal discrimination lawsuit argues for dismissal. *Masslive*. https://www.masslive.com/news/2016/05/lawyer_for_former_amherst_coll.html

Crable, A. D. (2009, August 29). Harrisburg area community college professor charged with stalking. *LNP/LancasterOnline*. https://lancasteronline.com/news/former-harrisburg-area-community-college-professor-charged-with-stalking/article_d4173d0d-d821-5e87-8646-6f0742afa0aa.html

Flynn, M. (2020, June 6). An art professor allegedly went to a colleague's home to admit her Feelings. She ended up attacking her with a fire poker, police say. *Washington Post*. https://www.washingtonpost.com/nation/2020/01/06/mount-holyoke-professor-attacks-colleague-with-fire-poker-garden-shears-rock-after-admitting-feelings-police-say/

Frisch, I. (2021, October 22). Shocking and violent crime that rocked Mt. Holyoke. *Town & Country*. https://www.townandcountrymag.com/society/tradition/a31942551/mount-holyoke-violent-assault-professor-true-story/

Gabbert, B. (2017, November 19). Professor accused of stalking hotshot crews. *Wildfire Today*. https://wildfiretoday.com/2017/11/19/professor-accused-of-stalking-members-of-hotshot-crews/

James, D. V., & MacKenzie, R. D. (2018). Stalking and harassment. In J. L. Ireland, P. Birch, & C. A. Ireland (Eds.), *The Routledge international handbook of human aggression: Current issues and perspectives* (pp. 170–182). Routledge.

Keatley, D. A. (2022). Time analysis of violence. In C. Martin, V. R. Preedy, & V. Patel (Eds.), *Handbook of anger, aggression, and violence* (pp. 1–16). Springer.

Keefer, W. (2018, January 25). Former prof suspended for sexual misconduct. *The North Wind*. https://thenorthwindonline.com/3878641/news/former-prof-suspended-for-sexual-misconduct/

Lakamp, P. (2013, September 1). University of Buffalo to pay Amherst woman in sex harassment Settlement. *Buffalo News*. https://buffalonews.com/news/local/crime-courts/university-at-buffalo-to-pay-amherst-woman-in-sex-harassment-settlement/article_cce087a2-7eeb-56c8-bbeb-526efb5321b2.html

Lim, C. (2021, July 11). LSU AgCenter researcher to return from paid leave after review of Title IX case against him. *Reveille*. https://www.lsureveille.com/news/lsu-agcenter-researcher-to-return-from-paid-leave-after-review-of-title-ix-case-against/article_bd331006-d9c8-11eb-85d0-932041fe2fa1.html

Mangan, K. (2023a, October 25). The harassment case that has Berkeley at a boil. *Chronicle of Higher Ed*. https://www.chronicle.com/article/the-harassment-case-that-has-berkeley-at-a-boil#:~:text=Clover%2C%20an%20emerita%20professor%20at,in%20front%20of%20her%20home

Mangan, K. (2023b, October 25). The harassment case that has Berkeley at a boil. *Chronicle of Higher Education*. https://www.chronicle.com/article/the-harassment-case-that-has-berkeley-at-a-boil

McDede, H. (2023, October 28). UC Berkeley students threaten hunger strike to reinstate Professor suspended for stalking. *KQED*. https://www.kqed.org/news/11965822/uc-berkeley-students-threaten-hunger-strike-to-reinstate-professor-suspended-for-stalking

Mohandie, K., Hatcher, C., & Raymond, D. D. (1998). False victimization syndromes in stalking. In J. R. Meloy (Ed.), *Psychology of stalking* (pp. 225–256). Academic Press.

Monastesse, T. (2021, November 9). Former professor Rie Hachiyanagi sentenced 10–12 years following Guilty plea. *Mt. Holyoke News*. https://www.mountholyokenews.com/news/2021/11/7/former-professor-rie-hachiyanagi-sentenced-10-12-years-following-guilty-plea

Mullen, P. E., Pathe, M., & Purcell, R. (2000). *Stalkers and their victims*. Cambridge University Press.

Mullen, P. E., Pathe, M., Purcell, R., & Stuart, G. W. (1999). Study of stalkers. *American Journal of Psychiatry, 156*, 1244–1249.

Purcell, R., Pathe, M., & Mullen. (2001). A study of women who stalk. *American Journal of Psychiatry, 158*, 2056–2060.

Quinn-Evans, L., Keatley, D. A., Arntfield, M., & Sheridan, L. (2021). *Journal of Interpersonal Violence, 36*(15–16), 6979–6997.

Sheridan, L. P., & Blaauw, E. (2004). Characteristics of false stalking reports. *Criminal Justice and Behavior, 31*(1), 55–72.

Sheridan, L., & Davies, G. M. (2001). Stalking: The elusive crime. *Legal and Criminological Psychology, 6*, 133–147.

Sheridan, L. P., Gillett, R., Davies, G. M., Blaauw, E., & Patel, D. (2003). "There's no smoke without fire": Are male ex-partners perceived as more "entitled" to stalk than acquaintances or strangers? *British Journal of Psychology, 94*(1), 87–98.

Siemaszko, C. (2015, December 1). Prof claims teaching assistants at Amherst College were urged to Seduce students to boost enrollments in Spanish classes. *NBC News*. https://www.nbcnews.com/news/us-news/prof-claims-amherst-college-used-sex-sell-students-spanish-class-n488521

Spitzberg, B. H., & Cupach, W. R. (2003). What mad pursuit? Obsessive relational intrusion and stalking related phenomena. *Aggression and Violent Behavior, 8*, 345–375. https://doi.org/10.1016/s1359-1789(02)00068-x

Spitzberg, B. H., & Cupach, W. R. (2014). *The dark side of relationship pursuit: From attraction to obsession and stalking*. Routledge.

Svluga, S. (2015, December 29). Lawsuit claims teaching assistants at Amherst were told to sleep With students to boost enrollment. *Washington Post*. https://www.washingtonpost.com/news/grade-point/wp/2015/12/29/lawsuit-claims-teaching-assistants-at-amherst-were-told-to-sleep-with-students-to-boost-class-enrollment/

Swenson, K. (2017, November 20). "Die at your next fire": Arizona professor accused of stalking firefighters and student. *Washington Post*. https://www.washingtonpost.com/news/morning-mix/wp/2017/11/20/die-at-your-next-fire-ariz-professor-accused-of-stalking-firefighters-and-student/

Tucker, K. (2016, February 17). GRCC professor resigns following sexual misconduct investigation. *The Collegiate*. https://thecollegiatelive.com/2016/02/grcc-professor-resigns-following-sexual-misconduct-investigation/

WLNS.com. (2017, July 15). *Woman says she was wrongfully terminated from MSU after Rejecting sexual advances from boss*. https://www.wlns.com/news/woman-says-she-was-wrongfully-terminated-from-msu-after-rejecting-sexual-advances-from-boss/

PART II

CHAPTER 7

Harassment Among Consenting Adults

Colleges and universities usually regard sexual activity between teachers and adult students as off-limits, even when the parties describe the relationship as consensual. Although many academic institutions do not have cohesive policies addressing student-faculty sexual relationships, those that do mainly focus on supervisory situations: for example, when instructors are sexually involved with students enrolled in their own classes. However, an increasing number of institutions, such as Harvard, Stanford, and Northwestern, ban all sexual relationships between students and faculty (Carrillo et al., 2019). That faculty/student and other supervisor/supervisee relationships involve consenting partners is often seen as immaterial (Coleman, 1988; Crittenden et al., 2021; DeChiara, 1987). What generally matters more to administrators and investigators—how they conceptualize avowedly consensual relationships between faculty and adult students as harassment—is that one of the parties has greater institutional power and authority than the other. The rationale behind disallowing sex between faculty and students is that such relationships interfere with students' learning, they reinforce female students' second-class status in the academy, and many believe that sexual relationships which occur under conditions of inequality are implicitly coercive: obtaining and giving sexual consent in a relationship in which one of the actors has more power may be impossible. The party with less power might feel obligated to

© The Author(s), under exclusive license to Springer Nature Switzerland AG 2024
L. Margolin, *Women Accused of Sexual Harassment*,
https://doi.org/10.1007/978-3-031-79021-8_7

engage in sex they do not want, and the other, the one with more power, might feel entitled to having sex regardless of the other's wishes.

At the same time, these rationales are far from unassailable. One need only consider that in many intimate relationships, perhaps in most, one partner occupies a more powerful position (e.g., makes more money) than the other. Mansnerus (1991) argued that prohibiting consensual relationships between students and faculty because they are susceptible to abuse implies that such a prohibition should be extended to other consensual relationships, such as marriage, given the prevalence of domestic abuse. Moreover, to make an exception of the academy or any other workplace—to say that women in these domains require special oversight—can be said to deprive (overwhelmingly) women of agency. Prohibiting women from making their own sexual choices can be said to invert the feminist anti-rape logic of "no means no" into the protectionist logic of "yes means no" (Srinivasan, 2020).

Women's Sample

That Nimrod Reitman was a student and Avital Ronell his professor—that he had less institutional power and authority than she—was one of the core arguments underlying Reitman's claim that Ronell had sexually harassed him. Because she, as his professor, had the power to advance or inhibit his professional development, he claimed he would have to pay a stiff price were he to refuse her sexual or romantic demands, an argument which shows how closely harassment based on the disparities in power and authority anticipates and overlaps with harassment based on quid pro quo deal-making. Your boss is your boss, and your professor is your professor: they don't need to make explicit threats or bribes, whether the assignment is writing a paper or accepting a kiss. Noncompliance is not an option.

According to institutions that disallow sex between adult students and faculty, the power disparity between them necessarily makes an intimate relationship unequal, illegitimate, and nonconsensual, regardless of what the parties who are involved claim. That is the reasoning behind the charges against Kristin Naca, Katie Rietkovich Browder, Jacqueline Hoffarth, and Anna Stubblefield. Cara Hale, an Iowa State psychologist, was also accused of sexual harassment for engaging in sex with a student despite the absence of evidence indicating coercion. The publicly available data in her case indicates only that, after the discovery that she had an intimate relationship with a male graduate student who was under her supervision, she was fired (Psychiatric Crime Database and Disciplinary Actions, 2013).

Another woman, Alice A. Parker, former chair of the women's studies department at the University of Alabama, was accused of having an "affair" with a female graduate student. The student initiated a civil suit against the University for failing to protect her from Parker, a professor who, she alleged, required her to "behave in a submissive and subservient role in their romantic and sexual relationship as a term or condition of [her] education" (Manger, 1996). In her defense, Parker claimed she recused herself from any involvement in the graduate student's academic career, disavowing quid pro quo, and other possible kinds of coercion. After a Title IX investigation, the University concluded that any psychological and educational distress or disadvantages the student may have experienced were not Parker's fault since the student initiated the relationship and went on to earn her master's degree in women's studies, and, so far as investigators could tell, Parker had not been overtly coercive (Manger, 1996). A lawyer for the University argued that the graduate student—who was 40 at the time of the complaint—"makes the situation different from that of some innocent young woman's being taken in by a lecherous professor." She's "not Rebecca of Sunnybrook Farm," the lawyer asserted but rather someone seeking an attractive settlement: she's "looking for a deep pocket." Nonetheless, Parker was punished with a pay cut and lost her position as department chair for violating the University's prohibition against amorous relationships with students (Manger, 1996).

Men's Sample

Among the 29 men randomly selected from the Academic Sexual Misconduct Database, four were accused of having sexual relationships with subordinates, employees, or students, without additional allegations of quid pro quo or any other type of verbal or physical coercion. For these men, the main harassment allegation—the one they publicly acknowledged—was that they engaged in a sexual relationship with someone with less institutional power and authority. This does not, of course, rule out the possibility that they engaged in quid pro quo bribes or threats, or other forms of sexually coercive behavior; rather, it is to say that the investigators—like the ones who handled the cases of Kristin Naca, Jacqueline Hoffarth, Alice Parker, and other women accused of sexually harassing adult students without evidence of overt coercion—either did not possess or chose not to reveal evidence of men's harassment beyond a disparity in power and authority.

To illustrate: in 1999, Mike DuBose, the head football coach for the University of Alabama, was charged with having a consensual sexual relationship with his secretary. The press referred to the relationship as an "extramarital affair"—implying consent and normality—though the relationship, in all likelihood, contained elements of overt coercion since the secretary subsequently sued DuBose and the University of Alabama for harassment, arguing that DuBose had mistreated her (Suggs, 1999). Nonetheless, potentially embarrassing details about DuBose's mistreatment of her, such as quid pro quo bribes or threats, never came to light. The secretary, who received a $350,000 settlement from Alabama, signed a nondisclosure agreement. So, while the allegations possess an objective referent—DuBose acknowledged that the sexual relationship with his secretary happened—they also possess gaps regarding the detail and depth of his culpability. In the aftermath, the Alabama board of trustees punished DuBose by shortening his contract from five years to 30 months and reducing his salary from $375,000 to $231,000 per year, penalties that may have been imposed as much because DuBose initially lied to them about the "affair," as from the affair itself. Immediately after the secretary's complaint about DuBose surfaced, he told reporters, "There is absolutely no truth or factual basis to any of these rumors involving me or other university employees. They are unfounded and hurting innocent people" (*Sun Sentinel*, 1999). Then, after the secretary sued and Alabama settled, he told reporters: "To say I am sorry is not enough. I was wrong but I cannot change the past today. Today I accept the university's discipline and punishment" (Associated Press, 1999). To register their displeasure with DuBose's failure to speak to them truthfully, the board of trustees amended his contract to stipulate that any further instances of duplicity could result in his termination (*Sun Sentinel*, 1999).

The harassment case against Richard Schneider, professor of biology from the University of California-San Francisco, concerns his covert sexual relationship with a graduate student that began in 2008 when she was 22-years-old and, as in the Dubose case, invites questions about the possibility that Schneider exercised coercion beyond his simply possessing greater institutional power. The student claimed the relationship with him began after he interrupted a conversation she was having with another professor: he pulled her aside and told her, "You don't want to work with that professor. You want to work with me." She followed his advice and chose him as her academic advisor, and at first thought their long talks indicated he was interested in her academic career. But then he started to schedule their meetings around lunch, which he called "lunch dates," and this eventually led to their first evening date, which was to a strip club, and then to their first sexual encounter (Panzer, 2019). "At the time, I felt like he valued me scientifically," the student recalled. "I felt like this is what a fun scientist would do" (Maxmen, 2020). Their sexual relationship, which they kept private, continued for the next two and a half years, but the student said she felt increasingly isolated and uncomfortable. "I didn't realize how dependent I was on his approval—what conferences I could go to, what projects I could work on, my references. He was my thesis advisor. I couldn't graduate without his approval" (Maxmen, 2020). Schneider, who was married, described the relationship as "welcome and consensual from beginning to end." The student, however, described the relationship differently: "I don't think it could be called consensual with that kind of power imbalance," an interpretation shared by the Title IX investigators who concluded that "although the relationship may have begun as consensual, the evidence supports a finding that the complainant, at some point, felt coerced to continue the relationship and reasonably believed that she had no choice but to continue the relationship lest it damage her career" (Maxmen, 2020). The student felt threatened by Schneider, given his greater power and authority, but because she did not report threats or bribes, the allegations did not rise to the level of quid pro quo harassment or overt coercion. As punishment, Schneider was demoted from professor to associate professor. Like DuBose, he managed to keep his job, he continued to supervise graduate students and, in 2016, he even received honors for his teaching, the "Mentor of the Year" award from UCSF. The student did not fare so well. "I went into a deep depression," she told *Nature* magazine. "I had panic attacks and crippling nightmares for years." She said that after Schneider was demoted, she lost her desire to become a scientist: "I floated around for a couple of years not doing anything because of the trauma. I would get panic attacks going to interviews. I didn't think I could survive in any place I had to work with a man" (Panzer, 2019).

The harassment case against former Alabama A&M professor of education and director of teacher certification, Edward Jones, given the sexual relationships between him and his students, also involved a disparity in institutional power and authority. But in his case, the disparity in power issue, while a fact acknowledged by all parties, was not identified by the school as Jones' main violation. Jones was fired in 2016 after videos were found on his university computer showing him engaging in oral sex with two male students. For the investigators, however, the issue of the students' possible coercion was secondary: Jones' letter of termination did not address the power differential between him and his students, nor did it address whether the sexual encounters were consensual or whether the students might have been harmed. Indeed, in Jones' lawsuit against Alabama A&M for firing him without cause, the University did not reference any investigation into the circumstances surrounding the students' participation in the sex acts. Instead, for Alabama A&M, another issue appeared paramount: that Jones had viewed and recorded "obscene material" on university-issued equipment. This is from Jones' termination letter:

> There is concerning evidence that you have engaged in sexual conduct below minimum standards of professional integrity and misused university computing/electronic assets in gross violation of well-established university policy.... ***You are charged with both using University resources to view obscene material and the production and/or creation of obscene materials*** (emphasis in the original) (Jones v. Alabama A&M, United States District Court, Northern District of Alabama, March 9, 2021, pp. 8–9).

In his defense, Jones did not disavow engaging in sex with students, nor did he argue that the sex was noncoercive. Rather, he argued that firing him was discriminatory; he was being fired, he said, because the sex acts in question were homosexual:

> Never before in the history of Alabama A&M University had any termination of faculty or staff had such wide-ranging broadcast by the University, and it is commonly known that several sexual scandals have occurred on the University campus, including scandals involving the highest leadership. But none involving homosexual activity, and none were publicized (Jones v. Alabama A&M, p. 9).

According to Jones, since he was fired, "at least two such sexual scandals have arisen, but both were heterosexual in nature and neither reached the public domain" (Jones v. Alabama A&M, p. 9). In support of Jones' contention that he was treated more harshly than other Alabama A&M employees because of his sexual orientation, he cited the fact that Alabama A&M suspended him months before the compromising videos were revealed: on Oct. 2015 he was placed on leave for making complaints about Alabama A&M. According to the suspension letter, he was seen as a "threat to the College of Education's Accreditation" (Jones v. Alabama A&M, p. 8). Also, supporting Jones' contention that he was treated more harshly than others due to his sexual orientation, only his name, among all other past or present Alabama A&M employees, is listed on the Academic Sexual Misconduct Database.

In the California State University-Long Beach sexual harassment case against psychology professor, Barry Singer, there were, likewise, no allegations of coercion and no mention of the power disparity between him and the students with whom he allegedly had sexual encounters, even though the school appeared to have grounds for such allegations, given Singer's admission that he had been "romantically involved" with several students. But in 1982, when the allegations against Singer first appeared, his teaching methods were treated as the central issue, in particular, his practice of giving academic credit to students in his psychology of sex course for engaging in homosexual, group, and extramarital sex, and for taking trips to gay bars, dressing in drag, and visiting nudist colonies. Singer shared that one of the benefits of an instructor having intimate relations with students is that those experiences could improve their teaching. As for encouraging his students to engage in homosexual, group, and extramarital sex, dressing in drag, etc., he said, "It can be a very powerful growth and learning experience.... The idea is not to go out and do some kinky things just to see what they're like, but to see change in your behavior and feelings." However, following public disclosure of his teaching methods, he received several death threats: "I've pretty much sunk to the basement level," he said. "I've 40 million people out there who are ready to kill me." California State suspended Singer on May 26, 1982; two days later, he resigned (UPI, 1982).

* * *

In a comparison of the handling of "disparities in power and authority" harassment in the sample of women with its handling in the men's sample, one of the seven women charged with this offense was exonerated (Rietkovich Browder), another was demoted (Parker), and five were either forced to resign or were terminated (Stubblefield, Naca, Hoffarth, Chatman, and Hale). Stubblefield was also sentenced to prison. Among the men, one of the four so identified received a pay cut (DuBose), another was demoted (Schneider), and two were forced to resign or terminated (Jones and Singer). As for gender overlap—points of similarity between the ways the men's and women's cases were handled—all the institutions that employed these individuals disapproved of their sexual activity with students and other subordinates, whether the putative perpetrators were men or women. The major gender difference—the main point of dissimilarity—is that the institutions appeared to come down harder on the women. Among the six women who acknowledged consensual sex with students and other subordinates, five were forced to resign or were terminated. By contrast, only two out of four men were terminated or forced to resign, and those two, Jones and Singer, had their penalties imposed for different reasons. Jones was fired, not for engaging in sex with students, but for his inappropriate use of university equipment and Singer was forced to resign for his incorporation of sexual activity into his course curricula. While Dubose's victim received a relatively large financial settlement, $350,000, as an acknowledgement of the magnitude of the abuse she suffered, DuBose was allowed to keep his position. None of the four men charged with the "disparities in power and authority" offense, unlike five of the women so charged, were terminated or forced to resign specifically for having a sexual relationship with a student or subordinate.

References

Associated Press. (1999, August 6). Settlement reached in harassment case. *New York Times*. https://www.sun-sentinel.com/1999/08/19/duboses-denials-prove-costly/

Carrillo, A., Crittenden, C., & Garland, T. (2019). Faculty perceptions of consensual sexual relationships between university faculty and students. *Journal of Academic Ethics, 17*, 331–343. https://doi.org/10.1007/s10805-019-09337-1

Coleman, P. (1988). Sex in power dependency relationships: Taking advantage of the fair sex. *Albany Law Review, 53*, 95–138.

Crittenden, C. A., Gimlin, A. M., Bennett, A., & Garland, T. S. (2021). Exploring faculty and students' attitudes about consensual sexual relationships and sexual harassment on college campuses. *Educational Policy, 35*(1), 41–66. https://doi.org/10.1177/0895904818810522

DeChiara, P. (1987). The need of universities to have rules on consensual sexual relationships Between faculty members and students. *Columbia Journal of Law and Social Problems, 21*, 137–162.

Manger, D. K. (1996, June 7). Professor-student affair leads to lawsuit at U. of Alabama. *The Chronicle of Higher Education*. https://www.chronicle.com/article/professor-student-affair-leads-to-lawsuit-at-u-of-alabama/

Mansnerus, L. (1991, April 7). Colleges break up dangerous liaisons. *New York Times*. https://www.nytimes.com/1991/04/07/education/colleges-break-up-dangerous-liaisons.html

Maxmen, A. (2020, February 24). Biologist exits prestigious post years after violating sexual harassment policy. *Nature*. https://www.nature.com/articles/d41586-020-00491-w

Panzer, A. (2019, March 12). Sexual harassment process troubles complainants. *Synapse*. https://synapse.ucsf.edu/articles/2019/03/12/sexual-harassment-process-troubles-complainants

Psychiatric Crime Database and Disciplinary Actions. (2013, July 11). *State places university psychologist Cara Hale on probation over sex with a graduate student*. https://www.psychcrime.org/news/index.php?vd=2062&t=State%20places%20university%20psychologist%20Cara%20Hale%20on%20probation%20over%20sex%20with%20graduate%20assistant

Srinivasan, A. (2020). Sex as a pedagogical failure. *The Yale Law Review, 129*(4), 1100–1145.

Suggs, W. (1999, August 10). U. of Alabama at Tuscaloosa settles sexual harassment accusation, fines coach. *Chronicle of Higher Education*. https://www.chronicle.com/article/u-of-alabama-at-tuscaloosa-settles-sexual-harassment-accusation-fines-coach/

Sun Sentinel. (1999, August 19). Dubose's denials prove costly. *Sun Sentinel*. https://www.sun-sentinel.com/1999/08/19/duboses-denials-prove-costly/

UPI. (1982, June 3). Sex professor resigns post. *UPI*. https://www.upi.com/Archives/1982/06/03/Sex-professor-resigns-post/4188391924800/

CHAPTER 8

Quid Pro Quo Sexual Harassment

The Equal Employment Opportunity Commission's (EEOC) definition of sexual harassment includes what is commonly known as *quid pro quo* workplace sexual harassment, a term Catherine MacKinnon introduced in her 1979 book, *Sexual Harassment of Working Women*. This kind of harassment takes two forms: in the first, involving a bribe, the harasser leads the target person to believe they will receive professional benefits (e.g., a promotion) in exchange for sexual favors. In the second, involving a threat, the harasser leads the target person to believe they will suffer negative career outcomes (e.g., lose their job) if they refuse to engage in sexual activities. However, even when the unwelcome sexual advances and requests for sexual favors come without an explicit reference to a bribe or threat, the target person can still argue (or feel) that a bribe or threat is in play. In the case of a bribe, they can say, "My professor (or boss) hasn't said anything, true enough, but they're acting as if they want me, as if I'm special and important. They're acting like, if I go along, if I let them date me, I might get the promotion I've been seeking." Or in the case of a threat, they can say, "My professor (or boss) has been swarming me with compliments, acting like I'm irresistible. What scares me is what happens if I tell them to back off. What if I tell them I'm not interested? Will I have to pay a price of some kind? Could I be fired or lose my chance of getting a scholarship or positive work reference?"

© The Author(s), under exclusive license to Springer Nature Switzerland AG 2024
L. Margolin, *Women Accused of Sexual Harassment*,
https://doi.org/10.1007/978-3-031-79021-8_8

Women's Sample

Nimrod Reitman may have been thinking something like this when Avital Ronell mentioned her plan for him to get a "super job wherever or whenever you want," which shows, again, how difficult it can be to distinguish between quid pro quo harassment and harassment which appears implicit, based only on the actors' disparities in power and authority. Because Ronell's compliments and encouragement, as represented in court documents, contain no evidence of an explicit quid pro quo bargain, that bargain, to the extent it existed, appears to have depended on Reitman's subjective assessment: how he rightly or wrongly imagined that he would receive a reward for complying with his advisor's demands. A similar kind of dynamic is apparent in the Jane Gallop harassment case, as illustrated by the accuser's claim that, while she was visiting Gallop's home to drop off a paper, as Gallop walked by her bedroom, she seemed to pause suggestively, which the accuser took as a sign that Gallop was looking for a sexual hook-up. The accuser also noted that, at one point, Gallop's bare foot reached over and rocked the rocking chair on which she was sitting. These behaviors, the pause by the bedroom and the bare foot on the rocker, although they may not have represented Gallop's explicit or implicit intention to initiate a sexual bargain, formed the basis of the accuser's quid pro quo allegation; in the accuser's mind, because she had spurned Gallop's sexual advances, Gallop retaliated by refusing to write the letters of recommendation the student believed she deserved.

The Academic Sexual Misconduct Database lists only one woman who was accused of making *explicit* quid pro quo threats. In that case, an assistant dean from Shippensburg University, identified as Dr. Jane Roe, allegedly told her supervisee, identified as Jane Doe, that she should participate in a threesome with her. Doe refused and then complained to the dean, Dr. Roe's supervisor. However, Doe claimed that the dean turned her away, saying she "did not want to hear about it" (Doe v. Shippensburg U., United States District Court, Middle District of Pennsylvania, March 7, 2022). Three months later, Dr. Roe allegedly showed her supervisee nude photos of herself acting as dominatrix with various men. When Jane Doe said she did not need to see these kinds of photos, Dr. Roe, refusing to take "no" for an answer, allegedly warned her supervisee that she would be terminated if she did not show more respect and cooperation. Then, during a work-related conference in New Orleans, Dr. Roe allegedly asked her supervisee to go on a date with her and a person from an online dating site. She also asked for her supervisee's room key. The supervisee refused both requests. The following day, Dr. Roe allegedly told Jane Doe she would not have a job when she returned to Shippensburg. When Doe did return to Shippensburg, she claimed she again notified the dean, and that the dean again refused to get involved. A few days later, the Shippensburg University vice president of human resources informed Doe that her supervisor, Dr. Roe, had accused her of "unprofessional behavior" during the New Orleans conference. When Doe told the vice president about her supervisor's sexual harassment, the vice president allegedly responded by telling Doe she was at fault for not having reported the harassment earlier. Jane Doe was then terminated. At that point, Doe filed a formal complaint to the Title IX coordinator, following which Dr. Roe was forced to resign (South, 2020).

Men's Sample

While the explicit quid pro quo threat from Dr. Roe is the only one on the Academic Sexual Misconduct Database from a woman and the only one from Shippensburg University, it is far from the only case of explicit sexual harassment attributed to an administrator: the Database lists 216 administrators who did not hold dual faculty-administrator positions (e.g., department chairpersons), who were accused of sexual harassment (17% of all cases). Seven were women and 209 were men, with most accused of making sexual advances to their staff. The earliest case of sexual harassment on the Database involves the former president of Colorado College, who allegedly harassed female staff from 1888 to 1917 (Jaschik, 2018). A substantial portion of the male administrators accused of sexually harassing their staff allegedly did so by offering quid pro quo deals for sexual favors, and many, like Dr. Roe, were accused of firing or threatening to fire staff who refused to accept those deals. For example, in 1995, Lee E. Monroe, the former president of Paul Quinn College, was sued by the College's vice president of enrollment for demoting her after she refused to travel with him to Mexico, and then for firing her after she "made it clear that she wasn't at all interested in a relationship with him." Unlike, Dr. Roe, who was forced to resign, Monroe managed to keep his position and did not receive a reprimand (*Chronicle of Higher Education*, 1995). In two more recent cases, however, male administrators accused of quid pro quo harassment did not fare as well. In 2018, the former acting president of Spokane Falls Community College, Darren Pitcher, was forced to resign after his subordinates accused him of threatening demotion or termination should they refuse his sexual advances (Criscione, 2018). Also in 2018, the former assistant dean of student programs at Bellevue College, Faisal Jaswal, retired under pressure after one of his staff accused him of sexually assaulting her, under the threat of termination should she reject or report him (Manandic, 2018).

Among the 29 men randomly selected from the Academic Sexual Misconduct Database, Bruce Conforth, a musician and founding curator of the Rock & Roll Hall of Fame, one of the most popular faculty at the University of Michigan until his retirement in 2017, was accused of threatening a student in exchange for sexual favors. Five years earlier, he had allegedly threatened another student in one of his classes with dire consequences if she did not submit to his sexual demands. She told investigators he required her to

> ...report anything I did with outside friends, scorning me for it, and then requiring that I service Bruce sexually as a way to redeem myself.... I grew scared, fearful to take missteps. I came to the university to learn and grow and instead one of the most popular professors used his knowledge, authenticated and raved about by the university, to stunt my growth, violate my body and to ruin my life out of jealousy (Dodge, 2022).

A prior harassment allegation against Conforth occurred in 2007, when a student in his seminar on blues music said he accosted her one evening in the back hallway of a bar, grabbed her, and repeatedly asked her to go home with him. “He said that he was sure his bed was better than mine,” the student said. “I was finally able to push him off and say no” (Dodge, 2022). She reported his conduct to the school authorities but claimed they did not take her allegations seriously: “We trust that the university has our best interests at heart,” she said, “but the university swept it under the rug” (Jesse, 2022). Consistent with Dziech and Weiner’s (1990) observation that faculty who are very popular—those regarded as stars—tend to be protected by their institutions, the University of Michigan appeared to have had a standing policy of excusing allegations against Conforth. But by February 2022, after eight former students filed lawsuits against Conforth for harassment and against the University of Michigan for tolerating his abusive behavior, protecting him no longer seemed feasible. Conforth admitted the allegations, which included unwelcome sexual advances, touching and groping, and retired after Michigan said it was prepared to initiate termination proceedings should he refuse to resign (Jesse, 2022).

In a second case of quid pro quo harassment from the men's sample, William E. Korf, associate professor of music at Ball State University, was terminated in 1981 after several current and former male students accused him of attempting to bribe them for sexual favors—offering good grades, money, and other gifts in exchange for sex. While Korf acknowledged that he had sexual relationships with his students, he insisted that those relations were "private and consensual," and that Ball State was not terminating him for these sexual encounters, but rather, for his "untraditional sexual preferences." He argued that faculty who have had consensual heterosexual sexual relationships with students have not been investigated nor charged as he was (Korf v. Ball State University, United States Court of Appeals, Feb. 8, 1984), an argument which may have been true in 1981, when Korf was terminated.

In a third case of quid pro quo harassment from the men's sample, a graduate student, referred to as Jane Doe in court filings, claimed that her professor at the Art Institute of Chicago, John Phillips, threatened her at first, not with physical harm, nor with undermining some dimension of her artistic/academic career. Rather, he threatened to harm himself if she did not do his sexual/romantic bidding. The student alleged, for example, that to make her visit his apartment, he showed her the rope he intended to hang himself with if she did not show. Later, he sent her pictures of people jumping off buildings to insinuate that he would do the same. He would also end his life, he told her, if she were to complain about him or charge him with harassment. According to the court filing, "Phillips told Doe she would never be able to live with herself if he committed suicide" (Jane Doe v. School of the Art Institute of Chicago, United States District Court, June 18, 2018, p. 18). Among his subsequent threats, he told her that he intended to circulate nude photographs of her and would sue her, should she claim their sexual relationship was nonconsensual. On one occasion, the student claimed that after she found nude photographs of other students on Phillips' computer and confronted him about the photographs, he locked her out of the apartment. The student also claimed that the Art Institute was complicit in the abuse she sustained (Jane Doe v. School of the Art Institute of Chicago), an allegation she supported by citing her mother's meeting with the Art Institute's dean of faculty who, the mother claimed, refused to discuss the sexual harassment with her. In fact, the student claimed that the dean called Phillips to alert him to the mother's complaint, as well as to reassure him that he would not be charged with harassment so long as his student did not herself file a complaint against him. However, the student did eventually file a formal complaint, as well as a civil suit against Phillips and the Art Institute, referencing the latter's failure to protect her. As a result, the Art Institute fired Phillips.

In two other cases, from 2004 and 2015, male administrators were accused of dangling the prospect of a job or promotion as a sexual lure. In the first of these cases, shortly after Loretta Grado became a program specialist at the University of Phoenix, one of her superiors, Manuel Ortiz, the campus director, began making surprise visits to her cubicle, asking personal questions and sharing unwelcome details about his sexual preferences, such as the fact that, for him, "partying" meant kissing and having sex. That was followed by Ortiz asking her if she liked to party and then by his trying to kiss her and run his fingers through her hair. She also claimed that Ortiz encouraged her to apply for a promotion to a position that had recently become available and said that because he had final say over who could be hired, he would waive the University's standard requirement that an employee occupy their position for at least six months before applying for a promotion. Grado followed Ortiz's lead and interviewed for the position. But the day before her promotion was to be announced, she claimed Ortiz asked her to "party" with him. After she refused, Ortiz selected someone else for the coveted position. In the aftermath, Grado testified that Ortiz's attempt to trade a promotion for sex resulted in nightmares, sleep loss, and emotional distress. At her deposition, she said that Ortiz's behavior was so disturbing it "took away her ability to care for her children." The University's investigation into the allegations against Ortiz uncovered other harassment complaints against him, such as this anonymous letter from a subordinate:

> Lately Manny has been behaving very rude and mean to me and the others (but mostly us women) here at work.... Some of us have seem him bullying different women in different departments, using sex and the fact that he is stronger than them. We are scared. I know I am not the only one to see this happen (Equal Employment Opportunity Commission, Plaintiff, and Lorena Pinon and Loretta Grado, Intervenors. v. University of Phoenix, United States District Court, District of New Mexico, April 18, 2007).

At the conclusion of the Title IX investigation into Ortiz's quid pro quo harassment, he was fired. Later, Grado sued the University of Phoenix for tolerating Ortiz's harassment and ignoring her complaints, which led to a settlement of $225,000 (Intervenors. v. University of Phoenix).

Todd Durham, director of online admissions at Belhaven University, was implicated in another case of a quid pro quo harassment based on his comments during an interview with a female job applicant, Erica Stewart. After she asked if she would need a degree for the job, he allegedly replied, "Not really, I can work something out" (Fowler, 2016). Stewart claimed that following the interview, Durham made sexual advances through social media which included a text photo of his erect penis. The photo was accompanied by the question, "Can I get something for the interview?" (Stewart v. Durham, United States District Court, Southern District of Mississippi, Feb. 9, 2017). Stewart's allegation of quid pro quo harassment was supported by the text message he sent her after the job interview: "I'm the boss ... you better be nice then. Lol." Her allegation was further supported by the fact that, after Stewart refused his sexual advance, she did not get the job. On February 11, 2017, two days after Stewart sued Durham for harassment, he was fired (Adams, 2017).

* * *

One of the main differences between the allegations against the five men (Conforth, Korf, Phillips, Ortiz, and Durham) and those against the three women (Gallop, Ronell, and Dr. Roe) accused of quid pro quo harassment, is that men's threats and bribes, in each case, appeared explicit, ranging from a professor threatening to kill himself if his student failed to comply with his demands, to an administrator offering a woman a promotion in exchange for sex and another professor offering students good grades, money, and other gifts to induce sexual payback. The institutional response in each of the men's cases was either termination or forced resignation. By contrast, among the three women accused of quid pro quo harassment, only one, Dr. Roe, was charged with making explicit quid pro quo threats; she was also the only one terminated. According to their accusers, the other two women (Gallop and Ronell) communicated their designs implicitly and indirectly. Another difference between women's and men's harassment allegations is that three of the men accused of explicit quid pro quo harassment had prior records of harassment—they were accused of committing offenses repeatedly, over extended periods—while none of the women had prior records of harassment.

References

Adams, R. (2017, September 29). Attorney releases new details about Belhaven University sexting lawsuit. *WAPT.* https://www.wapt.com/article/belhaven-university-leader-accused-of-sending-obscene-picture/3618875

Chronicle of Higher Education. (1995, November 10). $5-million lawsuit accuses college president of Harassment. *Chronicle of Higher Education.* https://www.chronicle.com/article/5-million-lawsuit-accuses-college-president-of-harassment/

Criscione, W. (2018, March 16). Former SFCC president Darren Pitcher exposed his genitalia And coerced sex from subordinates, attorney says. *Inlander.* https://www.inlander.com/Bloglander/archives/2018/03/16/former-sfcc-president-darren-pitcher-exposed-his-genitalia-and-coerced-sex-from-subordinates-attorney-says

Dodge, S. (2022, March 23). Rock "n" roll professor, University of Michigan finally served in Sexual harassment lawsuit. *MLive.* https://www.mlive.com/news/ann-arbor/2022/03/rock-n-roll-professor-university-of-michigan-finally-served-in-sexual-harassment-lawsuit.html

Dziech, B. W., & Weiner, L. (1990). *The Lecherous Professor: Sexual harassment on campus.* University of Illinois Press.

Fowler, S. (2016, September 21). Belhaven hit with sexual harassment. *Clarion-Ledger.*https://www.clarionledger.com/story/news/2016/09/21/belhaven-hit-sexual-harassment-suit/90801844/

Jaschik, S. (2018, March 14). Colorado College's own Harvey Weinstein. *Inside Higher Ed.* https://www.publicopiniononline.com/story/news/local/2020/08/14/title-ix-shippensburg-university-sued-dean-accused-sexual-harassment/5585384002/

Jesse, D. (2022, February 1). 8 former students sue u-m over sexual harassment claims against music lecturer. *Detroit Free Press.* https://www.freep.com/story/news/education/2022/02/01/university-michigan-sexual-misconduct-music-bruce-conforth/9283814002/

Manandic, K. (2018, August 29). Ex-Bellevue College dean allegedly raped assistant for years. *Bellevue Reporter.* https://www.bellevuereporter.com/news/ex-bellevue-college-dean-raped-assistant-for-years/

South, A. (2020, August 14). Grad student sues Shippensburg University over asst. dean's alleged Sexual advances. *Public Opinion.* https://www.publicopiniononline.com/story/news/local/2020/08/14/title-ix-shippensburg-university-sued-dean-accused-sexual-harassment/5585384002/

CHAPTER 9

Offensive Fun and Games

Harassment is not a single type of behavior, motivated by a singular goal. It can take a variety of forms and have a variety of goals, and, in one of its more benign forms, can be described as jokes that misfired, teasing that went too far, or play that felt aggressive or inappropriate (Brunner & Costello, 2002). It may not always be clear when jokes, teasing, and play rise to the level of harassment, but one of the clearest signs is the targets' overt and repeated expressions of displeasure: when they inform perpetrators that they find their behaviors offensive and want them to stop.

Women's Sample

A male assistant professor from the University of Florida claimed that two female administrators listed on the Academic Sexual Misconduct Database, Sheena Pryce Fegumps, a community outreach coordinator, and Christy Ewing, an academic programs specialist, were responsible for making repeated unwanted sexual advances to him. However, the women claimed their so-called sexual advances were not serious. They were only joking. Whether their sexual advances were serious or not, they were distinctive in that they were directed at the same man, and often at the same time. They were also distinctive because of people's readiness to dismiss them as inconsequential, to believe that the central motivation behind them was neither overtly sexual nor hostile, but rather, to have fun, for the

© The Author(s), under exclusive license to Springer Nature Switzerland AG 2024

L. Margolin, *Women Accused of Sexual Harassment*,
https://doi.org/10.1007/978-3-031-79021-8_9

presumptive harassers to entertain themselves, albeit, at the target's expense. Indeed, every time the presumptive victim reported the harassment to administrators, he was met with their refusal to see it as anything more than a joke. According to the University of Florida Ethics and Compliance Hotline incident assessment, it is "only because he is male that this behavior has continued and not been taken seriously" (Dean, 2020)

On December 11, 2018, the target of the harassment, an assistant professor of epidemiology and former director of educational programs at the University of Florida, sent an email to one of the University of Florida deans, in which he said that, as a result of continuing sexual harassment from Fegumps and Ewing, his blood pressure had sky-rocketed and he had been having "four or five panic attacks a day." "I am ready for the 'endgame' on these issues," he wrote. "I am tired of the fight. I want to start 2019 with a clean slate" (Dean, 2020).

He said the harassment began in 2017 during a conference in Atlanta. According to the professor, he, Fegumps, and Ewing were eating dinner at a Greek restaurant when Fegumps and Ewing began touching his upper thigh under the table; that was followed by Fegumps and Ewing suggesting that the three of them go back to one of their rooms. The professor said he tried to explain that he was married and was not interested. On another occasion, Ewing allegedly asked for a hug. After he refused, he claimed Ewing told him, "I just wanted to feel you against me." On yet another occasion, Fegumps allegedly told the professor that she could "relieve his stress" by getting under his desk with him; she said they could use the condoms she kept in her office as handouts for students. Then, while waiting for a meeting to begin, Fegumps allegedly asked him, "Do you want me to lay down on the conference table so you can ravage me" (Dean, 2020). The following year, the professor, Fegumps, and Ewing went to another conference in San Diego. This time the professor brought his wife. However, during a dinner that the professor shared with Fegumps and Ewing, he claimed that Fegumps began rubbing his lower back and then whispered into his ear that she wished his wife was not there so they could have some fun.

After the San Diego conference, the professor met with two University of Florida deans to say he could not work with Fegumps and Ewing any longer because of their continuing sexual advances. But, according to the professor, the administrators blamed him. "Why didn't you stop this?" they asked. When he tried to explain that he did try, the administrators allegedly interrupted to say that maybe he didn't try hard enough. It is unclear whether the deans ever reported the professor's allegations to Title IX, even though, as mandatory reporters, that was their responsibility. Then, in July 2019, the professor brought his sexual harassment complaints to Title IX on his own, claiming that Fegumps' and Ewing's harassment had recently taken a new and decidedly hostile turn. He said that they had started a rumor that he was forcing one of his subordinates to babysit his children and were telling people that he went out drinking with his students. Ewing later acknowledged to investigators that she had indeed started the babysitting rumor—she had talked about it with some colleagues—but insisted that the professor really was forcing a subordinate to babysit for him (Dean, 2020).

To date, the University of Florida has not reported any disciplinary action against either Fegumps or Ewing. Their putative victim, however, although still teaching at the University of Florida, was demoted from his administrative position. He speculated that he lost his administrative post because he cursed at one of the deans out of frustration stemming from their apparent unwillingness to intervene in his sexual harassment case (Dean, 2020). It is also possible that the University of Florida punished him, rather than Fegumps and Ewing, because investigators thought his allegations were not credible. They might have had difficulty understanding why two women would proposition the same man simultaneously. And they might have had difficulty understanding why he would find their sexual comments so distressing, producing, as he claimed, "four or five panic attacks a day."

While University of Florida administrators might have dismissed Fegumps' offer to have sex with him under his desk "to relieve his stress" and then, to "lay down on the conference table so you can ravage me" before a meeting began, on the grounds that they were jokes—that they were merely efforts to tease—they should have recognized that such behaviors, whether jokes or not, could still be construed as sexual harassment under the EEOC definition. They could be construed as "unreasonably interfering with an individual's work performance, or creating an intimidating, hostile or offensive working environment."

The University of Florida's forgiving attitude toward Fegumps and Ewing can be attributed to the fact that they are women. As women, they might have been seen as less predatory than men who behave in similar ways. Another possible explanation for the absence of disciplinary action is that, in comparison to the seven male employees at University of Florida who were accused of sexual harassment during the same period, all of whom lost their jobs, the presumptive victims in the men's cases were all subordinates; in each instance, the alleged harasser had institutional authority over the victims. In the Fegumps and Ewing cases, by contrast, their presumptive victim was a colleague—an institutional equal.

Men's Sample

University of California-Berkeley diving coach, Todd Mulzet, was accused of making unwelcome sexual comments to a student-athlete from 2014 through August 2015. These comments appeared to reflect sexual interest in the student-athlete, but they also appeared to have a snarky, teasing quality, reminiscent of some of the comments attributed to Fegumps and Ewing. For example, at the beginning of August 2015, with several students present, Mulzet asked the student for a "blow job." After the student refused, Mulzet responded, "I'll give you $300. You don't have to blow me. I'll blow you. We can put a board up with a hole in it like a glory hole." A witness overheard Mulzet later say, "when I get a big bonus check I can pay you." Following a swim meet, with several students close by, Mulzet allegedly announced in a loud voice, "This is my boyfriend," indicating the student-complainant. On another occasion, when the student was bending over, Mulzet allegedly stated, "Oooh, that's the position I like you in," to which the complainant responded, "Jesus Christ, shut up." On other occasions, when Mulzet saw the complainant bending over or stretching, he allegedly made similar sexually provocative comments, such as, "I'd love for your legs to be over my shoulders" and "Oh that's perfect, stay just like that." And on numerous other occasions, Mulzet allegedly asked him, "When are you coming to the dark side?" Mulzet denied making these comments and suggested that the complaints against him were a form of discrimination—homophobia (Anderson, 2016). However, after investigating the allegations, the University concluded that, by a preponderance of evidence, Mulzet had indeed committed sexual harassment. His penalty: a five percent pay cut for two months (Peter, 2016).

A second report of what might be interpreted as "offensive fun and games" from the men's sample involves a professor who sent unsolicited "dick pix" to a student. The student, Rebecca Farley, from New River Community and Technical College, alleged that, in December 2012, her psychology professor, Michael Curry, sent her an email which was accompanied by a photo of his erect penis. That was soon followed by a second email containing a photo of his "naked and hairy legs" (Asbury, 2016). While some men who send unsolicited "dick pix" might be motivated by hostility and misogyny, many others who send photos of this kind do not appear interested in harming their targets (Oswald et al., 2020). At the same time, the photos Curry sent his student appeared to have a negative impact on the student, as well as on her husband who saw them before his wife did. Suspecting she was having an affair with Curry, the husband confronted his wife about them. After she denied having an affair with her professor, her husband called the College to demand an investigation. But the College refused on the grounds that the husband was not a student at the College. Rebecca Farley then called the school herself to complain but said she "did not press her complaint" because Curry was teaching a course the following semester that she needed for graduation and "feared that pressing her complaint … would harm her ability to succeed in Professor Curry's class." As far as she knew, the College never investigated her allegations. Then, on September 14, 2014, Curry sent another text message to Farley's phone. The husband found the text before his wife did, became angry, and began responding to Curry's texts, pretending to be his wife, "in order to further draw out Professor Curry." Curry did, in fact, respond to the husband's texts: he described how aroused he was by Mrs. Farley, said he wanted to "jump her bones," and included another photo of his erect penis. This prompted the husband to again complain to New River about Professor Curry. At that point, the school initiated an investigation, but, according to Rebecca Farley, the investigators only interviewed her. And because investigators asked her whether she had experienced these kinds of incidents before, without also interviewing Curry, she assumed they believed that she was the one at fault. That prompted her to file a lawsuit against New River and Curry in which she alleged that the College failed to support her, in effect, leaving her on her own to endure rumors and speculation circulating throughout the campus community that she had behaved inappropriately. The net effect for Farley: she claimed she lost interest in her education, her attendance suffered, and her grades declined. The net effect for Curry: he resigned from New River under pressure (Farley v. New River Community and Technical College, United States District Court, Southern District of West Virginia, Feb. 1, 2017).

In a third case of verbal harassment that may have aspired to a flirtatious, playful tone, a student, Maria Currie, alleged that Boston University music professor, Eric Ruske, began harassing her after she arrived at music rehearsal in Nov. 2013: upon seeing that she was wearing high heel shoes, Ruske allegedly raised his eyebrows, looked her up and down, and said "Ooh, heels!" Then, the following month, after she failed her music evaluation, Ruske emailed her, stating, "I will certainly miss hearing and working with you in the quintet next semester (and of course seeing the concert heels)." The next day, when she met with Ruske in his office, he compared her performance to the two of them having sex: he said that listening to her play made him feel like they were engaging in sexual intercourse, but that Currie, while beautiful, "simply lay there and did nothing to enhance the sexual experience." Soon after the meeting, Ruske sent her this text message: "Fabulous chatting … and great blouse!" (Shyr v. Trustees of Boston University, United States District Court, Massachusetts, March 1, 2017). Since she had not yet received a grade from Ruske for her coursework, she said she felt obligated to send a polite response: "Have a great break!" Three hours later, Ruske texted her: "Without being too grossly inappropriate, I hope Santa brings you nice big high heels." Currie thanked him, and Ruske texted back, "It's such a shame that I won't ever get to see them/you." Currie's response: "I'll be having a recital next semester!" to which Ruske texted, "And the last thing you need is some creepy old guy in the front row…. You can always send pix." Currie interpreted the "pix" request as a solicitation for nude pictures. Because Ruske was due to grade her coursework, she again felt compelled to respond, "Ha, no promises!" to which Ruske responded, "Of course not … a girl can dream though." In December 2013, Ruske sent this text: "I probably owe you an apology…. I'm really sorry if I made you uncomfortable. Have a fabulous holiday and a happy New Year!" Currie did not respond, and in January, she withdrew as a student from Boston University, although she continued to practice at the school's fine arts facilities. Subsequently, on Jan. 30, 2014, Currie shared the text messages she received from Ruske with a Boston University student services coordinator, who, instead of encouraging her to file a harassment complaint against Ruske, appeared to accuse her of allowing Ruske's offensive behavior to continue: she suggested that she should have told him to stop texting her (Shyr v. Trustees of Boston University).

During the 2014 spring semester intermission, another music student, Erin Shyr, claimed she had a similar experience with Ruske. She said she received an email message which she interpreted as a request, like the one sent to Currie, for nude photographs: "Maybe you'll share a cute pic with me," he wrote. She pretended to not understand what he meant, and so wrote back: "I haven't taken many pictures in NYC, but here is a picture of my sister and I after her concert, and the other is a picture of a stray cat we fed leftovers to!" Ruske responded: "Forgive me for being a bit prejudiced, but although your sister and the kitty … are cute, you are amazing and do have something truly unique. Please don't be offended by [my] honesty … as I think you already know, I am rather blunt. Thanks for sharing … I like that." Later that month, Ruske sent Shyr this email message: "You are so damn bright and also wicked adorable." Shyr further claimed that when she ran into Ruske, he often gave her kisses on the cheek and hugs during which his hand skimmed across her lower back. She discussed Ruske's behavior with her mentor, who informed her that Ruske had a well-known reputation for harassing young women and advised her to stay away from him. She also contacted the Boston University Title IX coordinator who, like the student services coordinator Currie contacted, discouraged Shyr from filing a harassment complaint, suggesting, instead, that she should not take him seriously. She said that it was possible that Ruske has no idea that his behavior constituted sexual harassment: his problem, she suggested, may simply be that he has a "vibrant and effusive" personality (Shyr v. Trustees of Boston University).

In 2021, two more students complained of Ruske's online harassment—this time over dating apps, Bumble and Tinder. One of the students, whose age on his Tinder profile is 19-years-old and educational status is current Boston University student, claimed that Ruske sent this message, accompanied by a grinning face emoji: "We boys just aren't f— creative, are we? Too easily distracted by shiny things …and big boobs." The student's complaint: Ruske is "teaching undergraduate students and he knowingly messaged me with Boston University being in my bio." To date, Ruske continues to teach at Boston University and has not received any disciplinary action (Suarez, 2021; Suarez & Yehiya, 2021).

Retired MIT professor Walter Lewin, winner of multiple teaching awards, including being named to *The Princeton Review's* "Best 300 professors," also allegedly asked his female students to send nude photographs. According to an *Inside Higher Education* report, one of his students, Faiza Harbi, an English tutor living in France who enrolled in Lewin's online physics course, was at first flattered that such a well-regarded professor seemed to take an interest in her (Strausheim, 2015a, b). After about a year, however, she discovered that Lewin's interest in her was not strictly academic. She claimed that he began pushing her to engage in online sexual role-playing, which included requests for nude pictures and videos. Harbi, who takes medications for anxiety and depression, and has a history of self-mutilation, said she felt "trapped" by Lewin, and felt compelled, against her better judgment, to continue contacting him. Finally, to extricate herself, she attempted to locate other women through Facebook who enrolled in Lewin's course and had experiences like hers. She found ten who were willing to discuss Lewin's questionable behavior on the condition that their names be withheld. She then forwarded the chat logs, pictures, recordings, and screenshots she'd compiled, which included evidence of nudity and sexually explicit language, to MIT and *Inside Higher Ed.* (Strausheim, 2015a, b). After reviewing these materials, in December 2014, MIT concluded that Lewin had in fact "engaged in online harassment." The University then cut ties with him, stripped him of his emeritus title, and removed his physics course from MIT's online learning platform, with the admonition that Lewin's courses "Presented a [real] danger for people... expecting a student-teacher relationship and getting something inappropriate" (Strausheim, 2015a, b).

Michael O'Mahony, former professor of food science from the University of California-Davis, did not send or solicit nude photos from students, but his students did accuse him of repeatedly making sexually suggestive, inappropriate jokes since the 1980s. As in the Multzet, and Fegumps and Ewing cases, some of O'Mahony's offensive comments may have been intended as humor, albeit with a sneering, disdainful quality. Then, in 2007, a student filed a formal complaint against him, alleging that he shared pornographic cartoons with students in one class and explained how "lingua," Latin for tongue, is the root of our word "cunnilingus." Four years later, a student filed another formal complaint that a comment O'Mahony made to her suggested that she had offered him sex for better grades. O'Mahony contended that his comment was merely a joke. Whether his comment was serious or intended as a joke, his student's reaction was markedly negative: she claimed she was quite upset. At the time, he was also accused of making inappropriate comments about another female student's appearance, which led her to believe he was "hitting on her." Then, in 2012, he was accused of staring at the breasts of a female staff member. He denied the charge, claiming that he had only been staring at her unusual V-neck sweater. However, he said he soon realized that someone might misconstrue his intentions, and so tried to avert his glance. But too late, he said, because she caught his eyes. He attempted to explain that he was only staring at her sweater, but she was unconvinced.

In 2013, he again allegedly suggested that a student "put out" for good grades, and, during that same year, allegedly called another female student "gorgeous" and "exotic." After each of these allegations, University officials warned O'Mahony that his behavior was unacceptable. But he "consistently played down the past allegations, professing to be completely mystified at the reputation he has developed for harassing female students" (Romik & Theodossy, 2016). He claimed his sexual remarks were intended as irony, and added that he, unlike "most Americans who do not 'get' irony," knew how to appreciate its value, which Tile IX investigators interpreted as a demonstration either of his "inability or unwillingness to cease introducing subjects of a sexual nature into his interactions with students."

Then, in 2016, he allegedly told a student in front of her adviser to leave his lab because of her inappropriate sexual activity: he accused her of making love on the lab tables. Witnesses said the student became visibly distressed and cried after the comment. For the next week to 10 days, she said she did not feel like herself: she was quiet, depressed, and worried that she might have overreacted due to lack of sleep; however, she seemed to return to normal after learning that O'Mahony had been suspended. In February 2017, O'Mahony resigned in lieu of termination.

A final example of men's verbal harassment that may have lacked overt malice is the case of a Morehouse administrator, Demarcus Crews, who was accused of repeatedly teasing two male students about their claim to be heterosexual, suggesting they needed to come out of the closet. One student claimed Crews told him, "You need dick." A second student claimed that Crews teased him with comments, such as, "I don't know if you'll marry a male or female" and "All the girls want your pussy, huh?" To the student, these comments implied that "men at Morehouse College are physically interested in me and want to have sexual relations with me." The student said that Crews' comments made him so anxious and depressed, he no longer felt comfortable going to class or to other campus activities, and, as a result, "I isolated myself completely from everybody" (Blackmon, 2018). Morehouse suspended Crews in response to the allegations and initiated an investigation whose outcome is not yet publicly available (McLaughlin & Coffman, 2019).

* * *

Some offensive comments can be dismissed initially as infelicitous efforts to get a laugh—as a form of play or jokes. But on closer inspection, they seem to convey a quality of malice and exploitation. Two cases in the women's sample (Fegumps and Ewing) and six in the men's (Mulzet,

Curry, Ruske, Lewin, O'Mahony, and Crews) fit that description. Although Marybeth Gasman from the University of Pennsylvania and Donna Laird from St. Phillips College were reprimanded for sharing bawdy jokes and inappropriate satirical links with their staff, their attempts at humor, as noted in Chap. 5, were not aimed at individual staff members, and none of the recipients of their humor claimed injury. By contrast, the male and female perpetrators described in this chapter directed their so-called "humor" at specific targets and those targets claimed injury.

One of the most striking differences between men's and women's offensive joking and play is men's interest in nude photos: of the six men so accused, two allegedly requested nude photos of their students and one sent nude photos of himself. If we add Todd Durham to the list, a man charged with sending nude photos of himself as part of a quid pro quo scheme, a total of four men, 7% of the men's sample, were accused of either sending or requesting nude photos from subordinates, a type of harassment with only one counterpart among women. In the women's sample, a supervisee, Jane Doe, accused her supervisor, Dr. Jane Roe, of sharing nude photos of herself acting as a dominatrix with various men.

A second difference is that the women accused of offensive fun and games—Fegumps and Ewing—were treated as blameless: they were not punished even though their accuser provided multiple examples of their offensive behavior and how they harmed him. In fact, he may have been punished for lodging complaints: he claims he lost his administrative position because administrators became fed up with his protestations of victimhood. Other differences: the two women accused of offensive joking and flirtation targeted the same man, a faculty member, and appeared to work together, coordinating their harassment. In the men's sample, by contrast, the men allegedly harassed on their own with students as targets.

References

Anderson, J. (2016, April 6). Cal diving coach punished for sexual harassment, per school report. *Swim Swam*. https://swimswam.com/cal-diving-coach-punished-sexual-harrassment-per-school-report/

Asbury, K. (2016, October 11). Couple sues New River Community & Technical College for professor's harassment. *West Virginia Record*. https://wvrecord.com/stories/511017847-couple-sues-new-river-community-technical-college-for-professor-s-harassment

Blackmon, M. (2018, July 18). Two Morehouse College students said a male staffer sexually Harassed them, prompting an investigation. *BuzzFeed News*. https://www.buzzfeednews.com/article/michaelblackmon/morehouse-college-sexual-harassment-demarcus-crews

Brunner, P. W., & Costello, M. L. (2002, spring). Where's the joke? The meaning behind sexual humor. *Advancing Women in Leadership Journal*. www.advancingwomen.com/awl/spring2002/BRUNN%7E37.htm

Dean, H. (2020, January 17). Male professor harassed. *Independent Florida Alligator*. https://issuu.com/floridaalligator/docs/alligator01172020-pdf/1

McLaughlin, E. C., & Coffman, J. (2019, July 23). Staffer put on leave while school investigates sexual misconduct accusations. *CNN*. https://www.cnn.com/2019/07/22/us/morehouse-sexual-misconduct-allegations/index.html

Oswald, F., Lopes, A., Skoda, K., Hesse, C. L., & Pedersen, C. L. (2020). I'll show you mine so You'll show me yours: Motivations and personality variables in photographic exhibitionism. *Journal of Sex Research, 57*(5), 597–609.

Peter, J. (2016, April 6). Cal diving coach fined $455.30 for sexual harassment. *USA Today*. https://www.usatoday.com/story/sports/college/2016/04/06/cal-diving-coach-accused-sexual-harassment/82705088/

Romik, D., & Theodossy, M. M. (2016, July 20). *Confidential investigator report*. University of California-Davis. https://theaggie.org/wp-content/uploads/2019/06/160142_UCDID.pdf

Strausheim, C. (2015a, January 22). We all felt trapped. *Inside Higher Ed*. https://www.insidehighered.com/news/2015/01/23/complainant-unprecedented-walter-lewin-sexual-harassment-case-comes-forward

Strausheim, C. (2015b, March 9). Lewin's legacy. *Inside Higher Ed*. https://www.insidehighered.com/news/2015/03/10/despite-mits-decision-delete-walter-lewins-lecture-videos-live

Suarez, J. M. (2021, September 24). Second BU student comes forward with evidence of inappropriate Online communication from professor Eric Ruske. *Daily Free Press*. https://dailyfreepress.com/2021/09/24/second-bu-student-comes-forward-with-evidence-of-inappropriate-online-communication-from-professor-eric-ruske/

Suarez, J. M., & Yehiya, M. (2021, September 8). Students question University's commitment to sexual misconduct prevention after accused CFA professor messages student through Bumble. *Daily Free Press*. https://dailyfreepress.com/2021/09/08/students-question-universitys-commitment-to-sexual-misconduct-prevention-after-accused-cfa-professor-messages-student-through-bumble/

CHAPTER 10

Overtly Hostile Verbal Harassment

Workers in both public and private organizations sometimes make insulting and offensive remarks on gender and sexuality with an undisguised aim of causing harm and stimulating fear (Aquino & Thau, 2009; Einarsen, 2000). Consider, for example, the message Ivonne del Valle sent to a colleague, "I can do whatever the fuck I want piece of shit," and this message from Melissa Ann Santana to a group of firefighters, "You are [so] worthless that they don't really care if a whole crew [of] the granite mountain guys die.... Be a success ... and die at your next fire." In this chapter, I compare the overtly hostile verbal harassment attributed to another woman listed on the Academic Sexual Misconduct Database, Lavonette Bartley, to the overtly hostile comments attributed to men in the sample randomly selected from the Database.

Women's Sample

Bartley, an administrator from Alabama State University, was accused of repeatedly directing overtly hostile comments to her supervisees over a seven-year period, beginning in 2002. Verbal abuse, like that of del Valle and Santana, can be defined as stalking when it appears intentional, when it occurs over a protracted time period, and the abusive comments are directed at a specific person or persons with the goal of making them fear for their safety (Owens, 2016). Bartley's hostile comments to her

© The Author(s), under exclusive license to Springer Nature Switzerland AG 2024

L. Margolin, *Women Accused of Sexual Harassment*,
https://doi.org/10.1007/978-3-031-79021-8_10

supervisees, by contrast, appeared more like a series of spontaneous outbursts of contempt and loathing than a premeditated pattern of intimidation (Weatherly v. Alabama State, United States District Court, Alabama, Northern Division, April 30, 2010). For example, when Bartley was displeased with her supervisees' work, she was said to make comments such as, "I'm sick and tired of this nigger shit," "Bitch, you need to do what I asked you to do," and "These stupid bitches can't do anything right. And they ain't nothing but some niggas." She was accused of calling her supervisees "nigger," "white bitch," and "fat bitch," and was even accused of calling her supervisee's seven-year-old son "a nigger," a name which upset him so much he crawled under his mother's desk and assumed a fetal position. One of her supervisees accused her of telling her to "talk to the nigger side of the hand because the white side does not want to hear it" and "we got to dress professional; we don't dress like niggers." She allegedly called her supervisees' breasts "melons," their buttocks "hams," referred to their underwear and panty lines in the presence of others, and once reportedly told a supervisee to "strip to see how many other tattoos [she] had and where." When she asked one of her supervisees what race she was, and her supervisee answered that she was biracial and did not wish to be identified as either white or Black, Bartley allegedly "looked [her] up and down and curled her lip and walked away" (Weatherly v. Alabama State).

Bartley's supervisees described their responses to Bartley with terms such as "stunned," "humiliated," "hurt," "degraded," "embarrassed," "worthless," and "scared." They also described the physical costs—migraines, anxiety, loss of appetite, insomnia, and high blood pressure (Weatherly v. Alabama State).

When the supervisees took their complaints to Bartley's supervisor, John Knight, the University's chief operating officer and interim president, they claimed that he was dismissive: he told them that he was not interested and that he "was not going to walk on eggshells around his office … nobody can tell him how to run his office." He also allegedly warned them against taking their complaints to the EEOC: "No one was to speak to the EEOC and if they did, they would be dealt with. Terminated." After the supervisees defied him and forwarded their complaints to the EEOC, two were in fact terminated. But following their civil suit against Alabama State, the women who were terminated were awarded back pay, and the three women received a settlement from the University that collectively exceeded a million dollars (Weatherly v. Alabama State).

John Knight, who was also a state legislator—he called the lawsuit a political ploy to embarrass him during an election year—is listed on the Academic Sexual Misconduct Database alongside Bartley. He was accused of sexually harassing one of Bartley's supervisees by commenting on how attractive she is: he told her he "liked his coffee sweet like [her] and the color of [her] complexion." He was also accused of asking her to dance for him, the way he had once seen her dance at a party, and of calling her at home and asking her what the "wildest thing" was she wished she could do for her birthday.

The most controversial feature of this case—and what stands out most—is not the harassment attributed to Bartley, but the ways Bartley's harassment was treated by her institution. As in the Fegumps and Ewing cases, we have no record of Bartley's university reprimanding her for harassment. So far, Alabama State University has refused to confirm whether Bartley or her supervisor, John Knight, had been disciplined in connection with the harassment complaints levelled against them (Moon, 2013); this is despite the U.S. District Court of Appeals' strongly negative reaction to the University's handling of the case: "We are unnerved by the apparent acquiescence to, if not downright condoning of, the abusive work environment created by its high-level employees" (Weatherly v. Alabama State University, p. 12). Far from being judged more harshly than comparable male harassers, as appeared true of several of the women whose cases were reviewed in the previous chapters, Alabama State University appeared to allow Bartley to harass her supervisees with impunity.

Men's Sample

Christopher Dustin, a former professor of philosophy from the College of the Holy Cross, allegedly called a student "a real bitch" along with other aspersions, after working with her for more than a year (Sanders, 2019). Dustin and his student became acquainted in 2015 when the student was a junior. He selected her for a work-study position in his department for which, she claimed, she was ineligible. She alleged that the following year, Dustin pressured her to write her senior honors thesis under his direction. Her relationship with him, she said, felt positive at first: "Professor Dustin would compliment me all the time. He did a good job at making me feel special." In hindsight, however, she said she should have recognized that his compliments were a form of psycho/sexual grooming. That only became apparent to her when he began making sexual advances. "He repeatedly suggested we go on 'dates' or get drinks together. He bought me gifts, two of which included a bouquet of pink flowers and an item which had the message 'I love you' inscribed on it." As more time passed, she said his comments became increasingly sexual: "He told me I was 'hot' and said that he would 'love to see' my body. He told me he didn't want to 'share me' with anyone else and to stay away from certain other people." She also said that, in response to her continued resistance, his attitude shifted to hostility and he began insulting her. In the meantime, she said, he never mentored her or helped her with her thesis: "The year culminated in the total waste of an academic opportunity and a humiliating thesis presentation. It was a heartbreaking way to leave Holy Cross." In March 2017, Dustin was appointed dean of the Holy Cross faculty. The following month, the student whom Dustin allegedly called "a real bitch" reported his behavior to the Title IX office. During the 20-month investigation which followed, Dustin's work status did not change: he remained the dean of faculty, taught classes, advised theses, and continued to work with female students. However, at the completion of the investigation, his interaction with female students was restricted—he was no longer permitted to conduct private, one-on-one meetings with women—and he was stripped of his deanship. The release of a news article which quoted the allegations against Dustin prompted a series of student protests, culminating in a two-day sit-in (Sanders, 2019). Among students' demands was for Holy Cross to acknowledge "that for 20 months while Christopher Dustin was under investigation for alleged sexual misconduct, the college failed to alert the student body, faculty, and Board of Trustees of Professor Christopher Dustin's misconduct and to continue to interact with students." However, one of the students' other demands, that Dustin should be terminated, was honored in September 2020 (Hanson, 2020).

* * *

Among the 29 men randomly selected from the Academic Sexual Misconduct Database who were accused of overtly hostile verbal harassment, none appeared to express the level of malice and bitterness on display in the Bartley case. Her rudeness crossed all lines, from racial and gender insults to fat shaming and maligning peoples' intelligence. Only one man, Christopher Dustin, was charged with overtly hostile verbal abuse, according to the available records, but he did so only after he had known the student-victim for longer than a year; prior to his outburst of insulting language, the student claimed he behaved in a superficially supportive, albeit manipulative way. A second difference between the Bartley and Dustin cases is that Bartley, while reprimanded in court, was not reprimanded by her university. She managed to keep her job without loss of benefits. By contrast, Dustin was eventually fired. A third difference is that while Dustin attempted to engage in sexual activity with his target, the complaints against Bartley did not include sexual advances.

References

Aquino, K., & Thau, S. (2009). Workplace victimization: Aggression from the target's perspective. *Annual Review of Psychology, 60*, 717–741.

Einarsen, S. (2000). Harassment and bullying at work: A review of the Scandinavian approach. *Aggression and Violent Behavior, 5*(4), 379–401.

Hanson, M. (2020, September 11). Christopher Dustin, Holy Cross professor accused of sexual misconduct, no longer employed by college. *MassLive*. https://www.masslive.com/worcester/2020/09/christopher-dustin-holy-cross-professor-accused-of-sexual-misconduct-reportedly-no-longer-employed-by-college.html

Moon, J. (2013, September 4). Appeals court blasts Ala. university in harassment ruling. *USA Today*. https://www.usatoday.com/story/news/nation/2013/09/04/alabama-sex-harassment-n-word/2762491/

Owens, J. (2016). Why definitions matter: Stalking victimization in the United States. *Journal of Interpersonal Violence, 31*, 2196–2226. https://doi.org/10.1177/0886260515573577

Sanders, S. C. (2019, January 24). Sexual allegations raise concerns at Holy Cross. *WM*. https://www.worcestermag.com/story/news/2019/01/24/sexual-misconduct-allegations-raise-concerns-at-holy-cross/6213612007/

CHAPTER 11

Physical Sexual Intrusions

Physical sexual intrusions can range from unwelcome hugs or kisses to sexual assault and murder. They can occur as an isolated incident, as in Rie Hachiyanga's murderous assault of a colleague and Nicole Rovig's drunken efforts, one night at bar, to kiss and grope anybody who would stand still. Or they can occur over an extended time-period and represent a series of offensive behaviors. They can also occur alongside other kinds of harassment. In Ellerth v. Burlington Industries, for example—the case discussed in Chap. 2—a corporation vice president was accused of making demeaning comments to a prospective employee, but he was also accused of touching her without her consent. Individuals who commit one kind of sexual harassment may feel entitled to and capable of harassing their targets in any number of ways, combining bribes and threats with hectoring and hounding, unwelcome touching, and, on occasion, physical force.

Women's Sample

Rie Hachiyanagi and Nicole Rovig were accused of highly unusual, single-incident physical sexual intrusions. A third woman listed on the Academic Sexual Misconduct Database, Ellen Lemley, a former professor of criminology from Arkansas State University, was also accused of a highly unusual single-incident physical sexual intrusion: raping a 25-year-old female student with her husband, Gregory Russell, also a former professor of

© The Author(s), under exclusive license to Springer Nature Switzerland AG 2024

L. Margolin, *Women Accused of Sexual Harassment*,
https://doi.org/10.1007/978-3-031-79021-8_11

criminology from Arkansas. According to the student, they drugged her at a restaurant and then sexually assaulted her at their home on April 19, 2007. She said she "blacked out" during the assault, and afterwards did not "remember anything from sitting at the table to waking up naked" in Lemley's and Russell's home, covered in blood from her waist to her thighs. She added that after she woke up, Lemley joined her in bed and that Russell later drove her back to her apartment (Epstein, 2007). Lemley and Russell resigned from Arkansas State two weeks after the alleged assault. But University officials, citing confidentiality, declined to say whether they had been contemplating firing or reprimanding them before they quit. And two months later, after the assault allegations were forwarded to the police, the police said that they did not find any evidence corroborating the student's allegations (Epstein, 2007).

No other sexual assault in which two or more individuals worked in tandem appeared in the comparison sample of 29 men randomly selected from the Academic Sexual Misconduct Database. However, that kind of assault appears twice in the Database as a whole. In one of the cases involving men, music professor David Daniels and his husband, William "Scott" Walters, were charged with sexually assaulting the same victim, on the same night. The graduate student victim shared that he met his assailants at a Houston Grand Opera Reception, was invited back to their apartment where he was given a drink that made him lose consciousness (Flaherty, 2019a, b). "Yes, men are raped," the graduate student said. "I did not know that the word 'rape' applied to what happened to me until I lethargically went to tell a friend, and told her through tears and emptiness what happened to me. In fact, I was so naïve that I didn't know that I should have gone to the hospital or even what a 'rape kit' is" (McAboy, 2018). Daniels and Walters were subsequently charged with sexual assault, pleaded guilty, and were sentenced to eight years probation. Daniels also lost his faculty position at the University of Michigan (Veltman, 2023). In a second multi-assailant assault attributed to men listed on the Database, a student claimed she met three professors from Truman State University at a bar and accompanied them home. She told the police she was sexually assaulted at their home, but because she could not say what exactly had happened—the drugs they gave her made her lose consciousness—prosecutors dropped the case. However, two of the professors later resigned (Wilson, 1997).

A fourth woman accused of physical sexual intrusions, Denise Gabriel, a theater professor from the University of North Carolina-Greensboro, was listed on the Academic Sexual Misconduct Database following accusations that she touched her students in ways that were both sexual and deceptive. The touching attributed to Gabriel appeared rooted in the power differential between her and her students, but also in the ways Gabriel concealed her intentions, instilling doubt and confusion in victims. Like the assaults committed by Larry Nasser, the former physician for the United States Women's National Gymnastics Team who was charged with abusing hundreds of girls and young women, Gabriel's physical sexual intrusions were accomplished without overt physical coercion or quid pro quo bargains: her victims appeared to endure the assaults because they imagined that, given Gabriel's status as a well-respected professor, she was following legitimate pedagogical procedures.

To illustrate: one of Gabriel's accusers, a dance and theater student at UNCG, described how, one evening, Gabriel invited her to dinner at a restaurant, and then, just before driving her home, invited her to her apartment for one-on-one instruction (Green, 2021). "Once at Gabriel's apartment, she told me we could do some 'body work,'" the student said. "I didn't really understand what this meant, and she didn't exactly explain what it would entail. My relationship with Gabriel was extremely centered around the fact that I am a dancer and how she wanted me to unlearn everything I knew about my dancing training to be a more successful actor."

The student thought that the after-hours instruction at Gabriel's home would be no different from the kinds of instruction Gabriel provided in class. She soon learned that it was not the case. "She instructed me to shower in her bathroom attached to her bedroom," the student recalled. "She said to take as much time as I wanted and when I finished, to come out in whatever dress I felt comfortable in and lay on her massage table. I was taken aback. I couldn't believe that my teacher was asking me to do something like this." The student's next comments reveal that an individual in a position of power and authority can intimidate an adult subordinate without threatening, bribing, or persuading: "I couldn't believe that my teacher was asking me to do something like this. But for whatever reason, I felt compelled to say yes and proceeded with this request."

The student followed her professor's instructions "while panicking about what was to come." She showered, emerged from the bathroom in her bra, underwear, and a towel, and then walked to the massage table, where she slipped under the blanket and waited face down. What Gabriel did next, the student said, was both frightening and numbing: She "proceeded to perform a full body massage on me with various creams and oils. She touched every inch of my body, moaning at points while doing so. While there never was any penetration, I did feel extremely uncomfortable and violated.... I also distinctly remember feeling that I would get caught and kicked out of the BFA program if I told anyone about what Gabriel and I did during our 'body work'." Her last recollection was of "a small voice in my head [which] just kept telling me to lay quiet and wait for it to be over." The student and six other survivors reported Gabriel to the UNCG Title IX director and soon after, Gabriel resigned (Green, 2021).

To illustrate the "nonexceptional" nature of Gabriel's harassment, another UNCG faculty member, a man, appears on the Academic Sexual Misconduct Database accused of sexually harassing his male students in ways, locations, and circumstances closely resembling Gabriel's offenses. Preston Lane, an award-winning playwright, director, and co-founder of Triad Stage resigned from the UNCG theater department in 2020, only months before Gabriel, and under similar circumstances. Like Gabriel, he allegedly gained students' sexual compliance by virtue of their respect for this position and authority: "Everyone was in awe of him," a student shared with the *Triad City Beat.* Also, like Gabriel, Lane allegedly concealed his sexual advances under the guise of legitimate academic instruction. According to the student-reporter, Lane would invite theater students to work on their breathing or their monologues (Green, 2020). Then he would say, "Let's strip down to your underwear. Let's get naked." To those who hesitated, he said, "Are you homophobic?" "Are you a pussy?" The sexual activity which followed included oral and manual genital play without reports of penetration, and soon after these allegations came to light, Lane resigned. The main difference between him and Gabriel, the student-reporter said, is that during the sexual encounters, he encouraged students to drink alcoholic beverages: "these men were completely inebriated and passed out when Preston made it physical" (Green, 2020).

The fifth woman to appear on the Academic Sexual Misconduct Database following accusations of physical sexual intrusions is Amy C. Wilkins, former professor and director of the sociology department graduate program at the University of Colorado. That Wilkins' accusers waited 12 years before coming forward can be explained, in part, by the fact that Wilkins had power over graduate student teaching assignments and students' academic progress and was, in several ways, someone whom students had reason to fear. Ironically, she also chaired the committee tasked with the responsibility of processing students' internal complaints. According to students' testimony, Wilkins used this power to (1) have sexual relations with multiple students, (2) discuss their sex lives with them, (3) share this information with other students, (4) publicly discuss and rate students' attractiveness, (5) have sexual intercourse in close proximity to her students, (6) expose her naked body to students without their consent, (7) pressure students to touch her body while clothed, partially clothed, and fully naked, and (8) "retaliate against students who 'stepped out of line,' who did not defer to her, who changed advisors, who did not put her on their committees, who did not defend her to others..." (Hackett, 2018). While Wilkins was fired two years after these accusations surfaced—more than a dozen years after her abusive behavior supposedly began—her case illustrates how occupying a position of power can make it possible to commit a broad range of harassment violations, while at the same time shielding the presumptive offender from accountability (Klamann, 2020).

Men's Sample

Among the 29 cases involving harassment by men in the random comparison sample, intrusive physical sexual contact appeared the most common type of allegation, with a total of 13 cases. The assailants were identified as 10 faculty, one administrator, one coach, and one student. The victims, almost all of whom occupied lower ranks, were identified as 12 students and one university employee. Five of the physical sexual intrusion cases appeared to involve a single, seemingly isolated incident, four involved multiple incidents, and another four involved delayed allegations—allegations of intrusions which did not come to light until 30 or more years had elapsed (discussed in the next chapter).

Single-Incident Physical Sexual Intrusions by Men

In the first single-incident case, the president of Drexel University, William S. Gaither, was accused of putting his hand on the knee of a female subordinate and squeezing her knee repeatedly at a business dinner held in 1987. She said she tried to move her chair away from him but could not because there was not enough room. After he placed his hand on her knee a second time, she excused herself and stayed in the restroom for the remainder of the meal (Stevens, 1987). Gaither acknowledged touching the woman in the way she described but said "It is completely beyond my personal philosophy or ethical code or instincts to do anything that would be regarded as what I understand to be sexual harassment." Then, when asked why he squeezed her knee in the first place, he said: "I have on occasion, and I'm sure there will be future occasions, touched people without sexual intent. Human contact need not have absolute sexual connotations. In some churches people shake hands. In my church we mill around and hug each other" (Saunders et al., 1987). He added that his behavior could be explained in part as the result of his efforts to emerge from the guarded persona of an engineer. His goal, he said, was to become a more emotionally expressive human being (Stevens, 1987). In October 1987, after the Drexel faculty approved a motion of "no confidence" in Gaither by a vote of 229 to 14, asserting that his ability to lead the University had been "irreparably damaged," he resigned.

In a second single incident of alleged physical sexual harassment, Zamir Bavel, former Kansas University professor of information processing studies, was accused of touching and groping a student during a study session at a Perkins restaurant. According to the student, Bavel sat next to her, rubbed her knee, then placed his arm around her and rubbed her shoulder for half an hour as he helped her study for one of his courses. She also alleged that after she leaned over to pick up her backpack, Bavel grabbed her breast and pulled her up toward him until they were facing each other (Shepherd, 2014). Bavel denied the student's allegations, and in his defense, provided medical records documenting several of his ailments—e.g., arthritis, fused neck vertebrae, and degenerated lumbar discs—which he claimed would have made it physically impossible for him to move his arm in the ways the student alleged. On the other hand, the email message he sent to the student the following day ("Please tell me if I misinterpreted, if I assumed too much") seemed to corroborate the student's allegation, as did a second email he sent her a few days later: "From your lack of answer and your demeanor (the Mona Lisa smile is gone), I gather that I did, indeed, misinterpret. I apologize. Please erase." Further corroborating the student's version of events was the testimony of a witness interviewed by the Title IX investigator (Shepherd, 2014). At the conclusion of the investigation, Kansas University found that Bavel had violated the school's harassment policy, and as punishment, was suspended two weeks without pay, ordered to take sexual harassment training, and denied a raise for the following year. Among the other costs of the allegations, Bavel reported "Now, anytime a student asks to sit next to me in a booth, I'll refuse" (Blanton, Dec. 7, 2014).

In a third single-incident case involving a male assailant, a University of Florida student claimed that in September 2010, music professor, Arnold Irchai, grabbed her face and forcibly kissed her in his office during a private lesson. She said she pushed him away, left his office in tears, and then shared what happened with her undergraduate adviser and the music school director. Two previous harassment complaints had been lodged against Irchai, but one was dropped by the student and the other yielded inconclusive results. Irchai denied the most recent allegations and attributed them to the student being nervous about her upcoming concert performance. After the Title IX investigation, he was fired (Crabbe, 2011).

In a fourth single-incident case, Tracy McIntosh, a former professor of neurosurgery at the University of Pennsylvania, was convicted of sexually assaulting a woman who was enrolling in Penn's School of Veterinary Medicine. McIntosh had been the college roommate of the victim's uncle, and in September 2002, had agreed to show her around the campus. On the night of the assault, as McIntosh and the victim discussed a possible job working in his lab, they went out for drinks at several bars and restaurants near campus. At one of them, the victim claimed she started to feel sick, "strange" and "out of it," her vision blurred, and she could not hold her food down. McIntosh suggested smoking marijuana as a possible cure for her nausea. They then went to his office and smoked marijuana. The victim testified that he advanced on her sexually, but she felt unable to resist, physically immobilized as if she had been drugged on Nembutal, the "date rape" drug. "I absolutely remember him putting his penis inside of me," she said, adding that the following day, "My first reaction [when I woke up] was, 'I was just raped….' This was no mistake. This was a plotted, calculated, manipulated act." After McIntosh was charged with sexual assault, several women came forward to claim that he had also made "unwanted sexual advances" on them (Garrett & McBride, 2008). McIntosh pleaded guilty, and the judge, after factoring in his spotless academic record, including his "important work with stroke victims and brain injuries," sentenced him to fines, probation, and house arrest. However, following public outcry over what seemed an inordinately lenient sentence and an appeal by prosecutors, a new sentencing judge was assigned to his case who described McIntosh's crime as "breathtaking in its vileness." He increased McIntosh's sentence to a maximum of seven years in prison (ABC Action News, 2008).

The fifth and last single-incident case of physical sexual intrusion from the men's sample, occurred in 2017, when Cassandra Strickland, a star volleyball player at the University of Washington, was offered a ride by Roy Shick, an athletic department administrator. She had just returned from a fundraising event where she had been drinking. Her vision was "blurry," she said, she was worried about driving home on her own, and so got into Shick's truck. However, instead of driving her home, she claimed he drove behind the campus baseball fields, parked, and began kissing her. Stickland reported that she shook her head "no" when Shick asked for oral sex but otherwise felt "frozen" as he took off her shorts, groped her, and then penetrated her with his fingers and penis. In the days that followed, she told a friend what happened and confided to the athletic department's sports psychologist. But she did not file a formal complaint, not only because she found it hard to talk about the assault, but also because she said she was worried about her family's reaction, as well as how Shick's wife and children would respond. Finally, the athletic department's sports psychologist arranged for Strickland to speak anonymously with the University of Washington's Title IX investigators. Strickland followed through, Shick was placed on administrative leave, and in January 2018, he resigned. The University of Washington completed its investigation in March 2018, after interviewing 29 witnesses, including five people Strickland had spoken to about the incident, and concluded that Strickland's account was "extremely credible." The University reached a settlement with Strickland, agreeing to pay her up to $20,000 for therapy in exchange for her promise to waive any future claims against the University. And because the investigation findings were only disclosed to the University of Washington president, the UW athletic director, and a handful of employees, no record of Schick's alleged misconduct followed him. He was therefore free to apply for, and gain, the position of vice president of Grand Canyon University without that blemish on his record. However, after *The Seattle Times* alerted Grand Canyon, which, till then, knew nothing of the assault allegations, the school fired him (Fields, 2019).

Multiple-Incident Physical Sexual Intrusions by Men

In cases involving multiple physical intrusions by men, in October 2014, an Indiana University dental student alleged that Matthew C. Moeller, a professor of dentistry, touched her back and massaged her shoulders without her permission. She described three incidents. The first occurred in

July 2014, after she asked Moeller about a radiograph; she claimed that while he answered, he patted her on the back. At first, she said she dismissed it as just simple encouragement, but then he said something that struck her as odd: he mentioned that another faculty member told him that "Indian girls don't like to be touched." The second incident occurred two months later in a classroom: Moeller positioned himself in front of her while she sat in a chair; she thought he intended to greet her, but then he bent down and placed his hand on the top of her leg close to her thigh, a touch that lasted a couple of seconds. She described her reaction as stunned; she said she "froze" in her chair until the class was over. The third incident was similar: Moeller spotted her sitting in a classroom and dragged a chair over to sit next to her; next, he allegedly began massaging her back. She said this made her feel very uncomfortable, and a male student, who observed what was happening, approached and asked her if she wanted to change seats with him. Moeller then asked if he had offended her. She claims she said "no" because she was afraid of retaliation. In investigating the allegations, the University of Indiana interviewed a total of 12 students, with six of the eight female students reporting that Moeller had also touched them inappropriately: rubbing, patting, and massaging their backs and shoulders without permission. One of Moeller's former students reported that several years before, while Moeller was standing behind her as she showed him something on her laptop, he placed his hands on her shoulders, and then reached down and touched the top of her bra near her breast. Moeller acknowledged that he did on occasion touch his students in the manner they described but denied the touches were sexual and unwelcome; rather, he said he was simply trying to encourage his students and that he was, by nature, a touchy person. He added that his practice of touching students arose, in part, from his longstanding clinical depression. In his words.

> This has been a particularly difficult year, but with professional help I am learning much, and this needed change in my behavior can be part of my continued growth. I always have, and probably always will, strongly associate affectionate gestures with caring and support. About two weeks ago a student thanked me for something and gently touched my forearm. I smiled inside and out. I share my medical history not as a bid for sympathy or leniency, but rather as a factual disclosure of a significant influence on my personality/behavior (Moeller v The Board of Trustees of Indiana University, United States District Court, Southern District of Indiana, Dec. 27, 2017, p. 12).

While Moeller characterized his behavior as well-intended, he also acknowledged that he needed to change, and that the kind of touching described in the allegations "must never happen again." Nonetheless, on March 26, 2015, after completion of the University of Indiana Title IX investigation, Moeller was terminated (Russell, 2016).

In a second case involving multiple incidents, in 2019, four graduate students complained that University of Michigan computer science professor Walter Lasecki touched them sexually without obtaining consent at off-campus academic conferences. One student, who was referred to as Jane, reported that Lasecki encouraged her to drink excessively, at one point asked the waiter to bring her a "double," and then briefly placed his hand on her thigh. Later in the evening, he helped her return to her apartment, at which time she claimed he again touched her sexually. Jane reported: "When it first happened, I felt violated and disturbed but thought perhaps it was a miscommunication or misunderstanding. I also didn't know what to do about it, since we were not (and still are not) at the same institution" (Molina & Sussman, 2021). A second graduate student, referred to as Rachel, reported that Lasecki was sexually intrusive with her at four conferences: "I can't count the number of times he touched me in intimate and inappropriate ways. I'm anxious at events that he will come up to me and start touching me—it bothers me so much that I've started scanning the room at poster sessions, receptions, and parties to watch where he's at" (Molina & Sussman, 2021). A third graduate student reported that, at another conference, while she and Lasecki were talking to other people, he "leaned closer to me and essentially reached his hand between my legs. I was uncomfortable the whole time, but I distinctly remember knowing he was faculty and well-regarded, and so thinking I should be flattered. At the point where he groped my crotch, though, I knew that was past the line" (Molina & Sussman, 2021). The fourth student to allege harassment recalled how Lasecki encouraged her to drink at a social gathering: "Come on, one more," he'd say. She also recalled Lasecki touching her under her shirt despite her repeated efforts to stop his advances. Later, he tried to excuse himself: "Oh, sorry, from the way you were angling your body towards me during our meeting before, I figured you wanted me to." After 22 additional students came forward with accounts of sexual harassment by Lasecki, he resigned, effective August 2021 (Weykamp et al., 2021).

In a third multi-incident case, in 2019, University of Georgia professor of biogeochemistry, John Seaman, was suspended for two weeks without pay, following charges that he sexually harassed his former post-doctoral research associate. While allegations against him included unwelcome touching and kissing, he was also called out for intrusive comments: when the research associate began working in Seaman's lab in 2015, he allegedly told her that, "it was common ... for researchers to date or become romantically involved with students or technicians who worked in their labs." Eventually, he began inviting her for drinks and meals. After she told Seaman that she had a boyfriend, he allegedly replied that the boyfriend "was not the right kind of person for her." She also alleged that Seaman commented on how she should dress, recommending that she "should wear a skirt more often." Early in 2017, Seaman and the research associate attended a conference in Europe, with Seaman asking her to take him sightseeing since she was familiar with the area. She said she only agreed because he was her supervisor, but then found out to her surprise that Seaman, who had been tasked with making hotel reservations, booked only one room with two beds for the two of them. She said she was uncomfortable with that arrangement but could not afford a separate hotel room. So, on the nights they spent at the hotel, she waited until Seaman had fallen asleep before entering their room (Riggall, 2019).

According to Seaman's research associate, the physical sexual intrusions first occurred during meetings: when Seaman turned to talk with her, he would "often incidentally touch her leg or back." He also intruded on her physical space, she said, by making frequent, unwelcome visits to her office, a claim corroborated by witnesses. She went on to say that Seaman's most significant physical sexual intrusion—an attempted kiss—occurred outside a pub frequented by members of Seaman's lab. She also accused Seaman of attempting to sabotage her career, first, by discouraging her from applying to jobs at other universities, and second, by firing her from his lab while she waited for her new position to begin at another university. After another research professional whom Seaman supervised complained that he asked her out on a date (Riggall, 2019), Seaman sent an email to the University of Georgia newspaper, *The Red & Black*, in which he acknowledged that the incidents had occurred to his "greatest and professional regret." He went on to explain, "I am not a perfect person and I didn't always handle things in the best manner. I cooperated fully with the investigation and accepted the recommended punishment." In addition to a two-week suspension, Seaman's punishment included prohibitions "from initiating one-on-one interactions outside of work with any employee whom he supervises ... [and] from verbally commenting on or otherwise outwardly expressing his views about the physical appearance of women in the workplace" (Riggall, 2019).

The fourth multi-incident case involves a former professor of veterinary toxicology at Oregon State University, A. Morrie Craig, who, like John Seaman, was accused of making both verbal and physical sexual intrusions. In one of these cases, a freshman student whom Craig hired as a clerical assistant complained that while they were working together, he would rest his head on her shoulder and his hands in her lap or on her upper thigh. She claimed he also invited her to dinner at expensive restaurants, asked about her boyfriend, researched a male acquaintance she mentioned, and told her that when he was her age, he would go on dates with multiple women on the same night. At the same time, the clerical assistant complained that if she resisted his orders to work nights or weekends, or more hours than she was contracted to work, he would punch her arm and, in the presence of other students and coworkers, call her names such as "ornery" and "brat." The clerical assistant said that his behavior had a negative effect on her schoolwork and caused her to have nightmares and panic attacks. In his defense, Craig claimed the student never said she felt "bullied" or "sexually harassed" (Harbarger, 2018). A faculty colleague also complained about Craig: she said he came by her office so often that, to avoid him, she would turn off her office lights and lock her door, pretending she was not in. She said that while she never told him to stop coming to her office, she did tell him to stop discussing her body after he called her "zipper belly," a reference to her appendectomy scar. Still, he continued to call her "zipper belly" and even tried to touch her scar. She said he also touched her shoulders on multiple occasions in a way she felt was sexually charged. Again, Craig defended himself by saying she never told him she felt "sexually harassed" (Harbarger, 2018). Nonetheless, on May 24, 2018, the OSU board of trustees voted to terminate (Manning, 2018).

* * *

One of the main similarities between women's and men's physical sexual intrusions is that both women and men chose targets who occupied less powerful positions. Most of the presumptive perpetrators were faculty and most of their victims were students—female students. The only exceptions are Hachiyanagi's attack on a faculty colleague and Gaillardetz's alleged rape of a fellow grad student (to be discussed in the next chapter). A second similarity is that female perpetrators can appear as cunning and predatory as any man, as in the Gabriel and Wilkins' cases. They can also appear as brutal, as in the Lemley rape allegation and the Hachiyanagi attempted murder.

The main difference is the sheer volume of physical intrusions attributed to men. While only five women (Hachiyanagi, Gabriel, Wilkins, Lemley, and Rovig), 17% of the women's sample, were charged with physical sexual intrusions, 13 men, 45% of the men's sample, were so charged.

A second difference is in the serial nature of the physical sexual intrusions. Only two women, Gabriel and Wilkins, were alleged to have a history of repeated physical sexual intrusions, compared to seven men (Moeller, Lasecki, Seaman, and Craig, as well as Shipps, Moretti, and Roma who are discussed in Chap. 12 on delayed allegations).

A third difference: each of the five women accused of physical sexual intrusions chose same-sex targets—women. In comparison, each of the 13 men accused of physical sexual intrusions chose opposite-sex targets—women.

A fourth difference: each of the five women accused of physical sexual intrusions lost their academic positions following the allegations: four were fired outright and one—Lemley—resigned immediately following the assault allegations. Among the 13 men accused of physical sexual intrusions, five kept their positions: two, Seaman and Bavel, received a brief suspension, and three, discussed in the next chapter, received no penalty.

References

ABC Action News. (2008, February 13). Up to 7 years for professor. *ABC Action News*. https://6abc.com/archive/5955240/

Crabbe, N. (2011, September 14). Bassoonist ends UF career on a sour note. *Gainesville Sun*. https://www.gainesville.com/story/sports/college/2011/09/14/bassoonist-ends-uf-career-on-sour-note/64272004007/

Epstein, J. (2007, June 12). 2 professors resign amid rape charges. *Inside Higher Ed*. https://www.insidehighered.com/news/2007/06/13/2-professors-resign-amid-rape-charges

Fields, A. (2019, June 12). UW finds star athlete's sexual assault allegation credible, but athletic Executive quietly moved on. *Seattle Times*. https://www.seattletimes.com/subscribe/signup-offers/?pw=redirect&subsource=paywall&return=https://www.seattletimes.com/seattle-news/uw-athletic-executive-quietly-leaves-after-sexual-misconduct-investigation-finds-new-job-at-another-college/

Flaherty, C. (2019a, January 30). U of Michigan music professor arrested for assault. *Inside Higher Ed*. https://www.insidehighered.com/quicktakes/2019/01/31/u-michigan-music-professor-arrested-assault

Flaherty, C. (2019b, August 26). A culture of sexual harassment. *Inside Higher Ed*. https://www.insidehighered.com/news/2019/08/27/star-scholar-minority-serving-institutions-was-accused-fostering-hypersexualized-and

Garrett, E., & McBride, M. A. (2008, February 14). Ex-prof gets prison sentence for sex assault. *The Daily Pennsylvanian*. https://www.thedp.com/article/2008/02/exprof_gets_prison_sentence_for_sex_assault_w_interactive_feature#:~:text=Former%20Neurosurgery%20professor%20Tracy%20McIntosh,of%20his%20college%20roommate's%20niece.

Green, J. (2020, November 24). UNCG investigating Preston Lane, former instructor accused of sexual abuse. *Triad City Beat*. https://triad-city-beat.com/uncg-investigating-preston-lane-former-instructor-accused-sexual-abuse/

Green, J. (2021, January 22). UNCG theater professor resigns following accounts of abuse by former Students. *Triad City Beat*. https://triad-city-beat.com/uncg-theater-professor-resigns-abuse/

Hackett, C. (2018, November 5). Reclaiming our voices: Victims' statement on Amy Wilkins' abuse of students. *Medium*. https://medium.com/@colleenfirehawk/reclaiming-our-voices-victims-statement-on-amy-wilkins-abuse-of-students-99e8b39a5792

Harbarger, M. (2018, September 14). OSU professor's firing for sexual harassment, bullying upheld by Benton County judge. *Oregonian*. https://www.oregonlive.com/education/2018/09/osu_professors_firing_for_sexu.html

Klamann, S. (2020, November 13). CU board of regents votes to dismiss professor accused of sexual harassment. *Denver Gazette*. https://medium.com/@colleenfirehawk/reclaiming-our-voices-victims-statement-on-amy-wilkins-abuse-of-students-99e8b39a5792

Manning, J. (2018, May 25). OSU trustees uphold dismissal of professor accused of sexual harassment, bullying. *The Oregonian*. https://www.oregonlive.com/education/2018/05/osu_trustees_upholds_sex_haras.html

McAboy, K. (2018, August 24). University of Michigan professor accused of rape. *All about Ann Arbor*. https://www.clickondetroit.com/all-about-ann-arbor/2018/08/24/university-of-michigan-professor-accused-of-rape/

Molina, N., & Sussman, S. (2021, May 19). Daily investigation finds divergence in U-M, outside organizations' handling of allegations against CSE professor. *Michigan Daily*. https://www.michigandaily.com/news/daily-investigation-finds-divergence-in-u-m-outside-organizations-handling-of-allegations-against-cse-professor/

Riggall, H. (2019, November 11). UGA professor suspended after sexual harassment investigation, Records show. *The Red & Black*. https://www.redandblack.com/uganews/uga-professor-suspended-after-sexual-harassment-investigation-records-show/article_e109855e-0423-11ea-a1c0-575a7f890481.html

Russell, J. (2016, February 26). Former dentistry clinic director sues IU over firing. *Indianapolis Business Journal*. https://www.ibj.com/articles/57407-former-dentistry-clinic-director-sues-iu-over-firing

Saunders, J., Hartnett, E., & Blackney, K. (1987, May 8). Gaither interviewed: Will not resign. *Triangle*. https://services.library.drexel.edu/static_files/triangle/Drexel-Triangle_1987-05-08.pdf

Shepherd, S. (2014, October 19). 85-year-old professor accused of sexual harassment battling KU And its policies in court. *Lawrence Journal-World*. https://www2.ljworld.com/news/2014/oct/19/85-year-old-professor-accused-sexual-harassment-ba/

Stevens, W. K. (1987, June 7). Harassment charge poses threat to leadership of Drexel U. Head. *New York Times*. https://www.nytimes.com/1987/06/07/us/harassment-charge-poses-threat-to-leadership-of-drexel-u-head.html

Veltman, C. (2023, August 4). Opera singer David Daniels pleads guilty in sexual assault trial. *NPR*. https://www.npr.org/2023/08/04/1192210280/opera-singer-david-daniels-pleads-guilty-sexual-assault

Weykamp, G., Sussman, S. & Molina, N. (2021, May 28). Walter Lasecki resigns effective Aug. 30 amid new sexual harassment allegations. *Daily Michigan*. https://www.michigandaily.com/news/walter-lasecki-resigns-effective-august-30-amid-new-sexual-harassment-allegations/

Wilson, R. (1997, January 17). 2 Truman State professors resign after assault complaint. *Chronicle of Higher Education*. https://www.chronicle.com/article/2-truman-state-professors-resign-after-assault-complaint/

CHAPTER 12

Delayed Allegations

Accusations of sexual harassment often surface decades after the harassment episodes occurred, a phenomenon illustrated in the cases of several prominent individuals, including U.S Republican politician Roy Moore, Supreme Court Justice Brett Kavanaugh, and film producer Harvey Weinstein, each of whom was accused of sexual offenses dating back more than 30 years. Delays of this kind can be explained by victims' fear of harasser retaliation, their fear that they will be blamed or will not be believed, as well as by their fear of negative responses from family, friends, co-workers, and employers. They may even fear that if they were to tell others about the harassment they experienced, they might be forced to move or change jobs (Balogh et al., 2003; von Sikorski & Saumer, 2021). This chapter examines the cases of four men identified in the subsample of 29 men randomly selected from the Academic Sexual Misconduct Database whose accusers came forward more than 30 years after the harassment occurred.

"Recent Events in the News Have Sparked Memories."

In October 2017, the *New York Times* published allegations of sexual misconduct against Harvey Weinstein, which reminded a woman, identified only as Jane, that she had been sexually assaulted by her music professor,

© The Author(s), under exclusive license to Springer Nature Switzerland AG 2024

L. Margolin, *Women Accused of Sexual Harassment*,
https://doi.org/10.1007/978-3-031-79021-8_12

Stephen Shipps, more than 40 years earlier, when he was on the faculty of the University of North Carolina, and she was 16-years-old. This is the email in which Jane notified an administrator from the University of Michigan, where Shipps was currently a professor of music, that she had been assaulted by him:

> Recent events in the news have sparked memories from my past. Honestly, I've written letters/emails in the past but have not sent them because I didn't see the point. I guess I'm emboldened now. Who knows. Of course I expect absolutely nothing to come from this email. I don't know you and there's nothing you or anyone could do at this point anyway. So, here's the thing … Stephen Shipps raped me when I was sixteen. Over the years, I've heard stories similar to mine regarding Mr. Shipps, and, believe me, I've met many men who were cut from the same cloth as Prof. Shipps. I was telling [redacted] about all the incidents of sexual harassment or abuse I have encountered, and I was shocked that I have endured so much.
>
> Really, I should have spoken up years ago, because I'm sure my encounter was not anything new for him. At this point, I'm just a statistic that can't be proven. Plus, he's probably not really a danger anymore, given his age. He's still the same predator. Just look him in the eyes for me and know who he is. And maybe even keep an eye on his female students. Probably too late …
>
> Thanks for listening (Sussman, 2019).

Although university employees are required to report sexual harassment allegations to Title IX "as soon as possible upon learning of the behavior," more than a year elapsed before Jane received an email acknowledging her complaint. It's unclear why it took so long for the University of Michigan to respond, but what is clear is that such a delay affirms and supports victims' reticence to speak out. In the words of one of Shipps' victims, "Reporting and discussing these painful events takes a significant personal toll on those who report, and having those statements ignored reinforces victim's conditioning that it is not ok to talk about abuse, and if you do you will be ignored" (Sussman, 2019).

After waiting 408 days, Jane finally heard from Title IX, an investigation ensued, and shortly thereafter, the student newspaper, *The Daily Michigan*, followed up by interviewing Shipps' current and former students, one of whom, Maureen O'Boyle, shared what happened when, at the age of 17, in the spring of 1977, she began studying violin with Shipps and babysitting his children. O'Boyle claimed that one evening, during a party at Shipps' home, he poured strong alcoholic drinks for her, and then, after the other guests left, he sexually assaulted her. "I was very drunk, and very high, incoherent." She said that was how she lost her virginity. "I do vaguely remember that moment, though most of it is a blackout. [I] remember knowing what was happening with the feeling that my life was already horribly off course" (Sussman, 2018, p. 25). O'Boyle's studies with Shipps did not end there, nor did her job as his children's babysitter. "I babysat regularly, often spending the night in the spare bedroom," she said. "Sometimes we had violin lessons; sometimes Steve just wanted a blowjob on the couch" (Sussman, 2018, p. 26). Although O'Boyle went on to become a professor of music at the University of Tulsa, she said her experiences as Shipps' victim had profound negative effects on her professional life, especially regarding her relationships with students:

> I have never socialized with my students, other than at public, post-concert events. There is no couch in my office at TU or at home. I don't even hug my students, except after degree recitals in front of their parents (Sussman, 2018, p. 37).

During the 1980s, another young violinist, identified as Anne, began studying with Shipps at North Carolina. She also babysat his children and claimed that she was 16-years-old, when, in his car, as he drove her home from babysitting, he first sexually assaulted her. "For the next few months, I sometimes had a lesson during my scheduled slot. Other times we were engaged in heavy petting and he taught me how to perform oral sex on him" (Sussman, 2018).

The Michigan Daily's investigation into Shipps' background unearthed a whole network of current and former students dating back four decades who claimed that they had been sexually assaulted by him. *The Daily* also found evidence that at least one music department faculty member knew of the allegations against Shipps before he began teaching at Michigan in 1989 (Sussman, 2018). Within 48 hours of the appearance of *Daily's* first article on Shipps, he withdrew from his chairmanship of the school's string department and resigned as director of the Strings Preparatory Academy, a pre-college program at the University. A criminal investigation soon followed which led, ultimately, to Shipps' criminal conviction, and in April 2022, he was sentenced to five years in prison for transporting a minor across state lines with the intent to engage in sexual conduct (AP News Wire, 2022).

"Now 30-odd Years Later, I Know He Can't Hurt Me."

A second case involving delayed harassment allegations involved complaints against Franco Moretti, a professor whom the *New York Times* described, on Oct. 30, 2017, as the brilliant literary critic responsible for "promoting a ruthlessly impersonal idea of both scholarship and literary history" (Schuessler). Then, a week later, on Nov. 5, Kimberly Latta, Moretti's former graduate student, much like Jane in the Shipps' case, cited the #MeToo movement as the inspiration for sharing the details of her victimization. In her essay, she described Moretti as a predator who "stalked, pressured, and raped" her while she was studying at UC-Berkeley more than 30 years earlier (Latta, 2017). Latta said her relationship with Moretti was at first consensual ("He was cool. He was hip.... Franco demonstrated a great deal of interest in me, and I foolishly believed it was because he found me intelligent"), but after three or four months, she claimed the relationship shifted into psychological and physical sexual coercion. She recalled how he assaulted her in her apartment, pushing her down onto her futon, and how she tried to resist:

> I remember I said, "no." I remember I said I'm not comfortable with this "I don't want to." I remember him saying "Oh, you American women, when you say no, you mean yes." I remember leaving my body and hovering somewhere around the ceiling, looking down and telling myself, "This is not happening to me. It is happening to her, to that body, not to me, not to me, not to me."

She said he also raped her on campus, "where he would push me up against a wall in his office, right next to the window that looked out at the library, and push up my skirt and bra and forcibly kiss me, against my will." When she tried to resist, she alleged that he told her that "professors in Italy routinely slept with graduate students, so why was I being such a prude?" Latta claimed she reported him in 1985 to Title IX, but that the officer she spoke to, a colleague of Moretti's, discouraged her: she knew him quite well, and urged Latta not to file—"She was on his side." When Latta told Moretti that she had spoken with the Title IX officer, he allegedly threatened to ruin her career if she were to press charges against him. "He said he had powerful friends who were attorneys who would ruin my name." Latta explained why she waited so many years: "I wanted to speak out long ago but was afraid," she wrote. "He threatened me, after all.

Now, 30-odd years later, I know he can't hurt me." What also motivated her to finally come forward, she said, is "the hundreds of women who have spoken out—including Anita Hill, and all the women who exposed Bill Cosby, Harvey Weinstein, Louis C. K., and others ... [they] inspired me to tell my story" (Latta, 2017).

Following Latta's allegations against Moretti, two new allegations against him surfaced, one from a former graduate student who claimed that, in 1995, during a six-week summer seminar at Dartmouth, she had to set her dog on him to get him to stop chasing her around her house: "He acted as if it were a game, but I was alarmed.... He scared the hell out of me." The second allegation originated at Johns Hopkins, in 1997, when Moretti was applying for a position in the English department. A graduate student reported that during his visit, Moretti touched her inappropriately and, after she shared this information with members of the department, they decided against hiring him (Liu & Knowles, 2017).

Moretti denied Latta's allegations, claiming their sexual relationship was consensual, and while the Title IX coordinator for Stanford expressed interest in Latta's allegations, no formal investigation was launched, and Moretti, who retired from Stanford in 2017, was never reprimanded.

"My Brother, My Colleague, My Rapist. Thou Art the Man."

Like Jane's allegations against Shipps and Kimberly Latta's against Moretti, Laura Grimes' allegations against Richard Gaillardetz, former chair of Boston College's theology department, concerned assaults that occurred more than 30 years earlier. She posted her allegations in YouTube videos (2021), asserting, "Richard R. Gaillardetz, Joseph Professor of Systematic Theology at Boston College; my brother, my colleague, my rapist. Thou art the man." A second similarity to the Shipps and Moretti cases is that Gaillardetz was a highly successful academic: the author and editor of 13 books, he was the past president of the Catholic Theological Society of America, the largest professional association of Catholic theologians in the world. A third similarity: the allegations against Gaillardetz, like those against Shipps and Moretti, involve sexual encounters witnessed only by the two principals. There were no third-party observers who could have testified for or against Gaillardetz. A fourth similarity is that Gaillardetz, like Moretti, denied the assaults occurred. (Shipps finally acknowledged the assaults in court as part of a plea agreement.)

A major difference is that Gaillardetz and his accuser occupied the same institutional positions: both were graduate students at the time of the alleged assaults. Moreover, Gaillardetz, unlike Shipps and Moretti, had no record of other sexual offenses. Grimes was his only accuser. Finally, only Gaillardetz's accuser, Laura Grimes, was charged with lying: her allegations against Gaillardetz were portrayed as malicious fabrications.

Laura Grimes alleged that Gaillardetz assaulted her in her apartment on Halloween night 1987, and did so again in her apartment, less than two months later. At the time, they were both doctoral students at Notre Dame University and had become friends, according to Grimes, through their shared interest in theology and spirituality. On the night of the first incident, Grimes claims that Gaillardetz invited her to his apartment to share dinner with a few friends. After the friends left, she alleged that Gaillardetz assaulted her in his bedroom. Her initial response to the assault, she said, was a sense of personal shame; she felt she was responsible. At the time, she believed that she participated in the sex act voluntarily and had given Gaillardetz her consent. So, after she shared what happened in confession, she decided to ask Gaillardetz for forgiveness. "I think we were sitting in the Huddle [a Notre Dame food court] … talking over lunch, and I was gagged out apologizing to him," she said. "And now I think I apologized to my rapist." The second assault allegedly occurred in early December, the same year. She said that Gaillardetz, despite her repeated refusals, "bullied" her into going upstairs to her bedroom. There, she said he performed oral sex on her and then demanded that she do the same for him. She said she complied: "It made me gag but I went along with it" (Zacharias, 2021). What motivated Grimes, after so many years, to come forward with assault allegations was hearing Gaillardetz speak about sex abuse scandals in the clergy. She claimed she was struck by the hypocrisy: "he's everything he's pointing his finger at." She went on to say that Catholic theologians, like Gaillardetz, "instead of cleaning up their own house—their very serious problems—they're instead pretending they're the heroes and they're gonna save us from the bad bishop and the bad priests." She added that she finally came forward because she had come to recognize that her sexual encounters with Gaillardetz were not consensual, as she once thought: "Over the past several years, I've started to see more and more what he did to me was really horrible and was not consensual and realized, 'Oh, I need to speak about this'" (Kelly et al., 2021).

Boston College responded to Grimes' allegations by hiring an independent law firm to investigate (White, 2021). The law firm concluded, after claiming to have considered "the totality of the evidence gathered," that Grimes' allegations were without merit. In investigators' words, her allegations were "not only not credible but are also false" (Kelly, 2021).

Previous chapters discussed allegations against women which appeared unclear, exaggerated, and/or contrived. In the Gaillardetz case, the allegations appear similarly questionable on three levels: (1) they concern assaults that occurred more than 30 years earlier, (2) there were no third-party witnesses, and (3) there was no rape-kit evidence. What may appear even more questionable in the Gaillardetz case, however, is the definitiveness of the investigative conclusion—the finding that Grimes' allegations were "not only not credible but are also false." Such a conclusion appears suspect for the same reasons that the allegations against Gaillardetz might appear suspect: the 30-year time lapse between the alleged assaults and their investigations, as well as the absence of third-party witnesses and material evidence. How could investigators prove that no sexual activity occurred between Grimes and Gaillardetz? Alternatively, if investigators were to acknowledge that sexual activity had occurred, as Grimes contended, how could they have proven that she gave her consent? Even if Gaillardetz had insisted that Grimes consented to sex, how could he have known, definitively, that she consented, given the reality that individuals often experience the same sexual encounter in different ways: what appears to one person as knowing, voluntary, and clear permission to proceed, can be experienced by the other as confusing, abhorrent, and coercive. Casting further doubt on the definitive dismissal of the assault allegations is the absence of transparency—no evidence was publicly shared regarding how the "not credible and false" investigative conclusion was accomplished. A final concern: Grimes' claim that the investigators patronized her, interviewing her in a "hostile" and "cursory" manner (Kelly, 2021). In Grimes' estimate, the conclusion that her allegations were not credible was absurd and vindictive, as well as "dangerously misleading given the implication that the sexual incidents never occurred—which I doubt Dr. Gaillardetz alleged—rather than the more probable defense of supposed consensuality" (Kelly, 2021).

For his part, Gaillardetz opined that, given the investigation's "decisive findings ... I do not think it is necessary or appropriate to engage in a point-by-point response to the specific allegations" (Catholic News Service, 2021). This, of course, raises the question: how is it possible to arrive at "decisive findings" without responses to the specific allegations? How can the truth or falsity of the allegations be established without a "point-by-point" analysis?

While awareness of sexual exploitation and harassment may have changed in the wake of the #MeToo movement, many informal practices have not, including victim-blaming (Bongiorno et al., 2020; Whiting, 2019). Which may explain why, after Boston College published its conclusion that Grimes' allegations were false, Grimes was denounced. She was called hateful and insane, and critics argued that she should be held legally responsible for slandering Gaillardetz. "While it may seem the height of uncharity to initiate legal proceedings against a woman as unfortunate as yourself," one observer (O'Leary, 2020) messaged Grimes, "I think that were your victims to do so, they would be doing a service to the civil and ecclesial communities." Gaillardetz's response appears intended, on one level, to reflect compassion for Grimes, a woman whose life he characterized as difficult and troubled. "I am sorry for her suffering," he said. But, in keeping with a long-standing norm of sexual harassment, he blamed her for claiming victimization (Abrams et al., 2003; Ask & Landstrom, 2010; Dawtry et al., 2019; Grubb & Turner, 2012; Von Sikorski & Saumer, 2021). He blamed her for making contrived and unjust allegations that imposed pain and suffering on many people, including his wife and family, and "the cause of true victims everywhere. They undermine the privileged concern that victims rightly deserve and expect" (Kelly, 2021).

"It Should Not Have Been Allowed to Happen"

The fourth case of delayed allegations involves another female accuser, Mozhan Marno, who, like Grimes, was blamed for coming forward with sexual assault allegations: the Columbia University panel responsible for investigating her allegations determined that she had "provoked and contributed to" her professor's sexual advances (O'Connor & Alba, 2018). In 1998, when her harassment allegedly occurred, Columbia did not have policies which would have prohibited 48-year-old professor Thomas Roma from engaging in sexual activity with his 18-year-old student. Such policies were not enacted until 2012. With sexual relationships between faculty and students permissible, it was up to the Columbia panel to determine whether the sexual activity was coercive and predatory, and not whether sexual activity occurred. Marno claimed that Roma's advances began in his office, which she had to visit for her final one-on-one photography critique. She claimed that Roma told her that he did not need to see the seminude self-portrait she submitted, since he had been thinking about her nude body and "knew exactly what she looked like." The following semester, she claimed that Roma began pursuing her aggressively, at one point inviting her to his office, where, she said, he kissed her, put his mouth on her breast, undressed her, and then unzipped his fly and placed her hand on his penis. She said the experience "freaked me out ... I came to the realization that I should never have been put in the place to have experienced any of those things, and thus, it should not have been allowed to happen" (O'Connor & Alba, 2018). In her senior year, in 2000, Marnò filed her complaint against Roma. After Columbia investigators became aware of three other Columbia students who said Roma had sexually harassed them, they concluded that, even though Marno may have "provoked" Roma, he was partly responsible and was ordered to see a therapist. He was also ordered to attend "workshops or courses" specific to "increas[ing] his understanding of the developmental issues extant with late adolescent/early adult undergraduate students, especially with regard to their sexual and cognitive identities" (O'Connor & Alba, 2018). But he was allowed to continue teaching and was told that if no new harassment complaints were lodged against him, the previous complaints would be expunged from his record. As for Marno, the complainant, Columbia told her that if she wanted to keep studying photography, she should do so at another university, a penalty which, combined with the trauma of her harassment, made her lose faith in the educational system: "I didn't forge personal relationships with teachers. I didn't invest in the place as a whole," and from then on, viewed having a professional mentor relationship with men impossible (O'Connor & Alba, 2018).

According to interviews conducted by the *New York Times* as well as documents obtained by the *New York Times* and *BuzzFeed News*, additional harassment allegations surfaced against Roma, some dating back to the 1980s (Sutton, 2018). In 1985, for example, one of Roma's former students, then a 19-year-old undergraduate at Yale, claimed he invited her to his apartment where he got down on his knees and propositioned her for sex in a way she found "coercive" and "abusive." Another former student told *BuzzFeed News* that Roma would sometimes interrupt class to tell her to meet him in the hall, where he would ask her to kiss him. Two other former students said that Roma had them place their hands on his crotch; one described him touching her breast, and asking her to have sex with him, which she declined. During a *New York Times* interview, one of his students from the 1990s revealed that on one occasion, while she was sitting alone at a desk, Roma suddenly began advancing toward her with his erect penis exposed. She claimed that he put his penis in her mouth, committing "oral rape against me," a charge that, to this day, has not been acknowledged either by Columbia University or by Roma (Sutton, 2018).

The interviews and documents reveal that Columbia University knew that Roma had a reputation for making sexual advances to his female students which began with flattering them, then pressuring them, and then, as he advanced sexually, reminding them of his professional stature. But Columbia, except for the Marno allegations, chose not to investigate. In fact, Roma's lawyer said he was "shocked" by the new allegations which, he said, are "replete with inaccuracies and falsehoods. All … have been isolated, innocent incidents, none of them predatory, and have created fictitious versions of reality that are libelous and in the present political climate [a reference to the #MeToo Movement] designed to damage his career and personal life" (Alexander, Jan. 6, 2018). Roma retired "voluntarily" in 2018 without receiving an official reprimand.

* * *

Two of the key differences between physical sexual intrusion cases in the women's and men's samples are delayed allegations and the kinds of penalties which followed. At one extreme, Amy Wilkins, from the women's sample, was formally accused of sexual harassment after a lapse of 12 years following reports of physical sexual intrusions. Her penalty: termination. However, four men were formally accused of physical intrusions after a much greater lapse—more than 30 years. Their penalty: one was fired, convicted, and sentenced to prison. The other three received no formal penalty.

References

Abrams, D., Viki, T., Masser, B., & Bohner, G. (2003). Perceptions of stranger and acquaintance rape: The role of benevolent and hostile sexism in victim blame and rape proclivity. *Journal of Personality and Social Psychology, 84*(1), 111–125. https://doi.org/10.1037/0022-3514.84.1.111

AP News Wire. (2022, April 15). Ex-Michigan music professor gets prison on child sex charges. *Independent*. https://www.independent.co.uk/news/ap-university-of-michigan-detroit-ann-arbor-nebraska-b2058796.html

Ask, K., & Landström, S. (2010). Why emotions matter: Expectancy violation and affective response mediate the emotional victim effect. *Law and Human Behavior, 34*(5), 392–401. https://doi.org/10.1007/s10979-009-9208-6

Balogh, D. W., Kite, M. E., Pickel, K. L., Canel, D., & Schroeder, J. (2003). The effects of delayed report and motive for reporting on perceptions of sexual harassment. *Sex Roles, 48*(7/8), 337–348. https://doi.org/10.1023/A:1022990530657280C

Bongiorno, R., Langbroek, C., Bain, P. G., Ting, M., & Ryan, M. K. (2020). Why women are blamed for being sexually harassed: The effects of empathy for female victims and male perpetrators. *Psychology of Women Quarterly, 44*(1), 11–27. https://doi.org/10.1177/0361684319868730

Catholic News Service. (2021, April 6). Investigation finds claims against Boston College theologian not credible. *Crux*. https://cruxnow.com/church-in-the-usa/2021/04/investigation-finds-claims-against-boston-college-theologian-not-credible

Dawtry, R. J., Cozzolino, P. J., & Callan, M. J. (2019). I blame therefore I was: Rape myth acceptance, victim blaming, and memory reconstruction. *Personality and Social Psychology Bulletin, 45*(8), 1269–1282. https://doi.org/10.1177/0146167218818475

Grubb, A., & Turner, E. (2012). Attribution of blame in rape cases: A review of the impact of rape myth acceptance, gender role conformity and substance use on victim blaming. *Aggressive and Violent Behavior, 17*(5), 443–452. https://doi.org/10.1016/j.avb.2012.06.002

Kelly, M. (2021, April 5). Investigation finds allegations against theology chair false and not credible. *The Heights*. https://www.bcheights.com/2021/04/05/investigation-finds-allegations-against-theology-chair-not-credible-and-false/

Kelly, M., Kiersznowski, J., & Stefanescu, V. (2021, March 21). BC theology department chair accused of sexual assault. *The Heights*. https://www.bcheights.com/2021/03/01/bc-theo-chair-accused-of-sexual-assault/#:~:text=Boston%20College%20is%20investigating%20allegations,the%20University%20of%20Notre%20Dame

Latta, K. (2017, November 17). What happened? *Stanford Politics*. https://stanfordpolitics.org/2017/11/17/op-ed-latta-what-happened-franco-moretti/

Liu, F., & Knowles, H. (2017, Nov. 16). Harassment, assault allegations against Moretti span three campuses. *Stanford Daily*. https://stanforddaily.com/2017/11/16/harassment-assault-allegations-against-moretti-span-three-campuses/

O'Connor, E., & Alba, D. (2018, March 1). She "provoked" him: Columbia's old policies let a Professor off the hook for sexual harassment. *BuzzFeed News*. https://www.buzzfeednews.com/article/emaoconnor/columbia-thomas-roma-professor-student-sexual-harassment

O'Leary, J. (2020). *@josepholeary3286. Ecclesial rape culture #1: Introduction.* https://www.youtube.com/watch?v=4w40saeWZZQ

Sussman, S. (2018, December 10). Former students bring 40 years of misconduct allegations against SMTP professor. *Daily Michigan.* https://www.michigan-daily.com/news/community-affairs/former-students-bring-40-years-misconduct-allegations-smtd-professor/

Sussman, S. (2019, February 5). Sexual misconduct complaint about U-M professor goes unanswered for more than a year. *Michigan Daily.* https://www.michigandaily.com/news/focal-point/sexual-misconduct-complaint-about-u-professor-goes-unanswered-over-year/

Sutton, B. (2018, January 3). Thomas Roma, photographer and Columbia University professor, accused of sexual harassment [updated]. *Hyperallergic.* https://hyperallergic.com/419929/thomas-roma-sexual-misconduct-accusations/

von Sikorski, C., & Saumer, M. (2021). Sexual harassment in politics. News about victims' delayed sexual harassment accusations and effects on victim blaming: A mediation model. *Mass Communication and Society, 24*(2), 259–287. https://doi.org/10.1080/15205436.2020.1769136

White, C. (2021, February 25). Boston College investigates prominent theologian after sexual assault allegation. *National Catholic Reporter.* https://www.ncronline.org/boston-college-investigates-prominent-theologian-after-sexual-assault-allegation

Whiting, J. (2019, January 16). How denial and victim blaming keep sexual assault hidden. *Psychology Today.* https://www.psychologytoday.com/us/blog/love-lies-and-confict/201901/how-denial-and-victim-blaming-keep-sexual-assault-hidden

Zacharias, S. (2021, March 9). "I apologized to my rapist": ND alumna accuses former classmate, chair of BC theology department of sexual assault. *BishopAccountability.Org.* https://www.bishop-accountability.org/2021/03/i-apologized-to-my-rapist-nd-alumna-accuses-former-classmate-chair-of-bc-theology-department-of-sexual-assault/

CHAPTER 13

Conclusions and Recommendations

Research Limitations

In the spirit of transparency, I would like to share a note of caution about the findings. First, there is the matter of the inconsistency/unevenness of the data. At one extreme, the cases of famous individuals, including those charged with sensational violations and individuals, like Jane Gallop (1997), who have written or spoken extensively about their cases, provide much more detailed and elaborate records than do cases involving individuals who are relatively obscure. In some instances, individuals charged with sexual harassment refused to make public statements about the allegations and in others, where those charged with harassment did give statements, the investigators redacted them to protect the reputations of the victims and alleged harassers. Victims' statements are similarly uneven, some rich and detailed, while others are fragmentary and redacted.

A related limitation is that the Academic Sexual Misconduct Database does not provide a definition of "sexual harassment." As a result, academic institutions, in making referrals to the Database, can define "sexual harassment" in any way they wish, which, of course, makes the data less reliable and comparable.

A further limitation has to do with unknown possible reporting biases. Many cases of sexual harassment on college and university campuses go unreported or unrecorded. Observers often claim they failed to come

© The Author(s), under exclusive license to Springer Nature Switzerland AG 2024

L. Margolin, *Women Accused of Sexual Harassment*,
https://doi.org/10.1007/978-3-031-79021-8_13

forward because they did not think anything would be done about the harassment, they feared retaliation, doubted that people in authority would believe them, or they dismissed their experience as "small stuff," not the kind of thing worthy of their or anyone else's attention (Fisher, 2000; Ilies et al., 2003; Pershing, 2003; Vohlidalova, 1999). And many fail to come forward because they believe it would diminish their chances of career advancement (Hart, 2019). The problem for this research is not only that we have no way of estimating the number of these unreported, unrecorded cases, it is that the propensity to observe, report, or record sexual harassment by women may differ markedly from the propensity to observe, report, or record sexual harassment by men.

Finally, some colleges and universities may report all or most sexual harassment investigations to the Academic Sexual Misconduct Database, but many do not—an additional unknown. To illustrate how arbitrary this reporting can appear, consider that Northwestern University referred two male professors to the Database who were accused of sexual harassment, but did not refer to the Database, Laura Kipnis, a female professor also accused of sexual harassment and investigated by Title IX. Charges against her came from a student who claimed that an essay Kipnis (2015a) wrote about sexual politics on campus for the *Chronicle Review* had a "chilling effect" on students' ability to report sexual misconduct and from a second who claimed that Kipnis had created a hostile campus environment by briefly mentioning her name in connection with a sexual harassment lawsuit. As in Jane Gallop's case, students staged a protest against Kipnis and the campus newspaper broadcast students' demands for "a swift, official condemnation" of Kipnis' alleged wrongdoing (Kipnis, 2015b). Again, the problem for this research is that we have no way of estimating the number of Title IX investigations that are not submitted to the Database, and we have no way of knowing whether the propensity to submit records pertaining to women's sexual harassment may differ from the propensity to submit records pertaining to men's harassment.

The Knowns

The Sexual Harassment Attributed to Women Appears Different from Harassment Attributed to Men

Allegations of women's harassment, unlike men's, target behaviors that appear wide-ranging and heterogeneous. They defy predictability. Illustrating this heterogeneity, several harassment allegations against women appeared to have no counterpart in harassment allegations against men—neither in the random sample of men accused of harassment, nor in the entire Academic Sexual Misconduct Database. In one case, for example, a female Spanish instructor was charged with harassment for pressuring her female TAs to date male students. Why? She thought that would be an effective way of increasing male students' enrollment in Spanish classes. In a second case, a female professor attempted to intimidate and terrorize an elite group of firefighters known as "hot shots," a group deployed by the Forest Service and National Park Service to battle wildland forest fires. She is the only individual on the Academic Sexual Misconduct Database accused of stalking an entire community. In a third case, a female professor stalked and harassed a male professor whom she insisted was stalking and harassing her; she insisted, despite Title IX's failure, after multiple investigations, to find any evidence that the male professor was, in fact, stalking and harassing her. Her sexual misconduct appeared to be a case of "false victimization syndrome," a rare disorder unmatched by anyone else listed on the Academic Sexual Misconduct Database. In a fourth anomalous case, a professor showed up unannounced at the home of her friend and colleague, saying she needed to talk to her "about feelings" because her boyfriend had just broken up with her. However, as soon as she stepped inside, she hit her colleague with something hard, and continued to rain blows down on her with anything she could find, including a rock, a fire poker, and garden shears, proclaiming for the next four hours—the duration of the attack—her intention to blind, disfigure, and finally murder her victim.

The value of these strange stories—their theoretical importance—is that they reveal the randomness of women's sexual harassment behavior. They reveal not only that sexual harassment attributed to women is rare compared to men's, but also, unlike men's, it lacks a dominant logic or pattern. To say this another way, the unpredictability—the randomness—of harassment allegations levelled against women highlights the contrasting predictability of harassment allegations against men. It highlights how men's sexual harassment can be expected to possess a familiar set of features long associated with sexual harassment—sexual desire, sexual objectification, aggression, and antagonism—while among women, neither sexual desire nor antagonism (the desire to put targets down) appears as the primary incentive driving sexual harassment. Consider that only nine out of the 29 cases in the women's sample appeared to include evidence of sexual desire as part of the harassment allegation (Naca, Hoffarth, Hale, Chatman, Parker, Rovig, Wilkins, Gabriel, and Lemley), a figure that could be increased by three if Avital Ronell, Anna Stubblefield, and Roxana Recio are added. However, those additions would be controversial. First, because it is unclear whether Ronell, a lesbian, had a sexual or merely affectionate/platonic preoccupation with her male graduate student. The same applies to Anna Stubblefield and Roxana Recio. For while Stubblefield admitted to engaging in sexual activity with her presumptive victim, a 30-year-old man with severe cerebral palsy who could not talk or walk, no one claimed she found him physically attractive, no one claimed she had a sexual interest in his body, and no evidence emerged to contradict her claim that the sexual activity she had with him was primarily *for him*—to meet his needs. And while Roxana Recio may have sent a seemingly endless series of email messages professing affection for her target, no evidence surfaced which pointed to Recio's sexual, as opposed to platonic, interest.

Consider also that only four women accused of sexual harassment appeared primarily motivated by feelings of hostility with no admixture of sexual desire (e.g., the woman who attempted to kill a colleague, another who called her supervisees names such as "nigger," "bitch," "white bitch," and "fat bitch," a third who stalked a team of firefighters, and a fourth who stalked an academic colleague she believed was stalking her). That leaves 25 cases involving women as possible harassers (84% of the women's sample) lacking evidence of significant hostile motivation. Anna Stubblefield may have been found guilty of sexual coercion and sentenced to 12 years in prison, but it was without evidence of hostile motivation. The Maillo case, in which an instructor was accused of attempting to coerce graduate teaching assistants to date undergraduates in a scheme to increase course enrollments, and the Recio case, involving a faculty member's seemingly ceaseless expressions of affection and longing for another faculty member, although clearly troubling to their targets, also appeared to lack evidence of hostile motivation. The same applies to the Rovig case in which a female administrator was accused of indiscriminately kissing and groping several of members of her staff at an off-campus bar. Her presumptive victims may have been disturbed by her behavior, but they also appeared willing to see it as a fluke resulting from extreme intoxication.

What stands out in allegations of men's harassment—why it is so much more predictable and homogeneous than women's—is the prominent role played by sexual desire: men's tendency to evaluate targets in terms of their physical characteristics and sexual appeal. Among the 29 cases of harassment attributed to men randomly selected from the Academic

Sexual Misconduct Database, none showed that the desire to diminish, deprecate, or harm their targets was their *primary* motivation. While many men accused of harassment may have felt contempt for their targets, and may have even desired, on some level, to diminish, deprecate, and harm them, those hostile feelings did not appear as prominent as their sexual ones. Specifically, four men (Dubose, Schneider, Jones, and Singer) were accused of having sexual relations with subordinates—students or staff—without allegations of coercion beyond the fact that they occupied higher institutional positions and thus appeared to possess greater power and authority. Five more men (Conforth, Korf, Phillips, Ortiz, and Durham) were accused of bribing or threatening students and other subordinates for sexual favors, with one accused of texting a photo of his erect penis to a target. Three other men (Curry, Ruske, and Lewin) were also accused of sending or requesting nude photos from subordinates. Among the 13 men accused of physically intrusive sexual harassment (sexual assaults) in the men's sample, one professor (Irchai) was accused of forcefully grabbing a student's face in his attempt to kiss her. An act of aggression, to be sure, but aggression that appeared to be in the service of his sexual desire. The other professors, coaches, and administrators accused of forcing themselves on students also appeared motivated less by a wish to diminish or injure their targets than by their wish to take sexual advantage of them—their wish to use their bodies for sex. Consider the case of Roy Shick, an athletic department administrator who offered a ride to an intoxicated student-athlete. Instead of driving her home, as he agreed to do, he forced her to have sex with him. He assaulted her because she was defenseless; he assaulted her because he felt he could. His motivation, in other words, was not to take her down from her high perch—he did not assault her because she threatened his social status—rather, he assaulted her to take advantage of the fact that she was intoxicated and unable to resist. The same can be said of professor Tracy McIntosh's assault of a woman, who, as a prospective student, he was showing around campus. He had no reason to feel threatened by her. His motivation for sexually assaulting her, like Shick's, was her defenselessness. After he drugged her, she could not resist.

A second feature of sexual harassment allegations targeting men that distinguishes them from allegations targeting women is men's interest in nude "pix." While two men were accused of sending photos of their erect penises to their targets, and two men were accused of requesting nude photos from theirs, only one woman was accused of sharing nude photos.

A third way to distinguish men's harassment allegations from women's is its recurrent pattern. A total of 17 men, more than half of the men's random sample, were accused of harassing multiple targets (Jones, Singer, Conforth, Korf, Phillips, Ortiz, Ruske, O'Mahony, Lewin, Crews, Moeller, Shipps, Lasecki, Seaman, Craig, Roma, and Moretti); they were accused of making use of the same or similar repertoire of offensive and sexist comments and gestures to harass multiple targets over extended periods. Lucero et al. (2003) referred to this type as "persistent pursuers" and Lengnick-Hall (1995) referred to them as "hard-core harassers." By contrast, only seven women were accused of having multiple targets (Gallop, Rovig, Wilkins, Bartley, Maillo, Gabriel, and Santana), but among the seven, two did not appear to go from sexual target to sexual target, but rather, appeared to go from hostile target to hostile target: specifically, Bartley's name-calling and racist slurs, and Santana's attacks on firefighters. Two other harassment allegations against women appeared to have nothing to do with sexual desire or feelings of hostility: Maillo's creative efforts to boost Spanish class enrollments and Gallop's conversations with students on the topics of sex and gender. Finally, Rovig's drunken efforts to kiss and grope staff members at a bar appeared to represent a one-time event.

Lengnick-Hall's (1995) term for the kind of sexual harassment characteristic of women is "insensitive harassment," a type marked by ignorance and a lack of social sophistication. In this type of harassment, the perpetrator does not intend to make others uncomfortable; but once they understand—when confronted with how their behavior impacts others—they stop. This difference—the fact that women appeared less likely than men to be accused of hard-core, serial sexual harassment motivated by sexual desire—appears as one of the most distinctive features of harassment allegations levelled against women and men.

Women Who Do Not Conform to Traditional (Subordinate) Gender Roles Appear More Likely to Be Accused of Harassment

More than half of the women accused of sexual harassment, 17 out of the 29 (59%), identified either as lesbian and/or were accused of targeting other women. By comparison, among the randomly selected sample of men listed on the Database, same-sex sexual orientation and activity played a significantly smaller role, with only five (17%) men cited for harassment who identified as gay and/or were accused of targeting other men. Which is not to say that women who are oriented to other women are more likely to *commit* sexual harassment; rather, it is to say that women who are oriented to other women appear more likely to be *accused* of sexual harassment (see D'augelli, 1992). That only five men in the men's sample identified as gay or were accused of targeting other men, compared to 17 in the women's sample who identified as lesbian or were accused of targeting other women, may reflect the fact that women are much more likely than men, by a margin of almost two to one, to be victims of sexual harassment and assault (Kearl, 2018).

The overrepresentation of same-sex harassment in the women's sample might also suggest that charging women for same-sex harassment has more cultural support than charging men for same-sex harassment. It might suggest a bias which reflects a hypervigilance, as well as a broadening/loosening of the definition of sexual harassment, when the concept is applied to gender nonconforming women such as Gallop, Ronell, Stubblefield, provost Rosalyn Templeton, distinguished professor Marybeth Gasman, director of radiology Donna Laird, chair of kinesiology Karen Lopez and coaches Pokey Chatman and Joanna Warmington—women who also appear highly successful. Consistent with Berdahl (2007a, b) and several others (Dall'Ara & Maass, 1999; Maass et al., 2003) who argued that men are most likely to harass women who are perceived as ambitious and aggressive—women perceived as challenging male dominance—the 14 women listed on the Academic Sexual Misconduct Database who were charged with false or exaggerated harassment allegations (Gallop, Ronell, Stubblefield, Naca, Rietkovich Browder, Buchanan, Hoffarth, Chatman, Gasman, Warmington, Templeton, Laird, Austen, and Woytowicz) might have been seen as threatening to men. They might have been singled out, first, because they were perceived to be violating existing gender hierarchies and, second, because they were perceived to possess agentic personality qualities (i.e., confidence, competence, independence) deemed undesirable in women. Their accusers might have wanted to show them that they cannot get away with ignoring conventional versions of feminine virtue and delicacy. They might have been singled out for their "status incongruity" (Rudman et al., 2012).

Researchers have argued that victims of sexual harassment and third-party observers are often lax when it comes to identifying harassment; they experience decreased awareness or "motivated blindness," a failure to see harassment for what it is, thus decreasing the likelihood that harassment will be reported, which, in turn, increases the likelihood that it will continue unchecked (Stockdale et al., 1995; Tenbrunsel et al., 2019). However, the many questionable cases in the sample of women accused of sexual harassment—cases in which women appear to be charged based on false or exaggerated evidence—suggest that the opposite is true. Instead of sexual harassment being subjected to "motivated blindness," the sexual harassment attributed to the gender nonconforming women listed on the Academic Sexual Misconduct Database might have resulted from hypervigilance or "motivated awareness." Consider, for example, that in none of the 14 cases described in the book's first chapters did the harassment allegations against women include evidence of *unwelcome* sexual advances or requests for sexual favors. While Anna Stubblefield acknowledged sexual activity with D.J., there was no evidence that that activity was unwelcome. In the case involving Avital Ronell, a self-described lesbian accused of harassing a gay man, she acknowledged touching him but claimed the touching was strictly affectionate: no *sexual* activity occurred. Moreover, she provided material evidence—emails and voicemails—showing that her presumptive target may have welcomed (or pretended to welcome) the physical contact. The only exception might be the case of Rosalyn Templeton, the former provost of Montana State Northern-University, who was accused of touching her supervisee—"slow and lingering" sexual touches—without his consent. But that allegation appeared disingenuous for two reasons: (1) the supervisee-accuser, a Montana State Northern dean, had applied for Templeton's job; he was seeking to replace her; and (2) the "slow and lingering" sexual touches he described in greatest detail and which immediately preceded his decision to report Templeton, occurred under the most unlikely circumstances: in the home of the University's chancellor, at a dinner party, while Templeton and her alleged target were selecting food on a buffet line.

If a would-be harasser is not accused of making unwanted sexual advances or requests for sexual favors—if the question is no longer simply, "How has sexual harassment occurred?"—what other kinds of verbal or physical conduct can be—and are—used as evidence of sexual wrong-doing under conditions of "motivated awareness"? Consider a female professor-administrator's decision to wear an apron that displays the joke, "I keep the best snacks under my apron" (the Gasman case) or a track coach's decision to send a photo to her student-athletes in which she is dressed in running gear (the Warmington case). Under "motivated awareness," a female instructor who exchanges texts with a student on the topics of sex and sexuality can be said to have an inappropriate "sexual relationship" with him (the Woytowicz case), a female professor who discusses gender and sexuality with her graduate students without first getting permission from her dean, can be said to have violated her institution's prohibition against "amorous relationships" with students (the Gallop case), a female professor who has an ambiguous sexual relationship with a nonverbal adult student can be charged with rape (the Stubblefield case), and a female professor can be fired for choosing to discuss her student's sexual feelings in the wrong place—in her home instead of "an office space or a public place" (the Naca case). Under "motivated awareness," LSU's harassment report on Teresa Buchanan could include the charge that she used the word "pussy" three times during a meeting with student-teachers. Under "motivated awareness," Montana State University-Northern, in its harassment report on Rosalyn Templeton, could include the charges that she "doesn't communicate," "comes to work late," and "she's trying to get into the curriculum" (Rivard, 2014); and Weatherford College, in defending its decision to fire Karen Austen for sexual harassment, could report that she not only "forced students off treadmills during class time" but also compelled a department secretary "to do an assignment that would require her leaving her desk even though her boss had instructed her to answer an important phone call" (Austen v Weatherford College). Under "motivated awareness" women can be charged with sexual harassment for sharing satirical YouTube links, telling bawdy jokes, making "improper comments," or for having an "improper sexual relationship," without the need for finding evidence that the improper comments or improper sexual relationship have in fact occurred—when facts do not seem to matter.

In essence, Title IX investigators gathered a wildly divergent, idiosyncratic set of evidence for the purpose of charging 14 out of 29 women with sexual harassment without gathering a comparable set of divergent idiosyncratic evidence in charging any of the 29 men in the randomly selected comparison sample. The problem here is that, not only do the kinds of evidence used to charge the gender-norm-defying women with sexual harassment bear only the most tenuous relationship to the EEOC definition of harassment, but the unarticulated premise of their investigations is that gender-norm-defying women should be judged differently than men under investigation for sexual harassment. Another unarticulated premise: gender-norm-defying women charged with sexual harassment are guilty.

Women Appear More Likely Than Men to Be Victims of False or Inflated Sexual Harassment Allegations

Academic research on the credibility of women in cases of sexual harassment has focused, to date, on flawed efforts to blame the victim—on how women, as victims of harassment, are often denied credibility because they are seen as provoking their alleged victimization. "She was asking for it" (Australian Human Rights Commission, 2008; Bergman et al., 2002; Bongiorno et al., 2020; Dawtry et al., 2019; De Judicibus & McCabe, 2001; McDonald et al., 2010; Von Sikorski & Saumer, 2021). This research found that women are denied credibility in sexual harassment in another way: when they are charged as perpetrators. The finding that 14 cases in the women's sample, almost half of women's cases, appeared to be based on allegations which were exaggerated, contrived, and lacking in evidence, shows that investigations into women's suspected sexual harassment were subject to negative biases unobserved in the 29 randomly selected cases representing men's harassment.

Women Accused of Sexual Harassment Appear More Likely to Receive Severe Penalties

If we compare the penalties dispensed to women accused of sexual harassment to the penalties dispensed to the randomly selected group of men accused of harassment without looking at the contexts of the harassment allegations, we find few differences. Following accusations of sexual harassment, for example, 19 women and 19 men were terminated or forced to resign; similarly, in the relatively few instances in which individuals charged with sexual harassment were not reprimanded or punished, there was little difference between the numbers of women (three) and men (four) who came away without sanction. However, when we look at the contexts of the penalties, when we take into consideration how the penalties or their absence were matched to allegations, a very different picture emerges. In general, women accused of sexual harassment were not only penalized for less serious offenses than their male counterparts but their less-than-serious offenses were punished more harshly.

To illustrate: only three of the 19 women who were fired or forced to resign following allegations of sexual harassment were accused of harassing multiple victims over an extended period (Santana, Gabriel, and Wilkins). The other 16 women were fired or forced to resign either for first-time offenses involving a single target or for offenses which were murky and indeterminate (e.g., Teresa Buchanan for using words such as "pussy" and "fuck" in front of students). In the men's sample, by contrast, among the 19 men who were fired or forced to resign, the majority (Jones, Singer, Conforth, Korf, Phillips, Ortiz, Lewin, O'Mahony, Irchai, McIntosh, Moeller, Lasecki, Craig, and Shipps)—14 cases in all—were accused of making unwanted sexual advances against multiple victims over extended periods. In other words, the decision to fire or force a woman to resign following allegations of harassment tended to be immediate and involve her alleged harassment of a single target, compared to the decision to fire or force a man to resign, which tended to occur after an extended period of investigative indecision and involved cases with multiple targets. In short, men's academic survival did not hinge on a single offense—a difference that is particularly apparent in the cases where men accused of sexual harassment were able to retain their faculty positions more than 30 years after the first harassment allegation against them. What stands out in the latter cases is that three of those men (Moretti, Gaillardetz, and Roma) received no penalty at all, even though they were accused of sexual assault, while none of the women who came away with no penalty (Fegumps, Ewing, and Bartley) were accused of assault.

The incongruity between women's and men's penalties is particularly apparent when we compare how women and men accused of harassment were punished by their own institutions. To illustrate: (1) Jane Gallop was reprimanded for having a "consensual amorous relationship with a student" though her institution offered no evidence that such a relationship existed, while one year later, that same institution failed to reprimand a male professor for having what his presumptive student-victim described as a demeaning and exploitive sexual relationship with her. (2) Pokey Chatman, the highly successful coach of the LSU basketball team, was accused of having a consensual relationship with a student-athlete but was given only two hours to resign, while several men accused of multiple sexual assaults at LSU were allowed to remain on campus indefinitely. (3) Anna Stubblefield from Rutgers was sentenced to 12 years in prison for having sex with a man with disabilities despite the absence of evidence that she violated his sexual consent or that he had been harmed by the sexual activity. The only other sexual harassment case from Rutgers that ended in criminal court involved a male professor who acknowledged filming as many as 30 women in a bathroom, but those charges were dropped as part of his agreement to plead guilty to a series of other, non-sex-related crimes such as burglary, computer theft, and illegal possession of an assault weapon, which resulted in a sentence of 300 days in jail. (4) NYU charged Avital Ronell with making inappropriate non-violent demands on her male graduate student's time and attention, and suspended her for a year, while two male professors from NYU listed on the Academic Sexual Misconduct Database for allegations of groping and gender-demeaning slurs received no more than a letter of reprimand in one case, and no reprimand at all in the other. (5) Jacqueline Hoffarth, charged with having a consensual relationship with a student (which she announced publicly after he graduated), was immediately fired, while a male professor from Hoffarth's institution (from the very same department), who was accused of orally raping a student, received only a year's suspension, implemented more than 12 months after the assault allegation came to light. (6) Teresa Buchanan was terminated after allegedly making offensive comments to students such as, "Well, he [the student's fiancé] might support you when the sex is good, but trust me, he won't support you in five years when it's not so good," while the same institution retained male faculty who allegedly threatened and assaulted female students. (7) Coach Joanna Warmington was fired after she was charged with sending a "sexual picture" to her student-athletes consisting of her wearing a running bra, while two male employees from the same institution, one of whom was accused of soliciting personal relationships with female students and the other of making unwelcome sexual advances that included nuzzling students' necks and tickling their stomachs, were retained. The inevitable caveat is the incompleteness of the data: in coach Warmington's case, for example, while her student-athletes reportedly accused her of behaving in an inappropriate "sexualized" manner, we do not have access to their testimony; the words student-athletes used to describe Warmington's so-called inappropriate, "sex charged" behavior were never disclosed. What we do know, however, is that there were no reports of Warmington making unwelcome sexual advances on student-athletes—no reports of intrusive kissing, touching, groping, or other kinds of inappropriate sexual behavior. The same holds true of the other cases involving questionable sexual harassment allegations against women—no reports of intrusive kissing, groping, or other kinds of inappropriate sexual contact.

While this book's title, *Women Accused of Sexual Harassment*, suggests that it is about female perpetrators, the book can just as easily be understood as a study of female victims; it can be understood as a study of how the mechanisms of sexual harassment investigations—often cited as resources for protecting women—can be turned against women by falsely labelling them sexual harassers. Sexual harassment allegations against women, in other words, as well as responses to the allegations, can represent another way of sexually harassing women. That gender nonconforming women accused of sexual harassment tend to be treated more harshly than men who commit similar or more severe offenses, suggests that, when it comes to penalties, the severity of the offense may be less important than the gender performance of the offender. Men may have greater power to frighten, provoke, injure, and humiliate their harassment victims, but a double standard favoring men continues to affect how harassment allegations are judged and processed.

Victim Vulnerability Is Associated with Sexual Harassment

Researchers have argued that the primary targets of men's harassment are women who demonstrate power (e.g., Folke et al., 2020; McLaughlin et al., 2012), women who are outspoken, ambitious, and confident (e.g., Bai et al., 2014; Berdahl, 2007a, b)—so-called agentic, "uppity women"—but the findings from the Academic Sexual Misconduct Database suggest otherwise: the primary targets of sexual harassment are women with relatively little power. Confirming the lecherous professor stereotype (Dziech & Weiner, 1990), the most common victim/perpetrator dyad noted in the samples drawn from the Academic Sexual Misconduct Database is student-victim/faculty (or coach)-perpetrator (see Uggen & Blackstone, 2004), a relationship that prevailed in 13 cases of women and 22 cases of men accused of harassment. Among the randomly selected male perpetrators, only one case involved harassment allegations against a peer (Laura Grimes vs. Richard Gaillardetz). The remaining 28, or 98% of the men's sample, involved harassment of a subordinate, none of whom claimed they were targeted due to their accomplishments or behavior (cf. Fischer, 2011; Miceli & Castelfranchi, 2018; Roseman, 2001). None claimed they were targeted because they were perceived as insubordinate, belligerent, or threatening. And none claimed they were targeted because their harassers wanted "to keep them out of, or down in, male-dominated jobs, roles, and spaces" (Berdahl & Bhattacharyya, 2021, p. 478).

That so many victims, most of whom were women, claimed they had been harassed by male faculty when they were students—and thus belonged to a population unlikely to pose a professional threat to their harassers—provides strong support for the vulnerable victim hypothesis. At the same time, victim vulnerability cannot fully explain why sexual harassment occurs since many individuals who are relatively powerless do not experience harassment, and many who are relatively powerful do. Clearly, other factors need to be present to account for sexual harassment. Still, the perception of a victim's vulnerability appears to play an important role. Harassers may target their victims at times because they may feel threatened by them, but as the data from this research suggests, they also target victims for the opposite reason: because they feel they can get away with it. A would-be harasser, like the slave master who fathered multiple children with an enslaved woman, may decide to go ahead with sexual harassment because he believes that the possible costs are relatively minor.

What About Harassment Committed in Workplaces Dominated by Women?

Michael Crichton suggested that workplaces dominated by women should have more sexual harassment by women. "Whoever is behind the desk has the opportunity to abuse power." That prediction does not appear to fit the data collected for this study—not even close. Since women represent almost half of all college and university faculty, they can be expected to have a lot of power. Yet they are accused of committing only a minute portion of sexual harassment. Why don't women commit a larger share of sexual harassment in the academy if they have so much power? One answer is that men are more violent and sexually aggressive than women, in general, and college and university workplaces, even though they employ many women in high-status, high-paying positions, are not sites where that gender difference is somehow magically reversed. The data from this study show that some women commit sexual harassment, but that the perpetrators of sexual harassment are overwhelmingly men. Moreover, the randomness of the sexual harassment committed by women—the absence of a discernible pattern—suggests that, unlike men, women are not inclined to commit sexual harassment. Whether women have more workplace power appears irrelevant: it's a behavioral style that's either not in women's nature or is not part of the behavioral profile they've been taught to emulate.

The Unknowns

Does Harassment by Women Have the Same Effects on Female Victims as Harassment by Men?

Following gender stereotypes, scholars agree that sexual harassment by women is less threatening than harassment by men. However, this research has not been able to affirm or disconfirm that difference. While men and women sometimes harass in similar ways—for example, the two cases involving professors from the theater department of the University of North Carolina-Greensboro who committed almost identical sexual intrusions with students at about the same time—we don't know if similar intrusions committed by male and female perpetrators have similar or different effects on their targets.

When Are Men Denied Credibility in Harassment Investigations?

As noted in Chap. 5, the quid pro quo harassment allegations against Jeffrey Menaker, the former Hofstra University tennis coach, were unsubstantiated. He denied all the allegations and provided the names of multiple witnesses who could support his denials, but the witnesses were never interviewed, and despite the absence of evidence supporting the complainant's allegations, he was terminated. The University's grounds for termination were vague and indeterminate: Menaker's "unprofessional conduct" and "the totality of circumstances." Menaker then sued Hofstra, alleging discrimination, and won (see Menaker v. Hofstra University, on appeal from United District Court for the Eastern District of New York, Aug. 15, 2019). What remains unknown is how often, and in what ways, men are denied credibility in harassment investigations. What factors lead to or predict discrimination against men accused of sexual harassment?

How Do Sexual Harassers Explain Their Behavior?

Most sexual harassers do not acknowledge their offenses or minimize their responsibility (Blagden et al., 2014; Happel et al., 1995; Reinicke, 2022; Ware et al., 2015), a gap reflected in this research. What we lack—what we need to better understand—is perpetrators' perceptions of harassment, how they view their motivations and behavior. This gap in our knowledge may account for the uncertainties and competing theories surrounding why men harass—whether it's primarily to protect and enhance their social status, to convey contempt and hostility, or express sexual desire—or whether sexual harassment arises, not from a single or primary motivation but rather from varieties and combinations of motivation which vary from perpetrator to perpetrator, circumstance to circumstance, and workplace to workplace (see Lucero et al., 2003).

Biases in Sexual Harassment Research

The main unknown in sexual harassment research based on publicly available sexual harassment documents is the generalizability of the findings. The propensity to observe, report, or record sexual harassment by women may differ from the propensity to observe, report, or record sexual harassment by men. The problem here is that we have no way of knowing how to measure these possible differences or even whether such differences exist. We do not know if women are more likely than men to be charged with inflated or false harassment allegations or if that is an artifact of gender biases in reporting. We know, for example, that a former Stanford University student recently posted an article about her affair with a Stanford dean which occurred more than a decade ago (Haas, 2024), but we do not know why she waited so long to report the affair—whether that had something to do with the fact that the former dean is a woman. Nor do we know why, after the affair was reported and acknowledged by the former dean (Toohey, 2024), it was not included in the Academic Sexual Misconduct Database.

Some colleges and universities may report all or most sexual harassment investigations to the Academic Sexual Misconduct Database, but many do not. Who knows how many women (or men) could have been included in the Database but were not because their sexual misconduct was unnoticed, dismissed, or concealed?

Where Do We Go from Here?

The biggest advances in locating and reducing racial discrimination in criminal sentencing have come from the availability in the 1980s and 1990s of large, post-conviction datasets disseminated by sentencing commissions (Ulmer, 2012, 2019). To make similar advances in locating and reducing gender discrimination in sexual harassment investigations—to find ways to standardize investigations—the U.S. Department of

Education's Office of Civil Rights (OCR) should require educational institutions receiving federal financial assistance to collect post-investigation data. Once these kinds of data are available, they can be studied for the purpose of helping us understand whether and/or how harassment allegations are processed differently when the accused is a man or woman. If we are to reduce gender discrimination in sexual harassment investigations, we need to develop a set of norms regarding how such investigations should proceed. We need to make the investigative system predictable and coherent. By assembling Title IX investigation data involving men and women, and by examining how they are produced and processed, we may be in a position to develop guidelines for identifying and preventing gender discrimination in harassment investigations.

The finding that sexual harassment is more likely to occur when harassers feel they can offend with little or no cost to themselves also has important implications for reducing gender discrimination and improving deterrence. Consider, for example, the kinds of prevention recommendations and quagmires that might emerge from the belief that sexual harassment can be reduced to a single cause: men's sense that women are threatening them. If women who present themselves as "feminine," as opposed to "masculine," are less likely to experience sexual harassment (see Eagly et al., 1992; Rudman, 1998), those tasked with preventing harassment may very well wonder whether their efforts should focus on encouraging women to behave and appear more feminine. If women who threaten men are more likely to be harassed, some may wonder whether women should be encouraged to accept more passive, non-threatening workplace postures and outcomes.

The "women-are-too-threatening" explanation of sexual harassment is, of course, flawed empirically, given research consistently showing that female students who have the least power, members of sexual and racial minorities, younger students, and students with disabilities, are at greatest risk of harassment (D'augelli, 1992; Fedina et al., 2018; Ong, 2005; Vladutinu et al., 2011). And it is flawed as a guide to prevention, since the "women-are-too-threatening" model moves us closer to the idea that women are to blame for their own harassment. That model, instead of promoting women's upward mobility and career aspirations—instead of promoting women's equality and strengths—suggests that women put themselves at risk when they are successful at work, when they do their jobs well and behave assertively, with skill and confidence.

If women's perceived success plays less of a role in sexual harassment than their perceived defenselessness and vulnerability, it follows that, at the organizational level, promoting women's workplace success and advancement, and their access to the kinds of career opportunities available to men should be recognized as keys to combatting the sexual harassment of women. In the words of Dobbin and Kalev (2017, p. 687), "Training programs and reporting systems won't end sexual harassment. Promoting more women will."

If we find additional support for the connection between sexual harassment and victim vulnerability, then it follows that the central goal of prevention should be less about protecting the vulnerable (cf. Chamberlain, 2008) and more about empowering them. It should be more about encouraging would-be victims, at the interactional and behavioral levels, to resist, repel, and report harassment (see Langelan, 1993; Scott & Martin, 2006), goals which require considerable support from organizational personnel and decision-makers (Dobbin & Kalev, 2017; Foote & Goodman-Delahunty, 2021; Gruber & Smith, 1995; Roehling & Huang, 2018). The hope is that, if organizations encourage employees to file harassment complaints and those complaints are followed by timely and aggressive investigations, which are applied uniformly and fairly, even in the face of public pressure, sexual harassment and gender discrimination will decline.

References

Australian Human Rights Commission. (2008). *Sexual harassment: Serious business*. www.humanrights.gov.au/sexualharassment

Bai, F., Berdahl, J. L., & Schieman, S. (2014). The "ambition gap" explained: Workplace mistreatment as a function of gender, ambition, and rank. In *Academy of management proceedings, 2014* (p. 17425). Academy of Management.

Berdahl, J. L. (2007a). Harassment based on sex: Protecting social status in the context of gender hierarchy. *Academy of Management Review, 32*(2), 641–658. https://www.jstor.org/stable/20159319

Berdahl, J. L. (2007b). The sexual harassment of uppity women. *Journal of Applied Psychology, 92*(2), 425–437. https://doi.org/10.1037/0021-9010.92.2.425

Berdahl, J., & Bhattacharyya, B. (2021). Four ways forward in studying sex-based harassment. *Equality, Diversity and Inclusion: An International Journal, 40*(4), 477–492. https://www.emerald.com/insight/2040-7149.htm

Bergman, M. E., Langhout, R. D., Palmieri, P. A., Cortina, L. M., & Fitzgerald, L. F. (2002). The (un)reasonableness of reporting: Antecedents and consequences of reporting sexual harassment. *Journal of Applied Psychology, 87*(2), 230–242. https://doi.org/10.1037/0021-9010.87.2.230

Blagden, N. J., Winder, B., Gregson, M., & Thorne, K. (2014). Making sense of denial in sexual offenders: A qualitative phenomenological and Repertory Grid analysis. *Journal of Interpersonal Violence, 29*(9), 1–13. https://doi.org/10.1177/0886260513511530

Bongiorno, R., Langbroek, C., Bain, P. G., Ting, M., & Ryan, M. K. (2020). Why women are blamed for being sexually harassed: The effects of empathy for female victims and male perpetrators. *Psychology of Women Quarterly, 44*(1), 11–27. https://doi.org/10.1177/0361684319868730

Chamberlain, L. (2008). *A prevention primer for domestic violence: Terminology, tools, and the public health approach.* The National Online Resource Center on Violence Against Women.

D'augelli, A. (1992). Lesbian and gay male undergraduates experiences of harassment and fear. *Journal of Interpersonal Violence, 7*(3), 383–396. https://doi.org/10.1177/088626092007003007

Dall'Ara, E., & Maass, A. (1999). Studying sexual harassment in the laboratory: Are egalitarian women at higher risk? *Sex Roles, 41*(9), 681–704.

Dawtry, R. J., Cozzolino, P. J., & Callan, M. J. (2019). I blame therefore I was: Rape myth acceptance, victim blaming, and memory reconstruction. *Personality and Social Psychology Bulletin, 45*(8), 1269–1282. https://doi.org/10.1177/0146167218818475

De Judicibus, M., & McCabe, M. P. (2001). Blaming the target of sexual harassment: Impact of gender role, sexist attitudes, and work role. *Sex Roles, 44*(7/8), 401–417.

Dobbin, F., & Kalev, A. (2017). Training programs and reporting systems won't end sexual harassment. Promoting women will. *Harvard Business Review, 70*(4), 687–702.

Dziech, B. W., & Weiner, L. (1990). *The Lecherous Professor: Sexual harassment on campus.* University of Illinois Press.

Eagly, A. H., Makhijani, M. G., & Klonsky, B. G. (1992). Gender and the evaluation of leaders: A meta-analysis. *Psychological Bulletin, 111*, 3–22.

Fedina, L., Holmes, J. L., & Backes, B. L. (2018). Campus sexual assault: A systematic review of prevalence research from 2000 to 2015. *Trauma, Violence & Abuse, 19*(1), 76–93. https://doi.org/10.1177/1524838016631129

Fischer, A. (2011). Contempt: A hot feeling hidden under a cold jacket. In R. Trnka, K. Balcar, & M. Kuska (Eds.), *Re-constructing emotional spaces: From experience to regulation* (pp. 77–87). Prague College of Psychosocial Studies Press.

Fisher, B. (2000). *The sexual victimization of college women.* US Department of Justice, Office of Justice Programs, National Institute of Justice.

Folke, O., Rickne, J., Tanaka, S., & Tateishi, Y. (2020). Sexual harassment of women leaders. *Daedalus, 149*(1), 180–197. https://doi.org/10.1162/daed_a_01781

Foote, W. E., & Goodman-Delahunty, J. (2021). *Understanding sexual harassment: Evidence-based forensic practice.* American Psychological Association Press.

Gallop, J. (1997). *Feminist accused of sexual harassment.* Duke University Press.

Gruber, J. E., & Smith, M. D. (1995). Women's responses to sexual harassment: A Multivariate analysis. *Basic and Applied Social Psychology, 17*(4), 543–562. https://doi.org/10.1207/s15324834basp1704_7

Haas, O. S. (2024, July 10). I had an affair with my college dean. *First Person.* https://www.autostraddle.com/i-had-an-affair-with-my-college-dean/

Happel, T. M., Joseph, J. A., & Auffrey, J. J. (1995). Sex offender assessment: Interrupting the dance of denial. *American Journal of Forensic Psychology, 13,* 5–22.

Hart, C. G. (2019). The penalties for self-reporting sexual harassment. *Gender & Society, 33*(4), 534–559.

Ilies, R., Hauserman, N., Schwochau, S., & Stibal, J. (2003). Reported incidence rates of work-related sexual harassment in the United States: Using meta-analysis to explain reported rate disparities. *Personnel Psychology, 56*(3), 607–631.

Kearl, H. (2018). *The facts behind the #metoo movement: A national study on sexual harassment and assault.* https://www.nsvrc.org/resource/facts-behind-metoo-movement-national-study-sexual-harassment-and-assault

Kipnis, L. (2015a, February 27). Sexual paranoia strikes academe. *Chronical of Higher Education, Chronical Review.* https://www.chronicle.com/article/sexual-paranoia-strikes-academe/

Kipnis, L. (2015b, May 29). My title IX inquisition. *Chronicle of Higher Education.* https://www.google.com/search?q=my+title+IX+inquisition+kipnis&rlz=1C1GCEB_enUS882US882&oq=my+title+IX+inquisition+kipnis&gs_lcrp=EgZjaHJvbWUyBggAEEUYOTIHCAEQIRigATIHCAIQIRigATIHCAMQIRigATIHCAQQIRigATIHCAUQIRigAdIBCTE5NzA0ajBqNKgCALACAQ&sourceid=chrome&ie=UTF-8

Langelan, M. J. (1993). *Back off! How to confront and stop sexual harassment and harassers.* Simon & Schuster.

Lengnick-Hall, M. L. (1995). Sexual harassment research: A methodological critique. *Personal Psychology, 48,* 841–864.

Lucero, M. A., Middleton, K. L., Finch, W. A., & Valentine, S. R. (2003). An empirical investigation of sexual harassers: Toward a perpetrator typology. *Human Relations, 56,* 1461–1483.

Maass, A., Cadinu, M., Guarnieri, G., & Guarnieri, A. (2003). Sexual harassment under social identity threat: The computer harassment paradigm. *Journal of Personality and Social Psychology, 85*(5), 853–870. https://doi.org/10.1037/0022-3514.85.5.853

McDonald, P., Graham, T., & Martin, B. (2010). Outrage management in cases of sexual harassment as revealed in judicial decisions. *Psychology of Women Quarterly, 34*(2), 165–180.

McLaughlin, H., Uggen, C., & Blackstone, A. (2012). Sexual harassment, workplace authority, and the paradox of power. *American Sociological Review, 77*(4), 625–647. https://doi.org/10.1177/0003122412451728

Miceli, M., & Castelfranchi, C. (2018). Contempt and disgust: The emotions of disrespect. *Journal for the Theory of Social Behaviour, 48*(2), 205–229. https://doi.org/10.1111/jtsb.12159

Ong, M. (2005). Body projects of young women of color in physics: Intersections of Gender, Race, and Science. *Social Problems, 52*(4), 593–617. https://doi.org/10.1525/sp.2005.52.4.593

Pershing, J. L. (2003). Why women don't report sexual harassment: A case study of an elite military institution. *Gender Issues, 21*(4), 3–30.

Reinicke, K. (2022). *Men after #MeToo: Being an ally in the fight against sexual harassment.* Springer Nature.

Rivard, R. (2014, June 12). Unwelcome touch. *Inside Higher Ed.* https://www.insidehighered.com/news/2014/06/13/female-provost-accused-repeatedly-touching-her-male-colleagues

Roehling, M. V., & Huang, J. (2018). Sexual harassment training effectiveness: An interdisciplinary review and call for research. *Journal of Organizational Behavior, 39*(2), 134–150. https://doi.org/10.1002/job.2257

Roseman, I. J. (2001). A model of appraisal in the emotion system: Integrating theory, research, and applications. In K. R. Scherer, A. Schorr, & T. Johnstone (Eds.), *Appraisal processes in emotion: Theory, methods, research* (pp. 68–91). Oxford University Pres.

Rudman, L. A. (1998). Self-promotion as a risk factor for women: The costs and benefits of counterstereotypical impression management. *Journal of Personality and Social Psychology, 74*, 629–645.

Rudman, L. A., Moss-Racusin, C., Phelan, J. E., & Nauts, S. (2012). Status incongruity and backlash effects: Defending the gender hierarchy motivates prejudice against female leaders. *Journal of Experimental Social Psychology, 48*, 165–179. https://doi.org/10.1016/j.jesp.2011.10.008

Scott, G., & Martin, B. (2006). Tactics against sexual harassment: The role of backfire. *Journal of International Women's Studies, 7*(4), 110–125. https://vc.bridgew.edu/jiws/vol7/iss4/7

Stockdale, M. S., Vaux, A., & Cashin, J. (1995). Acknowledging sexual harassment: A test of Alternative models. *Basic and Applied Psychology, 17*(4), 469–496.

Tenbrunsel, A. E., Rees, M. R., & Diekmann, K. A. (2019). Sexual harassment in academia: Ethical climates and bounded ethicality. *Annual Review of Sociology, 70*, 245–270.

Toohey, G. (2024, July 15). Former Stanford dean, now local council member, apologizes for Affair with student. *Los Angeles Times.* https://www.latimes.com/california/story/2024-07-15/former-stanford-dean-student-affair-apology

Uggen, C., & Blackstone, A. (2004). Sexual harassment as a gendered expression of power. *American Sociological Review, 69*(1), 64–92. https://doi.org/10.1177/000312240406900105

Ulmer, J. T. (2012). Recent developments and new directions in sentencing research. *Justice Quarterly, 29*(1), 1–40.

Ulmer, J. (2019). Criminal courts as inhabited institutions: Making sense of difference and similarity in sentencing. *Crime and Justice, 48*, 483–522.

Vladutinu, C. J., Martin, S. L., & Macy, R. J. (2011). College- or university-based sexual assault prevention programs: A review of program outcomes: Characteristics and recommendations. *Trauma, Violence & Abuse, 12*(2), 67–86.

Vohlídalová, M. (1999). The perception and construction of sexual harassment by Czech university students. *Sociologický časopis/Czech Sociological Review, 47*(6), 1119–1147. https://www.jstor.org/stable/23535017

Von Sikorski, C., & Saumer, M. (2021). Sexual harassment in politics. News about victims' delayed sexual harassment accusations and effects on victim blaming: A mediation model. *Mass Communication and Society, 24*(2), 259–287.

Ware, J., Marshall, W. L., & Marshall, L. E. (2015). Categorical denial in convicted sex offenders: The concept, its meaning, and its implication for risk and treatment. *Aggression and Violent Behavior, 25*, 215–226. https://doi.org/10.1016/j.avb.2015.08.003

Appendix

Women's sample & allegations	*Men's random sample & allegations*
Gallop, Jane Inappropriate conversations and quid pro quo threats with female students.	Dubose, Mike Consensual sexual relations with female supervisee
Ronell, Avital Amorous relations and quid pro quo threats with male student	Schneider, Richard Consensual sexual relations with female student
Stubblefield, Anna Sexual relations with nonverbal student	Jones, Edward Sexual relations with male students
Naca, Kristin A sexual pass at female student	Singer, Barry Sexual relations with students
Rietkovich Browder, Katie Sexual relations with female student	Conforth, Bruce Quid pro quo threats
Hoffarth, Jacqueline. Consensual amorous relations with male student	Korf, William E. Quid pro quo bribes
Buchanan, Teresa Inappropriate language with female students	Phillips, John Quid pro quo threats
Chatman, Pokey Consensual sexual relations with female student	Ortiz, Manuel Quid pro quo bribes
Warmington, Joanna Inappropriate language with female students	Durham, Todd Quid pro quo bribes and "dick pix."

(*continued*)

© The Author(s), under exclusive license to Springer Nature Switzerland AG 2024

L. Margolin, *Women Accused of Sexual Harassment*,
https://doi.org/10.1007/978-3-031-79021-8

(continued)

Women's sample & allegations	*Men's random sample & allegations*
Templeton, Rosalyn	Mulzet, Todd
Touching male supervisee	Teasing male student
Gasman, Marybeth	Curry, Michael
Inappropriate humor with staff	"dick pix"
Laird, Donna	Ruske, Eric
Inappropriate humor with staff	Inappropriate language with female students
Austen, Karen Lopez	Lewin, Walter
Inappropriate language with students/staff	Inappropriate language with female students
Woytowicz, Catherine	O'Mahony, Michael
Inappropriate language with male student	Inappropriate language with female students
Rovig, Nicole	Crews, Demarcus
Touching staff members at a bar	Inappropriate language with male students
Hachiyanagi, Rui	Dustin, Christopher
Attempted murder of colleague	Offensive language with female student
Maillo, Victoria	Gaither, William S.
Asking supervisees to have sex with students	Touching female staff
Recio, Roxana	Bavel, Zamir
Stalking female colleague	Touching female student
Santana, Melissa Ann	Irchai, Arnold
Stalking male firefighters	Sexual assault of female student
Del Valle, Ivonne	McIntosh, Tracy
Stalking male colleague	Sexual assault of female student
Hale, Cara	Shick, Roy
Consensual sexual relations with male student	Sexual assault of female student
Parker, Alice A	Moeller, Matthew C.
Consensual sexual relations with female student	Touching female students
Dr. Jane Roe	Lasecki, Walter
Quid pro quo threats against female supervisee	Touching female students
Fegumps, Sheena Pryce	Seaman, John
Teasing male colleague	Touching female students
Ewing, Christy	Craig. Morrie A.
Teasing male colleague	Touching female student
Bartley, Lavonette	Shipps, Steven
Offensive language with female supervisees	Sexual assault of female students
Lemley, Ellen	Franco, Moretti
Sexual assault of female students	Sexual assault of female students
Gabriel, Denise	Gaillardetz, Richard R.
Sexual assault of female students	Sexual assault of female colleague

References

Alexander, J. (2018, January 6). Photographer and professor of photography at Columbia, Thomas Roma, accused of sexual assault. *FStoppers*. https://fstoppers.com/legal/photographer-and-professor-photography-columbia-thomas-roma-accused-sexual-210781

Assuncao, M. (2021, October 23). Montana professor Rob Smith quits over controversial posts. *New York Daily News*. https://www.nydailynews.com/2021/10/23/montana-professor-resigns-amid-investigation-into-alleged-homophobic-and-misogynistic-views/

Blanton, C. (2014, December 7). Professor who violated sexual harassment policy is still working to appeal KU's decision. *University Daily Kansan*. https://www.kansan.com/news/professor-who-violated-sexual-harassment-policy-is-still-working-to-appeal-kus-decision/article_f4d8a590-7e65-11e4-8783-9fc5e755dfd1.html

Buist, C., & Lenning, E. (2015). *Queer criminology*. Routledge.

Cantalupo, N. C., & Kidder, W. C. (2018). A systematic look at a serial problem: Sexual harassment of students by university faculty. *Utah Law Review, 2018*(3), 671–786.

Chodorow, N. J. (2023). *The reproduction of mothering: Psychoanalysis and the sociology of gender*. U. of California Press.

Connell, R. (2009). *Gender* (Vol. 14). Polity.

Cornelius, T. L., & Resseguie, N. (2007). Primary and secondary prevention programs for dating violence: A review of the literature. *Aggression and Violent Behavior, 12*(3), 364–375. https://doi.org/10.1016/j.avb.2006.09.006

© The Author(s), under exclusive license to Springer Nature Switzerland AG 2024

L. Margolin, *Women Accused of Sexual Harassment*,
https://doi.org/10.1007/978-3-031-79021-8

Grimes, L. (2021). https://www.youtube.com/watch?v=4w40saeWZZQ&t=140s; https://www.youtube.com/watch?v=AK421NB6Onk

Jin, Y., Sun, C., Wu, J., An, J., & Li, J. (2021). Precarious manhood and its effects on aggression. *Journal of Personality and Social Psychology, 36*, 9–10. https://doi.org/10.1177/0886260518800312

LaRocca, M. A., & Kromrey, J. D. (1999). The perception of sexual harassment in higher education: Impact of gender and attractiveness. *Sex Roles, 40*, 921–936.

Loofbourow, Lili. (2018, August 30). The Avital Ronell case: Some things aren't complicated. *Slate*. https://slate.com/news-and-politics/2018/08/avital-ronell-harassment-case-some-things-arent-complicated.html

Lucero, M., Allen, R., & Middleton, K. (2006). Sexual harassers: Behaviors, motives, and change over time. *Sex Roles, 55*, 331–343.

Mahoney, J., & Goertz, G. (2004). The possibility principle: Choosing negative cases in comparative research. *American Political Science Review, 98*(4), 653–669.

Mailman D. (2021, August 28). Ole Miss Softball coach caught fucking one of her players. *Total Frat Move*. https://totalfratmove.com/tfm/ole-miss-softball-coach-got-caught-fucking-one-of-her-players/

Manne, K. (2023). Moral gaslighting. *Aristotelian Society Supplementary volume, 97*(1), 122–145. https://doi.org/10.1093/arisup/akad006

Marino, J. J. (2018). *Judith Butler must resign as MLA President-Elect*. https://www.thepetitionsite.com/750/313/841/judith-butler-must-resign-as-mla-president-elect/

McKinney, K. (1992). Contrapower sexual harassment: The effects of student sex and type of behavior on faculty perceptions. *Sex Roles, 27*, 627–643.

Robinett, M. W. (2015, July 6). *Letter*. https://workplacebullying.org/multi/pdf/Austen.pdf

Robinson, A. E. (2018, August 18). On power and aporia in the academy. *Medium*. https://medium.com/@amyelizabethrobinson/on-power-and-aporia-in-the-academy-a-response-in-three-parts-f7387c346ffa

S. H. (2005, May 1). Former neurology professor sentenced to house arrest for sexual assault. *Pennsylvania Gazette*. https://thepenngazette.com/former-neurology-professor-sentenced-to-house-arrest-for-sexual-assault/

Schuessler, J. (2017, October 30). Reading by the numbers: When big data meets literature. *New York Times*. https://www.nytimes.com/2017/10/30/arts/franco-moretti-stanford-literary-lab-big-data.html

Sweet, P. (2019). The sociology of gaslighting. *American Sociological Review, 84*(5), 851–875. https://doi.org/10.1177/0003122419874843

Węziak-Białowolska, D., Białowolski, P., Mordukhovich, I., & McNeely, E. (2020). Work, gender and sexual harassment on the frontlines of commercial travel: A cross-sectional study of flight crew well-being. *The International Journal of Aerospace Psychology, 30*(3/4), 171–189.

Index

© The Author(s), under exclusive license to Springer Nature Switzerland AG 2024
L. Margolin, *Women Accused of Sexual Harassment*,
https://doi.org/10.1007/978-3-031-79021-8

E

F

G

T

The manufacturer's authorised representative in the EU is Springer Nature Customer Service Centre GmbH, Europaplatz 3, 69115 Heidelberg, Germany. If you have any concerns regarding our products, please contact ProductSafety@springernature.com

Printed and bound by CPI Group (UK) Ltd, Croydon, CR0 4YY

01/10/2026

02225967-0005

Labour in History and Society

Series Editors
Stefano Bellucci, Institute for History, Leiden University, Leiden, The Netherlands
Andrea Caracausi, DiSSGeA, University of Padua, Padua, Italy
Larissa Correa, Department of History, Pontifical Catholic University, Rio de Janeiro, Brazil
Chitra Joshi, Delhi, India

This series explores various forms of labour relations across the world, and over a broad temporal period from antiquity to the present. The editors invite contributions from researchers in a range of disciplines, including history, sociology, economics, anthropology and philosophy, and encourage an interdisciplinary approach which will make use of historical and social science methodologies. Covering different types of labour relations, from commodified labour for the market, to tributary labour for the polity and reciprocal labour for the household, the series aims to examine dominant classes such as masters, rulers and capitalists in order to unveil the dialectical relationship not only between employers and employees, but also between elites and the 'subaltern'. Providing insights from multiple disciplines, the series will examine aspects of race, gender and caste, as well as trade unionism, unpaid labour and precarious work. It will present a range of perspectives: both global and local; regional and national; micro and macro, and will include case studies and contributions from across the globe.

Samuel Andreas Admasie

The Ethiopian Labour Movement

Trade Unions, Collective Action, and Contestation, 1960–2020

palgrave
macmillan

Samuel Andreas Admasie
International Institute of Social
History
Amsterdam, The Netherlands

Swedish Labour Movement's Archives
and Library
Stockholm, Sweden

ISSN 2731-9474 ISSN 2731-9482 (electronic)
Labour in History and Society
ISBN 978-3-031-72840-2 ISBN 978-3-031-72841-9 (eBook)
https://doi.org/10.1007/978-3-031-72841-9

© The Editor(s) (if applicable) and The Author(s), under exclusive license to Springer Nature Switzerland AG 2025

This work is subject to copyright. All rights are solely and exclusively licensed by the Publisher, whether the whole or part of the material is concerned, specifically the rights of translation, reprinting, reuse of illustrations, recitation, broadcasting, reproduction on microfilms or in any other physical way, and transmission or information storage and retrieval, electronic adaptation, computer software, or by similar or dissimilar methodology now known or hereafter developed.
The use of general descriptive names, registered names, trademarks, service marks, etc. in this publication does not imply, even in the absence of a specific statement, that such names are exempt from the relevant protective laws and regulations and therefore free for general use.
The publisher, the authors and the editors are safe to assume that the advice and information in this book are believed to be true and accurate at the date of publication. Neither the publisher nor the authors or the editors give a warranty, expressed or implied, with respect to the material contained herein or for any errors or omissions that may have been made. The publisher remains neutral with regard to jurisdictional claims in published maps and institutional affiliations.

Cover illustration: Mahlet Birhanu Gebre (kuku's pencil)

This Palgrave Macmillan imprint is published by the registered company Springer Nature Switzerland AG
The registered company address is: Gewerbestrasse 11, 6330 Cham, Switzerland

If disposing of this product, please recycle the paper.

ወዛደራዊ ዓለምአቀፋዊነት ይለምልም

(inscription on trade union statue, Addis Ababa)

To Carin and Daniel, with endless affection.

Acknowledgements

This book is the outcome of a decade of research. Initially, it was undertaken within the framework of doctoral studies at the Centre for African Studies of the University of Basel, which evolved into a joint enrolment at the former and the Department of Political and Social Sciences of the University of Pavia. The research has, in various stages, benefited from funding from the Graduate School of Social Sciences of the University of Basel, the University of Pavia, the Freiwillige Akademische Gesellschaft Basel, and the Swedish Research Council. I am deeply grateful to all these institutions. I am particularly thankful to Elisio Macamo, Veit Arlt, Julia Büchele, Manuela Rossini, and Günter Schmidt-Gess at the University of Basel; and Massimo Zaccaria, Pierluigi Valsecchi, Marina Tesoro, and Virginie Gallati at the University of Pavia.

Other institutions have hosted me and provided me a platform from which to conduct research, teach, or write during the course of the production of this book. They include the Department of Political Science and International Relations of Addis Ababa University, the International Institute of Social History, the Institute for Peace and Conflict Studies of the University of Hargeisa, and the Swedish Labour Movement's Archives and Library. I would like to thank all colleagues at these institutions, not limited to, but in particular Kassahun Berhanu, Fekade Terefe, Shiferaw Bekele, Girma Negash, and Abdiwasa Abdilahi at Addis Ababa University; Stefano Bellucci, Marien van der Heijden, Jacqueline Rutte, Marcel van der Linden, Karin Hofmeester, and Filipa Ribeiro da Silva at the

International Institute of Social History; Nasir Ali at the University of Hargeisa; and Silke Neunsinger, Jonas Söderqvist, and Håkan Nilsson at the Swedish Labour Movement's Archives and Library.

Ten different archives in six countries were consulted as part of the research for this book. Numerous individuals helped facilitate my stays at the various institutions and acquire access to the archives. Special thanks go to Measho Berihu, Biniyam Negash, Kassahun Follo, Ayalew Ahmed, Berhanu Deriba, Diribsa Legesse, Fisehatsion Biadgilign, Assefa Belay, Masho Legesse, Zenebech Eguale, and Tewabech Kifle at the Confederation of Ethiopian Trade Unions; Issayas Tesfamariam, Jim Sam and Lisa Miller at the Hoover Institution Library and Archives; and Benjamin Scott Blake and Alan Wierdak of the University of Maryland Special Collections and University Archives.

I would also like to thank Kiflu Tadesse, Alemu Abebe, Dawi Ibrahim, Hailu Ourgessa, Demmelash Tebekew, Beyene Solomon, and the numerous contemporary trade unionists interviewed, for being so generous with their time and so earnest in their recollections. And Abrhaley Tesfagergs, Belayhun Hailu, Meriam Daniel, and Mattis Jalakas for research and statistical assistance.

Others who, in various ways, have contributed to this book coming into being, and deserve my sincere thanks, include Assefa Admassie, Maurizio Atzeni, Katrin Bromber, Eric Burton, Davide Chinigò, Demessie Fantaye, Elleni Centime Zeleke, Eyob Balcha, Ephrem Shiferaw, Adam Fishwick, Valentina Fusari, Valeria Guarneros-Meza, Pierre Guidi, Ezana Haddis, Jenny Jansson, Julian Tadesse, Geresu Tufa, Daniel Mains, Mahlet Birhanu, Fouad Makki, John Markakis, Mark Mcquinn, Hilma Mote, Immanuel Ness, Marco Di Nunzio, Supriya Roy Chowdhury, Melakou Tegegn, Mesfin Aman, Camille Pellerin, Craig Phelan, Ian Scott Horst, Uoldelul Chelati, Ella Verkaik, Maaike Westra, Jacob Wiebel, Yared Abayneh, Yeraswork Admassie, and Zelalem Yilma.

Finally, with utmost devotion, I would like to express my immense gratitude to my family, friends, and comrades.

CONTENTS

Abbreviations

AALC	African American Labor Center
AATUF	All-African Trade Union Federation
ACILS	American Centre for International Labor Solidarity (Solidarity Center)
AETU	All-Ethiopia Trade Union
AFL-CIO	American Federation of Labor and Congress of Industrial Organizations
AFRO	ICFTU's African Regional Organisation
AID	Agency for International Development (United States)
ATUC	African Trade Union Confederation
AUCCTU	All-Union Central Council of Trade Unions (of the Soviet Union)
CBA	Collective Bargaining Agreement
CBE	Commercial Bank of Ethiopia
CDE	Ethio-Djibouti Railway Enterprise
CELU	Confederation of Ethiopian Labour Unions
CETU	Confederation of Ethiopian Trade Unions
CFE	Franco–Ethiopian Railway Enterprise
CFELU	Confederation of Free Eritrean Labour Unions
CIA	Central Intelligence Agency
CLC	Canadian Labour Congress
COPWE	Commission to Organise the Party of the Working People of Ethiopia
CSA	Central Statistical Authority
EELPA	Ethiopian Electric Light and Power Authority
ELAMA	Ethiopian Workers' Revolutionary Union
EPRDF	Ethiopian People's Revolutionary Democratic Front

EPRP	Ethiopian People's Revolutionary Party
ETA	Ethiopian Teachers' Association
ETB	Ethiopian Birr
ETU	Ethiopian Trade Union
FDGB	Free German Trade Union Federation (of the German Democratic Republic)
FEE	Federation of Ethiopian Employers
FES	Friedrich Ebert Foundation
FTO	Full-Time Official
HIP	Hawassa Industrial Park
HVA	Handelsvereniging Amsterdam
ICFTU	International Confederation of Free Trade Unions
IEG	Imperial Ethiopian Government
IFPAAW	International Federation of Plantation, Agricultural and Allied Workers
ILO	International Labour Organization/Office
IMF	International Monetary Fund
ISF	International Solidarity Fund (of the ICFTU)
ITUC	International Trade Union Confederation
LO	Danish Confederation of Trade Unions
LRB	Labour Relations Board
MEISON	All-Ethiopia Socialist Movement
MNCD	Ministry of National Community Development (and Social Affairs)
MoLSA	Ministry of Labour and Social Affairs
NTC	National Textile Corporation
OATUU	Organisation of African Trade Union Unity
PFTUSM	Peace and Free Trade Union Seeking Members of CETU's Supreme Council
PMAC	Provisional Military Administrative Council
POMOA	Provisional Office for Mass Organisational Affairs
PWC	Provisional Workers' Committee
SAP	Structural Adjustment Programme
TGE	Transitional Government of Ethiopia
TPLF	Tigray People's Liberation Front
UEMLO	Union of Ethiopian Marxist-Leninist Organisations
WCL	World Confederation of Labour
WFTU	World Federation of Trade Unions
WPE	Workers' Party of Ethiopia

List of Figures

CHAPTER 1

Introduction

In Ethiopia, the last few years of the 2010s were marked by escalating social turbulence. An initially popular protest movement, coupled with spiralling levels of inter-ethnic tensions and violence, resulted in the collapse of the ruling coalition, the ascent of a new paramount leader, and the formation of a new ruling party. The advent of the new regime was followed by intense political violence on multiple levels—ranging from political assassinations, military clashes between rival ethnic militias, mass atrocities against civilians, and insurgencies. Then, in 2020, two even greater calamities occurred. First, the arrival of the global COVID-19 pandemic led to global trade and transport disruptions, which seriously impacted the Ethiopian economy. However, far worse was the military assault on the regional state of Tigray by the combined armed forces and militias of the federal government, the Amhara regional state, Eritrea, and other foreign entities. This led to a full-scale civil war, a humanitarian catastrophe, and the destruction of the regional economy of Northern Ethiopia.

For Ethiopian workers, these were trying years. The hardship that followed the breakdown of political order and security across the country was aggravated by the already difficult economic conditions that they laboured under. Wages had sunk to rock-bottom levels, and working conditions were harsh. Ethiopia was drawing global attention for the exceptionally low—by wide comparative margins—wages in its newly

© The Author(s), under exclusive license to Springer Nature Switzerland AG 2025

S. A. Admasie, *The Ethiopian Labour Movement*, Labour in History and Society, https://doi.org/10.1007/978-3-031-72841-9_1

established textile industries and plantations. Workers in such establishments were frequently super-exploited, in the sense that incomes were insufficient to cover even basic nutritional needs. This led to reports of workers collapsing from malnutrition on the factory floor,[1] or, more frequently, relying on support from family members in the agrarian sector to meet their most basic needs.[2]

At the same time, the second half of the 2010s saw the emergence of green shoots of hope for Ethiopian wage workers, manifested in a conspicuous revival and growth of the Ethiopian labour movement. Collective action by Ethiopian workers in the final years of the decade occurred more frequently than at any time since the 1970s. Moreover, the increasing mobilisation and militancy of workers and trade unions impacted workplace regimes and conditions, as well as legislation. Fuelled by rising union membership and an uptick in strike activity and labour unrest, the trade union movement grew more assertive. The central trade union confederation challenged the state in a high-profile dispute over a new labour bill, and was successful in having the bill withdrawn and revised. It also campaigned for workers in industrial parks to have the right to organise—a right that foreign investors and colluding state institutions had illegally denied them—and again succeeded. By the end of the decade, Ethiopian trade unions had regained a level of relevance and clout they had lacked for decades, their numbers had multiplied, and their membership had reached an all-time high.

Labour Movements

Strikes, which formed the basis of the movement's clout in these episodes, and the institutions of the trade unions which channelled that clout, constitute principal examples of the two *concrete* aspects that compose a labour movement: practice and organisation. The first aspect includes all those collective practices undertaken by workers—formally organised or not—that aim to affect change in their position and conditions, whether

[1] P.M. Barrett and D. Baumann-Pauly, *Made in Ethiopia: Challenges in the Garment Industry's New Frontier* (New York: NYU Stern Center for Business and Human Rights, 2019).

[2] See S.A. Admasie, S.A. Admasie "Work and Exploitation in Ethiopia and Beyond," *in Handbook of Research on the Global Political Economy of Work*, ed. M. Atzeni, D. Azzellini, A. Mezzadri, P. Moore, and U. Apitzsch (Cheltenham: Edward Elgar, 2023).

on a local, national, or international level. Strikes, work-to-rule, slowdowns, and absenteeism are examples of practices that aim to do so by withholding labour. But protests, rallies, sabotage, and even violent insubordination are also examples of practices that occasionally appear in the repertoire of labour movements. The second aspect includes all those organisational constellations based on the membership of workers which operate with the aim of increasing workers' collective leverage. They may include mutual self-help associations, cooperatives, educational, cultural and sports societies, strike committees, political organisations, and even armed formations. The most prominent example of such organisations is trade unions, which Richard Hyman has defined in the following manner:

> A trade union is, first and foremost, an agency and a medium of power. Its central purpose is to permit workers to exert, collectively, the control over their conditions of employment which they cannot hope to possess as individuals; and to do so largely by compelling the employer to take account, in policy- and decision-making, of interests and priorities contrary to his own. As the vehicle of workers' interests against those of the employer, the union is involved in external relationships of control. (Such relationships are essentially two-way; as unions seek to affect the decisions of employers and governments they are themselves subject to influence and pressure from a range of external agencies.) But at the same time, process of control pervade the internal relationships of the unions.[3]

The term 'conditions of employment' in this definition appears excessively restrictive. Trade unions frequently seek to have an impact on broader social, political, and economic affairs. When Beatrice and Sidney Webb revised their definition of trade unionism between the first and second editions of their seminal work *The History of Trade Unionism*, it reflected such concerns. While their first definition referred to 'maintaining and improving the condition of their *employment*', the second edition, in response to criticism raised on the grounds mentioned above, instead referred to *working lives*—a significantly broader term.[4] It is,

[3] R. Hyman, *Industrial Relations: A Marxist Introduction* (London and Basingstoke: Macmillan, 1975), 64–65.

[4] S. Webb and B. Webb, *The History of Trade Unionism* (New York: Longmans, Green and Co., 1920), 1.

however, important to retain Hyman's insistence on the dualism of trade unionism—as both channelling and constraining workers' agency.

The relative order of importance between strikes and trade unions has been explained by Marcel van der Linden, who has noted that whereas 'large and successful strikes are perfectly possible *without* unions… unions cannot exist without (the ultimate threat of) the strike weapon'[5]—at the very least not as mediums of power for workers. This is because it is the threat of unrest that provides unions with the leverage required to compel employers (or the state) to take into account those interests and priorities contrary to their own which Hyman noted. If the ultimate threat of the strike weapon and other forms of unrest is relinquished, the formal organisations may well survive or even expand, but they are rendered useless as vehicles of workers' empowerment. Instead, such 'pseudo-unions'[6] serve only the interests of external entities (such as those of employers or the state) in constraining the agency of workers. These are termed *yellow unions*. But, as van der Linden has noted, 'sometimes trade unions mutate'.[7] Vibrant and militant unions can become yellow unions, and vice versa, over time—primarily as a result of the internal contestation that takes place within them. Trade unions are thus not merely vehicles of empowerment and control, but also constitute arenas and objects of struggle. *Contestation*, in the title of this volume, therefore refers not only to the struggle between trade unions and workers, on the one hand, and external agencies (such as employers and the state), on the other, but also the internal struggles *within* trade unions and the broader labour movement—between, for example, proponents of a militant line and advocates of moderation and appeasement.

Finally, as indicated by the previous point, labour movements must also be considered to encompass an ideational dimension: the aims, strategies, and methods deemed most prudent and therefore adopted in the collective effort, or, put in another way, their orientation. These aspects—the collective practices, organisational constellations, and ideational dimensions that constitute labour movements—are intimately interlinked. For example, it is often a trade union (formally or informally)

[5] M. van der Linden, *Workers of the World: Essays Toward a Global Labor History* (Leiden & London: Brill, 2008), 179.

[6] Ibid, 228.

[7] Ibid, 229.

that organises a strike, while a strike can strengthen a union, bolstering its position in collective bargaining. Meanwhile, the ideational dimension is dialectically unified with practice in the category of *praxis*. Just as a successful strike is likely to bolster a trade union, it can also alter workers' perceptions of the type of practice that is feasible, desirable, and advantageous. A successful and victorious strike is thus likely to increase the militancy of workers, which in turn increases the probability that other strikes will occur—within the same establishment, or elsewhere.

The Ethiopian Labour Movement in the Literature

The Ethiopian labour movement has largely escaped serious scholarly attention. In the scarce literature that exists, there has been a tendency to treat it schematically, dismissively, and disparagingly. Scholars have tended to characterise the movement as too small and weak to have had any meaningful influence, or so subservient or closely controlled by authorities as to render it a mere instrument of the state.[8] Scholarly accounts depicting the labour movement in pre-revolutionary Ethiopia were strongly characterised by this tendency. 'Since union membership was small and workplace-based, the unions were far less significant than the local neighbourhood associations, known as *iddir*', Christopher Clapham has suggested,[9] while Edmond Keller has written that the movement 'was never able to present a serious militant challenge to the status quo in the industrial sector'.[10] According to René Lefort, the labour movement 'was apolitical, heterogeneous and atomised',[11] while Gebru

[8] Dessalegn Rahmato, "Civil Society Organizations in Ethiopia", in *Ethiopia: The Challenge of Democracy from Below*, ed. Bahru Zewde and S. Pausewang (Uppsala: Nordic Africa Institute, 2002), 114; Paulos Milkias, "The Role of Civil Society in Promoting Democracy and Human Rights in Ethiopia" (paper presented at the Ethiopian Americans Council Conference, Los Angeles, CA, 2006); Sisay Gebre-Egziabher, "The Role of Civil Society Organisations in Democratisation Process in Ethiopia" (paper presented at the Fifth International Conference of the International Society for the Third-Sector Research, Cape Town, 2002).

[9] C. Clapham, *Transformation and Continuity in Revolutionary Ethiopia* (Cambridge: Cambridge University Press, 1990), 35.

[10] E.J. Keller, *Revolutionary Ethiopia: From Empire to People's Republic* (Bloomington and Indianapolis: Indiana University Press, 1991), 149.

[11] R. Lefort, *Ethiopia: An Heretical Revolution?* (London: Zed Press, 1983), 27.

Tareke has dismissed the emerging working class altogether as 'small, factional, and inconsequential, both qualitatively and quantitatively'.[12]

In terms of detail, only Tom Killion's exceptional 1985 dissertation *Workers, Capital and the State in the Ethiopian Region, 1919–1974* has treated the movement as warranting serious attention. Killion's account described an 'incipient' and 'incomplete' process of working-class formation that culminated in a decade of organised trade unionism between 1963 and 1973,[13] and, ultimately, its 'denouement' in the revolution that followed.[14] Killion documented numerous strikes, increasing difficulties for the imperial state seeking to contain the movement, and growing radicalism within the movement. Yet, in his assessment, the labour movement was always, and remained, subordinated to the state.

Several other scholarly accounts have treated the pre-revolutionary national trade union centre—the Confederation of Ethiopian Labour Unions (CELU)—as little more than a government tool. 'The Emperor was patron to the CELU with the close collaboration of the American Federation of Labor and Congress of Industrial Organizations (AFL-CIO). The CELU leadership was usually handpicked by the Emperor himself and advised by AFL-CIO representatives', Makonen Getu has written. 'It was therefore more of an agent of the Government than of the working class. Due to this state of affairs and the fact that the CELU did not embrace the whole of the working class, the CELU was never in a position to lead a militant labor struggle', he concluded.[15] Ian Scott Horst's recent account generally supports this view, but offers a more dynamic understanding of the movement's development. CELU, Scott Horst wrote, 'was created with the sponsorship of pro-imperialist forces in world labor, that is to say, the [...] AFL–CIO, who hoped to create a captive, docile labor organization with whom the "business community" could cooperate, forestalling more militant working class organizing

[12] Gebru Tareke (2009: 23).

[13] T. Killion, "Workers, Capital and the State in the Ethiopian Region" (PhD diss., Stanford University, 1985), 2–4.

[14] Ibid., 545.

[15] Makonen Getu, *Socialism, Participation, and Agricultural Development in Post-Revolutionary Ethiopia: A Study of Constraints* (Stockholm: Almqvist & Wiksell International, 1987), 62.

while claiming to promote the free organization of workers'.[16] Horst cites a radical Ethiopian student movement publication from the time that 'described it as an organization built to put the brakes on popular struggle: "[B]ureaucratic leaders and traitors to the working class (leaders of CELU) restrict the working class's struggle and slow down the process whereby it becomes the class conscious vanguard of the revolution"'.[17] 'Of course it wasn't CELU's original intention to become a breeding-ground for Ethiopian Bolsheviks', Scott Horst rightly notes. 'And yet', he remarks in more appreciative terms, 'by March 8, CELU—with all its compromised history—initiated a general strike'.[18] This captures the crux of the problem with much of the scholarly literature, which describes the pre-revolutionary labour movement in static terms: its inability to explain the radical change that occurred in the movement's disposition.

As a consequence of the labour movement's participation in the Ethiopian 1974 revolution, the standard scholarly view of the movement underwent a slight alteration. However, scholarly accounts generally remained quite sceptical, particularly towards the movement's prior history. Bahru Zewde, for example, has written that prior to March 1974, 'CELU had been notable for its lethargy rather than its militancy',[19] while Gebru Tareke has claimed that it was 'relatively placid and dormant throughout the 1960s' and that 'the torpor was shattered only amid the dramatic circumstances of the 1970s'.[20] Makonen Getu, meanwhile, has opined that 'although at later stages the CELU began to raise political demands, its major struggle was economistic and directed by an ill-functioning leadership'.[21] Among the accounts that described the labour movement's genuine contribution towards the revolutionary movement of the mid-1970s, on the other hand, are John Markakis and Nega Ayele's

[16] I. Scott Horst, *Like Ho Chi Minh! Like Che Guevara! The Revolutionary Left in Ethiopia*, 1969–1979 (Paris: Foreign Languages Press, 2020), 119.

[17] Ibid., 119.

[18] Ibid., 119.

[19] Bahru Zewde, *A History of Modern Ethiopia: 1855–1991* (Addis Ababa: Addis Ababa University Press, 2002), 231.

[20] Gebru Tareke, *The Ethiopian Revolution: War in the Horn of Africa* (New Haven and London: Yale University Press, 2009), 23.

[21] Makonen, *Socialism, Participation, and Agricultural Development*, 62.

Class and Revolution in Ethiopia,[22] Kiflu Tadesse's[23] two books on the history of the Ethiopian People's Revolutionary Party (EPRP),[24] and Ian Scott Horst's work on the revolutionary left in Ethiopia.[25] But Markakis and Nega's account is rather unique in having noted that labour militancy actually had a history that preceded the revolution by quite some time: that strikes and industrial unrest were relatively frequent throughout the 1960s and early 1970s. This is an important but underappreciated point, which is almost entirely neglected elsewhere in the literature.

Other scholars, such as Marina Ottaway, have been openly dismissive of the labour movement's role in the revolution, downplaying the radicalism the movement exhibited as mere pretension. The labour movement, she argued, functioned as a vehicle for petty bourgeois and white-collar interests, which opposed the newly installed military government from a conservative position masked in radical rhetoric.[26] This is a position that she and David Ottaway reasserted in their 1978 volume *Ethiopia: Empire in Revolution*. The Ottaways characterised the trade union movement as a vehicle for narrow and moderate corporate interests of a privileged segment of the workforce, accused it of being unable to compromise,[27] and described its leadership as 'incompetent', 'confused' and 'opportunist'.[28] Their account is not alone in treating labour opposition to the military regime as inauthentic and illegitimate. The radicalisation of the labour movement in the 1970s and its opposition to the military government has frequently been dismissed as unconnected to the views and interests of workers. Instead, it has been interpreted as the outcome

[22] J. Markakis and Nega Ayele, *Class and Revolution in Ethiopia* (Nottingham: Spokesman Books, 1978).

[23] A former politburo member of the EPRP and a central committee member of the EPRP's labour front.

[24] Kiflu Tadesse, *The Generation: The History of the Ethiopian People's Revolutionary Party, part I: From the Early Beginnings to 1975* (Silver Spring, MD: Independent Publishers, 1993); Kiflu Tadesse, *The Generation: The History of the Ethiopian People's Revolutionary Party, part II: Ethiopia, Transformation and Conflict* (Lanham, MD: University Press of America, 1998).

[25] Scott Horst, *Like Ho Chi Minh*.

[26] M. Ottaway, "Social Classes and Corporate Interests in the Ethiopian Revolution," *Journal of Modern African Studies* 14, no. 3 (1976).

[27] M. Ottaway and D. Ottaway, *Ethiopia: Empire in Revolution* (New York: Africana Publishing Company, 1978), 101–105.

[28] Ibid., 106–107.

of 'infiltration' by radicals in general, or, more frequently, the EPRP in particular.[29] Not only does the concept of infiltration denote a mechanical and external form of control, but it also carries an implication of normative illegitimacy. In other words, these accounts reflect the view that the Ethiopian trade unions had no business in opposing the coming of a military-bureaucratic dictatorship. Despite the multiple calamities this would cause for Ethiopian workers.

Scholarly discussions on the labour movement in post-revolutionary Ethiopia, particularly after the 1980s, have been exceptionally rare. Such discussions have been conducted with a similarly schematic, dismissive, and disparaging attitude towards it. Dessalegn Rahmato's 2002 account stands out as a pertinent example. The trade union movement, Dessalegn contended, 'has been kept as a docile instrument of state policy by successive governments since the 1960s'. Yet, he argued, even this degradation reflects governments having assigned 'the trade union movement a significance and power far beyond its actual potential'. Ethiopian trade union history, he claimed, actually merited far less importance than accorded, and was rather 'the result of false perceptions and an exaggerated sense of worth'.[30]

In this volume, this flattened and almost entirely negative depiction of the Ethiopian labour movement is challenged. Instead, a more fluid, multifaceted, and dialectical account of a movement that has always been prone to drastic changes is presented. These changes have emerged through contradictions within the movement itself, and between the movement and external agencies. The account presented here builds on

[29] Andargachew, *The Ethiopian Revolution*, 141–142, 175; Negussay Ayele. "The Ethiopian Revolution: Political Aspects of the Transition from PMAC to PDRE," in *The Political Economy of Ethiopia*, ed. M. Ottaway (New York: Prager Publishers, 1990), 11–29; Lefort, *Heretical Revolution*, 30. Mengistu Hailemariam, "Speech Delivered to the Second Congress of the All Ethiopia Trade Union" (Addis Ababa: Commission for Organizing the Party of the Working People of Ethiopia), 1982, 31; Teferra Haile Selassie, *The Ethiopian Revolution 1974–1991: From a Monarchial Autocracy to a Military Oligopoly* (New York: Routledge, 2011), 134.

[30] Dessalegn, "Civil Society Organizations," 114.

a decade of research conducted in archives in Ethiopia,[31] the Netherlands,[32] the United States,[33] Switzerland,[34] and Denmark.[35] It draws on work by the International Institute of Social History in digitising additional relevant African labour archives, as well as interviews with key Ethiopian trade union officials, militants, and state officials conducted in Ethiopia, Uganda, the Netherlands, Switzerland, and the United States. It seeks to place the movement's contemporary shape—at the time of writing, the country's largest membership-based mass organisation by a considerable margin, with an extensive geographical reach across the country—in its accurate historical context, and examine the factors behind its varying fortunes and misfortunes.

Structure of the Book

The next chapter examines the history of the Ethiopian labour movement during the period of the country's imperial regime. The antecedents of the movement; its formation on a countrywide level during the late 1950s and the beginning of the 1960s; its development in the long decade that followed; and the divisions and conflicts that embroiled it, are elements that are explored. The chapter describes how a widening rift developed within the movement, and how external entities tried to control and subvert it. The common scholarly depiction of the labour movement in imperial Ethiopia as entirely subservient to the state is refuted, in favour of a more fluid picture of a movement whose relationship with the state was always tense, and within which different tendencies competed for dominance. They included a radical strand in opposition to the moderate leadership, which progressively grew stronger from the 1960s onwards

[31] The archives of the Confederation of Ethiopian Trade Unions and the Ministry of Labour and Social Affairs.

[32] The archives of the International Confederation of Free Trade Unions (ICFTU), hosted by the International Institute of Social History.

[33] The African American Labor Center (AALC) Records, the Lester N. Trachtman Papers, and the AFL-CIO International Affairs Department's archives, hosted by the University of Maryland's Hornbake Library; as well as the Tom Killion Papers, hosted by the Hoover Institution.

[34] The International Labour Organization (ILO) archives.

[35] The Danish Confederation of Trade Union's archives, hosted by the Danish Labour Movement's Library and Archive.

and eventually became dominant. The period ended with the Ethiopian Revolution, which led to the abolition of the monarchy in 1974.

Chapter 3 discusses the hitherto highest tide of labour mobilisation in Ethiopia, which occurred in close temporal proximity to the 1974 revolution and in the years that followed. The growing militancy and radicalisation of the movement is examined, against the grain of the prevailing tendency in the literature to subsume it under the historiography of the Ethiopian revolution. However, this subsumption is rejected. Instead, the wave of militancy around the years of the revolution is placed within a longer arc of internal contestation and radicalisation that originated in the 1960s. The chapter also examines the collapse of the movement against the backdrop of severe repression by the military regime, as well as the subsequent decade of yellow unionism, during which the trade unions were made formally subservient to the state.

Chapter 4 examines the labour movement during the period of the federal republic, which was established in a process that began with the Ethiopian People's Revolutionary Democratic Front's military victory over the previous regime in 1991. The chapter discusses an initial, ultimately failed, attempt to revive an autonomous labour movement in the early-to-mid 1990s; the repression of this attempt by the ruling party and state; and another decade of yellow unionism that followed. It also discusses the most recent re-emergence of a buoyant and relatively autonomous labour movement, which became apparent in the 2010s. Finally, the situation and state of the movement at the dawn of the 2020s is described.

In Chapter 5, attention is turned to the impact of foreign and international trade union organisations on the Ethiopian labour movement. The chapter focuses on the period of the most intense international attention to the Ethiopian trade unions, which occurred in the 1960s and 1970s. It examines the different elements of relationships that developed between the Ethiopian trade union movement and the International Confederation of Free Trade Unions, the African American Labor Center, and the Danish Confederation of Trade Unions. These elements included genuine and appreciated assistance, but also interference, obstruction and subversion. Finally, the chapter discusses later engagements between Ethiopian and international trade union organisations.

Chapter 6 shifts attention from the organisational aspect of the labour movement to its militant practices—namely strikes and labour unrest. It also explores the impact of those practices on the conditions and position of labour by measuring and comparing shifting levels of unrest and the movement of real wages in Ethiopia since the 1960s. The first section of the chapter examines aggregate levels of unrest in the waged sector, while the second section does the same for the movement of real wages. The two consecutive sections consist of case studies on wages and unrest in two large companies: the Bahir Dar Textile Factory and the Ethio-Djibouti Railway Enterprise. In the concluding section, the findings derived from the aggregate data and the case studies are summarised. This feeds into a model of how the labour movement has impacted the Ethiopian wage labour regime and conditions of workers—and how such an impact has fed back on the further development of the movement.

The final chapter contains a summary of findings and conclusions.

References

Admasie, S. A. "Work and Exploitation in Ethiopia and Beyond." In *Handbook of Research on the Global Political Economy of Work*, edited by M. Atzeni, D. Azzellini, A. Mezzadri, P. Moore, and U. Apitzsch, 614–624. Cheltenham: Edward Elgar, 2023.

Andargachew Tiruneh. *The Ethiopian Revolution, 1974–1987: A Transformation From an Aristocratic to a Totalitarian Autocracy*. Cambridge: Cambridge University Press, 1993.

Bahru Zewde. *A History of Modern Ethiopia: 1855–1991*. Addis Ababa: Addis Ababa University Press, 2002.

Barrett, P.M. and D. Baumann-Pauly. *Made in Ethiopia: Challenges in the Garment Industry's New Frontier*. New York: NYU Stern Center for Business and Human Rights, 2019.

Clapham, C. *Transformation and Continuity in Revolutionary Ethiopia*. Cambridge: Cambridge University Press, 1990.

Dessalegn Rahmato. "Civil Society Organizations in Ethiopia." In *Ethiopia: The Challenge of Democracy from Below*, edited by Bahru Zewde and S. Pausewang), 103–119. Uppsala: Nordic Africa Institute, 2002.

Gebru Tareke. *The Ethiopian Revolution: War in the Horn of Africa*. New Haven and London: Yale University Press, 2009.

Hyman, R. *Industrial Relations: A Marxist Introduction*. London and Basingstoke: Macmillan, 1975.

Keller, E.J. *Revolutionary Ethiopia: From Empire to People's Republic*. Bloomington and Indianapolis: Indiana University Press, 1991.

Kiflu Tadesse. *The Generation: The History of the Ethiopian People's Revolutionary Party, part I: From the Early Beginnings to 1975*. Silver Spring, MD: Independent Publishers, 1993.

Kiflu Tadesse. *The Generation: The History of the Ethiopian People's Revolutionary Party, part II: Ethiopia, Transformation and Conflict*. Lanham, MD: University Press of America, 1998.

Killion, T. "Workers, Capital and the State in the Ethiopian Region." PhD diss., Stanford University, 1985.

Lefort, R. *Ethiopia: An Heretical Revolution?* London: Zed Press, 1983.

Linden, M.v.d. *Workers of the World: Essays Toward a Global Labor History*. Leiden & London: Brill, 2008.

Makonen Getu. *Socialism, Participation, and Agricultural Development in Post-Revolutionary Ethiopia: A Study of Constraints*. Stockholm: Almqvist & Wiksell International, 1987.

Markakis, J. and Nega Ayele. *Class and Revolution in Ethiopia*. Nottingham: Spokesman Books, 1978.

Mengistu Hailemariam. "Speech Delivered to the Second Congress of the All Ethiopia Trade Union." Addis Ababa: Commission for Organizing the Party of the Working People of Ethiopia, 1982.

Negussay Ayele. "The Ethiopian Revolution: Political Aspects of the Transition from PMAC to PDRE." In *The Political Economy of Ethiopia*, edited by M. Ottaway. New York: Prager Publishers, 1990.

Ottaway, M. "Social Classes and Corporate Interests in the Ethiopian Revolution." *Journal of Modern African Studies* 14, no. 3 (1976): 469–486.

Ottaway, M. and D. Ottaway. *Ethiopia: Empire in Revolution*. New York: Africana Publishing Company, 1978.

Paulos Milkias. "The Role of Civil Society in Promoting Democracy and Human Rights in Ethiopia." Paper presented at the Ethiopian Americans Council Conference, Los Angeles, CA, July 2006.

Teferra Haile Selassie. *The Ethiopian Revolution 1974–1991: From a Monarchial Autocracy to a Military Oligopoly*. New York: Routledge, 2011.

Webb, S. and B. Webb. *The History of Trade Unionism*. New York: Longmans, Green and Co., 1920.

Scott Horst, I. *Like Ho Chi Minh! Like Che Guevara! The Revolutionary Left in Ethiopia*, 1969–1979. Paris: Foreign Languages Press, 2020.

Sisay Gebre-Egziabher. "The Role of Civil Society Organisations in Democratisation Process in Ethiopia." Paper presented at the Fifth International Conference of the International Society for the Third-Sector Research, Cape Town, July 2002.

CHAPTER 2

The Labour Movement in Imperial Ethiopia: Emergence and Ascent, 1960–1974

Formation

The Ethiopian labour movement was formed on a countrywide scale around the turn of the decade between the 1950s and 1960s. Its emergence was stimulated by a number of factors. Railway workers of the *Compagnie du Chemin de Fer Franco-Ethiopien* (CFE), who operated the Djibouti-Addis Ababa line, had been the first to organise. European workers of the company, with prior experience in organising, established the first workers' organisation and staged strikes in the years immediately following the First World War. But it was only in the aftermath of the Italian occupation that Ethiopian workers came to play a leading role, and in 1947 CFE workers staged the first large-scale Ethiopian-led strike. Another early stimulus came from dock- and maritime workers in the neighbouring port of Djibouti, who established a number of organisations and engaged in collective action and bargaining. Furthermore, the organised workers on the Djiboutian section of the railroad—which was administered separately from the Ethiopian section—won concessions that significantly improved their conditions compared to those on the

© The Author(s), under exclusive license to Springer Nature Switzerland AG 2025

S. A. Admasie, *The Ethiopian Labour Movement*, Labour in History and Society, https://doi.org/10.1007/978-3-031-72841-9_2

Ethiopian section of the line, and thus demonstrated the potential benefits of labour movementism. However, of more direct importance for the emergence of the Ethiopian labour movement was the experience of trade unionism in Eritrea, a territory which was federated with—and later incorporated into—the Ethiopian Empire in 1952. Prior to the federation, the British military administration of the territory had issued a law that permitted workers to organise. Owing to guarantees offered at the inception of the federation, this law was initially respected by the Ethiopian government, and organised labour, while banned in Ethiopia proper, continued to be permitted in Eritrea.

The Eritrean labour movement was relatively small and urban. By 1958, the Confederation of Free Eritrean Labour Unions (CFELU) united some 10,000 workers.[1] However, although the confederation was grudgingly tolerated, Ethiopian authorities were uneasy with its existence. Free association in Eritrea threatened to spark both imitative practices among workers in Ethiopia proper and centrifugal political mobilisation in Eritrea. The emerging link between Eritrean and Ethiopian workers at that time, and the inspiration the former exercised on the latter, was demonstrated by the immediate way in which a strike of Eritrean dockworkers in Massawa and Assab in 1954 was followed by a strike of Ethiopian workers on the Ethio-Djiboutian railway. In 1958, the situation in Eritrea came to a head when the CFELU organised a general strike. Repression followed, claiming the lives of several strikers and protesters.[2] In the aftermath, the confederation was banned, and its offices were closed. Although the organisational structure was thereby dismantled, the ideas propelling collective organisation had taken root among Eritrean workers. Through inspiration and social intercourse, those ideas were to spread further south and into Ethiopia proper. Meanwhile, southward labour migration from Eritrea, particularly in the waged sectors where labour movementism was about to emerge in earnest, provided the emerging Ethiopian labour movement with an infusion of workers with organisational experience. Some very important leaders of

[1] R. Stutz, "The Developing Industrial Relations System in Ethiopia" (mimeo, Haile Selassie I University, Addis Ababa, 1967), 112.

[2] The official figure of casualties was 535 wounded and nine killed. T. Killion, "Workers, Capital and the State in the Ethiopian Region" (Ph.D. diss., Stanford University, 1985), 379.

the Ethiopian labour movement, including CELU's eventual president, would be drawn from this group.

By the end of the 1950s, the objective conditions for the emergence of an Ethiopian labour movement had ripened, as developmental efforts had created a mass of wage labourers capable of sustaining an economy-wide movement. The poor conditions under which these workers entered wage employment created immediate friction. Meanwhile, local initiatives reinforced the external stimuli, combining to demonstrate the feasibility of collective action. Mutual aid associations—*iddirs*—were already a popular feature among Ethiopia's emerging urban population. These organisations, however, were generally limited in scope to aiding their members in times of extraordinary stress—most typically in the organisation of burials. In the 1940s and 1950s, however, workplace *iddirs* began to be formed by wage workers in a number of establishments. The scope of activities of these early workers' associations was limited to collective self-help and petitioning. Yet, in autonomously organising workers, they carried the seed of what was to evolve into the trade union movement. Initial attempts to sway the workplace power balance included 'many instances where workers simply joined together and, with a flag waving, marched to the palace to submit their petition in the form of complaints'.[3] Eventually, and where the conditions permitted, workers' associations turned into unions in all but name, and some of them—such as that at the Dutch enterprise *Handelsvereeniging Amsterdam*'s (HVA) Wonji-Shoa sugar refinery—came to stage successful strikes. With the genie out of the bottle, workers' associations multiplied and mushroomed across the empire, and strikes—a previously relatively rare and limited phenomenon—became frequent.

In 1960, a cooperative forum for workers associations around Addis Ababa was formed under the auspices of the workers' association of the Ethio-fibre Factory and its chairman, Aberra Gemu. In 1962, this forum was to form an umbrella organisation comprising twenty workers' associations. Although there was no legal basis for it, and its application for registration with authorities was therefore ignored, the actual existence of an emerging centre was warily tolerated by the imperial government. It was considered a lesser evil than the alternatives. In 1962, a senior official of the imperial government told a visiting representative of the

[3] Syoum Gebregziabher, "The Rise of CELU and the EFE Under Haile Selassie's Regime," (mimeo, 2005), 17.

International Confederation of Free Trade Unions (ICFTU) that the government was aware of the 'growing agitations among the workers who had staged several down-tools and walk-out actions recently'.[4] The official disclosed that a 'good number' of workers' organisations had already been established and that 'some of them had already started creating trouble with employers', including staging strikes. The government's concern, he admitted, was magnified by the fact that 'workers went on strike without [first] discussing with the employers their grievances', and by the fear that 'communist elements' existed among the workers. Another senior official of the Ministry of National Community Development's (MNCD) Labour Department concurred that 'the existing workers organisations were now growing into restless movements'.[5] Because the government 'was worried about the possible consequences of such illegal and "unwarranted" actions', the ICFTU representative reported, it was compelled to move faster to pass legislation regulating the formation and operation of trade unions. 'The problem of establishing trade unions and grievance and negotiating machineries had become acute and the government was eager to get things done as quickly as possible', the ICFTU's representative concluded.[6] The legalisation of trade unionism in Ethiopia was thus precipitated by urgent pressures asserted by the emergent labour movement, and was based on the expressed calculation that legalised trade unionism would stem the growing level of restiveness.

The heightened activity among workers and the growing number of workplace disputes combined with internal and external political pressures to convince the imperial state of the need to address the problem. In most of Ethiopia's newly independent continental neighbours, trade unions were not only permitted but also often served as important allies of ruling parties. As Addis Ababa had been selected as the capital of the Organisation of African Unity, and as Ethiopia was a long-standing member of the ILO, the absence of a national trade union centre posed an embarrassing problem to the international image the imperial government sought to project. Internally, moreover, a 1960 coup attempt had

[4] Serge Claverie to His Imperial Majesty Haile Selassie, April 1962, ICFTU/ITUC archives, collection ARCH00622, International Institute of Social History, Amsterdam.

[5] Ibid.

[6] Ibid.

exposed the political fragility of the imperial regime and made it somewhat more susceptible to pressure to initiate reform. These factors added to the pressure from workers to force a change in the government's position on trade unions, and a labour proclamation was finally issued in 1962 and enacted the following year. The proclamation permitted the legal establishment and registration of trade unions. In March 1963, they formed the Confederation of Ethiopian Labour Unions (CELU). It was recognised by the government the following month.

Right from the outset, the emergent movement was beset by a number of problems. The 1963 labour proclamation barred large sections of the workforce from organising, including agricultural workers and civil servants. In addition, the effective ban on unionism in Eritrea remained in force until 1966. Funds were scarce at the level of individual unions, particularly in terms of what they could afford to share with the national centre. As a result, the new confederation faced financial constraints from the outset. Size was another constraining factor. It was a relatively small confederation that came into existence: only 15,000 workers were trade union members in April 1963.[7] However, such limitations did not prevent the imperial state from closely monitoring the movement and enforcing control at the level it was most cost-effective: the central leadership.

The limits to CELU's autonomy were almost immediately tested and demarcated by the state. Within a year of its formation, the confederation's elected leadership—headed by HVA union head Abraham Mekonnen—had become impatient with the government's lack of interest in addressing concerns it had raised. Such concerns included the state's failure to safeguard rights established in the 1963 labour proclamation, its disregard for persistent harassment and dismissals of union representatives[8], and the growing backlog of cases referred to the Labour Relations Board (LRB), which meant that workers whose rights had been violated were left indefinitely suspended without pay. In order to enforce a resolution of these problems, CELU threatened to call a general strike. This constituted an intolerable act of insubordination, and the imperial government immediately moved to force a change in

[7] Emmanuel Fayessa Negassa, "The Confederation of Ethiopian Labour Unions and its First General Strike (March 7–11, 1974): Causes and Impact" (master's thesis, Cornell University, 1977), 65.

[8] Killion discusses the repression of a number of unions in the intervening time. Killion, "Workers, Capital and the State," 465.

CELU's leadership, threatening the dissolution of the young confederation.[9] Abraham Mekonnen resigned in response to the government's ultimatum, and Aberra Gemu was found shot to death.[10] According to confidential government communication to the ICFTU, the importance attached to having Abraham Mekonnen removed was not only motivated by his role in issuing the strike threat. He was also accused of having contacts with 'various Eastern countries' and having discussed funding for a literacy campaign with Soviet and Yugoslav officials[11]—a serious offence in the eyes of the equally intense anti-communists of the imperial government and the ICFTU. Whatever the precise factors prompting the purge, 'the illusion of CELU's autonomy was destroyed', as Tom Killion has written.[12] From this point on, it has correctly been noted, 'the leadership knew that the threat of violent suppression was always hanging over its head',[13] as the imperial government continued to keep a watchful eye over its activities.

While the strike threat had demonstrated the movement's potential power to both the government and workers, attracting new members to the trade unions in the process,[14] it had come at a price. It was a deferential and obedient leadership that replaced Abraham Mekonnen's, careful about keeping amicable relations with both the government and employers. Indeed, many years later, an official of the Federation of Ethiopian Employers (FEE) could testify to having 'always enjoyed excellent relationships and understanding with both the government and CELU'.[15] CELU's new president was Beyene Solomon, a trade unionist

[9] "Mission to Ethiopia 31 August–31 September 1963," H. Robinson, report, 1963, ICFTU/ITUC archives.

[10] Whether Aberra Gemu was assassinated or committed suicide has been a matter of debate. In Tom Killion's assessment, 'the cause of his death was state repression', either way. Killion, "Workers, Capital and the State," 467.

[11] "Mission to Ethiopia 31 August–31 September 1963," H. Robinson, report, 1963, ICFTU/ITUC archives.

[12] Killion, "Workers, Capital and the State," 467–468.

[13] Dessalegn Rahmato, "Civil Society Organizations in Ethiopia", in *Ethiopia: The Challenge of Democracy from Below*, ed. Bahru Zewde and S. Pausewang (Uppsala: Nordic Africa Institute, 2002), 114.

[14] A.M. Zack, "The New Trade Unions of Africa's Oldest Country," *Analyst* no. 3 (1965): 36.

[15] Syoum Gebregziabher, "The Rise of CELU and the EFE," 83.

and former shoe factory worker from Eritrea who lacked the merit of being an elected representative of any constituent union of CELU. Beyene surrounded himself with several young university-educated staff members, out of whom four were eventually co-opted into CELU's top executive leadership: Fissehatsion Tekie, Mesfin Gebremichael, Gebreselassie Gebremariam, and Tesfa Gebremariam [NB: no familial relation]. They were dubbed 'CELU's four horsemen' by American labour advisors and diplomats. As Killion noted, the young graduates would play an increasingly important role in CELU's organisation and administration, acting 'as intermediaries between the state and union leaders', while developing 'close contacts with the ICFTU and US labour advisors'. 'Together with Beyene Solomon', Killion wrote, 'these four university graduates dominated CELU's central administration between 1965 and 1973'.[16] In doing so, they provided Beyene with his most crucial source of support and instrument of control over the movement. Just like Beyene, they did not represent any constituent union, but unlike him, they also had no authentic experience of shop floor work. It has been alleged—even by sympathetic observers—that these staffers had little contact with workers and aimed 'only to develop a new labour profession'—that they 'tended to use their positions within CELU as a spring board for career development'.[17] Because non-elected employees did not represent any constituent union, they were prohibited from standing for election to executive positions in the confederation. However, as Beyene's and his staffers' influence increased, they arranged for CELU's statutes to be amended. A 1965 amendment permitted non-representative staff members to be co-opted and elected to CELU's top leadership—and all four eventually joined it in the senior-most positions immediately under Beyene.

CELU's new leaders enjoyed a level of government tolerance that had eluded their predecessors, and they earned it by suppressing radical impulses within the movement. The leadership's willingness to engage in manipulation to serve this end can be seen in Beyene's criticism of Abraham Mekonnen for allowing a vote on the proposal to issue a strike threat in 1963. Although a majority of workers' representatives supported

[16] Killion, "Workers, Capital and the State," 462–463.

[17] Killion, "Workers, Capital and the State," 64; Seleshi Sisaye, "Urban Migration and the Labor Movement in Ethiopia," in *Proceedings of the Fifth International Conference of Ethiopian Studies (Session B)*, (Chicago: University of Illinois, 1979): 689, 698.

the proposal, Beyene argued that it should have been rejected on procedural grounds or delayed through stalling tactics. Beyene remarked that Abraham 'should have handled the matter more delicately… he was in error when he asked all workers for a vote [and] could have easily evaded the problem by saying that he needed to study the complaint first or something to that effect'.[18] Such stalling tactics and procedural manipulation would henceforth be employed whenever the leadership was seriously challenged. But because of its timid approach and the bureaucratic subversions it engaged in, according to a CELU insider, the leadership 'alienated a significant [share] of the workers' and eventually came to cause 'a rift in the Ethiopian labour movement'.[19]

External Influences and Internal Bureaucratisation

Soon after its formation, CELU joined the ICFTU as an affiliate. As discussed in the fifth chapter of this book, this provided the confederation with crucial material relief. But it also provided individual members of CELU's top leadership with a range of personal benefits, as well as resources to be used to shore up the leadership's position vis-à-vis contenders.

For the confederation, relations with ICFTU provided access to funds, transfers of skills, and an international affiliation that could provide a certain level of protection against state encroachment. Financial support was particularly important considering CELU's poor internal finances. CELU's leadership, moreover, was adept at exploiting funds provided by the ICFTU and allies to its own best advantage. However, CELU came to grow more dependent on the ICFTU than what the latter was comfortable with. The ICFTU was also not alone in supporting CELU financially, but a host of other allies in the anti-communist strand of the international trade union movement that clustered in Addis Ababa provided additional assistance. They included the AFL-CIO's regional arm, the African American Labor Centre (AALC), and Danish *Landsorganisationen*. To gauge the relative importance of such funding, CELU's 1969 statement

[18] Beyene Solomon, *Fighter for Democracy: The Saga of an Ethiopian Labour Leader* (Baltimore: Publish America, 2010), 72.

[19] Emmanuel, "Confederation of Ethiopian Labour Unions and its First General Strike," 66–67.

of income, expenditure and balance revealed that, out of a total income of 140,000 Ethiopian Dollars, 38,000 came from ICFTU assistance, 54,000 from the AALC, and only 47,000—quite precisely one-third—was funds generated by CELU itself.[20]

Individually, CELU's top leaders were rewarded with a number of perks that came with holding high office. This played the role of very suddenly and drastically separating the top layer of officialdom from the rank-and-file socially and materially, in a process that bred the bureaucratisation of the movement. ICFTU documents reveal that as early as 1963, the *monthly* salary of CELU's president was 600 Ethiopian Birr (ETB),[21] while that of the general secretary was 450 ETB.[22] This amounted to a *yearly* salary of a very well-paid worker.[23] CELU's president, Beyene, owned a private villa, two cars and a film projector during his incumbency.[24] This illustrates a lifestyle far beyond the means of regular workers at the time. Indeed, by the time they were ousted, Beyene and his closest

[20] CELU, "CELU Statement of Income, Expenditure and Balance, From January 1st to December 31st, 1969," report, 1969, ICFTU/ITUC archives.

[21] "Mission to Ethiopia 31 August–31 September 1963," H. Robinson, report, 1963, ICFTU/ITUC archives. While Ethiopian currency has been known as *Birr* (ETB) in Amharic since its introduction, it was referred to as Ethiopian Dollars in English until 1975, when the name Birr was officially adopted in English as well. Since the Ethiopian Dollar was converted to Birr at an equal rate, the abbreviation ETB is used throughout this text for simplicity.

[22] In a report by ICFTU representative Robinson, it is stated that 'the president and general secretary agreed to draw only one-half of their salaries until the Confederation is in a better financial position'. However, only a few months later, this commitment was omitted from funding requests. In fact, the monthly salary of the president had by then been increased to 650 ETB. In addition, a dozen other salaries were mentioned in 1964, including monthly 400 for an education officer; 300 for an organiser; and 300 for a typist. The size of this representative and non-representative layer of relatively well-paid FTOs and staffers was only to continue to increase in the decade that followed. "Mission to Ethiopia 31 August–31 September 1963," H. Robinson, report, 1963, ICFTU/ITUC archives. "Mission to Ethiopia 31 August–31 September 1963," H. Robinson, report, 1963, ICFTU/ITUC archives; Beyene Solomon to Omer Becu, 29 November 1963, ICFTU/ITUC archives; Omer Becu to George Meany, 6 October 1964, ICFTU/ITUC Archives.

[23] In fact, a monthly wage of 25–30 Ethiopian Birr was common at the time.

[24] Beyene, *Fighter for Democracy,* 174.

lieutenant, Fissehatsion Tekie, each earned a regular salary from CELU that was over fourteen times higher than that of some confederation staff members.[25] Moreover, high salaries constituted only one aspect of the many perks they enjoyed.[26] CELU's top officials had access to extensive travel opportunities to the ICFTU and its member federations in Europe and North America, as well as funding for studies and training programmes abroad—opportunities that often came with generous *per diem* payments. These opportunities were evidently highly appealing. According to the ICFTU representative in Addis Ababa, senior CELU officials displayed an 'eagerness to get every possible chance to travel abroad'.[27] Social elevation was another benefit of holding high positions within the confederation. In his memoirs, Beyene[28] recounted rubbing shoulders with ministers, international officialdom, ambassadors, and the economic elite of Ethiopian society of the time. The American ambassador to Ethiopia thought very highly of Beyene, whom he considered 'a strong anti-Communist',[29] and Beyene could count Ethiopian aristocrats as well as top international labour officials among his personal friends. Eventually, Beyene and CELU's General Secretary Fissehatsion Tekie were themselves co-opted into an elite circle of international labour officialdom. Beyene was elected as a board member and a vice president of the ICFTU, as well as a member of the governing body of the ILO, whereas Fissehatsion served as the General Secretary of the ICFTU's African Regional Organisation (AFRO) between 1972 and his arrest in 1974. Their stature was evident from the substantial material support their international allies

[25] CELU, "ከሚያዝያ 1 ቀን 66 እስከ መጋቢት 30 ቀን 1967 ዓ.ም ባጀት ዝርዝር መግለጫ," memorandum, 1974, Confederation of Ethiopian Trade Unions (CETU) archives, CETU, Addis Ababa.

[26] According to former CELU employee Emmanuel Fayessa Negassa, other carrots extended by the government included duty free privileges and funded 'travel at will'. But it also included sticks, in terms of threat and surveillance. Emmanuel further claims that concealed government stipends to CELU constituted another control mechanism, but notes that the CELU leaders were unwilling to admit this. Emmanuel Fayessa Negesa, interviewed by Tom Killion, 1983, microcassette, Tom Killion Papers, collection 2017C40, Hoover Institution Library and Archives, Stanford University Stanford, CA.

[27] Lennart Kindström to P.H. de Jonge, 2 February 1966, ICFTU/ITUC archives.

[28] Beyene, *Fighter for Democracy*.

[29] William O. Hall to Dean Clowes, 12 July 1968, African American Labor Center (AALC) Records, collection 0547-LBR, Hornbake Library, Special Collections and University Archives, University of Maryland Libraries, College Park, MD.

continued to provide them and their families long after their eventual ouster from CELU.

The administration of support funds allowed significant leeway. For example, projects in Eritrea, personally overseen by Beyene, were withheld from CELU's board's scrutiny. Beyene had informally asked the ICFTU's representative in Addis Ababa to provide funds for these projects, without revealing their nature.[30] He explained that he refrained from disclosing the activities to CELU's board because 'some board members were against any activity in Eritrea'. Although this was probably partly true—such regional and ethnic animosities existed within CELU's leading bodies—his own deep involvement in factional struggles within CELU's Eritrean branch, where he used available resources to award loyalists and punish contenders, was facilitated by access to external funds with little oversight. The opportunity to travel abroad was another means used by the leadership to reward loyalists and punish union officials deemed disloyal. Those who opposed the leadership claimed that only its cronies—including individuals with spurious connections to the labour movement—were sent abroad.[31] CELU's international allies were aware that the leadership exploited funded training and travel opportunities in this manner.

As these examples illustrate, the provision of external funds allowed CELU's leadership—especially its president—to create clientelist relationships with CELU officials, staff, and basic union representatives, so as to secure their loyalty. This, however, required the leadership to keep exclusive control over relationships with funders and the revenue streams they provided. The Danish Confederation of Trade Unions (*Landsorganisation*, or LO for short), which ran projects in Eritrea in the 1960s, were made aware of this necessity when CELU's headquarters instructed them that *all* correspondence and contacts with the Ethiopian trade union movement had to be conducted *solely* with CELU's headquarters in Addis Ababa. In other words, they were prohibited from engaging directly with the branch office in Asmara, as well as with basic union officials and workers in Eritrea, except when acting on CELU's leadership's explicit instructions. This aggravated LO's concerns that travel,

[30] Lennart Kindström to P.H. de Jonge, 2 February 1966, ICFTU/ITUC archives.

[31] "CELU Radical Faction (Disaffiliated Unions) Critique," translation by Awetu Simesso and Tom Killion, Tom Killion Papers.

training, and job opportunities funded by LO were being used to reward loyalists rather than being allocated where they were most needed. 'If I know CELU well', an LO advisor responded to the suggestion of having CELU's headquarters select participants for a seminar on cooperatives abroad, 'it will be people from Addis that they send (where they do not have any cooperatives)'.[32] Similarly, in 1971, Beyene instructed the AALC, which had dozens of staff in Ethiopia, 'to assure that *all* communications to any officer or member of CELU be addressed directly to the President, the Chief executive officer of CELU' [NB: "all" underlined in the original].[33] The reasons were clear to the AALC's regional representative:

> Beyene is quite successfully displaying a new get-tough, take-charge attitude, and I support his efforts, as do key people in the IEG [Imperial Ethiopian Government].
>
> It is now obvious that Beyene not only intends to run for Presidency again next year, but that he has every possibility of winning quite decisively. Whereas one year ago Beyene was thinking in terms of "retiring" to the Senate, he now has openly decided he wants to be President-for-Life, and he is executing all the right political moves to see that he is.

By centralising all communication with international allies, CELU's president seized personal control over CELU's external relationships and the funding that came through them. This allowed him to eliminate any doubt his contenders or loyalists may have had about who it was that determined the allocation of externally provided resources: that prerogative belonged to the president.

The lack of transparency in the allocation and use of funds, however, remained a serious source of friction within the movement. This issue was not confined to the top level, but caused problems throughout the structures of the labour movement, extending down to the constituent enterprise unions. Many of the conflicts that developed within CELU were marked by allegations of improper use of funds, with charges of

[32] Kaj Jensen to Per Carlsen, 2 November 1968, Landsorganisationen i Danmark (LO) archives, Arbejdermuseet & Arbejderbevægelsens Bibliotek og Arkiv, Copenhagen.

[33] "Subject: Communications with CELU", Memorandum from Jerry Funk to AALC Staff, 25 August 1971, AALC Records.

outright corruption being common. 'They are all some bandits', a Danish LO advisor exclaimed in 1967, suspecting that a translator hired with Danish funds was forced to relinquish a share of his salary to a top union official in the Eritrean branch.[34] But it was the charges levelled against the top leadership that most severely damaged the unity of the movement. These charges were brought forward by oppositional labour groups from the mid-1960s onwards, and by radical left publications in the 1970s. They were subsequently instrumentalised and exaggerated for political reasons by the military regime that came to power in the 1974 revolution. However, they were not unfounded. As discussed in the fifth chapter, there is ample archival evidence documenting illicit use of funds, including instances of direct corruption of officeholders by CELU's international allies. Private, unaccounted-for loans were provided to influence top government policy makers, and lavish sums of secret, similarly unaccounted-for funding was used to prop up embattled top CELU officials and fund their re-election campaigns. The result was the erosion and subversion of the movement's internal democratic processes.

Support from CELU's allies in the ICFTU camp came at another cost to CELU. In return for their assistance, they demanded an unflinching commitment to anti-communism, and a level of exclusivity that prohibited CELU from establishing any relationships with the national trade union centres organised in the World Federation of Trade Unions (WFTU). Archival documents make it abundantly clear how the ICFTU, the AALC, and their allies viewed their engagement with CELU as motivated by, and essential to, preventing socialist bloc influence and labour radicalism from developing in Ethiopia. The ways in which this was policed is discussed in the fifth chapter. Suffice it to say here that assistance from ICFTU and the international 'free' trade union movement came with certain constraints on CELU's autonomy. The additional reputational damage this caused for CELU and its top officials has been acknowledged by Beyene, who has written that 'CELU has sometimes been accused of being less militant due to its affiliation to the ICFTU and its close relationship with AFL-CIO'.[35] To make matters worse the ICFTU established a close working relationship with the imperial state

[34] Daniel Pedersen to Villy Pedersen, 9 November 1967, LO archives.

[35] "A Brief History of the Genesis, Development, Decline and Future Prospect of the Ethiopian Labor Movement," Beyene Solomon, report written for the AALC, Addis Ababa, 1992, AALC Records.

and gained access to its highest officials, including the Emperor. Any radical impulse would henceforth be caught between and checked by, on the one hand and internally, a moderate leadership within a bureaucratised setting, and, on the other hand and externally, an international anti-communist trade union movement working in mutual understanding with the imperial state.

Structure and Development

CELU's structure essentially consisted of two tiers. At the lower end of the structure were the basic constituent unions. In the Ethiopian case, these consisted almost exclusively of enterprise unions, meaning that each company had one separate union, but that large enterprises with multiple branches united the workers of various workplaces into one union. This generated the first set of peculiarities of Ethiopian trade unionism. Instead of a few large sectoral industrial unions, Ethiopia had a plethora of minuscule enterprise unions. The underdeveloped nature of the waged Ethiopian economy ensured that most enterprises were small, and consequently, so were most unions. But not all. There were significant discrepancies in the size, capacity and finances between the few large unions and the many smaller ones. Moreover, the enterprise union model meant that constituent unions brought together employees of all different ranks: shopfloor workers, white-collar workers and even some managerial staff members. During CELU's early years—this was to change subsequently—it was not uncommon for managerial staff members to serve as presidents of constituent unions, even though the law did not permit it. Belatedly, there were also attempts to form industrial unions, as the typically minuscule size of the enterprise unions was recognised as a problem from the outset. However, these attempts were largely unsuccessful during the CELU period.

A second peculiarity arose from the Ethiopian trade unions' origin in self-help associations—*iddirs*. Constituent unions, supported by CELU, engaged in activities that reflected this origin, although what was called 'the secondary role – that of mutual help' was considered to be gradually diminishing by 1965.[36] Such activities included revenue-raising efforts, the organisation of credit and savings cooperatives, and consumer

[36] "Progress Report and Future Projected Activities of CELU", CELU report to the ICFTU, 22 October 1965, CETU archives.

cooperatives. Unions also established charitable and welfare initiatives, including a major literacy campaign, provided unemployment benefits, organised sports and entertainment activities, and vocational training for union members and their families. 'On the level of the individual unions, quite a surprising range of services are being offered to the members', the ICFTU noted in 1964. 'This includes benefits in the case of death or sickness, [and] providing some unemployment pay'.[37]

Finally, it should be noted that even while the waged section of the workforce was relatively small, significant parts of it were prohibited from organising into unions. Those included civil servants, seasonal workers, domestic workers, and farm workers—except those on the largest commercial farms. This exclusion of large segments of the workforce from union membership accounted for a third peculiarity of Ethiopian trade unionism.

The upper tier of the Ethiopian trade union movement's structure consisted of the confederation—CELU—or, more specifically, its headquarters, board, and primarily its topmost officeholders. Because resources were concentrated at the highest level and CELU did not have any large cross-country industrial unions to contend with, a tendency common to trade unionism, in general, was amplified in the Ethiopian case: the centralisation of power among a few central officials, and a concomitant top-down approach to the running of the confederation. 'CELU leadership had been no different than many African Labor Centers', the AALC's regional representative in Addis Ababa would later write,[38] 'there being just one or two people who really ran the organization. In the case of CELU it was Beyene and Fisseha'. The separation of this top layer of officialdom from the rank-and-file, and the degree to which power was concentrated in the former, fostered undemocratic attitudes and practices. Jerry Funk, another AALC representative and a personal friend of Beyene, acknowledged that CELU's top officials, and particularly Beyene, had engaged in a 'stubborn and hopeless attempt to control everyone and everything from the top'. Beyene was 'regarded generally as having a "big man complex"' and 'accused of being

[37] "ICFTU ISF meeting minutes," 17–19 June 1964, Geneva, ICFTU/ITUC archives.

[38] "BAR/LES No.3," Richard Baurmann to Lester Trachtman, 25 October 1974, AALC Records.

dictatorial, unresponsive, and unreasonable'.[39] 'Beyene takes the mildest criticism as a direct attack on him personally, and as a frontal assault on all his currently sacred principles', Funk continued. 'He tends to feel that he has been chosen and anointed as leader of the workers, much in the same manner as HIM [His Imperial Majesty, additionally titled "Elect of God"] was given somewhat broader responsibilities, and that like HIM, he should not be challenged'.[40] However, other senior CELU officials imposed themselves on lower levels and basic unions in similar undemocratic ways. Mesfin Gebremichael, CELU's Deputy General Secretary, for example, caused outrage in the HVA union when, in 1973, he intervened in its election process to steer the outcomes. 'Mesfin, over the past few months, has been mucking about with the plantation workers at Meta Hara and Wonji', Funk wrote. 'His engineering of elections, in which he manipulated in childish and pointless ways, has left a huge reservoir of discontent'.[41] The manner in which the top officials wielded the power that was concentrated in their hands would eventually lead to the emergence of strong opposition and the division of the movement into two averse strands.

Despite the widening separation of the leadership from the rank-and-file, the Ethiopian labour movement continued to make organisational progress over the 1960s and early 1970s. Between 1963 and 1965, the number of affiliated unions grew from 29 to 42. It reached 104 in 1966, 201 in March 1974, and 225 a year later. Although the membership numbers that CELU reported were somewhat unreliable—prone to inflation 'for political reasons'[42] and to attract greater ICFTU funding[43]—they nevertheless reflected a real and relatively rapid growth. The official number of members tripled from 10,000 to 30,000 between 1963 and 1964, reaching 38,000 in 1966, 55,000 in 1968, 56,000 in 1970, 73,000 in 1973, 90,000 in March 1974, and around 200,000 in

[39] "Report No. 233: CELU, CONFIDENTIAL", Jerry Funk to Irving Brown and Patrick O'Farrell, 6 February 1973, AALC Records.

[40] Ibid.

[41] Ibid.

[42] "Labor Education Project: Report, Dec. 1968–July 1971," John Kilhefner, 1971, AALC Records.

[43] Inactive unions and non-paying members were typically not removed from membership sheets for the same reasons.

1975. The pace of growth, a German labour advisor to the Ethiopian government acknowledged, 'exceeded every expectation'.[44]

The multiplication of basic unions—combined with their typical small size—created severe strains on CELU's capacity to service its affiliated unions. CELU made significant efforts to keep pace with these developments. From initially having only two salaried full-time officials (FTO), the number of FTOs and salaried staff reached 13 by 1965. By 1972, CELU employed no fewer than 50 staff members and advisors—several of them funded by the AALC—in addition to FTOs. During the same period, CELU moved its offices from a small mud house it had rented into spacious and top-modern facilities that the AALC had constructed for it. CELU branches were established in several cities and regions—including Eritrea, Addis Ababa and its vicinity, and Dire Dawa—and within a few years, the confederation constructed office buildings to house its branches in Asmara and Dire Dawa. In other places, such as Massawa, local constituent unions operated joint offices. But despite these developments, CELU faced severe financial and capacity constraints. The membership fees it collected from affiliates remained low, and its inability to raise sufficient revenue from members was a significant source of concern for CELU and its international allies throughout CELU's existence. It was calculated that for the full year of 1967, CELU received less than one ETB per three members.[45] Two years later, CELU's own income covered only about one-third of the budget for its activities, with the other two-thirds coming from its international allies.[46]

The fact that most unions were small and not vertically connected to one another, but only individually to CELU, amplified this problem. There was no cadre from sectoral cross-country unions to draw upon, since each constituent union only replicated the same board member roles. A few unions were nevertheless relatively large and comparatively well-off. A 1973 list of CELU-affiliated unions in and around Addis Ababa illustrates this by combining unions with less than 30 members, such as the Food and Bar Workers' Union by Mexico Square, with unions

[44] G. Graf von Baudissin "Labour Policy in Ethiopia," *International Labour Review* 89, no. 6 (1964): 564.

[45] Villy Pedersen to Per Carlsen, 28 September 1967, LO archives.

[46] "CELU Statement of income, expenditure and balance, From January 1st to December 31, 1969," ICFTU/ITUC archives.

that had over 4,000 members, such as the HVA's. It included both financially struggling unions and those that were in a better position. For example, while the Diabaco Cotton Workers' Union, a union with 660 members, had only 200 ETB in its account, the HVA union had saved 20,000 ETB.[47] Some of the financial discrepancies were the results of differences between unions that had negotiated payroll check-off systems for union dues with employers and those that had not. But the extreme variances in size, along with a large share of unions that were nearly too small to be viable, posed a fundamental problem.

To tackle these problems, CELU sought to create nine national industrial unions that would vertically integrate the various enterprise unions and create a mid-tier level of organisation. Several meetings were convened to this end. For example, in 1969, all the heads of unions in textile industries were brought together in a seminar, which was supposed to be the first step towards the creation of a country-wide industrial union. One national general union—for workers in enterprises employing fewer than 50 workers—was established for leather and shoe manufacturing workers. However, due to divisions within the movement and the reluctance of basic union bosses to hand over their power to these proposed structures, it was difficult to get constituent unions to sufficiently commit to the project. The plan to create industrial unions, which had been discussed as early as CELU's foundation in 1963, was not to materialise until 1977, when it was enforced by the military regime.

Eventually, CELU's inability to properly service its numerous unions led to many smaller unions becoming dormant, or even permanently inactive. This was particularly likely among those located far away from Addis Ababa or a CELU branch office. CELU's officers and staff were overburdened with the tasks of settling grievances and helping negotiate collective agreements. Very little time and resources remained available for organising activities. The lack of attention and service that constituent unions received was raised by the emerging opposition as a key example of the leadership's failures. As a result, several unions eventually refused to pay their affiliation fees, further aggravating CELU's precarious finances.

The situation was somewhat relieved by the introduction of CELU field workers. In a programme organised and funded by the AALC,

[47] "Annual Report II", CELU Research Department, September 1973, AALC Records.

six field workers were recruited, trained, and deployed in wage-work-intensive areas across the country. Primarily, they engaged in workers' and trade union education, but they also helped basic unions settle disputes with employers, engage in collective bargaining, and organise workers. In this way, the field workers became indispensable to the movement, and constituted an important factor behind CELU's increased potency and extended geographical reach in the first half of the 1970s. Two of the field workers, furthermore, would individually go on to play important roles in the radicalisation of CELU, albeit in different ways: Tedla Fantaye, who became a member of the labour opposition, and Alem Abdi, who became CELU's acting president following the 1974 revolution. But despite the important contributions of the field workers, CELU remained stretched and low on resources. The AALC viewed CELU as having 'outgrown itself' by the early 1970s, and its staff resources as having been rendered woefully insufficient by this growth.[48]

Activities and Strategy

The training of union leaders was a task that the CELU leadership and its international allies took very seriously. Rather than merely constituting a capacity-building exercise, such training included a crucial restraining aspect: it inculcated perceptions of the type of unionism deemed legitimate by CELU's leadership and its allies—moderate business unionism. An example of this reasoning is found in the archives of the ICFTU. Reporting on 'a serious wild cat strike in the course of which violence occurred', a West German labour advisor at the MNCD wrote that 'fortunately, it could be proved that in the pertinent undertaking no union activities whatsoever had been started before'. From this, he concluded that the conviction that 'education is primordial' had been reinforced.[49]

The concern with limiting wildcat strike activity continued to drive the provision of training. In the aftermath of CELU's 1963 general strike threat, the same German MNCD labour advisor wrote with concern that although the risk of a general strike had been overcome—and, in his view, an entirely positive purge of the leadership had taken place—it had

[48] "Semi-annual report (November 1972–April 1973)," Dick Arnold, 14 May 1973, AALC Records.

[49] Georg Graf von Baudissin to H.A. Tulatz, 10 January 1963, ICFTU/ITUC archives.

revealed an urgent need to promote 'better co-ordination, cooperation with educational and other agencies and practical advice'. To this end, he urged the ICFTU to step in and provide immediate assistance to intensify training efforts. 'We cannot afford to leave the Ethiopian labour leaders alone for any longer period which would lead only to a repetition of past frustration and even radicalisation', he wrote.[50] In 1966, moreover, the ICFTU's representative in Addis Ababa reported that he had been able to use a volatile situation—widespread labour unrest had led the Ethiopian Employers' Federation to call for government intervention—to convince CELU's leaders of the importance of conducting more intensive training of local union leaders. Neglect of trade union education, he wrote, was 'in all simplicity the big reason to most of the trouble and grievances we are now afflicted with'.[51] Labour unrest, in other words, was seen merely as an expression of ignorance of essential trade union values and principles, for which a strong dose of training and education—inculcating these values and principles—would serve as the most effective antidote.

It has been claimed that prior to 1974, 'the whole energy of the confederation was absorbed in arranging training seminars for trade union leaders'.[52] Indeed, this remained an important priority. Between 1970 and mid-1973 alone, CELU conducted no fewer than 128 training seminars across the country—typically lasting a week to ten days—for 4,572 union officials and members, while also organising educational film shows for 71,950 trade unionists.[53] However, CELU was by no means confining itself to this task. It undertook a wide range of other activities, including campaigning for legislative changes, participating in tripartite bodies, providing legal and practical services to unions, assisting in collective bargaining efforts, mediating disputes between local unions and employers, and supporting unions engaged in legal disputes. 'CELU, by virtue of its wide coverage is looked upon to by many unions as conciliator and advocate', CELU reported to ICFTU.[54] It stated that 'about 40

[50] Georg Graf von Baudissin to H.A. Tulatz, 25 September 1963. ICFTU/ITUC archives.

[51] Lennart Kindström to H.A. Tulatz, 3 May 1966, ICFTU/ITUC archives.

[52] Teketel Wegayehu, "Union Structure under Proclamation No. 222/82 and its Impact on Labour Movement," (Bachelor's thesis, Addis Ababa University, 1983), 13.

[53] "Semi-annual report (November 1972–April 1973)," Dick Arnold, 14 May 1973, AALC Records.

[54] Ibid.

percent of [active unions] have involved CELU in their negotiations with management'. 'Furthermore, almost all seek the help of CELU when the case goes to the Labour Department for conciliation and mediation', it reported, with 90 per cent of 1,644 cases lodged with the department allegedly involving CELU.[55]

The confederation also published the newspaper *Voice of Labour*. Despite the imperial government's crippling and time-consuming censorship regime—requiring texts to be submitted for careful scrutiny and approval before publication—*Voice of Labour* became an important vehicle for CELU to popularise its views. Launched in 1963 as a mimeographed paper, it was initially intended for biweekly publication. Due to staff and financial shortages, as well as the cumbersome censorship process, new issues were generally published far less frequently. By 1969, however, an AALC project revived the publication as a printed paper, and it eventually became a monthly publication. New editorial staff were recruited in 1974, and that year it achieved a record distribution, with of 20,500 copies of its June issue printed and circulated.[56]

As noted, a good deal of CELU's officials' and staff's efforts went into assisting basic unions in collective bargaining. During the long decade that CELU existed, this resulted in the completion of around 100 negotiated collective agreements,[57] which by the end of the decade covered around 30 per cent of CELU's members.[58] A number of generalities characterised collective bargaining during this period. First, most enterprises were unconvinced about the necessity of entering into collective negotiations. They typically had be pushed into this realisation by workers through strikes and other forms of unrest. Since striking legally was more or less impossible under the imperial labour law, such actions almost exclusively took the form of nominal wildcat strikes—even though the concerned union frequently organised or supported them covertly. Due to the leverage that comes with numbers, this strategy was most

[55] "Progress Report and Future Projected Activities of CELU", CELU report to the ICFTU, 22 October 1965, CETU archives.

[56] "Project activity #24: Research, Administration and Publications Project, Ethiopia", report, 5 September 1974, AALC Records.

[57] "Semi-annual report (November 1972–April 1973)," Dick Arnold, 14 May 1973, AALC Records.

[58] Emmanuel, "Confederation of Ethiopian Labour Unions and its First General Strike," 70.

effective in large enterprises. In smaller ones, strikers—and particularly strike leaders—were more easily identified and dismissed. Second, almost all basic unions lacked the technical skills and resources to negotiate on their own behalf and, therefore, required CELU's assistance in bargaining with employers. Additionally, they needed CELU's help to enforce their rights to engage in bargaining and to uphold existing agreements in the Labour Relations Board. By the early 1970s, for example, the LRB had over 60 such cases pending.[59] As a result, CELU was compelled to prioritise assigning its scarce staff to where they would have the greatest impact. Third, a few large state-owned and foreign-owned companies were among the exceptions that willingly entered into collective bargaining with unions. For all these reasons, large enterprises were typically the first ones to conclude collective bargaining agreements (CBAs). They included HVA, Ethiopian Airlines, the Ethio-Djibouti Railway Enterprise, a number of large textile factories, and other major manufacturing, transport, and trading establishments. The agreements entered into were often quite beneficial to workers. They included significant wage increments that often reached between 10 and 15 per cent,[60] and occasional additional benefits such as medical care. These improvements were direct outcomes of effective pressure from workers, underpinned by a willingness to engage in conflict when required. Most of the enterprises where workers secured such betterments, through the establishment of CBAs and adherence to them, had relatively strong unions and a history of strikes and unrest.

In smaller enterprises, unions found it more difficult to muster the strength to force employers into collective bargaining. And when they did, securing significant concessions in the content of the CBAs was even more difficult. Lynn Morehouse, an American industrial relations scholar who conducted research in Ethiopia in the late 1960s, found that 'many of the collective agreements [offered] little more than the law requires or what the employees had previously been receiving'[61]—a point also corroborated by a former official of the Federation of Ethiopian

[59] "Semi-annual report (November 1972–April 1973)," Dick Arnold, 14 May 1973, AALC Records.

[60] See Chapter 6 for a discussion on the cumulative effect of such pay rises on aggregate wages during this period.

[61] L.G. Morehouse, "Ethiopian Labour Relations: Attitudes, Practice and Law" (research project paper, Northwestern University, 1969), 70.

Employers.[62] Due to this reluctance to grant anything beyond what the law already required, he argued, the labour movement had been compelled to shift its attention towards the state, seeking legislative and institutional changes rather than solely pursuing enterprise-level agreements. This sentiment was reflected in a speech delivered by CELU President Beyene Solomon in 1972, in which he stated that 'the unions have come to the conclusion that the fate of the Ethiopian worker does not so much depend on the day-to-day activities of individual employers, but more on [the] government', and, as a result, CELU aimed to acquire greater influence at that level.[63]

Because Ethiopian labour law lacked provisions for a minimum wage, its institution had been a demand raised by CELU in its first, unsuccessful attempt to have the law revised in 1963. With the repression that followed, the issue was put on the back burner. But in 1966, CELU had been strengthened by numerical growth and an increasing record of successfully handled disputes and negotiations—all within a generally restive industrial scene characterised by growing numbers of wildcat strikes. At the same time, CELU had come to recognise that collective bargaining was not as effective a tool in increasing wages in the many very small enterprises that dominated the economy as it was in the large ones. To make matters worse, a number of factors combined to reduce the bargaining strength of workers in large parts of the economy: unionisation levels remained low, much of the waged economy consisted of only unskilled jobs, and unemployment was high. Consequently, CELU resumed campaigning for a revision of the labour law that would include the introduction of a minimum wage. At a tripartite industrial relations conference in 1966, Beyene made a passionate plea for its institution by law, asserting that industrial peace would not exist until that was in place[64]. Two years later, CELU presented a memorandum of its position on the question. However, it faced strong opposition from both employers and state officials, whose roles frequently overlapped. 'One has to understand that the head of [the Ministry of National Community

[62] Syoum Gebregziabher, "The Rise of CELU and the EFE," 99.

[63] "Speech on the occasion of CELU's ninth anniversary," Beyene Solomon, 1972. International Labour Organization (ILO) archives, International Labour Office, Geneva.

[64] "The First National Industrial Relations Conference, August 1966," Imperial Ethiopian Government Ministry of National Community Development and Social Affairs, Department of Labour, Addis Ababa, AALC Records, 17.

Development, in charge of labour affairs] is himself an employer. There is not the necessary neutrality', a Danish advisor to CELU wryly noted[65]. CELU would not make any significant progress in pushing the imperial state to initiate labour law reform before the 1974 revolution broke out.

Repression and Subversion

The Ethiopian labour movement encountered a number of profound challenges and obstacles in the long decade that followed the foundation of CELU. One major challenge was the repression of organised labour that occurred at the level of the workplace. Morehouse's contemporaneous investigation found that 'the area of dismissal remains the most litigated [and] the most important in the eyes of employees' among individual rank-and-file workers and union officials. The fear of being dismissed—'all-pervasive' as it was found to be—constituted the 'dominant characteristic of employment relations'.[66] There were few limitations on employers' prerogative to arbitrarily dismiss workers, and in cases where severance pay was prescribed, it was frequently simply ignored.

To pre-empt union formation, workers who were in the process of forming one were often dismissed. And where unions had already been formed, targeted dismissals of union officials and members occurred frequently. Morehouse took note of a number of examples that indicated 'the extent to which some companies have gone to thwart a union'.[67] They included 'one bottling company [whose management] refused to recognise the right of its workers to form a union until a short strike was staged coinciding with a visit to the company by officials of the MNCD'; 'the managing director of another company freely [admitting] that if the union pushed too much [for] a collective agreement, he would simply dismiss its leaders'; and one garage where 'workers were told that since they were now working for different employers, they could not mix, the one objecting employee being summarily dismissed'. Other examples included the banning of all discussion among employees at work,

[65] "Rapport over den senste tids udvikling omkring projektet, dækkende perioden 2- maj—29 august 1968," report from Kaj Jensen to Udenrigsministeriet, Sekretariatet for teknisk samarbejde med udviklingslandene [Danish Ministry of Foreign Affairs, Secretariat for technical cooperation with developing countries], 29 August 1968, LO archives.

[66] Morehouse, "Ethiopian Labour Relations," 51, 69.

[67] Ibid., 66.

and several employers who 'openly admitt[ed] that an employee who complains too much will be dismissed'.[68] In the city of Dire Dawa, the enterprise union of the Chandris meat canning factory reported that no fewer than 132 of its members had been arbitrarily dismissed by 1973.[69] Large state- and foreign-owned or managed enterprises tended to be more accommodating of unionisation. This, however, did not constitute a universal rule. The Lazaridis textile factory, A. Besse & Co, and Banco di Roma were among the several large foreign-owned companies that were engaged in disputes after having fired union leaders in the year 1971 alone. At the Diabaco Cotton Company, moreover, the union was repressed vigorously. All members of the executive committee of the company union had been fired in the 1960s, and in 1972 union representatives reported that 'every time there is a general [union] meeting the management calls for the police and workers are jailed for no reason'.[70]

As the above suggests, state bias presented another significant obstacle to the labour movement. Individual unions considered to be engaged in 'unfair practices'—when calling a strike, for example—could be forcefully dissolved by the Labour Relations Board. This was the fate of the union of Lazaridis Cotton Mills in 1963. Displeasing the LRB, moreover, could have other deleterious effects, 'since any declaration of illegality'—its typical ruling on any strike—would 'entitle management to dismiss all the strikers'.[71] Because of the unlevel playing field this presented, basic union leaders frequently complained that the government was 'anti-labour' and that the LRB was 'anti-employee and anti-union'.[72] This was most emphatically expressed in its failure to safeguard the rights of union leaders. 'The Board's reported tendency to allow dismissal', Morehouse

[68] Ibid., 70.

[69] This figure is found on CELU's union summary sheet for Chandris. Although 132 dismissed workers is an exceptionally high number, many unions reported, in the same set of summary sheets compiled in 1973, being at loggerheads with the employer over dismissed workers. "Confidential Data: Summary of Unions", CELU research department, 1974, CETU archives.

[70] CELU, *3ኛው በየሦስት ዓመት የሚከናወን ጠቅላላ ጉባዔ/3rd Triannual Conference* (Addis Ababa: Confederation of Ethiopian Labour Unions, 1972).

[71] Morehouse, "Ethiopian Labour Relations," 65.

[72] Ibid., 60.

noted,[73] 'has placed a deep sense of insecurity on all present and potential union leaders'.[74]

According to a former CELU staff member, state intervention in industrial conflict was frequent and tended, 'in most cases', to be 'in support of the employers'.[75] Seleshi Sisaye, an Ethiopian industrial relations scholar at the time, concurred and described the imperial government as altogether 'anti-labour'.[76] The manner in which the boundaries of permissible union activity were policed was indicative of this. In regular times, trade unionists were habitually harassed when conducting organising campaigns. Union officials were vetted by authorities and occasionally purged or arrested. The whole movement was subject to surveillance and the confederation needed to adhere to strict guidelines and directives, which included a tight censorship of its newspaper. But in cases where component parts of the movement nevertheless transgressed the boundaries of what was deemed acceptable, a stronger reaction could be expected. Strike leaders were routinely arrested, and strikes, particularly larger ones, often resulted in the deployment of strike-breaking security forces. Police were, for example, called in during the 1973 strikes of Diabaco cotton factory and Central Printing Press workers.[77] In the course of the 1971 Assab port strike, moreover, an army officer in charge of port security threatened 'to shoot any worker who did not report to work'.[78] In another example, efforts to organise plantation workers in Nurahera and Melka Sedi were banned by the authorities, and the union treasury was confiscated. As the workers staged a strike in protest,

[73] Ibid., 81.

[74] As a compendium of cases reviewed by the LRB up to 1967 indicates, however, the LRB was not averse to rule in favour of reinstating or compensating workers in individual cases. This, however, was never the case when a strike was involved. And the huge backlog of the LRB in any case meant that the effect of the selective justice it dispensed was undermined. Moreover, in several cases where the LRB ruled in favour of reinstating fired workers, the ruling was simply ignored by employers. Compendium on labour disputes and Labour Relation Board rulings, Federation of Ethiopian Employers, n.d., CETU Archives.

[75] Emmanuel, "Confederation of Ethiopian Labour Unions and its First General Strike," 71.

[76] Seleshi, "Urban Migration and the Labor Movement," 688.

[77] Ibid., 698.

[78] Beyene, *Fighter for Democracy*, 107.

police fired on them and killed several.[79] A subsequent attempt by the plantation workers to march to Addis to petition the emperor was also prevented by the police. Lethal repression was suspected in other cases too. According to Kenyan labour leader and ICFTU official Tom Mboya, foul play was possibly involved in the death of two leaders of the railway workers' union, from allegedly the very same cause—a ruptured spleen—only days apart.[80] Equally suspicious was an alleged 1965 attempt on the life of CELU President Beyene, the reasons for and perpetrators of which were never established.[81]

Even where repression was not open and apparent, state presence made itself felt routinely and casually. Danish advisors to CELU in the 1960s were bothered by the way police officers tended to break up even the most innocuous meetings of workers without any stated reasons. Moreover, they were convinced that the trade unions they worked with were heavily infiltrated by security agents. 'There undoubtedly are people from the security services among our board members in the trade union movement', one advisor in Eritrea wrote. 'We recently had our suspicion confirmed [when we] were invited to the officers' club in a military facility. Our inviter was an excellent, active member of the board of one of the trade unions, but in addition to his day job, he was a detective for the security service and a former officer in the army', he reported[82]. In a similar vein, an ICFTU visitor to Addis Ababa in 1963 reported that 'three men were always behind me to watch my movements, record of the persons who come to meet me and report my speeches'.[83]

But there were also exceptions to the imperial state's hostility towards organised and assertive workers. When faced with nationalistic sentiments

[79] Killion, "Workers, Capital and the State," 537.

[80] "Report on Mission to Ethiopia, 2nd–10th October 1958," Tom Mboya, 1958, ICFTU/ITUC archives.

[81] ICFTU Representative Lennart Kindström had found Beyene 'very uncommunicative of his own opinion about the reason for the [attempt on] his life'. On the question of whether it was related to his position, Kindström reported Beyene as having answered in the affirmative, but this, Kindström noted, 'is all I get out of him'. Lennart Kindström to P.H. de Jonge, 12 February 1965, ICFTU/ITUC archives.

[82] "Rapport for perioden 21. April 1967–21. Oktober 1967," report from Villy Pedersen to Udenrigsministeriet, Sekretariatet for teknisk samarbejde med udviklingslandene, 1967, LO archives.

[83] Desigar Ramanujam to Stephan Nedzynski, 6 February 1963, ICFTU/ITUC archives.

and outrage against foreign employers who openly violated workers' rights, police sometimes sided with strikers. This, for example, was the case in relation to a wildcat strike in an Eritrean textile factory in 1968. 'The sentiments against the Italian employers and their harsh personnel policy create ever-greater bitterness among the population at large, which to an increasing extent is beneficial to the trade unions', Danish advisors to CELU noted. 'We received strong support from the police during the unlawful strike. We also received guidance covertly, and prominent police officers from the security services have more than once put great pressure on an employer to resolve the conflict'.[84] However, such police support for striking workers was exceptional.

State presence was not only felt in the relationship between workers and employers, but also penetrated the internal dynamics of the trade union movement. The imperial state would readily intervene to shore up the position of CELU's moderate leaders whenever assailed from within the movement. But it would also intervene to impress on the very same leaders the importance of remaining within the approved parameters. Where the leadership could or would not guarantee an outcome consistent with official expectations placed on it, the state did not shy away from employing repression to generate such outcomes. It repeatedly displayed its repertoire of repressive measures, which ranged from harassment, arrests, and violent dispersal, to the occasional use of lethal force. However, open state interference in union affairs often triggered an adverse reaction among workers and trade unionists, and contributed to radicalisation. In that sense, state repression was neither as reliable, cost-efficient, nor effective as the internal control outsourced and entrusted to the top labour bureaucracy.

With the emergence of a leadership with no direct links to, or origins in, any constituent unions, and which was also materially and socially quite radically separated from the rank-and-file, bureaucratism was an essential aspect of CELU's features from the outset. Its top officials were not elected representatives of any constituent unions. Nor did they, in most cases, possess any direct experience of wage work prior to being employed by the confederation. In that sense, the process of bureaucratisation within CELU was extraordinarily advanced. The fact that the

[84] "Rapport for Perioden 21 oktober–Juni 1968," report from Villy Pedersen to Udenrigsministeriet, Sekretariatet for teknisk samarbejde med udviklingslandene, 1968, LO archives.

number of top officials was relatively small does not change the fact that they were greatly privileged—socially and materially. These officials—the core group consisting of the president and the university-educated staff members co-opted into the leadership—wielded a significant amount of power over the confederation, and the basic unions. And they used it consistently to contain, subvert, and purge what was considered excessive radicalism and militancy.

Trade unionism had been legalised in Ethiopia in a conjuncture where labour unrest was becoming increasingly frequent. The imperial government assumed that open trade unionism under a moderate leadership and within a restrictive legal-institutional framework could provide more effective control mechanisms than external control and repression alone. The general success of this approach can be illustrated with a quote from a bakery union leader that appeared in *Voice of Labour*:

> Your union has tied our hands and feet. Before you organised us we used to get substantial concessions from employers by merely threatening a walkout. The employers knew that we did not kid when we threatened – the work, the flour even the equipment was not safe. Yet, now you have advised us that through the union we have first to discuss with our employers, then if we are not satisfied we have to submit our grievance to the labour relations section of the MNCD and that if we are not reconciled by the section we have to lodge our dispute with the LRB. The case does not stop there, either employers or employees can appeal to the Supreme Imperial Court [or even be referred] to His Majesty's [court]. Yes, your union has weakened our unity. We neither have the money, the time nor the manpower to follow up our disputes through these channels. Your union has only tied us to the benefit of our employers.[85]

A telling example of how state repression functioned in synergy with moderating pressures emanating from employers and CELU's own leadership can be found in the case of the Dire Dawa Textile Factory, where the assertive enterprise union leader Zeleke Woldemariam had been imprisoned for allegedly orchestrating an attack on a management representative. His successor Shiferaw Dessalegn, however, did not prove to be sufficiently compliant either, and was accused by CELU's leadership of

[85] "The Ethiopian Labour Movement: The Aftermath of Birth," *Voice of Labour/ የሠራተኛው ድምፅ* (special issue on the occasion of the 7th anniversary and the inauguration of its new headquarters, 9 April 1970): 11.

making excessive demands on the employer. CELU initially attempted to remove Shiferaw from his position by bureaucratic means, but when this move was opposed by the factory workers and thus failed, CELU's leaders called on the state to intervene and remove him[86]—which it subsequently did.[87]

The above does not detract from the achievements of CELU and affiliated unions but rather illustrates the dual role of trade unionism. Whether the pragmatism of CELU's leadership was determined by the privilege that came with office or not was initially a moot point. After the ouster of Abraham Mekonnen and the death of Aberra Gemu, it appeared evident that meaningful assertiveness would lead to removal from office in any case, and top labour and state officials were under the mutual assumption that it was likely to result in the forced dissolution of CELU altogether.[88] In appearance, external pressures seemingly fused privileged bureaucratic interests with the institutional imperative to defend the organisation. The fact that this conflation was largely illusory and that an assertive strategy could actually lead to far-reaching concessions from the state, securing greater autonomy for the labour movement, was a proposition that was not tested until 1973. By the time it became clear that this was the case, CELU's moderate leadership was doomed.

Internal Dissent and Factional Infighting

Internal opposition to CELU's central leadership emerged in the movement's early years. Such opposition 'is as old as the organisation itself and seems to gather momentum in course of time', a CELU employee wrote.[89] Internal dissatisfaction was evident on two levels: with the composition of the confederation's leadership and its undemocratic internal practices on the one hand, and with its external strategic orientation on the other. With respect to the former, Beyene and his closest allies in the leadership were viewed as illegitimate usurpers since they

[86] Fissehatsion Tekie, interviewed by Tom Killion, 1983, microcassette, Tom Killion Papers.

[87] Killion, "Workers, Capital and the State," 507–508.

[88] "Mission to Ethiopia 31 August–31 September 1963," H. Robinson, report, 1963, ICFTU/ITUC archives; Morehouse, "Ethiopian Labour Relations," 75.

[89] Emmanuel, "Confederation of Ethiopian Labour Unions and its First General Strike," 71.

were not elected representatives of any constituent unions. They were also accused of subverting internal democracy and of monopolising power among themselves. As for the latter, their timid and unassertive approach, which lacked any militant qualities, constituted a serious cause of discord. To their detractors, the leadership was needlessly compliant in its dealings with authorities and employers, and excessively concerned with acquiring the government's approval. Beyene himself was, even in the words of his allies, 'often regarded as a pawn of the IEG [Imperial Government of Ethiopia]'.[90] The leadership's socio-material separation from the rank-and-file fed into and fuelled criticisms of its composition and orientation. Dissent was further aggravated by the leadership's unwillingness to submit to and implement binding majority decisions. On two separate occasions—in July 1964 and December 1969—the leadership failed to honour General Assembly congress decisions to call general strikes and demonstrations. Such subversion could only further frustrate and antagonise dissatisfied members and representatives. In light of this, it became increasingly difficult for the leadership to retain control over the movement, which gradually began to exhibit tendencies of radicalisation.

The first serious challenge to Beyene's leadership came in 1965, merely a year after he assumed the presidency. When Beyene was out of the country, a group of union representatives attempted to have him replaced. They sought to establish an investigation committee and call a General Assembly meeting to oust him[91]. Two CELU employees allied with the president described the attempt as motivated by the desire of oppositional candidates to take over the presidency and the hefty pay that came with it, as well as by 'personal hatred against Beyene by some union leaders'. But they also acknowledged that there were substantial issues involved. Those issues included opposition to Beyene's close relationship with the government, and the irregular frequency of General Council meetings. At the time, the General Council had not met for a considerable period, and the oppositional representatives alleged that this was because of the leadership's fear of being held to account. Although the attempt ultimately failed, more challenges were to come. In the subsequent year, the ICFTU's representative in Addis Ababa noted that CELU's board was

[90] "Report No. 233: CELU, CONFIDENTIAL", Jerry Funk to Irving Brown and Patrick O'Farrell, 6 February 1973, AALC Records.

[91] Gebreselassie Gebremariam and Mesfin Gebremichael to Arnold Zack, December 1964, Tom Killion Papers.

'divided in different groups'.[92] However, divisions were not confined to any single level of the confederation. Tensions and disputes permeated all levels of CELU's structures.

Most fundamentally, opposition to the leadership was rooted in its reluctance to put the movement on an offensive footing. There were instances where CELU's leadership covertly and discreetely supported local strikes, officially calling on unions to adhere to legal procedures while simultaneously 'indirectly telling them to go [on strike]'.[93] CELU also sought to support workers affected by labour conflict—those locked out by employers and those whose employment was terminated. However, when strike activity and unrest broke out—which it frequently did—the leadership consistently sought to come to a speedy agreement with employers. 'I always chose the path of peace in my dealings with employers', CELU's president Beyene has recalled.[94] In doing so, the leadership worked to contain and displace militant pressure that was building from basic unions and rank-and-file workers. While it did so relatively effectively in CELU's initial years, the displaced pressures built up and exacerbated the rift within the movement.

By the mid-1960s, CELU's leadership had began expressing concern about being 'unable to cope with the demands of the workers', which, it claimed 'were often quite unrealistic'.[95] It acknowledged significant internal discord, noting that there had been 'much disagreements between CELU and its affiliates',[96] with 'one of the major criticism against CELU [being] that it was not doing enough for its membership'. Early internal opposition, however, occurred without structured coordination, and CELU's leadership skilfully combined a strategy of playing on external ties and resources it had access to with a degree of procedural and constitutional manipulation to retain overall control over the movement. One example of the former was the selective distribution and withholding

[92] Lennart Kindström to P.H. de Jonge, 2 February 1966, ICFTU/ITUC Archives.

[93] Beyene Solomon, in discussion with the author and Biniyam Negash, February 20, 2016.

[94] Beyene, *Fighter for Democracy*, 109.

[95] "Progress Report and Future Projected Activities of CELU", CELU report to the ICFTU, 22 October 1965, CETU archives.

[96] In fact, the same report referred to a 'perpetual strife between CELU and its affiliates', which the leadership had hoped that the constitutional changes of 1965 would put an end to. Ibid.

of services, assistance, and funds accessible at the central level—a tactic frequently used to compel constituent unions to fall in line with the leadership. The latter included the revision of CELU's constitution to allow for the promotion of key moderates that surrounded Beyene to high offices; interference in and manipulation of constituent unions' elections, including tactics and gimmicks to sway the vote against disfavoured candidates, or to stall and prevent elections; and the subversion of binding majority decisions where a vote could not be prevented or its outcome not predetermined.[97] Despite cries of foul play triggered by such manipulation, the leadership was re-elected at the congresses of CELU's General Assembly in 1965, 1967, 1969, and 1972— but not without contention.

In the lead-up to the 1965 congress elections, Beyene was challenged by CELU's Deputy General Secretary Alemu Bogale, but the latter failed to generate sufficient support and was removed from the ballot just before voting began. Beyene's re-election was then followed by constitutional amendments that shored up his position. As a result of these changes, two employees of the confederation, who were part of Beyene's moderate group, were promoted to the positions of General Secretary and Deputy Secretary, respectively: Fissehatsion Tekie and Tesfa Gebremariam. Following Beyene's own elevation to the presidency the year before, this constituted another key step towards the establishment of a layer of non-representative top officials. The move in this direction, however, generated its own tensions—'the opposition charged, and not without cause, that under the original CELU constitution anyone not directly linked or delegated by either a local or national union, cannot hold electoral office in the confederation', a CELU insider explained.[98] More constitutional engineering followed the second congress of CELU's General Assembly in 1967. Unlike in the past, when the incumbent

[97] Former CELU staffer Emmanuel Fayessa claims that refusal to intercede with the government when representatives it did not back were elected, thereby denying them registration and legal recognition, was another method by which CELU's leadership discriminated against undesirable candidates. Additionally, preferred candidates were sometimes supported by CELU's leadership directly campaigning in constituent union elections, and evoking the threat of government intervention—should its preferred candidate not prevail. Ironically, such state intervention was occasionally courted by the CELU's leadership itself, when its interventions failed to sway the outcome. Emmanuel Fayessa, interview, Tom Killion Papers.

[98] Emmanuel, "Confederation of Ethiopian Labour Unions and its First General Strike," 73.

president was barred from chairing CELU's board and the confederation's general secretary was ineligible to serve as secretary of its board, they were henceforth assigned to these positions mandatorily. Moreover, the task of electing officeholders was transferred from the General Assembly to the board, with the General Assembly's role reduced to providing ratification of the board's selections.[99] These measures significantly increased the powers of the top officeholders at the expense of the General Assembly, but they did not prevent the rising tide of opposition against the leadership.

Opposition to the top leadership of the confederation was directly linked to rank-and-file militancy. Alemu Bogale, for example, who left the confederation's leadership after his failed effort to unseat Beyene, returned to his basic union, where he was accused of instigating strikes and imprisoned.[100] The removal of Shiferaw Dessalegn, an opponent of CELU's leadership, from his position as the basic union president of the Dire Dawa Textile factory followed a similar trajectory. Shiferaw had taken a hard line in negotiations with the management following strikes at the factory. He raised demands that CELU's leadership considered excessive, and refused to moderate those demands at its request. CELU, therefore, intervened directly in the affairs of the enterprise union and sought to have the membership remove Shiferaw from the presidency. Having failed to convince the factory workers of their case, CELU's leaders instead called upon the government to remove him. As police arrived to remove Shiferaw, workers who supported him entrenched themselves in the union offices and began pelting the police with stones.[101] Just like Alemu, Shiferaw was also imprisoned, and another union leader opposed to CELU's leadership was thus removed.

In 1966, it was reported that 'harsh' power struggles within the movement were ongoing, which included several instances of gun violence. In one such incident, at the Koka hydroelectric power plant south of Addis Ababa, two trade unionists were shot to death, and one was injured.[102] By

[99] Lennart Kindström to Morris Paladino,31 May 1967. ICFTU/ITUC archives.

[100] Daniel Pedersen to Villy Pedersen, 11 December 1967, LO archives.

[101] Fissehatsion Tekie, interview, Tom Killion Papers; "ሪፖርት ከመጋቢት 11 እስከ ከመጋቢት 13 ቀን 1962 ዓ.ም," Beyene Solomon, report, 1970, CETU Archives.

[102] Daniel Pedersen to Eiler Jensen, 10 September 1966, LO archives.

1967, the general situation within the movement was described as 'something of a wasp's nest',[103] and by 1968 'deep disunity and great division' was reported to run across it.[104] Locally, conflict and turbulence erupted among and between unions around the Addis Ababa area that same year. Meanwhile, serious conflict had broken out among unions in Eritrea soon after the ban on trade unionism in that region had been lifted in 1966. CELU's leadership was heavily involved in both cases. In Eritrea, it used subterfuge and postponed elections to protect its unpopular branch president Emmanuel Kahsai—rumoured to be Beyene's relative—from being ousted by the representatives of the unions in the region. But in 1969, the threat of a total split in the Eritrean branch of the movement—most basic unions having stopped paying contributions to the branch—compelled CELU to allow new regional elections to be held. Emmanuel was duly voted out of office, marking an important victory for oppositional unions.

In April 1969, CELU held its third General Assembly congress, and Beyene stood for re-election as CELU president. The strong opposition Beyene faced at this congress astounded his American allies who were in attendance. The AALC's representative reported that CELU's leadership was severely criticised 'by the mass of the delegates who were demanding more vigorous action from CELU'. When it came to electing office-holders, 'Beyene started out the voting in real trouble, and apparently ***did not have*** a majority' [NB: underlined in original].[105] However, because the opposition was split in at least three ways—the strongest challenge presented by Alem Abdi—Beyene was re-elected for a third term. Even though all top officials in the moderate leadership retained their positions, they had received a serious warning. 'The opposition is still there', the AALC's representative observed, 'and if it can ever pull itself together to back one candidate, Beyene will lose'.

The election was followed by efforts to consolidate power further: two additional staff members who were considered loyal were co-opted to CELU's leadership. This meant that five members of CELU's central leadership—a solid majority of its executive body—henceforth represented no constituent unions, and four of them had no experience of

[103] Daniel Pedersen to Villy Pedersen, 11 December 1967, LO archives.

[104] "Rapport over den senste tids udvikling omkring projektet, dækkende perioden 2-maj—29 august 1968," LO archives.

[105] "Report No. 106: CELU Elections General Conference," Jerry Funk to Irving Brown, 8 May 1969, AALC Records.

shop floor work whatsoever. But consolidation also required CELU's leadership to win over, or at the very least to placate, some of the opposition. At the congress, the recurrent demand that CELU ought to press harder for a revision of the labour law was once again raised, receiving resounding approval from the delegates. To break the impasse and force the government's hand, it had been resolved that CELU would call a national work stoppage if no progress was made on amending the labour law. Partly because of CELU's leadership's increasingly tenuous position, it was compelled to take a more offensive approach and make a real attempt to achieve tangible progress on labour law reform.

In August 1969, CELU signalled its intent to treat the issue seriously. It sent a letter to the MNCD listing its demands on legislative changes, including the institution of a minimum wage, and threatened action unless they were urgently addressed.[106] This was followed by CELU's withdrawal from participating in three tripartite committees—the Labour Standards Advisory Board, the Manpower Advisory Committee, and the Labour Relations Board. At the same time, CELU's leadership signalled an increased assertiveness on other issues. When HVA fired some twenty trade unionists after workers at its Wonji-Shoa sugar plantation had downed tools, CELU resolutely came to its union's support and readied the workers for a confrontation. By threatening HVA with a strike it forced the enterprise to the negotiation table. Danish LO advisors subsequently helped to convince CELU to abort the strike. 'It seems that CELU was interested in a manifestation of the strength of the trade union movement', an advisor speculated.[107] In December, CELU sought clearance for such a manifestation of strength, applying for a permit to hold demonstrations on December 7, 1970—Christmas Day in the Ethiopian calendar. Simultaneous demonstrations of an estimated 15,000–20,000 workers were planned to be held in seven cities, including Addis Ababa, Asmara, Bahir Dar, Dire Dawa, and the two towns where HVA had

[106] "CELU demands Labour Legislation Threatens to Take Action," *Voice of Labour* 7, no. 4 (August 1969).

[107] "Rapport over projektets slutfase, dækkende perioden 1. Juli–4 december 1969," Kaj Jensen to Udenrigsministeriet, Sekretariatet for teknisk samarbejde med udviklingslandene, 12 December 1969, LO archives.

plantations: Wonji and Metahara.[108] However, while the government predictably rejected the application, it agreed to instead establish a joint committee to explore legislative reform and assured CELU that changes would be made. The committee first met in the immediate and tense aftermath of—a mere three days after—a particularly violent episode that had vividly demonstrated the government's capacity to engage in large-scale repression: the December 28, 1969 murder of the University Students' Union of Addis Ababa's president, and the subsequent day's brutal killing of students that were protesting the murder. Whether CELU's leadership was content that the government's promises to amend legislation in accordance with several of its demands would be honoured, or whether it feared the repression that would, in all likelihood, have occurred should it have pressed on, it nontheless cancelled the planned demonstration and returned to the tripartite committees. But the promised legislative changes never materialised, and the ultimate failure of CELU's efforts convinced the opposition that CELU's leadership had never been resolute in its commitment. Even more damning, by cancelling the demonstrations, CELU's leadership had failed to implement another General Assembly resolution. That failure was used against CELU's leadership by radical trade unionists in the years that followed.

'By the early 1970s', labour scholar Tom Killion has written,[109] 'the dissatisfaction among various groups within CELU had coalesced into a serious opposition movement to the entrenched national leadership'. Somewhat paradoxically, however, the increasing militancy from constituent unions and rank-and-file workers enabled CELU's leadership to take a more assertive approach towards employers. 'CELU has been steadily winning good [CBA] contracts from businesses in all sectors of the economy, and has been quite successful in a number of confrontations over contract enforcement, in situations that would have been a dead loss two years ago', the AALC's Addis Ababa representative reported in 1971.[110] At the same time, he noted that there had been a 'minor revolt' by unions around Addis Ababa dissatisfied with CELU's ability

[108] "A Brief History of the Genesis, Development, Decline and Future Prospect of the Ethiopian Labor Movement," Beyene Solomon, report written for the AALC, Addis Ababa, 1992, AALC Records.

[109] Killion, "Workers, Capital and the State," 478.

[110] "Report No 178: Six-month Progress Report, 1 January–30 June, 1971," Jerry Funk, 14 October 1971, AALC.

to service unions, and with 'Beyene's arrogant refusal to respond to small but pertinent criticism of CELU'.[111] 'CELU eventually handled it well arriving at a compromise', he noted, but warned 'that there will be increasingly threats to the present CELU leadership in the next year (prior to elections in late Spring 1972)'.[112] Working to pre-empt such threats, CELU's leadership suspended its staunch opponent Mesfin Abraha—with whom Beyene had allegedly 'been carrying on a personal grudge match… for the past 1 ½ years'[113]—from his elected post as the president of CELU's Eritrea branch. He was replaced with a Beyene supporter. Moreover, in order to eliminate another base of the most strident opposition, the mandate of CELU's regional branch committee for Addis Ababa and its vicinity was revoked. To the opposition, both actions were additional evidence of CELU's leadership inclination to centralise power, and its aversion to the notion of the regional branches exercising any real autonomy. The resulting outrage eventually forced CELU's president to reinstate Mesfin (albeit only as vice president, until elections could be held) and re-establish the regional committee for Addis Ababa and its vicinity. But in the meantime, Beyene secured a fourth term.

At CELU's fourth congress, held in April 1972, 'Beyene Solomon and the entire group of national officers came in for three days of strong criticism', the 'intensity and extensiveness' of which left them 'jarred'[114]. According to the AALC representative covering the congress, the opposition was spearheaded by two groups: '(1) possibly 1/3 of the Asmara delegation, angry over Beyene's suspension of the Asmara Branch Chairman, Mesfin; and (2) a fairly large group of people from Shoa [the area around Addis Ababa], still dissatisfied with their attempt of last year to gain more autonomy, presumably to ensure better services from CELU'.[115] Eighty delegates were suspended from the voting process, representing basic unions that had allegedly not fully paid affiliation fees.

[111] "Report No. 233: CELU, CONFIDENTIAL", Jerry Funk to Irving Brown and Patrick O'Farrell, 6 February 1973, AALC Records.

[112] "Report No 178: Six-month Progress Report, 1 January–30 June, 1971", Jerry Funk, 14 October 1971, AALC Records.

[113] "Report No. 233: CELU, CONFIDENTIAL", Jerry Funk to Irving Brown and Patrick O'Farrell, 6 February 1973, AALC Records.

[114] "Report No. 206: CELU 3rd Triannual Conference, Elections," Jerry Funk, 24 April 1972, AALC Records.

[115] Ibid.

The remaining 220 General Assembly delegates elected 25 members of the General Council. Despite Beyene and other top officials having received only around half of the eligible votes—'Beyene, Fisseha, Gebre-selassie and Mesfin [Gebremichael] were all bunched about 5 [to] 8th place, with 110–120 votes each'[116]—they were all re-elected. Beyene received between 50 and 60 General Assembly votes less than the basic union leaders of the Assab oil refinery and the HVA Metahara plantation, yet was nevertheless selected to remain president by the General Council. The opposition was convinced that the vote-counting process was flawed and subject to government interference, but the demand for a recount was turned down.[117]

In the aftermath, CELU's leadership moved to shore up its position. Tedla Fantaye, a CELU field worker accused of supporting the opposition, was dismissed from the confederation. Meanwhile, elections among the unions around Addis Ababa were 'engineered'—the term was used by an AALC advisor to describe brazen manipulation—by CELU's leadership to instal an ally as the branch chair and confederation vice president representing the area.[118] The opposition, in turn, grew more resolute. The charges brought against the leadership included 'gross negligence in running the affairs of the confederation', including financial maladministration, feeble organisational attempts, electoral irregularities, and mismanagement of internal disputes.[119] CELU's leadership, the oppositional movement claimed, 'neither represent the workers nor sees itself as representing workers; rather having never dealt with a boss, they actually regard themselves as akin to management rather than labour'.[120] The leadership was accused of colluding with employers and, it was alleged, had gone as far as sabotaging collective bargaining and blocking collective agreements drawn up by oppositional unions.[121] In terms of objectives,

[116] Ibid.

[117] Emmanuel, "Confederation of Ethiopian Labour Unions and its First General Strike," 74–75.

[118] "Report No. 233: CELU, CONFIDENTIAL", Jerry Funk to Irving Brown and Patrick O'Farrell, 6 February 1973, AALC Records.

[119] Emmanuel, "Confederation of Ethiopian Labour Unions and its First General Strike," 75.

[120] "CELU Radical Faction (Disaffiliated Unions) Critique," translation by Awetu Simesso and Tom Killion, Tom Killion Papers.

[121] Ibid.

the oppositional movement advocated a more politically assertive, offensive, and confrontational stance. It resolved that the most viable option was to leave CELU and form a new central organisation of Ethiopian labour altogether.

In response to the fallout from the disputed 1972 congress elections, 36 dissatisfied unions, representing some 15,000 workers, discontinued payment of their affiliation fees to CELU. Instead, they declared their intention to disaffiliate from the confederation and establish a separate trade union centre. The core group consisted of unions from around Addis Ababa and Eritrea, but the dissenting unions also included at least one union in the northwestern Gojam province. Their efforts were coordinated from the office of CELU's regional branch for Addis Ababa and its vicinity, located in the capital. 'Because of their disciplined organisation and commitment as well as their vigorous organising drives', a former CELU employee wrote,[122] they 'were soon to surface and shake CELU to its foundations'. Unsurprisingly, however, when they applied for recognition as a separate trade union centre with the Labour Department of the MNCD, their request was denied. Seeking greater leverage, the dissenting unions sought international recognition through affiliation with the Christian Democratic-oriented World Confederation of Labour (WCL)—a rival organisation to the ICFTU.

In February 1973, the General Secretary of the WCL arrived in Addis Ababa to hold discussions with the dissenting unions. Allegedly, he came with 'great expectations on his part, and on the part of several Eritrean and Shoan[123] unions, that CELU was about to split, form a new body, and join WCL'.[124] However, on his arrival at Addis Ababa's airport, he was singled out for 'a thorough and prolonged perusal' of his luggage by security agents, his documents were seized, and 'he was given a lengthy and stern lecture by Lt. Michael'[125]—the head of the MNCD's Labour

[122] Emmanuel, "Confederation of Ethiopian Labour Unions and its First General Strike," 76.

[123] The region surrounding Addis Ababa, at the time.

[124] "Report No. 243; February/March 1973: CELU General," Jerry Funk, 23 March 1973, AALC Records.

[125] Ibid.

Department, and a close confidant of the AALC.[126] The WCL official's scheduled arrival had been reported to security services by none other than CELU's president Beyene himself,[127] who in turn had been tipped off by Jerry Funk, the AALC's representative in Addis Ababa. This episode underscores the deep extent of collusion that existed between CELU's leadership, the imperial state and the AALC. As a result of the tip-off, 'the visit was a complete bust', the AALC reported. In the aftermath, the oppositional unions 'that had been flirting with WCL were given the message, in several ways, that they were dealing with the wrong people'. 'The Minister of MNCD; H.E. Ato Mulatu Debebe, together with Lt. Michael', an AALC report stated, 'has been knocking heads together, urging CELU officers to give way a bit, and telling dissidents that while they don't have to join in with CELU, they damned sure aren't going to join anyone else'. As a result, a compromise was reached, but this was merely taken to mean that 'the fractures and fissures which were threatening to tear CELU apart at the start of the year, have been papered over'.[128] 'Serious stresses and strains' were expected to persist.

Recognising that it would be impossible to establish a separate confederation under the incumbent imperial regime, the oppositional movement instead launched a campaign to bring about a change of orientation within CELU itself and to undermine and overthrow CELU's moderate and compliant leadership. Meetings between the dissenting unions and CELU, under MNCD's auspices, followed the failed attempt to have a separate trade union centre registered. Both parties agreed to binding arbitration by a conciliation committee, which led to the signing of a peace agreement in July 1973. In that agreement, CELU committed to calling an extraordinary congress of the General Assembly in March 1974, with a mandate to thoroughly review and revise the confederation's constitution. CELU also agreed, in the meantime, to reinstate Tedla Fantaye, the field worker who had been dismissed because of his support for the opposition. Additionally, the agreement formalised a procedure for filling vacant posts, barring CELU's leadership's practice of simply appointing by co-option top officeholders, and it stipulated a procedure

[126] See the fifth chapter for further discussion on this relationship.

[127] Beyene, *Fighter for Democracy*, 167.

[128] "Report No. 243; February/March 1973: CELU General," Jerry Funk, 23 March 1973, AALC Records.

for the regional committees of Eritrea and Addis Ababa and its vicinity—the two strongest bases of the opposition—to adopt by-laws and thus enable them to resume official activities. The dissenting unions, on the other hand, committed to paying outstanding arrears only up to May 1972—the moment of the split—until unresolved matters were settled.

The agreement essentially met the opposition's immediate demands for a new congress of the General Assembly under more transparent conditions than the 1972 congress and the curtailment of the national centre's scope to interfere in the affairs of constituent unions and regional branch committees. In doing so, it led to a temporary truce. Fundamental questions, including those relating to CELU's constitution, were postponed to the extraordinary congress. The open infighting was thus put on hold with the understanding that the factions would fight it out in 1974. With the two factions awaiting and preparing for the expected showdown, the agreement was 'honored reasonably well' in the months that followed.[129] The regional branch committee for Addis Ababa and its vicinity elected a new leadership. It was headed by Getachew Amare, the president of the trading company A. Besse's union and a veteran member of the labour opposition. Meanwhile, Tamyalew Eshete, a textile union president and 'a moderate',[130] was elected CELU vice president representing the area. 'The Shoa (hard-core) dissidents are still active, and even though their activities are no longer paralyzing CELU, they are still a problem', the AALC's representative reported. In Eritrea, however, the re-election of a representative leadership was delayed by CELU's leadership, which was hoping that time would allow its appointed interim branch head, Gidey Gebre, to improve his chances of defeating Mesfin Abraha, or another candidate supported by the opposition, in a branch election. It was a tense truce, and when Getachew Amare and the basic union president of the Mitchell Cotts trading company spoke to the government daily newspaper *Ethiopian Herald* in August 1973, they gave voice to their continued opposition without mincing their words.[131] 'CELU is diametrically opposed to the aims and objectives of the labour movement

[129] "Report No. 256: CELU General," Jerry Funk, 23 August 1973, AALC Records.

[130] Ibid.

[131] "Labour Confederation: What future?," retyped article from *Ethiopian Herald*, 21 August, 1973, AALC Records.

in Ethiopia', they said.[132] The whole organisation—which they alleged was being led by unrepresentative and occasionally unelected 'unionists without unions', including actual employers—was called 'rotten and in need of complete reshaping'. 'The [month of March] 1974', in which the extraordinary congress was scheduled to take place, 'will thus be a decisive month for the labour movement in Ethiopia', the reporter perceptively noted. That was to prove extraordinarily prescient. But not for the reasons the reporter would have presumed. Before CELU's constitutional issues could be resolved in the extraordinary congress, focus would shift to more urgent tasks in workplaces and broader society—as industrial conflict exploded.

The Labour Opposition Ascendant: Taking on the Imperial State

1973 saw a significant uptick in strike activity. That year, workers at the HVA plantations in Wonji-Shoa and Metahara, the Nura Hera plantation, and the Diabaco Cotton factory were among the many that had gone on strike—in some cases repeatedly. However, as the AALC's Addis Ababa representative Jerry Funk noted, Ethiopian strikes had up to this point tended to be 'of short duration, on local issues, not well-publicized, and usually settled on fairly good terms on the informal intervention of [Ministry of National Community Development]'.[133] For these reasons, Funk had not regarded strike activity as sufficiently serious to warrant coverage in his reports to the AALC's New York headquarters. But when the 300 employees of Addis Ababa Bank's offices across the country staged a strike, he was convinced that things were of a new magnitude of importance: 'CELU took on the Addis Ababa Bank (private share company), in a very visible (illegal) two-day strike of all branches all over the Empire. And they won – in the face of Labour Board and High Court rulings against them', he wrote. The surprise he expressed at the favourable outcome was enhanced by the fact that the Minister of the MNCD, Mulatu Debebe, was himself 'a very active shareholder and Director of the Bank'. In other words, the bank workers, with CELU's support, had taken on interests at the heart of the imperial state in a

[132] Ibid.

[133] "Report No. 256: CELU General," Jerry Funk, 23 August 1973, AALC Records.

highly visible manner—and they had prevailed. 'CELU won an impressive victory', Funk wrote. He added that it ought to be viewed as 'a benchmark in its history' that 'set the power structure to pondering'.[134] As impressive as the strike victory was, however, Funk worried that it was likely to enhance the momentum of the labour opposition, which had long argued that a more militant strategy was both possible and necessary. Moreover, he reasoned, 'while the strike can be called a victory, it also opens a new area of concern: how to keep the lid on a potential rash of ill-conceived wildcat strikes'. For, he reasoned, 'as with all "successes", problems don't go away, they merely shift from one order to another'.[135]

Jerry Funk's fears proved to be prescient. Within a couple of months, workers at the Melka Sedi banana plantation, the Central Printing Press, and several parastatal enterprises in Addis Ababa had launched strikes. 'Strikes are becoming more common and frequent', Funk wrote. His projection that 'strikes [in Ethiopia] would become more of a fad (the answer to anything)', he dryly noted, 'seems to be coming to the fore'.[136] But there was one major and notable strike—also of bank workers—that provided even more momentum to this turn of events than the strike at the private-owned Addis Ababa Bank: that of the workers of the large state-owned Commercial Bank of Ethiopia (CBE), which occurred in the immediate aftermath of the Addis Ababa Bank strike.

When the CBE's union called out its 1,200 workers across the country on strike, pressure piled on CELU's leadership to intervene in their support. The CBE union had two simple and compelling demands: that its legal existence be recognised by the MNCD and the CBE's management, and that its right to engage in collective bargaining with the employer be respected.[137] It was met with unanimous support among CELU's affiliates. On August 26, 1973, a CELU General Council meeting was convened. The council resolved to take solidarity measures with the striking bank employees, warned that it was ready to call out more workers in support, and vowed to remain in session until the issue

[134] Ibid.

[135] Ibid.

[136] "Report No. 11," Dick Arnold, 11 January 1974, AALC Records.

[137] Although civil servants were exempt from labour legislation, and therefore did not enjoy the rights to form trade unions and engage in collective bargaining, this exemption did not cover workers of public enterprises, such as CBE. The refusal to recognise the union was thus illegal.

was resolved.[138] The enthusiastic support that this confrontational stance received within the movement was apparent in dozens of letters from basic unions to CELU's president Beyene Solomon, expressing their determination and readiness to intervene.[139] Faced with such decisiveness, the imperial government yielded to the bank workers' demand. In addition to having the CBE union and its right to engage in collective bargaining recognised, it resulted in a collective agreement which included substantial retroactive wage increments.

The success of the bank strikes marked two important victories on behalf of the labour movement. They also put the cautious strategies hitherto pursued by CELU's leadership into sharp perspective, as it was made apparent that a more assertive stance could result in major gains. CELU's support for the 1973 bank strikes must partly be viewed as a result of the serious challenge the leadership had faced from the more militant labour opposition in February and March that same year, and the increasing militancy of the basic unions and the rank-and-file. For the leadership to remain on top of the evolving movement and retain any chance of riding out the challenge it faced, it needed to prove its mettle and discard its submissive image. In much the same way, the radical turn CELU would take in the following months, must be viewed in light of the militant momentum that the successful bank strikes had generated. As the 1974 February movement—an urban uprising in the form of demonstrations and strikes that would mark the beginning of the Ethiopian Revolution—commenced, the lessons of these successful strikes lingered heavily, and as

[138] "ስለ ኢትዮጵያ ንግድ ባንክ የሠራተኞች ማኅበር የተሰጠ ውሳኔ," CELU resolution, 26 August 1973, CETU archives.

[139] For example, from the unions of Ethiopian Petroleum Workers; Indo-Ethiopian Textile Factory; Michell Cotts; HVA; Ethiopian Airlines; Addis Ababa Bank; United Wood Workers; and Addis Ababa Hilton. "በኢትዮጵያ ንግድ ባንክ ሠራተኞች ማህበር ላይ ስለሚፈጸመው ተፅዕኖ," Hailu Yusuf to Beyene Solomon, 31 August 1973, CETU archives; "በኢትዮጵያ ንግድ ባንክ ሠራተኞች ላይ ስለተፈጸመው ተፅዕኖ," Sherefedin Musa to Beyene Solomon, 30 August 1973, CETU archives; "ስለኢትዮጵያ ንግድ ባንክ ሠራተኞች," Elias Mengesha to Beyene Solomon, 30 August 1973, CETU archives; "ስለንግድ ባንክ ሠራተኞች ሥራ ማቆም," Seid Mohamed to Beyene Solomon, 29 August 1973, CETU archives; "ስለንግድ ባንክ ሠራተኞች ማኅበር ሥራ ማቆም," Alemayehu Endalew to Beyene Solomon, 31 August 1973, CETU archives; "የኢ.ሠ.አ.ማ ጠቅላይ ምክር ቤት ስለኢትዮጵያ ንግድ ባንክ ሠራተኞች ነሐሴ 20 ቀን 65 ዓ.ም ያሳለፈውን ውሣኔ ይመለከታል," Gebremichael Woldemedhin to Beyene Solomon, 31 August 1973, CETU archives; Woldemariam Tato to Beyene Solomon, 31 August 1973, CETU archives; etc.

pressure from within the labour movement to join in the popular upsurge increased, CELU's top leadership was cornered.

At the same time, the increasing aloofness of CELU's leadership had played into the hands of the opposition movement. 'Beyene has lost a great deal of his touch with the workers and affiliated officers', Jerry Funk wrote, adding that Beyene appeared 'primarily concerned with his personal status in international circles'.[140] Other top officials around Beyene, who had played key roles in keeping CELU on a moderate path, were also increasingly exhibiting preferences for external engagements. By early 1974, former executive board member Gebreselassie Gebremariam had taken up alternate work for the MNCD and was 'withdrawing further from CELU affairs'.[141] Whereas Deputy General Secretary Mesfin Gebremariam was preparing to leave Ethiopia for an ILO position in Geneva with only paperwork remaining, CELU's General Secretary Fissehatsion was spending an increasing amount of time on his secondary role as the General Secretary of ICFTU's African Regional Organisation (AFRO)—a post he had been elected to the year before. Quite tellingly, Beyene was out of the country in the run-up to CELU's decisive 1974 congress, and was called upon to urgently return by Fissehatsion when the content of draft resolutions became clear to him.[142]

CELU's extraordinary congress of February 23 to March 1, 1974, was held in a radicalised mood. The opposition within the movement had strengthened with the previous year's victories. Outside of it, the February popular movement that would eventually topple the monarchy had begun. By this time, the labour opposition had developed a comprehensive and radical critique that included fundamental aspects of CELU's strategy. It accused the confederation's central leadership of 'economism', of betraying the labour movement, and of collaborating with a reactionary

[140] "Report No. 233: CELU, CONFIDENTIAL", Jerry Funk to Irving Brown and Patrick O'Farrell, 6 February 1973, AALC Records.

[141] "Report No. 261: CELU," Jerry Funk, 12 October 1973, AALC Records.

[142] Fissehatsion Tekie, representing the top leadership, has admitted being against the proposal that won the day: to launch a general strike. At most, he was willing only to repeat the practice of threatening to call one. Another member of the leadership, Gebreselassie Gebremariam, meanwhile, has contended that the general sentiment among delegates of the GA was that a strike had to be called, and that the strike would be a political strike announcing the arrival of the labour movement as a country-wide political force. Fissehatsion Tekie, interview, Tom Killion Papers; Gebreselassie Gebremariam, interviewed by Tom Killion, 1983, microcassette, Tom Killion Papers.

government. 'The opposition's basic argument was that the Ethiopian labour movement [had] not only the right, but also the duty and responsibility, to go beyond its own immediate interests and join the masses, if not lead them, in a popular resistance against [the emperor's] semi-feudal and oppressive regime', a former CELU employee has written.[143] The congress displayed the degree to which the opposition had won over the majority of the delegates of the constituent unions. It did so by issuing an extensive list of demands that were underlined by the commitment to launch a general strike should they not be immediately met. The demands have been characterised as 'primarily corporate' by unsympathetic observers.[144] This misinterpretation may emanate from the leadership's concomitant assurances of moderation and loyalty to the Emperor. By this time, however, the leadership was no longer in effective command of the movement, and the external mechanisms of repression and control that partly relied on that conduit had also broken down. A glance at the actual demands dispels their characterisation as purely corporate in nature. They include respect for the unconditional right of all workers to freely organise and to strike; the repealing of the old labour legislation and the implementation of a new progressive labour law; the establishment of a minimum wage and social security provisions, including pensions' funds; price controls; an end to censorship; and universal free education.[145] The fact that the demands were delivered as an ultimatum, and that government pleas for negotiation were turned down, further underlines the unprecedented political and rebellious nature of CELU's act of insubordination.

On March 7, when it had become clear that its demands could not or would not be met, CELU called a general strike for the following day. Close to 100,000 workers honoured the call, paralysing the waged economy and communications for three days. The number of strikers underscored the resonance of the strike call as it surpassed the number of members in CELU-affiliated unions. The strike also demonstrated the clout of the labour movement as it forced the imperial state to surrender.

143 Emmanuel, "Confederation of Ethiopian Labour Unions and its First General Strike," 1977: 77.

144 M. Ottaway, "Social Classes and Corporate Interests in the Ethiopian Revolution," *Journal of Modern African Studies* 14, no. 3 (1976), 477.

145 "የኢትዮጵያ ሠራተኞች አንድነት ማኅበር ጠቅላይ ምክር ቤት ውሳኔ," CELU resolution, 1 March 1974, CETU Archives.

The concessions extracted included government commitments to replace the labour law; to guarantee wage increments in all sectors and to establish a minimum wage; to allow all government workers to unionise; to punish managers who violated workers' rights; to introduce price controls; to postpone an unpopular reform of the educational sector and to make education free; to establish pension and disability schemes; to restrict the legal space for irregular labour contracts; and finally, to guarantee that no disciplinary actions were taken against any worker or union official participating in or leading the strike.[146] The fact that the government procrastinated on the implementation of the demands and attempted to backpedal in the months that followed only underlines the magnitude of concessions it had made. Something similar can be said of official statements forthcoming in the wake of the strike. In the week that immediately followed the strike, state media lauded workers for 'staying at home peacefully until their demands were met', for their 'gentlemanly behaviour', and their 'honest motives'.[147] That was a far cry from the threatening and scolding government rhetoric which had accompanied the practice of control and repression in previous decades, and it indicated the degree to which the balance of forces had shifted.

The strike was a stunning success in every respect, and it signalled the arrival of CELU as a central actor on the national political scene. The AALC's staff had been sceptical about CELU's capacity and ability to command the necessary level of support from workers to prevail. But in the aftermath of the strike, they were forced to recognise as much. 'The strike was a total success in every respect and the social reforms proposed will not only help the union membership but all citizens of Ethiopia', its representative reported. 'Neither the British TUC [Trades Union Congress] nor the AFL-CIO could hold a candle to the performance'.[148]

The success of the general strike had three immediate effects on the disposition of the labour movement. The first was that it irrevocably discredited the central leadership and the cautious strategy it had

[146] "Government, CELU, Reach Sixteen-Point Agreement," *Ethiopian Herald*, 12 March 1974.

[147] "What Others Write," *Ethiopian Herald*, 19 March 1974.

[148] "CELU Meeting," meeting minutes, appendix to "Report No. 2, East African Region," Richard Baurmann to Lester Trachtman, 29 March 1974, AALC Records.

pursued. Beyene only tendered his resignation a few months later,[149] and would remain in office until September 1974. But there was no question that effective control had been lost. This would also doom Beyene's efforts—conducted in close collaboration with the AALC—to select his own successor.[150] The central leadership was henceforth unable to arrest the movement's drift towards increasing militancy, and despite efforts to restrain the strike wave that followed, strikes multiplied.[151] The split between the ascendant radicals and the proponents of CELU's moderate tradition was deepening across the movement. 'Within CELU affiliates', the US embassy reported,[152] 'inner rivalries are causing quarrels to flare up, and moderates are having to contend with more aggressive and radical elements'. 'Fist fights', it added, were 'not uncommon'.

A second consequence of the strike was the sudden surge in both prestige and membership that CELU experienced in its aftermath. 'After the unqualified success of the recent general strike, CELU was catapulted to a position of great admiration and success. Thousands of workers began demanding immediate organization', the AALC's representative wrote.[153] Membership growth was further fuelled by the government's reluctant approval for employees in over 40 public enterprises to unionise. New unions were consequently formed, while several previously dormant ones were reactivated.[154] In the weeks following the strike, membership in CELU-affiliated unions increased by 40 per cent, adding some 35,000 workers to union ranks.[155] By July, another 10,000

[149] The content of Beyene's resignation letter suggests that his resignation indeed was due to his unpopularity in the movement. While not stating any direct reason, the short letter admitted that organisational performance had been far from satisfactory, and apologised 'for any hard feelings' caused. Beyene Solomon to the Executive Council of CELU, 31 August 1974, ILO archives.

[150] Described in more detail in the fifth chapter.

[151] See Chapter 6.

[152] P.D. Wyman, cable 1974ADDIS04184 from the US Embassy in Addis Ababa, 17 April 1974, Wikileaks Public Library of US Diplomacy (PLUSD), https://wikileaks.org/plusd/cables/1974ADDIS04184_b.html.

[153] "Impact Project Proposal No. 191: Expansion of Organization Program", 1974, AALC Records.

[154] Emmanuel, "Confederation of Ethiopian Labour Unions and its First General Strike," 104.

[155] "CELU Membership to Shoot Up by 40%," *Ethiopian Herald*, 28 March 1974.

new members had joined affiliated unions.[156] Workers also began physically gathering at CELU in large numbers. A US embassy cable from April 1974 reported that 'CELU headquarters has become [a] rallying point for workers whether unionised or not', where 'daily hundreds, often thousands, assemble' keeping the assembly hall 'in constant use'.[157] 'CELU has been besieged daily with people begging to join their ranks', the AALC's representative reported from inside the building.[158] 'It is impossible for anyone to visualize the activity around the CELU building during the last two months. Even on Sundays and holidays one has to fight his ways in and out of the building. Meetings take place all day long in the large conference hall downstairs, in the small offices and the corridors', he continued. 'Ato Tsegaye says the building is going to be wrecked, not deliberately but by overcrowding. Already a couple of windows have had to be replaced'.[159] The successful strike also won CELU significant international attention and respect. Its American advisors, who had previously tended to be somewhat reserved in their assessments of CELU, were notably impressed by the achievement. 'With a tremendous impetus from CELU a healthy seed of democracy has been planted in Ethiopia', the AALC's Addis Ababa representative acclaimed. 'CELU's future is really Ethiopia's future and … optimistically there is an opportunity now to make Ethiopia and CELU a model for Africa, or for that matter, the world'.[160]

A third and related consequence of the strike was that it triggered an explosive boost in the confidence of workers and union representatives vis-à-vis employers and the state. Five weeks after the settlement of the strike, the US embassy reported that the 'turmoil in [the] labour scene continues', with new cases arising 'almost daily'.[161] Throughout the following months, a flurry of strikes engulfed the economy—from

[156] "Organized Labour Grows in Strength in This Country," *Ethiopian Herald*, 25 July 1974.

[157] Wyman, cable 1974ADDIS04184, PLUSD.

[158] "Ethiopia—CELU, Future," Richard Baurmann to Lester Trachtman, 28 March 1974, AALC Records.

[159] '"Pre-Easter Interim April Report," Richard Baurmann to Lester Trachtman, April 1974, AALC Records.

[160] "Ethiopia—CELU, Future," Richard Baurmann to Lester Trachtman, 28 March 1974, AALC Records.

[161] Wyman, cable 1974ADDIS04184, PLUSD.

the smallest workplaces to the largest, from private to public, and across the country. Strikes large enough to warrant mention in the government's mouthpiece *Ethiopian Herald* included those by airport employees, tobacco monopoly workers, teachers, farm workers, import–export firm employees, civil aviation workers, staff of the Elementary School Building Unit, municipal employees, finance ministry employees, railway workers, bus firm employees and transport company workers, dairy industry workers, hospital staff, garment manufacturing workers, taxi drivers, university staff; postal workers, truck drivers, and telecommunication workers. The sheer magnitude of wildcat unrest and mobilisation worried CELU's leadership, which sought to have non-sanctioned striking workers return to work and to limit striking workers' use of CELU's building and meeting hall.[162] However, the unrest also enhanced CELU's leverage and enabled it to maintain pressure on the government to implement labour law reform. By April, CELU was already making plans to launch another general strike—should the right of all state enterprise workers, such as those of the Tobacco Monopoly, to unionise not be respected.[163] Moreover, even its moderate leadership began to publicly speculate that the time to form a political party representing labour was approaching. 'We cannot say that the labour movement is devoid of politics', Beyene stated, contradicting his prior positions. 'But before now we had been busy organising our members. I think we have now reached a stage where we can have an influence on the way the country is run'.[164]

By late April, however, a newly appointed government—whose tenure was to be short-lived—sought to stem militancy, reassert its authority, and impose industrial peace. Retroactively, CELU's general strike was ruled to have been illegal, and state media launched a campaign against striking workers for 'spreading anarchy', warning of stern measures against them.[165] The acute upsurge in labour unrest only began to recede

[162] Richard Baurmann to Lester Trachtman, 19 April 1974, AALC Records.

[163] Ibid.

[164] "Interview: Beyene Solomon: Leader of Ethiopia's trade union movement," photocopied article from *Africa*, no, 33 (May 1974) in "Press Clippings on Developments in Aftermath of General Strike," US Embassy Addis Ababa to US Department of State, April 17, 1974, AALC Records.

[165] See, for example, "Against Anarchy," *Ethiopian Herald*, 25 April 1974; "Government Issues Warning Statement," *Ethiopian Herald*, 25 April 1974; "Government Gives Strong Warning Against Planned Strike," *Ethiopian Herald*, 30 April 1974.

when the government adopted a strategy of repression, including the deployment of security forces in workplaces, the disruption of workers' meetings, beatings, and arrest of workers and union leaders. On top of that, the Ministry of National Defence intervened, threatening that should CELU not cease its alleged agitation, the confederation would be shut down. 'It was obvious that the next move by the Ethiopian Government would be to bring to a screaming halt the rash of strikes that have plagued the country since the CELU general strike', the AALC's Addis Ababa representative reported. He continued as follows:

> By Tuesday, April 30, 1974 when it was apparent that the workers on strike were not going to return to work, and that others, especially the [public enterprise employees] were going to strike, the government, through the police, surrounded the CELU building at about noon. They broke up the meeting taking place and informed CELU officials that there were to be no more strike meetings of any groups in the building. The workers were to get back to work and if the CELU officials continued to allow the disruption of work, or continued to hold mass meetings in the building, the government could not be responsible for what might happen. This included a threat of coming in and tearing down the building piece by piece.
>
> The same afternoon, about five pm, when another small group started to gather, four trucks (GI type dodges) and two jeep loads of police drove up, surrounded the building and entered with their guns at the ready. Some of the striking men tried to escape over the back fence but were apprehended and apparently placed under arrest. …
>
> That evening the radio announced that the Ministry of Defense issued a warning to CELU, stating that they would close CELU down if CELU persisted in assisting the [public enterprise employees] groups and if CELU workers did not return to their jobs.
>
> The situation currently is sort of a Mexican stand-off. The bus drivers have not returned to work, even though the eight officials they wanted removed from office have been detained by the army. The drivers now say they want pay for the days they have been on strike. Some [public enterprise

> employees] are working with guns in their back and under protests. Others have stayed off the job. CELU is threatening another general strike.[166]

The shift in state rhetoric and practice towards labour denoted in this account illustrates a fourth effect of the general strike and the upsurge in strike activity that followed: it compelled the state to acknowledge the clout and potential of the labour movement and triggered the adoption of even tighter measures of supervision and repression. Although the repression was slightly relaxed in mid-1974, as a radical faction of the military came to challenge and paralyse the government, the importance of pacifying the labour movement had been recognised. Cumulatively, these outcomes set the labour movement and the state on a path of escalating confrontation over increasingly significant stakes.

References

African American Labor Center (AALC) Records. Collection 0547-LBR. Hornbake Library, Special Collections and University Archives, University of Maryland Libraries, College Park, MD.

Beyene Solomon. *Fighter for Democracy: The Saga of an Ethiopian Labour Leader*. Baltimore: Publish America, 2010.

Confederation of Ethiopian Labour Unions. *3ኛው በየሦስት ዓመት የሚከናወን ጠቅላላ ጉባዔ/3rd Triannual Conference*. Addis Ababa: Confederation of Ethiopian Labour Unions, 1972.

Confederation of Ethiopian Trade Unions (CETU) archives. CETU, Addis Ababa.

Dessalegn Rahmato. "Civil Society Organizations in Ethiopia." In *Ethiopia: The Challenge of Democracy from Below*, edited by Bahru Zewde and S. Pausewang), 103–119. Uppsala: Nordic Africa Institute, 2002.

Emmanuel Fayessa Negassa. "The Confederation of Ethiopian Labour Unions and its First General Strike (March 7–11, 1974): Causes and Impact." Master's thesis, Cornell University, 1977.

Ethiopian Herald. "Government, CELU, Reach Sixteen-Point Agreement." March 12, 1974.

Ethiopian Herald. "What Others Write." March 19, 1974

[166] Richard Baurmann to Lester Trachtman, 5 January, 1974, AALC Records.

Ethiopian Herald. "CELU Membership to Shoot Up by 40%." March 28, 1974.
Ethiopian Herald. "Organized Labour Grows in Strength in This Country." July 25, 1974.
Ethiopian Herald. "Against Anarchy." April 25, 1974.
Ethiopian Herald. "Government Issues Warning Statement." April 25, 1974
Ethiopian Herald. "Government Gives Strong Warning Against Planned Strike." April 30, 1974.
Graf von Baudissin, G. "Labour Policy in Ethiopia." *International Labour Review* 89, no. 6 (1964): 551–569.
ICFTU/ITUC Archives. Collection ARCH0062, International Institute of Social History, Amsterdam.
International Labour Organization (ILO) archives, International Labour Office, Geneva.
Killion, T. "Workers, Capital and the State in the Ethiopian Region." PhD diss., Stanford University, 1985.
Landsorganisationen i Danmark (LO) archives. Arbejdermuseet & Arbejderbevægelsens Bibliotek og Arkiv, Copenhagen.
Morehouse, L.G. "Ethiopian Labour Relations: Attitudes, Practice and Law." Research project paper, Northwestern University, 1969.
Ottaway, M. "Social Classes and Corporate Interests in the Ethiopian Revolution." *Journal of Modern African Studies* 14, no. 3 (1976): 469–486.
Seleshi Sisaye. "Urban Migration and the Labor Movement in Ethiopia." In *Proceedings of the Fifth International Conference of Ethiopian Studies (Session B)*, 679–700. Chicago: University of Illinois, 1979.
Stutz, R. "The Developing Industrial Relations System in Ethiopia." Mimeo. Haile Selassie I University, Addis Ababa, 1967.
Syoum Gebregziabher. "The Rise of CELU and the EFE Under Haile Selassie's Regime." Mimeo, 2005.
Tom Killion Papers. Collection 2017C40, Hoover Institution Library and Archives, Stanford University Stanford, CA.
Teketel Wegayehu. "Union Structure under Proclamation No. 222/82 and its Impact on Labour Movement." Bachelor's thesis, Addis Ababa University, 1983.
Voice of Labour/የሠራተኛው ድምፅ. "The Ethiopian Labour Movement: The Aftermath of Birth." Special issue on the occasion of the 7th anniversary and the inauguration of its new headquarters, April 9, 1970, 11–23.
Voice of Labour. "CELU demands Labour Legislation Threatens to Take Action." Vol. 7, no. 4 (August 1969).

Wyman, P.D. Cable 1974ADDIS04184 from the US Embassy in Addis Ababa, 17 April 1974. Wikileaks Public Library of US Diplomacy, https://wikileaks.org/plusd/cables/1974ADDIS04184_b.html.

Zack, A.M. "The New Trade Unions of Africa's Oldest Country." *Analyst* no. 3 (1965): 29–37.

CHAPTER 3

The Labour Movement in Revolutionary and Socialist Ethiopia: High Tide and Collapse, 1974–1991

Revolution and Aftermath

The Ethiopian Revolution began as a spontaneous eruption of demonstrations and strikes in urban centres in February 1974. CELU's general strike in March fed into this. Meanwhile, a soldiers' movement that had begun with a barrack mutiny in Negele Borana in January had politicised and mobilised the lower ranks of the armed forces in opposition to the imperial state. By June, the soldiers' movement had coalesced organisationally, with the establishment of the Coordinating Committee of the Armed Forces, Police, and Territorial Army—known as the *Derg*, meaning 'committee' in Amharic. The Derg was constituted by 126[1] elected representatives of the various units of the armed forces and police. From its formation, it began arresting high state officials and eroding the power of the monarchy. But it also took steps to sideline and eventually repress both the civilian popular movement and the soldiers' movement from which it had emerged—by declaring itself an autonomous institution whose members could neither be recalled, replaced, nor held to account by any external body. In September, with most senior imperial officials already behind bars, it deposed the emperor and seized power,

[1] Pliny the Middle-Aged [pseud.], "The PMAC: Origins and Structure, Part One," *Northeast African Studies* 2, no. 3 (1978–1979), 1. This number would subsequently decline as purged and killed members were not replaced.

© The Author(s), under exclusive license to Springer Nature Switzerland AG 2025
S. A. Admasie, *The Ethiopian Labour Movement*, Labour in History and Society, https://doi.org/10.1007/978-3-031-72841-9_3

renaming itself the Provisional Military Administrative Council (PMAC) in the process. Upon doing so, the PMAC suspended basic democratic rights, indicating that no opposition would be tolerated.

CELU's annual congress began only three days after the toppling of the imperial regime, with 250 union representatives from across the country in attendance. The delegates were split between adherents of the movement's different strands, but the momentum was with the more militantly inclined opposition. A 'fair amount of slogan shouting and occasional catcalls against CELU leadership' accompanied the proceedings.[2] US embassy official Wyman[3] reported that 'a degree of radicalism has appeared' in which some delegates 'are suggesting that foreign "exploiters" should be pushed out and that CELU must beware of too much Americanism'. The congress adopted a resolution that lent support to the dethronement of the emperor but opposed the PMAC's usurpation of power from the popular movement, of which CELU saw itself as a central component. It denounced the suspension of democratic rights, particularly the ban on strikes and demonstrations. And it demanded that the PMAC be replaced by a provisional people's government, in which CELU sought representation. Finally, it warned that any harassment or repressive measures from the government would trigger another general strike.[4] The PMAC rejected CELU's demands, but it also sought to convince CELU to retract the resolution.

CELU's weakened but conciliatorily inclined leadership was caught between contradictory necessities. It was already assailed from within the movement, and in the run-up to the congress, leaflets—whose authors were not known—accusing it of corruption and malpractice were being distributed around the capital city. Such leaflets had also begun calling for Beyene's arrest—something which, given the numerous arrests of officials, must have appeared a plausible threat. The leadership was thus facing

[2] P.D. Wyman, "CELU General Assembly Meeting," cable 974ADDIS11161_b from the US Embassy in Addis Ababa, 17 September 1974, Wikileaks Public Library of US Diplomacy (PLUSD), https://wikileaks.org/plusd/cables/1974ADDIS11161_b.html.

[3] P.D. Wyman, "Labor Situation," cable 1974ADDIS11122 from the US Embassy in Addis Ababa, 17 September 1974, PLUSD, https://wikileaks.org/plusd/cables/1974ADDIS11122_b.html.

[4] "የኢትዮጵያ ሠራተኞች ማኅበር ዓመታዊ ጠቅላላ ጉባዔ ያሳለፈው ውሳኔ," CELU resolution, 16 September 1974, Confederation of Ethiopian Trade Unions (CETU) archives, CETU, Addis Ababa.

the simultaneous threat of being ousted by CELU's membership and congress delegates for not being sufficiently assertive, and of incurring the wrath of the Derg either if appearing to challenge it or coming across as too closely tied to the old regime. Charting a path out of that conundrum required an impossible balancing act. While the top leaders, particularly Beyene and Fissehatsion, were unfavourably disposed towards calling of a strike[5] and sought to reach a compromise with the PMAC, they were powerless to retract the congress resolution.

When it became clear that the resolution would not be retracted, the PMAC arrested CELU's top leaders. In response, CELU's remaining leadership called a general strike. But the strike failed. Lack of clarity and coherence meant that it was largely pre-empted. According to ICFTU representative Andrew Kailembo,[6] the effort suffered from a lack of preparation. The fact that most union leaders were assembled for the congress in Addis Ababa meant that they were not able to lead the strike of their respective unions in person. In Eritrea, the regional branch—due to errors in communication—failed to convey the strike call to its member unions.[7] However, the most deleterious problem emanated from an internal rift within CELU's remaining leadership. Vice President Alem Abdi—a trade union leader from the Seferian trading company, a former CELU field worker, and a veteran CELU General Council member, who was also the highest-ranking CELU official that had not been arrested—actively contributed to the failure of the strike. Without any mandate or procedural right to do so, he issued a circular rescinding the strike call. Accompanied by military officers, moreover, he toured workplaces to announce to workers and union officials that the strike had been called off.[8]

[5] "Information and Suggestions on Current CELU Situation," Richard Baurmann to Lester Trachtman, 26 September 1974, African American Labor Center (AALC) records, collection 0547-LBR, Hornbake Library, Special Collections and University Archives, University of Maryland Libraries, College Park, MD.

[6] "Report on Ethiopia", Andrew Kailembo, 16 October 1974, ICFTU/ITUC archives, collection ARCH00622, International Institute of Social History, Amsterdam.

[7] G.B. Sherry, "CELU Strike," cable 1974ASMARA00784_b from the US Consulate General in Asmara, 24 September 1974, PLUSD, https://wikileaks.org/plusd/cables/1974ASMARA00784_b.html.

[8] Kiflu Tadesse, in discussion with the author, June 15–18, 2014. Kiflu was a member of the Politbureau of EPRP and the central leadership of its labour front, as well as editor of CELU's newspaper and head of CELU's educational department in the mid-1970s.

Despite being undermined by such factors, the call was nevertheless heeded in several workplaces during the morning of September 25. Workers of the Meta Abo Brewery were among those who did not show up for work.[9] A US embassy cable[10] reported that 'a few hotels and branches of Commercial Bank had none or small number of employees report for duty' while 'some 200–300 [striking] workers appeared mid-morning at CELU headquarters'. Soldiers soon arrived, however, and it was announced that all workers who had not returned to work by noon would be dismissed. By that time, the embassy noted, 'remaining CELU officials [were] obviously despondent and recognised the futility of further effort'. Tesfa Gebremariam, Assistant Secretary General of CELU and thus one of its most senior officials who had not been arrested, had appeared in the office 'visibly shaken' by the apparent failure of the strike that morning.[11] By noon, CELU called a press conference and announced that the strike had been postponed due to the many unions that it had not managed to notify, but that a new date for a strike would be set once the General Assembly had deliberated.

In the aftermath of the attempted strike, the subordination of the labour movement took on greater importance for the military authorities. The incident had made the PMAC aware that the trade union movement was a potential source of serious opposition, and as a result, it became determined to prevent that risk from materialising.[12] Initially, a mixture of repressive and co-optive measures was adopted.

The groundswell of militant energies from rank-and-file workers and representatives had continued unabeted. This expressed itself not only in strike activity, but also in turbulence at, among other places, the offices of the Labour Relations Board. 'Crowds of unemployed workers', reported

[9] Beyene Solomon, *Fighter for Democracy: The Saga of an Ethiopian Labour Leader* (Baltimore: Publish America, 2010, 148–153.

[10] P.D. Wyman, cable 1974ADDIS11576_b from the US Embassy in Addis Ababa, 25 September 1974, PLUSD, https://wikileaks.org/plusd/cables/1974ADDIS11576_b.html.

[11] "Information and Suggestions on Current CELU Situation," Richard Baurmann to Lester Trachtman, 26 September 1974, AALC records.

[12] Alemu Abebe, in discussion with the author, 31 January 2014. Dr Alemu was initially a POMOA official who, in 1977, became the mayor of Addis Ababa. He was later to become a politburo member of the WPE and serve as, among other positions, deputy prime minister.

the US embassy,[13] 'appear daily before [the] labour commissioner's office and block entrance'. Employers' representatives arriving at the offices were reported to 'have been beaten up' on several occasions, including a case of one being 'heaved over [the] compound wall'. Workers were said to have attempted to set the buildings of the board on fire, and it was allegedly 'not uncommon for [the] labour commissioner to be locked into his office, and frequently army and/or police called in to escort officials and members of LRB out of compound'. A violent crackdown occurred in October, when police opened fire on a congregation of several hundred unemployed workers in CELU's compound, killing one and wounding two. Following the shooting, workers were reported to have chanted in protest, 'we got rid of the Emperor but see how we are being treated', while parading the body of their killed comrade.[14] That same month, a demonstration by 'several hundred' unemployed workers was dispersed by 'several truckloads of troops with guns at the ready', and a commander who made clear his readiness to order fire.[15]

But meanwhile, the PMAC was exercising increasing influence over CELU's acting leadership and sought to cajole it into adopting a submissive approach. The arrest of most senior and long-standing members of CELU's leadership had created a vacuum at the top, which Alem Abdi, aided mainly by Tesfa Gebremariam, attempted to fill without holding fresh elections. Although these two senior officials were content with running the confederation along lines broadly supportive of and agreeable to the PMAC, they faced stiff opposition from within the movement. A few influential unions, such as those of the CFE, HVA's Metahara Sugar Plantation, and some from the industrial Akaki and Kality areas south of the capital, shared Alem's inclination to rally behind the new government. However, a larger share of union representatives was dismissive of what was seen as a simple continuation of the prior leadership's submissiveness to the government. Sensing this danger, the acting leadership ruled out

[13] P.D. Wyman, "Labor Situation," cable 1974ADDIS12489_b from the US Embassy in Addis Ababa, 18 October 1974, PLUSD, https://wikileaks.org/plusd/cables/1974ADDIS12489_b.html.

[14] "Report on Visit of Top-Level Delegation to Ethiopia, 19 to 27 October 1974," Andrew Kailembo, October 1974, ICFTU/ITUC archives.

[15] P.D. Wyman, "Labor Situation," cable 1974ADDIS12489_b from the US Embassy in Addis Ababa, 18 October 1974, PLUSD, https://wikileaks.org/plusd/cables/1974ADDIS12489_b.html.

holding new elections, using the pretext that it needed time to organise a congress of the General Assembly. The PMAC threw its weight behind the acting leadership and erected bureaucratic and logistical obstacles to prevent a General Congress from being held until such a time that the outcome could be expected to be more favourable to it. Union leaders from Eritrea—who generally sided with the opposition—were denied the necessary permits to travel to Addis Ababa to attend meetings. This only aggravated opposition and discontent within the movement.

Dissent against Alem's new—yet familiarly compliant—acting leadership was championed by the same labour opposition movement that had previously challenged Beyene's rule. Unions and regional branch committees in Eritrea and Addis Ababa and its vicinity continued to spearhead the opposition. When the ICFTU's representative Andrew Kailembo visited Ethiopia in October 1974, he was told by members of the General Council that they, and particularly those coming from Asmara, held Alem Abdi and Tesfa Gebremariam directly responsible for the arrest of CELU's leaders and were therefore seeking their dismissal.[16] But since the travel restrictions imposed by the Derg prevented Eritrean unions from actively participating in central matters, it fell upon unions clustered in and around Addis Ababa to coordinate efforts. A US embassy official in Addis Ababa reported that a 'committee of 15 dissidents in Addis [Ababa] CELU affiliates, headed by Getachew Amare from Besse Co' had taken the lead in the campaign to unseat Alem.[17] Beginning in October 1974, they demanded that new elections be held to replace the arrested office-holders. In January 1975, these efforts intensified when about 100 unions in and around Addis Ababa met and elected representatives to a coordinating committee of the dissident unions. The committee was headed by Marcos Hagos, a militant trade union leader from the insurance sector.[18]

That same month, CELU's acting leaders issued a statement endorsing the PMAC and its commitment to a vague programme of 'Ethiopian

[16] "Report on Visit of Top-Level Delegation to Ethiopia, 19 to 27 October 1974," Andrew Kailembo, October 1974, ICFTU/ITUC archives.

[17] P.D. Wyman, "Labor Situation," cable 1974ADDIS12489_b from the US Embassy in Addis Ababa, 18 October 1974, PLUSD, https://wikileaks.org/plusd/cables/1974ADDIS12489_b.html.

[18] Kiflu Tadesse, *The Generation: The History of the Ethiopian People's Revolutionary Party, part I: From the Early Beginnings to 1975* (Silver Spring, MD: Independent Publishers, 1993), 217.

Socialism' on the confederation's behalf.[19] In doing so, they further discredited themselves in the eyes of the opposition and, notably, CELU's own staff (including the trade union of CELU employees)—with whom the acting leadership was falling out completely. 'The relationships between the acting president and the CELU staff are not good', a recently arrived AALC advisor in CELU's offices reported.[20] 'The staff union has presented a list of grievances which in some aspects becomes a serious charge of inefficiency, if not actual mismanagement of CELU', he wrote. 'This is, of course, fuel for opposition elements. In turn, staff members are accused (in some cases quite justly) of campaigning for opposition groups. Staff morale is at an all-time low'. Alem and Tesfa, the advisor concluded, 'have not been able to unify and solidify the organization. Thus CELU is like a ship without a rudder'.[21] The writing was on the wall: the acting leadership had failed to deliver the labour movement to the PMAC and turn it into a bastion of government support. The PMAC would therefore need to seek other ways of controlling or appeasing it.

The oppositional unions continued to push for a general congress to be held, for a new leadership to be elected. By March 1975, the acting leaders had forbidden the Addis Ababa committee from meeting in CELU's offices. In response, the following month, the delegates detained Alem and Tesfa by locking them into a room in the CELU building, thus triggering the intervention of security forces to have them released. The May Day that followed was the first time the International Worker's Day was officially observed in Ethiopia, and a public parade was called on Addis Ababa's Revolution Square. This was an important opportunity for the PMAC to display its intention to seek a closer relationship with the bloc of socialist states—the Soviet consul receiving a far more central place under the canopy than American diplomats, who were seated 'out in the bleachers in the hot sun'.[22] Marking the historic occasion, CELU unfurled a new flag, on which its emblem had been set against a red background instead of the customary blue. 'The day was peaceful',

[19] "CELU Firmly Supports Ethiopian Socialism," Ethiopian Herald, 4 January 1975.

[20] "Report Project No. PA 24, Jan 1–Mar 31, 1975," David F. Summers, 16 April 1975, AALC records.

[21] Ibid.

[22] "BAR-LES No.7: Final Report," Richard Baurmann to Lester Trachtman, 24 May 1975, AALC records.

an American spectator observed,[23] but many oppositional demands were raised by parading workers. Among them were calls to respect the independence of CELU, to restore democratic rights, and to dismiss Alem Abdi from office. One report described workers going further than that, carrying placards 'calling for the hanging of Alem Abdi and accusing him of being a tool of the government'.[24] Alem was reportedly unable to complete his speech since it was drowned out by the noise from jeering workers.[25] The public display of discontent demonstrated the unpopularity of the acting leadership and the unlikelihood that it could defeat the proponents of a radical reorientation of CELU if genuine elections were to be held.

Nevertheless, in the weeks that followed the contestation over CELU continued. On May 18, the opposition forcefully took control of CELU's headquarters building with the aim of holding a congress, and banned Alem from entering it. This appears to have been the final straw for the military rulers, demonstrating the inability of Alem's leadership to reassert a semblance of control. The PMAC consequently closed down CELU's headquarters altogether and banned the confederation from holding meetings. In its statement announcing the closure, the PMAC bluntly stated that the 'so-called CELU' had 'outlived its usefulness, [and had] no place in Socialist Ethiopia'.[26] However, when the PMAC sent delegates to unions and workplaces to canvass support for its decision, it met tumultuous protests and sharp opposition from enraged workers.[27] This embarrassed the PMAC representatives and helped to convince the majority of them to reverse the position. Only a few days afterwards, the PMAC overturned its decision altogether.[28] It permitted CELU not

[23] Ibid.

[24] "ICFTU Executive Board meeting, Brussels, June 26–27, Agenda Item 11: Africa: (b) Ethiopia," Meeting minutes with supplement, ICFTU/ITUC archives.

[25] Kiflu Tadesse, discussion.

[26] "Government Announces Temporary Closure of CELU Headquarters", *Ethiopian Herald*, 20 May 1975.

[27] Andrew Kailembo to ICFTU General Secretary, 3 June 1975, ICFTU/ITUC archives.

[28] In a rather apologetic tone contrasting with the PMAC's statement from the week before, an *Ethiopian Herald* writer claimed that '[the] temporary closure of the headquarters of the Confederation of Ethiopian Labour Unions last month was mistaken by some to be an indication of the government to emasculate organised labour'. This, the writer

only to reopen its offices, but also to hold new elections—thus meeting the principal demand the labour opposition had insisted on for the past seven months. But the PMAC was far from united in finally acquiescing to this demand, and the permission to hold elections came with a strong flavour of conditionality: that CELU would be closely monitored in the future too.

Delegates to CELU's General Assembly who could travel to the capital met there between May 31 and June 4, 1975, to elect a provisional leadership. The elections were reported to have taken place in good order with minimal state presence—represented by one single security officer. Observers acknowledged that 'democratic processes were being followed' and that the outcome was consistent with the will of the majority.[29] The elected officeholders were mandated to lead CELU until a full congress of the General Assembly could be held. Reflecting its temporally limited mandate, the leadership body was named the Provisional Workers' Committee (PWC). It was chaired by a workers' representative who had long participated in the labour opposition movement: Marcos Hagos.

The Labour Opposition Comes to Power

The formation of the PWC marked a critical turning point that brought an end to Alem Abdi's tenure and to the moderate faction's control of CELU. After nearly a decade of dissent and strife, the labour opposition had finally emerged triumphant. It also marked the establishment, for the first brief (as it proved to be) time in CELU's history, of genuine freedom from state interference in the confederation's affairs. These shifts constituted a fundamental break with CELU's past orientation. This was reflected in the content of the resolution the meeting adopted. 'After many years of working class struggle', it read, 'the assembly of Ethiopian

rather unconvincingly assured readers, 'of course, was a totally erroneous assumption' as demonstrated by later events. Rahel Teshome, "The week that was," *Ethiopian Herald,* 8 June 1975.

[29] US Embassy in Addis Ababa, "Provisional CELU Executive Committee Selected—CELU Headquarters Reopened," cable 1975ADDIS06558_b from the US Embassy in Addis Ababa, 3 June 1975, PLUSD, https://wikileaks.org/plusd/cables/1975ADDIS06558_b.html. Fissehatsion Tekie also acknowledged that Marcos' group had the support of the majority. Fissehatsion Tekie, interviewed by Tom Killion, 1983, microcassette, Tom Killion Papers, collection 2017C40, Hoover Institution Library and Archives, Stanford University Stanford, CA.

union leaders that met from 31 May to 4 June, marked the historic occasion of the rebirth of the CELU into a democratic organization'[30]:

> CELU has reached its present stage of development after many struggles, strenuous endeavors and the sacrifices of its contending leaders. Many years have passed since the progressive (union) leaders within the fold of CELU started their struggles to organize the CELU to the benefit of the working class. The glowing struggles prevailed thereby driving out the reactionary elements who were enemies of the working class and reinstate CELU under the direction and control of the toiling masses. The misinterpretation of this factual sequence of events as power struggle for leadership has been opposed by the totality of the working class.

However, there was also a fair degree of continuity with the tradition of CELU's more militant strand, as evidenced by this excerpt from the resolution. Although most PWC electees represented what had up to this point been the oppositional movement, they were nevertheless, for the most part, experienced workers' representatives and veteran trade unionists and included some very senior CELU officials. The PWC was chaired by Marcos Hagos, who himself had been an elected workers' representative and a member of CELU's General Council for many years by that time, and its vice chairman was Mesfin Abraha, the former president of CELU's Eritrea branch. It also included what was described as 'trade unionists of established reputation', such as Elias Mengesha of HVA, Shumiye Teferra of Hilton Hotel, and Ibrahim Ahmed of Amropa Motors,[31] as well as the experienced leaders of two trading and retail companies' unions—Gebremichael Gebremedhin of Mosvold and Getachew Amare of A. Besse.[32]

[30] CELU resolutions of the newly elected PWC leadership, passed and dated June 5, 1975, translated by an ILO regional officer in ILO's regional office in Addis Ababa, attachment to memorandum from ILO's Regional Meshack Ndisi Archive to H. Dunning and H. Hammar, 13 June 1975. ILO archives, International Labour Office, Geneva. International Labour Organization (ILO) archives, International Labour Office, Geneva.

[31] US Embassy in Addis Ababa, "Provisional CELU Executive Committee Selected—CELU Headquarters Reopened," cable 1975ADDIS06558_b from the US Embassy in Addis Ababa, 3 June 1975, PLUSD, https://wikileaks.org/plusd/cables/1975ADDIS06558_b.html.

[32] CELU resolutions, 5 June 1975, ILO archives.

In establishing CELU's new positions, the June 1975 resolution reflected the radicalised mood of the General Assembly. It 'strongly warned' the PMAC against repeating the closure of CELU's offices, demanded the release of its arrested leaders, and an end to the exercise of censorship over its publications. It denounced the management of nationalised corporations and demanded that workers, 'through leaders of their own choosing, in an atmosphere of equality and freedom', should participate in the management of these enterprises. It further called for government inspectors to be removed from state enterprises to create a democratic workplace atmosphere; an end to the wage-freeze policy imposed by the PMAC; the establishment of a minimum wage; the promulgation of a new progressive labour law, to include provisions for job security, extensive social security, and the abolishment and replacement of the LRB; and the free organisation of all workers. By this point, CELU had begun tilting towards positions of the clandestine leftist Ethiopian People's Revolutionary Party[33] (EPRP), and although no formal alliance was ever proclaimed a certain convergence of views was to become apparent.[34] The US embassy in Addis Ababa reported that the resolution contained 'the first specific appearance of [a] communist line'.[35]

[33] The organisation that was to become the EPRP had still not announced its existence, nor adopted the name EPRP. That was only to occur two months later. But the existence of a pole organised around its popular newsletter *Democracia* had become apparent.

[34] Note however, that while the EPRP's signature demand for a provisional people's government was featured in the September CELU's 1974 resolution (a year before the emergence of that party), that particular demand was conspicuously absent from both its June and September 1975 resolutions.

[35] P.D. Wyman, "CELU Provisional Executive Committee First Actions; Severance of CELU/AALC Relations," cable 1975ADDIS06634_b from the US Embassy in Addis Ababa, 4 June 1975, PLUSD, https://wikileaks.org/plusd/cables/1975ADDIS06634_b.html.

Mesfin Gebremichael of CELU's old leadership was quoted as having told the embassy that four technical advisors led by Kiflu Tadesse and Girmachew Lemma were responsible for drafting the CELU resolution attacking the PMAC, but another member of the ousted CELU leadership—Gebreselassie Gebremariam—added that 'many of those elected do indeed oppose the [PMAC]'. Mesfin would not have known that Kiflu and Girmachew were EPRP members at the time. Kiflu has concurred that Girmachew probably drafted the resolution. P.D. Wyman, "1. Two of CELU's 'Four Horsemen' Discuss Developments 2. AALC Office to Close by June 30," cable 1975ADDIS06929_b from the US Embassy in Addis Ababa, 11 June 1975, PLUSD, https://wikileaks.org/plusd/cables/1975ADDIS06929_b.html; Kiflu Tadesse, discussion.

To US officials, the probably most unpalatable aspect of CELU's June resolution was the announcement of CELU's disaffiliation from ICFTU and the severing of relations with the AALC and AFL-CIO, which included the eviction of both organisations from CELU's premises, alongside the denouncements that accompanied it. The Americans' understanding of how the labour opposition had defeated the moderates and seized power within the confederation—and its implications—was coloured by the intense mutual hostility. But it was nevertheless strikingly well-informed, in most parts remarkably accurate, and reflective of the views of CELU's former leadership and its international allies. For these reasons, it must be recounted in some extensiveness.[36]

> The events of April and May, leading up to the General Assembly resolution were not unexpected. ...
>
> In 1973 CELU lost two of its leaders almost at the same time. Mesfin G/ Michael, Director of Organization and Education went to the ILO, and Gabre Selassie G/Mariam, General Secretary went to the Ministry of the Interior. This left the leadership of CELU in a seriously weakened position. Opposition elements increased their efforts.
>
> About the same time, perhaps a little earlier, CELU had turned down an offer of assistance from the WCL (Christian Unions) on the grounds that the results could promote divisions within the Ethiopian trade union movement. It is believed that this assistance was in fact given to dissident elements, thus enabling the opposition to create an organization. ...
>
> It appears that a cell had been working in the trade union movement for some time. Girmachew (a former president of the University Students Union) was hired as an assistant legal advisor. Kiflu Tadesse was taken on as Assistant Editor of the Voice of Labour. During October, November, and December (probably with outside financial assistance) [a] carefully planned campaign to visit local unions was intensified.
>
> Dissatisfaction with the leadership of the Acting President, Alem (who had been the elected Vice President) and acting General Secretary Tesfa

36 "Background Report to All Ethiopian Projects," David F. Summers, Quarterly report, 6 July 1975, AALC records.

(elected the Deputy General Secretary) became a major issue of trade union politics.

The leadership given by Alem and Tesfa was weak. They made several bad judgements. ... Their major misjudgement was the neglect of large sections of their electorate. They prevented CELU staff from visiting and servicing the locals. Evidently they were aware of the successful campaign going on, but did not realize it was organized by a small, well organized and well financed group. They suspected their own staff (some of whom were directly involved – and many of whom became involved as a result of the poor personnel relationships which developed) and thus erected as many hurdles as possible to prevent direct contact between local trade unions or their leaders and most CELU staff members.

Instead of enlarging their base of popular support, Alem and Tesfa tried to base their position on the support of strong local leadership factions, on an appeal to constitutional ways of solving problems, on the support of the Ministry of National Community Development for constitutional and legal ways of doing things, and on the promises of persons in, or close to, the Derg.

The various factions of opposition and dissidents formed a tight coalition with one common objective: "Get rid of Alem and Tesfa!".

By itself, the weak leadership given by Alem and Tesa would not have led to their downfall. But with opposition co-ordinated and stimulated by a cell which was not identified and isolated, the results were catastrophic for the administration. ...

[T]he cell was able to plant suspicion of the AALC in the minds of CELU administration, and to play up a feeling of incompatibility between [AALC representative] Summers and Tesfa Alem, until it became a major factor in AALC-CELU relationships.

During January to April CELU staff made several attempts (progressively becoming more extreme) to take over CELU and to depose Alem, and Tesfa. They created (probably stimulated by the cell) confusion and conflicts, leading to the order of the Derg, in mid-April, to close CELU headquarters, and to suspend CELU activities, while leaving the local unions freedom to continue operations.

It was only after the closure of CELU that Tesfa and Alem began to lose confidence in their ultimate victory. They had close contacts within, or close to, the Derg. They were sure that the Government (derg) would support the constitution, and deal with the extreme dissidents.

However, during the period of CELU closure it became very clear that the opposition elements too had close contact with members of the Derg (whether direct or indirect is not known).

When the Assembly was called for May 31st, the Derg made it clear that it opposed the 'old' leadership and wanted new leaders elected. This played into the hands of the cell. Somehow 'old' opposition leaders were not under the shadow of objection.

The Assembly which met in the Grand Palace on Saturday morning and moved to the Parliament in the afternoon, paved the way for the reopening of CELU building, the holding of elections, thus releasing the bank account, and for the re-organization of CELU on 'revolutionary lines'. The Assembly reconvened in the CELU building on Monday, June 2, and continued till June 4.

The membership of this Assembly was largely new inexperienced trade unionists.[37] A few experienced leaders were specifically prevented from attending. For example Tesfa and Alem were prohibited on the grounds that they did not represent local unions, and the President of Indo-Ethiopian Textile Workers [Tamyalew Eshete] was prohibited by name. Several other experienced leaders deliberately did not attend, as a mark of protest, sending junior unknown persons largely as observers. A few experienced leaders did attend, but found themselves outnumbered and out-maneuvered.

The Assembly was practically unanimous in ousting Alem and Tesfa. … Techniques of manipulation of democratic process were skillfully used to put through a series of decisions. Some of them were popular and used to carry others with them. …

The clause of the resolution severing relations with ICFTU and with AFL-CIO was one of the sections that had a great deal of debated. Several argued that the question was premature – that the Assembly did not know

[37] Note the difference between the General Assembly *delegates* and the PWC *electees*.

the roles played (by AALC in particular) nor did it know the consequences, financially or otherwise.

However the arguments that Americans are CIA agents, and that the reason for AALC 'intervention' in CELU affairs was to promote the interests of foreign capitalists created an emotional appeal that carried the day. It appears the majority of the delegates voted against Capitalist, Imperialist and CIA interests without any knowledge or understanding of the objectives, methods or programs of AALC...

The fact that AALC works with the constitutionally elected officials, in this case Tesfa and Alem, clinched the case. Delegates suspected that AALC was making secret contributions which had financed the old administration.[38]

Since the Provisional Workers Council has assumed power, there has been a tightening up of some administrative procedures. ... However, the unanimous desire of the Assembly to accept the financial sacrifice of rejecting AALC aid, and to make sure that the local unions pay their per capita assessments regularly is not resulting in quick action. ... CELU will be facing a serious financial problem when the accumulated funds of their recently released bank accounts are spent. ...

The united front of the dissident opposition groups is crumbling now that the common objective of ousting Alem and Tesfa is achieved. The cell that thought it was using Getachew Amare and his group now finds that Getachew has a mind of his own. Getachew, who thought he is using the cell is now seriously vying with them for power. The four technical advisors (self or cell appointed CELU staff members) are not showing the degree of unanimity they formerly did.

There is passive resistance emerging within influential sections of the trade unions ... It would appear that the possibility of the emergence of elements of free trade unionism is so linked up with national political questions that prediction at this time is quite unreliable. ... Thus, the decision to suspend all AALC/CELU project support as of May 31, 1975, appears to be a wise decision, even if forced on the delegates.

[38] These were allegations that were later to proven to be true. See Chapter 5 for details.

The PWC Period and the September 1975 General Strike

The election of the PWC temporarily created political space in which a relatively autonomous labour movement could operate without significant direct state intervention. The emergence of a free and militant trade union centre—for the first time in Ethiopian history[39]—led to immediate gains. Organisationally, the PWC was successful in re-establishing and expanding the network of unions in the months that followed. Its autonomy and combativeness enabled it to attract large numbers of previously unorganised workers and establish new unions. This much was reluctantly admitted by the US ambassador, who reported that although '[the] PWC is suffering internal strains and rivalries [it] seems to be making some progress towards its stated objective of re-establishing CELU HQs as [a] genuine national centre for affiliated unions and workers'.[40] The PWC's three-month report leading up to the September 1975 General Assembly congress noted that inroads had been made in new sectors—for example, in organising tailors and sewers, tea house and bar employees, taxi and tractor chauffeurs, and mission employees—leading to the establishment of 41 new unions with 8,500 members, while also reviving a number of dormant unions and recruiting additional members to existing unions.[41] Progress was also made politically, in acquiring the release of imprisoned former CELU leaders and obtaining official permission to hold a General Assembly congress, with the delegates of Eritrean unions finally granted permission to travel to Addis Ababa for the occasion.

The General Assembly congress held in September 1975 demonstrated the level of support the radical leadership had acquired. The previously provisional leadership was re-elected for a regular term, on an explicitly Marxist-Leninist platform.[42] A special issue of *Voice of Labour* featuring

[39] Kiflu Tadesse has convincingly argued that the three months that followed constituted 'the first time in Ethiopian history that there was an independent [trade union confederation]'. Kiflu Tadesse, discussion.

[40] A.W. Hummel, "Ethiopian Labor Scene," cable 1975ADDIS08716_b from the US Embassy in Addis Ababa, 22 July 1975, PLUSD, https://wikileaks.org/plusd/cables/1975ADDIS08716_b.html.

[41] "ከሕግና ቀሬታ ክፍል የቀረበ ክንውን ሪፖርት," CELU Report. CETU Archives.

[42] "ከመስከረም 8-11-1968 ዓ.ም. ድረስ ተሰብሰቦ የነበረው የኢ.ሠ.ማ. ልዩ ጠቅላላ ጉባኤ ያሳለፋቸው ውሳኔዎች," CELU Resolutions, CETU Archives.

a study compendium of *The Communist Manifesto* was published the same month. Although clearly unsympathetic to CELU's new political line, the US embassy viewed the congress as having been conducted legitimately and the outcome as consistent with the prevailing mood of the membership. 'CELU's rank-and-file was well represented at its General Assembly by individual union leaders', it stated, 'and we have no doubt that the resolution's bread and butter demands accurately expressed labour's needs'.[43] The large number of unions represented at the congress, furthermore, was viewed as indicative of the extent to which the PWC 'had done its work well in re-establishing links between affiliated unions and national centre'.[44] However, the resolutions passed included demands that the Americans deemed to be 'obviously unacceptable' to the PMAC.[45]

Most of the demands contained in CELU's September 1975 resolutions were similar to those that had been raised in the June resolution—and subsequently ignored by the Derg. However, they were now articulated in a more assertive manner.[46] The September resolution expressed support for a popular democratic form of socialism—under the leadership of a proletarian party guided by Marxisn-Leninism—and voiced strong opposition to the prevailing authoritarianism and the bureaucratic nature of Derg's state capitalism. It demanded the restoration of civil and democratic rights—including the right to demonstrate and strike—and the release of arrested progressives. Having had its previous demands for the democratisation of workplace relations ignored, CELU now called for the complete removal of state-owned enterprises' managements, and their replacement with workers' representatives. It further stipulated that if its demands were not met within a month, 'all necessary measures' would be taken. Given that the PMAC's rejection of these demands was somewhat of a foregone conclusion, and as this rejection would likely result

[43] A.W. Hummel, "Dirg's Confrontation with Ethiopian Workers; Embassy's Further Views," cable 1975ADDIS11756_b from the US Embassy in Addis Ababa, 2 October 1975, PLUSD, https://wikileaks.org/plusd/cables/1975ADDIS11756_b.html.

[44] A.W. Hummel, "Trade Union Situation," cable 1975ADDIS11934_b from the US Embassy in Addis Ababa, 8 October 1975, PLUSD, https://wikileaks.org/plusd/cables/1975ADDIS11934_b.html.

[45] Ibid.

[46] "ከመስከረም 8-11-1968 ዓ.ም. ድረስ ተሰብስቦ የነበረው የኢ.ሠ.ማ. ልዩ ጠቅላላ ጉባኤ ያሳለፋቸው ውሳኔዎች," CELU Resolutions, CETU Archives.

in repressive measures, CELU's resolution included a provision that any harassment or repression would automatically trigger a general strike. Accordingly, preparations were made for a strike committee to take charge in the event of arrests. However, as subsequent events would reveal, these preparations were inadequate.

The PMAC responded to the demands contained in the September resolution mercilessly. An infamous event of brutality occurred at Addis Ababa's Bole International Airport, where picketing airline workers were distributing leaflets containing CELU's resolution. Upon arrival, security forces found several hundred Ethiopian Airlines employees who, according to the government, 'tried to obstruct the officers performing their duty, refused to disperse peacefully, and in fact encircled the security officers'.[47] What followed was a massacre, in which around a dozen workers were killed, while many more were beaten and teargassed.[48] The wave of repression and violence subsequently spread across the capital rapidly. The ICFTU's assistant general secretary reported that 'over a hundred people have been shot and it is reported that some 1,600 people have been arrested'. Among the detained were most members of CELU's executive committee. Marcos Hagos was so badly beaten up during his arrest that he was initially assumed to have sustained permanent injuries.[49] In addition, security agents attempted to track down each of the General Assembly delegates and the 175 union representatives who had signed the

[47] ILO, *155th Report of the Committee on Freedom of Association* (Geneva: International Labour Office, November 1975).

[48] M. Ottaway and D. Ottaway, *Ethiopia: Empire in Revolution* (New York: Africana Publishing Company, 1978), 9.

The official number of casualties was four, while the number of injured was 29, whereas the AALC reported seven dead and 17 injured. In the government's account of events, the soldiers responded to 'someone from the crowd [firing] a shot at them'. "Four Killed, Twenty-Nine Others Injured at Bole Airport", *Ethiopian Herald*, 26 September 1975; "Visit to Addis Ababa From 20 to 24 October 1975," D.J. O'Laughlin to Patrick.J. O'Farrell and John Gould, 25 October 1975, AALC records; ILO, *155th Report of the Committee on Freedom of Association*.

[49] "Visit to Addis Ababa From 20 to 24 October 1975," D.J. O'Laughlin to Patrick.J. O'Farrell and John Gould, 25 October 1975, AALC records; Francis L. Luyimbazi, "Report on the Main Activities of ICFTU Research Office and General Labour Situation in Ethiopia, From October 1974 to date," report 9 January 195, ICFTU/ITUC archives.

resolution, arresting most of them.[50] Reports indicated that 'at least 150 union leaders' were imprisoned as a result.[51] Workplaces were combed by agents seeking to identify rank-and-file workers who had been absent during the strike. Those deemed to have been responsible for organising or participating in the strike were arrested, subjected to beatings, and in some cases 'reportedly shot'.[52]

During the strike a bomb detonated outside Addis Ababa's telecommunications office, where the workforce was known for its strong opposition to the Derg.[53] This incident was swiftly exploited as another pretext for clamping down on the labour movement. A state of emergency was declared: strikes, slow-downs, public gatherings and the distribution of leaflets were prohibited. This was enforced in the strictest manner as security forces were granted the right to shoot offenders on sight.[54] In Akaki, detained strikers and union leaders were allegedly massacred.[55] With much of CELU's leadership forced underground, the strike was left without a coordinating body and failed to rally a critical mass. The US embassy in Addis Ababa[56] provided a detailed account of how it unravelled: 'In the wake of [the Ethiopian Airlines] incident', it reported, the 'strike call was assumed by some, but others awaited notification'. As a

[50] John Vanderveken to L. Murray [Trades Union Congress], n.d [1975]. ICFTU/ITUC archives.

[51] "Visit to Addis Ababa From 20 to 24 October 1975," D.J. O'Laughlin to Patrick.J. O'Farrell and John Gould, 25 October 1975, AALC records.

[52] A.W. Hummel, "Trade Union Situation," cable 1975ADDIS11934_b from the US Embassy in Addis Ababa, 8 October 1975, PLUSD, https://wikileaks.org/plusd/cables/1975ADDIS11934_b.html.

[53] As late as March 11, 1977, an article published in *Ethiopian Herald*'s 'Revolutionary Forum' column ostensibly written by a telecommunication worker, found it necessary to exhort colleagues to 'clean our unions from EPRP traitors'. Tele Progressive [pseud.], "Abiot Forum. Let Us Clean Our Union From EPRP Traitors," *Ethiopian Herald*, 11 March 1975.

[54] "PMAC Declares State of Emergency," *Ethiopian Herald*, 1 October 1975; C. Clapham, *Transformation and Continuity in Revolutionary Ethiopia* (Cambridge: Cambridge University Press, 1990), 55.

[55] Kiflu Tadesse, discussion; Fissehatsion Tekie, interviewed by Tom Killion, 1983, microcassette, Tom Killion Papers; "Visit to Addis Ababa From 20 to 24 October 1975," D.J. O'Laughlin to Patrick.J. O'Farrell and John Gould, 25 October 1975, AALC records.

[56] A.W. Hummel, "Trade Union Situation," cable 1975ADDIS11934_b from the US Embassy in Addis Ababa, 8 October 1975, PLUSD, https://wikileaks.org/plusd/cables/1975ADDIS11934_b.html.

result, 'hesitation, confusion and lack of communications doomed action from start'. The AALC's representative similarly concluded that 'because of poor planning, timing and communication, [the strike] had little chance of succeeding'.[57]

But the commitment to strike in the event of repression was far from universally ignored. Workers of the Motor and Engineering Company (MOENCO), Crown Cork, Sabean Metals, Darmar Shoes, and Ethiopian Airlines, among others, were reported to have responded to the prearranged call, and wildcat strikes continued for a full week at workplaces such as the Berhanena Selam Printing Press, Addis Tyre Company, Addis Shoe Factory, Fiat Company, Lazaridis Company, Addis Ababa's grain storage depot, Ethiopian Cider, Cement factory, Sadaolin Paints, Vaskin Company, as well as among petroleum workers, bank workers and insurance employees.[58] The US embassy[59] estimated that between 8,000 and 10,000 workers participated in the strike, but significantly higher figures have also been suggested, based on an assessment that at least 80 to 120 basic unions fully took part in the strike.[60] It has been claimed that participation in the September 1975 strike was relatively greater among white-collar workers. 'Those who eventually walked off their jobs seem to come primarily from labour's most regarded elite', a US embassy cable read.[61] However, the same cable also noted that the September 1975 strike was a landmark event, marking 'the first time that substantial numbers of workers have translated their opposition to the [PMAC] into overt and united action'. The strong support the strike call received

[57] "Visit to Addis Ababa From 20 to 24 October 1975," D.J. O'Laughlin to Patrick.J. O'Farrell and John Gould, 25 October 1975, AALC records.

[58] A.W. Hummel, "Addis Airport and Labor Developments: Sept. 30," cable 1975ADDIS11623_b from the US Embassy in Addis Ababa, 30 September 1975, PLUSD, https://wikileaks.org/plusd/cables/1975ADDIS11623_b.html; A.W. Hummel, "Wildcat Strikes Appear to Wane," cable 1975ADDIS11720_b from the US Embassy in Addis Ababa, 1 October 1975, PLUSD, https://wikileaks.org/plusd/cables/1975ADDIS11720_b.html; Hummel, "Dirg's Confrontation with Ethiopian Workers".

[59] A.W. Hummel, "Trade Union Situation," cable 1975ADDIS11934_b from the US Embassy in Addis Ababa, 8 October 1975, PLUSD, https://wikileaks.org/plusd/cables/1975ADDIS11934_b.html.

[60] Kiflu Tadesse, discussion.

[61] Hummel, "Dirg's Confrontation with Ethiopian Workers".

in many workplaces in Akaki—an important industrial hub just south of the capital, where blue-collar unions were predominant—and the ensuing violence which lasted for days in the district, lends credence to this.

The September 1975 general strike turned out to be, the AALC commented, 'an expensive failure'.[62] 'CELU is now entirely without elected leadership', it reported. 'All are either in detention or in hiding'.[63] The same applied to CELU's employees: except for clerical staff, only three employees remained free and at liberty to continue overt work. Reeling from the blow suffered, activists that remained at large were forced to adopt clandestine ways of coordinating activity to sustain the movement. The experience of using clandestine networking to augment pressures on the PMAC before the formation of the PWC provided a blueprint for constructing a new organisational structure. This was made up of mushrooming groups of labour activists coordinated by an underground CELU Resurrection Committee. Funds were collected to support the dependents of arrested workers and labour leaders, and a covert network was created to coordinate resistance against attempts to impose control over the movement. By December 1975, a relatively strong organisational foundation had been created.[64] At around this time, EPRP activists in the labour movement, along with workers who had become sympathetic to the party's line, formed the Ethiopian Workers' Revolutionary Union (ELAMA).[65] ELAMA represented a distinct organisation from the EPRP but maintained horizontal ties to the party structures. It functioned as the labour wing of the united front the EPRP was seeking to build. Its establishment provided both an organisational asset for radicalised workers determined to continue to resist state control,

[62] "Visit to Addis Ababa From 20 to 24 October 1975," D.J. O'Laughlin to Patrick.J. O'Farrell and John Gould, 25 October 1975, AALC records.

[63] Ibid.

[64] Notably, the organisation even came to publish its own clandestine newspaper, *CELU Resurrection*. Kiflu Tadesse, *ኢትዮጵያ ሆይ: ቅጽ 1* (self-pub., Addis Ababa, 2016).

[65] The organisation is known by its Amharic acronym ELAMA, which reads የኢትዮጵያ ላባደሮች አብዮታዊ ማኅበር, literally translating to Ethiopian Proletarians' Revolutionary Association, but since the translation Ethiopian Workers' Revolutionary Union has been used elsewhere, this translation will also be used here. Kiflu Tadesse, *The Generation: The History of the Ethiopian People's Revolutionary Party, part II: Ethiopia, Transformation and Conflict* (Lanham, MD: University Press of America, 1998).

and a political asset for the EPRP that allowed it to recruit workers in large numbers. This influx of workers provided the party with some of its most dedicated militants in the violent confrontations that lay ahead.[66]

The Derg's Counter-Offensive

In December 1975, the PMAC proclaimed a new labour law. The proclamation effected the legal dissolution of CELU and its replacement with a new central trade union body: the All-Ethiopia Trade Union (AETU). It also restructured the trade union movement by introducing a three-tier configuration. At the base of this structure were the constituent unions formed at the enterprise level, or, in cases where enterprises employed fewer than twenty workers, general craft unions. Basic enterprise unions within the same sector would then join each other to form mid-tier industrial unions, which, in turn, would constitute the AETU.

The new legal regime was geared towards the imposition of industrial and institutional control rather than empowering workers. While individual rights, such as provisions for job tenure security, overtime pay, and annual, maternity, and sick leave were improved, collective rights were further constrained. Organising a legal strike remained essentially impossible. The law permitted strikes only where a collective trade dispute had been referred to the labour division of the high court, and where the court had not taken any decision nor ruled against a strike being permitted: essentially, striking still required the explicit permission of authorities—a nearly impossible proposition. But wildcat striking, 'lack of good faith in a collective negotiation', failure to immediately execute 'an agreement, decision or order given at any level', or 'to obstruct or be the cause of a delay of the speedy settlement of a trade dispute', were acts assigned the status of criminal offences punishable with imprisonment. Moreover, the law introduced a centralised and hierarchical logic on trade union structures, which stipulated that 'lower trade unions shall be subordinate to higher ones' and 'shall be obliged to accept and implement the decisions of higher trade unions'. The top leadership of the central confederation—the AETU—was assigned the function of overall control and to 'issue directives to unions to ensure their functioning in line with socialist principles'. Basic enterprise unions, meanwhile,

[66] Kiflu, *The Generation, part II.*

were to 'encourage and stimulate workers to increase production, and to participate and render services to voluntary community activities'—a euphemism for the requisition of free labour from workers, who in turn were 'required to maintain strict discipline'. The thrust of the law was so top-down and restrictive that even the name of the confederation was determined by it. Only on one point did the law nominally improve collective rights: it included provisions for paid union leave for elected officeholders. But such officeholders were, in any case, ordained to act on the directives of higher levels, rather than on the will of union members.

If there were any doubts as to the nature of the labour regime the proclamation sought to establish, official rhetoric,—neatly exemplified by an *Ethiopian Herald*[67] editorial entitled 'Do more, ask less'—quickly dispelled them. 'Under the canon now in force', it read, 'organised labour is no longer saddled with the burdensome [sic] task of airing workers' grievances and engaging in invariably acrimonious wrangling with invariably materialist management'. Rather, workers' representatives were now expected to 'bring their weight to bear on other areas where action is of the essence... meaning, essentially, ***hard work*** [emphasis added] for the common good'. 'Then and only then', it claimed 'will organised labour find justification'. In another editorial, it was added, should anyone have gotten a contrary impression, that 'discipline is more indispensable than the luxury of "democracy"'. The US ambassador in Addis Ababa[68] remarked that the law, 'stripped of its socialist jargon', was essentially 'moderate', while the EPRP and ELAMA denounced it as a 'proclamation of slavery'.[69] Its promulgation has been interpreted as having sounded the death knell of the labour movement as an autonomous force.[70] However, this could not be achieved by legislation alone, but would require meticulous scrutiny and culling of eligible candidates, recurrent purges and

[67] "Do More, Ask Less," *Ethiopian Herald*, 24 December 1975.

[68] A.W. Hummel, "Comment on New Labor Law," cable 1975ADDIS14564_b from the US Embassy in Addis Ababa, 19 December 1975, PLUSD, https://wikileaks.org/plusd/cables/1975ADDIS14564_b.html.

[69] Ethiopian Workers' Revolutionary Union (ELAMA), "የፋሺስቶች መፍጨርጨር የላብ አደሩን ትግል አይገታውም" (mimeo. leaflet, Addis Ababa, 1976); Kiflu, *The Generation, part II*.

[70] T. Killion, "Workers, Capital and the State in the Ethiopian Region" (PhD diss., Stanford University, 1985); M. Ottaway and D. Ottaway, *Ethiopia: Empire in Revolution* (New York: Africana Publishing Company, 1978).

re-elections, and sustained heavy repression that would continue for the next several years. The immediate result of the dissolution of CELU was twofold: first, the focal point of conflict shifted to the systemic purging of oppositional labour leaders within basic enterprise unions and their replacement with more compliant candidates; second, opposition gradually relocated into clandestine structures.

Through the latter part of 1975 and the first half of 1976, ELAMA coordinated a campaign of union and labour activists that demanded respect for labour and democratic rights, an end to state interference in union elections, and the release of imprisoned labour leaders. This campaign generated a flurry of defiant petitions and protest notes, stamped and signed by unions, representatives, and workers.[71] Workers were encouraged to refuse to re-register their unions according to the requirements of the new labour law and to hold fresh elections under the authorities' auspices. As the protest and petition movement was conducted by and carried the seals of basic unions—or in some cases simply signatures of workers—the campaign appeared to be spontaneous rather than coordinated by clandestine structures. In March 1976, the PMAC yielded to pressure and released several imprisoned labour leaders, including Marcos Hagos, Beyene Solomon,[72] and Fissehatsion Tekie, just in time for union elections to be held before the stipulated deadline expired. This, however, proved to be the last major concession the labour movement extracted from the state, as the PMAC was simultaneously preparing to subdue it once and for all.

In the PMAC's attempts to enhance its influence and ability to penetrate new social layers, the Provisional Office for Mass Organisational Affairs (POMOA) played an important role. POMOA—formally established in April 1976 but having operated unofficially since the previous year—was intended to serve as a platform for the part of the civilian left that was willing to work with the PMAC. It also intended to provide the latter with a cadre that could extend its social reach and assist it in establishing and asserting influence over broader segments of society and mass

[71] See, among the plenty examples in the CETU archives, various trade unions to the PMAC, 2 September 1976, CETU archives; and Workers' Union of the National Tobacco and Match Corporation to PMAC, *Hamle* (Ethiopian calendric month) 1976, CETU archives.

[72] Beyene would later be re-arrested and spend several additional years in prison. He was released in 1981.

organisations. POMOA was predominantly led and staffed by members and sympathisers of the All-Ethiopia Socialist Movement (known by its Amharic acronym MEISON) and, to a somewhat lesser degree, several smaller Marxist-Leninist groups,[73] which all had their own reasons for wanting to establish influence over and within the labour movement. POMOA played an important role in the drafting of the 1975 labour proclamation—which a MEISON official would subsequently describe as 'one of the most important landmarks of the Ethiopian revolution'[74]—and in reorganising trade unions. Jealous of EPRP's influence within the labour movement, the POMOA-aligned groups saw the restructuring of the trade unions as a vital opportunity to secure that precious foothold among the working masses that their Marxist-Leninist credentials required.

From April 1976 onwards, participation in workplace discussion clubs known as Workers' Revolutionary Forums was made compulsory for all employees in mid- and large-scale establishments. The ostensible reason was to facilitate 'free and democratic exchange of views'.[75] In reality, they were meant to guide the election of desirable representatives, disseminate official policy among workers, and to identify and expose oppositional workers. A painstaking process of weeding out and purging so-called 'anarchists' and 'reactionaries' within the workforce in general and among labour representatives in particular ensued. The 'guided' elections of labour leaders to the emerging structures—the basic enterprise unions and the industrial unions to begin with—of the AETU proceeded in tandem with this process. Despite the intimidation and the 'coercive manner'[76] in which the process proceeded, it proved very difficult to ensure that regime-loyal representatives won the votes. This resulted in frequent incidents of dismissals, arrests, and even executions of union

[73] *Waz* (Labour) League, Ethiopian Oppressed Peoples' Struggle (ECHAAT), Marxist-Leninist Revolutionary Organisation, and, at a later stage, Revolutionary *Seded* (flame).

[74] Frewe Abayneh, "Full Text of the Interview Given to Two Foreign Journalists by Frewe Abayneh, a Representative of the Leadership of MEISONE, The All Ethiopian Socialist Movement at a Meeting in Addis Ababa, Ethiopia, in September 1979," *New Ethiopia* (March 1980), 5.

[75] "PMAC Issues Clarification on Function of Workers Forums," *Ethiopian Herald*, 10 April 1976.

[76] A.T. Tienken, "Assassination of Cabinet Official," cable 1976ADDIS11591_b from the US Embassy in Addis Ababa, 10 November 1976, PLUSD, https://wikileaks.org/plusd/cables/1976ADDIS11591_b.html.

leaders; cancellations of election results; forced re-elections; disrupted meetings; arrests of meeting participants; and postponements. Workers in enterprise unions and their representatives in industrial unions would be compulsorily summoned to seminars in which the opposition was denounced and the desirable electoral outcome was outlined. However, through a combination of workers' defiance and ELAMA coordination, elections were often either not held or, quite frequently, resulted in the re-election of the very same representatives that they were meant to replace.[77] In the case of the organisational congress of the industrial union of manufacturing workers, for example, 200 out of 250 delegates walked out of the meeting to protest attempts to rig the voting process. Subsequent attempts led to turmoil, physical altercations and the arrest of eleven delegates—some of whom were imprisoned for years and some of whom were later executed.[78] The frustrations experienced by authorities were palpable. 'There were not enough pro-government candidates to be promoted', a senior POMOA official later acknowledged. Although the authorities had rigged the platform and overseen elections with the sole intent of transferring offices to loyalists and blocking the labour opposition from representative posts, oppositional workers kept winning them: 'the people who were elected were still those that the labourers knew', the POMOA official noted.[79]

Condemnations published in state media made clear that slow-downs, strikes, sabotages, and other forms of industrial unrest were occurring with such frequency that it evidently was considered a pressing problem. The 1975 labour proclamation and the wrangling over control of the unions it had set in motion had only aggravated this problem. Nor did the workers' forums and other control mechanisms prove to be particularly successful in bringing workers into line. May Day demonstrations in 1976 saw ranks of workers raising oppositional demands on banners smuggled in and unfolded on Addis Ababa's main parading square. While demonstrators had been carrying government and POMOA-approved placards in the procession to the square, many had discarded them and replaced them with concealed placards displaying oppositional demands upon

[77] Kiflu Tadesse, discussion.

[78] Ibid.

[79] Alemu Abebe discussion.

entering the square.[80] Photographs from the demonstrations show participants marching across Revolution Square having unfurled a large banner proclaiming that 'CELU and ELAMA are companions in the struggle'.[81] Others were carrying placards that demanded the establishment of a provisional people's government.[82] But once on the square, they were met with armed repression, as security officers opened fire. Around twenty demonstrators were killed,[83] and many more were wounded or arrested.

Yet, labour unrest continued unabated in the months that followed. On May 28, 1976, *Ethiopian Herald* voiced exasperation, stating that 'undue advantage is being taken of the opportunity provided by the discussion forums', and reported that POMOA was expressing, 'its dismay over this unfortunate drift'.[84] The next day, the PMAC issued a stern warning alleging that 'some discussion forums have been turned into tools serving the interests of reactionaries desirous of causing production slowdowns'.[85] In July, the US embassy[86] reported that postal workers in Addis Ababa were protesting and demanding the release of their arrested union leaders. Port workers in Eritrea, sugar estate workers at Wonji, and casual coffee-cleaning workers were also reported to have been involved in the unrest.

The state responded to these frustrations with escalating levels of violence. Executions of suspected EPRP members had begun in 1976, and open confrontation with the latter was becoming increasingly likely. By September, the labour movement became embroiled in the violence. At around the same time, the EPRP began to assassinate PMAC,

80 Kiflu Tadesse, discussion.

81 "May Day 1980: The Long Struggle of the Ethiopian Proletariat," *Abyot* 5, no. 4 (1980).

82 J. Markakis and Nega Ayele, *Class and Revolution in Ethiopia* (Nottingham: Spokesman Books, 1978).

83 One account alleges that an initial shot had been fired by the demonstrators, provoking the massacre, but this appears an implausible excuse. Andargachew Assegid, በአጭር የተቀጨ ረጅም ጉዞ፡ መኢሶን በኢትዮጲያ ሕዝቦች ትግል ውስጥ (self-pub., Addis Ababa, 2020).

84 "Against Shadow-boxing," *Ethiopian Herald*, 28 May 1976.

85 "PMG Urges Vigilance Against Reactionaries," *Ethiopian Herald*, 29 May 1976.

86 A.T. Tienken, "Post Office Workers Strike in Addis Ababa," cable 1976ADDIS08471_b from the US Embassy in Addis Ababa, 16 July 1976, PLUSD, https://wikileaks.org/plusd/cables/1976ADDIS08471_b.html.

POMOA and MEISON cadres it alleged were responsible for the heightened repression. The debate on the relative responsibility for the turn to violence is not resolvable here.[87] However, a senior leader of EPRP and ELAMA—Kiflu Tadesse—has suggested that the PMAC's inability to subordinate the labour movement constituted an immediate trigger of the violent repression that eventually spiralled into the so-called 'Red Terror'.[88] This interpretation is noteworthy, at the very least because it calls attention to the central role of the labour movement in the convulsions that Ethiopia was in the midst of. In Kiflu's interpretation, mass repression was initially launched against the labour movement in Dire Dawa in mid-1976. Correspondence from Dire Dawa and its twin city Harar through 1975 and 1976 seems to corroborate the notion that the levels of unrest, contestation, and harassment of the labour movement were particularly severe there. Frequent strikes, layoffs and arrests of labour leaders and workers were reported.[89] Regardless of the merits of this interpretation of the origins of the terror, mass repression soon replaced administrative measures as the authorities' preferred means of subjugating the oppositional labour movement throughout the country.

Meanwhile, the state went to great lengths to ensure that new and loyal structures were formed. The purging of oppositional workers' representatives and the identification of reliable candidates was only one side of this process—the other was the wholesale reorganisation of the unions and federations in anticipation of the re-establishment of a national centre. Re-elections, as noted, however, continued to create frustratingly uncertain outcomes. Eight industrial unions—uniting the constituent unions within their sectors—had been formed and elected officeholders by mid-1976. By the end of the year, however, half of the new officeholders had been replaced, either by intimidation or forceful eviction. The constituent

[87] See, for instance, F. Halliday and M. Molyneux, *The Ethiopian Revolution* (London: Verso, 1981); R. Lefort, *Ethiopia: An Heretical Revolution?* (London: Zed Press, 1983); Kiflu, *The Generation, part II;* Negede Gobezie, ይድረስ ለግንቦት ከየካቲት (Washington, DC: AESOP Publishers, 2014); Fikreselassie Wogderes, እኛና አብዮቱ (Los Angeles: Tsehai, 2014); and Fisseha Desta አብዮቱና ትዝታዬ (Los Angeles: Tsehai, 2015).

[88] Kiflu Tadesse, discussion.

[89] See, for example, various trade unions to CELU PWC, 28 June 1976, CETU archives; "የሐረር ላብ አደሮች በሙሉ" ("All Harar's Proletarians") to the Hararge Regional Administration, June 21 1976, CETU archives; and various trade unions to the to the Hararge Regional Administration, 24 May 1976, CETU archives.

unions of banking and insurance workers had refused to partake altogether, and therefore had not elected any industrial union leadership in the first place. Despite intense efforts, only the leaders of four out of the eventual nine industrial unions were deemed sufficiently reliable to participate in the foundation of a new confederation.[90] In December 1976, MoLSA called a meeting of a select group of thoroughly vetted and trusted trade union leaders in the town of Ambo, quite some distance away from the ferment of urban and industrial scenes, and 'free from any possible lobbying by union members'.[91] This meeting was attended by the senior political leadership at the time, including the PMAC's vice chairman, Mengistu Hailemariam, and the POMOA leadership. The session evolved into the founding congress of AETU, which officially occurred in January 1977, after sufficient preparations had been made to allow for the stage-managing of the elections. Basic enterprise unions were not directly represented, so as to assure that each representative had been sufficiently vetted. As a result of the stringent requirements of the vetting procedure, only 65 industrial union representatives participated in the congress, and few individuals on the roster, if any, were prominent union leaders. Those industrial unions that had failed to generate unmistakably loyal candidates were denied representation at the congress.[92]

With the formation of the AETU, the PMAC had finally managed to establish a confederation that appeared sufficiently loyal at the top level. However, the authorities recognised that they had not begun to penetrate the lower levels and basic unions in earnest yet, and even their hold over the top leadership was tenuous. Out of 12 executive committee members, ten were reportedly affiliated with the four organisations[93] that,

[90] A.T. Tienken, "Recent Ethiopian Labor Developments," cable 1976ADDIS12645_b from the US Embassy in Addis Ababa, 30 December 1976, PLUSD, https://wikileaks.org/plusd/cables/1976ADDIS12645_b.html.

[91] Ibid.

[92] Ibid; A.T. Tienken, "All-Ethiopian Trade Union Formed," cable 1977ADDIS00126_c from the US Embassy in Addis Ababa, 10 January 1977, PLUSD, https://wikileaks.org/plusd/cables/1977ADDIS00126_c.html.

[93] These were the All-Ethiopia Socialist Movement (*MEISON*), the *Waz* League, Oppressed Peoples' Revolutionary Struggle (*ECHAAT)*, Marxist-Leninist Revolutionary Organisation *(MALERID)*, and *Abyotawi Seded*/Revolutionary Flame. Together, they made up the joint front Union of Ethiopian Marxist-Leninist Organisations (*EMALEDH*).

for the time being, supported the PMAC.[94] Only three were associated with the organisation that was closest to the Derg—*Abyotawit Seded/* Revolutionary Flame. The others were affiliated with organisations whose relationships with the PMAC were already becoming increasingly strained, and with whom it would fall out in the coming couple of years. This included the AETU's chairman, Tewodros Bekele—who, however, would be assassinated before the split occurred. Moreover, despite every measure to weed out EPRP and ELAMA sympathisers, two executive committee members were nevertheless later found to exhibit such sympathies. There was, consequently, factional disunity within AETU's executive committee from the outset. Whereas its chairman was assassinated, an additional two of its members would depart in the months that followed—one of whom sought asylum while abroad on a confederation assignment.

Confrontation and Subjugation

September 1976 marked the last serious attempt by the oppositional labour movement to resolve the conflict industrially and politically, although this attempt was accompanied by insurrectionary tactics and means. Repression and arrests had taken their toll on the movement in the preceding months, and in many places the structures of the movement had already been depleted or rendered defunct. Having concluded that the movement faced destruction if things proceeded along the prevailing trajectory, ELAMA's third congress decided to call a general strike as a desperate gamble.[95] In response to ELAMA's general strike call, the PMAC released a statement warning that it had ordered security forces 'to take appropriate revolutionary measures on the spot against all those individuals and/or groups who either instigate work stoppage or go on strike'. 'All anti-revolutionary forces who trade on the struggle of workers', it vowed, 'will perish'.[96] The strike nevertheless commenced on September 22. Simultaneously, demonstrators and stone-throwers appeared on the streets of the capital, pelting buses and vehicles that

94 "A Brief History of the Genesis, Development, Decline and Future Prospect of the Ethiopian Labor Movement," Beyene Solomon, report written for the AALC, Addis Ababa, 1992, AALC records.

95 Kiflu Tadesse, discussion.

96 "Revolutionary Justice Awaits Plotters: Government Warns Anarchist Elements," *Ethiopian Herald,* 22 September 1976.

were deemed to defy the strike call. On the second day of the strike, the EPRP conducted a failed assassination attempt on the PMAC's chairman, Mengistu Hailemariam. This reinforced the Derg's commitment to crush the unrest, whatever the price.

The US embassy in Addis Ababa estimated that between 20 and 50 strikers, demonstrators, and stone-throwers were killed on September 22 and 23, and that between 500 and 650 persons were arrested in the week that followed.[97] The state's violence included seemingly random atrocities, such as the killing of seven people in a raid on a popular hotel, but it also involved systematic and targeted repression, including the execution of somewhere between 100 and 600 of the arrested strikers and protestors.[98] Before the strike was smothered by such repression, it had effectively caused power and water supply failures in parts of Addis Ababa, as well as transportation stoppages.[99] Strikes, which occurred throughout the city, included those of bank, utility, and transportation workers, as well as workers at the tobacco monopoly and in two textile factories. Shooting and stone-throwing were reported across the city for several days, but in the face of the tense atmosphere and the intensifying repression, the momentum could not be sustained.

After the failure of the strike, conventional industrial unrest and contestation began to peter out. It became less difficult for state agents and allies to achieve desirable electoral outcomes in the reorganisation of remaining unions and federations—although not yet in all—as anything resembling opposition was now considered a serious crime punishable by death, and most of those identified as radical labour activists had either been arrested or gone underground. The imprisoned allegedly included 'thousands of first, second and third generation labour leaders'.[100] Coordinated resistance, in this context, was no longer viable. Furthermore, a number of

[97] A.T. Tienken, "Tensions in Addis Ababa," cable 1976ADDIS10880_b from the US Embassy in Addis Ababa, 8 October 1976, PLUSD, https://wikileaks.org/plusd/cables/1976ADDIS10880_b.html.

[98] Ibid.

[99] A.T. Tienken, "New Outbreaks of Violence in Capital," cable 1976ADDIS10494 from the US Embassy in Addis Ababa, 23 September 1976, PLUSD, https://wikileaks.org/plusd/cables/1976ADDIS10494_b.html; A.T. Tienken, "EPMG To Clamp Down on Possible Strikes," cable 1976ADDIS10465_b from the US Embassy in Addis Ababa, 22 September 1976, PLUSD, https://wikileaks.org/plusd/cables/1976ADDIS10465_b.html.

[100] Kiflu Tadesse, discussion.

additional safeguards were introduced to ensure that only vetted representatives were elected at the various levels. Instead of dispersed workers' resistance, the still very prevalent contradictions increasingly manifested themselves in armed conflict. Workplaces were militarised, and workers deemed loyal were organised in pro-government militias, armed, and unleashed on perceived enemies within and outside their own ranks. Oppositional workers were a primary target of these militias and other security forces, and the campaign to expose and weed out real and imagined opponents within the workforce was intensified. In workplace after workplace across the country, 'mercenaries', 'anarchists', and 'reactionaries' were identified, denounced, imprisoned, and, with increasing frequency, executed.

The opposition also militarised its strategy. Workers played a prominent role in the EPRP's urban military squads, and ELAMA established its own armed squads of workers.[101] Victims were claimed on both sides, although the opposition bore the brunt. A US embassy cable from March 1977[102] depicts a war-like situation in the Akaki industrial area, where workers organised in opposing constellations were involved in hostilities that included assassinations and the use of explosive devices.[103] It was to become a bloody month for the radical labour movement as well as the opposition in general. In one of the most infamous incidents of the revolution, ELAMA central committee member and Berhanena Selam Printing Press union representative Daro Negash, who was eight months pregnant at the time, along with eight of her colleagues from the printing press, were killed by an armed squad working under the command of

[101] Ibid.

[102] A.T. Tienken, "All-Ethiopian Trade Union Formed," cable 1977ADDIS00126_c from the US Embassy in Addis Ababa, 10 January 1977, PLUSD, https://wikileaks.org/plusd/cables/1977ADDIS00126_c.html.

[103] 'Not all trade unionists were opposed to the new regime', Christopher Clapham has correctly noted: 'the main industrial area of Addis Ababa, around Kaliti and Akaki to the south of the city, provided some of its most active and violent supporters'. Clapham, *Transformation and Continuity*, 55.

From a perspective supporting the oppositional workers, the EPRP Foreign Committee's journal *Abyot* claimed that in March, state atrocities against workers in Addis Ababa alone—many of them in the mentioned district Akaki—included the killing of 25 employees of the cement factory; 15 employees of the Lazaridis company; 20 employees of Indo-Ethiopian textile factory; 5 customs employees; 7 railway workers; 23 workers of the Pepsi Cola factory; and an unknown number of weaving workers in the Kolfe district. "News," *Abyot* 2, no. 2 (1977).

a local Urban Dwellers' Association[104] chairman.[105] They had allegedly been identified as 'anarchists' in the workers' discussion club.[106] The same month, the following account was reported in the *Washington Post*:

> The government's arming of workers and the neighbourhood associations immediately led to bloody strife last week in the Akaki industrial sector of the city and to widespread night-time shootings. Unconfirmed reports said that as many as 70 workers died in fighting inside half a dozen factories... Meanwhile, six more assassinated labour officials were buried here this weekend.[107]

May Day celebrations in 1977—called by ELAMA to begin two days before the actual occasion, in order to circumvent expected repression—turned into the single most bloody episode of the urban violence of the revolutionary period. Protesters were met by machine-gun-equipped jeeps firing into the crowds, and large groups of demonstrators that had been rounded up were summarily executed the very same night. Estimates of the number of dead vary between several hundred and over a thousand.[108] Although far from all, or even a majority, of the victims of this massacre were organised workers, it is telling that the episode occurred in response to demonstrations for the International Workers' Day called by a workers' organisation. Exposures and purges would continue for several years, but by the end of 1977, what was left of the oppositional labour movement had been vanquished and destroyed.

Aside from scores of other rank-and-file workers and workers' representatives, the militarised struggle within and over the labour movement

[104] Known by their Amharic name, *Kebeles*.

[105] The public outrage sparked by the killings and other atrocious excesses of the squad proved too much for the PMAC: its members—as well as the two colleagues of the murdered workers from Berhanena Selam Printing Press who had 'identified' them and called on the squad—were themselves in turn executed. See J. Wiebel and S.A. Admasie, "Rethinking the Ethiopian Red Terror: Approaches to Political Violence in Revolutionary Ethiopia," *Journal of African History* 60, no. 3 (2019), for a broader contextualisation and discussion of the meaning of this incident within the campaign of state-sanctioned terror.

[106] "Six Persons Executed for Dastardly, Inhuman Murder of 24 persons," *Ethiopian Herald*, 3 April 1977.

[107] D. Ottaway, "Fighting Up Sharply in Ethiopia," *Washington Post*, 14 March 1977.

[108] Markakis and Nega, *Class and Revolution*.

took the lives of the last chairman of CELU, Marcos Hagos, and the first two chairmen of the AETU, Tewodros Bekele and Temesgen Madebo—the former killed by agents of the state and the latter two assassinated by ELAMA squads. Apart from the chairmen, the AETU's treasurer Kebede Gebremichael; first deputy vice president Gezahegn Kassahoun; vice president Gezahegn Teklearegay; and executive committee member Kebede Tekle also perished. Other victims of executions and assassinations included Tessema Deressa, secretary general of the PWC and representative of the Awash Valley Project union; Ali Hussein, PWC member[109] and union representative of the Indo-Ethiopian Textile Factory; Tsegaye Yehwalashet, secretary of the Transport and Communication Workers' industrial union; Teferra, chairman of Electricity, Water and Gas Workers' Industrial Union; Wondimu Woldemedhin, first deputy chairman of the manufacturing industry workers' federation; Ademe Seifu, president of the Metahara Sugar Factory Workers' Union; Orion Adamutu, vice chairman of the plastics factory workers' union; and Kassahun Ambaye, chairman of the union of Awassa Farm Development Enterprise.[110] At the Ministry of Labour and Social Affairs, victims of assassination included Permanent Secretary Guetnet Zewde—allegedly an important officer in the reorganisation and wresting control over the trade unions.[111] The rank-and-file members of the Ethiopian labour movement who died are countless. That the violence of the period disproportionally involved workers is something that is acknowledged by former POMOA officials as well as EPRP leaders.[112] The PMAC's chairman Mengistu seemed to share this view too when, decrying 'infiltrators' within the labour movement that had 'inflicted heavy damage', he spoke of the 'death blow' dealt to them by 'revolutionary defence squads in residential areas as well as in

[109] A fourth PWC member, Mekonnen Tesfaye, was reportedly executed in a later round of purges of MEISON-affiliated labour activists. Mekonnen was the assistant general secretary of the PWC, representing the union of Addis Ababa Cement Factory.

[110] Negede, *ለግንቦት ከየካቲት*, 253; Beyene, *Fighter for Democracy*, 170–171; Fikreselassie, *እኛና አብዮቱ*, 290; Kiflu Tadesse, discussion; Andargachew Assegid, *ረጅም ጉዞ*, 409.

[111] A.T. Tienken, "Assassination of Cabinet Official," cable 1976ADDIS11591_b from the US Embassy in Addis Ababa, 10 November 1976, PLUSD, https://wikileaks.org/plusd/cables/1976ADDIS11591_b.html.

[112] Negede Gobezie, "Interview with the BBC," *New Ethiopia* (May 1980); Kiflu, *The Generation, part I*; *The Generation, part II*; discussion.

production centres'.[113] In fact, a death blow had been landed on the labour movement as a whole.

The Radical Left and Labour Radicalism

Labour radicalism and the coming of the high tide of workers' and trade union militancy during the 1970s have frequently been viewed solely as the consequence of influence from external parties and events. Some authors have gone to the extent of dismissing CELU's increasing radicalism as nothing more than the simple and direct outcome of 'infiltration' by leftist radicals.[114] Since labour radicalism and militancy peaked during the conjuncture that also produced the Ethiopian Revolution, the former has unfortunately and erroneously come to be subsumed under the historiography of the latter. It is only in this context that the idea of 'infiltration' has any meaning, as it is only in this context that an infiltrating agent can be identified: Marxist-Leninist groups that emerged within the same conjuncture in general—and the EPRP in particular. But labour radicalism and militancy preceded the revolution and the formation of the EPRP by many years. To explain the former as a consequence of the latter is thus not just to deny endogenous actors in the labour movement their agency, but is also ahistorical. A longer arc of endogenous radicalisation within the labour movement had taken place since the mid-1960s, at the very least. This was evident not only in the contention between militant and moderate strands within the trade union movement, but also in continuous grassroot unrest and strike activity. By 1972, the momentum and the balance of forces in the movement had shifted in favour of labour radicals, and CELU's opposition was in ascendancy. This was two full years before the revolutionary movement began and the group that was to become the EPRP became active in Ethiopia. Nevertheless, although it did not constitute a factor that propelled the labour movement's longer arc of radicalisation, the EPRP eventually—but only

[113] Mengistu Hailemariam, *Speech Delivered to the Second Congress of the All Ethiopia Trade Union* (Addis Ababa: Provisional Military Government of Socialist Ethiopia/ Commission for Organizing the Party of the Working People of Ethiopia, 1982), 36.

[114] See, for example, Andargachew Tiruneh, *The Ethiopian revolution, 1974–1987: A Transformation From an Aristocratic to a Totalitarian Autocracy* (Cambridge: Cambridge University Press, 1993), 141.

at a late stage—came to exercise actual influence within the movement. For this reason, the subject requires a more substantial treatment.

In mid-1974, two staff members were recruited to CELU, as a part of the AALC's project to revive *Voice of Labour*: Seyoum Kebede, as its Editor and Director of Publications, and Kiflu Tadesse, as its Assistant Editor. Both were members of the antecedent organisation of the EPRP[115]—the latter a member of its Politburo—although they were not known as such by either CELU's leadership, the AALC (which financed the appointments), or the authorities. Girmachew Lemma, a former president of the University Students' Union of Addis Ababa who would join the same organisation as Seyoum and Kiflu later that year, was already employed as CELU's legal advisor at that time. Kiflu and Girmachew, together with CELU field worker and veteran labour opposition activist Tedla Fantaye, then formed a minuscule workers' committee of the EPRP.[116] By mid-1974, however, what was to become the EPRP was a very small organisation, and its structures were in a rudimentary state. It was not in a position to exercise direct influence over or within CELU, except on an individual basis. Priority was given to securing legal and occupational cover for its members and returnees from abroad—such as Kiflu[117]—in order to avoid drawing the attention of the authorities. Since EPRP member Samuel Alemayehu was a former CELU board member who retained helpful contacts in the confederation's leadership, he personally recommended the two EPRP members for the positions.

Initially, given the roles of the EPRP members, it was the content of *Voice of Labour* that was most prone to their influence. Because the government censorship apparatus, which restricted any radical voice on domestic political affairs, the impact was initially subtle and mostly ideological—as the *Voice of Labour* began publishing more Marxist-oriented content. In August 1974, the newspaper's increasingly assertive tone dovetailed with CELU's growing confidence—by which even the confederation's old leadership had begun to publicly advocate for the formation of a political party representing labour—but added a more elaborate ideological dimension to it. 'Trade unions cannot, through economic

[115] Which was still operating clandestinely under the name Ethiopian People's Liberation Organisation. It was not to adopt the name EPRP and declare its existence for another year.

[116] Kiflu Tadesse, discussion.

[117] Kiflu had returned from the Soviet Union, where he had studied journalism.

struggle alone, resolve the recurring conflicts between the workers and the capitalists',[118] an editorial read, and continued:

> The resolution of the worker-capitalist conflict can be effected only with the elimination of classes. The elimination of the exploiting classes necessitates a political struggle which in turn requires a political party. In other words, a political party of the working class and of the oppressed masses in general is absolutely essential if a just, democratic and egalitarian society is to be brought into being. This political party of the working class and other exploited sections of the population, such as peasants, soldiers, small merchants, the lumpen proletariat, etc., will be joining hands with other democratic political organizations in the burial ceremony of feudalism and imperialism, the twin enemies of the Ethiopian people.

Of course, what the chief editor and assistant editor already knew was that a political party that sought to conform precisely to that description already existed. Few others, however, were aware of this. While the AALC was correct in identifying 'a cell' that 'had been working in the trade union movement for some time' by 1975,[119] it did not know to which entity this cell belonged. Meanwhile, a senior private-sector manager in Addis Ababa expressed, in a meeting with the US ambassador and senior labour department officials, being 'concerned about radicals in the trade unions' whose numbers he felt had grown in the preceding years, and who he believed had 'brought back crazy ideas from brief trips to Russia and Eastern Europe'.[120] In September 1974, it was Girmachew Lemma who drafted CELU's congress resolution, which was subsequently endorsed by the General Assembly—a clear indication that the EPRP cell members had become important resources and allies of the oppositional movement.

Yet, the type of influence exerted by EPRP cell members at the time was not direct—it was primarily ideological, rather than operational. They held no elected positions, and were therefore capable only of lending support and advice to radical trade union leaders. None of the prominent oppositional labour leaders—including Marcos Hagos—were initially EPRP members, nor did they exhibit any traits that would distinguish

[118] "Editorial: The Necessity of Political Parties," *Voice of Labour*, August 1974.

[119] See quote from David F. Summer's report to the AALC on pages 80 to 83 of this chapter.

[120] "Meeting with Bob Caldwell," meeting minutes, 30 August 1974, AALC records.

them as partisan to any political faction. They were seasoned labour activists and workers' representatives, nearly all of whom had been elected officials in CELU, CELU's branches, and/or constituent unions for years. Many had accumulated experience going back to the 1960s. Moreover, the demands that attracted the rank-and-file to the labour opposition and eventually made it dominant were pragmatic issues related to the immediate conditions of labour, freedom of association, and the independence of trade unions from the state, rather than ideologically flavoured questions of state power. This consensus is shared by both former ELAMA and POMOA insiders.[121]

However, in the fertile conditions of the revolutionary upsurge, workers' and trade union demands were instrumentalised by the EPRP in order to acquire broader influence in the movement and attract members. The Derg's authoritarian approach further facilitated the EPRP's ability to do so. At that point, a few key leaders joined the party, and a few additional EPRP members were eventually employed by CELU.[122] EPRP's workers' committee members in CELU also began playing more important roles in the internal and external contention over CELU's line. When, in April 1975, the dissident committee briefly seized control of CELU's headquarters and detained its erstwhile leaders, the AALC reported that the take-over was led by Girmachew Lemma, whom it called a 'ring leader against the Alem-Tesfa regime'.[123] It also reported that the demonstration on May 18, which triggered the Derg's intervention—first by closing CELU's offices, and later by permitting the election of a new

[121] Alemu Abebe, discussion; Kiflu Tadesse, discussion.

[122] They included EPRP militant Mezgebnesh Abayu, editor of the party-aligned *Goh* journal. Her story was retold in former EPRP militant Mohamed Yimam's book *Wore Negari,* in which Mohamed also described how he and another EPRP member was recruited by CELU to hold classes on socialism for workers at HVA's Wonji Shoa site. Mezgebnesh's personnel file in CETU's archives confirms that her date of employment with CELU was September 1, 1975, and she remained a CELU employee until at least March 1976. She was, in numerical order, the fifth EPRP militant to have been employed by CELU's headquarters, following Samuel Alemayehu (who had left CELU by this time), Girmachew Lemma, Seyoum Kebede, and Kiflu Tadesse. This was in addition to the many members recruited from among the rank-and-file workers and representatives, and a few EPRP militants like Mohamed Yimam who were engaged for short-term tasks. Mohamed Yimam, *Wore Negari: A Memoir of an Ethiopian Youth in the Turbulent 1970s* (n.p.: Xlibris), 2013.

[123] "BAR-LES No.7: Final Report," Richard Baurmann to Lester Trachtman, 24 May 1975, AALC records.

leadership that the dissidents had demanded—was organised by Girmachew.[124] Although this may somewhat exaggerate his role and understate the role of the dissident committee of trade unionists that coordinated this struggle, the reports underline the growing influence of EPRP's workers' committee in CELU.

Once the radical opposition took over the leadership of CELU, and both the trade union confederation and the EPRP found themselves targets of state repression, a certain unity of purpose was established. However, although never openly proclaimed, it is far more correct to describe the two organisations' relationship as an alliance than as a case of infiltration—whereby one controls the other. 'EPRP's ties with the CELU leadership were ties between two distinct organizations, one student-based, the other a trade union body', Fred Halliday and Maxine Molyneux have correctly observed.[125] The organisational skills and resources that the EPRP could offer, particularly in establishing and operating clandestine networks, constituted a key aspect of this alliance. In return, militant and radicalised workers and trade unionists provided the EPRP with its first real bastion of support among the working masses. 'The EPRP-CELU alliance reflected the growth of a new consciousness among CELU members, both blue- and white-collar, after the PMAC came to power, a very real if delayed politicisation that gave the EPRP its broader popular following', the same authors have written.[126] Politically, the confrontation between labour and the PMAC pushed CELU further towards the party's position. By mid-1975, there was a broad convergence of views. But they never became identical. The EPRP was not the only radical political organisation to have sympathisers in CELU's leadership and the PWC. And the majority of CELU's leadership never joined the EPRP or ELAMA. In October 1975, however, after the PWC had been repressed by the Derg, Teferra Haile Selassie, the Minister of Labour, discussed CELU's radicalisation with the AALC representative in the following terms:

> Girmachew [Lemma] and Yilma Tiruneh (former cooperative field worker) apparently played major and radical roles in CELU during the past few

[124] Ibid.

[125] F. Halliday and M. Molyneux, "Ethiopia's Revolution from Above," *MERIP Reports* 106 (June 1982).

[126] Ibid.

> months. The 13 members of the Provisional Labor Council [PWC] were greatly influenced by the radical ideas of Girmachew and his role in the removal of Alem and Tesfa from CELU.
>
> On different occasions Girmachew led CELU delegations to Tafera Haile Selassie's office with various grievances. According to Tafera, Girmachew refused to discuss the points at hand in any logical manner and insisted, instead, upon repeating communist rhetoric – which was supported by the other CELU representatives. Girmachew reportedly maintained an office in his house where he effectively influenced the thinking of many labor leaders.
>
> Because of his personality and apparent sincerity, Yilma had considerable influence over certain leaders. (He was good with his communist and socialist rhetoric when he worked with me [the writer of the report, Dan O'Laughlin of the AALC] in Ethiopia, but in the beginning he always did his job well). He was also very active in organizing the general strike in September and he was taken into detention when he came out of hiding and went to the CELU building on about the 17th of October.[127]

The account above was coloured by the fact that it came from a senior cabinet member, and therefore reflected the government's position. It ought to be noted that whereas Girmachew Lemma was an EPRP member, Yilma Tiruneh was only recruited to the party later. However, in the months that followed the closure of CELU, the EPRP members' direct influence grew as the clusters of workers they helped to organise became the organisational building blocks of a clandestine network. This network was eventually built upon to establish ELAMA—the EPRP's labour front. In ELAMA's most successful campaigns (such as the coordination of constituent unions' efforts in the 1976 campaign to have arrested leaders released, and to have union representatives opposed to the reorganising of CELU into the AETU elected or re-elected), clandestine party-organised structures and activists helped restructure, revitalise and coordinate the labour movement. But they did not necessarily create militant energies where none existed in the first place.

This exposition suggests that there is evidence of only late external influence—whether framed as infiltration or vanguardism—in generating

[127] "Visit to Addis Ababa From 20 to 24 October 1975," D.J. O'Laughlin to Patrick.J. O'Farrell and John Gould, 25 October 1975, AALC records.

militancy within the movement. Labour militancy and radicalism generally developed outside of, and for most of the 1960s and 1970s, in the complete absence of, influence from political organisations operating within the labour movement. The militant labour opposition movement, moreover, was led by experienced workers' representatives, rather than infiltrating external agents. The fact that some of these representatives were later recruited to political organisations does not alter this fact. But most importantly: labour militancy and radicalism; wildcat unrest; rank-and-file dissent and rebelliousness; violent contention within the labour movement; and the emergence of a full-fledged oppositional movement within it, were all phenomena that predated the establishment of political parties in Ethiopia altogether. To seek to explain the radicalisation of the former as a consequence of the latter is, therefore, to place the cart before the horse. Equally, the trajectory of growing militancy and radicalisation of the labour movement was considerably longer than its subsumption under the historiography of the revolution would permit.

But if not simply the effect of external agencies, what then were the factors that kindled the emergence of a radically assertive and militant Ethiopian labour movement in the 1960s and 1970s? The strongest factor appears to have been internal pressures from the lower levels of the movement: from rank-and-file workers and workers' representatives. There are several ways to substantiate this claim. Contemporaneous research showed that workers themselves identified massive injustices in their relations with employers, sparking an increasing willingness to engage in industrial contention. Lynn Morehouse, an American industrial relations scholar who conducted research on workers' attitudes in Ethiopia at the time, found that 'unwillingness to give a wage increase is viewed only as an attempt by the employer to squeeze more of an already *outrageous* [emphasis added] profit from the workers' toil'.[128] Morehouse's findings also vividly illustrated that by 1969, workers and basic union representatives had begun to view employers, the state, and even the central confederation leadership as being inimical to their interests.

Another way in which militant pressure from below came to express itself was in recurrent wildcat unrest. In fact, it was largely due to the desire to control such unrest that trade unionism was legalised in Ethiopia in the first place in 1963. In the long decade that followed, CELU's

[128] L.G. Morehouse, "Ethiopian Labour Relations: Attitudes, Practice and Law" (research project paper, Northwestern University, 1969), 70–71.

president Beyene acknowledged, pressures from the rank-and-file often led to strikes, whether union officials wanted it or not.[129] Morehouse found that rank-and-file pressures produced an inclination among union leaders to frequently call strikes during negotiations. Union leaders, she claimed, accepted this as a concession to the 'the militancy of the mass of union members'.[130] 'CELU has always been a restraining force, because usually the workers would want to use force', former CELU Secretary General Fissehatsion Tekie stated,[131] corroborating this view.

A final, most definite, expression of how militant pressures from below radicalised the movement over time was the emergence of the oppositional movement, the protracted campaign it pursued against the submissive approach of CELU's moderate leadership, and its eventual ouster of that leadership, placing the movement on an offensive footing. In the words of CELU insider Emmanuel Fayessa,[132] the radicalisation of CELU's demands in 1974 occurred 'due to the pressure from the breakaway unions and also the growing militancy among the rank-and-file members of the organisation itself'. Whichever level examined then, militant pressures from below appear to be the main determinant and propelling force of the drift towards greater radicalism through the 1960s and the first half of the 1970s.

The emergence of a separate layer of labour bureaucracy, while helpful in checking militant impulses from below, was simultaneously an attendant factor that fostered resentment and anger. The submissive orientation of the top bureaucracy only reinforced this tendency. Morehouse[133] has described how CELU's leadership drew 'a great deal of criticism from union leaders and employees' and how its role 'as an intermediary earned it some of its most bitter criticism'.[134] This included allegations of

[129] Beyene, *Fighter for Democracy,* 109.

[130] Morehouse, "Ethiopian Labour Relations," 71.

[131] Fissehatsion, interview, Tom Killion papers.

[132] Emmanuel Fayessa Negassa, "The Confederation of Ethiopian Labour Unions and its First General Strike (March 7–11, 1974): Causes and Impact" (master's thesis, Cornell University, 1977), 97.

[133] Morehouse, "Ethiopian Labour Relations," 72–74.

[134] Similarly, Killion has stated that 'the very connections between CELU leaders, capital and the state created distrust of the national leaders on the part of rank-and-file workers'. Rather than lessened, he claimed, this was only reinforced by reliance on international financial aid. Killion, "Workers, Capital and the State," 486–487.

'giving in and siding with the employer too soon'. According to Syoum Gebre Egziabher[135]—a prominent Ethiopian intellectual at the time, but also a senior official of the employers' federation—union leaders faced the constant danger of being labelled as 'pro-management' by rank-and-file workers. Typically, union officials were 'distrusted by a substantial number of union members'. This distrust often stemmed from the perception that union officials were 'too friendly with the management':

> Whenever a leader opposes the demands of the majority, even when on some reasonable ground, the workers accuse him of selling out to the company. After seeing the previous leaders removed from office for this reason, one union leader refused to compromise an outrageous wage demand with which he disagreed, but rather waited for the Labour Relations Board to rule against the union, thus preserving his image in the eyes of the members.[136]

Collusion between CELU's leadership and the state provided another source of mounting rank-and-file anger. It was even found to have 'earned some of the CELU officials the name of government agents'.[137] For while rank-and-file militancy was sometimes deftly displaced by CELU's leadership through bureaucratic means and subterfuge, its collusion with authorities and employers, subversion of democratic decisions, arbitrary and punitive allocation of resources, and the unaccountability of its top officials simultaneously served to reinforce militant opposition as often as it thwarted it. Blatant state interference, repression, and bias were equally double-edged swords. The recurrent denial of basic rights—to organise, to hold a general congress, to assemble and strike, and to elect representative officials—became points of the most vociferous opposition from the militant strand of the labour movement. In this manner, the high-handedness of the state inadvertently provided fuel for further radicalisation.

A final and intriguing aspect of labour militancy, radicalisation, and assertiveness during the period is the degree to which it appeared to

[135] Syoum Gebregziabher, "The Rise of CELU and the EFE Under Haile Selassie's Regime," (Mimeo, 2005), 60.

[136] Morehouse, "Ethiopian Labour Relations," 72.

[137] Morehouse, "Ethiopian Labour Relations," 75.

display attributes of a completely different dynamic. This dynamic—arguably at least as important as the ones mentioned but hitherto neglected in the literature—can be viewed as a factor driving much of the cyclical growth in militancy and assertiveness discussed in this chapter: the process appears to exhibit traits of path dependence in the way that assertiveness and readily identifiable achievements—in terms of outcomes of militant practices—played into and fuelled one another. In the course of the late 1950s, the 1960s, and the early 1970s, a string of major achievements resulted from Ethiopian workers' struggles. This began with the establishment of the first workers' associations and the undertaking of the first successful strikes; continued with the legal recognition of trade unionism and the establishment of a confederation; a progressive shift in the workplace balance of forces and the institution of collective bargaining; and the development of the labour movement into a national social-political force capable of extracting significant concessions from employers and the state, which ultimately generated a confrontation with the latter. At each step of this process, prior achievements appear to have further energised the movement and ratcheted up its militancy and strength. The best and most direct example of this took place in the two years leading up to the revolution. 'CELU's political clout, (small perhaps, but growing) has become a recognized factor in Ethiopia', an AALC representative acknowledged in early 1973.[138] But such hard-earned clout exposed the leadership to mounting pressures to put the movement on an even more offensive footing, resulting in a spiral of increasing contention. First, it led CELU to support the bank strikes later that year. Second, the successful outcome of the 1973 bank strikes demonstrated the feasibility of militancy and, through the momentum it created, paved the way for the March 1974 general strike. Third, the successful general strike triggered a strike wave through the following months, and thus generated a proletarian insurgency—a term coined by political economy scholar Ernesto Screpanti[139] to describe sudden and spectacular surges of strike activity and labour unrest—that

[138] "Report No. 233: CELU, CONFIDENTIAL", Jerry Funk to Irving Brown and Patrick O'Farrell, 6 February 1973, AALC records.

[139] E. Screpanti, "Long Economic Cycles and Recurring Proletarian Insurgencies," *Review (Fernand Braudel Center)* 7, no. 3 (1984).

lasted for the following couple of years, despite severe repression. Moreover, it propelled the labour movement into a head-on collision course with the state.

Interregnum: A Decade of Yellow Unionism

Despite the defeat of the labour opposition in 1977, dispersed trouble remained or re-emerged in the constituent enterprise-level unions. More purges were also to follow as the POMOA coalition broke apart, one group at a time. First, beginning in the second half of 1977, MEISON-associated trade unionists and representatives were purged, arrested, and occasionally killed. Subsequently, those affiliated with the remaining smaller parties were subjected to the same fate. On May 25, 1978, the full membership of the executive committee of AETU was dismissed and replaced.[140] This led to another round of purges in the constituent unions, which also involved violent repression. At the Metahara sugar factory, for example, the AETU reported that an unstated number of 'right roaders'[141] in the leadership of the union and revolutionary guard committee had been ousted, brought before a newly established 'Red Terror Committee', and had 'revolutionary measures' taken against them.[142] According to a senior member of MEISON's leadership, over 600 MEISON-affiliated workers and labour leaders were purged, imprisoned, or executed in this round of repression.[143] Among those killed were leaders of the Dire Dawa textile and cement factories' unions, as well as 15 workers' representatives from the Wonji sugar factory union and a trade union chairman in the city of Adama.[144] This repression led a MEISON official[145] to claim that 'the vanguard elements and elected leaders [of the working class] have been thrown in the [PMAC]'s prisons in their

[140] Walker, "Ethiopian Labor Union Replaces Entire Leadership," cable 1978ADDIS02387_d from the US Embassy in Addis Ababa, 26 May 1978, PLUSD, https://www.wikileaks.org/plusd/cables/1978ADDIS02387_d.html.

[141] The derogatory label used for MEISON in the aftermath of its falling out with the PMAC.

[142] "ከግንቦት 11 እስከ ሐምሌ 29 ቀን ድረስ ምን ተሰራ? ሪፖርት," AETU Report, CETU Archives.

[143] Negede, *ለግንቦት ከየካቲት*, 253.

[144] At the time known as Nazret.

[145] Frewe, "Interview Given to Two Foreign Journalists," 7–9.

thousands'. Another former MEISON cadre—who served as the Mayor of Addis Ababa and remained loyal to the Derg after its split with his former party—has noted that 'the moment MEISON went underground, [the AETU] was taken over by another organisation with *literally with no resistance* [emphasis added]',[146] but this seems only partially accurate. In the aftermath of the purge, the AETU reported that labour unrest, sabotage, and subversion remained persistent problems for the constituent unions at the Metahara sugar factory, Wonji plantations, the Ethio-Fibre factory, the Commercial Bank of Ethiopia, the Upper Awash Agricultural Development Enterprise, church-owned enterprises, and the Edget yarn factory.[147]

In November 1978, a new round of arrests took place at the AETU's headquarters, as a couple of smaller Marxist-Leninist groups—including *Waz* League—fell out of official favour. In December of that year, this was followed by another purge of the full leadership of the AETU, and two officials were reported to have been executed.[148] The reasons for this purge were related to another bout of inter-party rivalry over control of the AETU, but the ousted leadership was also accused of having proven insufficiently committed to preparing the workers for the 'extensive sacrifices' that the upcoming National Revolutionary Development Campaign would require. 'The failure of the AETU leadership to cooperate fully' was allegedly 'seriously threatening the government's ability to impose its will upon the workers',[149] indicating that whatever residues of autonomy that remained were now being removed.[150] This time, it appears, no resistance emerged from the rank-and-file. Ethiopian workers whom the US embassy reported to have been in contact with were resigned to 'the

146 Alemu Abebe, discussion.

147 "ከግንቦት 11 እስከ ሐምሌ 29 ቀን ድረስ ምን ተሰራ? ሪፖርት," AETU Report, CETU Archives.

148 F. Chapin, "Arrests of Ethiopian Trade Union Officials," cable 1979STATE005993_e from the US Embassy in Addis Ababa, 9 January 1979, PLUSD, https://wikileaks.org/plusd/cables/1979STATE005993_e.html.

149 F. Chapin, "New Leadership for Ethiopian National Labor Union," cable 1979ADDIS00125_e from the US Embassy in Addis Ababa, 10 January 1979, PLUSD, https://wikileaks.org/plusd/cables/1979ADDIS00125_e.html.

150 This conclusion was also drawn by the Department of State (1980: 70), which claimed that by 1979, 'the modest level of independence enjoyed by unionists even a year ago has disappeared', with the unions now having become '*entirely* [emphasis added] controlled by the government, and serve only to mobilise and control workers'.

seeming impossibility of any real labour union representation' and were 'well aware of the extensive political manipulation by the government of the AETU'. 'There is a widespread feeling that the organisation is a charade', the ambassador concluded.

Indeed, by the early 1980s, few independent-minded labour leaders remained in high positions. A new degree of control over the labour movement, unprecedented in scope, had been established. Unlike the earlier stages, this phase was marked by 'more or less absolute control' over its structures. 'Everything was manipulated—there was no room for mistakes', former Addis Ababa Mayor and subsequently ruling party Politburo member Alemu Abebe has acknowledged. 'Before anybody was nominated, he was scrutinised'.[151] Trade union structures had, for all intents and purposes, been rendered impenetrable to and insulated from opposition, militant labour activism and rank-and-file influence alike. But this came at the cost of widespread disillusionment among workers, who never displayed anything remotely comparable to the enthusiasm that the radicalised CELU had generated. After the purges, 'the loyalty of the mass of wage earners to this new imposed structure was bound to be suspect' it has rightly been noted.[152]

The Derg had initially lacked a party-organisation that provided it with a cadre and an organisational reach capable of penetrating mass institutions such as the trade unions. This was the reason it established POMOA, as a means to draw on the cadre of civilian leftist parties. The formation of *Abyotawi Seded* followed a similar logic, and in 1977, the Union of Ethiopian Marxist-Leninist Organisations (UEMLO) had been established as a joint front of the parties, with the espoused aim of eventually merging into a unified party. By 1979, however, the Derg's alliance with the civilian parties was in tatters: all the original constituent members of UEMLO, save for Seded, had been purged. Meanwhile, Mengistu Hailemariam had emerged as the country's undisputed ruler. At this stage, Mengistu's loyalists inside and outside the Derg decided to end the pretence of establishing a ruling party by the merger of existing leftist parties, and instead build a party centered entirely around the person of Mengistu. The first step in this process was the establishment of the Commission for Organising the Party of the Working People of Ethiopia

[151] Alemu Abebe, discussion.

[152] Halliday and Molyneux, "Ethiopia's Revolution from Above".

(COPWE)—a pre-party formation whose central committee and politburo members were directly appointed by Mengistu himself. Upon its formation, COPWE established that an immediate priority was to assert control over the various mass organisations. With regard to the labour movement, it inherited responsibility from POMOA and UEMLO—which were both dissolved—to oversee elections and to assess and select candidates for official posts across the AETU's structures, from basic unions to industrial unions and the confederation. Party control would strengthen further over the following years, as COPWE's cadre and party committees multiplied, culminating in its transformation into a ruling party proper in 1984: the Workers' Party of Ethiopia (WPE).

Nevertheless, there were early signs that COPWE's leadership lacked confidence in the officialdom of the AETU, despite the repeated cycles of purges and re-selections the it had undergone. 'The most surprising omissions from the Central Committee [of COPWE] in 1980 were workers and peasants, even though representatives from the AETU and AEPA [All-Ethiopia Peasants' Association] were delegates to the congress', a scholar observing the process noted.[153] 'Both bodies had been organized at the national level before COPWE was set up, and the PMAC evidently considered their loyalty to be in doubt'. Within a year, COPWE had become openly dissatisfied with the performance of the AETU in delivering the type of control over workplaces and rank-and-file workers it coveted. On the one hand, it viewed the confederation as ineffective, lacking the necessary manpower, and excessively occupied by resolving disputes (i.e., ironically, actually representing individual workers). On the other hand, it lacked trust in the AETU's cadre and leadership—which had come of age during the UEMLO joint front period, when affiliation with any one of the competing civilian parties had sufficed. 'Workers were made to engage in unnecessary bickering due to the prevailing narrow and cliquish outlooks, which also had an impact on the AETU leadership', COPWE's ideological journal *Meskerem* argued in May 1981.[154] This, it reasoned, was aggravated by a structure that 'itself hinders the thorough practical implementation of democratic centralism on a national

[153] P. Gilkes "Building Ethiopia's Revolutionary Party Patrick Gilkes," *MERIP Reports* 106 (June 1982).

[154] "History of the Struggle of the Ethiopian Working Class," *Meskerem* 1, no 4 (1981), 38.

scale'.[155] It was for these reasons that COPWE's central committee, in its second regular plenary meeting in February 1981, resolved to reorganise the confederation. Reorganisation was deemed necessary to guarantee 'proximity of working localities and similarity of professions', but more importantly 'to facilitate work and control', and to bring the confederation under the firm leadership of COPWE.[156] 'In order to advance the practical implementation of COPWE's mission, the organizational structure of AETU will have to conform to those of COPWE', *Meskerem* declared.

In May 1982, the Trade Unions Organization Proclamation[157] was issued by the PMAC, formally turning the trade union movement into a regimented vehicle of COPWE rule, and, by extension, the state executive. The proclamation further strengthened the hierarchical centralist logic that had been introduced with the 1975 labour proclamation which had made lower trade union instances answerable to higher ones. From 1982 onwards, trade unions were also made subordinate to the state and obliged to 'implement decisions, directives and orders transmitted to it from higher authorities'. They were assigned responsibility for tasks such as to 'educate and agitate workers to implement the development plans of the Government, and, in cooperation with mass organizations in the area, promote the participation of members in development activities'; 'disseminate Marxism-Leninism among workers'; 'encourage and consolidate further struggle of workers to protect the gains of the Revolution... and preserve the territorial integrity of the Revolutionary Motherland'; and to 'ensure the observance and proper implementation by members of, laws, regulations, government directives and statements'. But the task of instituting control to increase the intensity of work and to boost output was also emphasised. Unions were to 'politicize, agitate and educate members with a view to promoting the dignity of labour, labour discipline and productivity' and 'fight against abuse and wastefulness'; 'create the appropriate conditions for, encourage and assist workers to familiarize themselves with modern science and technology with a view to upgrading their skills and increasing their productivity'; and 'encourage, assist and

[155] Ibid., 38.

[156] Ibid., 38.

[157] "Trade Unions Organization Proclamation," Proclamation number 222/1982, *Negarit Gazeta*, 24 May 1982.

guide every worker to promote socialist emulation in his trade'. All in all, the proclamation transformed the trade union structure into a vehicle of unidirectional top-down control over workers.

The process of reorganising the trade union movement had begun in the first months of the year, with meetings and elections held in constituent enterprise and industrial unions, as well as the confederation's local and regional branches, under COPWE supervision. The month after the proclamation was issued, AETU convened its second general congress to complete this process at the highest level. At the congress—in which CELU's first president, Abraham Mekonnen, participated as a member of the presidium—a new central leadership was elected. Tadesse Tamrat from the Akaki Textile Factory's trade union—which has been described as 'the Derg's main source of industrial support during the terror'[158]—was elected chairman of the confederation. Between 1977 and 1982, the AETU's leadership had been subject to an astounding turnover of officials. In the year 1977 alone, two consecutive leaders—Tewodros Bekele and Temesgen Madebo—had been killed and a third interim head, Gedlu Tekle had assumed leadership after them. He had, in turn, been replaced by Mekonnen Tadesse, who led the confederation until Mulugeta Yimer took over in November 1978. But in appointing Tadesse Tamrat, the AETU's sixth leader in only five years, the Derg had found the pliant guardian it had been looking for. He would lead the organisation until its—as well as the regime's and his own[159]—demise occurred in 1991.

The AETU would hold a third and final congress under its original name in 1986, overseen directly by the ruling party. Two years prior to the congress, COPWE had become the Workers' Party of Ethiopia (WPE). As a consequence, the AETU was made to align with the new party's structure. The AETU was represented in the WPE's central committee, but not in its politburo. However, it is probably more accurate to say that the WPE was represented in AETU's leadership: henceforth, Tadesse Tamrat would use the title WPE CC member *before* the title of AETU Chairman in official correspondence, illustrating the order of hierarchy between the two organisations. At its third congress, the AETU was renamed the Ethiopian Trade Union (ETU), to remove the vestiges of MEISON's past influence that the former name could imply, but also to demonstrate

[158] Clapham, *Transformation and Continuity*, 136–137.

[159] Tadesse committed suicide in May 1991, days after Addis Ababa fell to insurgents.

commitment to the Derg's unitarian nationalist ideology: that there were no legitimate national sub-units of Ethiopia. The confederation, however, retained its essential structure, character, and functions.

The functions of the AETU and ETU continued to revolve around the core aim of controlling labour. Outside of ensuring political domination, such control was sought for a number of additional purposes. Raising productivity was, according to COPWE's journal *Meskerem*, 'the cardinal objective' of the 1975 labour proclamation and the 1982 trade union organisation proclamation, to which 'singular importance is attached'.[160] Various directives on collective agreements and remuneration stressed the primary importance of this objective and linked potential wage increments to output. The AETU/ETU was tasked with implementing such agreements, but also with whipping up productivity through campaigns, agitation, and material incentives. However, due to an actual wage freeze, collapsing real wage levels,[161] and, in the late 1980s, suspension of collective agreements, trade unions had to rely on agitation, emulation campaigns and intangible star prizes to cajole workers into increasing efforts and output. 'In the absence of pay rises, the unions have to encourage their members with symbolic rewards, and the press frequently records the distribution of certificates to meritorious workers. One star worker, at the main Addis Ababa printing press, was made a member of the WPE Central Committee', a scholar observed.[162] Vocational training constituted another aspect of this. But none of these measures led to much success in raising productivity.[163]

At the lower levels, trade unions also began playing a role in the management of state enterprises, participating in committees related to personnel administration and disputes committees. Due to the patronage offered by the state, the institution of obligatory union membership and check-off systems, the scope of activities unions undertook grew. They set up political discussion forums and reading rooms in workplaces across the country, organised work teams for development activities, as well as workers' militias for the regime's many wars and for providing local security.

[160] "The Ethiopian Working Class Yesterday and Today," *Meskerem* 3, no. 13 (1983), 62.

[161] See Chapter 6.

[162] Clapham, *Transformation and Continuity*, 137.

[163] See Chapter 6.

But at the same time, their capacity to deliver services to members was also greatly expanded. They employed a cadre that was in better shape to check the worst forms of breaches of occupational safety and health provisions, and their position as an intermediary between state, management, and labour at the shop floor enabled them to resolve disputes between individual workers and management. They operated subsidised shops for union members, in which coveted goods were scarce but prices were low. They built and managed recreational centres to which well-performing workers and union representatives were treated to vacations, and organised an extensive network of sporting activities. Unions of most large enterprises operated cafeterias and after-work leisure centres. In some cases they also operated nurseries and even schools.

After the reorganisation of the AETU, its structures deepened and expanded. Both the central confederation and sectoral industrial unions cascaded into branches at the region, *awraja* (sub-province), and *wereda* (district) levels, in cases where a sufficient number of members were found. Partly because membership in the AETU and the ETU was mandatory for production and state enterprise workers, and partly because the threshold for unionisation was lowered to a workplace minimum of 20 members, the number of workers in affiliated unions grew from around 200,000 in 1977 to over 300,000 members in the 1980s.[164] They were organised in over 1,500 constituent unions, clustered into nine industrial unions.[165] The number of employed staff also increased. The number of employees of the central confederation reached 644.[166] And, more significantly, all levels—constituent unions, industrial unions, and confederation—had a large number of full-time officials (FTOs) set aside for union duties. By 1982, the trade union cadre consisted of 26,133 officials, constituting a massive bureaucratic layer of officialdom—almost exactly

[164] Desta Alemu, "The Ethiopian Trade Union Movement Pre and Post Revolution," in *Proceedings of the Ninth International Conference of Ethiopian Studies*, vol 1 (Moscow: Africa Institute, 1988), 140–142; Clapham, *Transformation and Continuity*, 136–137. For Andargachew, who cites a slightly higher number of unionised workers in 1977, this expansion alone constituted a 'great victory of the Ethiopian workers', and that was indeed how it was officially presented. Andargachew Assegid, *ረጅም ጉዞ*, 340.

[165] "A Brief History of the Genesis, Development, Decline and Future Prospect of the Ethiopian Labor Movement," Beyene Solomon, report written for the AALC, Addis Ababa, 1992, AALC records, 77.

[166] "የኢሠማኮ ሥራ አስፈጻሚ ኮሚቴ የአቋም መግለጫ አወጣ," *Voice of Labour*, new series 1 no. 3 (1994).

a tenth of the membership—largely released from productive work.[167] The Akaki Textile Factory alone, for example, had eleven FTOs with full wages paid by the company.[168] The funding for this massive machinery came from the—often state-owned—enterprises, as the 1982 trade union organisation proclamation granted union officials the conditional right to 'devote their regular hours of work on the activities of the union on a permanent basis' with salaries maintained. Moreover, this layer was privileged and protected as the political cadre it was, the 1982 proclamation having established that no member of any trade union representative body could be dismissed, suspended, or transferred by the employer, for whatever reason, without the explicit approval of the concerned minister.

As the above number of confederation employees indicates, the central confederation developed into a relatively wealthy institution during the COPWE and WPE period. New branch offices were opened around the country, including in the cities of Mekelle, Bahir Dar, Gondar, Dessie, Jimma, Assab, and Awassa, and new for-profit enterprises—such as hotels and resorts, gas stations, restaurants, and bakeries, among others—as well as rental properties were established. The greatest potential rental income came from the old three-storey headquarters building constructed with funding from the AALC in the 1970s, as the AETU and the industrial unions relocated to a brand-new 11-storey headquarters building in central Addis Ababa in 1984—constructed with material and financial aid from socialist bloc confederations. However, at the lower levels, unions were under severe budgetary constraints. They were generally deprived of their own resources and the leverage that would have come with those resources, while all intermediary levels were dependent on budgetary allocations from the top. In all aspects, the AETU and the ETU remained top-down institutions in which hard centralism prevailed, and they were, in turn, subordinated to COPWE, the WPE, and the state. Christopher Clapham, a scholar of Ethiopian affairs, summarised their situation within this matrix in 1988, stating that 'there is nothing at all to indicate that either [ETU or its senior officials] have any policy-making role; they are

167 Ibid, 77; Beyene Solomon, የኢትዮጵያ ሠራተኞች አንድነት ማህበር: ውልደት ዕድገት ውድቀት. (self-pub., Addis Ababa, 2012), 245–246.

168 "Report on the Mission to Ethiopia, 14–19 May, 1993," Robinson H. Sikazwe, ICFTU/ITUC archives.

seldom referred to in the press, save for their appearance at official functions. However, the political quiescence of the trade unions during the 1980s, compared with their activism during the later 1970s, presumably indicates their successful discharge of their main function'.[169]

Renewed Stirrings

The pacification and subjugation of the labour movement had been achieved by the close of the 1970s. Unions and workplace discussion forums, reinforced by party committees and armed squads, enforced industrial peace and discipline, disseminated government policy, and intercepted early signs of discontent and opposition quite effectively throughout the 1980s. For most of the remaining period of WPE rule, the labour movement remained docile. Industrial tranquillity was only occasionally disrupted by minor, localised outbreaks of discontent, additional state impositions on workers, or new purges of labour representatives not deemed sufficiently reliable. In 1990, for example, it was reported that several trade union leaders had been arrested, including the secretary general of the Construction Workers' Union, the ETU secretary for the south-western Kaffa region, and ETU central secretary Alemayehu Tadesse.[170] A notable exception to industrial tranquillity—in terms of strikes—took place at the Asmara (known as Barattolo before nationalisation) textile factory in 1983. Workers at the plant refused to work extended extra hours without compensation—a recurring demand—and when wage penalties were imposed, they called a strike. The strike was met with a response that would strongly discourage any other group of workers from contemplating a similar course of action. First, the factory was surrounded by soldiers, and 65 workers were arrested.[171] The committee tasked with investigating the incident then declared the strike illegal and warned that any such industrial action was 'anarchist' and 'anti-revolutionary'—two foreboding labels in the aftermath of the high terror of the 1970s. In addition to administrative punishment meted out against the workers, the ruling authorised the government to take 'legal

[169] Clapham, *Transformation and Continuity*, 137.

[170] Hassan A. Sunmonu to ICFTU General Secretary, 6 June 1990, ICFTU/ITUC archives.

[171] "Important dates in the history of Eritrean workers," translation of an article by Goitom [pseud.] in ፍጻሜታት 180, 15 May 1985, 3–7, Tom Killion Papers.

"measures"'[172] [N.B. citation marks from the original text of the ruling] against strike leaders, who were accused of being followers of 'secessionists', and warned that in the future 'measures' would be taken 'without hesitation' in similar cases.[173] No large-scale industrial action reoccured in the years that followed. That was the case until, in the final years of the 1980s, the WPE's authority began to rapidly erode.

As the civil wars in Eritrea and Tigray intensified in the second half of the 1980s, and as the economic situation worsened, working conditions deteriorated accordingly. In 1988, collective bargaining agreements were suspended, overtime pay was cancelled, and wages were frozen. Moreover, increasing numbers of workers were drafted into the militias—organised with the ETU's active and enthusiastic participation. Swaths of them—probably many thousands—were killed or maimed in the intensifying wars. These factors led to growing discontent among workers, for which the state-controlled union structures provided no outlet.

Although open industrial conflict was rare, a few episodes of unrest occurred during the final years of WPE rule. When and where the opportunity arose, workers displayed their resentment towards the structures imposed upon them. In 1989, some 400 workers who had been transferred from the Akaki Textile Factory[174] to the Adey Abeba factory without prior consultation walked off the job and took their grievances to the labour ministry. The lenient and careful manner in which they were handled by authorities and ETU officials indicated the beginning of a shift in the balance of forces.[175] In early 1991, when the rapid erosion of the WPE's authority, its repressive capacity, and its already shallow legitimacy became increasingly obvious, signs of renewed labour combativeness multiplied. Workers in the industrial district of Akaki repeatedly protested

[172] What these 'measures' consisted of can only be speculated on. It is noteworthy, however, that the word 'measures' was the standard euphemism for execution. The reservation that the measures would be legal is not very reassuring since the emergency law operational in Eritrea at the time, and referred to in the ruling, permitted the use of lethal force.

[173] "በአሥመራ ጨርቃ ጨርቅ ፋብሪካ በ22.6.75 ተደርጉ የነበረው የሥራ ማቆም አድማ በማስመልከት በኢ.ክ.ሀገር ከፍተኛ ባለሥልታኞች ያሉበት ኮሚቴ መርምሮ በ26.6.75 የፋብሪካው ጠቅላላ ሠራተኞች በተገኙበት የተሰጠ ውሳኔ," ruling by committee of senior officials, CETU archives.

[174] Prior to its nationalisation, this factory was known as the Indo-Ethiopian textile factory.

[175] "በቤሐራዊ ጨርቃ ጨርቅ ኮርፖሬሽን የአደይ አበባ ድርና ማግ ፋብሪካ የስብሰባ ቃለ ጉባኤ," meeting minutes, 21 September 1989, CETU archives.

against their working conditions and the unpopular labour bureaucracy. On multiple occasions, over a period of several months, workers from the Akaki Textile Factory and youth from the area demonstrated outside, throwing stones at the villa of ETU Chairman Tadesse Tamrat.[176] Among workers and residents of the area, mythical stories about the extravagant luxuries of the house included rumours of facilities that allowed a car to be driven into the bedroom,[177] and the perception among the workers was that the villa had been built with money that was rightfully theirs.[178] In one case, they were reported to have caused significant damage to parts of the building.[179]

Beyene Solomon[180] has described what he calls an 'uprising' taking place among workers in and around Addis Ababa in the waning years of WPE rule. According to Beyene, the uprising was precipitated by the arrest of numerous workers and representatives who had protested poor pay and intensified requisitions of 'voluntary contributions' to support the war effort.[181] As unrest spread through the industrial corridor leading south from the capital, it was joined by workers at the Ethiopian Cargo Transport Corporation, on construction sites, at the Wholesale and Resale Trading Corporation, the Alcohol Corporation, the Metahara and Wonji sugar factories, the Akaki Textile Factory, and the Ethio-Fibre Factory. At the Akaki Textile Factory, workers' grievances included complaints over postponed annual wage revisions and the collective agreement. But they also charged union leaders with being mere tools of the WPE who did not represent workers, and demanded that workers be allowed to freely elect genuine representatives. Eventually, the dispute became sufficiently

[176] Geresu Tufa, online communication with the author, 16 June 2017.

[177] Ibid.

[178] Hailu Ourgessa, in discussion with the author, 28 May 2017. Hailu Ourgessa was the President of the Federation of Commerce, Technical and Printing Industry Trade Unions.

[179] Ibid.

[180] Beyene, የኢትዮጵያ ሠራተኞች አንድነት ማህበር, 250–254.

[181] Contributions to the war effort did not only take the form of cash contributions. The AETU/ETU also drafted members to the wars with various insurgent movements that continued unabated throughout the period of PMAC/WPE rule. According to a sympathetic observer, 'AETU was able to arm and dispatch tens of thousands of volunteers [sic] from its ranks when Ethiopia was attacked by counter-revolutionaries and imperialist aggression' in 1977/78 alone. Desta Alemu, "Ethiopian Trade Union Movement," 140.

serious to trigger the intervention of a WPE delegation led by Deputy Prime Minister Fisseha Desta. He promised to address some 'minor economic questions urgently' in order to pacify the workers. Meanwhile, however, Beyene claims that the chairman of the WPE and the president of the country, Mengistu Hailemariam, had clarified that action would be taken against the ETU leadership should there be any further incidents of worker disobedience. In any event, the slow-burning 'uprising' was said to have lasted until the WPE government fell in 1991. Since Beyene's account is not backed up by any sources, and no dates are given for the events, it is difficult to substantiate in detail. The documentation and recollections available on the rumblings of discontent, petitioning, protesting, and repression that took place in the final years of WPE rule seem to suggest that the term 'uprising' is an exaggeration. Nevertheless, Beyene's account corroborates the impression that stirrings of open discontent had again begun to emerge among workers and within the labour movement.

The archive of the Ministry of Labour and Social Affairs in Addis Ababa contains evidence of a number of additional disputes. In April 1991, for example, a bitter conflict erupted between the management of the fuel company Total Mer Rouge and its union. On April 3, the union, alarmed by seemingly wanton disciplinary actions taken against workers in the context of negotiations for a new collective agreement, passed a resolution threatening to go on strike.[182] During a meeting with the company's management, the workers' representatives invoked the possibility of 'bloodshed' should the latter stick to its intransigence.[183] The menacing choice of words triggered strong protests from the company management and intervention by the ETU and authorities, forcing the union to back down from some of its bluntest threats.[184] However, the grievances had not been addressed, and the conflict was far from resolved

[182] Paul Graf to Ministry of Labour and Social Affairs, 23 April 1991, ICFTU/ITUC archives; "November 21 meeting about the Total company problem," meeting minutes. Ministry of Labour and Social Affairs (MoLSA) archives, MoLSA, Addis Ababa; Tadesse Tamrat to Total Mer Rouge Company, 29 March 1991; MoLSA archives; Kedeme Teshome to Total Mer Rouge Company, 7 May 1991, MoLSA archives.

[183] P. Graf to Ministry of Labour and Social Affairs, 23 April 1991, ICFTU/ITUC archives; Kedeme Teshome to Total Mer Rouge Company, 7 May 1991, MoLSA archives.

[184] Paul Graf to Total Mer Rouge Workers' Union, 17 May 1991, MoLSA archives.

when the insurgent army of the Ethiopian People's Revolutionary Democratic Front entered Addis Ababa in May 1991, ending WPE rule. The WPE was declared illegal, and its senior officials were ordered to report to the victorious front. Rather than doing so, Tadesse Tamrat, the ETU's chairman, elected to end his life.

References

Abyot. "News." *Abyot* 2, no. 2 (1977): 5–10.

Abyot. "May Day 1980: The Long Struggle of the Ethiopian Proletariat." *Abyot* 5, no. 4 (1980):6–16.

African American Labor Center (AALC) records. Collection 0547-LBR. Hornbake Library, Special Collections and University Archives, University of Maryland Libraries, College Park, MD.

Andargachew Assegid. *በአጭር የተቀጨ ረጅም ጉዞ፡ መኢሶን በኢትዮጲያ ሕዝቦች ትግል ውስጥ*. Self-published, Addis Ababa, 2020.

Andargachew Tiruneh. *The Ethiopian revolution, 1974–1987: A Transformation From an Aristocratic to a Totalitarian Autocracy*. Cambridge: Cambridge University Press, 1993.

Beyene Solomon. *Fighter for Democracy: The Saga of an Ethiopian Labour Leader*. Baltimore: Publish America, 2010.

Beyene Solomon. *የኢትዮጵያ ሠራተኞች አንድነት ማህበር: ውልደት ዕድገት ውድቀት*. Self-published, Addis Ababa, 2012.

Chapin, F. "Arrests of Ethiopian Trade Union Officials." Cable 1979STATE005993_e from the US Embassy in Addis Ababa, 9 January 1979. PLUSD, https://wikileaks.org/plusd/cables/1979STATE005993_e.html.

Chapin, F. "New Leadership for Ethiopian National Labor Union." Cable 1979ADDIS00125_e from the US Embassy in Addis Ababa, 10 January 1979. PLUSD, https://wikileaks.org/plusd/cables/1979ADDIS00125_e.html.

Clapham, C. *Transformation and Continuity in Revolutionary Ethiopia*. Cambridge: Cambridge University Press, 1990.

Confederation of Ethiopian Trade Unions (CETU) Archives, Confederation of Ethiopian Trade Unions, Addis Ababa.

Desta Alemu. "The Ethiopian Trade Union Movement Pre and Post Revolution." In *Proceedings of the Ninth International Conference of Ethiopian Studies*, vol 1, 135–144. Moscow: Africa Institute, 1988.

Emmanuel Fayessa Negassa. "The Confederation of Ethiopian Labour Unions and its First General Strike (March 7–11, 1974): Causes and Impact." Master's thesis, Cornell University, 1977.

Ethiopian Herald. "Disreputed Leadership." September 19, 1974.
Ethiopian Herald. "CELU Firmly Supports Ethiopian Socialism." January 4, 1975.
Ethiopian Herald. "Government Announces Temporary Closure of CELU Headquarters." May 20, 1975.
Ethiopian Herald. "Four Killed, Twenty-Nine Others Injured at Bole Airport." September 26, 1975.
Ethiopian Herald. "PMAC Declares State of Emergency." October 1, 1975
Ethiopian Herald. "Do More, Ask Less." December 24, 1975.
Ethiopian Herald. "PMAC Issues Clarification on Function of Workers Forums." April 10, 1976.
Ethiopian Herald. "Against Shadow-boxing." May 28, 1976.
Ethiopian Herald. "PMG Urges Vigilance Against Reactionaries." May 29, 1976.
Ethiopian Herald. "Revolutionary Justice Awaits Plotters: Government Warns Anarchist Elements." September 22, 1976.
Ethiopian Herald. "Six Persons Executed for Dastardly, Inhuman Murder of 24 persons." April 3, 1977.
Ethiopian Workers' Revolutionary Union (ELAMA). "የፋሺስቶች መፍጨርጨር የላብ አደሩን ትግል አይገታውም." Mimeo. leaflet. Addis Ababa, 1976.
Fikreselassie Wogderes. እኛና አብዮቱ. Los Angeles: Tsehai, 2014.
Fisseha Desta. አብዮቱና ትዝታዬ. Los Angeles: Tsehai, 2015.
Frewe Abayneh. "Full Text of the Interview Given to Two Foreign Journalists by Frewe Abayneh, a Representative of the Leadership of MEISONE, The All Ethiopian Socialist Movement at a Meeting in Addis Ababa, Ethiopia, in September 1979." *New Ethiopia* (March 1980): 1–14.
Gilkes, P. "Building Ethiopia's Revolutionary Party Patrick Gilkes." *MERIP Reports* 106 (June 1982): 22–28.
Halliday, F. and M. Molyneux. *The Ethiopian Revolution*. London: Verso, 1981.
Halliday, F. and M. Molyneux. "Ethiopia's Revolution from Above," *MERIP Reports* 106 (June 1982): 5–15.
Hummel, A.W. "Addis Airport and Labor Developments: Sept. 30." Cable 1975ADDIS11623_b from the US Embassy in Addis Ababa. 30 September 1975, PLUSD, https://wikileaks.org/plusd/cables/1975ADDIS11623_b.html.
Hummel, A.W. "Wildcat Strikes Appear to Wane." Cable 1975ADDIS11720_b from the US Embassy in Addis Ababa, 1 October 1975. PLUSD, https://wikileaks.org/plusd/cables/1975ADDIS11720_b.html.
Hummel, A.W. "Ethiopian Labor Scene." Cable 1975ADDIS08716_b from the US Embassy in Addis Ababa, 22 July 1975. PLUSD, https://wikileaks.org/plusd/cables/1975ADDIS08716_b.html.

Hummel, A.W. "Comment on New Labor Law." Cable 1975ADDIS14564_b from the US Embassy in Addis Ababa, 19 December 1975. PLUSD, https://wikileaks.org/plusd/cables/1975ADDIS14564_b.html.

ICFTU/ITUC archives. Collection ARCH00622, International Institute of Social History, Amsterdam.

International Labour Organization (ILO) archives. International Labour Office. Geneva.

ILO. *155th Report of the Committee on Freedom of Association*. Geneva: International Labour Office, November 1975.

Kiflu Tadesse. *ኢትዮጵያ ሆይ: ቅጽ 1*. Self-published, Addis Ababa, 2016.

Kiflu Tadesse. *The Generation: The History of the Ethiopian People's Revolutionary Party, part I: From the Early Beginnings to 1975*. Silver Spring, MD: Independent Publishers, 1993.

Kiflu Tadesse. *The Generation: The History of the Ethiopian People's Revolutionary Party, part II: Ethiopia, Transformation and Conflict*. Lanham, MD: University Press of America, 1998.

Killion, T. "Workers, Capital and the State in the Ethiopian Region." PhD diss., Stanford University, 1985.

Lefort, R. *Ethiopia: An Heretical Revolution?* London: Zed Press, 1983.

Markakis, J. and Nega Ayele. *Class and Revolution in Ethiopia*. Nottingham: Spokesman Books, 1978.

Mengistu Hailemariam. *Speech Delivered to the Second Congress of the All Ethiopia Trade Union*. Addis Ababa: Provisional Military Government of Socialist Ethiopia/Commission for Organizing the Party of the Working People of Ethiopia, 1982.

Meskerem. "History of the Struggle of the Ethiopian Working Class." *Meskerem* 1, no 4 (1981): 20–39.

Meskerem. "The Ethiopian Working Class Yesterday and Today." *Meskerem* 3, no. 13 (1983): 45–71.

Ministry of Labour and Social Affairs Archives (MoLSA) archives, MoLSA, Addis Ababa.

Mohamed Yimam, *Wore Negari: A Memoir of an Ethiopian Youth in the Turbulent 1970s*. N.p.: Xlibris, 2013.

Morehouse, L.G. "Ethiopian Labour Relations: Attitudes, Practice and Law." Research project paper, Northwestern University, 1969.

Negarit Gazeta. "Trade Unions Organization Proclamation." Proclamation number 222/1982. *Negarit Gazeta*, May 24, 1982.

Negede Gobezie. "Interview with the BBC." *New Ethiopia* (May 1980): 6–9.

Negede Gobezie. *ይድረስ ለግንቦት ከየካቲት*. Washington, DC: AESOP Publishers, 2014.

Ottaway, D. "Fighting Up Sharply in Ethiopia." *Washington Post*, March 14, 1977.

Ottaway, M. and D. Ottaway. *Ethiopia: Empire in Revolution*. New York: Africana Publishing Company, 1978.

Pliny the Middle-Aged [pseud.]. "The PMAC: Origins and Structure, Part One." *Northeast African Studies* 2, no. 3 (1978–1979): 1–18.

Rahel Teshome. "The week that was." *Ethiopian Herald,* June 8, 1975.

Screpanti, E. "Long Economic Cycles and Recurring Proletarian Insurgencies." *Review (Fernand Braudel Center)* 7, no. 3 (1984): 509–548.

Sherry, G.B. "CELU Strike." Cable 1974ASMARA00784_b from the US Consulate General in Asmara, 24 September 1974. Wikileaks Public Library of US Diplomacy (PLUSD), https://wikileaks.org/plusd/cables/1974ASMARA00784_b.html.

Syoum Gebregziabher. "The Rise of CELU and the EFE Under Haile Selassie's Regime." Mimeo, 2005.

Tele Progressive [pseud.]. "Abiot Forum: Let Us Clean Our Union From EPRP Traitors." *Ethiopian Herald*, March 11, 1975.

Tienken, A.T. "Post Office Workers Strike in Addis Ababa." Cable 1976ADDIS08471_b from the US Embassy in Addis Ababa, 16 July 1976. PLUSD, https://wikileaks.org/plusd/cables/1976ADDIS08471_b.html.

Tienken, A.T. "New Outbreaks of Violence in Capital." Cable 1976ADDIS10494 from the US Embassy in Addis Ababa, 23 September 1976. PLUSD, https://wikileaks.org/plusd/cables/1976ADDIS10494_b.html.

Tienken, A.T. "EPMG To Clamp Down on Possible Strikes." Cable 1976ADDIS10465_b from the US Embassy in Addis Ababa, 22 September 1976. PLUSD, https://wikileaks.org/plusd/cables/1976ADDIS10465_b.html.

Tienken, A.T. "Tensions in Addis Ababa." Cable 1976ADDIS10880_b from the US Embassy in Addis Ababa, 8 October 1976. PLUSD, https://wikileaks.org/plusd/cables/1976ADDIS10880_b.html.

Tienken, A.T. "Assassination of Cabinet Official." Cable 1976ADDIS11591_b from the US Embassy in Addis Ababa, 10 November 1976. PLUSD, https://wikileaks.org/plusd/cables/1976ADDIS11591_b.html.

Tienken, A.T. "Recent Ethiopian Labor Developments." Cable 1976ADDIS12645_b from the US Embassy in Addis Ababa, 30 December 1976. PLUSD, https://wikileaks.org/plusd/cables/1976ADDIS12645_b.html.

Tienken, A.T. "All-Ethiopian Trade Union Formed." Cable 1977ADDIS00126_c from the US Embassy in Addis Ababa, 10 January 1977. PLUSD, https://wikileaks.org/plusd/cables/1977ADDIS00126_c.html.

Tom Killion Papers. Collection 2017C40, Hoover Institution Library and Archives, Stanford University Stanford, CA.

Voice of Labour. "Editorial: The Necessity of Political Parties." *Voice of Labour*, August 1974.

Voice of Labour. "የኢሠማኮ ሥራ አስፈጻሚ ኮሚቴ የአቋም መግለጫ አወጣ." *Voice of Labour*, new series 1 no. 3 (1994): 1–5.

Walker. "Ethiopian Labor Union Replaces Entire Leadership." Cable 1978ADDIS02387_d from the US Embassy in Addis Ababa, 26 May 1978. PLUSD, https://www.wikileaks.org/plusd/cables/1978ADDIS02387_d.html.

Wiebel, J. and S.A. Admasie. "Rethinking the Ethiopian Red Terror: Approaches to Political Violence in Revolutionary Ethiopia." *Journal of African History* 60, no. 3 (2019): 457–475.

Wyman, P.D. "CELU General Assembly Meeting." Cable 974ADDIS11161_b from the US Embassy in Addis Ababa, 17 September 1974. Wikileaks Public Library of US Diplomacy (PLUSD), https://wikileaks.org/plusd/cables/1974ADDIS11161_b.html.

Wyman, P.D. "Labor Situation." Cable 1974ADDIS11122 from the US Embassy in Addis Ababa, 17 September 1974. Wikileaks Public Library of US Diplomacy (PLUSD), https://wikileaks.org/plusd/cables/1974ADDIS11122_b.html.

Wyman, P.D. "Labor Situation." Cable 1974ADDIS12489_b from the US Embassy in Addis Ababa, 18 October 1974. Wikileaks Public Library of US Diplomacy (PLUSD), https://wikileaks.org/plusd/cables/1974ADDIS12489_b.html.

United States Embassy in Addis Ababa. "Provisional CELU Executive Committee Selected—CELU Headquarters Reopened." Cable 1975ADDIS06558_b from the US Embassy in Addis Ababa, 3 June 1975, Wikileaks Public Library of US Diplomacy (PLUSD), https://wikileaks.org/plusd/cables/1975ADDIS06558_b.html

CHAPTER 4

The Labour Movement in the Federal Republic: New Beginnings, 1991–2020

In the previous chapter, it was discussed how, in the waning years of WPE rule, new stirrings within the labour movement had begun to emerge. Although these early signs of revival were real, they were soon nipped in the bud. With the Ethiopian People's Revolutionary Democratic Front's (EPRDF) military victory over the WPE regime in May 1991, and the formation of the EPRDF-dominated Transitional Government of Ethiopia (TGE), a process of state restructuring began. This process was to culminate in the foundation of the Federal Democratic Republic of Ethiopia in 1995 (Eritrea having acquired independence the year before), over which the EPRDF became the incontestable ruling entity. But by 1991, this was not yet the case. Conceiving itself as representing rural masses and marginalised nationalities, the new ruling party was intolerant of anything that could be perceived as urban opposition. Moreover, it was ready to use such force as had brought it to Addis Ababa to bear on any expression of such opposition. The labour movement did not constitute an obvious source of support for the EPRDF in this scheme of things,[1] but its very size and strategic location made the control of

[1] While the peasantry was considered the mainstay of EPRDF support, and was indeed the social force that had brought it to power, the relationship the EPRDF claimed to enjoy with workers was more ambivalent. 'Though the aim of our Revolutionary Democracy is not to completely free the proletariat from exploitation', an internal party document was reported to read EPRDF, "Our Revolutionary Democratic Goals and the Next Steps,"

© The Author(s), under exclusive license to Springer Nature Switzerland AG 2025

S. A. Admasie, *The Ethiopian Labour Movement*, Labour in History and Society, https://doi.org/10.1007/978-3-031-72841-9_4

it—or, at the very least, its pacification, preventing it from becoming a base of opposition—an important task. An EPRDF document stated that 'without compromising [the trade unions'] organisational independence, we should try to control them and lead them through indirect organisational links'.[2] This turned out to be a prescient description of the route that was to be followed. Similarly to the Derg and the WPE, the TGE set out to reorganise the labour movement into a shape that would ensure pacification, neuter internal opposition, facilitate control, and possibly even render it a vehicle of government support. But just like the Derg, it met unexpected resistance.

Breaking Up the Old Dispensation

As Addis Ababa fell to the insurgents in May 1991, the high-rise headquarters building of the trade unions, which offered an unparalleled vantage point from which to monitor the capital's centre, was initially occupied by the EPRDF army and turned into a command centre.[3] The national trade union centre ETU—tainted as it was by its close organisational and political attachment to the WPE—and its industrial unions were dissolved by the interim authorities. Several ETU and industrial union leaders ended up in prison, and a few fled the country. The basic enterprise unions, however, were not abolished but were subjected to a leadership purge and mandatory re-elections.

Initially, the incoming government had not formulated a coherent strategy for dealing with workers and the trade unions, except for purging the latter of WPE remnants and perceived oppositional holdouts. In July 1991, the TGE established grievance hearing committees in all public enterprises and some large private companies. In principle, they were meant to identify individuals guilty of corruption, mismanagement and abuse of power. In practice, however, they became highly politicised and were prone to being used as vehicles to settle all kinds of grudges, not only against managers and supervisors but also trade

excerpts published in "TPLF/EPRDF's Strategies for Establishing its Hegemony and Perpetuating its Rule," *Ethiopian Register* (June 1996), 23. 'it is still the only approach that best serves its interests now'.

[2] Ibid., 28.

[3] Dawey Ibrahim in discussion with the author, 20 May 2015.

union officials and workers' representatives.[4] Since the grievance committees assumed the power to dismiss or detain alleged wrongdoers, and since many excesses were noted in this respect, their presence in workplaces created a fearsome environment. Meanwhile, senior trade union officials—including some who had fallen afoul of the WPE regime—were made political examples of. For instance, Alemayehu Tadesse, the ETU secretary whose arrest was mentioned in the previous chapter, was released from prison when the WPE fell in May 1991, only to be re-arrested by the TGE in August that same year.[5] All this served to demonstrate the EPRDF's determination to break up the old dispensation. But it was not yet clear what it would be replaced with.

During the same month that the grievance committees were established—in July 1991—the TGE began to organise new elections in all enterprise unions. Former WPE members and security personnel of the old regime were banned from standing as candidates.[6] In combination with the politicised mood of the grievance committee processes, this brought about significant change in the trade union leaderships. A majority of the former union leaders were either banned or discouraged from standing for re-election, and a new crop of leaders consequently emerged.

Reflecting the lack of a broader government strategy, however, the purge and reorganisation of basic unions was not initially combined with hostility towards rank-and-file workers' activity. The TGE initially appeared to believe that such activity was primarily directed against vestiges of the old regime. 'In the absence of official guidelines Transitional Government officials have been tolerant of strikes and protests in the workplace' a report from 1992 stated.[7] Frequent demonstrations and protests against enterprise management by aggrieved workers were reported in government press, and several strikes took place during the

[4] J. M. Cohen, W. Hammink and E. Simmons, "Evaluation Report: Ethiopia Democracy/Governance Support Project", Draft Report Prepared for Ethiopia Mission, United States, Agency for International Development, Addis Ababa, May 10, 1994, https://pdf.usaid.gov/pdf_docs/pdabk181.pdf.

[5] Hassan A. Sunmonu to Meles Zenawi, 30 August 1991, ICFTU/ITUC archives, collection ARCH00622, International Institute of Social History, Amsterdam.

[6] Department of State, *Country Reports on Human Rights Practices for 1991* (Washington DC: Joint Committee Print, 1992), 130–131.

[7] Ibid. 130–131.

transitional period. To employers and managers, this initial tolerance of strikes seemed to imply that 'the TGE [was] being indulgent with labour demands'.[8] But for workers, mass retrenchments and selective dismissals of trade union leaders appeared to seriously contradict this interpretation.

Economically, wage workers came under intense pressure during the initial years of EPRDF rule. The TGE's policies ushered in a wave of retrenchments, which contrasted starkly with the high degree of job security workers had enjoyed under the previous regime. While no conclusive total figure is available, an ILO study estimated that over 17,500 workers in state-owned enterprises alone were dismissed or forced into early retirement between 1991 and 1997.[9] That figure did not account for the likely much higher number of workers retrenched from private companies and newly privatised enterprises. Moreover, the 1992 decision of the TGE to drastically devalue the Ethiopian Birr—cutting its value against the USD by more than half in one fell swoop—in combination with the liberalisation of food prices, led to the erosion of the real wages of those workers who were fortunate enough to retain their jobs.[10] This was only partially offset by the TGE's decision to raise nominal wages in the public sector. But renewed attacks on the position of labour did not only come from the state. Employers were also eager to take advantage of the disorganisation of workers and the shifting workplace balance of power that it entailed.

The 1982 Trade Union Organisation Proclamation, discussed in Chapter 3, included the provision that no member of any leading body of any trade union could, without the prior explicit approval of the Minister of Labour and Social Affairs, be suspended or transferred from his or her place of work. In line with these provisions, the Ministry of Labour and Social Affairs (MoLSA) established a file containing cases of union leaders who had been dismissed or transferred by their employers. These files, entitled 'dismissed or transferred union leaders',[11] were kept open

[8] Ibid. 130–131.

[9] International Labour Organization, *The Situation of Laid-Off Women Workers in Ethiopia* (Addis Ababa: ILO, 2005), 21.

[10] This point is examined in more detail in Chapter 5.

[11] Three volumes, labelled ማህበር መሪዎችን ከሥራ አገዱ ወይም የሥራ ዝውውር መመሪያ, were compiled before the files were closed in 1993, and are kept in MoLSA's archive. These contain only the cases sent to MoLSA's head office. Cases resolved at the workplace or through the mediation of local MoLSA branches did, therefore, not reach the central level. However, as any case that could not be solved locally or regionally in amicable terms

between the passage of the proclamation in 1982 and its repeal in January 1993. They contain valuable evidence of what can only be described as a renewed crack-down on workers' representatives in the later years of this period. Ostensible reasons for termination and transfer ranged from disciplinary issues such as lateness, absence, embezzlement and corruption, to more explicit expressions of discontent, such as protesting and arguing, minor acts of sabotage, organising unrest, and 'fomenting anarchy'. But they also contain documented cases of violence against management personnel and colleagues. Chart 4.1 illustrates the number of documented cases of terminations and transfers of union leaders over the years these files were open.

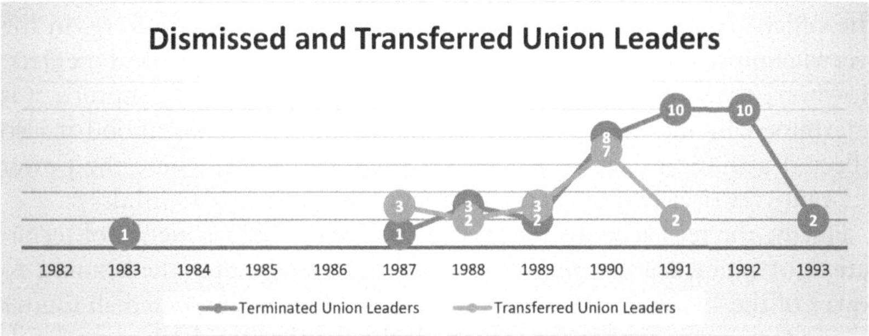

Chart 4.1 Dismissed and transferred union leaders 1982–1993 (*Source* Compilation of data from the three volumes of files from MoLSA's archives[12])

This compilation illustrates three aspects of the worsening workplace balance of power for workers. First, it is clear, given the scarce numbers of cases dated before 1989, that union leaders possessed a considerable level of job security under the period of stable WPE rule. There was only a single case of termination of a union official in the years between 1982

was transferred to the Ministry, it nevertheless accounts for the most significant cases and those which actually ended in termination. Ministry of Labour and Social Affairs archive, MoLSA, Addis Ababa.

[12] Note that the data for the years 1982 and 1993 does not cover those full years. Since the 1982 law only came into force in the month of March of that year, any cases prior to that would not have been registered. More importantly, the law was repealed in the very first month of 1993. The few cases reported in that year are thus an outcome of the fact that only incidents during the 21 days of the year were registered.

and 1986. This should, of course, not be confused with tenure security, as there were other mechanisms—internal to the trade unions or based on the external directives of the WPE—to remove union leaders from office. But it was extremely rare that union leaders were dismissed or transferred by the employer. To take such action was simply not a prerogative that employers and managers enjoyed.

Secondly, however, there was a sharp increase in the number of dismissed and transferred union leaders during the last couple of years of WPE rule. This indicates an increasing power of employers and management vis-à-vis trade unions that coincided, on the one hand, with the weakening of WPE power and, on the other, with its 1990 introduction of a reform agenda intended to establish a liberalised 'mixed economy'. The official reasons cited for the terminations and transfers were, in the overwhelming majority, related to workplace indiscipline and neglect. However, that cannot be assumed to have meant that the upturn was determined by increasing indiscipline alone, but in all likelihood it also reflected a shifting balance of power in the workplace, where the power of employers over labour increased as the state somewhat withdrew.

Finally, the files account for another upturn in the frequency of termination of union leaders that occurred immediately after the coming to power of the EPRDF. As already noted, the EPRDF instructed all unions to conduct new elections in which WPE members and labour officials associated with the old regime were prohibited from standing. Since this thorough purge, which affected *all* unions, ostensibly took place within the trade unions and did not involve employers, it was not registered in the files examined. The renewed purge of labour leaders illustrated in the graph was thus not directly connected to the political purge of the unions, but took place *in addition* to it and originated in employer-employee relations. Again, the reasons given for dismissals did not refer to activities of unionism or politics, but rather workplace transgressions. As the case of the Total Mer Rouge workers illustrated, however, disciplinary pretexts were often used to dismiss labour leaders when relations with management became antagonistic. Though it is clear from the correspondence of the management of Total Mer Rouge that the enterprise's union leader was fired for union activities, a belated and unconvincing attempt was nevertheless made to justify his dismissal by accusing him of embezzlement.[13] Certainly, this is likely to have been the case in many more instances. But the importance of the new wave of harassment of trade union leaders that began in 1990 lay in how it reflected a major shift in the workplace balance of power: the weakening of the labour movement vis-à-vis employers and managers.

Once it became obvious that workers would not have a real say in the TGE's new dispensation, it resulted in resentment, anger, and, eventually, dispersed resistance. 'What surprised me', a young resident of the Akaki industrial area at the time recalled, '[was that] two years after EPRDF came to power, protests erupted and people became nostalgic about the Mengistu time'.[14] In August 1991, 2,500 workers of the Ethiopian Mines Resources Development Corporation staged an eight-day strike in Southern Ethiopia, demanding pay increases and improvements in conditions. Two months later, the Prime Minister of the TGE acknowledged that several other strikes had occurred as workers were demanding better remuneration. In the following month and a half, workers at printing presses, an animal fodder factory, and the Ethiopian Freight Transport Corporation also went on strike.[15] In late 1991 and early 1992, moreover, two large strikes took place among skilled and comparatively privileged workers: those of the Commercial Bank of Ethiopia[16] and Ethiopian Airlines. The frequency and scale of strikes indicated that the government and employers were facing increasing problems in taming labour. This problem manifested itself in other ways too, including a wave of agitation, protests, and demonstrations.

In 1993, 'numerous actions taken by former employees of state agencies who had been laid off in the process of economic restructuring' were reported.[17] But it was not only retrenched workers who protested.

[13] Wolde Mikael Miquele to S.D.G.M., Total Mer Rouge, memorandum, 13 August 1991, MoLSA archives.

[14] Geresu Tufa, online communication with the author, 16 June 2017.

[15] "Goldmines' Workers End Strike," *Ethiopian Herald*, 20 August 1991; "Prime Minister Urges Serious Attitude to Work," *Ethiopian Herald*, 16 October 1991; "Factory Workers End Strike," *Ethiopian Herald*, 23 November 1991; "Corporation Employees End Strike," *Ethiopian Herald*, 5 December 1991.

[16] More on this strike in the below.

[17] Department of State, *Country Reports on Human Rights Practices for 1993* (Washington DC: Joint Committee Print, 1994), 99.

Workers who had staged public demonstrations and protests against poor salaries and injustices in the two previous years included, among others, those of the Kaliti Food Factory, Assab and Massawa docks, Addis Ababa Fuelwood Plantation, the Addis Tool Machine Factory, the Ethiopian Building Construction Authority, the Merchandise Wholesale Trade and Import Enterprise, and employees of six hospitals around Addis Ababa.[18] Some of these protests were related to the politicised grievance committee processes. But many were nevertheless motivated by real industrial and class grievances. The most visible protest of workers during this period took place among retrenched workers of the Ethiopian Maritime Transport Authority, who erected makeshift shelters and camped on Addis Ababa's central Mesqel Square while conducting a hunger strike.

Meanwhile, workers scrambled to reorganise in such a manner that would allow them to establish some form of collective defence against the most pressing danger—the threat of mass dismissals. The situation in 1991 was described by a newly elected leader of the union of the Ethiopian Domestic Distribution Corporation in the following way:

> The government was trying to sell every enterprise. Workers were losing their jobs on a daily basis. Our enterprise, EDDC, was one of the high -risk priorities for the government. They were openly declaring that they [were] going to retrench everybody and sell the company. That was the time that I became a trade union leader, and it was a very risky time to get this responsibility. But in a few ways, we started to get organised and started to talk to authorities, to talk to our managers on this issue and on how to save the families of the workers. For us, the priority was to get job security.[19]

The revival of reorganised basic unions added some momentum to attempts to resist new impositions and threats. At Total Mer Rouge, for example, the conflict between workers and management had not yet come to a conclusion. Workers continued to petition against the company's management, demanding redress for the perceived injustice they had

[18] "Prime Minister Urges Serious Attitude," *Ethiopian Herald*. Workers of a significantly higher number of other enterprises demonstrated against management officials accused of corruption and embezzlement. However, since it is difficult to decipher the degree to which these demonstrations were related to government-instigated purges of management, they have been left out of this discussion.

[19] Hailu Ourgessa, in discussion with the author, 28 May 2017.

suffered.[20] Their reorganised union, which had continued to demand a resolution to their grievances—including a greater say in management decisions and a 20 per cent wage increase as part of a new collective agreement—became the target of renewed harassment by the management in mid-1991. The union's executive committee was refused recognition by management and was denied permission to meet during working hours or on company premises.[21] While the union instructed all workers to refuse any transfers and disciplinary actions pending discussions between management and the union, its chairman, Debebe Haileselassie, was accused of 'attempting to foment anarchy' and suspended.[22] He was only rehired after significant pressure from the workers—a petition signed by 91 workers threatened a strike should he not be reinstated[23]—and the intervention of the government, which recognised the volatility of the situation.[24]

At the Akaki Textile Factory, problems began when the government arrested the union leader Legesse Bajeba and subsequently refused to recognise his election as union chairman, alleging that he was a participant in the inappropriately named 'red' terror of the 1970s. According to more sympathetic accounts, however, Legesse had in fact been imprisoned for several years by the previous government, and it was suspected that it was rather his outspokenness against plans to privatise the factory and retrench workers that drew the government's ire.[25] At the Ethiopian Electric Light and Power Authority (EELPA), meanwhile, the union leadership was dismissed for allegedly having attempted to organise a strike.[26]

[20] Petition by Total Mer Rouge workers to whom it concerns, 6 August 1991, MoLSA archives.

[21] Paul Graf to MoLSA, 1 August 1991, MoLSA archives.

[22] Debebe Haileselassie to Total Mer Rouge Company, 23 October 1991, MoLSA archives; "November 21 Meeting About the Total Company Problem," meeting minutes, Ministry of Labour and Social Affairs Archives, MoLSA archives; Paul Graf to Debebe Haileselassie, 3 August 1991, MoLSA archives.

[23] Petition by Total Mer Rouge workers to whom it concerns, 6 August 1991, MoLSA archives.

[24] Dawit Gutema to Negasso Gidada, 20 November 1991, MoLSA archives.

[25] Dawey Ibrahim, discussion.

[26] Ibid.

Bank workers were at the forefront of the renewed stirrings in the labour movement and in the government's efforts to rein them in. At the Commercial Bank of Ethiopia, wages had largely been frozen since the 1970s.[27] This had significantly eroded the real income of employees. The union's demand to revise these wages—as well as to overturn a unilateral managerial decision to discount compensation for annual leave forfeited—triggered a confrontation with management and, by extension, the EPRDF government.[28] Despite the CBE union having been reorganised and having held officially sanctioned elections, its leadership proved anything but submissive on this point. A series of meetings was held to avert the union's threat to launch a strike, but they came to naught as the management refused to negotiate the union's demands. In the absence of dialogue, a strike was called, and the workers walked off the job on December 12, 1991. MoLSA denounced the strike as illegal, and the government announced that all strikers would be dismissed. Two days into the strike, several union leaders, including the president of the union, were arrested.[29] Responding to these measures and management promises to address the grievances, workers in provincial branches began to return to work. In the capital, the strike continued for 11 days before the High Court intervened, declaring the strike illegal and threatening workers who failed to report back to work immediately with both dismissal and criminal prosecution.[30] 54 workers and trade union representatives were labelled instigators and were banned from returning to work.[31] Despite the unsuccessful outcome for workers, the strike had revealed the degree to which a large share of the workforce had come to view its conditions as intolerable, the determination it had developed

[27] Andu-alem Aragie, "A Short History of the Employees of the Commercial Bank of Ethiopia from 1964 to 1997 (with Special Emphasis on the Employees in Addis Ababa)," (bachelor's thesis, Addis Ababa University, 1999).

[28] Andu-alem, "A Short History," 51–52; Etana Geleta to Meles Zenawi, 14 December 1991, ICFTU/ITUC archives.

[29] Andu-alem, "A Short History," 51; Ethiopian Human Rights Council, *Democracy, Rule of Law, and Human Rights in Ethiopia: Rhetoric and Practice* (Addis Ababa: EHRCO, 1995), 58.

[30] Andu-alem, "A Short History," 55–56.

[31] 46 of them were rehired two years later, following negotiations between a new union leadership and the government. Andu-alem, "A Short History," 58; EHRCO, *Democracy, Rule of Law, and Human Rights in Ethiopia*, 58–59.

to struggle to change those conditions, and the intolerance the incoming government displayed towards the demands of labour.

A New Confederation

While most enterprise unions continued to operate—under newly elected officials—no industrial federations or national trade union centre existed between 1991 and 1993. It has been alleged that the TGE initially was planning to transfer the ETU's assets to a committee rehabilitating its former combatants.[32] However, employees of the confederation helped to persuade the government that such an action would have been considered inimical to free trade unionism and damaging to its democratic reputation.[33] A caretaker committee was established in 1991 to administer the ETU's assets, help reorganise the unions, and prepare the ground for the re-establishment of a national trade union centre.[34] The caretaker committee consisted of seven members: one government official who chaired it, Dawit Yohannes; one former ETU Executive Committee member, Yohannes Teferi, its former head of international relations; and several employees of the former ETU, among whom Tedla Fantaye[35] was one. However, the caretaker committee's mandate was restrictive, and it was dismissed as 'a committee of bureaucrats carried over from the past regime'[36] by visiting AALC representative Gebreselassie Gebremariam[37].

Outside of the government-sanctioned process represented by the caretaker committee, basic unions and labour activists networked in impromptu constellations. They began what a participant has described

[32] "Trade Union Situation in Ethiopia: Factual Documentation," CETU memorandum, 1995, MoLSA archives.

[33] Ibid.

[34] "Report on the Mission to Ethiopia, 14–19 May, 1993," Robinson H. Sikazwe, ICFTU/ITUC archives.

[35] A veteran confederation employee and former participant in the labour opposition of the 1960s and 1970s, who had spent several years in prison due to his involvement in the movement. See Chapters 2 and 3.

[36] "Report on Egypt and Ethiopia, September 30, 1992," Gebreselassie Gebremariam to Patrick O'Farrell, African American Labor Center (AALC) Records, collection 0547-LBR, Hornbake Library, Special Collections and University Archives, University of Maryland Libraries, College Park, MD.

[37] A former member of CELU's senior leadership. See Chapter 2.

as a 'clandestine movement', which was 'informal, with no structure' and which was essentially geared towards exchanging information and coordinating responses.[38] An ad-hoc network of workers' representatives was formed soon after the enterprise unions elected new leaders in 1991. 'Once we were elected and started leading the basic trade unions, we went into this clandestine fight to bring back the banned confederation', one union leader has recalled.[39] 'We started connecting to other trade unionists everywhere, within the city [Addis Ababa] and outside the city. We started a kind of chain around the country. That's how we started the clandestine arrangement to bring back the national [confederation]', he stated. Eventually, a network committee of around twenty leaders of the most influential unions around Addis Ababa—including the CBE, the railway corporation, and the Berhanena Selam printing press—was formed, and it added to the pressure on the government to vacate the headquarters buildings and permit the re-establishment of a central confederation.[40]

Another, more formalised, constellation that emerged around this time was the Unity Association[41], which has been described as 'an activist core' and 'a rival force against the illegitimate caretaker committee'.[42] The Unity Association established contacts with ETU employees and set up an office inside the disbanded confederation's building.[43] The fact that it was permitted to do so indicates that authorities had granted it some form of permission—explicit or implicit—to conduct its activities. Purportedly, the government saw an opportunity to draw in leading members into its orbit (as it eventually would).[44] However, it is also plausible that the joint pressure these developments exerted on the government contributed to the TGE's decision to speed up the re-establishment of a national centre.

[38] Hailu Ourgessa, discussion.

[39] Ibid.

[40] Dawey Ibrahim, discussion.

[41] አንድነት ማህበር, which also translates to Union.

[42] "The Legal Aspect of the Dispute Between the Two Factions of the Confederation of Ethiopian Trade Unions (CETU) and the Position of the Transitional Government of Ethiopia in this Respect," Dessalegn Mesfin, 1995, MoLSA archives.

[43] Hailu Ourgessa, discussion.

[44] Ibid.

In August 1992, the TGE organised a conference to present and discuss a draft of a labour law. The conference was chaired by the TGE's Prime Minister, Tamrat Layne, and 3,000 trade unionists were in attendance. Workers reacted with anger against the draft presented, which included reduced job security provisions. 'Unfortunately, the conference was too unwieldy to evoke much other than complaints about the draft law', the US embassy reported from the conference.[45] However, Gebreselassie Gebremariam, who attended the conference as an observer of the AALC, identified two major tendencies. 'One group, and it looked to be the majority or at least the most vocal, wanted to keep the labor law of the previous regime because it is more favorable to workers than the new draft', he reported. 'The second group had specific amendments on the proposed draft'. But it was not for the workers to ultimately decide. 'The government's position was that keeping the old law was out of the question, but they would entertain proposals for amending the provisions of the draft law', Gebreselassie wrote.[46] Having included a few such amendments, the revised bill was put before the Council of Representatives and promulgated into law in early 1993.

The 1993 labour law retained the most unpopular provision from the draft that had been discussed and rejected by the workers' representatives. It granted employers the right to terminate contracts on relatively loosely defined grounds—and permitted employers to select less productive workers for dismissal when retrenchments were made. In doing so, it ushered in a labour regime in which the threat of termination and unemployment, after years of assured job safety under the Derg, again became potent. For organised labour, the law retracted a number of the most unwelcome centralising aspects of the Derg's code, released trade unions from formal state control, and made it theoretically possible to establish contending trade union centres. But the law also removed the provisions protecting trade union leaders from dismissal. This was not coincidental. The government acknowledged that the law was designed to remove provisions that were deemed to constitute a disincentive to private

[45] "Ethiopian Labor Scene: The Latest Update," photocopy of cable from US Embassy in Addis Ababa, August 1992, AALC Records.

[46] "Report on Egypt and Ethiopia, September 30, 1992," Gebreselassie Gebremariam to Patrick O'Farrell, AALC Records.

investors and were believed to stifle productivity.[47] The promulgation of the law kick-started the process of re-establishing a central confederation. But once again, external entities came to play important interfering roles in that process.

The ICFTU-aligned international trade union movement reinvolved itself in the reorganisation of an Ethiopian national trade union centre from the outset. Expressing quite striking continuities in aims and priorities, some of the very same institutions as those that were active in Ethiopia in the 1960s and 1970s returned to Addis Ababa. And they, in turn, were represented by some of the very same key individuals from that era. In 1992, Fissehatsion Tekie and Gebreselassie Gebremariam[48] returned to Addis Ababa representing the AALC, and Andrew Kailembo, who had been sent to Addis Ababa by the ICFTU in the 1970s, also returned on a mission representing that organisation. These two organisations—and particularly the AALC—again inserted themselves right into the process of re-establishing a national centre. Right after the national trade union conference to discuss the draft labour law had been held, the AALC arranged a seminar for one hundred specially invited labour representatives. It was decided that this, in turn, was to be followed by an ICFTU-held two-week intensive course for selected participants. The ICFTU also joined a panel set up by the caretaker committee, that provided input on modes of trade union organisation, in preparation for the re-establishment of a national centre.[49]

The Ethiopian government involved itself as another central player in the reorganisation of the labour movement. As early as December 1991,

[47] Council of Representatives, *Ethiopia: The Process of Transition to Democracy: Special Report (From July, 1991 to August, 1993)* (Addis Ababa: Secretariat of the Council of Representatives, 1993), 49.

[48] Fissehatsion was, as discussed in the second chapter, CELU's former Secretary General, and Gebreselassie was a former CELU Deputy Secretary and board member. Both had been key members of the group of young graduates that Beyene Solomon had brought into the leadership of CELU in the mid-1960s. Fissehatsion would stay on as the AALC representative in Addis Ababa for a couple of years, and would play a role in the struggles over the new confederation. A third member of 'CELU's four horsemen', Mesfin Gebremichael, was dispatched as an ILO observer to a 1993 national conference of trade unionists in preparation for the formation of a national centre. "Report on the Mission to Ethiopia, 14–19 May, 1993," Robinson H. Sikazwe, ICFTU/ITUC archives.

[49] "Report on the Mission to Ethiopia, 14–19 May, 1993," Robinson H. Sikazwe, ICFTU/ITUC archives.

the ICFTU's regional representative reported having 'learnt of moves within the EPRDF government to tame the trade unions'.[50] Several sources confirm that the EPRDF government was initially considering the establishment a trade union confederation composed of ethnic/regional sub-components rather than sectoral/industrial ones.[51] The ICFTU, the ILO, and the US embassy in Addis Ababa, however, lobbied for the adoption of a conventional trade union structure based on sectoral divisions. They argued that an ethnic/regional compartmentalisation would entail a politicisation of ethnicity that 'contradict the trade union spirit'.[52] When ICFTU AFRO's President Andrew Kailembo met with Prime Minister Tamrat Layne in 1992, they discussed the suggestion of trade union federations being formed along ethnic lines. 'Kailembo cautioned Dawit that such notions are dangerous', a US Embassy cable reported, adding that 'we, too, are apprehensive about such ideas. The concept of an Oromo Labor Federation has been batted around for several months now—we have disagreed with the idea from the start'.[53] While international pressure on the TGE and opposition from labour activists themselves did much to dissuade the government from imposing such a configuration, the issue was only conclusively resolved at the founding congress of the new confederation.

[50] "Report on Mission to Ethiopia, 4–8th November," Robinson H. Sikazwe, 1994, ICFTU/ITUC archives.

[51] "Report on the Inaugural Congress of the Restructured Ethiopian Trade Union Movement, Addis Ababa, 26–29 November, 1993," Robinson H. Sikazwe, ICFTU/ITUC archives; Dawey Ibrahim, discussion; Hailu Ourgessa, discussion; "Mission to Addis Ababa, Ethiopia, 18–20 January 1996," H.J. Schwass, ICFTU/ITUC archives.

According to Hailu Ourgessa, the idea was based on the experience of the largest constituent party of the EPRDF—the TPLF—during its years of armed struggle. In Tigray, it had organised workers in the ማሕበር ሸቃሎ ትግራይ (Proletarian/Workers' Association of Tigray, or Trade Union of Tigray). In Tigray, which is nationally/ethnically relatively homogenous, this form of organisation faced no obvious limitation, but when transplanted to a multinational setting such as those of workplaces around Addis Ababa, things would be insurmountably more complicated. The idea was eventually dropped, but according to Hailu, the separate structures of ማሕበር ሸቃሎ ትግራይ were not absorbed into the re-established CETU.

[52] "Report on the Mission to Ethiopia, 14–19 May, 1993," Robinson H. Sikazwe, ICFTU/ITUC archives.

[53] "Ethiopian Labor Scene: The Latest Update," photocopy of cable from US Embassy in Addis Ababa, August 1992, AALC Records.

Originally, the congress to re-establish a central confederation was scheduled to be held in March 1992. But just as had been the case in the 1970s, the process of reorganisation—in which the government sought to ensure that it would yield acceptable outcomes—took longer than expected. In mid-1993, however, the caretaker committee finally called a national conference. The conference was attended by 400 representatives of basic enterprise unions. It was tasked with determining the structure of the new confederation and electing an organising committee that, in turn, would oversee the establishment of federations and prepare the ground for a general congress. The committee that was elected consisted of 28 members and was chaired by Mekuria Gebremedhin. However, there were allegations that both the selection of delegates and the election process were flawed and that the committee was, therefore, illegitimate.[54] Among other things, it was alleged that some of the largest unions had been excluded and that, as a result, 'preorganised stooges' of the government had prevailed.[55] To some participants, it became obvious that there was an organised hand behind the selection of delegates.[56] It was suspected that it belonged to the Unity Association, which had allegedly placed supporters in key positions, allowing it to exercise control over the meeting and the elections.[57] However, despite such alleged manipulation, the conference nevertheless spelled the end of overt and direct government control over the affairs of the labour movement. It dissolved the caretaker committee and replaced it with an elected committee.

In the months that followed, the organising committee drafted a constitution and oversaw the preparations for the general congress. This included another round of reorganisations of basic unions in accordance with the 1993 labour law, ensuring that they were legally recognised and registered. However, suspicion that covert and indirect external control

[54] EHRCO, *Democracy, Rule of Law, and Human Rights in Ethiopia,* 56.

[55] "Trade Union Situation in Ethiopia: Factual Documentation," CETU memorandum, 1995, p. 3, MoLSA archives.

[56] Hailu Ourgessa, discussion.

[57] Dawey Ibrahim, discussion. According to Dawey, the majority of the 28 members of the Organising Committee were unaffiliated trade unionists, while he characterised 11 as 'out-right members' of the ruling party and its proletarian branch. Hailu Ourgessa corroborates the existence of such a divide by stating that 'in the organising committee [there were] quite obvious divisions on what should be done, how it should be done and on a vision towards a national trade union'. Hailu Ourgessa, discussion.

was being exercised continued to linger. There were allegations that the process was directed from above and that the leading body continued to report to the government.[58] In some cases, where workers refused to cooperate with the committee and hold government-supervised elections, their unions were denied recognition by the authorities.[59] This was the case for the large unions of EELPA, CBE, and the Akaki textile factory—where, as noted, friction and conflict between the government and workers had already developed.[60] In November 1993, however, the organising committee declared that the process of reorganising basic unions in accordance with the law had been completed and called a general congress.

That month, 1,500 delegates representing all duly registered basic unions met for a four-day congress in Addis Ababa to form the Confederation of Ethiopian Trade Unions (CETU). The confederation was constituted by nine industrial federations, which incorporated 482 basic unions with a total membership of over 200,000 workers.[61] The suggestion to structure the movement along ethnic/regional lines was rejected by an overwhelming majority of delegates.[62] Instead, a conventional structure of sectoral sub-units was adopted. CETU's nine sectoral industrial federations were themselves constituted by basic unions—almost exclusively of the enterprise type. Industrial federations thus, to some extent, replaced the industrial unions of the ETU, but they lacked the hierarchical top-down logic of the former and were nominally constituent of CETU rather than subordinated to it. Basic union representatives elected the councils and executive committees of the industrial federations, and the industrial federations, in turn, selected delegates to CETU's General Assembly Congress and General Council. The General Council[63] was the body of 107 delegates tasked with supervising the activities of

[58] Hailu Ourgessa, discussion. According to Hailu, the organising committee, in fact, continued to function 'under [advisor to the prime minister] Dawit Yohannes'.

[59] EHRCO, *Democracy, Rule of Law, and Human Rights in Ethiopia*, 57.

[60] EHRCO, *Democracy, Rule of Law, and Human Rights in Ethiopia*, 57–60.

[61] "Trade Union Situation in Ethiopia: Factual Documentation," CETU memorandum, 1995, p. 7, MoLSA archives; "ETUC to Ask for Council Seat," *Ethiopian Herald*, 4 December 1993.

[62] "Trade Union Situation in Ethiopia: Factual Documentation," CETU memorandum, 1995, MoLSA archives.

[63] Also referred to as the Supreme Council.

the Executive Committee. The number of delegates to the Congress and General Council was determined by quotas derived from the size of membership. CETU's Executive Committee members and its senior-most officeholders were elected directly by the General Assembly for four-year terms. Each federation elected one executive committee member. All of them were salaried by the confederation. The weight that federations received in the constitution of CETU thus imbued them with significant power and autonomy, which was intended to counterbalance the confederation's executive body and escape the excessive centralism of the AETU/ETU years. However, such power and autonomy in the hands of the federations also carried the risk of enhancing centrifugal dynamics and encouraging divisions within the movement.

CETU's foundation was immediately followed by congresses of the industrial federations, and, subsequently, the first congress of CETU's General Assembly. Members of the confederation's General Council and Executive Committee were elected in what observers reported was 'a free and fair election'.[64] The candidate for the presidency allegedly preferred by the government, Mekuria Gebremedhin, was defeated in the vote, and Dawey Ibrahim of the National Industrial Federation of Tourism, Hotel and General Service Workers' Trade Unions was elected CETU president. Dawey was a former EPRP member who had left the organisation a decade earlier. During the rule of the WPE, he had made a civil career as an employee of the Ethiopian Red Cross, whose union he was subsequently elected leader of. After the fall of the WPE regime, he had participated in *Forum 84*, a platform of former EPRP members willing to work with the new government. As such, he was initially said to have had at least the tacit approval of the government.[65] If this was ever the case, that approval was withdrawn shortly following his election. The decisively pro-government faction Mekuria represented, on the other hand, failed to secure a majority in either the General Council or the Executive Committee. The defiant mood and outcome of the congress were described by a delegate to it:

[64] "Report on the Inaugural Congress of the Restructured Ethiopian Trade Union Movement, Addis Ababa, 26–29 November, 1993," Robinson H. Sikazwe, ICFTU/ITUC archives.

[65] B. Praeg, *Ethiopia and Political Renaissance in Africa* (New York: Nova Science, 2006).

> From the outset, it was a fight. It seemed as if everybody was informed through the informal structure. We had already discussed what the government was doing, and everybody was angry about what the government tried – on the issue of organising the confederation on ethnic lines [and] that the government was trying to control the trade union movement. They tried all their best to control the [congress]. They failed.[66]

'From the informal discussions I had with several delegates', the ICFTU's representative Sikazwe noted, 'it was obvious that the conclusions including the election results were to the satisfaction of the vast majority'.[67] However, this would not prevent the emergence of a dissenting group, clustered around former members of the organising committee, who advocated for closer adherence to government policies. Despite having been outvoted on issues pertaining to the constitution and key positions in the confederation's leading bodies, they were more successful in the elections to the leading bodies of the various industrial federations. The majority of federation presidents were drawn from this group. Mekuria, its most prominent member, was elected president of the Federation of Food, Beverages and Tobacco, and Allied Trade Unions and also secretary general of the confederation.

Long before the congress, the ruling party had attempted to 'influence election results' within basic unions that were to send delegates to it, thus controlling its composition.[68] One way of doing so was through the EPRDF's 'proletarian branches', whose central institution purportedly established its headquarters in the building of Bole Printing Enterprises in Addis Ababa. Its leader was allegedly a former EPRDF commander named Tesfamariam Faris.[69] An internal EPRDF document described the envisaged rationale and role of the proletarian branches.[70] It argued that while workers, in principle, required an organisation that enhanced class unity,

[66] Hailu Ourgessa, discussion, abridged.

[67] "Report on the Inaugural Congress of the Restructured Ethiopian Trade Union Movement, Addis Ababa, 26–29 November, 1993," Robinson H. Sikazwe, p. 2, ICFTU/ITUC archives.

[68] Praeg, *Ethiopia*, 186; "Trade Union Situation in Ethiopia: Factual Documentation," CETU memorandum, 1995, MoLSA archives.

[69] Dawey Ibrahim, discussion.

[70] "EPRDF's Organizational Structure & Operation (PART V)," photocopy of an article from *Ethiopian Register*, February 1998, pp. 20–24, ICFTU African Regional Organization (ICFTU-AFRO) archives, ITUC Africa, Lomé.

in the Ethiopian case, the various nationality-based fronts that together made up the EPRDF would have to play that role. There would be no separate country-wide proletarian political party, or mass organisation attached to the EPRDF, but, the document established, different parties would vie for the support of workers. 'Like any other party, EPRDF can win over the support of the workers on the basis of its capacity to generate ideas which serve the interests of the proletariat and its ability to disseminate these among the workers', it stated. For this reason, an intermediate organisational form—not quite an open component of the front—was deemed to be required. The role of the EPRDF's proletarian branches was described as 'enabling the workers' struggle to acquire short-term and long-term benefits without disturbing the industrial peace; closely monitoring anti-proletarian activities which are carried out in the name of the proletariat in order to benefit a minority; making the workers understand the aims and orientation of these movements and mobilizing it to counter them; increasing the productivity of the workers and spearheading the combat of corruption and other anti-development activities; [and] striving to attain the constructive and continuous participation of the workers in all the political, social and economic activities in the country'.[71] In other words: the purpose was to ensure that no opposition to the EPRDF was allowed to take hold in the trade unions or among workers, and to integrate them—broadly speaking, not as directly as the Derg intended—with the aims of the new regime.

The proletarian branches were led by a Country-Wide Labour Leadership Committee, formed by seven to nine professional EPRDF cadre drawn from its former fighters and 'assigned to lead the proletariat', as well as 'EPRDF members assigned to the leadership of the [trade union] confederation'. However, the election of trade union leaders, the EPRDF document argued, nevertheless required procedural freedom. 'The labor organisations which are established at any level will be formed freely and not under the direct leadership of the government or any political party'. However, it stated, the country-wide committee would seek 'to provide an overall and day-to-day leadership to the labour movement'. It would 'draw plans for the activities of confederation as well as the trade unions and strive to persuade the leaders to adopt them'. And to the extent that it was successful in persuading 'leaders of the labor unions at the various

[71] Ibid.

levels [to] endorse them', it was also tasked with ensuring the implementation of its plans. In other words, the Country-Wide Labour Leadership Committee of the EPRDF was designed to play the role of a concealed hand of the ruling party manipulating the trade union movement. The proletarian branches constituted its instrument.

Beneath the country-wide committee, there were to be regional leadership committees in Ethiopia's various regional states and, where possible, district-level labour leadership committees. However, in individual enterprises and workplaces, workers were to be encouraged to join the primary organisations of the different parties of the front: 'The Primary [party] Organizations will have the responsibility of leading our activities in the specific trade union as well as among unorganized factory workers', the EPRDF's document stated. By the proletarian branches' arrangement, trade unionists from workplaces across the country would be vetted, selected, recruited, given courses in party policy, prepared for elections to offices in the labour movement, and instructed on which candidates to vote for.[72] This strategy was successfully implemented in the elections to the leadership of numerous basic unions and most industrial federations. However, it failed to generate firm control over the majority of delegates to CETU's General Assembly.

Despite the EPRDF's attempt—using its proletarian branches—to enhance its influence over the movement, a relatively autonomous national trade union centre reappeared temporarily after CETU's founding congress. It was a quite well-resourced confederation that came into existence, having inherited the most important assets of the ETU. This included both its former and its newer headquarters buildings, vehicles, and income-generating enterprises such as hotels and gas stations, which combined 'generated quite a bit of money for CETU'.[73] It also managed to secure the return of some of the deposited funds that belonged to the defunct ETU, although allegedly not all.[74] The new

[72] "Trade Union Situation in Ethiopia: Factual Documentation," CETU memorandum, 1995, MoLSA archives.

[73] "Mission to Addis Ababa, Ethiopia, 18–20 January 1996," H.J. Schwass, ICFTU/ITUC archives.

[74] According to CETU leaders, the EPRDF had seized 29 vehicles, 20 furnished offices, and above one million USD of funds that belonged to the labour movement. "Speech Delivered by Mr Hailu Ourgessa, Representative of the Confederation of Ethiopian Trade Unions, At the 82nd Session of the International Labour Conference Workers' Group

confederation attracted a growing number of workers in the short period during which it remained relatively autonomous. Within the 14 months that followed its establishment, CETU grew to incorporate 506 basic unions with 258,000 members.[75]

The question of CETU's international alignment was not resolved by CETU's founding congress, instead, it was assigned to the newly elected leadership to determine. Soon after the congress, CETU's president wrote to the WFTU announcing the confederation's disaffiliation from the latter and intent to 'maintain neutrality'.[76] The ICFTU, however, actively courted CETU from the outset and pledged a donation of 10,000 USD to cover immediate educational needs of the new confederation.[77] Six months after the founding congress, neutrality ceased to be a priority, as the General Council decided to reapply for affiliation with the ICFTU.[78] The application was expected to be approved at the ICFTU's Executive Board meeting scheduled for December 1994. But before that could occur, CETU came under siege. Meanwhile, its relationship with the AALC had grown increasingly close, with the AALC purportedly extending 'unreserved assistance' to CETU.[79] However, as later events would reveal, this assistance was far from unconditional.

Tacit government hostility towards the new confederation was apparent to top CETU officials from the outset of their tenure. There were strong suspicions that the ruling party continued to interfere in the affairs of the movement by orchestrating the removal of basic union leaderships—such as that of the Ethio-Djibouti Railway—which were deemed insusceptible to influence from the pro-government faction.[80]

Meeting, June 15, 1995, Geneva," transcription of speech, Hailu Ourgessa's private collection; "Trade Union Situation in Ethiopia: Factual Documentation," CETU memorandum, 1995, MoLSA archives.

[75] "Trade Union Situation in Ethiopia: Factual Documentation," CETU memorandum, 1995, p. 7, MoLSA archives.

[76] Dawey Ibrahim to Alexander Khorikov, 23 December 1993, ICFTU/ITUC archives.

[77] "Report on Mission to Ethiopia, 4–8th November," Robinson H. Sikazwe, 1994, ICFTU/ITUC archives.

[78] "Application for Affiliation," CETU to ICFTU 7 June 1994, ICFTU/ITUC archives.

[79] "የኢሠማኮ ሥራ አስፈጻሚ ኮሚቴ የአቋም መግለጫ አወጣ," *Voice of Labour* 1 (new series), no. 3 (1994).

[80] Hailu Ourgessa, discussion.

The factional division that had emerged before and during the foundational congress became more pronounced in its aftermath. As early as May 1994, a UN agency that was renting office space within CETU's headquarters building reported that 'it became clear from commotions on the eleventh floor... that there were difficulties in a meeting of CETU', and that such commotion had introduced 'a great sense of insecurity' among its staff.[81] CETU's leaders, meanwhile, spent the months following the congress focused on efforts to rebuild the movement while seeking to fend off the challenges presented by the dissenting faction. It re-established dissolved unions, conducted seminars and workshops for trade union leaders, and planned for cooperative efforts to purchase firms slated for privatisation and generate employment for retrenched workers.[82] However, there was no major effort to mobilise workers, no major victories over employers, no groundbreaking advances in the relationship with the state, nor even much success in mitigating the worsening conditions for much of the wage-working force. CETU remained on the defensive in an increasingly hostile environment.

Although there had been several sources of friction between the government and CETU,[83] it was the government's economic policies that eventually led to the complete breakdown of relations. The TGE had launched a programme of liberalisations that created pressures on the income and job security of workers. Privatisations and efforts to improve the profitability of state-owned enterprises led to massive retrenchments, which had already triggered a number of spontaneous protests by workers. In 1992, the TGE entered into an agreement with the International Monetary Fund (IMF) that saw it adopt a structural

[81] Miriam K. Were to Hussen Abdula, 18 October 1995, MoLSA archives.

[82] "Priority Needs of CETU: Points for Discussion with ICFTU Appraisal Mission, Sept., 14–15, 1994," M. Svartbekk, ICFTU/ITUC archives.

[83] The most serious issue was CETU's demand that the government and ruling party return requisitioned CETU property. But other issues included the refusal of the government to make customary courtesy calls and engage in dialogue with CETU; its insistence on minor changes in CETU's constitution—replacing the word 'nation' with 'countrywide' in order for it to adhere to the ruling party's definition of the concept of nation; and its refusal to recognise the election of an industrial federation president who was dismissed from his job in the aftermath of his election. One exception to the fraught relationship was the handover to CETU-backed cooperatives of around 40 trucks that had belonged to the dissolved public enterprise Ethiopian Freight Transport Corporation, as well as several shops. Dawey Ibrahim, discussion.

adjustment programme (SAP) supported by loans from the latter. In addition to shrinking the budget deficit, devaluing the national currency, removing subsidies, liberalising prices and trade, the SAP included further privatisations, triggering legitimate fears that they would result in more retrenchments. The government admitted that it was 'well aware' that the implementation of the programme would be 'painful' and entail 'massive hardships'.[84] Those fears were later corroborated.[85] While CETU did not oppose economic adjustment in principle, it demanded a say in the implementation of the process and was critical of SAPs due to the social costs generated by such programmes elsewhere on the continent. In mid-1994, these concerns prompted CETU to plan a symposium to 'come up with a concrete trade union position… as to how to deal with the social costs of SAP affecting its members'.[86] However, before the symposium, scheduled for October that same year, could be held, open conflict erupted within the movement and between its leadership and the government.

CETU's leaders were also coming under increasing pressure from the membership to act, as the effects of structural adjustment policies started to take a toll:

> Workers' representatives were coming to the national centre. Even those that were not retrenched. Those who had heard that the government was going to close their factory. They were coming to [CETU's] office, to Dawey's office, from everywhere. Workers were ready to go for a strike.[87] Workers were coming to the office and asking us what we were doing. Some were asking us to go for a general strike. Some were asking us [the leadership] to go for a demonstration. We discussed, and what we said was, 'look, let us stay our ground – what we should do is to make it public that we oppose what the government is doing'.[88]

[84] Council of Representatives, *Transition to Democracy*, 51–53.

[85] Hishe Hailu, "An Assessment of the Process of Privatization in Ethiopia" (master's thesis, Addis Ababa University, 2005).

[86] Dawey Ibrahim to Andrew Kailembo, 7 July 1994, ICFTU/ITUC archives.

[87] Hailu Ourgessa, discussion.

[88] Ibid.

On August 10, 1994, having concluded that no meaningful dialogue with the government was forthcoming, but that the negative consequences of the programme and the pressures from the membership were becoming acute, CETU called a press conference to lay out its position and concerns. CETU's president, Dawey, outlined the problems and concerns of the trade union movement. They included the government's refusal to return the entirety of the confederation's confiscated properties, the bureaucratic obstacles the government erected to CETU's operations, its neglect in addressing cases of labour rights transgressions lodged with government bodies, and its refusal to engage in policy dialogue with CETU.[89] But the most damning charges were levelled against the government's SAP-aligned policies. Dawey stated that the policies had aggravated unemployment, eroded job security and led to 6,000 arbitrary dismissals, undermined the position of Ethiopian industry, and, through the devaluation of the Ethiopian Birr and the abolishment of subsidies, led to rampant inflation.[90] CETU demanded a say in the planning and implementation of SAP policies to alleviate their negative social effects and that the government reduce the 'rushed' pace of programme implementation. The statement called on workers 'to struggle without opportunism and hesitation with the leadership of CETU'. It declared that the duty to 'fight and fend off' the threats the SAP posed to all of society would have to fall upon the workers.[91] Whether intended as such or not, CETU's call could very easily be interpreted as an act of opposition against the EPRDF government, and the EPRDF government thus reacted with the same unconditional hostility that it invariably responded to other acts of opposition with. This set the stage for open conflict and the eventual destruction of the relative autonomy that CETU briefly had enjoyed.

Resubjugation

Speaking at CETU's press conference, Dawey hinted at the internal divisions that existed within CETU when condemning 'some trade union leaders [who] give statements blessing the inflictions caused on the workers'. He demanded that the industrial federations, several of which

[89] "የኢሠማኮ ሥራ አስፈጻሚ ኮሚቴ የአቋም መግለጫ," *Voice of Labour.*

[90] Ibid.

[91] Ibid., 5.

were controlled by his opponents, fall in line with CETU's Executive Committee and its willingness to 'struggle to protect and preserve the rights and interests of the workers'.[92] Dawey's announcement 'provoked immediate reaction from both his opponents and supporters'.[93] A group of industrial federation leaders issued statements distancing themselves from Dawey and his criticism of the government. The fault lines were unsurprisingly identical to those that had become apparent during CETU's founding congress. The group of trade unionists aligned with the government—affiliated with or under the sway of the ruling front's proletarian branches—led six of the nine industrial federations. With the schism developing between CETU's leadership and the government, they formed what has been described as 'a splinter group from within the Confederation with the objective of making it dysfunctional'.[94]

The dissenting faction charged Dawey with issuing a statement without the approval of CETU's Executive Committee and the industrial federations. It also accused him of turning down a government offer to meet with CETU's General Council. It characterised the leadership as 'confrontational' and accused it of exhibiting a discriminatory attitude towards trade unionists of Tigrayan origin.[95] A weeklong meeting of the General Council failed to resolve the differences. Rather, it led to further acrimony and an open split. The sessions were preceded by government harassment and intimidation,[96] and were reportedly interrupted by 'unruly behaviour and walk-out of some members of the council during the meeting, including the brandishing of a pistol'.[97] Some members of the dissenting faction had come dressed in military jackets and carrying arms, and one

[92] Ibid.

[93] "Report on Mission to Ethiopia, 4–8th November," Robinson H. Sikazwe, 1994, p. 3, ICFTU/ITUC archives.

[94] Praeg, *Ethiopia*, 187.

[95] Tamene, "Officials Prepare to Dismiss Labor Leaders as Confederations Nears Losing Legal Status," *File* newsletter 1, no. 8 (18 November 1994); "Report of Mediation in the Crisis Within the Leadership of the Confederation of Ethiopian Trade Unions (CETU): By Hassan A. Sunmonu, Secretary-General, Organisation of African Trade Union Unity (OATUU): Addis Ababa; 19–23 October, 1994", ICFTU/ITUC archives.

[96] Ages Mukupa to Andrew Kailembo, 5 October 1994, ICFTU/ITUC archives.

[97] "Report of Mediation," Sunmonu, ICFTU/ITUC archives.

of them had allegedly threatened the chairman of the audit commission at gunpoint.[98] Following a walkout by 29 dissenting members of the council, including Mekuria, Dawey suspended them on disciplinary grounds.

In the executive committee, the majority—six out of nine members—sided with CETU's president.[99] This was also the case in the General Council, where 79 out of 108 delegates sided with the leadership.[100] But among the leaders of the industrial federations, six out of nine remained within the dissenting group.[101] The dissenters created a parallel structure of pro-government unionists, labelling themselves the 'Peace and Free Trade Union Seeking Members of CETU's Supreme Council' (PFTUSM). They asserted that under the prevailing circumstances of open division, no one was mandated to act or speak in the name of CETU. The dissenting group sought MoLSA's intervention, assuming correctly that the government would support it. Five federation presidents[102] affiliated with the group even suggested that MoLSA should intervene and cancel CETU's registration altogether,[103] thus nullifying the organisational efforts and gains of the prior years.[104] The dissenting faction produced a document listing its grievances, which included the allegation that Dawey was seeking to 'direct the labour movement to

[98] Dawey Ibrahim, discussion.

[99] "Report on Mission to Ethiopia, 4–8th November," Robinson H. Sikazwe, 1994, ICFTU/ITUC archives.

[100] "Crisis in the Union and Arrests," *Indian Ocean Newsletter* 640 (October 1, 1994).

[101] Ibid.

[102] Namely those of the Energy Chemicals, Petroleum and Minerals Trade Union Federation; Food, Beverages and Tobacco Trade Unions Federation; Transport and Communications Trade Unions Federations; Tourism, Hotels and General Service Trade Unions Industrial Federation; and Agriculture, Fishery and Agro-Industrial Trade Unions Federation.

[103] This account was given by the Minister of Labour and Social Affairs in the court. The Ethiopian Human Rights Council corroborated the claim that the dissenting federation presidents petitioned for the cancellation of the Confederation. However, in spite of such evidence, the presidents of the dissenting federations would later claim that they had been opposed to deregistration in principle. EHRCO, *Democracy, Rule of Law, and Human Rights in Ethiopia*, 63; Haileselassie Abraha et al. to ILO Director General, letter from presidents of six industrial federations, 20 January 1995, ICFTU/ITUC archives.

[104] "Report of Mediation", Sunmonu, ICFTU/ITUC archives; "Civil Case No 4/94, December 12, 1994," translation of court order from the Central High Court, ICFTU/ITUC archives.

serve the interests of the opposition forces',[105] that their suspension from the Executive Committee were motivated by ethnic discrimination, and that CETU's leadership had embarked on a campaign 'mobilising support of rank and file members travelling throughout the country, dividing the movement on the ground of ethnic grouping'.[106] The open split did indeed generate activity on both sides. CETU's leadership decided to call an extraordinary congress to resolve the situation, and this required coordination with unions throughout the country. The leadership claimed that it had secured a quorum and a majority in the General Council for suspending the 29 dissenting members, rendering the minority's opposition irrelevant to its legal right to call a congress. But instead of a congress, what followed was a prolonged court process punctuated by repeated mediation attempts and accompanied by a government prohibition on CETU from conducting any activities.

According to one observer, 'prolonged litigation suited the members of the pro-system faction', and the manner in which they acted seemed to corroborate that interpretation.[107] OATUU's Secretary General Hassan Sunmonu, who travelled to Ethiopia in late October 1994 to seek to mediate differences, returned frustrated by the group's obstructive tactics. 'I observed', Sunmonu reported, 'that the CETU president and his group were genuinely ready and willing to negotiate with the other group in order to peacefully resolve the crisis'.[108] 'On the other hand', Sunmonu noted, 'the dramatis personae of the other group, namely, Mekuria Gebremedhin, CETU secretary general, did not attend the two sessions of the reconciliation meeting'. From Mekuria's reluctance to attend the meetings and the dissenting group's unwillingness to agree even on an agenda for the discussions, Sunmonu concluded that 'it was apparent that [the dissenting group's delegation] either had no full mandate to negotiate or they were negotiating in bad faith'.[109] Such a mandate could

[105] The fact that opposition parties released statements in support of CETU's independence may have contributed to this interpretation. "Report on Mission to Ethiopia, 4–8th November," Robinson H. Sikazwe, 1994, ICFTU/ITUC archives.

[106] National Committee of Peace and Free Trade Union Seeking Members of CETU's General Council to Andrew Kailembo, 1 November 1994, ICFTU/ITUC archives.

[107] Praeg, *Ethiopia*, 187.

[108] "Report of Mediation," Sunmonu, ICFTU/ITUC archives.

[109] This interpretation was supported by ICFTU representative Sikazwe, who opined that 'it can be safely concluded that covert government support to Dawey's rivals is

only have come from the EPRDF's proletarian branches' leadership—but that was an institution whose existence Sunmonu was not aware of. Meanwhile, the dissenting group encouraged all constituent unions to boycott the upcoming extraordinary congress of CETU, and several basic union leaders under its sway publicly announced their intention to do so.[110] It was becoming obvious that the group that called itself the Peace and Free Trade Union Seeking Members was seeking neither a negotiated resolution nor a resolution based on a congress majority. Instead, it sought direct government intervention.

The failure of attempts to reconcile the groups meant that the point of dispute shifted to the question of whether to bring the issue to the General Assembly for resolution. While CETU's leadership argued that this was the most procedurally correct and democratic option, the dissenting faction sought to prevent a General Assembly meeting by all means. The government, perhaps unsurprisingly, intervened on the dissenting group's side. Four days before an extraordinary congress was to be held, uniformed and plain-clothed police, sent by the Ministry of Internal Affairs, arrived at CETU's headquarters. They occupied the president's office and forbade CETU's General Council from conducting a preparatory meeting that its members had already arrived for.[111] This intervention was followed, a few days later, by a complete prohibition on CETU from conducting any form of activities, including holding meetings or accessing its offices, vehicles, and funds.[112] Sources claimed that government intervention was triggered by the expectation that a

responsible for their belligerent conduct'. "Report on the Mission to Ethiopia, 30th January to 1 February 1995," Robinson H. Sikazwe, p. 6, ICFTU/ITUC archives.

[110] See Tamene, "Officials Prepare"; and "Trying to Get Them Into Step," *Indian Ocean Newsletter* 646 (November 21, 1994). The overwhelming evidence and documentation (see, for example, the explicit statements to this end in "Trade Union Federation Calls for Boycotting General Assembly," *Ethiopian Herald* 26 October 1994;. "Federation of Trade Unions Opposes Convening of General Assembly," *Ethiopian Herald* 27 October 1994; and "Federation Voice Opposition to CETU General Assembly," *Ethiopian Herald* 28 October 1994) of the dissenting group's opposition to the holding of the proposed congress did not stop its representatives from attempting to convince visiting foreign trade unionists, a few years later, that it was CETU's leadership that refused to call a congress. "Mission to Addis Ababa, Ethiopia, 18–20 January 1996," H.J. Schwass, ICFTU/ITUC archives.

[111] Dawey Ibrahim to Enzo Frizo, 31 October 1994, ICFTU/ITUC archives; EHRCO, *Democracy, Rule of Law, and Human Rights in Ethiopia*, 64.

[112] Dawey Ibrahim to Enzo Frizo, 3 November 1994, ICFTU/ITUC archives.

majority of delegates 'would have called for strikes against the structural adjustment, and would have endorsed the expulsion of the government group'.[113] Whether that would have occurred or not is not known, but the government's action clearly demonstrated that it was operating under the assumption that the outcome of a congress would be detrimental to its interests, as represented in the labour movement by the PFTUSM faction.

An ICFTU representative, arriving at CETU's headquarters on the morning of the scheduled congress, learned that no fewer than 30 police officers and MoLSA officials had locked and sealed CETU's offices.[114] The officials argued that they were enforcing a court order suspending CETU's activities, which had been issued at the request of MoLSA. MoLSA, in turn, had been petitioned to request the court order by the dissenting PFTUSM group.[115] According to MoLSA's vice minister, 'the intervention was required to keep industrial peace'.[116] However, MoLSA issued an additional threat of its own, announcing its intention to cancel CETU's registration altogether if the matter was not speedily resolved.[117] In the absence of a congress, however, such a resolution never seemed likely, and the government's intervention only strengthened the resolve of the dissenting faction, which now explicitly insisted on government mediation alone. This unhelpful stance, a visiting ICFTU representative reported, 'gives merit to the fear that the group may be buying time so as to allow the one-month suspension notice to elapse and therefore give the government an excuse to withdraw CETU's registration and establish a "conformist" organisation'.[118]

[113] Tamene, "Officials Prepare".

[114] Robinson H. Sikazwe to ICFTU General Secretary, 4 November 1994, ICFTU/ITUC archives; "Report on Mission to Ethiopia, 4–8th November, 1994," Robinson H. Sikazwe, ICFTU/ITUC archives.

[115] "A Reply to an Allegation Submitted by OATUU Against the Transitional Government of Ethiopia Regarding the Confederation of Ethiopian Trade Unions (CETU)," Ministry of Labour and Social Affairs memorandum, MoLSA Archives; "Report on Mission to Ethiopia, 4–8th November," Robinson H. Sikazwe, 1994, ICFTU/ITUC archives.

[116] Tamene, "Officials Prepare".

[117] Robinson H. Sikazwe to Bill Jordan, 6 March 1995, ICFTU/ITUC archives.

[118] Ibid.

Before cancelling CETU's registration, MoLSA engaged in a mediation attempt. But the government was hardly a credible arbitrator. It was openly accusing CETU's leadership of being agents of the opposition. Meanwhile, representatives of its favoured PFTUSM faction were in the habit of turning up to meetings in government-plated vehicles and issued with permits to carry arms.[119] Unsurprisingly, MoLSA's mediating efforts failed—not least because the ministry insisted that CETU must first acknowledge that its suspension of the 29 Supreme Council members was illegal and reinstate them.[120] This demand played directly into the dissenting faction's purposes. At the expiration of the one-month notice period, MoLSA announced the deregistration of CETU.[121] Although a court order ruled that MoLSA's actions were 'inappropriate' and instructed the ministry to allow CETU to reopen its offices,[122] the government simply refused to heed the court order.[123]

MoLSA henceforth refused to recognise the legality of CETU's higher bodies, since the organisation was considered dissolved,[124] and opted instead to only interact with the federations, where a majority of leaders

[119] "Conclusion of the ICFTU AFRO Mission to Ethiopia, 9–12 May, 1995," Andrew Kailembo, report, ICFTU/ITUC archives; "Mission to Addis Ababa, Ethiopia, 18–20 January 1996," H.J. Schwass, ICFTU/ITUC archives.

[120] The argument was that after the walkout of the dissenters, the necessary quorum of three-fourths of delegates was not present. That argument was rejected by CETU, which pointed out that the meeting began with 94 out of 106 delegates present. "Trade Union Situation in Ethiopia: Factual Documentation," CETU memorandum, 1995, MoLSA archives; "The Legal Aspect of the Dispute Between the Two Factions of the Confederation of Ethiopian Trade Unions (CETU) and the Position of the Transitional Government of Ethiopia in this Respect," Dessalegn Mesfin, 1995,p. 2, MoLSA archives.

[121] "The Legal Aspect of the Dispute Between the Two Factions of the Confederation of Ethiopian Trade Unions (CETU) and the Position of the Transitional Government of Ethiopia in this Respect," Dessalegn Mesfin, 1995, MoLSA archives.

[122] Wossenyeleh Denekew to CETU Federations, 30 Jan 1995, MoLSA archives; "Trade Union Situation in Ethiopia: Factual Documentation," CETU memorandum, 1995, p. 34, MoLSA archives; "Civil Case No 4/94," Central High Court, ICFTU/ITUC archives.

[123] This indifference to a court decision convinced OATUU that the government 'aimed, without any doubt, at repressing CETU and finally, subjugating the trade union movement at a time when the situation of Ethiopian workers is seriously threatened'. Organisation of African Trade Union Unity to the Director General of the ILO, 10 February 1995, MoLSA archives.

[124] A couple of weeks after it had criticised the minister for acting outside of his jurisdiction in closing CETU offices and requested it to be reopened, however, the court,

were dissenters. Without any basis in either CETU by-laws or labour legislation, MoLSA instructed the federations to establish a joint interim committee to administer the confederation's assets.[125] This measure marked the beginning of efforts to reorganise CETU into an 'appendage confederation', according to its president at the time.[126] An ICFTU representative on a mission to Ethiopia appeared to be of the same view, writing that 'the setting up of an interim committee by the Ministry of Labour is a clear sign of government's intention to reorganise CETU in order to install its own people into trade union leadership'.[127] MoLSA would face frustration as the legality of this open intervention was rejected by the courts, but it nevertheless indicated the extent to which the government was willing to go to see to it that CETU was subjugated.

Meanwhile, supporters of CETU's autonomy faced persecution. In mid-November, Dawey wrote to the ICFTU claiming that CETU delegates had been refused exit visas to attend meetings abroad.[128] Moreover, he reported that harassment of workers' representatives by police and security forces was ongoing across the country. This included arrests, dismissals, suspensions, and forced removals of labour leaders, as well as surveillance and intimidation of representatives, and even physical

faced with the deregistration of CETU, closed the case on the basis of the dissolution of the latter.

[125] Wossenyeleh Denekew to CETU Federations, 30 Jan 1995, MoLSA archives.

The leadership of the three industrial federations aligned with CETU's leadership rejected the call to join the interim committee, and the court eventually ruled to affirm that MoLSA had no legal grounds to ask CETU to set up such a body. "Report on the Mission to Ethiopia, 30th January to 1 February 1995," Robinson H. Sikazwe, ICFTU/ ITUC archives; Robinson H. Sikazwe to Elias J. Mashasi, 28 November 1995, ICFTU/ ITUC archives.

[126] Dawey Ibrahim to ILO Director General, 3 January 1995, MoLSA archives.

[127] "Mission to Ethiopia, 30th January to 1 February 1995," Sikazwe, p. 7, ICFTU/ ITUC archives.

[128] Dawey Ibrahim to ICFTU, 14 November 1994, MoLSA archives.

assault.[129] Combined with the ban preventing CETU from holding meetings or calling a congress, these measures were aimed at 'paralysing the trade union movement'—a purpose for which the government had allegedly 'mobilised all its resources'.[130]

In early 1995, Dawey had concluded that MoLSA was 'waging a war of annihilation against the confederation'.[131] By this time, 80 out of 108 Supreme Council members had reported being subjected to harassment or intimidation.[132] At least nine union leaders had been victims of unlawful dismissals, and in EELPA alone, some 80 rank-and-file union members had also been let go. But the occurrence of repression and the gravity of the threat it posed would only increase in the months that followed. By early 1995, two senior CETU officials had fled abroad, citing 'persistent persecution', and in March that year, two labour leaders from EELPA also crossed the Kenyan border into exile.[133] A few months later, the president of the Federation of Commerce, Technical and Printing Industry Trade Unions presented the following testimony to the workers' group of the International Labour Conference in Geneva:

> [The government] has removed trade union leaders from their positions in unions forcefully, through political means, dismissal, forced resignation etc. Up to now 73 trade union leaders have lost their leadership without the consent and willingness of members. It has waged [a] massive terrorisation campaign, has physically assaulted the vice president of the confederation, has interrogated, harassed, intimidated, surveyed and imprisoned

[129] Ibid.; "Trade Union Situation in Ethiopia: Factual Documentation," CETU memorandum, 1995, MoLSA archives.

The vice president of CETU had been attacked on his way home from the office in May 1994 and spent a week hospitalised. Fekadu Tenkir, a CETU Executive Committee member and president of the union of the Ethiopian Insurance Corporation, claimed to have been beaten by eight opponents while presiding over the annual congress of the union in March 1997. Fekadu Tenkir to Protection Office, UNHCR Branch Office Kenya, Nairobi, 7 May 1997, ICFTU/ITUC archives; "Trade Union Situation in Ethiopia: Factual Documentation," CETU memorandum, 1995, p. 15–16, MoLSA archives.

[130] Dawey Ibrahim to ICFTU, 14 November 1994, MoLSA archives.

[131] Dawey Ibrahim to OATUU, 16 February 1995, MoLSA archives.

[132] Dawey Ibrahim to ICFTU, 10 October 1994, ICFTU/ITUC archives.

[133] "Mission to Ethiopia, 30th January to 1 February 1995," Sikazwe, ICFTU/ITUC archives; Robinson H. Sikazwe to Bill Jordan, 6 March 1995, ICFTU/ITUC archives.

> union leaders and their families. As a result of this campaign some of our colleagues are forced to leave their country and run into exile.[134]

CETU's application for ICFTU-affiliation, lodged in June 1994, was left pending. Because of the turmoil that engulfed CETU in the following months, the ICFTU's Executive Board meeting in December that year decided to suspend the admission process. The ICFTU had 'strongly condemned' the deregistration of CETU, which it argued represented 'a naked aggression by the authorities against the autonomy and independence of the Ethiopian trade union movement'.[135] It had also protested the government's non-adherence to court orders obliging it to reopen CETU's offices, allow its officials to carry out their tasks, return requisitioned property, and unfreeze its bank accounts.[136] In early 1995, the ICFTU began extending relief and legal support funds to CETU.[137] However, the provision of such funds was limited, both in terms of volume and duration. Moreover, it was apparent that the international trade union movement was split on the issue. While the ICFTU, the Canadian Labour Congress, and initially the OATUU offered CETU some financial and political support, the AALC, represented by Fissehatsion Tekie, was considered sympathetic to the pro-government faction, and was financing activities of its six federations.[138]

Similarly to what transpired in the 1970s, a protracted process of establishing new submissive and government-aligned trade union structures ensued. The one significant difference was that in the 1990s it was accompanied by considerably less violence. First, the government backed

[134] "Speech Delivered by Mr Hailu Ourgessa, Representative of the Confederation of Ethiopian Trade Unions, At the 82nd Session of the International Labour Conference Workers' Group Meeting, June 15, 1995, Geneva," transcription of speech, Hailu Ourgessa's private collection.

[135] "Statement on the Deregistration of the Confederation of Ethiopian Trade Unions (CETU)," ICFTU statement, ICFTU/ITUC archives.

[136] Bill Jordan to Meles Zenawi, telefax via Embassy of Ethiopia in Brussels, 21 February 1995, ICFTU/ITUC archives.

[137] "Acknowledgement and Report on Relief Fund," Dawey Ibrahim to ICFTU AFRO, 1 February 1995, MoLSA archives. "Legal Assistance Reference Confederation of Ethiopian Trade Unions (CETU)," André Dewil to Dessalegn Mesifin, 27 January 1995, ICFTU/ITUC archives.

[138] "Mission to Ethiopia, 30th January to 1 February 1995," Sikazwe, p. 5, ICFTU/ITUC archives 5.

the dissenting faction in establishing an ad-hoc committee at the level the latter was dominant: among the leaders of the industrial federations. Then, state-aligned actors began to campaign for the ouster of workers' representatives deemed disloyal at the basic union level. 'New committees were set up in factories' throughout the country, it was reported.[139] A representative of the International Federation of Employees, Technicians and Managers visiting Ethiopia at the time reported that the government was using every means, including 'intimidation, harassment and bribes' in order to 'capture' resistant unions.[140] At the Fincha sugar plant, for example, local authorities removed nine members of the trade union's executive committee for having refused to denounce CETU's leadership.[141] By 1995, resistant workers' representatives were reported to have been removed, dismissed, arrested, or transferred from dozens of workplaces.[142] The dismissed and arrested representatives included members of CETU's Supreme Council and Executive Committee. CETU's president Dawey was himself briefly detained in 1995.[143] He was subsequently ousted from the leadership of the basic union and federation he represented, in decreed re-elections he was not permitted to stand for. For the ICFTU's representative, this indicated 'that the government [was] making serious inroads in the trade unions and swaying the rank and file support to its side'.[144] At the federation level, the leaders who remained aligned with CETU's Executive Committee also came under additional pressure. The following excerpts from an Ethiopian Human Rights Council report illustrate the type of subterfuge and force that facilitated the take-over of the remaining federations:

[139] Praeg, *Ethiopia*, 187.

[140] "Mission to Addis Ababa, Ethiopia, 18–20 January 1996," H.J. Schwass, ICFTU/ITUC archives.

[141] "Trade Union Situation in Ethiopia: Factual Documentation," CETU memorandum, 1995, MoLSA archives.

[142] "Trade Union Situation in Ethiopia: Factual Documentation," CETU memorandum, 1995, p. 21–26, MoLSA archives; Dawey Ibrahim to ILO Director General, 3 January 1995, MoLSA archives.

[143] Dawey was detained three times that year, on each occasion between 8 and 10 hours. Dawey Ibrahim to Protection Office, UNHCR Branch Office Kenya, Nairobi, 8 May 1997, ICFTU/ITUC archives.

[144] Robinson H. Sikazwe to Andrew Kailembo, 5 October 1995, ICFTU/ITUC archives.

> On October 19, 1996, the [Commerce, Technical and Printing Industry] Federation's 152 Council members representing 47 member plant unions held a meeting. … [On] October 20, about 30 factionalists began to stir trouble by demanding that the Federation's Executive Committee give up the podium and submit themselves to a *gimgema* (assessment) of their performance. When the other Council members rejected their unprocedural demand, the former began shouting and prevented the meeting from proceeding smoothly. In order to avoid the break-out of violence, it was decided to adjourn the meeting. However, 30 of these factionalists remained behind and tried to proceed with the discussion on their own. At this time the Executive Committee of the Federation reported the matter to [a] police station and the latter evicted the factionalists from the meeting hall. On the evening of October 21, however, Ethiopian Radio and Television reported an incredible piece of news. The official media falsely claimed that at its meeting of October 19–21, the Federation of the Commercial, Technical and Printing Federation rejected the reports of the Executive Committee as well as Audit Committee, replaced these committees' members by newly elected ones and passed a resolution demanding that CETU be newly re-organised. Following this false report on the official media, [the] deputy minister of labour and social affairs, wrote a letter on November 4, 1996 giving recognition to the newly "elected" leaders.[145]
>
> Having secured the government's support, the "new federation leaders", accompanied by two policemen, went to the head office of the Federation where they found Ato Mulatu Gurmu, the legitimate treasurer, working alone in his office. They assaulted him physically, took away from him the keys of his drawers and office, his personal notebook and money, and then evicted him by force from the office. They also broke into the other offices of the Federation and thus staged their coup. Surprisingly though, two of these "new federation leaders" do not belong to any member plant union and hence are not even members of the Federation.

On the level of basic unions too, foul play facilitated the process of removing resistant leaderships. In several cases, MoLSA and its bureaus simply refused to recognise elected leaders of basic unions or asserted that their terms had expired. MoLSA also prohibited some basic unions

[145] Ethiopian Human Rights Council, *The Violation of Human Rights in Ethiopia: 11th Report of* EHRCO (Addis Ababa: EHRCO, 1996), 5–6.

from meeting, or carrying out activities altogether, until the election of an approvable leadership was arranged.

In January 1997, sufficient preparatory work in overturning resisting unions and federations had been conducted to ensure that the government-sanctioned process of reorganising CETU could commence in earnest. That month, eight of the nine industrial federations met and formed a coordinating committee to do so. Between April 22 and 24, these eight federations held a general congress and reconstituted CETU with a new leadership. A new confederation, devoid of any assertive ambitions, was born. Its novelty was illustrated by the fact that its entire executive committee—save one member—consisted of new electees.[146] An observer to the congress concluded that 'manoeuvres from the Ethiopian government have paid off'. But while 'on the surface everything seemed rosy', it was also reported that 'a lot of behind-the-scene moves' took place.[147] The risk that an unpleasant surprise, like that of the 1994 congress, would reoccur in the elections of officeholders was thus eliminated. Rather than a celebration of trade union democracy, the ICFTU's observer of the congress reported that it marked 'the climax of interference by the Ethiopian government into CETU affairs'.[148]

By the time of the congress, some parties of the international trade union movement had begun to argue that since the supporters of the dissenting group were now in the majority, they could no longer be ignored.[149] The AALC had made its approval of what transpired explicit, delivering an address to the congress and pledging to work with the new confederation.[150] But OATUU[151] and ILO had also 'in effect given

[146] "The 8th General Congress of the Ethiopian Trade Unions (CETU) (Addis Ababa, 22–24 April, 1997)," report, Lawrence Egulu, ICFTU/ITUC archives.

[147] Andrew Kailembo to Bill Jordan General Secretary, 5 June 1997, ICFTU/ITUC archives.

[148] "The 8th General Congress," Egulu, ICFTU/ITUC archives.

[149] Andrew Kailembo to Bill Jordan, 10 April 1997, ICFTU/ITUC archives.

[150] Andrew Kailembo to Bill Jordan General Secretary, 5 June 1997, ICFTU/ITUC archives; "The 8th General Congress," Egulu, ICFTU/ITUC archives.

[151] With regard to OATUU, the change of heart of its general secretary, Sunmonu, appears to have been sudden and spectacular. He was reported to have told congress delegates not to 'disappoint Africa, *your government* and OATUU' [emphasis added], and to have promised them to assert pressure on the absent Bank and Insurance Federation to join them and to work with the government. "The 8th General Congress," Egulu, p. 2, ICFTU/ITUC archives.

recognition to the new leadership'.[152] And some officials in the ICFTU, such as its regional secretary Andrew Kailembo, were likewise keen to mend fences.[153] 'We should also recognise', Kailembo wrote, 'the fact that the government has succeeded in breaking up CETU and making it a pro-government organ'.[154] It would take the ICFTU another five years to fully normalise relations with CETU.

A False Dawn

The re-establishment of a national trade union centre in 1993 had been hailed by those present as the culmination of years of efforts by workers and representatives. Senior leaders believed that the government's attempts to control the new confederation had been defeated at CETU's formative congress. The establishment of CETU was expected to usher in an era of genuine and independent Ethiopian trade unionism. However, this optimism proved short-lived. Within just a few years, all that had been achieved was reversed, and firm government control had been restored. In fact, whereas CETU may not have been as directly tethered to the state apparatus as the AETU/ETU was, by 1997 its relationship with the government was not fundamentally different from that of its predecessor. The reasons why the attempt to create an autonomous trade union centre failed require explanation.

The most apparent explanation emerges from the role of the state. 'History repeats itself', Dawey presciently observed in 1994.[155] 'The confederation at its inception, is confronted with such difficulties as infringements of trade union rights [and] violent repression of its activities'.[156] 'Unfortunately', he continued, 'the Transitional Government

[152] Andrew Kailembo to Bill Jordan General Secretary, 5 June 1997, ICFTU/ITUC archives.

[153] "Mission to Addis Ababa, Ethiopia, 18–20 January 1996," H.J. Schwass, ICFTU/ITUC archives; Andrew Kailembo to Bill Jordan General Secretary, 5 June 1997, ICFTU/ITUC archives; Andrew Kailembo to Bill Jordan, 10 April 1997, ICFTU/ITUC archives.

[154] Andrew Kailembo to Bill Jordan General Secretary, 5 June 1997, ICFTU/ITUC archives.

[155] Dawey Ibrahim to ICFTU, 10 October 1994, ICFTU/ITUC archives.

[156] The references to the past and to events discussed in the previous chapter were manifold. According to Hailu Ourgessa, members of Mekuria's PFTUSM faction referred to the seventh floor of the CETU building—where the intransigent Federations of

of Ethiopia and/or the party in power has [since the beginning] been engaged in outright suppression of the confederation with a view to make it its own wing'. The motive of the government, he alleged, was to 'formally subordinate the confederation to the control of the party in power so that it will play the role of a transmission belt'. Indeed, in this respect, there was a strong sense of history repeating itself.

The methods of re-establishing state control were also well-tested. They included the refusal to register or recognise large unions—such as those of the Akaki Textile and Garment Factories and the Ethio-Fibre factory—that were considered resistant; interference in the internal processes of constituent unions; dismissal of union representatives; refusal to turn over union property held by the government; derogatory mass media campaigns; and harassment and intimidation of workers' representatives. They also included support for a dissenting faction from within the movement, exploiting and fomenting internal divisions. The TGE 'had done all its preparatory job to draw its stooges in the movement so that it [would] fight from within to pursue its political ends' a CETU document read.[157] 'By monopolising the leadership of the Organising Committee the pro-government members succeeded in holding federations executive leaderships through rigged elections', it stated. 'Among the nine federations they succeeded in holding majority positions in five, which now sparked the split'. However, as plausible as these allegations appeared, the methods were old. CETU's predecessor, CELU, had been subjected to the same tactics in the 1970s, when Alem Abdi had played the role of the internal spoiler, providing the pretext for government intervention. However, Alem Abdi was ousted, and the government was forced to retreat. Externally driven divisions and splits alone, at least, are not sufficient to explain the demise of the autonomous labour movement.

CETU had no effective external allies in the 1990s and was not part of any broader social coalition or popular movement. There were occasional

Commerce, Technical and Printing Industry and of Banking and Insurance had their offices—as 'Assimba', the name of the mountain base of the EPRP's army in the 1970s, denoting the accusation that those federations were somehow linked to the latter. Moreover, Hailu recalls that members of the government-aligned faction 'reminded us many times that this area, this building, this trade union movement, is used to blood, telling us that blood might flow if we follow the same line'. Hailu Ourgessa, discussion.

157 "Trade Union Situation in Ethiopia: Factual Documentation," CETU memorandum, 1995, p. 10, MoLSA archives.

symbolic expressions of support for trade union freedom from opposition groups, but the weakness and vulnerability of those groups was so glaring that any affiliation—even by association—was deemed likely to become a liability rather than an asset by CETU's leadership. That is not to say that there were no individual labour representatives who came to join these groups—just as some would join the ruling party. However, real support from these groups was neither deemed plausible nor desirable. CETU's leaders were informed by what they considered the pitfalls of the past. Excessive proximity to political parties—both the EPRP and the ruling WPE, albeit in different ways—was considered to have brought disaster to the movement in the 1970s and 1980s. The leaders were therefore convinced that they needed to jealously guard whatever autonomy the trade union movement had acquired. When opposition parties sought to call a demonstration against government attacks on the movement, CETU's leadership interpreted it as an attempt by politicians to 'hijack' the struggle over the labour movement and therefore refused to participate.[158] Autonomy was considered a virtue and a strength that was dependent on organisational detachment, and any relationship with opposition groups would have likely invited immediate repression in any case. But organisational detachment could also be viewed as an obvious weakness that led to isolation.[159]

When the eventual assault on the trade union movement began in earnest, the latter offered little resistance. The isolated and vulnerable strategic position the movement occupied likely contributed to the cautiousness and restraint exercised by the leadership—including its reluctance to call a general strike. There had been strong support for such a course of action from some basic unions. CETU leaders acknowledged that they were coming under intense pressure 'from every direction' in the movement, including rank-and-file members and representatives, to call a strike.[160] Several basic unions expressed their willingness to call out their members. And there were corresponding government fears that a general strike was looming. CETU received repeated warnings and threats from authorities that should it call such a strike, it would 'be the end of

[158] Hailu Ourgessa, discussion.

[159] There were common initiatives with the ETA, but nothing that moved much beyond the issuance of joint press statements.

[160] Hailu Ourgessa, discussion.

it'.[161] But in the end, the decision against calling a strike came down to the leadership. 'On our part', one federation president acknowledged 'we were not ready to call a general strike because we had just been in office for few months [and] we had not even finished going to the basic trade unions to introduce ourselves when the government started attacking us'.[162] Calling a strike, the leadership reasoned, was an 'ultimate' option for which it did not consider itself ready.[163]

CETU's leadership was convinced that it needed to pursue a legal path, even when making tentative plans for the possibility of a strike. The General Council decided to do so by collecting union representatives' signatures in support of action.[164] However, several of CETU's messengers responsible for gathering signatures from basic unions were arrested. The legal path to a strike was further narrowed when the ban was imposed on CETU. However unlikely it was that the concerned judicial institutions would ever have permitted CETU to organise a strike in the first place, the option of calling an extra-legal general strike was never seriously entertained. 'We [were] the ones who said "do not do it"', one member of the central leadership acknowledged. 'We were not strong enough to go in that direction'.[165]

Once the repression had begun, a senior official has claimed, workers 'mounted a very determined resistance to keep their local trade unions'.[166] However, this resistance lacked the central coordination that CELU's resurrection commmittee and ELAMA had provided in the 1970s. Rather, workers and trade union representatives were left to fend for themselves in dispersed local struggles where the balance of forces was tilted decisively against them. In most cases, this bred resignation, defeat, and eventual surrender to imposed trade union structures, employers, and management.

In the early 1990s, the labour movement had autonomously and spontaneously produced networks and informal mechanisms. These networks bore striking similarities to those that emerged before the founding of

[161] Ibid.

[162] Ibid.

[163] Ibid.

[164] Dawey Ibrahim, discussion.

[165] Hailu Ourgessa, discussion.

[166] Ibid.

CELU in 1963, during the labour opposition of the late 1960s and early 1970s, and after the dissolution of CELU in 1975. However, the spontaneity of these networks and their failure to crystallise into proper organisational structures contributed to CETU's failure to exhibit the same kind of tenacity and dynamism that the labour movement had in the 1960s and 1970s. The absence of central coordination atomised resistance, rendering it ineffective once the formal institutions of CETU had been incapacitated. That facilitated the process of asserting government control over the movement.

Meanwhile, the ruling party was also organising clandestine networks—primarily through its proletarian branches—and it was intervening in the affairs of the movement long before it had developed a determination to suppress it outright. Much as in previous decades, this did not immediately generate the outcomes intended. Instead, the government's high-handedness fostered resentment and determination among the workers. One union leader reflected on this period:

> The agenda that the government pushed on labour united labour itself. They went from union to union with the same agenda. Every union was angered, every union was against this. We did not want [a dependent confederation]. The previous trade union of the Derg – we hated it. It was not a trade union. Did we want to have the same thing again? That was the issue. We didn't want to have a party-controlled trade union. That was basic. That was the thing that united us.[167]

State intervention, then, again created its own counterforce in moving workers to resist. As workers began to organise, state-aligned actors commenced a process of restructuring, purging old officials, and selecting new candidates, which was strikingly similar to the process that preceded the formation of AETU, even if less violent. Just like in the initial phases of the reorganisation of the trade union movement under the AETU in 1975 and 1976, however, the government's aims initially proved elusive. The representatives elected by basic unions and the national leadership appointed by these representatives proved unwilling to submit and go against the most basic interests of the workers: retaining their jobs and pay.

[167] Ibid., abridged.

'It is not known', a journalist reporting on the tribulations of CETU in the mid-1990s wrote, 'why the government has been so determined to oust a popularly elected leader'.[168] But determined it was. And it is probably not too far-fetched to assume that its determination was related to the potential of an autonomous labour movement. Not necessarily only, as the journalist speculated, 'for it to become a conduit for opposition groups', but also for it to become an effective instrument for the defence of workers' interests, at a time when government policy aligned with the IMF's notorious SAP programmes.

Another Interregnum

The reassertion of control over the trade union movement had repercussions. The Ethiopian government was severely criticised for its actions, both domestically and internationally.[169] But judging by its subsequent use of similar methods against other organisations it disapproved of,[170] it appeared that the government considered the outcome well worth the price. For CETU, however, the fallout from its resultant lack of legitimacy would continue to linger. 'New CETU' appeared fundamentally illegitimate. There were palpable doubts over the degree to which it represented the interests of Ethiopian workers at all. In 2001, an Ethiopian newspaper ridiculed CETU's president Amare Alemayehu's assertion that CETU 'does not believe that strikes can resolve industrial disputes'.[171] This standpoint of CETU, the author argued, hollowed the constitutional right to strike, 'outrageously disparage[d] the great sacrifices of workers in Ethiopia', and posed questions as to whose interests CETU's leadership really represented.[172]

168 Tamene, "Officials Prepare".

169 See EHRCO, *Democracy, Rule of Law, and Human Rights in Ethiopia*; EHRCO, *The Violation of Human Rights in Ethiopia*, and the reports and protest letters from OATUU (1995) and ICFTU cited in the above.

170 In subsequent years, both civil society organisations—such as the Ethiopian Teachers' Association—and a number of legally registered political parties found themselves having offices closed, bank accounts blocked, splits fomented, and courts' rulings favouring the dissenting faction issued against them, in a similar fashion.

171 John W. [pseud.], "An Opponent of Strikes in Charge of a Labour Union," *Reporter* 5 no. 241 (18 April 2001).

172 Ibid.

As a result of its lack of legitimacy and its unwillingness to make any assertive stands, the confederation remained unpopular with workers. Aggregate membership in affiliated unions declined over the 1990s and the first half of the 2000s. When the ICFTU sent a mission to Ethiopia in 2000, they found that membership in the Industrial Federation of Banking and Insurance Trade Unions alone had decreased from 21,000 to 9,000 following the repression it had faced.[173] The industrial scene was tranquil. But the tranquillity was not rooted in contentment but in dispirited and disarmed workers. The nadir was probably reached in the first couple of years of the 2000s, when the US Department of State reported that 'allegations of widespread corruption within CETU's leadership ranks and of CETU's close ties to the Government [had] paralysed the organisation'.[174] The ICFTU's *Annual Survey of Violations of Trade Union Rights* for 2002 found that 'the government blatantly interferes in trade union affairs in all sectors', with 'many trade union leaders [having] been removed from their posts and/or forced to leave the country'.[175] It stated that 'trade union leaders are still being sent to prison because they sought to protect their rights, while many more are sacked simply for forming a trade union'.[176]

By 2003, however, it appeared that the forceful removal of basic union leaders had come to a halt. The US Department of State reported that 'government interference in unions' nevertheless continued. It was described in the following terms:

> CETU leadership was aligned with the ruling party and did not fight vigorously for workers' rights. Findings of widespread corruption in 2002 within CETU's leadership had not resulted in any disciplinary actions by year's end. In January, four members of CETU's nine-member executive committee, who criticised the majority five member block's decisions

[173] This federation was disproportionally severely affected, given that it had been the last one of the nine to resist a pro-government takeover. See "Report of the ICFTU mission to Ethiopia from 16 to 18 November 2000," Peer Coret to Members of the ICFTU Mission to Ethiopia, 17 December 2000, ICFTU AFRO archives.

[174] Department of State, *2002 Country Reports on Human Rights Practices*, (Washington DC: Joint Committee Print, 2003).

[175] This precise wording would reappear in each consecutive issue of the annual survey until, at the very least, 2012.

[176] ICFTU, *Annual Survey of Violations of Trade Union Rights 2003* (Brussels: ICFTU, 2003).

were forced from office and replaced by four members hand-picked by the Government.[177]

Simultaneously, however, there were signs that CETU was finally being aroused to some form of action, or at least a realisation that its continued silence was untenable. The pariah status it had acquired internationally was a source of embarrassment that became a factor propelling change. As CETU sought to regain membership in the ICFTU, it became obvious that it needed to improve its reputation. Meanwhile, the rank-and-file workers' disillusionment with the confederation also demanded addressing, which could only come in the form of greater assertiveness. A final factor pulling CETU in a more assertive direction was the political thaw that the end of warfare on the Ethio-Eritrean border[178] in 2000 ushered in. The government's intolerance and repressive practices were subsequently slightly relaxed, giving independent associations—temporarily at least—a somewhat greater degree of space. There was a pressing need to utilise the space that had presented itself. The organisation had lost all semblance of credibility and was the subject of ridicule. Membership was falling, and it was at severe risk of being rendered completely irrelevant.

CETU's 10th General Congress, held in July 2001, marked the beginning of this process. It issued a resolution condemning violations of workers' rights and cautiously requesting the government to initiate reform in a number of labour-related areas. These included the amendment of the labour law; expansion of the number of labour courts and labour relations boards; revision of salaries in government enterprises; dismissal of managers guilty of violating labour rights; an end to police interference in workers' activities; inclusion of workers in the privatisation process; and workers' representation in management boards.

A few months later, on November 2, 2001, CETU's Executive Committee met and issued a press statement. Reacting to several incidents of retrenchments and extra-legal dismissals, it argued that CETU was being forced into action 'by the worsening unlawful actions against

[177] Department of State, 2003 *Country Reports on Human Rights Practices* (Washington DC: Joint Committee Print, 2004).

[178] In June 2000, Ethiopia and Eritrea signed a cessation of hostilities agreement that put an end to the Ethio-Eritrean border war that had begun in May 1998.

the workers' and 'continue[d] violations of the rights of the workers'.[179] It condemned the 'evil deeds' of 'greedy and self-centred' employers and managers, who were accused of inflicting illegal damage on workers. 'Certain private enterprises owners and managements have continued in their violation of workers' rights more than ever before. These individuals have gone to the extent of using policemen... to suppress the workers' constitutional and labour proclamation rights', it lamented. In that respect, there was a novel political undertone in the statement. 'Workers and union leaders that are put to prison without due process of law simply because they raised protection of their rights and benefits, are not few in number', it stated. 'This situation', it read, 'indicates as if few individuals at the top of the hierarchy are mandated to suppress others'. The Executive Committee's statement ended with a warning. 'If our demands are to be neglected, we will be forced to advance our [constitutional] struggle to the next stage'. 'We call upon all Ethiopian workers to stand alongside of the struggles of CETU'.

Two days after CETU issued its statement, the Federation of Food, Beverages, Tobacco and Allied Trade Unions staged an unprecedented rally in Addis Ababa—with 7,000 workers participating. The federation warned the government that it would call a strike unless its demands were met. Those demands included the reinstatement of illegally dismissed employees; the protection of freedom of association; the revision of the labour law; and greater workers' participation in decision-making.[180] Then, on November 9, CETU's General Council held an extraordinary meeting to follow up on events. It reasserted the demands issued by CETU's July General Congress. The Council 'strongly urge[d] the government' to consider CETU's proposal for labour law amendment and likewise demanded that 'thousands of those workers unlawfully fired' should be reinstated or compensated. Moreover, it lent support to the demands raised by the Federation of Food, Beverages, Tobacco and Allied Trade Unions during its rally a few days earlier and demanded that they be addressed. Finally, it requested 'the immediate arrangement of a tripartite

[179] "Press Release by the Executive Committee of CETU", 9 November 2001, ICFTU AFRO archives.

[180] "Informing about the peaceful demonstration by the Federation of Food, Beverage, Tobacco and Allied Trade Unions," Wondafrash Tuffa to the International Union of Food, Agricultural, Hotel, Restaurant, Catering, Tobacco and Allied Workers' Associations' (IUF) Regional Secretariat, Nairobi, received 7 January 2002, ICFTU AFRO archives.

consultation forum to find out a common response to these demands'. 'Or else', it warned, CETU would 'be obliged to advance to the next legal protest for the respect of our rights'.[181] The General Council resolution and Executive Committee press statement of that month—combined with the rally organised by the Federation of Food, Beverages, Tobacco and Allied Trade Unions—marked the first real sign that CETU was earnestly attempting to shed its image of yellow unionism. At least it was beginning to sound like a genuine trade union organisation again.

CELU insisted that plans to call nationwide rallies were still in the making in 2002. However, they were cancelled after the government had initiated a process of revising the labour law and given the confederation a consultative role in handling privatisations. Plans that had purportedly been made for a strike were also abandoned. But although a CETU-backed general strike may not have been a realistic proposition, the mere mention of such plans had marked a clear change in CETU's language and in its playbook. In a similar shift towards a gradually more assertive approach, the confederation cautiously reopened the debate on the institution of a minimum wage—a demand that had been left to linger without a champion since the 1970s. CETU commissioned Addis Ababa University's economics department to conduct a study on the topic, which was released in 2004. The study argued for the institution of a minimum wage but recommended a floor that it would not allow workers to meet minimum nutritional needs.[182]

Meanwhile, in 2003, a revised labour law was promulgated by parliament. It included provisions that strengthened the position of individual workers facing dismissal or retrenchment, such as stipulations for severance pay and compensation. It also removed the prerogative of the government to dissolve trade unions, and it introduced changes that were designed to make dispute settlement easier and the Labour Relations Boards more effective. While the law thus implied somewhat of a strengthening of the position of individual workers, it included several stipulations that CETU interpreted as weakening collective labour rights and, therefore, leaving the overall balance of legislation tilted in favour

[181] "Final Resolution of the CETU General Council Extra-Ordinary Meeting," 9 November 2001, ICFTU AFRO archives.

[182] Addis Ababa University Economics Department, "Minimum Wage for Ethiopia: A Report for the Confederation of Ethiopian Trade Unions By Economics Department of Addis Ababa," (unpublished final report, June 2004).

of employers. Whereas CETU took credit for having influenced the government to some limited extent, the confederation was not entirely content.

On May Day 2004, CETU's cautiously growing assertiveness—albeit admittedly from a low base—was again on display. In all probability, this was also related to the fact that the process of being readmitted into the ICFTU was gathering pace—something that CETU's habit of translating its more assertive resolutions into English and sending them to the ICFTU's African Regional Organisation's office in Nairobi suggested. CETU objected that the law treated slowdowns as strikes and that it rendered non-renewed collective agreements legally void shortly upon their expiration. This, CETU warned, 'could result in industrial chaos'.[183] CETU's demands had evolved to encompass that new revisions to the recently promulgated labour law be made; that pension rights for workers in private firms be introduced; that government clamp down on violations of workers' rights and enforce the freedom of association; and that it intervene to rescue failing state-owned enterprises. To mark the International Workers' Day, rallies were held in the cities of Addis Ababa, Dire Dawa, Adama, Jimma, Bahir Dar, Mekelle, and Awassa on May 1. According to CETU, 100,000 workers participated[184]—the greatest number of attendants since the ETU had been dissolved. All in all, events during the year 2004 indicated that CETU had made some progress towards becoming an authentic trade union organisation again. It culminated in CETU's readmission into the ICFTU at the end of the year.

However, even if CETU's efforts could be viewed as genuine, it was not bargaining from a position of strength. Workers retained very low confidence in its leadership, and the government and ruling party remained prone to manipulating the election of its officeholders. In fact, the majority—if not all—executive committee members of CETU remained members of the constituent parties of the EPRDF. Moreover, CETU remained a very isolated organisation. In a workshop of its leaders

[183] "Sending a copy of request submitted to government", Haileselassie Abraha to Kelly Zidana, with attachment, 6 May 2004, Confederation of Ethiopian Trade Unions (CETU) archives, CETU, Addis Ababa.

[184] "The CETU stands on questions raised by ICFTU", attachment to Amare Alemayehu letter to Guy Rider, 6 September 2004, CETU archives.

and ICFTU representatives in 2004,[185] CETU officials acknowledged that CETU's 'poor relationship with professional associations' constituted a weakness. The relationship between CETU and other civil society organisations was also described as limited. This was, of course, largely of CETU's own making: it had, for example, refused to offer support to the Ethiopian Teachers' Association when the latter came under government repression during the 1990s. In fact, it had even sought to justify the government's excuses for the repression. Other weaknesses identified by CETU's leaders in the frank discussions that took place with the ICFTU included financial constraints; an inability to collect dues in a timely manner; a lack of strike funds; a shortage of skilled manpower; and an unstable leadership with high turnover of individuals.

The trade union movement was, moreover, neither liberated from continued government interference in its internal affairs nor from occasional repression. In 2005, the US Department of State alleged that 'complete government control of the Confederation of Ethiopian Trade Unions (CETU)'s executive committee continued throughout the year'. Serious infringements on trade union rights were reported in 2007 and included harassment, intimidation, and imprisonment of union leaders by security forces that collaborated with employers. In one case, militia and police allegedly killed labour activists on a sugar plantation in the Afar region.[186] Harassment continued to be reported by the end of the decade, targeting union members and organisers. It included frequent dismissals of activists. In 2008 alone, it was reported that ten workers, including three union officials, at the Bole Printing Enterprise in Addis Ababa had been suspended, and that similar dismissals had taken place at the Kaliti Food Factory[187] and the Dashen Brewery.[188] These allegations represented only the tip of the iceberg of reported infringements on

[185] "Report on CETU & ICFTU-AFRO Joint National Workshop on Capacity Building for Trade Union, Addis Ababa, 21–23 April 2004," CETU Archive.

[186] Department of State, *2007 Country Reports on Human Rights Practices*, (Washington DC: Joint Committee Print, 2008).

[187] The problems faced by the Kaliti Food Factory union in its relationship with management—it was a state-owned enterprise at the time—were confirmed by the union chairman, who claimed that the management 'tried to divide the union'. Teshome and Teklemedhin, in discussion with the author, Kassahun Berhanu, and Assefa Admassie, 2015.

[188] ITUC, *Annual Survey of Violations of Trade Union Rights 2009* (Brussels: ITUC, 2009).

union rights by both employers and the state.[189] Moreover, many newly established corporations refused their workers the right to organise altogether, contravening labour legislation but only rarely facing sanctions from the pertinent authorities or courts. Harassment and dismissals of union organisers occurred across the waged economy. Generally speaking, the first decade of the twenty-first century was as bleak for the Ethiopian labour movement as the last two decades of the twentieth century had been.

Yet, in the shadow of repression and denied rights, the slow but incremental process of growing trade union assertiveness continued. That process was sped up by a change in the confederation's leadership. Kassahun Follo, a CETU Executive Committee member and former industrial relations department head, was elected its president in early January 2006, whereas the old guard that had engineered the pro-government faction's takeover of the confederation in the mid-1990s was retired. The process of incrementally growing assertiveness would eventually lead to the revival of the trade union movement, and its restoration as a relatively autonomous force.

Revival: Two Victories

By the mid-2010s, CETU had replaced its entire leadership and acquired a new batch of leaders less tethered to the ruling party. Meanwhile, external factors also created conditions favourable to greater trade union autonomy. Following the death of its long-standing leader, Meles Zenawi, in 2012, the ruling front became embroiled in increasingly severe internal factional conflicts. This led to the gradual weakening of the coalition, until it ultimately broke up in 2019. Its mechanisms for exercising control over the trade union movement also atrophied, and the proletarian branches withered away. However, long before that final dissolution, CETU had taken advantage of the opportunities that presented themselves and embarked on a process of revitalisation and growth. Over the course of the 2010s, the trade union movement gradually acquired greater relative autonomy and displayed increasing assertiveness.

This took place within a political-economic context that was characterised by rapid economic growth and an even faster growth of the

[189] See, for example, the numerous reports from ILO's Committee on Freedom of Association and ICFTU's/ITUC's Annual Survey of Violation of Trade Union Rights.

wage-working population—the number of Ethiopian wage workers nearly tripled between 2005 and 2019.[190] However, this period was also marked by growing inequality and stagnant—or even declining—real wages.[191] Working conditions in many of the major establishments that sprang up in the 2010s were abysmal, and wages were often so low that workers could not even afford the costs of their individual upkeep.[192] Partly in response to this situation, industrial unrest began to rapidly increase from the mid-2010s onwards and exploded into a wave of wildcat strikes in the final years of the decade. The unrest was occasionally, but not generally, coordinated by formal trade unions. More frequently, it was organised by spontaneous constellations and informal networks of workers. Nevertheless, the heightened level of unrest imbued trade unions with increasing strategic leverage, as they emerged as the only credible interlocutors between management and workers.

At the same time, rank-and-file militancy and unrest provided bottom-up pressure on CETU to act with greater determination. Throughout the 2010s, the trade union movement's advocacy for legal reform and efforts to acquire greater respect for workers' rights grew in intensity and assertiveness, as did its activity in seeking redress for disaffected workers. Meanwhile, organising efforts and campaigns began to grow the numbers of basic unions affiliated with CETU and boost the ranks of their membership. In the second half of the decade, the trade union movement had grown confident enough to directly take on the state and employers in two high-profile cases in areas of significant strategic importance. In doing so, it achieved two remarkable victories. It managed to block a new labour law bill proposed by the government and alter its content to the considerable advantage of workers, and it overturned an illegal ban on unionisation in the country's largest industrial park, securing freedom of association for the tens of thousands of workers employed there.

[190] Compare the estimated 2,478,000 in paid employment in Central Statistical Agency, Statistical Report on the 2005 National Labour Force Survey, Addis Ababa, 2006, p. 215., with 6 912,000 derived from ILOSTAT and World Bank data in S.A. Admasie, "Trade Union Resurgence in Ethiopia," *Global Labour Journal*, 13 no. 2 (2022), 180. These estimates are low, but the growth trajectory is real.

[191] See chapter 6.

[192] For a discussion on the conditions of exploitation, see S.A. Admasie "Work and Exploitation in Ethiopia and Beyond," *in Handbook of Research on the Global Political Economy of Work*, ed. M. Atzeni, D. Azzellini, A. Mezzadri, P. Moore, and U. Apitzsch (Cheltenham: Edward Elgar).

With regard to the contestation over the revised labour law, tripartite discussions on its amendment had begun in 2011. They were conducted in the Labour Advisory Board, which included representatives of the Ministry of Labour and Social Affairs, the employers' federation and CETU. The government had initiated the process to revise the law, seeking to make Ethiopia more attractive to foreign investors. Eventually, in 2015, a draft law was agreed upon by all parties and sent to the Cabinet of Ministers. However, the cabinet rejected the draft on the grounds that it was not considered sufficiently investment-friendly and purportedly did not adequately incorporate employers' interest. Instead, the government—with significant input from its most investor-friendly institutions, the Ministry of Industry and the Ethiopian Investment Commission—unilaterally changed 25 articles that had been agreed on in the tripartite board and presented it as a new draft. This bill, a CETU executive committee member commented, 'was anti-union and anti-worker'.[193] 'Only clauses that were favourable to employers were added'. CETU protested against both the procedural violation of the tripartite principle and the 'anti-workers' content of the draft. It was subsequently returned to the tripartite advisory board, where it was deliberated upon for another two years. In the resultant document that was resubmitted to the cabinet in 2017, CETU objected to 42 articles. The draft bill remained abysmal to the interests of workers. It included provisions that doubled the length of the probation period and reduced annual leave days. The draft law would also have legalised the termination of employment contracts on the flimsiest grounds, including for reporting late to work on few and far-between occasions, and would have thus eliminated all traces of job security for workers. CETU concluded that the effort to safeguard workers' interests through dialogue alone had reached its limits and that another, more assertive, approach was required.

CETU's Executive Committee held broad consultations among all levels of the trade union movement—the confederation, the federations, branch offices, the basic unions, and their membership across the country. Thirteen seminars were arranged throughout all regions, to which every basic union was invited. The confederation's leadership received strong support for its position from aggrieved workers and workers' representatives. On each level of consultation and in each seminar, the Executive

[193] Measho Berihu, in discussion with the author, 27 June 2019. CETU Executive Committee Member and Head of CETU's Foreign and Public Relations Department.

Committee's objections to articles of the draft were agreed on, and its proposal to therefore reject the draft and resist its promulgation into law was adopted. One proposal that emerged from the membership also received widespread support: to prepare for a general strike and for rallies should CETU's objections be ignored. Workers' representatives present at the seminars vowed 'to give any kind of support' required of them in this regard.[194] There appeared to be unanimous support for the proposal to resist the imposition of the draft bill, come what may. This strengthened the position and resolve of the confederation's leadership.

Equipped with and propelled forward by this show of support and readiness from the grassroots, CETU's General Council wrote to the government, issuing a final warning: if the bill was not withdrawn, CETU would call demonstrations and a general strike. After having ignored CETU's previous objections and pleas, this finally forced the government to back down. The Prime Minister hurriedly established a tripartite ad-hoc committee to defuse the immediate threat, and after the government had accepted that the draft needed to be amended, it referred the draft back to the Labour Advisory Board. After almost two years of additional wrangling—which, this time around, included a real say for CETU—a final bill was agreed upon and enacted by parliament in June 2019.

The content of the law that was ultimately passed was very different from the bill the government had proposed two years earlier and was significantly more favourable to workers. CETU only retained one reservation against provisions in the new law: that civil servants remained ineligible to unionise. On the other hand, it had managed to remove the provisions most inimical to workers in the draft and secured new stipulations which had been long-standing demands of CETU. They included an extension of the maternity leave period—from 90 to 120 days—and the institution of a board to set minimum wages. The trade union movement's achievement—in having had the bill withdrawn and renegotiated, before being passed with the inclusion of some of its key demands—was nothing short of historic. Although the Ethiopian trade union movement had, for most of its history dating back to the early 1960s, consistently demanded revisions to labour legislation and a say in its drafting, it had never before been successful in achieving this demand. Moreover, for over four decades prior to this landmark event, Ethiopian unions had

[194] Ibid.

not managed to push a government to make any major concessions and had not successfully wielded the threat of a general strike. In fact, only a few years earlier, the government would habitually ignore trade union complaints over violations of workers' rights, or respond with reproach and ridicule.[195] The struggle over the labour law between the early 2010s and 2019, in other words, generated the greatest impact Ethiopian trade unions had achieved on the legal field since 1963, and their most successful challenge to a government since the 1974 strike. But even if this demonstrated how the government was amenable to its pressure, employers, in many cases, remained unyielding.

Employers tended to frequently ignore legally mandated workers' rights. Occasionally, they collaborated with authorities in denying workers their rights. This was particularly common among investments in areas that were deemed to be of strategic importance. One prominent case serves as an illustrative example of this. In the 2010s, the Ethiopian government began to establish a chain of industrial parks across the country to facilitate foreign investments in manufacturing. Hawassa Industrial Park (HIP), which was the largest, was opened in 2016. It was designated for textile and apparel production, and hosted foreign firms that produced for export markets. Immediately upon its opening, employers formed a de-facto wage cartel, paying uniformly low wages for all workers in the park, irrespective of workplace. Moreover, employers' collusion in wage-fixing was supplemented by a joint refusal to permit workers to unionise. Starting wages were set at around the equivalent of 26 USD monthly. The government had a direct role in establishing such poverty wages—which were not nearly sufficient to cover the costs of satisfying basic needs. It assured investors and sourcing firms that workers would readily accept such wages. In fact, a team of researchers concluded that the Ethiopian 'government's eagerness to attract foreign investment led it to promote the lowest base wage in any garment-producing country'.[196] It had also assured investors that they would not face any 'labour problems', which meant that investors could illegally prohibit

[195] See, for example, Tamrat G. Giorgis, "Indignant Labor Rebuked by Aspirant Administration," Addis Fortune 14, no. 714 (5 January 2014).

[196] P.M. Barrett and D. Baumann-Pauly, *Made in Ethiopia: Challenges in the Garment Industry's New Frontier* (New York: NYU Stern Center for Business and Human Rights, 2019).

unions without risking any intervention from authorities. The government would 'turn a blind eye' to such union-busting practices among investors, as Ethiopian employers' representatives acknowledged.[197] In fact, it did more than that: authorities actually policed the ban by prohibiting union organisers from entering the park. However, while the government could aid investors in preventing unionisation, it could not ensure industrial peace.

The employers in HIP faced two serious labour-related problems in the years after the park's establishment: a high level of turnover, as workers quit the low-paying jobs in droves—and sustained unrest in the form of wildcat strikes and walkouts. Over time, labour activists inside the park also formed networks, and occasionally, simultaneous strikes in multiple workplaces appeared to be coordinated. Efforts by CETU to send organisers into the park were rebuffed by the park authorities, but CETU retained contacts with the networks of labour activists present inside them and continued to campaign for their rights. In 2019, CETU increased efforts to pressure authorities and employers inside the park to permit workers to organise. CETU vowed to organise the workers in the park at any cost—including the option of calling out workers on strike if this demand was not met. By doing so, CETU and the Industrial Federation of Textile, Leather and Garment Workers' Trade Unions invested much prestige in the issue. The outcome was a resounding success. In combination with the exigencies the recurrent wildcat unrest inside the park created, sustained trade union pressure from outside eventually forced employers in the park—as well as the government institutions that colluded with them—to overturn their illegal ban and accept unionisation as a lesser evil. Although the global pandemic and the war on the regional state of Tigray that broke out in 2020 delayed the implementation, CETU and the federation began organising basic unions in most enterprises in the park the following year.[198] Another symbolically and strategically important victory had been achieved.

The contestation over the labour law and the struggle to overturn the illegal ban on unions in HIP took place at a time when intense but decentralised workplace unrest had become common. Wildcat strikes and

[197] Asmera Defa, in discussion with the author, 1 August 2019. Chief Executive Officer of Ethiopian Employers' Federation.

[198] Solomon Zena, "የሐዋሳ ኢንደስትሪ ፓርክ ሠራተኞችን የማደራጀት እቅዴ በስኬት ተጠናቀቀ, *Voice of Labour* 1 (Digital Series), no. 3 (25 September 2021).

walkouts grew precipitously in frequency between the mid-2010s and the end of the decade in workplaces across the country and particularly in foreign-owned ones. The strikes were legally unsanctioned but often successful in extracting significant concessions from employers. To force employers to permit unionisation in the high-profile case of HIP required sustained pressure, wildcat action, and significant risks of confrontation. Such unrest forced many additional reluctant foreign owners of newly established companies across the country to tolerate unions. In another set of cases, employers eventually came to support the formation of unions as a way out of the restive status quo—the trade unions serving as representative institutions with whom they could cooperate to reduce unrest. In a similar manner, CETU's involvement in solving companies' problems with recurring wildcat strikes was increasingly being requested by employers themselves.[199] This further enhanced CETU's clout and prestige. However, those advances were directly premised on the willingness of workers to engage in industrial conflict—without the nominal legal right to do so—in the first place.

Rank-and-file militancy was equally important when it came to overturning the 2017 labour law bill. CETU's resolve and leverage in compelling the government to withdraw its initial bill was built on the momentous wave of wildcat strikes and unrest that took place simultaneously. Moreover, CETU's leadership was given an open and militant mandate by its grassroots when consulting and canvasing them for support. It was, in fact, instructed to do anything in its powers—including calling strikes and demonstrations—to stop the bill from becoming law, and it was promised the full-hearted support of the basic unions and their membership in the campaign. The readiness of rank-and-file workers and basic union representatives to confront employers and the government was essential to the credibility and viability of CETU's firm line on the issue, as well as to the potency of the general strike threat. There is thus conclusive evidence that CETU's growing assertiveness in the latter half of the 2010s was made possible by the increasing willingness of the rank-and-file membership and basic union representatives to engage in militant practices and unrest. At the same time, CETU's successful contestation of unpopular edicts and practices bolstered this willingness and resonated with the workers.

[199] Measho Berihu, discussion; Asmera Defa, discussion.

One way of illustrating this resonance is through the unprecedented growth in the number of CETU-affiliated unions and the increasing membership of these unions. Between the years 2015 and 2019, the number of CETU-affiliated basic unions more than doubled, from 918 to 1,901, and the number of workers who were members of these unions grew from 415,000 to around 750,000.[200] As Fig. 4.1 illustrates, this represented the greatest numerical growth of trade union membership in Ethiopian history. In terms of the relative pace of growth, the only prior period that comes close to comparison was the years between 1973 and 1975, when CELU—as the national trade union centre at the time was called—was radicalised by the ascendancy of the labour opposition movement, and openly confronted employers and the state in an intense flurry of strikes (Fig. 4.1).

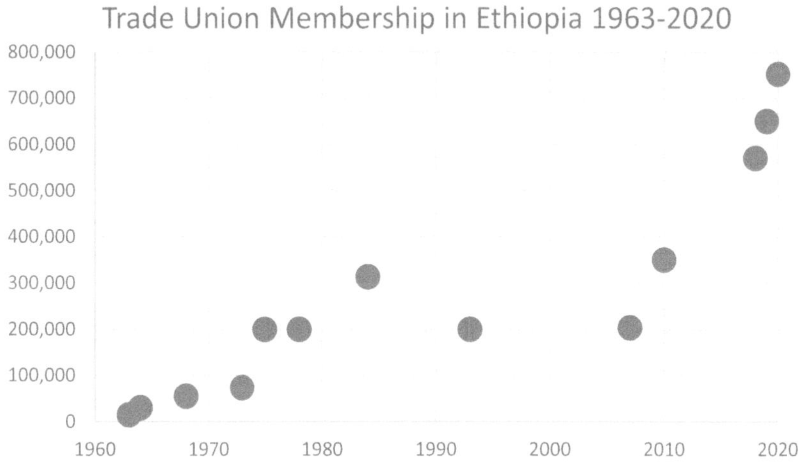

Fig. 4.1 Reported membership in Ethiopian trade unions, 1963–2020 (*Source* Author's compilation from various archival sources)

[200] Biruk Tsegaye, "የኢሠማኮ የአምስት ዓመታት ጉዞ *Voice of Labour* 13 (new series), no. 113 (21 October 2019). 4; Dereje Gebriel "ኢሠማኮ በአንድ ዓመት ከመንፈቅ"*Voice of Labour* 13 (new series) no. 102(10 October 2018); CETU, *የኢሠማኮ ጠቅላይ ምክር ቤት የሁለት ዓመት ተኩል የሥራ አስፈጻጸም ሪፖርት,* CETU 18th General Congress, (Addis Ababa: CETU, 2019): 14; Measho Berihu, in discussion with the author July 2019; October 2022.

The Trade Union Movement at the Dawn of the 2020s

At the beginning of the 2020s, the Ethiopian trade union movement was more relevant and in better shape than it had been for decades. CETU had acquired a real say in domestic labour affairs, and its reputation as a genuine representative of Ethiopian workers appeared more credible than it had in a long time. CETU-affiliated unions had a membership that was far larger than at any time in the trade union movement's prior history, and it was poised for further growth—set to surpass the one-million mark in the near future.[201] However, it remained a movement starved of resources across its structures, and in a politically vulnerable position.

The configuration of CETU's structure was adopted in 1994, although these structures expanded with the numerical and geographical growth of the membership in subsequent years. The rank-and-file membership of CETU consisted of individual workers joining basic unions. The basic unions in Ethiopia have almost exclusively been of the enterprise-union type. Together, these basic unions formed nine sectoral industrial federations, which, in turn, came together to constitute the confederation. The confederation operated specialised departments and branch offices. These components, along with the interrelationship between them, formed the organisational structure of the Ethiopian trade union movement (Fig. 4.2).

The basic building block of the Ethiopian trade union movement has remained the basic constituent union. The two types of basic unions that have been prescribed by Ethiopian law are the enterprise union and the general union. Unlike in the typical case, the general union has in Ethiopia been legally confined to very small enterprises. The structural organisation of the Ethiopian trade union movement has thus remained rather peculiar and unique in the sub-region. The enterprise union model has imposed certain structural characteristics on the Ethiopian trade union movement. While it has generated a structure of officialdom which is relatively flat hierarchically, it has also produced a large horizontal base composed of a high number of individually small basic unions.

Since the enterprise model of unions was adopted in Ethiopia (at the time of the formation of CELU in 1963), the number of basic unions

[201] Which it subsequently did in the years that followed.

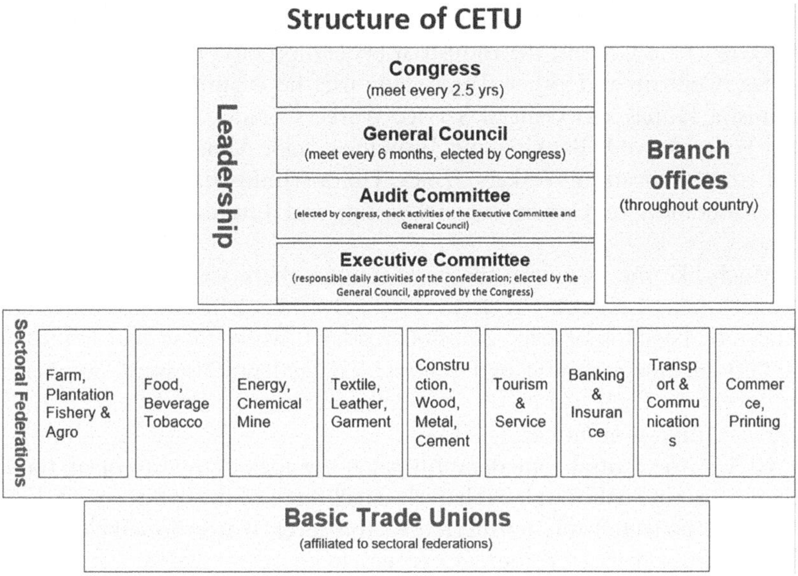

Fig. 4.2 CETU's structure in 2021 (*Source* CETU)

grew from a few dozen to over 2,000 by the dawn of the 2020s. By that time, each of these basic unions had an average of around eight elected executive committee members, including auditors, which amounted to a total of over 18,000 elected officials.

Because of the enterprise union model, there were also significant differences in the size and capacity among the various basic unions. A few basic unions were extraordinarily well-endowed. An example is the union of the Commercial Bank of Ethiopia, which had 32,000 members, assets that included buildings and vehicles, and large savings in bank accounts. But at the same time, there was a plethora of minuscule unions, which possessed none of these resources.

The basic unions were served by nine sectorally defined industrial federations of which they were part, and geographically by CETU's eight branch offices. The industrial federations included the National Federation of Farm, Plantation, Fishery and Agro-Industry Trade Unions; the Federation of Food, Beverage, Tobacco and Allied Trade Unions; the National Federation of Energy, Chemical and Mine Trade Unions;

the Industrial Federation of Ethiopian Textiles, Leather and Garment Workers Trade Unions; the Industrial Federation of Construction, Wood, Metal, Cement and other Trade Unions; the National Federation of Tourism, Hotels and General Service Workers Trade Unions; the Industrial Federation Of Banking and Insurance Trade Unions; the Transport and Communication Workers' Trade Unions Industrial Federation; and the Federation of Commerce, Technical, and Printing Industry Trade Unions.

Much like the case with the basic unions, there were significant variations in size between the federations. By the early 2020s, some had total memberships of over 200,000 workers, while some had less than 40,000 members in affiliated unions. The federations were nominally autonomous. Each had its own general congress, which elected councils and executive committees.

CETU, the central confederation, sat at the apex of the Ethiopian trade union structure. Although a relatively small share of the membership dues that were collected was transferred to this level, it was nonetheless here that a critical mass of resources existed. In the early 2020s, CETU had over 170 staff members. The vast majority were clustered in its Addis Ababa headquarters. Only 10 staff members were classified as expert staff, whereas another ten were full-time officials. CETU owned a significant stock of real estate and received significant rental income, as well as a slighter smaller amount from its income-generating enterprises. Revenue from membership dues were dwarfed by income from rents and donations. The basic funding model was that basic enterprise unions collected union dues from their members. Workers paid one per cent of their wages as membership dues. The basic unions then shared 40 per cent of the collected dues with the federations which, in turn, transferred a quarter of what they received to CETU.

CETU invested much time in tripartite activities and dialogue, representing Ethiopian workers at the national and international level—including in the national tripartite Labour Advisory Board. Most organising and dispute settlement activity occurred at the level of the branch offices or industrial federations, but CETU assisted the various offices and federations in the more complicated cases. CETU also conducted training and workers' education for basic union representatives. Given the size of the elected officialdom in the basic unions, this constituted an important but challenging task.

CETU operated eight branch offices in the early 2020s. Their geographical locations were based on the historical spatial development of the Ethiopian waged economy and the labour movement. Their establishment had therefore occurred without an original grand plan. They were located in the cities of Addis Ababa, Bahir Dar, Mekelle, Hawassa, Dire Dawa, Jimma, Kombolcha, and Adama, respectively. Their reach was, in principle, supposed to encompass the whole country. But because they were relatively few and, in most cases, far apart, the catchment areas of nearly all the branch offices were very large. The Dire Dawa office, for example, represented CETU's only office in the eastern part of the country, and the Hawassa office covered the entire area south to the Kenyan border. The total number of staff posted to the branch offices was slightly fewre than 50, and they, too, operated on a tight budget.

The Ethiopian labour movement appeared to face several apparent risks and vulnerabilities at the dawn of the 2020s. It remained relatively isolated socially and institutionally. It had not developed sturdy and consistent relationships with workers in non-unionised sectors, and it did not enjoy close relations with any other mass organisation or political party. It was not part of any broader popular coalition, leaving it vulnerable in case of conflict with the government. The worsening political situation in Ethiopia aggravated such risks. As evident in the previous pages, the Ethiopian government has repressed independent-minded trade unions and workers repeatedly in the past—most notably in 1964, 1975, and 1994. In that respect, history has tended to repeat itself. The federal government's atrocious war on the regional state of Tigray that began in 2020—which CETU defiantly refused to voice any support for, despite facing intense pressure to do so and despite being nearly entirely alone in its refusal to submit to this pressure—and the government's increasing authoritarianism further aggravated that risk. State repression of the trade union movement remained a potent threat.

A second set of obvious threats and vulnerabilities stemmed from employers. The intolerance of some employers towards unionisation—particularly among recent foreign entrants to the Ethiopian scene—combined with the government's tendency to tolerate or even facilitate illegal union-busting practices, to create a hostile environment. This risk was amplified in cases where a sector or a particular employer was deemed strategically important to the government's plans. These two factors combined to produce illegal bans on unions in at least two industrial parks. While the bans were enforced by employers, they were facilitated by state agencies. In general, it was reported that 'strong resistance of private employers, including those in textile and garment sector, against unionization and collective bargaining' prevailed.[202] But the situation was typically better in older, Ethiopian-owned, and public enterprises, in which unions were almost universally tolerated. On a central level, relations between CETU and the employers' federations were generally cordial and characterised by mutual willingness to resolve disputes. This was partly because—unlike in the 1960s and 1970s—Ethiopian employers played dominant roles within the federations. However, amicable institutional relations did not necessarily translate into mutual understanding between trade unions and employers on the enterprise level, as the prevalence of industrial conflict demonstrated.

Financial constraints remained another major vulnerability—with particularly income from dues remaining alarmingly low. Nearly half of CETU's income in 2019 came from real estate rents, whereas membership dues only accounted for around seven per cent of the central confederation's income.[203] Although the share of income from dues was somewhat greater for basic unions and industrial federations, it nevertheless remained low. Members contributed one per cent of their income as dues. However, the basic problem was that this contribution was based on wages that were very low in the first place. This problem was aggravated by the fact that, despite the impressive growth in trade union membership, union density remained very low. The primary factor behind this was the legal obstacles that prevented large parts of the Ethiopian workforce from organising. Categories of workers that were excluded from the relevant legislation, and whose freedom of association was therefore denied, included civil servants, teachers, and domestic workers.

At the same time, several opportunities for the movement's further development also appeared to exist. The breakthrough in having provisions for a minimum wage included in the 2019 labour law meant that should the minimum-wage-setting board provided for in the 2019 law eventually be established, it would open another front and arena on which to campaign and struggle for better conditions for Ethiopia's workers. Considering how low Ethiopian wages typically were, this could serve

[202] International Labour Organization, "Improving Industrial Relations for Decent Work and Sustainable Development of Textile and Garment Industry in Ethiopia," (unpublished programme document, July 2015).

[203] CETU, *የሁለት ዓመት ተኩል የሥራ አስፈጻጸም ሪፖርት*.

as an obvious social justice cause, around which the support and solidarity of broader parts of the population could be mobilised, and social coalitions formed. In a similar manner, CETU's campaign to pressure the Ethiopian government to ratify the ILO's Domestic Workers Convention and the trade union movement's cooperation with a newly formed domestic workers' association on that issue, held the potential to create broader coalitions around the rights of excluded workers. The rights of such workers to organise, if granted, could also increase the ranks of organised workers further.

Other opportunities resided in the political context. In the final years of the 2010s, the trade union movement internally debated a proposal to form a political party representing labour. The idea attracted broad support from workers' representatives. In November 2020, shortly before the war on Tigray began, the proposal was discussed by the General Council of the Industrial Federation of Tourism, Hotels and General Service Workers. In this meeting, the delegates insisted that the federation leadership should work for the prompt formation of a labour party.[204] Even if such a process would naturally involve many pitfalls, the support the proposal received highlighted the confidence the movement had developed, and the potential for the formation of new organisational vehicles, as well as new social and political coalitions, to overcome the movement's relative isolation.

Finally, significant opportunities existed for substantial further growth. The Industrial Federation of Ethiopian Textiles, Leather and Garment Workers Trade Unions, for example, estimated that it had only organised 15 per cent of the workers engaged in the sector in 2019.[205] Similar figures prevailed in other sectors. The increasing prestige and self-confidence the trade union movement enjoyed at the beginning of the 2020s, and the successes it had accomplished in the final years of the 2010s, combined with a reacquired readiness of workers to engage in militant industrial contestation to make its plans to organise considerably more workers increasingly realistic. The Ethiopian trade union movement entered the 2020s with tangible forward momentum.

[204] Dereje Gebriel, "የሠራተኛው የፖለቲካው ፓርቲ ማቋቋም እና የዝቅተኛ ደሞዝ ወሰን ጉዳይ ለምን ቸል ተባለ?" *Voice of Labour* 14 (new series), no. 120 (12 November 2020).

[205] Angessom Yohannes, in discussion with the author, July 2019. President, Industrial Federation of Ethiopian Textile, Leather and Garment Workers Trade Union.

References

Addis Ababa University Economics Department. "Minimum Wage for Ethiopia: A Report for the Confederation of Ethiopian Trade Unions By Economics Department of Addis Ababa." Unpublished final report, June 2004.

Admasie, S.A. "Trade Union Resurgence in Ethiopia." *Global Labour Journal*, 13 no. 2 (2022): 171–186.

Admasie, S. A. "Work and Exploitation in Ethiopia and Beyond." In *Handbook of Research on the Global Political Economy of Work*, edited by M. Atzeni, D. Azzellini, A. Mezzadri, P. Moore, and U. Apitzsch, 614–624. Cheltenham: Edward Elgar, 2023.

African American Labor Center (AALC) Records. Collection 0547-LBR. Hornbake Library, Special Collections and University Archives, University of Maryland Libraries, College Park, MD

Andu-alem Aragie. "A Short History of the Employees of the Commercial Bank of Ethiopia from 1964 to 1997 (with Special Emphasis on the Employees in Addis Ababa)." Bachelor's thesis, Addis Ababa University, 1999.

Barrett, P.M. and D. Baumann-Pauly. *Made in Ethiopia: Challenges in the Garment Industry's New Frontier*. New York: NYU Stern Center for Business and Human Rights, 2019.

Biruk Tsegaye. ""የኢሠማኮ የአምስት ዓመታት ጉዞ." *Voice of Labour* 13 (new series), no. 113 (21 October 2019): 4.

CETU. *የኢሠማኮ ጠቅላይ ምክር ቤት የሁለት ዓመት ተኩል የሥራ አስፈጻጸም ሪፖርት*. CETU 18th General Congress report. Addis Ababa: CETU, 2019.

Cohen, J.M., W. Hammink and E. Simmons. "Evaluation Report: Ethiopia Democracy/Governance Support Project." Draft Report Prepared for Ethiopia Mission, United States. Agency for International Development, Addis Ababa. May 10, 1994. https://pdf.usaid.gov/pdf_docs/pdabk181.pdf.

Confederation of Ethiopian Trade Unions (CETU) archives, CETU, Addis Ababa.

Council of Representatives. *Ethiopia: The Process of Transition to Democracy: Special Report (From July, 1991 to August, 1993)*. Addis Ababa: Secretariat of the Council of Representatives, 1993.

Dereje Gebriel. "ኢሠማኮ በአንድ ዓመት ከመንፈቅ." *Voice of Labour* 13 (new series) no. 102 (10 October 2018): 11.

Dereje Gebriel. "የሠራተኛው የፖለቲካው ፓርቲ ማቋቋም እና የዝቅተኛ ደሞዝ ወሰን ጉዳይ ልምን ቸል ታብለ?" *Voice of Labour* 14 (new series), no. 120 (12 November 2020): 2, 15.

Department of State. *Country Reports on Human Rights Practices for 1991.* Washington DC: Joint Committee Print, 1992.

Department of State. *Country Reports on Human Rights Practices for 1993.* Washington DC: Joint Committee Print, 1994.

Department of State. *2002 Country Reports on Human Rights Practices*. Washington DC: Joint Committee Print, 2003.
Department of State. *2003 Country Reports on Human Rights Practices*. Washington DC: Joint Committee Print, 2004.
Department of State. *2007 Country Reports on Human Rights Practices*. Washington DC: Joint Committee Print, 2008.
EPRDF. "Our Revolutionary Democratic Goals and the Next Steps." Excerpts published in "TPLF/EPRDF's Strategies for Establishing its Hegemony and Perpetuating its Rule," *Ethiopian Register* (June 1996):20–29.
Ethiopian Herald . "Goldmines' Workers End Strike." August 20, 1991.
Ethiopian Herald. "Prime Minister Urges Serious Attitude to Work." October 16, 1991.
Ethiopian Herald. "Factory Workers End Strike." November 23, 1991.
Ethiopian Herald. "Corporation Employees End Strike." December 5, 1991.
Ethiopian Herald. "ETUC to Ask for Council Seat." December 4, 1993.
Ethiopian Herald. "Trade Union Federation Calls for Boycotting General Assembly." October 26, 1994.
Ethiopian Herald. "Federation of Trade Unions Opposes Convening of General Assembly." October 27, 1994.
Ethiopian Herald. "Federation Voice Opposition to CETU General Assembly." October 28. 1994
Ethiopian Human Rights Council. *Democracy, Rule of Law, and Human Rights in Ethiopia: Rhetoric and Practice*. Addis Ababa: EHRCO, 1995.
Ethiopian Human Rights Council. *The Violation of Human Rights in Ethiopia: 11th Report of EHRCO*. Addis Ababa: EHRCO, 1996.
Hishe Hailu. "An Assessment of the Process of Privatization in Ethiopia." Master's thesis, Addis Ababa University, 2005.
Indian Ocean Newsletter. "Crisis in the Union and Arrests." *Indian Ocean Newsletter* 640 (October 1, 1994).
Indian Ocean Newsletter. "Trying to Get Them Into Step." *Indian Ocean Newsletter* 646 (November 21, 1994).
Indian Ocean Newsletter. "Trade Union Mission to Addis." *Indian Ocean Newsletter* 786 (May 24, 1997).
ICFTU/ITUC archives. Collection ARCH00622, International Institute of Social History, Amsterdam.
ICFTU. *Annual Survey of Violations of Trade Union Rights 2003*. Brussels: ICFTU, 2003.
ICFTU African Regional Organization (ICFTU-AFRO) archives. ITUC Africa, Lomé.
International Labour Organization. *The Situation of Laid-Off Women Workers in Ethiopia*. Addis Ababa: ILO, 2005.

International Labour Organization. “Improving Industrial relations for Decent Work and Sustainable Development of Textile and Garment Industry in Ethiopia.” Unpublished programme document, July 2015.

Ministry of Labour and Social Affairs archives, MoLSA, Addis Ababa.

Praeg, B. *Ethiopia and Political Renaissance in Africa*. New York: Nova Science, 2006.

Solomon Zena. “የሐዋሳ ኢንደስትሪ ፓርክ ሠራተኞችን የማደራጀት እቅዱ በስኬት ተጠናቀቀ.” *Voice of Labour* 1 (digital series), no. 3 (25 September 2021): 1–2.

Tamene. “Officials Prepare to Dismiss Labor Leaders as Confederations Nears Losing Legal Status.” *File* newsletter 1, no. 8 (18 November 1994): 1.

Tamrat G. Giorgis. “Indignant Labor Rebuked by Aspirant Administration.” *Addis Fortune* 14, no. 714 (5 January 2014).

Voice of Labour. “የኢሠማኮ ሥራ አስፈጻሚ ኮሚቴ የአቋም መግለጫ አወጣ.” *Voice of Labour* 1 (new series), no. 3 (1994): 1–5.

W., John [pseud.]. “An Opponent of Strikes in Charge of a Labour Union.” *Reporter* 5 no. 241 (18 April 2001): 11.

CHAPTER 5

The International Dimension

An important aspect in the development of the Ethiopian trade union movement has been its relationships with foreign and international trade union organisations. The international anti-communist trade union movement, spearheaded by the International Confederation of Free Trade Unions (ICFTU), played a key role in the birth of CELU and in its development in the decade and half that followed. During the period of the ETU and AETU, relations with trade union centres of the socialist bloc countries and the World Federation of Trade Unions (WFTU) were important. Each of these periods of cooperation made its mark on Addis Ababa's skyline, as both CELU's and the AETU's headquarters were constructed with the assistance of their respective allies. After a period of hiatus in the 1990s and early 2000s, when CETU was widely viewed as an inauthentic and government-controlled yellow union, international trade union organisations and their affiliates again began to render assistance to CETU after the latter's readmission to the ICFTU in 2004. Meanwhile, the ILO was present in Addis Ababa providing technical assistance throughout, and organisations such as the Friedrich-Ebert-Stiftung (FES) have at different times operated an office in the city, partly with an intent to assist the trade union movement.

However the provision of resources and assistance has represented only one side of the Ethiopian trade union movement's relations with its international counterparts. The other side has consisted of attempts by

© The Author(s), under exclusive license to Springer Nature Switzerland AG 2025

S. A. Admasie, *The Ethiopian Labour Movement*, Labour in History and Society, https://doi.org/10.1007/978-3-031-72841-9_5

the latter to influence the former in various ways and directions. This has included efforts to monitor the Ethiopian trade union movement, constrict it, interfere in its internal processes, and even subvert it. At no time were both aspects—aid and influence—more important than over the course of CELU's first decade. During this period, entities in the international anti-communist trade union movement considered it strategically highly important that the young Ethiopian trade union movement was guided to a path of moderation. Its representatives and affiliates descended on CELU in high numbers, and CELU's officers were courted around the world, so as to cement the relationship. At different times during this period, the ICFTU, the African American Labor Center (AALC), the Danish Confederation of Trade Unions (LO, for *Landsorganisationen*) and the FES operated offices in Ethiopia. The FES' stay in the country was to be the shortest, beginning in the mid-1960s and ending, for that time being, in 1967. The other organisations remained in Ethiopia longer, and influenced events more profoundly.

In this chapter, CELU's experience of close relations with the ICFTU, the AALC and Danish LO will be examined. There is a sound reason for selecting these three organisations: whereas they, much like CELU, were trade union organisations, the ILO and FES represent amalgamation of interests that includes states and employers (in the case of the former) and a political party (in the case of the latter). By focusing on CELU's relations with the three partnering organisations that operated offices in Ethiopia during the period when foreign attention and influence was most intensive, and the engagement between the parties was the closest—with all the resultant frictions and tensions it brought about—pertinent insights into the nature and effects of the Ethiopian trade union movement's relationship with the international trade union movement can be obtained. These have not been relationships between real equals, albeit nominally so. But although highly asymmetric, they were relationships in which the Ethiopian trade union movement exercised important agency and, as we shall see, eventually the final say. They were also relationships from which the Ethiopian trade union movement benefited in many ways, despite attempts to constrict its autonomy and subvert it.

International Confederation of Free Trade Unions

The ICFTU was a Cold War creation. It was established on the initiative of American and British unions in opposition to the presence of Communist trade unions in the World Federation of Trade Union, from which they split in 1949. The word 'free' in its name was meant to convey a non-communist, or even anti-communist meaning. It brought together national trade union centres of different ideological orientation, from the staunchly pro-business AFL-CIO to reformist social democratic North European and Scandinavian confederations. What they had in common was their hostility to communism—which constituted the ICFTU's *raison d'etre* until the end of the Cold War. Its activities in Ethiopia were premised on this rationale from the outset.

The first contact between the ICFTU and Ethiopian trade unionists occurred before the formation CELU. In October 1958, the Secretary General of the Kenyan Federation of Labour and Chairman of ICFTU's African regional committee Tom Mboya had visited Ethiopia. In addition to meeting with the emperor and senior government officials, he made contacts with Ethiopian trade unionists. Upon receiving his report from the trip, and fearing an imminent threat from 'Communist activities' in the country, the ICFTU concluded that 'the question of organisation in Ethiopia should be treated as urgent'.[1] By 1962, the ICFTU viewed the trade union situation in the country as at once 'delicate' and 'extremely important to the ICFTU', given its—at the time baseless—fear of growing socialist bloc influence among Ethiopian workers.[2] The ICFTU therefore considered it necessary to urgently begin to work directly with the leaders of the emerging trade union movement.[3] The argument that ICFTU intervention and assistance was necessary to pre-empt rumoured but unsubstantiated 'communist' influence over the movement would be

[1] Serge Claverie to Charles Millard, 23 July 1959, ICFTU/ITUC archives, collection ARCH00622, International Institute of Social History, Amsterdam.

[2] No arguments of why Ethiopia specifically would be at risk for such influence—except normal diplomatic relations between its government and socialist bloc states—was ever proposed.

[3] Briefing report to Desigar Ramanujam, confidential, ICFTU, 1962, ICFTU/ITUC archives.

routinely invoked over the coming years to justify its growing involvement in Ethiopia.

Prompted by such fears, the ICFTU was present at CELU's birth. In fact, to some extent one can say it played the role of CELU's midwife. It was the ICFTU that organised the March 1963 seminar for trade union leaders which ended in the formation of CELU and the election of its initial officeholders. Moreover, the constitution adopted by CELU at this meeting had been drafted by ICFTU officers. Less than a month later, CELU applied for affiliation with the ICFTU—a request that was granted. On January 1, 1964, CELU became an official affiliate, and interactions intensified rapidly.

On CELU's request, the ICFTU stationed a permanent representative in Ethiopia in order to assist and liaise with CELU. Lennart Kindström, a former Swedish Miners' Union official with a background working for the ICFTU in Liberia, was selected for the role. He arrived in early 1964 and would remain in Ethiopia until May 1973. His primary responsibility was to manage the dispensation of ICFTU aid to CELU. Most of it was provided as annually set volumes of institutional budget support to help achieve organisational consolidation and development. Additional funding for specific purposes and projects was also regularly provided: for example for the purchases of vehicles and equipment; arrangement of campaigns, conferences and meetings; and the facilitation of overseas travel—whether paid for by ICFTU, or, through its facilitation, by affiliates in Europe and North America. But Kindström's role was not confined to providing material and organisational assistance. As will be described, he was also tasked with keeping a close eye on CELU, its officials, and the broader trade union movement in Ethiopia, so as to make sure that it abided to what was considered the only politically acceptable line: pro-West, non-radical unionism. He would report transgressions to the ICFTU's headquarters in Brussels, liaise with the imperial government and the ICFTU's international allies in Addis Ababa, and take even the senior-most CELU officials to task when failing to adhere to the line. He would also help to prop up CELU's leadership when challenged by more militant trade unionists. But to grasp how the ICFTU came to hold such leverage over CELU, one must first consider the dependence that CELU developed on the ICFTU.

Dependence

The ICFTU's relationship with CELU was marked by two conflicting tendencies. On the one hand, it was acknowledged that the development of a dependent relationship was a danger that ought to be avoided. The provision of direct financial support was rationalised as a short-term endeavour by both sides. 'It is only at the initial stages that the Ethiopian movement will need our unstinted support in essentials and within 6 months they will stand on their own resources',[4] an ICFTU officer in Ethiopia wrote as the administration of the first round of support was being prepared in 1963. Moreover, ICFTU efforts to 'avoid the habit of total dependency'[5] included an early insistence on the principle that CELU should match ICFTU contributions evenly, and cover the full costs of its own staff salaries and office rent. There was a sound rationale for this. 'Good trade unionists are developed and paid only after they have won the confidence of workers', the ICFTU's Assistant General Secretary wrote. He continued: 'our payment of officers' salaries interrupts this development and thus, in many cases, would provide a kind of trade union elite whom, in the final analysis, may not have the support of workers'.[6] But as prudent as the insistence on this principle may have sounded, there was a tendency to habitually override it by invoking the boogey of growing communist influence and/or radicalisation should the playing field be left open to other forces. Pressing needs and innumerable requests for assistance from Addis Ababa also contributed to the principle being overlooked. In this manner, the institutional support programme was considerably expanded in volume and extended in length beyond original conceptions. It took no more than a few months before ICFTU funds were dispensed to cover salaries of CELU officials in contravention of explicit principles, and the six months period until CELU was expected to be financially self-dependent turned into nearly 12 years.

The annual volumes of institutional budget support from the ICFTU's International Solidarity Fund (ISF)—the considerably largest of its several instruments of aid to CELU—was initially set at USD 5,800 for the years 1963 and 5,000 for 1964. By the latter year, however, an additional 15,000 USD was extended to establish an office and station Kindström

[4] Desigar Ramanujam to Stefan Nedzynski, 21 January 1963, ICFTU/ITUC archives.

[5] Stefan Nedzynski to Desigar Ramanujam, 10 January 1963, ICFTU/ITUC archives.

[6] Ibid.

in the country. The contribution was regularised as a monthly subsidy of 1,000 USD, paid out by Kindström. The ICFTU also elevated the status of its programme in Ethiopia and determined that 'quite a substantial part of the ICFTU's efforts should now be concentrated on Ethiopia'.[7] For the following year, 1965, the annual allocation grew to an extraordinary level of 23,075 USD, and covered salaries of officials and staff ranging from CELU's general secretary, to organisers, education officers, typists, clerks, drivers, messengers, and night guards. CELU's costs for office rent, transportation, publications, telephone bills, electricity and utilities were also covered.[8] At this point, if not before, CELU became entirely financially dependent on the ICFTU. According to Danish trade unionists stationed in Asmara, CELU received around 90 per cent[9] of its operative budget from the ICFTU at the height of its assistance. While that is probably somewhat of an exaggeration, the regular annual ISF allocation reached USD 16,000 in 1966, and remained at roughly this level until 1970, when a gradual decline in volumes began. In 1972 the ISF allocation was set to USD 11,000, before declining to USD 6,500 in 1973, and, finally, USD 3,500 in 1974.

External Control and Internal Subversion

This book's second chapter described how the ICFTU played into the bureaucratisation of CELU, and how it propped up the moderate leadership, helping it to overcome radical impulses and more militant challengers. The corrosive effects this had on the intra-union democracy of CELU and the internal legitimacy of its leadership has also been discussed. But ICFTU support also came at the steep price of undermining CELU's external autonomy. In return for its assistance, the ICFTU demanded an unflinching commitment to anti-radicalism, and a level of exclusivity that permitted no relationships whatsoever with the trade union centres organised in the World Federation of Trade Unions (WFTU). In fact, archival documents make it abundantly clear how the ICFTU—together with the AFL-CIO, AALC and its allies—viewed their

[7] Stefan Nedzynski to Lennart Kindström, 25 September 1964, ICFTU/ITUC archives.

[8] "ISF Emergency Procedure: Ethiopia," Omer Becu to George Meany, 6 October 1964, ICFTU/ITUC archives.

[9] Daniel Pedersen to Eiljer Jensen, 25 December 1966, Landsorganisationen i Danmark (LO) archives, Arbejdermuseet & Arbejderbevægelsens Bibliotek og Arkiv, Copenhagen.

engagement with CELU as a means to 'bar the way' for communist, radical and 'anti-free trade union forces'.[10]

The mechanisms by which adherence to 'free' and 'democratic' trade unionism—meaning anti-communist, ICFTU-affiliated, non-militant and anti-radical business unionism—was policed included continuous supervision. Kindström, the ICFTU representative to Ethiopia, was stationed—or embedded—inside the offices of CELU, from where he closely monitored the confederation's operations and its officers' movements. His correspondence reveals a great deal about the relationship between CELU, the ICFTU and the rest of the 'free' international trade union movement. Travels of CELU leaders to 'suspect' countries and contacts with trade unionists from outside the 'free' trade union movement were scrutinised, reported, and sometimes penalised. They constituted a source of repeated exasperation among ICFTU representatives and officials, and a point of friction between the former and CELU officials. In 1966, for example, having been informed that CELU's general secretary Fissehatsion had attended and given a speech at a WFTU meeting in Budapest, the ICFTU representative in Ethiopia was ordered to intervene by his Brussels headquarters. In response, Kindström[11] disparagingly opined that 'the CELU people do not really understand politics' but were acting out of perceptions that it would be impolite not to accept invitations. Nevertheless, he arranged a meeting with CELU's leadership to sternly lecture them on the unacceptability of having done so.

On hearing about the arrival of a Soviet trade union delegation to Ethiopia on another occasion, the ICFTU's General Secretary Omer Becu wrote to Kindström in Addis Ababa demanding that 'you take immediate initiative [for a] common approach among free trade union representatives to make clear to CELU [the] consequences of accepting aid from elsewhere',[12] adding that he was 'expecting firmness in handling this situation'. The ICFTU representative in Addis Ababa consequently assembled the representatives of the FES, Danish *Landsorganisationen*, and called on the advice of the AALC. Presenting a joint front of funders they called

[10] "ISF Emergency Procedure: Ethiopia," Omer Becu to George Meany, 6 October 1964, ICFTU/ITUC archives.

[11] Lennart Kindström to P.H. de Jonge, 1 February 1967, ICFTU/ITUC archives.

[12] Omer Becu to Lennart Kindström, 23 December 1966, ICFTU/ITUC archives.

CELU's president and secretary general to a meeting, of which Kindström gave the following account:

> In the discussions my colleagues and myself were blaming both [Beyene] Solomon and [Fissehatsion] Tekie very hard [for] their action. Brother Tekie said that if he had known our serious reaction he should not [have] arranged this visit without consulting us first. That gave us the opportunity to tell him that he always is unwilling to inform and consult us of his dealing with CELU affairs. For instance; of his going to Dakar we [were] informed just a few days before his departure but no one told about his intended trip to Europe after the Dakar Conference. That Brother Tekie had been to Budapest I got knowledge of by the cable from you. I told Brother Tekie that I knew of his visit to Budapest and asked him where else he had been and he told that he had been even to Bulgaria and Yugoslavia. I have had several private talks in this matter with Brother Solomon, and he has told me for sure that CELU is not going to accept any aid from the Russians.[13]

Having proceeded to discuss the matter with a representatives of the concerned Ethiopian government ministry—the Ministry of National and Community Development (MNCD)—and having received the latter's assurance that the government would not permit any aid from the Soviet Union to CELU in whichever case, the ICFTU representative laid the matter to rest for the time being. The archival records thus illustrate how the ICFTU and its allies demanded that CELU report on all its operations, and reserved the right to decide on matters concerning whom CELU officers could meet and where they could go. But despite CELU repeatedly bowing to pressure and conceding to ICFTU demands, the records also show that such high-handed interference bred resentment. This provoked attempts to circumvent and challenge ICFTU oversight through rather innocuous and sporadic contacts with WFTU parties. These contacts were sometimes concealed and other times conducted openly. Another 'serious complication' thus developed when the ICFTU's assistant general secretary, Morris Paladino, attended the 1970 CELU anniversary celebrations and noticed the presence of two representatives of the Soviet trade union centre. This is how he described what happened next:

[13] Lennart Kindström to P.H. de Jonge, 5 January 1967, ICFTU/ITUC archives.

> I officially protested the presence of the WFTU and reminded CELU officers… that since I was obliged to report to the general secretary and the Executive Board on my representation to the Conference, that I would require explanations on CELU's invitation to the WFTU. The explanations which were given were of a make-shift nature and contradictory. The CELU officers finally resorted to the implication that the WFTU had been invited as a result of Government pressure. When I offered to discuss this directly with the Government and the Emperor if necessary, this argument was withdrawn.
>
> Most of us who witnessed the activities of CELU officers and their treatment of the Russian and WFTU representatives during these days concluded that the decision to invite the WFTU was one calculated to balance the impression that CELU was heavily dependent on the family of free trade unions; that the invitation was manoeuvred by the secretariat officers of CELU, aided and abetted by the inability of the CELU president, Beyene Solomon, to cope with the situation.
>
> I advised CELU officers that the ICFTU would look sternly on any continuous relationship of the CELU with the WFTU, and that the CELU would have to be judged in the future by its acts as by its stated intentions. In my discussions with our representatives Kindström and Kanyago, I left instructions that from now on they would have to deal with CELU with a stronger hand. They agreed that the policy of caution which has been employed during the formative years of CELU would now have to be abandoned for more positive guidance.[14]

In other words, in response to what was admittedly a token gesture by CELU to demonstrate some level of autonomy, the ICFTU determined that the exercise of even stricter control was warranted. In light of CELU's heavy reliance on ICFTU funds, this determination came with leverage. The ICFTU and the international 'free' trade union movement thus imposed a major constriction on CELU's external autonomy. To make matters worse the ICFTU struck up a close working relationship with the imperial state, and was granted access to its highest offices, including that of the emperor. Any radical impulse would henceforth be caught between and checked by, on the one hand and internally, a moderate and bureaucratised CELU leadership, and on the other hand

[14] "Mission to Addis Ababa and Nairobi," Morris Paladino, ICFTU/ITUC archives.

and externally, an international trade union movement and the imperial state, working in close mutual understanding.

As is indicated by CELU's timid attempts to assert some level of autonomy, however, ICFTU's high-handedness generated resentment and created tensions. The internal opponents of CELU's leadership were critical of CELU's close international alignment with the ICFTU camp, which prohibited the confederation from cooperating with WFTU-affiliated organisations and accepting support from them. CELU's Deputy Secretary Alemu Bogale, who challenged Beyene Solomon in CELU's 1965 General Assembly congress, was considered to be close with such WFTU-affiliated unions. It was rumoured among ICFTU affiliates that upon resigning from his post in CELU, and before being imprisoned for leading strikes in his basic union, he received his salary from a socialist bloc embassy, so as to be able to serve his basic union for free.[15] During CELU's subsequent General Congress of 1967, its top leadership's was again challenged on the close and exclusive relationship it nurtured with the ICFTU camp. This time the challenge was spearheaded by the chairman of CELU's Executive Board, Abraham Gabre—a unionist 'known for his militant views and actions'.[16] In response to the challenge, CELU's international partners rallied to the support of its leadership. In accounting for how this challenge was averted with his direct assistance, the ICFTU's representative Kindström provided an illustrative example of the depth of ICFTU manipulation and interference in CELU's internal affairs:

> Abraham Gabre [chairman of the executive board of the CELU] has always been very fond of WFTU and AATUF[17] and adversary to the ICFTU, [FES], and AALC and the West in general and have argued for assistance and aid from the East instead of the West. He had support of some few members within [the] CELU board for the idea of aid from the East, and possibly of some other union leaders. However, some time before the

[15] Daniel Pedersen to Villy Pedersen, 11 December 1967, LO archives.

[16] "Ethiopia Visit: July 6th–15th," field report, John Gore, 28 July 1966, African American Labor Center (AALC) Records, collection 0547-LBR, Hornbake Library, Special Collections and University Archives, University of Maryland Libraries, College Park, MD.

[17] The All-African Trade Union Federation. A body that in 1973 was replaced by OATUU.

> annual Conference, Brother Beyene Solomon got knowledge of the intention of Abraham Gabre to raise the question about the foreign assistance to the CELU at the Conference without informing CELU in advance. Brother Solomon informed me what was going on and both of us agreed to the necessity of a counter-move to prevent the attempt of Abraham Gabre... I suggested Brother Solomon to have a flag made with CELU emblem and to present the flag to the CELU as a gift from the ICFTU, at the Conference. Brother Solomon found the idea good and, as the excellent policy maker he is, suggested that the flag should not be given at the opening ceremony but the time Gabre raised his matter. The flag was made, and in the afternoon on the second day of the Conference Brother Solomon called me to present the flag. Gabre had at that time raised his question but Brother Solomon suggested a break of the discussion for the 'flag ceremony'. I could never imagine that the flag should be of so great effect as it became. All the delegates were happy and applauded and cheered and many of them made speeches with thanks to the ICFTU and praising the ICFTU for all the support and assistance given to the CELU. As the whole afternoon became a 'thanksgiving day' to the ICFTU, Brother Solomon found afterwards there were neither time nor reason to continue the discussion of the matter raised by Gabre, and suggested the matter dismissed which was met with universal approval. Afterwards almost every delegate personally thanked me and the ICFTU for the grandiose gift. That proves again that things which can be seen with one's own eyes and touched with the hand is more appreciated by these people than things of abstract nature even if the latter is worth a million more.[18]

This example starkly demonstrates how the ICFTU colluded with the top leadership in subverting CELU's internal democracy—the ostensible protection of which constituted its official purpose for operating in the country. But although it also illustrates how close the relationship between ICFTU and CELU's leadership was, it was not a frictionless relationship.

Friction and Break

The rationale for CELU's leadership's close cooperation with ICFTU only partially overlapped with the ICFTU's ultimate motivations. In 1965, CELU outlined six mutually agreed objectives for the intensified

[18] Lennart Kindström to P.H. de Jonge, 8 February 1967, ICFTU/ITUC archives.

cooperation with ICFTU that began the year before. The fifth objective was to obstruct the efforts of 'some people with other interests than that of CELU who were trying to get into the labour movement to further their own ends'.[19] Only this objective was earnestly shared by the two partnering organisations. Indeed, CELU's leadership had a genuine desire to 'bar the way'[20] against potential challengers from within the movement. And given the ICFTU's aversion to anything radical, such challengers could henceforth conveniently be portrayed as radicals or communist-influenced. But CELU's leadership had a harder time to accept ICFTU-imposed restrictions to its own autonomy in dealing with foreign trade union confederations. For this reason, it developed ways of circumventing ICFTU control. 'CELU officers always try to keep secret for me their connections with the trade unions in communist countries as I am an adversary of it', Kindström acknowledged.[21]

Another source of friction concerned the volumes of ISF allocations and forms of assistance extended by the ICFTU. Despite the increasing volumes provided, CELU consistently requested more aid than what was forthcoming, and was not necessarily content with what was granted. Moreover, CELU often desired funding for activities in manners that the ICFTU was not willing to provide. In such cases, CELU's senior officials had no qualms about openly expressing their discontent, while ICFTU officers and officials were often uneasy about CELU's assertiveness in those regards. 'It has been no undivided pleasure to talk to [Beyene] Solomon, since he must obviously assume that we adopt a very negative attitude towards assisting CELU', one ICFTU official[22] wrote upon encountering Beyene's strident insistence that additional funding be extended for CELU's activities in Eritrea. Whereas ICFTU viewed their funding as 'rather lavish', CELU, sensing its own leverage and ability to

[19] "Progress Report and Future Projected Activities of CELU," CELU to ICFTU, 22 October 1965, ICFTU/ITUC archives.

[20] The role of the ICFTU and the AFL-CIO in Ethiopia, the ICFTU's General Secretary Omer Becu had written to the President of the AFL-CIO in 1964, was to 'bar the way' to 'anti-free trade union forces'. Omer Becu to George Meany, 6 October 1964, ICFTU/ITUC archives.

[21] Lennart Kindström to P.H. de Jonge, 21 February 1968, ICFTU/ITUC archives.

[22] "Visit of Mr. Beyene Solomon," P.H. de Jonge to Stefan Nedzynski, 17 July 1964, ICFTU/ITUC archives.

play prospective and mutually suspicious donors off against each other, was determined to extract a higher price for its loyalty.

Even before CELU's radical turn, its relationship with the ICFTU was, by the early to mid-1970s, beginning to appear less intimate. Volumes of ISF funding began to drop sharply in 1973 and 1974. There was a plan to phase out support altogether, and the ICFTU's resident representative Kindström left Addis Ababa in May 1973 without being replaced. From that time on, the ICFTU was only represented in Addis Ababa by Paul Kanyago of its small regional research office,[23] and occasionally visiting representatives. In parallel, CELU, while still firmly within the international camp of 'free' trade unions, began to develop more cordial relations with WFTU-affiliated confederations. In 1973, the All-African Trade Union Federation (AATUF) and the ICFTU-backed African Trade Union Confederation (ATUC) merged into the Organisation of African Trade Union Unity (OATUU). CELU was a founding member of OATUU—and the organisation's initiating conference was held in Addis Ababa. In the face of the emergence of a non-aligned pan-Africanist trade unionist camp, CELU's credibility required it to maintain a certain degree of autonomy from the pro-Western camp of trade unions represented by the ICFTU. In fact, OATUU repeatedly called on its members to disaffiliate from other international trade union alliances. But for CELU that would not occur before its moderate leadership was ousted.

Despite signs of a cooling relationship, the moment of break came suddenly. CELU had notified the ICFTU of its intention to disaffiliate from it during the interim leadership of Alem Abdi in early 1975—citing its commitment to internationalism and to overcome the division of the international trade union movement. The notification was dismissed by the ICFTU as being an illegitimate decision of a minority, and 'not regarded as the decision of CELU'.[24] However, in June of the same year CELU's elected leader, Marcos Hagos, backed by an extraordinary General Assembly Congress resolution informed the ICFTU of its decision to sever ties completely, and ordered the ICFTU to vacate the office space it had been making use of. 'What is the ICFTU?', CELU's General

[23] The ICFTU's regional research office—staffed by only one research officer, Paul Kanyago—had been moved from Kampala to Ethiopia in 1969. In 1974 Francis Luyimbazi succeeded Kanyago. After the ICFTU's expulsion from Ethiopia, it was moved to Nairobi.

[24] Francis Luyimbazi to Ott Kersten, 17 February 1975, ICFTU/ITUC archives.

Assembly resolution rhetorically asked[25]: 'When we get the answers to these questions it will not be difficult to determine, whether CELU should maintain relations with [it] or not'. The resolution answered its own question: 'It is certain that imperialism uses this organisation (ICFTU) to sabotage the international struggle of the working class'. The ICFTU reacted bitterly, challenging Marcos Hagos' credentials to represent CELU at the ILO's 1975 International Labour Conference. However, it could not ignore CELU's decision, and it departed from Addis Ababa altogether later that year.

The ICFTU had played a very important role in the formation and early development of CELU. It had aided CELU's evolution into a relatively competent organisations, firmly aligned with the anti-communist international trade union movement. To ensure that this alignment was maintained, it had supported and facilitated the survival of a moderate incrementalist leadership. However, its subversion of CELU's internal democracy and its restriction of its external autonomy had also held back CELU's organic development into a more assertive and militant movement, and generated friction between the two. Once its control mechanisms failed and the pent-up pressures were released, CELU would not merely move incrementally in a more radical direction, but leap into the revolutionary movement, fully negating its experience with the ICFTU.

African American Labor Center

The AALC was founded in 1964 as the American Federation of Labor and Congress of Industrial Organisations' (AFL-CIO) organ for working in African countries. Despite its name, there was nothing African-American about the origin of its officers: its representatives were exclusively, or near exclusive, White Americans. Its executive director was Irving Brown, a Cold Warrior with a long experience of, and a single-minded intent to, weed out and erase real or perceived communist influence in the international trade union movement. He had played a key role in the ICFTU's

[25] CELU resolutions, passed and dated June 5, 1975, translated by an ILO regional officer in ILO's regional office in Addis Ababa, attachment to memorandum from ILO's Regional Meshack Ndisi Archive to H. Dunning and H. Hammar, 13 June 1975. ILO archives, International Labour Office, Geneva. International Labour Organization (ILO) archives, International Labour Office, Geneva.

split from the WFTU, and he had developed strong links to the US Central Intelligence Agency (CIA).

From its outset, the AALC identified Ethiopia as a priority country. The year after its foundation—in 1965—it signed a memorandum of understanding with CELU to initiate a cooperation programme. It fell upon Jerry Funk, who was appointed the AALC's regional representative in East Africa and opened an office in Addis Ababa in 1967, to develop and manage the programme. He remained in this position until early 1974, when he moved to the AALC's New York office to serve as its deputy director, and was replaced by Richard Baurmann.

Funk was himself a CIA man. This is an accusation that is often—for probably good reasons—levelled against US and particularly AFL-CIO officials involved in the international trade union movement, though it is not always substantiated. In Funk's case, however, there is certainty in this fact, as he acknowledged it himself in his 2003 self-published memoirs.[26] Having been recruited by the CIA in 1961, he entered the AFL-CIO without any real experience of rank-and-file trade unionism, and became an official of United Steelworkers. He was soon dispatched to the International Federation of Petroleum and Chemical Workers, before being assigned to Ethiopia by the AALC.

Due to its working methods, its connections and experience in intelligence operations, and the funds and manpower it was ready to invest, the AALC became the best-informed international trade union organisation operating in Ethiopia. It knew significantly more about the intricacies of Ethiopian trade union politics than other organisations. For example, it reported intelligence that there was 'an active communist party operating in Ethiopia' as early as January 1975, and linked it to the prevalence of 'pro-Chinese' dissidents in CELU.[27] At that time, the group that was to become the EPRP, and its workers' committee in CELU, was still operating entirely clandestinely—so much so that even among informed insiders, few would have known of its existence. The AALC was not only the most intrusive and subversive of the organisations discussed here, but also the most unscrupulous. It did not hesitate to use funds to acquire influence in ways that can only be described as corrupt. As a result of

[26] J. Funk, *Life is an Excellent Adventure: An Irreverent Personal Odyssey Or: Trying to Decide What I Want to Be When I Grow Up* (Victoria: Trafford, 2006).

[27] "BAR/LES No. 1, 1975," Richard Baurmann to Lester Trachtman, 10 January 1975, AALC Records.

these factors, it wielded significant influence both within CELU and with the government and the MNCD, and it used its leverage to actively shape events. But it also contributed to CELU's development.

AALC programmes in Ethiopia

The AALC's programmes entailed a more hands-on approach than the ICFTU's did. The AALC did not generally provide CELU with budget support—except for a short period between 1968 and 1969 when the ICFTU failed to disburse its subsidy on time—but preferred to operate its own programmes. For that reason, the AALC had plenty more staff posted and employed in Ethiopia than comparable organisations. By 1974, it had stationed four American staff in Ethiopia and employed another 19 Ethiopian staff members for CELU.[28] Its budget was also significantly higher than comparable organisations. By 1974, it estimated that it had spent a total of 1.6 million USD on programmes supporting CELU during the years it had been active in Ethiopia.[29]

Its most notable undertaking was the construction of a new headquarters building for CELU, completed between 1968 and 1970. Previously, CELU had occupied a 'dimly lighted mud structure' with insufficient space.[30] The new building, which costed 300,000 USD to construct, comprised 40 modern office rooms spread across three floors, along with a large auditorium. It occupied 2,000 square metres of land around the capital's centrally located Mexico Square. The joint agreement that granted AALC assistance for the project included provisions that the AALC and other international trade union organisations would have the right to install their staff in the building. Each AALC officer was granted one office. Once CELU had moved into the building, AALC and ICFTU representatives were thus able to monitor CELU from very close proximity. But the primary importance of the new headquarters building lay in relieving CELU's lack of office facilities and space. It also relaxed some of the financial strains it was facing. Its completion meant that CELU was no longer forced to spend funds on renting offices, but could instead itself

[28] "BAR/LES No. 4," Richard Baurmann to Lester Trachtman, 28 October 1974, AALC Records.

[29] "Report on Ethiopia," Andrew Kailembo, 16 October 1974, ICFTU/ITUC archives.

[30] "Labor Education Project: Report: Dec. 1968–July 1971," John Kilhefner, AALC Records.

rent out a full floor of the new building, and thus acquire a new source of funding. The AALC also contributed 30,000 USD to the construction of a CELU branch office in Asmara, which was completed in 1973.

Other projects that the AALC ran in CELU's favour included provision of assistance to cooperatives and credit unions, vocational training, and literacy classes. It also revived and expanded the publication of CELU's newspaper *Voice of Labour* from 1969 onwards, making it a monthly publication with skilled editorial staff. As has been noted, Seyoum Kebede and Kiflu Tadesse—both EPRP members, a fact unknown to the AALC—assumed the roles of chief and assistant editor in 1974, and transformed the newspaper into a radical publication. That same year the AALC also launched a project to fund and capacitate a research department of CELU, and, once new members had started swarming to CELU in the aftermath of the general strike, initiated a union organisation campaign that employed four organisers.

However the major effort of the AALC was in the field of trade union education, and its most consequential intervention was its recruitment, training, deployment, and financing of field workers for CELU. Six field workers, each covering an assigned geographic area, were recruited for this purpose starting in April 1969. 'To CELU's credit they did pick 6 real fine trade unionists', the AALC officer in charge of the programme enthusiastically reported.[31] Those selected for the roles were Alem Abdi, the future acting President of CELU, covering the greater Addis Ababa area; Tedla Fantaye, who later became involved in the labour opposition and eventually the EPRP, also operating in the industrial centres around Addis Ababa; Abraham Ghilazghi covering Eritrea—a former employee of the Danish LO project discussed in the next section of this chapter; Seyoum Hailu, covering the eastern Dire Dawa area; Solomon Tekle Tsion, covering the vicinity surrounding the city of Adama,[32] south of Addis Ababa; and Aberra Tadesse, covering the area surrounding Bahir Dar. The selected field workers underwent seven weeks of training before being deployed. By early 1970, all six field workers had been dispatched to their assigned areas. The next year, CELU would hire another two field workers, bringing their total number to eight.

[31] Ibid.

[32] At the time known as Nazret.

The deployment of field workers was a great success that considerably enhanced CELU's reach and capacity. Although the confederation's capabilities and resources continued to be stretched, this constituted a major improvement in its ability to service unions across the country. Initially, the AALC's intention was that the field workers would concentrate on setting up programs in labour education and literacy, arranging seminars and film displays. But the field workers came to do much more than that. Just as CELU officers and branch office staff were compelled by necessity to become all-round union staff, so were the field workers. Before long they found themselves organising unions and helping them in handling grievances and disputes, in addition to arranging the intended labour education seminars. During 1970 and the first six months of 1971 alone, the field workers organised seminars—usually lasting a week, but sometimes two—for 1,955 trade unionists; displayed films shows attended by 58,641 workers; negotiated 19 collective agreements; and organised the establishment of nine new unions.[33] In 1970, Tedla Fantaye described a typical field work stay:

> During our stay in Kebre Mengist we were busy from dawn to night. Workers were coming to our bedrooms to tell us their grievances. In the morning from 8 to 12 we used to go to the four employers to settle grievances. Every afternoon of the day we used to give lectures to the participants. During every evening of the 3 days we were showing films.[34]

Using the example of seminars held in Dire Dawa and Bahir Dar, John Kilhefner of the AALC explained how the field workers' activities brought CELU closer to its constituent unions and rank-and-file workers, deeply resonating with them:

> The image of CELU has been helped by these seminars. Little activity existed in many of these areas before and the branches began to question the value of belonging to the national center. Now they are praising CELU.

[33] "Labor Education Project: Report: Dec. 1968–July 1971," John Kilhefner, AALC Records.

[34] Report by Tedla Fantaye from February 2, 1970, cited in "Labor Education Project: Report: Dec. 1968–July 1971," John Kilhefner, AALC Records.

> They are happy about the seminars and especially about a Field Worker being assigned to their areas. The Field Workers are doing a wonderful job, much better than I ever expected. Where political problems exist within a union, [CELU's director of education] Mesfin meets with the representatives between classes to try and help work these out.[35]

The growing intimacy between field workers and local unionists contrasted with CELU's leadership's perceived aloofness, and the latter's greater attention to international affairs than to basic union work in the provinces. The AALC's advisor in charge of the field worker programme put it in the following way:

> Through the seminars the workers are getting to know the Field-Workers and Mesfin. Other top officials should make more of an attempt to take part in the education program, even if it is just to present certificates. Some of the areas that are difficult to get to and uncomfortable to stay in must be paid more attention unless CELU is to lose more affiliates. The purpose of the union is to make life more comfortable for all workers but until that time comes the leaders of the workers must have to share some of the discomfort the workers face every day.[36]

The field workers would play an important role in the continuing growth of CELU-affiliated unions, and in the upsurge of radical unionism in the mid-1970s, contributing significantly to countering the centralising impulse of CELU's embattled leadership.

However the AALC was not in Ethiopia primarily to connect workers to union services. Its main concern was consistently to 'influence events',[37] and its officers believed that the AALC's influence would continue to grow and 'inevitably become stronger'.[38] What the AALC sought to achieve with such influence can be distilled into two main objectives. Its first priority, much like the ICFTU's, was to ensure that CELU remained within the anti-communist camp of international

[35] John Kilhefner to John P. Hannah, 17 February 1970, AALC Records.

[36] "Labor Education Project: Report: Dec. 1968–July 1971," John Kilhefner, AALC Records.

[37] See, for example, "Recent Events in (1) Ethiopia and (2) Nigeria", memorandum from Patrick J. O'Farrell to Ernie Lee (draft), 1975, AALC Records.

[38] "Letter No. 14," John Gore to Lester Trachtman 24 November 1967, AALC Records.

trade unionism. It's leading officers, particularly Brown and Funk, were adamant that CELU could not be allowed to entertain the idea of any form of cooperation with socialist bloc trade unions. Secondly, it sought to counter labour militancy and radicalism within the Ethiopian trade union movement. The rise of what Jerry Funk called 'the opposition movement' and 'the Shoa (hard-core) dissidents' greatly concerned him.[39] He was nearly equally worried about the spread of wildcat strikes. 'While the [Addis Ababa Bank] strike [of August 1973] can be called a victory', he wrote in August 1973, 'it also opens a new area of concern: how to keep the lid on a potential rash of ill-conceived wild-cat strikes'.[40] To achieve the AALC's twin aims in Ethiopia, labour education and the inculcation of anti-communist trade union doctrines were considered essential. But of higher practical and immediate priority was to seek to prevent any challenges to CELU's moderate leadership. 'I feel we have in Ato Beyene a strong anti-Communist', the US ambassador in Addis Ababa wrote to the AALC, 'but he cannot hope to contain the discontent and disenchantment with the western labor organisations which is likely to develop if CELU cannot count on assistance from us in a crisis'.[41]

Propping up CELU's Leadership and Playing Kingmakers

Most interventions that the AALC undertook were designed with an implicit or explicit goal to strengthen the internal position of CELU's leadership. The construction of CELU's headquarters, for example, was motivated partly by Beyene 'badly needing a start on the building as a means of recapturing lost prestige and momentum'.[42] The resources the AALC made available were also intentionally used to build or consolidate internal clientelist networks with favours flowing from higher levels, and to support the leadership's efforts to centralise communication and service delivery for this purpose. In 1971, for example, Funk instructed all AALC staff in Ethiopia that 'all communications to any officer or member of CELU [must] be addressed directly to the President', in order

[39] "Report No. 256 Subject: CELU General," Jerry Funk, 23 August 1973, AALC Records.

[40] Ibid.

[41] William O. Hall to Dean Clowes 12 July 1968, AALC Records.

[42] "Report No. 52," Jerry Funk to Lester Trachtman, 24 November 1968, AALC Records.

to support Beyene's 'new get-tough, take-charge attitude' and thus facilitate his campaign to be re-elected the following year. 'He now has openly decided he wants to be President-for-Life, and he is executing all the right political moves to see that he is', Funk wrote to the staff. 'I support his efforts as do key people in the IEG [Imperial Ethiopian Government]'.[43]

AALC and AFL-CIO resources were also used to keep senior CELU officials personally loyal to its president. In 1971, Funk asked Irving Brown, on Beyene's request, to redirect Beyene's invitation to that year's AFL-CIO convention to another senior member of CELU's leadership, extend the length of the trip for an additional month, and include the senior official's newly-wed spouse in the invitation so as to allow them to spend their honeymoon in the US. 'The trip request is in the nature of both a carrot and stick for [the senior official] Fisseha, who is working well with Beyene, and cooperating completely in the "new look"', Funk explained.[44]

When the increasingly coordinated labour opposition intensified in strength from 1972 onwards, the AALC stepped up its operations to support the assailed leadership. The 'revolt', Funk acknowledged,[45] stemmed from 'a crisis of leadership at the top'. 'The situation is critical, but not yet fatal' he wrote: 'Beyene is still viable, but he needs help, badly'. The AALC's key manoeuvre was to arrange for a shuffle of CELU officials. In Tsegay Abebe, the former HVA union president, they had identified 'the man who can bring some semblance of intelligent leadership back to CELU, working with and advising Beyene'.[46] Given the respect he commanded and his reputation of being clean and daring, Tsegay was considered ideally placed to 'to play a particular role in blunting the incipient Shoa[47]/Amhara revolt against CELU'. But first, he needed to return from the United States, where he was at the time.

[43] "Communications with CELU," memorandum to AALC staff from Jerry Funk, 25 August 1971, AALC Records.

[44] "NLRB and/or AFL-CIO, Convention Travel for Ato Fisseha, GEN. SEC., CELU," Jerry Funk to Irving Brown, 24 September 1971, AALC Records.

[45] "Report No 234. Subject: Second Half Report 1972," Jerry Funk, 13 February 1973, AALC Records.

[46] "Report No. 233: CELU, CONFIDENTIAL", Jerry Funk to Irving Brown and Patrick O'Farrell, 6 February 1973, AALC Records.

[47] Shoa (or Shewa) was the name of the central region in which Addis Ababa was located.

It was, in fact, the AALC that had sent Tsegay to the US in the first place. He had been dispatched there two years earlier to acquire experience in union affairs, working for the United Steelworkers union. By that time, the AALC had already identified him as a future asset to be 'groomed'—possibly to eventually replace Beyene.[48] But as Beyene's position had weakened precipitously, Tsegay's presence in Ethiopia had become needed sooner than expected. Tsegay, the AALC reasoned, was needed 'in elective office, either in CELU or a strong affiliate – this far in advance of April 1975 elections to insure his effectiveness', and the route to get him 'in a better position to get moving', was to bring him back to Ethiopia right away. 'We should encourage Ato Tsegay Abebe to return to Ethiopia, as soon as possible, to give Beyene badly needed support, advice and guidance', Funk wrote in a confidential report to Irving Brown.[49] In addition, Funk argued, Tesfa Gebremariam, who was also abroad at the time, should also be brought back sooner than originally planned. 'Tesfa, as the only Amhara in the original cast of characters', Funk wrote, 'will be most useful, should he return this summer, in acting as an honest broker between Beyene and the Amharas of Shoa (Addis)'.[50] Tesfa, like Tsegay, had been sent to the US in another AALC-initiated power manoeuvre. 'Regarding Tesfa, I am now very determined to push him to the States for a year as a counter-balance to [CELU Secretary General] Fisseha', Funk had explained in 1969[51]: 'he needs the tour and study for self-confidence as well as prestige'. Beyene, Funk noted, was 'somewhat nervous about Tesfa's loyalty and ambitions. But he needs him in Shoa… and has to take a gamble'. Brown and Beyene concurred on both points, and Funk proceeded to implement his plans.

In 1973, the AALC engineered the return of Tsegay through the offices of the International Federation of Plantation, Agricultural and Allied Workers (IFPAAW). Tsegay was employed within an IFPAAW project organising plantation workers. To facilitate this, the AALC had offered to pay a share of Tsegay's salary, but IFPAAW settled for a bartered exchange: the AALC donated a Landcruiser vehicle to the

[48] T. Killion, "Workers, Capital and the State in the Ethiopian Region" (PhD diss., Stanford University, 1985, 536.

[49] "Report No. 233", Funk, AALC Records.

[50] Ibid.

[51] "Report No. 97: CELU; General Comments," Jerry Funk to Lester Trachtman, 27 March 1969, AALC Records.

IFPAAW project, which in turn released the funds required for Tsegay's employment.[52] The word of Tsegay's return, Funk wrote, immediately 'gave the moderate dissident unions an intangible but nonetheless important feeling that changes could be possibly coming at some point in the foreseeable future'. His arrival was deemed an immediate success that 'made it possible for serious discussions of reconciliation to take place between CELU officers and several of the key dissidents', Funk wrote, 'discussions which would have been unthinkable a month ago'.[53] The real purpose of his return, however, to prop up Beyene, was to be concealed until he could be elected to a representative office: 'He has been playing, and will continue to play, a low-key, background role, not getting directly involved in day to day problems', Funk wrote. Although the strategy ultimately failed, and Beyene was forced to resign, Tsegay would continue to play the role of supporting a relatively moderate leadership, until he was ousted for his backing of Alem Abdi in 1975.

As the above illustrates, AALC officers played the role of king-makers in various ways. This continued beyond Beyene's downfall and subsequent arrest. In between Beyene's announcement of his resignation and his arrest, Beyene met with the AALC's newly appointed executive director Patrick O'Farrell. They discussed how to secure moderation and continuity in CELU beyond Beyene's tenure, and how to ensure that his designated successor was elected.[54] By late 1974, after Beyene and most of his allies in the senior leadership had been imprisoned, the AALC had come to the conclusion that Alem Abdi's pro-PMAC faction—supported by Tesfa Gebremariam, who had become CELU's deputy secretary—was its best remaining bet against the radical opposition. It therefore transferred its support to Alem's faction. Alem and Tesfa, the AALC's newly appointed regional representative Baurmann wrote in October, 'convinced me they could hold the organization together with some financial help'.[55] The AALC financed two CELU staff conferences that month, which, according to the AALC, 'kept the organization together and prevented the left wing elements [i.e. the labour opposition] from

[52] T. Killion, "Workers, Capital and the State", 538.

[53] "Report No. 243; February/March 1973: CELU General," Jerry Funk, 23 March 1973, AALC Records.

[54] Richard Baurmann to Lester Trachtman, 31 August 1974, AALC Records.

[55] "BAR/LES No.3," Richard Baurmann to Lester Trachtman, 25 October 1974, AALC Records.

exercising their plan'.[56] Alem was highly appreciative, and publicly praised the AALC at the conference for having 'saved the situation'.[57] However, that was not the greatest service rendered to him and his faction by the AALC. In February 1975, Alem requested that the AALC suspend all its seminars and programs until a General Assembly congress had been held. This allowed Alem Abdi, Baurmann acknowledged, to 'use AALC Field Workers for the political campaign'.[58] The AALC acquiesced to the request.

Covert Funds and Activities

The source of AALC funding was deliberately concealed. The AALC was keen on being seen as a 'private organisation' despite the fact that its funding came from the US government, and it therefore concealed the origin of the funds it dispensed. The US embassy in Addis Ababa deemed it essential that the funding was not construed as coming from state sources, 'in order to avoid the accusations that the US Government is meddling in Ethiopian labor'.[59] But that was false. The AALC's programmes were entirely funded by the US government, and this was known to CELU's higher officials, although not openly acknowledged. CELU's leadership 'were certainly aware of the AID/AALC relationship', Baurmann wrote to the AALC's New York headquarters in 1974. 'I cannot explain how they may have gained this knowledge', he continued, but noted approvingly their 'maturity' in withholding this information and his trust in their continued discretion to do so. This was especially important, he noted, 'in light of "foreign manipulation, CIA and other rumors" being castigated against labor'.[60]

The AALC's use of funds was occasionally even more opaque than their source. As has been discussed, resources were frequently used purposely to support the maintenance of clientelist relationships within the movement, which tied a diverse range of officials, union representatives and

[56] Richard Baurmann to Patrick O'Farrell, 23 October 1974, AALC Records.

[57] "BAR/LES No.3," Baurmann to Trachtman, AALC Records.

[58] Richard Baurmann to Lester Trachtman, 10 February 1975, AALC Records.

[59] William O. Hall to Dean Clowes, 12 July 1968, AALC Records.

[60] "BAR/LES No. 8," Richard Baurmann to Lester Trachtman, 20 November 1974, AALC Records.

staff to the top leadership. In other cases, the AALC displayed a relaxed attitude to means being diverted from their intended purposes, as long as it supported such clientelist networks. In late September 1974, for example, Beyene had been arrested and AALC officers worried that charges of misappropriation of funds would be levelled against him. 'I am aware of Beyene's covert operations but what African leader hasn't been involved at one time or another?', the AALC's representative in Addis rhetorically asked.[61] Earlier that month, the AALC had handed Beyene 13,000 Ethiopian dollars, to covertly fund CELU's leadership's doomed attempt to prevent the radical labour opposition from coming to power. This was reported by the AALC's representative in Addis Ababa:

> By [Beyene] resigning now, but making the date effective in February 1975, the more moderate CELU faction can build a candidate prior to any special election. There are some who believe however, that the left wing element may still try to push for a complete new CELU leadership during the coming September 17th meeting. *In this connection, I have written a check for cash in the amount of Ethie $3,000 for the current campaign. We wish no record of AALC help. Beyene believes that another Ethie $10,000 will be needed for an all-out campaign between the September meeting and February.* [NB: capitalised in the original].
> I wish approval to spend up to an additional ethio $10,000.00 as I believe thirteen thousand ethio is a small amount to hopefully secure what has been spent during the last ten or eleven years.[62]

In yet another type of cases, the disbursement of funds came close to entail the open corruption of officeholders and government officials. A prime example of this relates to the AALC's relationship with the Ministry of National Community Development and Social Affairs (MNCD) of the Imperial Ethiopian Government, and particularly the head of its Labour Department. Lt. Michael Amede—a member of a prominent aristocratic family, and a former recipient of a US government grant. For the AALC, it was important to enjoy a close, confidential and mutually trustful relationship with the imperial government, and particularly the MNCD. On the one hand, this facilitated cooperation in acquiring government permission for its various activities. But it also enabled intelligence sharing, and

[61] "Information and Suggestions on Current CELU Situation," Richard Baurmann to Lester Trachtman, 26 September 1974, AALC Records.

[62] Richard Baurmann to Lester Trachtman, 2 September 1974, AALC Records.

cooperation in preventing external actors from entering the Ethiopian labour scene, as well as in hindering radical Ethiopian trade unionists from acquiring the upper hand within the movement. The MNCD's Labour Department served as a final safeguard against CELU radicalisation.

Lt Michael played an important role in these designs. When CELU's General Secretary Fissehatsion, returning from a trip to the US in 1969, suggested that CELU would have a role to play in politics that was greater than AFL-CIO's conception of 'businesss unionism', the AALC's representative Jerry Funk contacted Lt Michael. The latter assured Funk 'that he was going to inform Fissehatsion that "it was the government's assumption that CELU's objective was to establish economic unionism"'.[63] In 1973, moreover, when the General Secretary of the World Congress of Labour (WCL) came to visit the oppositional trade unions, Lt Michael again came to the defence of the AALC's and the ICFTU's interests. On his arrival to Addis Ababa's airport, the WCL official was stopped, searched and had his documents confiscated. He was then taken to Lt Michael, who gave him 'a lengthy and stern lecture', and informed the opposition that 'they were dealing with the wrong people' by approaching WCL.[64] 'I am not concerned that the [WCL]'s ultimate objective could fully succeed', Funk wrote to Irving Brown. The government, he assured, 'can, and will, if necessary, crush any serious, open move by [the WCL]'.[65] But how could Funk and the AALC be so certain of the government's disposition towards a possible contender of theirs? There were two reasons for this self-assuredness.

On the one hand, the AALC had nurtured relationships with the imperial state on multiple levels. This included the Prime Minister's Office, which, at the time of the WCL's General Secretary's visit had become 'directly concerned about the whole situation'.[66] And the manner in which the Prime Minister's Office consulted Funk on issues of key importance testified both to the prevalence of a genuinely trustful relationship,

[63] "Report No 81: FISSEHA (Gen.Sec., CELU) trip to US, Student criticism of CELU", Jerry Funk, 6 February 1969, AALC Records.

[64] "Report No. 243", Funk, AALC Records.

[65] "Report No. 233", Funk, AALC Records.

[66] "Report No. 243", Funk, AALC Records.

and the extraordinary level of collusion that occurred between the imperial state and the AALC—a foreign organisation—in blatantly interfering in CELU's affairs.

> They [the Prime Minister's Office] are watching developments very closely, and have approached me about my assessment of CELU's internal problems, the role of WCL, etc. They have unofficially kept me very well informed about their information on WCL. They feel that it 'may be time for a change in leadership'. I have tried to convince them that, at minimum, Beyene must be retained for the foreseeable future. Their general feeling is that this may be acceptable.[67]

But the AALC's relationship with the Labour Department of the MNCD was even closerthan with the Prime Minister's Office. Not only was Jerry Funk and Lt Michael Amede, the Labour Department's head, personal friends, with the latter having played an honorary role in the former's wedding. But what was not publicly known was the fact that Lt Michael was privately indebted to the AALC. In early September 1974, as senior figures of the imperial government and aristocracy were hauled off to prison one by one by the Derg, on charges, among others, of corruption—the Minister of MNCD, Mulatu Debebe, was among them, and he would be summarily shot two months later—Lt Michael was in a vulnerable position. His situation was not made any better by the fact that the AALC—an institution he had colluded and cooperated closely with for the past seven years—was becoming a target of the underground leftist press that was proliferating in Addis Ababa, accused of being a CIA front. Early one Saturday morning that month, Lt Michael therefore called to the AALC's new representative Richard Baurmann, asking the latter to remove any documents linking him to the AALC from its offices. He was primarily concerned with documents pertaining to an unaccounted loan that he had received from the AALC a few years before.[68] In other words, while the Labour Department under Lt Michael's direction aligned itself fully with the objectives of the AALC, the relationship extended far beyond what could be publicly acknowledged or even legally justified. It included covert financial transactions to individual senior officials. The AALC did more than Lt Michael had requested. In fact, before departing

[67] Ibid.

[68] Richard Baurmann to Lester Trachtman, 2 September 1974, AALC Records.

from Addis Ababa the next year its representative destroyed nearly all of its archived records, to make sure that no compromising or sensitive information fell into the wrong hands. Only 'very mundane records' and some files related to the construction of CELU's headquarter building, that were deemed important for Beyene's court case, were spared.[69]

Tensions

In the end it was not external forces—which the AALC had feared—such as the Derg or socialist bloc influence,that doomed the AALC's relationship with CELU, but rather the internal tensions it generated. In particular, it was the AALC's intense meddling in CELU's internal affairs that strained it. There had been occasional tensions between the supposed allies going back to the first years of the relationship. Sometimes they emerged from strained personal relationships, and in the contrast between the patronising attitude of the AALC's officer—who were in the habit of frequently referring to CELU's senior elected officials as 'boys'—and CELU leaders' desire to be seen as equals. In early 1968, for example, CELU asked the AALC to recall one of its advisors, John Gore, from Ethiopia. 'These Americans are not diplomats and he [Gore] has stepped on too many toes, so CELU has asked to have him removed', a Danish trade union advisor in Asmara reported.[70] In that specific case, the AALC acquiesced. But different priorities, and the determination of the AALC to tether CELU's positions and worldview to its own, constituted the more fundamental factor behind the eventual fall-out.

CELU's leadership's reasons for nurturing ties with its international allies were entirely pragmatic. Its relations with the AALC, much like those with the ICFTU, were rooted in its need to acquire resources, skills, and stature. Its leadership did not shy away from using ICFTU and AALC resources to thwart perceived threats from internal or external challengers, which included the militant labour opposition. But internally, its officials were hesitant towards the virulent anti-communism of the AFL-CIO and unconvinced that CELU's interests were best served by severing all ties to

[69] "BAR-LES No.7; FINAL REPORT," Richard Baurmann to Lester Trachtman, 24 May 1975, AALC Records.

[70] Villy Pedersen to Per Carlsen, 26 February 1968, LO archives.

socialist bloc trade unions. On several occasions, they stated their reservations bluntly but casually to their American allies, to the latter's great chagrin. In fact, John Gore's expulsion was preceded by a number of incidents in which his reaction betrayed the real conflict of views.

In late 1967, Gebreselassie Gebremariam had returned to Addis Ababa from an ICFTU conference in Kampala with a book on the topic of the connection between AFL-CIO and the CIA. 'He is now playing the role of one filled with a reservoir of inside information and is actively spreading it about', John Gore wrote.[71] Gore requested that Irving Brown intervened to 'tell Beyene that certain individuals, the college boys, should not impede AALC's program by invoking "nationalistic sentiments"'. What Gore considered to constitute such impediment was an alleged attempt by Tesfa Gebremariam 'to stymie my efforts to obtain two unused offices at CELU for [AALC advisor] Thomas on the ridiculous grounds CELU should not be identified with the Americans (AALC)'. 'AALC will not rent offices separate from CELU', Gore made clear, and Tesfa's objections were overruled. To Gore, the strategical aspects of the disagreement—the difference in outlook between CELU and AALC officials—was a ruse. Instead, he reasoned, Tesfa was simply dissatisfied that power was shifting from CELU's officials towards the AALC:

> With each passing month as more unions come to deal directly with employers and Government, the college boys [CELU's university educated officials] are finding their once prominent positions of power and influence to be slowly withering away. And when considered in the future context that our presence will inevitably become stronger and more prominent, slight stirrings of what was once latent nationalism are beginning to emerge. For example, both [AALC advisor] Thomas and the Education Advisor will be dealing directly with rank and file leaders through intermediaries of their own choice and not the college boys. This is the rub.[72]

This statement exemplifies a disparaging attitude to CELU's staff and officeholders that was common in AALC officers' correspondence and reporting. But leaving that aside, the divergent strategical and political

[71] "Letter No. 14," John Gore to Lester Trachtman, 24 November 1967, AALC Records.

[72] Ibid.

priorities of the two parties could not be dispelled as easily as Gore's argument would suggest. The very same month the letter cited above was written, Gore had been informed by another AALC advisor that the officials Gore referred to as 'college boys' had expressed their disagreement with the AALC's rigidity at an informal luncheon. They 'took AALC to task for being overly "anti-Communist" in its policy and complained that "ICFTU is strictly political"', asking 'why couldn't CELU enjoy the best of two worlds'.[73] The real conflict of views this reveals did not end with the departure of John Gore. Jerry Funk, the long-time regional representative, repeatedly found himself at odds with the four younger and university-educated CELU officials and staff. He accused them of 'xenophobia', 'beeing coy', and of 'continu[ing] to think within a Marxist frame of reference'.[74] The latter accusation emerged in response to an interview, in which CELU's General Secretary Fissehatsion had rejected the relevance of US-style business unionism to CELU.[75] It indicated latent but real disagreement with the AALC and the AFL-CIO on the strategically most important question possible.

There is ample archival evidence demonstrating that the relationship between AALC and CELU officials was not always characterised by trust, even during its more harmonious phases. In 1967 a Danish trade union advisors in Ethiopia had developed the impression that, with regard to the AALC, 'there is much more love for American dollars than the Americans themselves'.[76] At the groundbreaking ceremony for the construction of CELU's new headquarters in 1968, CELU's insistence on reading out 'a lot of long greetings from communist countries', meant that the ICFTU's greeting had to be cut short. 'They are some strange men these CELU people', the Danish trade union advisor bemusedly noted. 'I have a feeling that once the centre is built they will kick the Americans out'.[77] One year into the construction, CELU sprang the idea upon the AALC that instead

[73] "Asmara visit—November 7–11th," John Gore to Lester Trachtman, 15 November 1967, AALC Records.

[74] "Report No. 97: CELU; General Comments," Jerry Funk to Lester Trachtman 27 March 1969, AALC Records.

[75] "Report No 81", Funk, AALC Records.

[76] "Rapport for Perioden 21. April 1967–21. Oktober 1967," report, Villy Pedersen to Danish Ministry for Foreign Affairs' Secretariat for Technical Cooperation with Developing Countries, October 1967, LO archives.

[77] Villy Pedersen to Per Carlsen, 9 April 1968, LO archives.

of building a three-storey building, they should build a five-storey one. This was rejected as implausible by the AALC, which triggered a serious disagreement between the parties. It was described by Jerry Funk in the following terms:

> [T]hings got pretty rough between me and CELU during the week prior [and] Beyene was leading the attack, but they were all united. I was ready to kill Beyene several times, and he was ready to reciprocate and we made no damned pretenses. He at one point demanded that I sign the building over to them as it was; at another, he thumped the table and said that they would never accept the building, never touch it, until it had 5 floors, and finally threatened to call security and tell them to refuse me exit visas. It was at this point that I lost my cool, informed Beyene that he was a small boy, was making a fool of CELU and Ethiopia, and that he could take the building as it was, break it into bits with a small hammer, and shove it up his ass, until it came out his ears bit by bit.[78]

The situation was ultimately resolved, but it betrayed a lingering sense of distrust. This was evident from Funk's report.

> I managed to get Beyene alone, for the first time, and he said that he was getting terrific pressure, unspecified, from within and without, but that he didn't want to make trouble for me or for [Irving Brown], that he now believed that I wasn't trying to screw CELU, and that he would absolutely guarantee that the dogs would be called off, but that he needed time to take care of things before this became public. We then went through the hugging and kissing routine…., and swore eternal friendship. This is fine, but I intend to keep my back to the wall for a while. As of this afternoon, the news is not yet public, but Beyene seems to be maneuvering in such a way that indicates he is keeping his word.[79]

By the mid-1970s, the AALC had begun to realise that their many advisor had overstayed their welcome. In the AALC representative Jerry Funk's assessment, CELU was, by early 1974, 'rapidly outgrowing its need for "advisors"', and had already, he added, 'outgrown my ever-present "lording" over their daily activities'. 'CELU', he stressed, 'does not need or want continuing advisorships, only intermittent counseling and financial

[78] "Personal", Jerry Funk to Patrick O'Farrell, 1 August 1969, AALC Records.

[79] Ibid.

assistance'.[80] The following month, Funk's newly arrived successor, Baurmann, found himself less than warmly welcomed by CELU, which did not invite him to meet with its leadership until six weeks had passed. 'I've been trying to rationalize CELU's indifference toward AALC', he wrote, suggesting that the accusations against the AALC of engaging in 'third party interference' was a possible factor in this.[81] Around the same time, the AALC noted that a *Voice of Labour* editorial had openly criticised 'the political strings attached to some Western foreign assistance' to CELU.[82] Although the relationship was clearly cooling, the sudden nature of its termination nevertheless took the AALC by great surprise.

Departure

By early 1975, the AALC was attempting to nurture a relationship with CELU's interim leadership, headed by Alem Abdi. In order to retain some of its influence, it was willing to consider adapting to the political changes underway in Ethiopia. 'If developments allow AALC to remain in Ethiopia, and permit CELU to operate a viable program, our intent is to work with CELU staff in articulating CELU's role in the new Ethiopian Socialist order', one of the AALC's more progressively inclined advisors wrote.[83] Alem Abdi, in turn, assured the Americans that CELU wished to maintain its relationship with the AALC.[84] For this reason, the AALC was convinced that the notification of disaffiliation that the ICFTU had received in early 1975 did not affect its own bilateral relationship with CELU. This abruptly changed with CELU's extraordinary congress in May-June 1975 and the election of the PWC. The congress voted to sever CELU's relations with both the ICFTU and the AALC. The AFL-CIO and the AALC were the subject of even sharper condemnation than

[80] "Report No. 13, Ethiopia," Dick Arnold to AALC head office, 12 February 1974, AALC Records.

[81] "CELU MEETING," minutes from meeting on 20 March 1974, appendix to "Report No. 2, East African Region," Richard Baurmann to Lester Trachtman, 29 March 1974, AALC Records.

[82] "Ethiopian Policy with Respect to CELU and AALC Viability", memorandum, Richard Baurmann, 12 March 1974, AALC Records.

[83] "P.A. 24, Ethiopia, July 1 to December 31, 1974," project report, John F. Summers, 25 January 1975, AALC Records.

[84] Richard Baurmann to Lester Trachtman, 15 March 1975, AALC Records.

the ICFTU. The congress resolution accused the AFL-CIO of a historical record of sabotaging and splintering the international labour movement. It included having been 'in the forefront of reactionaryly [sic] disaffiliation from the international organization (WFTU)', having 'participated in the anti-Bolshevik campaigns', supported imperialist war and colonization of the Philippines, and war against the people of Vietnam. But CELU also took the AFL-CIO to task for its activities in Africa, and particularly in Ethiopia, reflecting the resentment of CELU's radicals towards the AALC's history of interference in their movement's affairs:

> In Africa [the AFL-CIO] has been spreading its sabotage through its organ known as the AALC. Up to this date, this organization had been the supporter of Alem Abdi and his group and thereby spending the money that comes in the name of the workers, for anti-working class activities.

As a result, CELU's congress resolution announced that 'as of today 3 June 1975 the anti-imperialist workers of Ethiopia have severed their relations with AFL-CIO and AALC'. The resolution acknowledged that the severance of relations would lead to 'financial shortages', but insisted that it would be worth the 'sacrifice'.[85] The AALC was thus forced to immediately suspend all its programmes in Ethiopia and evacuate the offices it utilised in CELU's headquarters. It did not, however, abandon hope that it could retain some level of influence. The AALC's Addis Ababa office was well-informed about the deliberations that had taken place at the conference, and summarized the discussions and factors that led to their expulsion as follows:

> The clause of the resolution severing relations with ICFTU and with AFL-CIO was one of the sections that had a great deal of debate. Several argued that the question was premature that the Assembly did not know the roles played (by AALC in particular) nor did it know the consequences, financially or otherwise.
>
> However the arguments that Americans are CIA agents, and that the reason for AALC 'intervention' in CELU affairs was to promote the interests of foreign capitalists created an emotional appeal that carried the day.

[85] CELU resolutions, passed and dated June 5, 1975, ILO archives.

> It appears the majority of the delegates voted against Capitalist, Imperialist and CIA interests without any knowledge or understanding of the objectives, methods or programs of AALC. …
>
> The fact that AALC works with the constitutionally elected officials, in this case Tesfa and Alem, clinched the case. Delegates suspected that AALC was making secret contributions which had financed the old administration.[86]

Despite this understanding of the factors that had led to the break—and the deep resentment from which it sprung—the AALC retained hope that CELU's ordinary General Assembly congress, scheduled for September 1975, would overturn the decision to sever relations. The AALC moved into an externally rented office and retained a much-reduced number staff in Addis Ababa in order to 'listen to the various elements of the trade unions in Ethiopia, and await the development of opportunities'.[87] By contrast, the AALC's central directors in New York and the AFL-CIO shared a cruder, more hawkish understanding of events. 'CELU has been taken over by a small group of leftists, using Russian money and ideology, and with the approval and active support of an increasingly tyrannical and repressive military regime', the AALC's executive director wrote to the AFL-CIO's international affairs department.[88] The content of CELU's resolution was dismissed as 'lengthy Moscow-written polemics'. However, that assertion was patently false. It was also at odds with what had been reported by its Addis Ababa office, which knew that the resolution had been written exclusively by Ethiopians. In the short term, the AALC's executive director hoped to use the regional office 'to monitor events in CELU and keep whatever contacts we can with CELU affiliates'.[89] In the longer term, he argued, 'we must make every effort to maintain our presence… for as long as possible to enable us to influence events in any way we can'. Ultimately he was pessimistic about such possibilities, reasoning that trade union 'freedom' from state intervention could only result from another military coup:

[86] "Background Report to All Ethiopian Projects," John F. Summers, 6 July 1975, AALC Records.

[87] Ibid.

[88] "Recent Events in (1) Ethiopia and (2) Nigeria", O'Farrell to Lee, AALC Records.

[89] Ibid.

> [W]e must recognize that the only real hope for return of trade union freedom in Ethiopia is contingent upon a fairly dramatic change of policy by the [PMAC] – and that this can probably only be affected by some sort of coup by the moderate officers within the [PMAC] itself. There is some reasonable expectation that this could happen.[90]

In September 1975, CELU's General Assembly congress dashed the AALC's hopes by reaffirming the line established at the May/June extraordinary congress. That same month, the AALC relocated its regional representative to Nairobi. Its office in Addis Ababa was henceforth tasked only with liaisoning with the ILO's regional office and the UN Economic Commission of Africa, and retained just one secretary on its payroll. It was finally closed in May 1978.

In the end, the AALC's strategy of controlling the Ethiopian labour movements through the upper echelons of the trade union confederation—by acquiring the loyalties and indebtedness of CELU's most senior officeholders and key state officials—failed spectacularly. 'In a very real sense, we have been directly responsible for the creation of CELU and for its solid growth', the AALC's executive director concluded, summarising his organisation's experience in Ethiopia.[91] While that claim was factually incorrect, it betrayed the arrogance that what was to doom the AALC's efforts. Despite the very real contributions the AALC's assistance had made to the Ethiopian trade union movement, its patronising attitude and blatant interference in CELU's internal affairs had also provoked deep resentment and fostered hostility. When the labour opposition came to power in CELU, and the officeholders and state officials in whom the AALC had invested were ousted, its levers of influence over CELU vanished entirely.

Danish LO

Of the three interventions focused on here, the smallest in scale and shortest in duration was that of the Danish Confederation of Trade Unions—known by the abbreviation of its Danish name, *Landsorganisationen* (LO). Despite its brevity and the comparatively limited personnel and financial resources invested, it led to some significant outcomes.

[90] Ibid.

[91] Ibid.

Similarly to the AALC's intervention, it generated tensions and became embroiled in bitter conflict before its premature termination. In both aspects, it contains important insights into how CELU interacted with, benefited from and, occasionally, came into conflict with its partners in the international 'free' trade union movement.

LO's intervention—or the Danish mini-project, as the Danish trade unionists frequently called it in their internal correspondence—in Ethiopia began with a proposal from the ICFTU's Swedish representative in Addis Ababa, Lennart Kindström, that CELU invite LO to assist it. CELU accepted this, and in February 1965, Per Carlsen, LO's international secretary, travelled to Ethiopia to appraise fields in which assistance could be provided. On his return, he proposed four areas for such assistance: workers' education, promotion of workers' cooperatives, technical training, and education of workers' spouses. Out of these, workers' education came to be seen as the primary task.

LO's proposal was met with approval and funding from the Danish Ministry for Foreign Affairs' Secretariat for Technical Cooperation with Developing Countries, and it was agreed upon that a Danish officer should be sent to work with CELU for an initial period of a year. It was, at the time, the only such development cooperation project LO operated, highlighting the importance it assigned to trade union development in Ethiopia.

The Danes, like the ICFTU but unlike the Americans, assigned experienced trade unionists to their project. The first Danish advisor to CELU—a workers' education specialist named Daniel Pedersen—arrived in February 1966. He remained in Addis Ababa until October of that year, when CELU asked him to relocate to Eritrea to support the development of the trade union movement that had just been legally permitted in that province. The LO advisors were to remain in Eritrea until they encountered difficulties in their relationship with the local and central institutions of CELU in 1968. However, by that time, Daniel Pedersen had first been replaced by Villy Pedersen—another workers' education specialist from the Danish labour movement's bank who arrived in April 1967; and Villy Pedersen had also, in turn, been replaced. The final Danish advisor to CELU was Kaj Jensen of the Danish Seamen's Union. He arrived in May 1968 and would remain in Ethiopia until the end of December 1969.

By relocating their intervention to Eritrea, LO was submitting to plans designed and determined by CELU—in contrast to ICFTU and AALC.

From the outset, LO gave CELU an open mandate to assign its advisor to wherever it saw the greatest needs. Before Eritrea was decided upon, CELU had floated the idea of dispatching the Danish advisor to either Bahir Dar or Awash. Daniel Pedersen agreed with CELU's decision to move him out of Addis Ababa. He argued that CELU was already capable of servicing the unions around the capital, having its resources concentrated there. At the same time, he identified acute needs in Eritrea. Since the ban on trade unions in the region had been lifted a few months before his arrival, twenty unions encompassing 9,000 members had been formed—numbers that had grown to 37 and 13,000 respectively, three months later.[92] 'The swift recruitment of such a large number of members presents a risk that the process goes astray, unless an intervention to educate them on their rights and duties is conducted', he wrote.[93]

Although the Danish advisors were to focus on workers' education, the scarcity of CELU staff in the region meant that they soon became what they described as 'all-round advisors'.[94] By 1967, they were engaging in a range of activities: teaching office and trade union administration to trade unionists, organising new unions, assisting in establishing cooperatives, settling labour disputes and negotiating collective agreements. The fact that the Danish advisors were involved in hands-on tasks such as establishing unions and assisting them in labour disputes rendered LO assistance directly beneficial to CELU and its affiliate unions. In mid-1968, for example, the Danish advisor in Asmara reported that he and his Ethiopian colleague—also employed by LO—had successfully negotiated ten collective agreements, despite an industrial scene characterised by frequent wildcat unrest and employer intransigence. At the Barattolo textile factory, his efforts included setting up camp with 1,700 striking workers—the overwhelming majority of whom were women—to bring about a favourable end to the strike, as Villy Pedersen reported:

[92] Report for Period 8 August 1966 to February 1967, Daniel Pedersen to Danish Ministry for Foreign Affairs' Secretariat for Technical Cooperation with Developing Countries (henceforth Secretariat for Technical Cooperation, 2 February 1967, LO archives.

[93] Daniel Pedersen to Secretariat for Technical Cooperation, 13 November 1966.

[94] Report for Period 8 August 1966 to February 1967, Daniel Pedersen to Secretariat for Technical Cooperation, 2 February 1967, LO archives.

> Abraham [assistant of the Danish advisor] and I literally lived with the girls on the country road outside the factory for several days, since we had to create the necessary relationship of trust with them and have the strike brought to an end. After a month of negotiations, we reached an outstanding agreement with the enterprise, considering the circumstances, in which the girls' minimum demand for a daily wage of one Ethiopian Dollar was achieved, and fair salary increments for higher wages were also granted.[95]

Such results, Pedersen wrote, meant that Eritrean workers came to have high confidence in LO staff, and created a buoyant mood with 'the [CELU branch] offices in Asmara buzzing with activity from morning to evening'. According to the LO representative, their hands-on approach and closer proximity to workers compared favourably to that of the Americans:

> I do not think the Americans enjoy greater affection for their big projects than we do for our "little" project here in Asmara, where we provide a hand in the tiresome daily work, and to a completely different degree, share sorrows and joys with the trade union members and leaders. Our work in Eritrea is very accepted and appreciated, and I can also say respected.[96]

As this indicates, however, the LO advisors had developed a tendency to consider their own role in the developments of the Eritrean trade union movement in somewhat exaggerated terms. 'With the Danish expert as the motive and leading force, it has practically been a solo race', Villy Pedersen wrote in 1968.[97] This attitude would soon lead to strains that exacerbated the challenges the project encountered.

Trouble Begins

By the time Villy Pedersen had begun planning for his departure from Ethiopia in late 1967, his predecessor, Daniel Pedersen, expressed his

[95] "Rapport for Perioden 21 Oktober–Juni 1968," report, Villy Pedersen to Secretariat for Technical Cooperation, 23 June 1968, LO archives.

[96] "Rapport for Perioden 21. April 1967–21. Oktober 1967," report, Villy Pedersen to Secretariat for Technical Cooperation, October 1967, LO archives.

[97] "Rapport for Perioden 21 Oktober–Juni 1968," report Villy Pedersen to Secretariat for Technical Cooperation, 23 June 1968, LO archives.

worries that the situation within the country's trade union movement was 'something of a wasp's nest to send a new man into'.[98] Daniel Pedersen reasoned that it was unfortunate that Villy Pedersen was not able to stay for some additional time. The Eritrean trade unionists 'eternal intrigues against one another are quite deleterious to unity', he wrote, 'someone is always on the way up or down in the internal power struggle'.

Around this time, simmering tensions within and among Eritrean trade unions erupted into open conflict. There was 'serious internal infighting within the trade union movement in Asmara', the Danish advisor reported.[99] The division ran so deep that he feared that a complete split could occur in the movement, in which case he believed that the majority of Eritrean unions would likely seek to disaffiliate from CELU. What had divided the movement had been a challenge to unseat the leadership of the Asmara branch. The Danish project had, by this time, employed a local member of staff, Abraham Ghilazghi, to assist the Danish advisor in workers' education. However, during a temporary absence of the branch leaders, Abraham instead assumed the role of a de-facto coordinator of the daily activities of the branch office, and oppositional unions rallied around him as an alternative to the incumbent leadership. LO's representative estimated that 90 per cent of union leaders supported Abraham's apparent bid to remain in the branch office. Meanwhile, the incumbent branch committee president, Emmanuel Kahsai, had identified Abraham as a threat. According to the Danes, the branch president had 'set out to destroy Abraham, and if necessary have the Danish project closed, since he believed it was through the power of the project that Abraham had acquired his position'. The situation became acrimonious and potentially explosive. 'The threat of using weapons or other harsh means were latent', the Danish advisor reported.[100] However, by May 1968, tensions were temporarily reduced, as CELU's president Beyene Solomon visited Asmara and negotiated a truce.

It was this delicate situation that the third and final Danish advisor, Kaj Jensen, waded into in 1968. Having observed the Eritrean employee of LO becoming a party to the factional infighting, the Danish advisor

[98] Daniel Pedersen to Villy Pedersen, 11 December 1967, LO archives.

[99] "Rapport for Perioden 21 Oktober–Juni 1968," Pedersen to Secretariat for Technical Cooperation, LO archives.

[100] Ibid.

plunged right into it himself. In early August, CELU's president Beyene returned from Addis, suspended the branch office's constitution and ordered new elections of officeholders. These elections were allegedly rigged to generate outcomes favourable to Beyene. Around twenty unions were barred from voting, ostensibly for having withheld affiliation fees in protest. Members of the dissenting faction—whom Jensen called 'the progressives'[101]—were purged. Incumbent branch president Emmanuel, who was allegedly a relative of Beyene's and at least his close ally, came out victorious. In contrast, Abraham was accused of financial misconduct and suspended from CELU entirely. This infuriated LO's advisor Jensen, who circumvented CELU's decision by having Abraham continue working with the branch trade unions from Jensen's private residence. In a more serious error of judgement, he travelled to the port city of Massawa, where several oppositional unions were located, and began a series of evening classes. This was interpreted as an open challenge to the Asmara branch president. CELU accused Jensen of using the lectures to agitate against CELU's branch president and incite the dissenting unions to withdraw from CELU—allegations that Jensen denied.[102]

At the same time, increasing friction emerged between CELU and LO's advisor over the degree of the two organisations' respective control and ownership over the project. The latter believed that LO ought to have a bigger say in general matters and possess the standing right to participate in CELU's internal meetings. 'We need, in short, to have more influence than what CELU in Addis is willing to give us', he asserted. 'We cannot be interested in having an officer sitting and waiting for an invitation from CELU to advise. I am thinking of ICFTU's officer here in Addis—he does not participate in CELU's meetings but is called upon only when they desire his advice'.[103] CELU, however, was pushing in the opposite direction. Its senior officials wanted firmer control and ownership over the various programmes its foreign partner organisations funded and implemented. They also wanted Danish and ICFTU funds directly transferred to CELU's account, so that they could administer the programmes and employ the advisors directly. 'One is given to think',

[101] "Rapport Over den Senste Tids Udvikling Omkring Projektet, Dækkende Perioden 2-maj–29 august 1968," report, Kaj Jensen to Secretariat for Technical Cooperation, 29 August 1968, LO archives.

[102] Kaj Jensen to Per Carlsen, 8 October 1968, LO archives.

[103] Kaj Jensen to Per Carlsen, 13 August 1968, LO archives.

Pedersen wrote, 'that if we only transferred the funds, they would be happy to see us slide into the background'.[104]

Instead of acquiring greater influence, the Danish advisor found his role reined in. On 29 August 1968, CELU's president Beyene stopped by Asmara on his way abroad. He handed LO's advisor Jensen a letter calling him back to Addis Ababa and ordering him to report to CELU's headquarters there. 'I regret to inform you that your attitude and comportment you have recently shown contrary to the verbal directive given to you, has resulted in a very serious grievance in the branch office and among affiliated unions', it read. 'All your activities and assigned duty in this branch shall stop effective today'.[105] This infuriated Jensen, who believed that he was being treated as an 'on-call servant that can be hounded and pushed around'. CELU's conduct, he wrote, was 'utterly condescending, and strongly reminiscent of the [Stalinist] processes of the 1930s'.[106] Instead of returning to Addis as instructed, Jensen remained in Eritrea. Labour dissent in the province had intensified further since CELU's high-handed intervention in the branch elections and purge of the opposition. Twenty-five out of 44 trade unions attached to the branch office reportedly withdrew from its activities, and decided to withhold affiliation fees.[107] Jensen consequently assumed that CELU was on the verge of a split, and, on his own initiative, decided to try to mediate a settlement. While 'tacitly accepting that the Danish advisor will no longer observe nor directly participate in branch meetings', Jensen wrote to Copenhagen, he would 'seek to convince [CELU's leadership] to allow me to negotiate peace'.[108] 'It is only Abraham and I', he wrote, 'that have a chance – even if it is gradually declining – to bring unity to the forces again'.[109] He thereby further involved himself in CELU affairs, contrary to CELU's instructions.

In Copenhagen, the Ministry of Foreign Affairs and LO were alarmed by Jensen's reports. Per Carlsen, LO's international secretary, took Jensen

[104] Ibid.

[105] Beyene Solomon to Kaj Jensen, 29 August 1968, LO archives.

[106] "Rapport Over den Senste Tids Udvikling", Jensen to Secretariat for Technical Cooperation, LO archives.

[107] Ibid.

[108] Ibid.

[109] Kaj Jensen to Per Carlsen, 31 August 1968, LO archives.

to task for having acted so brazenly. The Ministry, he noted, was likely to conclude 'that you, with or without guilt of your own, are in conflict with the cooperation partner in Ethiopia'.[110] Carlsen instructed Jensen to avoid involvement in internal infighting, rebuild trust with CELU, and accept a reassignment outside of Eritrea. 'You cannot work without them', Carlsen found it necessary to point out.[111] In a follow-up letter, he instructed Jensen to stop attending meetings between trade unionists and employers and discontinue covert salary payments to Abraham—'a man that is deeply engaged in internal union matters'.[112]

But Carlsen's efforts did not seem to discourage Jensen, who by his own assessment was united with 12,000 Eritrean workers against an isolated regional branch committee constituted by 'five plotters'.[113] Contrary to Carlsen's advice, he admitted to having continued to 'carry out certain activities behind the curtain'.[114] He returned to Massawa, where he attended meetings with the dissenting unions and engaged in discussions with the trade unionists he had met on his prior visit. On Jensen's initiative, these trade unionists issued a statement addressed to the Asmara branch grievance committee, seeking to clear Jensen of any charges of misdoing. However, in doing so, they also confirmed that their discussions with Jensen had included at least one sensitive issue: a broken promise by Beyene to establish a CELU office in Massawa. On his return to Asmara, Jensen noted that 30 out of 44 Asmara branch-affiliated unions had now distanced themselves from the branch office, demanding the president's and the coordinating committee's removal—a situation that he remained convinced was due to support for his own persona and role.

Jensen's intransigence sealed the fate of the Danish project in Eritrea and, eventually, the cooperation between LO and CELU. When Jensen finally showed up in Addis Ababa in the final days of September, he claimed to have been met by CELU officials who exhibited visibly bad conscience and admitted that the whole affair had been a misunderstanding, arising from Jensen having got caught between infighting

[110] Per Carlsen to Kaj Jensen, 9 September 1968, LO archives.

[111] Kaj Jensen to Per Carlsen, 31 August 1968, LO archives.

[112] Per Carlsen to Jensen, 680911.

[113] Kaj Jensen to Per Carlsen, 12 September 1968, LO archives.

[114] Kaj Jensen to Per Carlsen, 8 October 1968, LO archives.

factions.[115] Beyene Solomon's letter to Jensen recounting their meeting gave another account. It repeated the charge that Jensen had been 'unnecessarily intervening in [CELU's branch's] internal affairs', and recounted a list of things that had been agreed upon.[116] That list stipulated that Jensen should arrange education seminars only at such places that CELU directed him. It explicitly forbade him from attending meetings without prior invitation or involving himself in disputes and strikes unless called upon for technical advice. It also directed him to take all his instructions directly from CELU's headquarters in Addis Ababa, report on his activities to it in writing every quarter, and notify it of any complaints or misunderstandings. There were no signs of restored trust in any of the enumerated points. CELU's dismissal of Abraham Ghilazghi only underlined this. The mistrust, moreover, was mutual. 'I believe it is imperative that CELU's President is replaced. He is really "a bad guy"', Jensen wrote soon after.[117] If Jensen had been hoping for greater influence and more autonomy for the Danish project, he had miscalculated. His missteps had hardened CELU's leadership's resolve to bring LO's activities in Eritrea under its own firm control. Despite some attempts to secure an extension, the project was wound up in December of 1969.

Summing up

What had been achieved by the 'Danish mini-project', as the LO staff called it? Jensen tried to grapple with this question in his report on the concluding phase of the project. A comprehensive assessment was difficult to conduct given that the project had no explicit goals at the outset, so implicit goals had to be assumed retrospectively. 'It is unknown to me whether, at the start of the project, there was an established actual goal', Jensen wrote.[118] 'If there was, and if this goal was to establish a self-operating forward-going organisational totality in the Eritrean region, one can say that the goal was achieved'. As noted, however, even the project's location was decided well after the first Danish advisor

[115] Ibid.

[116] Beyene Solomon to Kaj Jensen, 11 October 1968, LO archives.

[117] Kaj Jensen to Per Carlsen, 2 November 1968, LO archives.

[118] Report of the concluding phase of the project, covering the period 1 July–4 December 1969, Kaj Jensen to Secretariat for Technical Cooperation, 12 December 1969, LO archives.

had arrived. Jensen argued that the project also created awareness of trade unionism among unionists and government officials, and by the mere presence of the Danes, assuaged government hostility and suspicion towards the Eritrean trade unions. Initially, Jensen wrote, government institutions were not only ignorant of trade unions, 'but simply opposed to an organization that (as they perceived it) could develop into a mass movement against the existing system'. 'The presence of the Danish advisors by example showed the authorities they did not need to entertain such fearsome thoughts', he continued, highlighting a similar line of reasoning that motivated other Western interventions at the time.

In terms of concrete legacies, LO claimed that the field worker approach, which would play a vital role in CELU's future development, was designed based on LO's intervention. During the final year of the LO project, Per Carlsen informed the Danish Ministry of Foreign Affairs that one of CELU's six field workers who were being trained under the auspices of the AALC would take over the educational work done by LO in Eritrea.[119] In his concluding assessment, Jensen claimed that the field worker programme was an outcome of the Danish project, which had demonstrated CELU's need of field-based staff and the impact it could have. He was correct in arguing that the role of the field workers—essential in extending all types of services to basic unions across the country—was similar to LO 's staff in Eritrea. In that sense, the field worker programme could indeed be seen as a scaled-up version of the Danish project. Jensen also took part in the training of the initial batch of CELU/AALC field workers, sharing experiences from the project. The Danish project thus helped to identify the demand for and appropriate role of field workers. However, it was the needs identified among the trade unions themselves that shaped this role. LO's intention had been to provide workers' and trade union education, not to deliver comprehensive services to fledgling unions. Moreover, it was CELU that had assigned LO's staff to Eritrea, while CELU's own staff (increasingly aided by the AALC) already played similar roles elsewhere in Ethiopia, particularly in the areas bordering the capital. LO's contribution to the consolidation of trade unions in Eritrea was important, and that experience generated important lessons. CELU expressly appreciated it for those reasons. But

[119] Report from visit to Ethiopia concerning future of workers' education, attachment, Per Carlsen to Secretariat for Technical Cooperation, 18 March 1969, LO archives.

it was not as catalytically important as LO later suggested, and there were also negative lessons to be learnt from the experience.

However much appreciated the practical aspects of the Danish programme were from CELU's perspective, the Danish advisor in the field had overstepped his mandate and become party to the infighting. Per Carlsen, the project's initiator in Copenhagen, realised how sensitive such involvement was. In late 1968 he agreed to a new protocol which prohibited the Danish advisor from 'directly engaging in problems that must be considered internal Ethiopian affairs'.[120] As discussed previously in this chapter, the ICFTU and the AALC were guilty of interfering in CELU's internal affairs in very similar ways—and purposefully so. But what made things different for LO was that, unlike ICFTU and AALC, its representative Jensen had backed the wrong horse and unintentionally sided with what was crystallising into the labour opposition. LO was aware of and repeatedly reported on the heavy infighting among the Ethiopian trade unions. But unlike the ICFTU and the AALC, they were oblivious to the stakes involved, the nature of the congealing factions, and the intricacies of the infighting. For that reason, the Danes also never quite figured out why their local representative Jensen had come into sudden conflict—as the Ministry of Foreign Affairs had ostensibly concluded—with their cooperation partner CELU.

Jensen himself believed that the conflict was caused by the desire of CELU's leadership in Addis to eliminate the forward momentum of the trade union movement in Eritrea, by removing its most competent figures such as Abraham. In having strengthened the movement in Eritrea, he reasoned, a precedent had been created—primarily by the Danish project and Abraham, in his version of things—against which CELU's efforts in the rest of the country compared poorly. This, he concluded, created both jealousy and fear, and prompted CELU's leadership to support 'the plotters' in the Asmara branch office leadership, with an aim to rein in the development of the Eritrean trade union movement. This interpretation is readily falsifiable. CELU's senior leadership was dominated by men of Eritrean origin—including its president and its secretary general—and had itself requested LO to direct their intervention to assist the fledgling movement in Eritrea to begin with. CELU's president Beyene was personally invested developing the Eritrean trade union movement

[120] "Vedr. Ta.j.nr 104.P3. Æthiopien 11," Per Carlsen to Secretariat for Technical Cooperation 11 November 1968.

and constructing a CELU branch building in the regional capital. He was courting various CELU partners to invest in it, even to the extent of exposing himself to criticism within CELU for allegedly favouring his home province. Jensen's predecessor, Villy Pedersen, acknowledged that Beyene Solomon was 'the primus motor behind the [construction] project'.[121] While Jensen was correct that he, Abraham, and a majority of trade union leaders in Eritrea had come into conflict with CELU's and the branch office's leaderships, it was not because CELU's leadership was jealous of developments in Eritrea. It was rather because CELU was divided between opposing strands, each congealing into separate camps, and CELU's leadership sought to ensure that its allies remained in control of the Asmara branch.

Jensen had occasionally made this connection to the broader context. In August 1968, for example, he reported that 'in the same way they are dissatisfied with [branch president] Emmanuel in Asmara, they are dissatisfied with Beyene in Addis'.[122] Yet, when the opposition around Addis Ababa was struggling to form a branch, he opposed it.

> For the moment, there is a movement to establish a sort of 'joint organisation' for trade unions in the Shoa province.[123] They have a lot in common with the joint office in Asmara, and claim that the same form of organisation could be of great service and support the work in and around the capital, Addis Ababa.
>
> I am, however, somewhat hesitant about this development. It looks to me as if they want to establish this form of organisation because of provincial sentiments, in other words, for the sake internal infighting. To the extent possible, I have tried to restrain this development.[124]

Ultimately, Jensen believed that the conflict he was embroiled in had begun within the Asmara branch—suddenly in 1968—around Abraham's role, and that CELU's treatment of Abraham constituted evidence of

[121] "Rapport for Perioden 21. April 1967–21. Oktober 1967 Pedersen to Secretariat for Technical Cooperation, LO archives.

[122] "Rapport Over den Senste Tids Udvikling", Jensen to Secretariat for Technical Cooperation, LO archives.

[123] Which surrounds Addis Ababa.

[124] Report of the concluding phase of the project, Jensen to Secretariat for Technical Cooperation, LO archives.

its desire to have the Eritrean movement brought to a halt. That interpretation missed the bigger picture. The opposition against CELU's leadership was much older than that, and had an equivalent in unions in Eritrea that wanted to unseat the branch leadership. Abraham had advertently or inadvertently become involved in that conflict, either by backing the opposition or having the opposition rally around him as an opportunity to take the leadership to task. CELU's leadership's treatment of Abraham—his dismissal—was no different from how it treated employees who became affiliated with the opposition in other places, such as in the case of Tedla Fantaye. Moreover, the two strands of the movement in Eritrea had already clashed before the arrival of Abraham, and would continue to do so long after his dismissal. In August 1969, the branch president Emmanuel was ousted by the opposition—only for his successor, Mesfin Abraha, to be suspended by CELU's leadership in 1972, triggering another round of conflict. But since the Danes did not grasp this broader context of a movement-wide struggle between two congealing but pronounced strands, they came to erroneously believe that the cardinal issue was limited to Abraham's and their own projects' role, as a harbinger of CELU's leadership's perceived hostility to the rapid growth of the movement in Eritrea.

In conclusion, the history of LO's intervention in Ethiopia demonstrates not only the importance that Western trade union organisations attached to influencing the development of the Ethiopian labour movement, but also the difficulties they faced in navigating the terrains of a fracturing movement. However, in the meantime, they made a meaningful impact on the development of the Ethiopian trade union movement.

Generalities

By mid-1975, CELU had severed its ties to all the organisations of the international anti-communist trade union camp that had been operating in Ethiopia. For the prior decade, these organisations had sunk significant resources and efforts into seeking to ensure that CELU continued to develop on an anti-communist and non-radical path, and that its relations with socialist bloc trade union organisations were kept to a minimum. These efforts had failed spectacularly. By 1975, WFTU delegations had been dispatched to Addis Ababa, and CELU's president Marcos Hagos attended the WFTU's Executive Board meeting in Paris. The process of admission to the WFTU was delayed by the demise of CELU later that year, but its successor, the AETU, would join the organisation as a full member.

The three foreign and international trade union organisations discussed in this chapter had cooperated closely and coordinated their activities in Ethiopia 'as much as possible'.[125] Their mutual relationships were-described as 'informal, warm, friendly, [and] cooperative'.[126] The AALC found it useful to cooperate with the Scandinavians in Danish LO and in the ICFTU's regional office, who, despite belonging to the same 'pro-Western' camp, had the advantage of being considered relatively 'unburdened by the United States' bad reputation in large parts of the world'.[127] Presenting a united front against CELU while remaining in close contact and coordination with each other and the imperial government, the three organisations were capable of exercising significant leverage. CELU, which was dependent on the external funding the organisations provided, risked both defunding and government repression if it fell afoul of its international allies. This was partly because the imperial government considered the international organisations—particularly the AALC and the ICFTU—guarantors that CELU's activities remained non-subversive and non-militant. Additionally, key state officials had developed personal loyalties and indebtedness to the AALC in particular. The AALC thus considered itself assured of the 'complete and eager cooperation' of the imperial government.[128] When the various organisations decided to interfere in CELU's internal or external affairs, they thus did so from a position of significant leverage.

However, there was also competition and occasional tension between the foreign organisations. The sheer number of partner organisations and foreign advisors to CELU posed a challenge. The AALC believed that of the several organisations present in Ethiopia, 'only the ICFTU representative has sufficient funds to justify his presence'.[129] But there was also

[125] "Rapport for Perioden 21. April 1967–21. Oktober 1967 Pedersen to Secretariat for Technical Cooperation, LO archives.

[126] "AALC-CELU Programs, 1973", Jerry Funk to Ted Morse, 2 December 1972, AALC Records.

[127] Daniel Pedersen to Per Carlsen 8 December 1967, LO archives.

[128] "AALC-CELU Programs, 1973", Funk to Morse, AALC Records.

[129] "Ethiopia Visit: July 6th–15th", Gore, AALC Records.

a self-acknowledged 'interest game'[130] playing out between the ICFTU and the Danes on one side, and the Americans on the other—originating in their somewhat differing degrees of anti-communist virulence. At one point, the relationship between the AALC and the ICFTU was described as 'icy': 'the Americans want to conquer the initiative in Africa and work completely independently of the ICFTU', the Danes had concluded.[131] The Americans were equally suspicious of their partners in the ICFTU. In 1969, for example, they were convinced that ICFTU's representative Kindström was sharing articles with CELU—allegedly 'distributed through the good offices of ICFTU Brussels'—that revealed the role of CIA in providing funding and direction for the AFL-CIO's foreign activities, including the AALC's.[132] For these reasons, the foreign and international trade union organisations in Ethiopia consistently preferred running separate programmes instead of pooling resources. CELU's ambition to 'isolate' the donors from one another, and thereby acquire greater volumes of funding, also played a role.[133] 'The result', a Danish advisor reported, 'is that CELU applies from several instances at once for the same assistance'. In doing so, CELU attempted to increase its own leverage by playing its international partner organisations off against each other.

When CELU proposed building an Asmara headquarter for its Eritrean branch, it approached the Danes with a blueprint and a promise 'to hand over all Eritrea to Denmark [in matters of trade union cooperation]' if LO would fund its construction. The Danes were not convinced of the exclusivity of the offer. 'At least ten more countries in East and West Europe have received the same drawings – that is as sure as [the fact that] our old translator Fisseha was an under-cover agent of the security services', Daniel Pedersen wrote.[134] He was probably correct. The Americans had also been asked to fund the office, and agreed to do so partially with an amount matching that which CELU could raise. Using subterfuge, CELU took a temporary loan so as to give the AALC the impression that

[130] Kaj Jensen to Per Carlsen, 15 August 1969, LO archives.

[131] Villy Pedersen to Per Carlsen, 28 September 1967, LO archives.

[132] "Report No. 105: Publicity on AALC," Jerry Funk to Irving Brown, 9 May 1969, AALC Records.

[133] Daniel Pedersen to Per Carlsen, 26 March 1966, LO archives.

[134] Daniel Pedersen to Villy Pedersen, 9 November 1967, LO archives.

it had raised the necessary funds, whereby the Americans released a contribution of 25,000 USD.[135] Danish LO then contributed an additional 25,000 USD. However, CELU also had more direct ways of exercising influence over the content of the various cooperation programmes and the uses of funding. The factors that led to the recall of the AALC's John Gore and the re-stationing of LO's Kaj Pedersen to Addis Ababa are two good examples of this. In another example, the ICFTU was compelled to scrap plans, in 1968, to organise a seminar between employers and the government, because CELU opposed it.[136] But there were limits to CELU's influence. CELU's attempts to acquire full control over funds provided by the ICFTU and LO in the late 1960s tested those limits and ultimately failed.

On balance, CELU's close cooperation with the anti-communist international trade union organisations active in Ethiopia during the period yielded mixed results. These organisations had helped build CELU's capacity, develop its assets, and train and deploy the field workers who played a key role in the movement's expansion. However, their involvement had also fostered financial dependence. 'You will not be independent, as long as you must depend primarily on support of finances from the outside', Irving Brown had stated at the inauguration of CELU's AALC-built headquarters.[137] This was particularly true because the international partners Brown represented eagerly used the leverage stemming from CELU's financial dependence to impose strict limitations on its autonomy.

One such limitation was the suppression of militant trade unionism. The prevalence of militancy worried all partnering organisations, although to somewhat different degrees, and they deemed it vital that CELU remained under the leadership of officials considered moderates. Funds provided were used to prop up CELU's leadership internally and to effect moderation among constituent unions. One way of doing so was through the ubiquitous training programmes that inculcated principles of 'business unionism' or moderate economistic reformism among workers' representatives. However, since these attempts to internalise the values of 'free'

[135] Beyene Solomon, *Fighter for Democracy: The Saga of an Ethiopian Labour Leader* (Baltimore: Publish America, 2010), 195–196.

[136] Daniel Pedersen to Per Carlsen, 9 May 1966, LO archives.

[137] "Speech by Mr Irving Brown," opening of CELU headquarters, Addis Ababa, 7 April 1970, AALC Records.

trade unionism proved to be neither entirely effective nor nearly sufficient to halt militancy, more direct measures were introduced. Selective disbursement of funds and opportunities supplied by international partners was a key tool by which CELU's leadership exercised influence over the orientation of constituent unions and could force the latter to fall in line. Non-compliance led to funds and opportunities being withdrawn. The precarious finances of the movement enhanced the leverage exercised in this manner. Where this was insufficient, CELU's international allies colluded with its leadership to subvert and overturn democratic decisions and processes. Ultimately, the AALC and the ICFTU colluded with key state officials and offices to check militant impulses, relying, in the final instance, on the imperial state's repressive capacity to ensure control over the movement.

Another area in which the international partnering organisations imposed strict limitations regarded CELU's relationships with the WFTU and WFTU-affiliated organisations. The ICFTU and the AALC were particularly focused on keeping such contacts to a minimum. The high-handed ways this was policed—including by openly threatening and berating senior Ethiopian trade union officials—bred resentment. CELU's foreign allies appeared to have little understanding of CELU's leadership's desire to be seen as equals, but the prohibition they imposed on CELU from engaging with socialist bloc trade unions adversely affected the relationship. To CELU, it was not at all clear why it could not enjoy relations with both strands of the international trade union movement, and the strong reactions that even the most formal and innocuous exchanges triggered from its allies left CELU officials 'quite honestly shaken'.[138] For this reason, CELU concealed its sporadic contacts with socialist block unions—occasional visits and, at least once, the provision of a small amount of project funding—from its anti-communist allies. The high-handed approach to policing CELU's external relations ironically contributed to the eventual rift between CELU and the ICFTU camp. Moreover, just as cooperation between CELU and the WFTU camp had been kept to a minimum by the ICFTU and the AALC before their expulsion, the WFTU was to completely displace the ICFTU and its affiliates after the break.

[138] "Report No 148: Quarterly Report, 1st Quarter 1970," Jerry Funk, 18 May 1970, AALC Records.

Later Engagements

Soon after its its formation in 1977, the AETU joined the WFTU as a full affiliate. For the following decade and a half, the Ethiopian trade union movement remained within the WFTU fold. One aspect of the relationship consisted of frequent exchanges of visits by official delegations, mutual conference participation, and joint statements. However, technical and material assistance to Ethiopian trade unions and workers—including vehicles, building materials, medicines, clothes, tools, technical equipment such as typewriters and food aid—from WFTU-affiliated national confederations constituted its most tangible aspect. The Free German Trade Union Federation (FDGB) initiated a comprehensive programme that included multi-year degree and diploma programmes in the German Democratic Republic for selected Ethiopian trade unionists, and dispatched German trade union educatators to Ethiopia. Meanwhile, the Soviet All-Union Central Council of Trade Unions (AUCCTU) provided annual intensive training of large batches—typically 30 at a time—of Ethiopian trade unionists in the USSR, and academic education for others. It also provided ETU with vehicles and financial assistance. In 1988, for example, the AUCCTU donated 30,000 USD to ETU. By 1984, 118 Ethiopian trade unionists had completed educational programmes of between one and four months in socialist bloc countries, while another 700 had completed shorter courses abroad.[139] Most importantly, the WFTU-affiliated unions[140] funded the construction of a massive headquarters complex for the AETU in Addis Ababa, which was completed in 1984. The 11-storey building—for many years, it was the talest high-rise in Addis Ababa—accompanied by a four-storey annex, was erected on a large plot of land next to the capital's central Revolution square.[141] It constituted a valuable asset of the trade union movement—and remained so in the 2020s.[142]

[139] All-Ethiopia Trade Union, *የኢትዮጵያ ሠራተኞች እንቅስቃሴ፡ ክፍል ሁለት* (unpublished manuscript, Addis Ababa, 1984), 111.

[140] The trade union confederations of the USSR, the GDR, Hungary, Bulgaria, Czechoslovakia and Yugoslavia contributed funds and material to this project. AETU, *የኢትዮጵያ ሠራተኞች እንቅስቃሴ፡ ክፍል ሁለት*, 112.

[141] Renamed Meskel Square in the 1990s.

[142] After CETU was formed in 1993, it became an important source of rental income.

By the late 1980s, the ETU was a committed affiliate of the WFTU, and the ETU's president, Tadesse Tamrat, served as its Vice President. With the progressive decline of the political and economic situation in the countries of the socialist bloc, however, interactions decreased and assistance began to dwindle. The FDGB, as an example, informed the ETU of its decision to discontinue all ongoing educational programmes in early 1990. When the ETU was banned in 1991, the WFTU was itself experiencing a profound crisis resulting from the bloc's dissolution. Shortly after its formative congress, in December 1993, the ETU's successor organisation, CETU, announced its disaffiliation from the WFTU.

In the following years, CETU sought to rejoin the ICFTU and re-establish relations with the latter's affiliates. Although it was initially welcomed, blatant government interference in CETU's affairs beginning in 1994 and the subsequent take-over of the confederation by the pro-government faction undid these efforts and prompted the ICFTU to freeze relations with CETU.

The ICFTU and its affiliates had initially shown significant interest in the reemergent Ethiopian trade union movement. The AALC reacted to the 1991 change of government in Ethiopia by immediately dispatching CELU's former senior officials Fissehatsion Tekie and Gebreselassie Gebremariam—who, by this time, were both working for the AALC—on missions to the country and arranging seminars for Ethiopian trade union leaders. By 1993, the AALC had stationed Fissehatsion in Addis Ababa as its regional representative, leasing an office within CETU's headquarters building. In March that same year, a CETU delegation headed by its president visited the ICFTU in Brussels and was promised a donation of 20,000 USD to support CETU's organisational activities.[143] The Canadian Labour Congress (CLC) dispatched a representative of its own to the Ethiopian capital in September 1994. It subsequently entered into a bilateral agreement with CETU, which covered assistance in trade union development, workers' education, vocational training, cooperatives, and other related fields of activities.[144]

[143] "Assistance to CETU (Ethiopia) for Organisational Activities," Andrew Kailembo to Enzo Friso, 5 September 1994, CETU archives.

[144] "Agreement between the Confederation of Ethiopian Trade Unions and the Canadian Labour Congress", 31 May 1994, Confederation of Ethiopian Trade Unions (CETU) archives, CETU, Addis Ababa.

However, when the Ethiopian government began to heavily intervene in CETU's affairs, seeking the ouster of its leadership, the ICFTU-affiliated organisations took contrasting stances. The ICFTU and the CLC sided with the elected leadership and began to provide support for it. Such support included limited funding to cover costs for running expenses and legal fees. As a result of the CLC's position, the Ethiopian government expelled its representative, Betrand Bégin, from the country. The ICFTU, meanwhile, discontinued the appraisal of CETU's re-affiliation application, while protesting the government's interference in the confederation's affairs.

The AALC took a radically different approach, repeating its undue interference from two decades earlier and once again seek the role of the kingmaker in the Ethiopian confederation, while aligning itself with the government. By November 1994, the relationship between CETU's elected leadership and the AALC's regional representative Fissehatsion had soured. CETU's president claimed that Fissehatsion had violated the agreement between CETU and the AALC and worked against CETU's interests. Fissehatsion was accused of having funded meetings of the pro-government factionalists, and sided with the government when it cracked down on the unions of Ethiopian Airlines and EELPA.[145] In a workshop that the AALC had organised, Fissehatsion allegedly had sought to persuade trade union leaders to form a new confederation, entirely sidelining CETU, and had produced an action plan to this end. Because of this, CETU considered him to have openly sided with the pro-government side. It therefore expelled him from the CETU office the AALC had rented for him, with the intention to suspend CETU-AALC relations.

As an example of the subversive activities undertaken by the AALC, an industrial federation president who remained supportive of CETU's elected leadership has alleged that Fissehatsion—with the aim of removing what he considered one of the central troublemakers from the scene—offered him a scholarship abroad.[146] At least one other federation president is believed to have been won over to the side of the government-aligned faction by similar offers from the AALC's representative.[147]

[145] Dawey Ibrahim to Patrick O'Farrell, 2 November 1994, CETU archives.

[146] Hailu Ourgessa, in discussion with the author, 28 May 2017.

[147] Dawey Ibrahim in discussion with the author, 20 May 2015; Hailu 2017, discussion.

Moreover, the disbursement of AALC funds to dissenting federations, rather than to the confederation, weakened the national centre while strengthening centrifugal forces at a critical conjuncture. Eventually, the AALC's support for the federation-based interim committee of CETU—the body designed to take over the confederation after the ousting of its elected leadership—evolved into an open endorsement of these forces.

By 1996, Fissehatsion was based in Nairobi, where he served as the AALC's representative. From that position he continued to manage the AALC's interference in the affairs of the Ethiopian trade union movement and support the pro-government federation leaders in Ethiopia. This caused great dismay within CETU's elected leadership, which complained to the ICFTU-AFRO that 'the AALC is stubbornly working against the existence of free trade unions'.[148] CETU was far from alone in viewing the AALC's role as that of a spoiler. According to the FES representative in Addis Ababa, Fissehatsion had become known for 'his partisan support for the government faction'.[149] Disapproval of his activities had become so severe that 'a consensus among ICFTU and major affiliates to keep [him] out of Ethiopia (and Eritrea)' had developed, 'because', they had concluded, 'he cooperates with the government to keep trade unions in line'.[150]

When the CLC sent an official, Paul Puritt, on a fact-finding visit to Ethiopia in 1996, he confirmed this view in more detailed terms. 'Fisseha', he reported—'is obviously supporting the seven federations and the Ethiopian government'.[151] Fissehatsion had sought to persuade Puritt to meet with the pro-government federation leaders and 'not to judge Ethiopian trade unionists by North American standards', in an attempt to convince him of the merits of their position. He further sought to convince Puritt that all nine federations were 'working well together' and 'that the problem is [only CETU president] Dawey'. Puritt considered this an obvious falsehood, given his prior discussions with federation

[148] Dawey Ibrahim to Andrew Kailembo, 26 August 1996, CETU archives.

[149] "Visit to Addis Ababa, Ethiopia, January 19–21, 1996," report, Paul Puritt to CLC International Affairs Department, 12 February 1996, ICFTU African Regional Organization (ICFTU-AFRO) archives, ITUC Africa, Lomé.

[150] "Mission to Addis Ababa, Ethiopia, 18–20 January 1996," H.J. Schwass, ICFTU/ITUC archives.

[151] "Visit to Addis Ababa", Puritt to CLC International Affairs Department, ICFTU-AFRO archives.

leaders who supported the elected leadership. He declined to meet with the pro-government federation leaders, stating that 'any attempt (as the AALC is doing) to work with the seven federations (or even the nine) is to ignore this ongoing (and illegal, according to Ethiopian lower courts) violation of ILO convention 97 and other trade union rights'. But what Puritt found most peculiar was that, on the very day of his arrival in Addis Ababa—a visit few, other than the AALC's representative, were informed about—he was unexpectedly met at the gates of the Canadian embassy by two senior leaders of the pro-government faction. When he inquired how they knew of his presence, they explained that they had actually been waiting at the airport that morning , after having been informed of an important arrival. Given that the explanation did not account for how they would have found him at the Canadian embassy, Puritt concluded that Fissehatsion had likely informed them of his arrival.

The ICFTU and its affiliates, meanwhile, were generally supportive of the elected leadership, though not entirely unconditionally. One precondition was that CETU should not engage in any assertive activities that the government could view as provocative. When CETU, amidst of the government-backed campaign against it, in February 1995 planned 'a major demonstration', ICFTU-AFRO's General Secretary helped to persuade its leadership to cancel such plans, insisting that it would be counter-productive.[152] By 1997, some ICFTU officials and affiliates had begun to argue that CETU's newly installed, government-backed leadership could not be entirely ignored. The ICFTU sent a representative to CETU's 1997 reconstitutive congress as a non-committed observer. He found the congress to have been stage-managed by government-aligned actors, marking 'the climax of interference by the Ethiopian government into CETU's affairs'.[153] The AALC and OATUU also attended the congress, but took a contrasting stance. The AALC pledged that it would support CETU's new leadership, and in his address to the congress, OATUU's Secretary General urged the delegates not to 'disappoint Africa, your government, and OATUU'. 'It is the phrase "your

[152] Andrew Kailembo to Bill Jordan, 22 February 1995, ICFTU/ITUC archives.

[153] "The 8th General Congress of the Confederation of Ethiopian Trade Unions (CETU) (Addis Ababa, 22–24 April, 1997," report, Lawrence Egulu, 2 May 1997, ICFTU-AFRO archives.

government" that interested me' the ICFTU's observer wryly noted.[154] 'OATUU, AALC and ILO have in effect given recognition to the new leadership and have pledged to work with it', he concluded, '[but] the time is not ripe yet for AFRO to work with restricted CETU'.[155]

In 1998, CETU reapplied for affiliation with the ICFTU. But the ICFTU rejected its application, citing CETU's lack of independence. The failure of CETU to oppose the Ethiopian government's repression of the Ethiopian Teachers' Association was considered a particularly troubling indication of this. In 1998, war had broken out between Ethiopia and Eritrea, and Ethiopia had expelled thousands of Eritrean citizens. Former CELU president Beyene Solomon was one of them. CETU's attempts to justify this act in correspondence further damaged its relationship with the ICFTU, which subsequently declined an invitation to attend CETU's congress in September 1999. CETU's appeal to re-establish relations with the CLC the same year was rebutted, and the CLC made it clear that it did not consider CETU an independent organisation. 'We have followed with dismay the erosion of independent trade unionism in your country including the killing, arrest, and forcing into exile of real workers representatives' the CLC's response stated, '[and] we agree with the ICFTU/AFRO policy of isolating those inside the country who are collaborating with the current government and not speaking out against the violation of trade union rights'.[156]

However, the attitude of the ICFTU was slowly beginning to shift, with some affiliates and offices—particularly AFRO—being of the opinion that CETU could no longer be ignored. Meanwhile, CETU was beginning to sound somewhat less subservient to the government, and cautiously express some genuine trade union demands. In December 2000, ICFTU-AFRO sent a fact-finding mission to Addis Ababa. The delegation was sharply divided between ICFTU-AFRO's general secretary, Andrew Kailembo, who preferred a swift process of mending fences with CETU, and a Dutch representative of the ICFTU, Peer Coret, who believed that AFRO was seeking to sweep criticism under the rug and

[154] Lawrence Egulu to Andrew Kailembo, fax transmission instructions, 23 April 1997, ICFTU-AFRO archives.

[155] "The 8th General Congress of the Confederation of Ethiopian Trade Unions (CETU) (Addis Ababa, 22–24 April, 1997," Andrew Kailembo to Bill Jordan, 5 June 1997, ICFTU/AFRO archives.

[156] Robert White to Amare Alemayehu, 24 February 1999, ICFTU/ITUC archives.

sabotage attempts to meet with imprisoned trade unionists. Kailembo—and by extension ICFTU-AFRO—was accused of exhibiting 'strong pro-government and pro-CETU bias'.[157] 'There exists a government dominated trade union centre CETU, affiliated to OATUU and maintaining contacts with the ICFTU-AFRO, bilaterally supported by the American Centre for International Labor Solidarity'[158] (ACILS), Coret wrote.[159] 'On the other hand there also exists a CETU in exile, supported by a number of ICFTU affiliates, which has strong contacts with trade union leaders who are fighting for the principles of free, independent and democratic trade unions inside the Ethiopian trade union organisations'. While this division persisted, the supporters of Coret's position gradually became fewer.

CETU continued to court the ICFTU and contacts between the two organisations eventually became more regular. In 2001, CETU was invited as an observer to ICFTU-AFRO's congress in Nairobi. The Norwegian Confederation of Trade Unions (LO), an ICFTU-affiliated confederation, began to support a project to promote dialogue between CETU and Eritrean unions in 2003. Meanwhile, the ICFTU and CETU began to organise workshops together. In January 2004, ICFTU-AFRO sent a mission to Ethiopia to hold discussions with CETU. Later that year, it invited CETU to reapply for affiliation, which it promptly did. However, at the following ICFTU Executive Board meeting, CETU's readmission was opposed by the South African, Nigerian and Dutch trade union centres—who believed CETU had not sufficiently demonstrated its independence. CETU was asked to clarify its position on several questions raised by the ICFTU. CETU's answers seemed to suggest it had become more cognisant of the importance of not being seen as a government institution. After intense lobbying efforts by ICFTU-AFRO, the AFL-CIO and its Solidarity Center, as well as Kenyan trade union head Francis Atwoli, CETU's application for re-affiliation was finally accepted

157 "Report of the ICFTU mission to Ethiopia from 16 to 18 November 2000," Peer Coret to Members of the ICFTU Mission to Ethiopia, 17 December 2000, ICFTU-AFRO archives.

158 ACILS, or Solidarity Center as it later became known, encompassed the AFL-CIO's regional organisations. It thus succeeded the AALC.

159 "Report of the ICFTU mission to Ethiopia from 16 to 18 November 2000," Peer Coret to Members of the ICFTU Mission to Ethiopia, 17 December 2000, ICFTU-AFRO archives.

in December 2004. Amare Alemayehu and Haileselassie Abreha, CETU's president and its head of international relations, attended the ICFTU's congress in Japan that month. They were two prominent leaders of the pro-government faction who had played important roles in the demise of CETU's autonomy the decade before, leading to its subsequent isolation from the international trade union movement. It was a historic irony that they would oversee CETU's readmission into that movement, as one of their final acts as CETU officials. At the subsequent CETU congress, they were retired from office, marking the beginning of the process in which CETU would shed the yellow unionism they had imposed.

In the process described, the ICFTU and most of its affiliates played a role somewhat different from what they did in the 1960s and 1970s—supporting the independent-minded trade unionists rather than the subservient pro-government faction. However, the AALC and the AFL-CIO repeated their parts, doing the opposite. In the years that followed CETU's readmission to the ICFTU, several affiliates and global union organisations began assisting CETU through joint projects. These projects became an important source of revenue for CETU that dwarfed affiliation fees (although income from rents remained higher). They were also important in funding unionisation drives that grew CETU's ranks. Between 2015 and 2018, for example, Norwegian LO funded a 330,000 USD project with an emphasis on organising more basic unions. The number of CETU-affiliated unions grew by 45 per cent during this period—from 1,146 to 1,714.[160] But most support came in the form of significantly smaller projects which, in many cases, saw CETU and its affiliates compete with the growing number of NGOs that mushroomed in Ethiopia in the 1990s and 2000s, as one 'implementing partner' among many. Such projects—often in the form of campaigns or series of workshops—were incomparable in scope to the ambitions and importance that were attached to the programmes of the ICFTU, the AALC, and even Danish LO's 'mini-project' in the 1960s and 1970s.

Meanwhile, the Ethiopian trade union movement gradually became a respected member of the international trade union movement—which itself was slowly overcoming some of the divisions originating in the Cold War order, as global unions went through a wave of mergers. By 2020,

[160] G. Koyi, O. Andresen and M. Karimu, "LO—Norway—CETU Final Evaluation Report, 2015–2018," NORAD, April 2020, https://www.norad.no/om-bistand/publikasjon/ngo-evaluations/2020/lo---norway--cetu-final-evaluation-report-2015-2018/.

CETU enjoyed close and frequent relations with organisations affiliated with the ITUC (the product of the ICFTU's merger with the WCL), OATUU, and the WFTU.

References

African American Labor Center (AALC) Records. Collection 0547-LBR. Hornbake Library, Special Collections and University Archives, University of Maryland Libraries, College Park, MD.

All-Ethiopia Trade Union. *የኢትዮጵያ ሠራተኞች እንቅስቃሴ፡ ክፍል ሁለት*. Unpublished manuscript, 1984.

Beyene Solomon. *Fighter for Democracy: The Saga of an Ethiopian Labour Leader*. Baltimore: Publish America, 2010.

Confederation of Ethiopian Trade Unions (CETU) archives. CETU, Addis Ababa.

Funk, J. *Life is an Excellent Adventure : An Irreverent Personal Odyssey Or: Trying to Decide What I Want to Be When I Grow Up*. Victoria: Trafford, 2006.

ICFTU/ITUC archives. Collection ARCH00622, International Institute of Social History, Amsterdam.

ICFTU African Regional Organization (ICFTU-AFRO) archives. ITUC Africa, Lomé.

International Labour Organization (ILO) archives. International Labour Office. Geneva.

Killion, T. "Workers, Capital and the State in the Ethiopian Region." PhD diss., Stanford University, 1985.

Koyi, G., O. Andresen and M. Karimu. "LO - Norway - CETU Final Evaluation Report, 2015–2018." NORAD, April 2020, https://www.norad.no/om-bistand/publikasjon/ngo-evaluations/2020/lo---norway--cetu-final-evaluation-report-2015-2018/.

Landsorganisationen i Danmark (LO) archives. Arbejdermuseet & Arbejderbevægelsens Bibliotek og Arkiv, Copenhagen.

CHAPTER 6

Militant Practices and Effects: Strikes and Wages

A labour movement, as noted in the first chapter, consists of both organisational forms and sets of practices. In this chapter, attention is turned to the militant practices that Ethiopian workers engaged in between the 1960s and 2020, and the impact those practices have had on the conditions and position of labour within the waged political economy. Real wage levels are used to measure this. The chapter begins with a section examining shifting levels of strike activity and labour unrest in the Ethiopian waged economy. This is followed by a section examining the impact of the labour movement on the conditions of work—namely wages. The subsequent two sections consist of case studies examining the impact of the Ethiopian labour movement at the level where most activity occurs, which is at the basic enterprise union level—meaning the workplace. The chapter concludes with a discussion on the historical patterns identified in the relationship between the militant practices of the Ethiopian labour movement and shifting wage levels.

Strikes and Unrest

Continuous statistics on occurrences of labour unrest or strikes in Ethiopia do not exist. Neither are such incidents compiled in any existent archival register. Partly, this is a result of the fact that strikes in Ethiopia have almost exclusively been wildcat and informal in nature. The absence

© The Author(s), under exclusive license to Springer Nature Switzerland AG 2025

S. A. Admasie, *The Ethiopian Labour Movement*, Labour in History and Society, https://doi.org/10.1007/978-3-031-72841-9_6

of comprehensive data and statistics has made a multifaceted approach necessary. By combining numerous sources of fragmented data and references, the outlines of a general periodisation of shifting levels of intensity of unrest can be established. What is presented here has three parts. First, all substantial strike incidents[1] that have been found in the literature, in official and unofficial reports, in various archives and the correspondence of labour and state officials, and major newspapers and journals,[2] are compiled. Second, references to the general trends and levels of industrial conflict in the literature are reviewed. Finally, the limited data and short statistical time series that exist—such as mentions of short-term trends in industrial disputes—are presented to augment the above. Combined, this allows for a schematic periodisation of shifting aggregate levels of unrest between the 1950s and 2020. Chart 6.1 below illustrates the number of major strike incidents encountered, using the method described above.

[1] This is taken to mean incidences in which a number of employees, sufficient in number to disrupt regular workplace operations, have withheld labour by not showing up to work, by laying down tools, or by walking out of work. Only strikes where the workplace or sector, and year of occurrence—in the Gregorian, or the Julian calendar used in Ethiopia—have been established are included.

[2] Newspaper coverage constitutes a very incomplete source when it comes to measuring shifting levels of unrest in Ethiopia. During extensive periods of heavy censorship, industrial conflict has not been reported on. Relying on newspapers alone would generate a heavily skewed representation of shifting levels of unrest. Newspapers, therefore, only constitute a complementary source to the others mentioned.

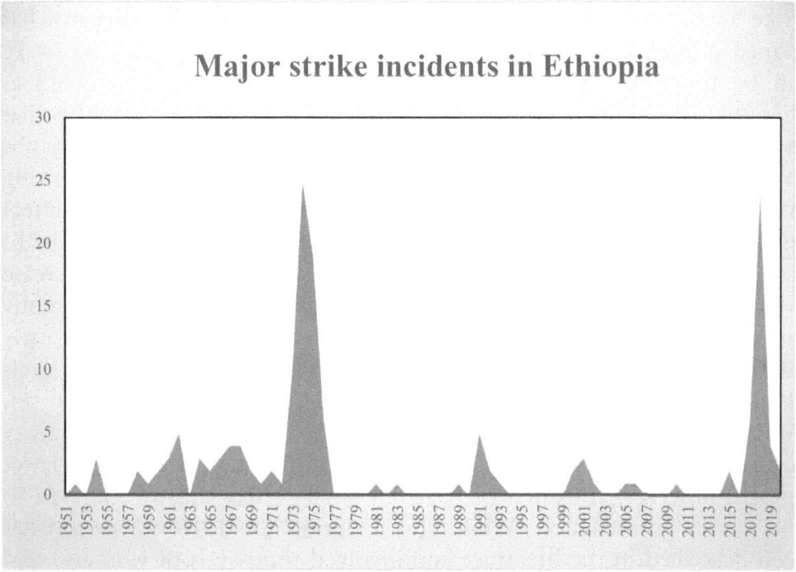

Chart 6.1 Major strike incidents in Ethiopia (*Source* Author's compilation[3])

The data presented in this chart is incomplete, and the majority of smaller strikes are omitted since no record of them has survived in the archives or the literature. Nevertheless, the compiled data on which the chart is based covers the most significant strikes in terms of the number of strikers, the longevity of strikes, and the disruption they have caused. Taking the cue from the method used by Beverly Silver in her seminal work *Forces of Labor*, 'the procedure is intended to produce a measure that reliably indicates *the changing levels* of labour unrest—when the incidence of labour unrest is rising or falling, when it is high or low—*relative to* other points in time', rather than attempting to 'produce a count of *all or even most* incidents of labour unrest'.[4] The aim here is the same.

Several findings can be derived from the data presented in the chart above. First, between 1973 and 1976, an unprecedented explosion of

[3] Deposited in the International Institute of Social History's Labour Conflicts Dataverse, https://datasets.iisg.amsterdam/dataverse/labourconflicts.

[4] B. Silver, *Forces of Labor: Workers' Movements and Globalization Since 1870* (Cambridge: Cambridge University Press, 2003), 37.

strike activity took place, corresponding to what Ernesto Screpanti has termed a ***proletarian insurgency***.[5] While references to this strike wave can be found in the literature, it has commonly been interpreted as an outcome of the revolution. In this context, it is noteworthy that the upsurge in activity preceded the 1974 revolution—strike activity was already increasing rapidly the year before the revolution began—putting into serious question the standard interpretation of cause and effect between labour unrest and the revolution. Second, the years immediately before the formation of CELU also saw a pronounced increase in labour unrest, and such unrest continued to occur consistently throughout the entire decade and a half spanning the 1960s and early 1970s. This is particularly conspicuous when compared to the low levels of unrest in the years preceding 1958 and following 1976. However, from the tranquil paucity of the latter period, brief episodes of activity occurred between 1989 and 1993, and again around 2000. The latter upturn, however, consisted of relatively small strikes mostly confined to one sector: construction. While unrest during the 1989–93 period has been described in the literature and involved thousands of workers, very few sources mention the incidents in the early 2000s. In other words, it is evident that the activity registered in the early 2000s was of a significantly lesser magnitude than in the 1990s—let alone the 1960s and 1970s. This situation, however, was to change with the wave of strikes that began in 2016 and lasted until the coming of the global coronavirus pandemic in 2020 and the outbreak of civil war that same year. Between the mid-2010s and 2020, another explosion in strike activity occurred across the waged economy. The intensity of this latest strike wave is comparable only to the 1973–1976 proletarian insurgency.

General references to unrest in the literature and archives broadly confirm the picture of shifting unrest levels outlined in Chart 6.1 above. One writer who worked for the employers' federation noted that 'wildcat strikes' had occurred 'in many industries around 1960'.[6] In 1962, Ethiopia's assistant foreign minister Getachew Makasha told a visiting ICFTU representative that some of the unions had 'started creating trouble with employers', including staging 'two strikes in the

[5] E. Screpanti, "Long Economic Cycles and Recurring Proletarian Insurgencies," *Review (Fernand Braudel Center)* 7, no. 3 (1984).

[6] Syoum Gebregziabher, "The Rise of CELU and the EFE Under Haile Selassie's Regime," (mimeo, 2005), 28.

shoe industry and in the textiles'.[7] Other senior officials informed the same ICFTU source about a number of 'concerning' strikes and 'growing agitations among the workers, who had staged several down-tools and walk-out actions recently'. In the following years, it has been noted that 'strikes were plenty'.[8] One writer reported 'numerous strikes since the legalisation of labour unions', with Ethiopian Airlines and Indo-Ethiopian Textile workers having 'conducted several work-stoppages over prolonged periods'.[9] In Eritrea, Danish advisors to CELU reported that 'countless labour disputes' were taking place in the second half of the 1960s,[10] including numerous wildcat strikes and slow-downs. At the HVA plantations and factories, recurring unrest was reported through the 1960s, and strikes were accompanied by episodes of sabotage. 'Wonji [sugar plantation and factory] has had series and series of strikes', senior CELU official Mesfin Gebremichael stated. 'If it was not in the plantation, it was in the factory; if it was not in the factory, it was in the plantation'.[11] By 1966, the president of the employers' federation, J.M.J. Prakken, was growing exasperated. Citing 'an increasing tendency of labour difficulties in many enterprises', he called on the government to exercise stricter control over unions and to do more 'to eliminate labour unrest and restore order'. 'Violation of the law by workers and unions', he noted, 'is a common feature now'.[12] Yet, by 1973, industrial conflict had not subsided. At the HVA's plantations, unrest climaxed in the period leading up to the revolution, and particularly the last couple of months of 1973 saw a remarkable number of strikes at the Wonji and Metahara sites, according to its union

[7] "Report on my Visit to Ethiopia" Serge Claverie, April 1962, ICFTU/ITUC archives, collection ARCH00622, International Institute of Social History, Amsterdam.

[8] J. Markakis and Nega Ayele, *Class and Revolution in Ethiopia* (Nottingham: Spokesman Books, 1978), 58.

[9] A.C. Suter, *Labor Law and Practice in the Empire of Ethiopia*, BLS Report No. 298 (Washington, DC: Bureau of Labor Statistics, 1966), 37.

[10] "Rapport for Perioden 21. April 1967–21. Oktober 1967," reports, to Danish Ministry for Foreign Affairs' Secretariat for Technical Cooperation with Developing Countries, October 1967, Landsorganisationen i Danmark (LO) archives, Arbejdermuseet & Arbejderbevægelsens Bibliotek og Arkiv, Copenhagen.

[11] Mesfin Gebremichael interviewed by Tom Killion, 1983, microcassette, Tom Killion Papers, collection 2017C40, Hoover Institution Library and Archives, Stanford University Stanford, CA.

[12] "Memorandum on Labour Developments," circular letter, J.M.J. Prakken, 1966, ICFTU/ITUC archives.

leader Elias Mengesha.[13] That year, Prakken's successor at the employers' federation lamented that Ethiopia was in the midst of a 'spat of illegal strikes', which included at least three strikes in 'very important establishments'. He concluded that 'industrial relations developments in Ethiopia seem to have taken a turn for the worse'.[14]

Strike activity exploded in 1973, and unrest continued unabated throughout the early years of the revolution. The extraordinary level of strike activity that occurred in 1974 was described in Chapter 3. In 1975, a representative of the employers' federation told an AALC advisor that management and labour relations had deteriorated further and that there had been 'been a lot of unannounced work slow downs'.[15] And in 1976, a senior POMOA official claimed that production was 'seriously hampered by slowdowns, attempted strikes, and other forms of sabotage'.[16] The PMAC's chairman, Mengistu Hailemariam, later acknowledged that widespread labour unrest had posed a serious threat to the regime during the early years of the revolution.[17] Two prominent economists claimed that such unrest was as important in explaining the poor performance of the early post-revolutionary economy as 'shortages, war and civil strife'.[18]

Before the most recent wave of unrest, it was not only in terms of the number of strikes or strikers that the period between the 1960s and early 1970s stood out. The intensity of the unrest that occurred during those decades also manifested itself in terms of the practices that accompanied the strikes. A few examples derived from Killion's research can

[13] Killion, "Workers, Capital and the State", 527.

[14] "Speech by Ato Bekele Beshah at the Annual General Meeting of the Federation of Employers of Ethiopia September 13, 1973," transcription of speech, Bekele Beshah, ICFTU/ITUC archives.

[15] "BAR/LES 2, 1975," report, Richard Baurmann to Lester Trachtman, 27 January 1975, African American Labor Center (AALC) Records, collection 0547-LBR, Hornbake Library, Special Collections and University Archives, University of Maryland Libraries, College Park, MD.

[16] Senay Likke, *The Ethiopian Revolution: Tasks, Achievements, Problems and Prospects*, (unknown publisher, Addis Ababa, 1976), 18–19.

[17] Mengistu Hailemariam, *Speech Delivered to the Second Congress of the All Ethiopia Trade Union* (Addis Ababa: Provisional Military Government of Socialist Ethiopia/ Commission for Organizing the Party of the Working People of Ethiopia, 1982).

[18] Mulatu Wubneh and Yohannis Abate, *Ethiopia: Transition and Development in the Horn of Africa* (Boulder, CO: Westview Press, 1988), 105.

serve to illustrate that point. At the Bahir Dar Textile Factory, unrest in the year 1967 alone included repeated strikes and the setting on fire of parts of the factory and warehouses.[19] At the Dire Dawa Cotton Factory, meanwhile, serious problems developed between the union and management, leading to the personnel manager being attacked and 'severely beaten' by assailants, before the state intervened and imprisoned the union chairman.[20] Throughout the waged sector of the economy, similar reports lend credence to the impression that unrest was not just extensive, intensive and recurring, but also very volatile and steadily escalating.

After repression and terror had subdued the labour movement in 1977, references to unrest in the literature became glaringly few. That remained the case until the years between 1989 and 1994. The emergence of renewed stirrings and unrest in the waning years of the WPE regime and the first years of the EPRDF regime included the process Beyene Solomon labelled an 'uprising' in the industrial corridor leading south from Addis Ababa.[21] It also included the relatively modest but substantive strike wave that occurred between 1991 and 1993. The US Department of State's *Country Report on Human Rights Practices* in 1991, for example, noted that there appeared to be a certain tolerance 'of strikes and protests in the workplace'.[22] In 1993 it reported that the Ethiopian labour scene had seen 'numerous actions' of retrenched workers.[23] Only a few rare cases with relatively few strikers were reported in the following two decades.

However, in the mid-2010s, sources and accounts indicated that widespread unrest had returned. In 2016, two scholars who conducted research on labour in Ethiopia noted that four wildcat strikes had recently taken place on flower farms and a shoe factory.[24] October 2017 alone,

[19] T. Killion, "Workers, Capital and the State in the Ethiopian Region" (PhD diss., Stanford University, 1985), 512.

[20] Ibid., 506–507.

[21] Beyene Solomon, *የኢትዮጵያ ሠራተኞች አንድነት ማህበር: ውልደት ዕድገት ውድቀት* (self-pub., Addis Ababa, 2012), 250–254.

[22] Department of State, *Country Reports on Human Rights Practices for 1991* (Washington DC: Joint Committee Print, 1992), 130–131.

[23] Department of State, *Country Reports on Human Rights Practices for 1993* (Washington DC: Joint Committee Print, 1994).

[24] C. Blattman and S. Dercon, "Occupational Choice in Early Industrializing Societies: Experimental Evidence on the Income and Health Effects of Industrial and Entrepreneurial Work" (working paper, National Bureau of Economic Research, 2016).

moreover, saw major strikes at a horticulture farm and a winery, involving a combined total of 5,200 workers. Additionally, CETU issued a general strike warning—for the first time in over 40 years.[25] By 2018, journalistic accounts had also begun speaking of a 'wave of strikes'.[26] Those strikes were accompanied by other militant practices, such as the enforced lock-out of managers and destruction of property. By the late 2010s, the image of industrial tranquility from the early decade had changed drastically. 'Strike action', two scholars wrote in 2019, 'is widespread in Ethiopia and near-universal among the firms we sampled'.[27]

The limited statistical data that exist from labour courts corroborate these general outlines. One labour scholar who conducted research in Ethiopia in the 1960s, for example, identified an upward trajectory in the occurrence of labour disputes during the 1960s. Individual labour disputes registered in courts grew from 137 in 1963; to 468 in 1964; and 776 in 1965.[28] Meanwhile, cases involving trade unions increased from 11 to 70, and disputes handled by the Labour Relations Board grew from 31 to 161 between 1962/63 and 65/66.[29] Figures in the Ministry of Labour and Social Affairs' 1979 *Labour Statistics Bulletin*—a one-off publication that was discontinued after the first issue—provides evidence of the strong effects of the militarisation of the industrial conflict in 1977—a period which saw the most intense violence in workplaces: between the years 1976/77 and 1977/78, the number of new labour disputes registered declined from 27,700 to 12,000.[30] A final conjuncture

[25] Fasika Tadesse, "Sher on Hot Plate: Heavy Tax, Labour Dispute," *Addis Fortune* 18, no. 911 (8 October 2017); Fasika Tadesse, "Castel Labour Suspends Strike after Pay Raise Vow," *Addis Fortune* 18. No. 914 (5 November 2017); "CETU Warns of Labour Strike," *Addis Fortune* 18, no. 913 (26 October 2017).

[26] Samuel Getachew, "Awash suspends production amid workers strike," *The Reporter* (8 September 2018), https://www.thereporterethiopia.com/6344/.

[27] F. Schaefer and C. Oya, *Employment Patterns and Conditions in Construction and Manufacturing in Ethiopia: A Comparative Analysis of the Road Building and Light Manufacturing Sectors*, IDCEA Research Report (London: SOAS, University of London, 2019).

[28] R. Stutz, "The Developing Industrial Relations System in Ethiopia" (mimeo, Haile Selassie I University, Addis Ababa, 1967), 90–91.

[29] Ibid., 95.

[30] Ministry of Labour and Social Affairs, *Labour Statistics Bulletin 1979* (Addis Ababa: MoLSA, 1980), 17.

for which statistical time series data exist is the aftermath of the implementation of the 1982 Trade Union Reorganisation Act. In the year of its promulgation—1982/83—labour disputes registered in Addis Ababa lower courts numbered 2,300.[31] By 1985/86, this figure had declined to 1,150, meaning that the number of registered disputes had halved in the three years since the legislation that turned trade unions into formal WPE instruments had been enacted.[32]

All of the above supports a periodisation of labour unrest levels that aligns rather well with the strike data presented earlier in this chapter (see Chart 6.1 on page 261). A schematic periodisation of shifting levels of unrest derived from these sources may, therefore, look something like Chart 6.2 presented below.

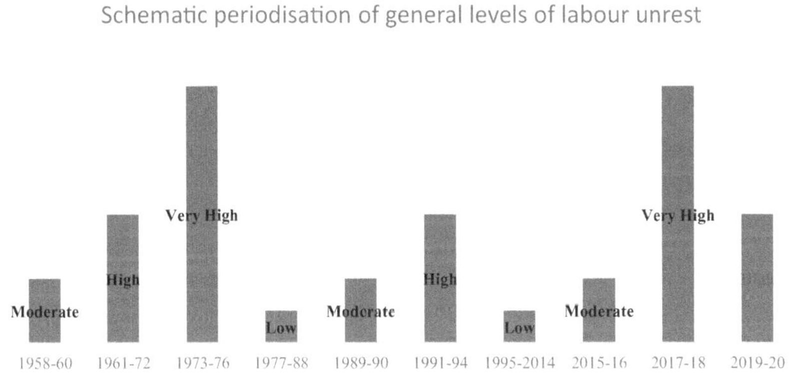

Chart 6.2 Schematic periodisation of general levels of labour unrest 1958–2020

A notable pattern is that the periods of relatively low levels of unrest have tended to coincide with periods when organised labour has been

The subsequent year—1978/79, which was the last one covered—saw an increase to 17,700 cases, but this is not to be taken to mean that there was any real re-emergence of industrial conflict. Instead, the Ministry of Labour and Social Affairs explained, this partial rebound was caused by an increase in the number of reporting branch offices that year. 'In general', the document states, 'labour disputes are reducing'. Ibid., 17.

[31] Ministry of Labour and Social Affairs, የሥራ ክርክር ሁኔታ ጥናት (Addis Ababa: Ministry of Labour and Social Affairs, 1987), appendix 1, 5.

[32] Ibid., appendix 1, 5.

thoroughly co-opted and controlled. In contrast, the periods of moderate, relatively high and very high levels of unrest have tended to coincide with the prevalence of a relatively autonomous trade union movement. Another noteworthy pattern is the cyclical pattern in which the shifting levels of unrest appear. An explanation for this is proposed in the final section of this chapter.

Real Wages

This section examines the movement of average real wages in Ethiopia's manufacturing sector. Real wage levels are taken as indicative of the conditions of labour, and their movement as expressive of the position of Ethiopian labour. The aim is to establish the degree to which the Ethiopian labour movement has been able to command influence over those conditions. In 1963, the Central Statistical Office—later renamed the Central Statistical Authority (CSA) and eventually the Central Statistical Agency—began to publish annual *Statistical Abstracts* in which manufacturing wages were measured. The *Statistical Abstracts* were published until 2012, after which they were discontinued. Two things must be noted regarding the wage data presented in what follows. First, it is derived from the manufacturing sector alone. Since, however, workers in that sector were the first to unionise to a comprehensive degree this is deemed appropriate for examining the impact of collective organisation and action. Second, while nominal wage data is available from 1955 onwards, comparable price index data—which is required to deflate nominal wages and calculate the value of real wages—is only available from 1963 onwards. It may be noted that in the full eight-year period between 1955 and 1963, nominal wages grew by only a total of 7.5 per cent. If later inflationary trends prevailed, this seems to indicate that real wages were stagnant or even decreasing in the period immediately prior to the emergence of the labour movement. However, in the absence of comprehensive inflation data, the real rate cannot be calculated with any precision. From 1963 onwards, however, deflated average real wages can be calculated by dividing the nominal wage by the annual price index. The resultant movement of average real wages is illustrated in Chart 6.3 below.

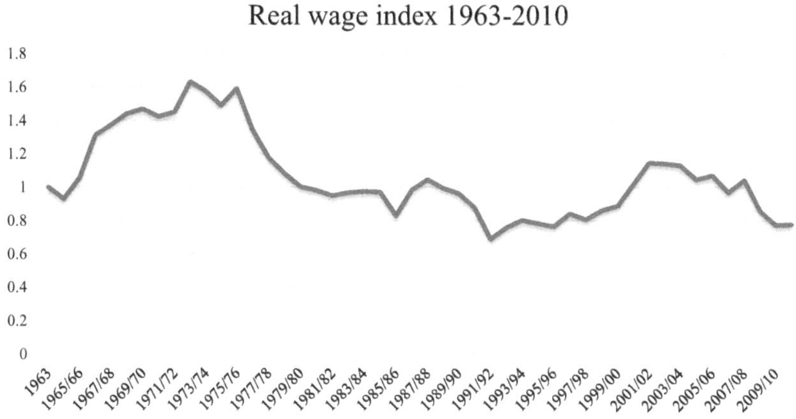

Chart 6.3 Deflated real wage index 1963–2010 (*Source* Author's computation from CSA's annual *Statistical Abstract* 1963 to 2012/13[33])

A few observations can be made from the data presented in the chart. To begin with, while real wages appear to have been stagnant or only slowly growing in the decade[34] prior to 1965, the pace picked up considerably in the mid-1960s. Real wages grew rapidly throughout the latter half of the 1960s and the early 1970s, peaking around the time of the 1974 revolution. But as much as the revolution coincided with the highest relative level of real wages recorded, it also constituted the conjuncture in which the Ethiopian labour movement was thoroughly subjugated, and the point where a catastrophic collapse of real wages began—during the second half of the 1970s wages declined sharply, consuming the entirety of wage gains in the prior decade. At the end of the decade, they stabilised at this significantly reduced level. In the following decades, two notable shifts occurred. The first was a renewed fall of the average wage to its lowest position—less than half of its 1975 levels—in the aftermath

[33] See conversion charts of nominal wages into real wages in S.A. Admasie, "Dynamics of Assertive Labour Movementism in Ethiopia: Organized Labour, Unrest and Wages in a Socio-Historical Perspective" (PhD diss., University of Pavia and University of Basel, 2018), 198.

[34] Due to the slow nominal wage growth in the years between 1955 and 1963 noted in the previous paragraph, and the stagnant real wage during the two first years covered in the chart.

of, first, the WPE's suspension of collective agreements and wage increments in its final years, and, subsequently, the seizure of state power and implementation of structural adjustment and liberalisation programmes by the EPRDF. Second, after what appeared to be the beginning of a recovery in the first years of the 2000s—coinciding with the beginning of a phase of expansion of the Ethiopian economy—real wages levelled out, before dropping back again at the end of the decade. At the end of the first decade of the twenty-first century, real wages thus remained considerably lower than in 1963, and quite catastrophically lower—still less than half—of their mid-1970s levels. In other words, the collapse of wages that coincided with the defeat of the labour movement in the 1970s had neither been reversed nor significantly ameliorated.

Before establishing the importance of class conflict and the labour movements' agency in determining wage movements during the period under discussion, two alternative explanations need to be considered. The first is the effects of inflation and the second is the role assigned to shifting productivity levels. Inflation has indeed exercised recurrent pressure on Ethiopian real wages. However, to assign a determinant significance to this factor would be to exaggerate its role. While inflation is typically—in any economy—the immediate factor that depresses real wages, it cannot do so effectively without relative nominal wage stagnation. Inflation has been a constant feature of the Ethiopian economy over the past six decades, yet it has not always resulted in falling real wages. In the 1960s and early 1970s, nominal wage gains were more than sufficient to compensate for this factor. Only with the stagnation of nominal wages did this factor becomes important, and then only as an attendant factor.

Another factor that could potentially have explained the decline of real wages is shifting productivity levels. It could, for example, have been suggested that the WPE's practice of overstaffing workplaces with relatively superfluous workers affected wages negatively. However, although overstaffing appears to have taken place,[35] this cannot adequately explain the collapse of wages. On the one hand, the sector-wide wage share—reflecting *total* wages as a share of the value of output—also declined.[36] Moreover, the connection, or lack thereof, between productivity and

[35] Mulatu and Yohannis, *Transition and Development*, 105.

[36] See the chart below.

wages can be examined in terms of the deflated average value of output per worker.

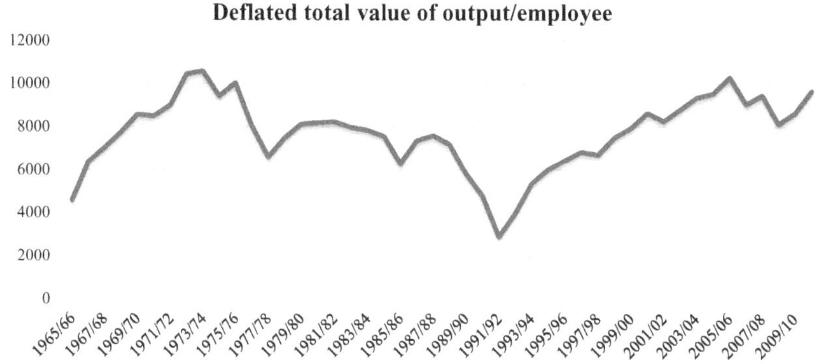

Chart 6.4 Deflated value of output per employee 1965–2010 (*Source* Author's computation from CSA's annual *Statistical Abstract* 1963 to 2012/13[37])

It is apparent in Chart 6.4 above that while overstaffing industries may have led to somewhat of a decline in labour productivity in the late 1970s, productivity remained significantly higher than in the early-to-mid-1960s. The sharp indention observable in the late 1980s/early 1990s, it needs to be noted, is a ruse. It is explained by a sharp but temporary drop in output that coincided with the acute phase of the Ethiopian civil war—where supply and distribution systems broke down, and an increasing number of industries found themselves cut off from the larger market—and the political-economic reconfiguration that followed. But this dip levelled out after a few years as the crisis receded. While it is evident that productivity began to increase again in the late 1990s, this did not result in any enduring real wage gains. In other words, the movement of real wages in Ethiopia during the period under examination has largely been disconnected from shifts in labour productivity. And since labour productivity has more than doubled since the 1960s, while real wages have fallen, the rate of exploitation[38] of labour has risen sharply. Much more so in later years, in fact, than what was the case in 1983, when the ILO warned that

[37] The value for 1967/68 alone is a proxy.

[38] Measuring the ratio between the value of output/surpluses and wages.

'wages were lagging far behind productivity increases, revealing a rapidly increasing rate of exploitation'.[39]

The data presented above indicates that ***absolute exploitation*** has increased in degree over time, but it is noteworthy that ***relative exploitation***[40] has done so at a significantly higher rate. The ***wage share*** consists of the total amount of wages paid, divided by the total value of output. Its decline in Ethiopia during the period under consideration is illustrated in Chart 6.5 below.

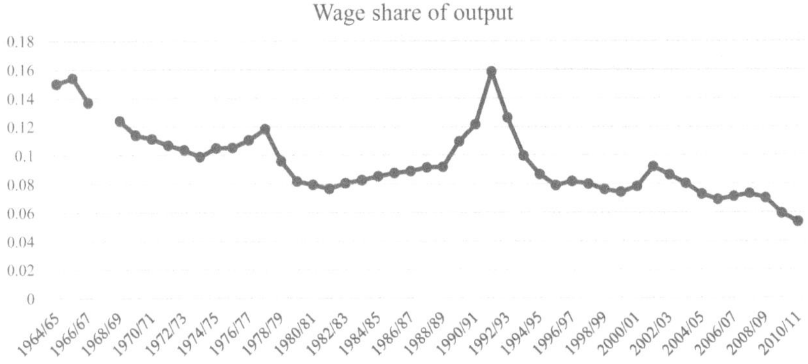

Chart 6.5 Wage share of total value of output 1964–2010 (*Source* Author's computation from CSA's annual *Statistical Abstract* 1963 to 2012/13)

Here, the secular trend of decline is striking, with the wage share descending from over 15 per cent of the value of output in 1966 to just over 5 per cent in the early 2010s. The upward movement in the late 1960s and early 1970s can largely be attributed to the rising real wages achieved during that period. However, the previously noted distorting and disrupting effect of the acute phase of the civil war is here expressed in an inverted shape, in the form of the sudden and temporary spike of the wage share in the period between 1988/89 and 1992/93. What the graph illustrates is that while workers lost around one-quarter of real

[39] International Labour Organization, "Memorandum to the Government of Ethiopia on Reform of the Wage System: Wage Regulation, Job Evaluation and Payment by Results" (confidential report, ILO, Geneva, 1983), 15–16.

[40] Denoting the degree to which increasing output is uncompensated for in wages.

wages between 1963 and 2020, they were, over the same period, deprived of almost two-thirds of the wage share they had previously commanded.

One pertinent question is to what extent these figures align with the representations in the literature and the archives. The literature has generally, and quite sweepingly, represented real wages in imperial times as stagnant and poor: 'extremely meagre' according to one scholar[41]; 'extremely low' in the words of another[42]; or even 'appealingly low' according to a third.[43] This impression is put into serious question by the data presented above—at least when wages in late imperial Ethiopia are compared to subsequent developments. Moreover, dispersed references to wages in specific workplaces and/or during specific conjunctures in the literature and archives, when assembled into an aggregate view of trends in wage movements, lend support to the validity of the data presented. They also explain the pathways through which the labour movement impacted wages and pushed them upwards.

By the mid-1960s, two researchers found daily wages to range between 0.65–1.50 ETB in the Ethiopian industrial sector, reaching up to 200 ETB/month in the service sector.[44] The figures seem to tally rather well with CSA data for that period. However, collective agreements and conflict settlements reached at one workplace after another over the course of the late 1960s and early 1970s cumulatively lifted overall wage levels. Whereas only a handful of unions had entered into collective agreements with employers by 1965/66, 92 new agreements were signed in the seven years that followed (See Chart 6.6 below).[45] Some examples may serve to illustrate the wage impacts of those agreements. At the Dire Dawa Textile Factory, workers' minimum daily wages were increased from 0.80 ETB to 1.25 ETB in 1963 alone, following an agreement

[41] Bekure Woldesemait, "The Industrial Labor Force in the Addis Abeba Region Before 1975: Origins, Expectations and Realities," in *Proceedings of the Seventh International Conference of Ethiopian Studies: University of Lund, 26–29 April, 1982*, ed. S. Rubensson (Addis Ababa: Institute of Ethiopian Studies; Uppsala: Uppsala University; East Lansing, MI: African Studies Center, Michigan State University, 1984): 611.

[42] Killion, "Workers, Capital and the State", 429.

[43] R. Lefort, *Ethiopia: An Heretical Revolution?* (London: Zed Press, 1983), 26.

[44] E. Ginzberg and H.A.S. Smith, *Manpower Strategy for Developing Countries: Lessons from Ethiopia* (New York: Columbia University Press, 1967), 98.

[45] See chart below.

between the newly established union and factory management.[46] Meanwhile, the collective agreement struck between the HVA and its union in 1964 increased daily minimum wages at the Wonji Sugary Factory—a site of fierce contestation and conflict—from 1.10 to 1.30 ETB.[47] More significantly, it increased the wages of permanent employees by some 70 per cent. Something similar occurred at the Bahir Dar Textile Factory, where collective bargained agreements increased daily wages from 0.80 to 1.40 ETB between 1963 and 1966.[48] In Massawa, the salt factory union entered into a collective agreement that assured wage increments varying between 15 and 50 per cent for all workers in 1968—after a year-long dispute with management over the issue.[49] In 1972, CELU celebrated the establishment of collective agreements at the S:t George Brewery, the Ethio-Synthetic Textiles, and the Chandris Meat Canning Factory, all of which had raised wages and set minimum wage rates.[50] This contrasted with the situation at the Diabaco cotton company, where the union had been subject to severe harassment and had failed to compel the company to negotiate a collective agreement. There, it was reported, ‘workers that have served for more than 15 years with the company still now get 0.75 [ETB] a day’.[51] However, individual employers could only resist the unions’ demands so far without risking serious disruption, and the wage movements in the economy at large testified to the overall trend. In the decade between 1964 and 1974, real manufacturing wages were found to have grown at an average annual rate of 7.4 percent.[52]

46 Killion, “Workers, Capital and the State”, 505–506.

47 Bahru Zewde, *Society, State and History: Selected Essays* (Addis Ababa: Addis Ababa University Press, 2008), 136.

48 Report for Period 8 February to 8 August 1966, Daniel Pedersen to Secretariat for Technical Cooperation, 10 August 1966, LO archives.

49 “Activity Report 3”, CELU Research Department, January 1975, AALC Records.

50 CELU, *3ኛው በየሦስት ዓመት የሚከናወን ጠቅላላ ጉባዔ/3rd Triannual Conference*, occasional publication (Addis Ababa: Confederation of Ethiopian Labour Unions, 1972).

51 Ibid.

52 Mulatu Wubneh, “State Control and Manufacturing Labor Productivity in Ethiopia,” *Journal of Developing Areas* 24, no. 3 (1990).

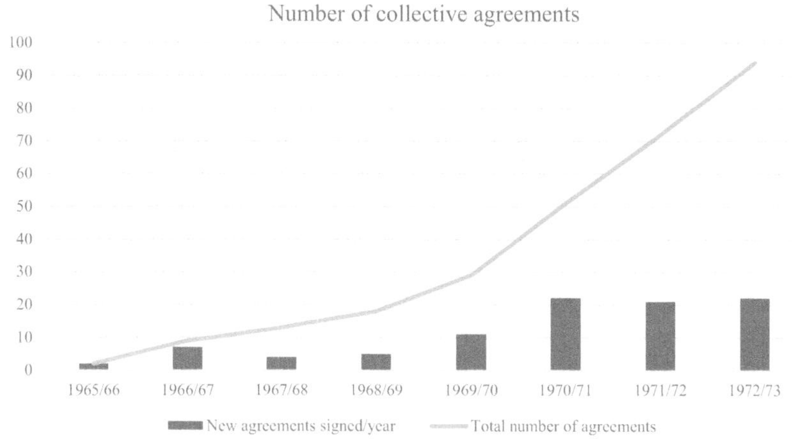

Chart 6.6 Number of collective agreements entered into per year/cumulative number of collective agreements established (*Source* CELU[53])

That Ethiopian employers were starting to feel the pinch of rising wages in the first half of the 1970s is a documented fact. In 1972, Bekele Beshah, the president of the Federation of Ethiopian Employers (FEE), wrote a letter to the minister in charge of labour affairs[54] stating that 'wages and fringe benefits are becoming more and more excessive and are not reciprocated with a commensurate rise in productivity'. 'Such a tendency of spiralling wages and cost', the FEE president continued, 'will, unless checked in time, damage the national economy [and] need in our view, countermeasures on a national scale'. CELU did not dispute the fact that wages were on the rise, but placed them in the context of the relatively small size of the workforce covered by collective agreements approximately 25,000 workers at the time—compared to the broader labour force and population.[55] Nevertheless, the contending parties shared the understanding that the trend of wages was one of rapid increase. That included the government, which was, perhaps surprisingly,

[53] "Activity Report 3", CELU Research Department, AALC Records.

[54] Letter from Bekele Beshah to Mulatu Debebe, January 31, 1972, reprinted in CELU, *3rd Triannual Conference*.

[55] CELU, "An Open Letter to the President of the Federation of Ethiopian Employers", by Solomon Tekle Tsion, reprinted *3rd Triannual Conference*.

not viewing such developments in entirely negative terms. The fact that the imperial state was not uniformly opposed to wage increases in the urban sector was affirmed by the Minister of Labour and Social Affairs, Getahun Tessema. Getahun explicitly asked employers to raise wages and condemned those 'in their zeal to amass greater profits have rejected demands for wage increases that could well be afforded'.[56]

The upward trajectory of wages and causes thereof was highlighted by an ILO report released in 1973. It warned that 'trade union pressure' and high civil service pay had possibly made urban wages 'too dear'.[57] While the ILO report found civil service wages the most concerning, it recommended imposing 'immediate wage restraint' in the manufacturing sector too.[58] Considering the source of the report, this recommendation was quite remarkable. In addition to confirming the degree to which wages had grown, the report highlighted the issue of pay differentials within the waged sector. 'The unionised sector', the ILO report stated, covered 'approximately 70 plants, largely owned by the government or by foreigners'. Union pressures in this sector, it observed, had resulted in a situation where 'high wages' prevailed, which for many workers entailed wages 'substantially in excess of ETB 2.00 per day'.[59] As long as relatively high wages only prevailed in a comparatively small share of the economy, this was deemed tolerable by the ILO. However, wages in the unionised sector, the report warned, nevertheless needed 'to be monitored carefully', to avert the danger that 'collectively bargained wage spills over into the non-unionised sectors'.[60] This concern was also evident from the government's prohibition of unionisation in larger sectors, such as the civil service and the waged part of the agrarian economy. The government's strategy had apparently been successful, because although there

[56] "Minister Addresses Conference", *Ethiopian Herald*, 10 April 1970.

[57] International Labour Organization, *Employment and Unemployment in Ethiopia*, report of the Exploratory Employment Policy Mission (Geneva: International Labour Office, 1973), 56.

[58] Ibid., 56.

[59] Ibid., 53.

[60] Ibid., 54.

were indications that rural wages were growing,[61] they were still assumed to amount to only 'around 40 percent of urban wages' in 1973.[62]

The collapse of wages following the revolution is as evident in the literature as in statistics. Scholars have observed that by 1981, real manufacturing wages had declined to 61 per cent of their 1974 level,[63] and by 1985 a US State Department report noted that 'while consumer prices have soared, wages have not risen in 10 years'.[64] The result, according to the report, was a dire situation in which 'wage earners at the bottom of the pay scale can no longer be said to earn a salary that provides a decent living for workers and family'. If this was true in 1985, it was all the more so in 2010, as real wages had slid even further in the intervening time.

Initially, the mechanism triggering the collapse of wages was a wage freeze imposed by the PMAC, which allowed high inflation to take its toll on the real value of wages. This was facilitated and exacerbated by the repression of unions and strikes. The wage freeze was eventually lifted, but real wages were not allowed to recover. The PMAC's and the WPE's ambition was to gradually narrow wage gaps by raising the lowest wages by the relatively highest percentages, while retaining a cap on the comparatively highest wages. That measure had some effect on wage distribution, but it was offset and dwarfed by the overall rise in the retail price index.[65] While wage differentials slightly narrowed, they only did so while *all* wages collapsed. The PMAC also introduced several additional non-waged forms of surplus extraction that immiserised workers further. They included nominally voluntary—but in reality requisitioned—contributions of free labour, and the equally 'voluntary' cash contributions solicited for the various war efforts and campaigns.

[61] Girma Negash, for example, found that wages for migrant agricultural wage labourers in Wondo Genet grew from 0.50 ETB/day in 1966 to 0.75 ETB around the time of the 1974 revolution. Girma Negash, "The Rise and Rise of Agricultural Wage Labour: Evidence from Ethiopia's South, c.1950–2000," *Africa* 87, no. 1 (2017), 47.

[62] ILO, *Employment and Unemployment in Ethiopia*, 55.

[63] Mulatu and Yohannis, *Transition and Development*, 108–109.

[64] Department of State, *Country Reports on Human Rights Practices for 1985* (Washington DC: Joint Committee Print, 1986), 112.

[65] D. Robinson, "Wage Guidelines," in *Socialism from the Grass Roots: Accumulation, Employment and Equity in Ethiopia, Vol II: Working Papers,* ILO Jobs and Skills Programme for Africa (Addis Ababa: ILO, 1982), 32.

A powerful mechanism for regulating the movement of real wages during the PMAC/WPE era was the government's issuance of guidelines for overall wage movement in the dominant state-owned sector. There was never any pretence as to the reasons for state intervention in wage setting. Tesfa Gebremariam, CELU's former Deputy Secretary, who by the 1980s had become a Ministry of Labour and Social Affairs official,[66] stated that under circumstances wherein underdevelopment and poverty prevailed, 'any social and economic planning of necessity has to constrain free collective bargaining'.[67] It should be noted that there was a significant upturn in the number of collective agreements established during the PMAC/WPE era—no less than a 20-fold increase in the first decade of PMAC/WPE rule, according to Tesfa.[68] However, the importance of this factor pales when the coercive atmosphere and the commandist manner in which the agreements were established are factored in. Not only were the unions hierarchically organised, but the wage-setting mechanism of the state lingered heavy. 'Nothing is regarded as outside the scope of negotiation *except*, of course, the areas where government regulations determine the parameters for the public sector for some negotiable issues like *the setting of the maximum increase in wages*' [emphasis added], Tesfa reported without a hint of irony.[69] Considering that these areas of government regulation and parameter-setting were quite extensive and, as noted, included wages, this, in effect, meant that most essential issues were outside the scope of bargaining. Moreover, the state reserved extensive rights to enforce collective agreements throughout the economy. It included the unilateral prerogative of the minister of labour and social affairs to 'declare the draft collective agreement proposed by one of the parties to be binding upon the [other] party' if he considered either side to be negotiating in 'bad faith'. Moreover, even on issues where the parties were in agreement, the minister had the right to refuse to register the agreement should it contravene any existing law, regulation, or policy

[66] Tesfa had been ousted from CELU in the mid-1970s, after having participated in Alem Abdi's attempt to put the confederation on a pro-government footing.

[67] Tesfa Gebremariam, "The Promotion of Collective Bargaining in Ethiopia," in *Collective Bargaining and Security of Employment in Africa: English Speaking Countries: Proceedings of and Documents Submitted To, a Symposium, Victoria Falls, Zimbabwe, 4–8 May 1987* (Geneva: International Labour Office, 1988), 147.

[68] Ibid., 149.

[69] Ibid., 149. Emphasis added.

of the government.[70] Throughout the PMAC/WPE era, the declining trend in real wages was embedded in government policy.

Neither the wage data presented above nor the literature indicates that the downward trajectory of wages was substantially altered, or that real wages were permitted to recover, after the fall of the WPE regime. By 1993, a public sector minimum pay of 105 ETB/month had been set, but many workers in the private sector earned far less than that. Meanwhile, the Office for the Study of Wages and Other Remunerations calculated that a family of five would require a monthly income of 430 ETB 'to maintain a bare minimum standard of living'.[71] 'Even with two family members earning the public sector minimum wage', a US Department of State report noted, 'the family receives only about 50 per cent of that needed for healthful subsistence'.[72]

Contrasting with the direct manipulation of nominal wages that had characterised the PMAC/WPE era, the mechanisms that undercut wages in the EPRDF period were subtler. They included a sliding decline reinforced by repeated devaluations of the ETB exchange rate, the removal of a range of subsidies on consumer goods, increasing taxation and introduction of new indirect taxes, and, partly resulting from this, recurring bouts of inflation. But although wage suppression was not as direct as during the WPE era, it was an equally important priority of the EPRDF government, and during the period between the 1990s and the mid-2010s, it was equally premised on the government's ability to subdue the labour movement—both its practices, as demonstrated by the low levels of unrest, and its organisational manifestations, as shown by the thoroughly yellow unionism that was imposed on CETU during the period. As World Bank researchers found, because of the large relative size of the public waged sector, inflation has been exceptionally effective in checking real wages in the Ethiopian economy, and the development of Ethiopian wages has therefore been 'particularly prone to political "manipulation"'.[73] In this manner, real wages were, whenever showing signs of recovery, pushed back down again. In 1998, a report found that wages in the public sector

[70] Ibid., 148.

[71] Department of State, *Country Reports on Human Rights Practices for 1993.*

[72] Ibid.

[73] World Bank, *Fifth Ethiopia Economic Update: Why so Idle? Wages and Employment in a Crowded Labor Market* (Washington, DC: World Bank Group, 2016), 51.

had not yet recovered from the 1991 'inflationary shock'.[74] Moreover, World Bank researchers found evidence that real wages had again dropped between 2003 and 2014, and that only a slight recovery had occurred in the last couple of years of that period.[75]

By 2016, Ethiopian wages were allegedly 'on average one tenth the price of those in China', with blue-collar manufacturing wages hovering around 700 to 800 ETB a month.[76] A plethora of accounts substantiated this depiction of the general level of wages,[77] with one author going as far as suggesting that Ethiopian manufacturing wages had become 'the lowest in the world'.[78] Even an institution as thoroughly wedded to the interests of capital as the World Bank found the situation concerning. It described manufacturing wages for unskilled workers as being so low that they could not possibly drop any further, thus 'preventing the market from clearing'.[79] What prevented wages from falling further was not, the World Bank argued, high 'reservation wages', but rather 'because they [were] already clustered below the food poverty line' any further downward movement would render workers incapable of meeting 'minimum nutritional requirements'. In other words, they had hit rock bottom at precisely the same time that the vitality of the labour movement had.

[74] P. Krishnan, Tesfaye Gebreselassie and S. Dercon, "The Urban Labour Market During Structural Adjustment: Ethiopia 1990–1997," (working paper, Centre for the Study of African Economies, University of Oxford, 1998).

[75] World Bank, *Why so Idle?*, 51.

[76] G. Mills, "Ethiopia's Hailemariam Desalegn: Growth has to be shared to be sustainable," *Daily Maverick*, 7 June 2016, https://www.dailymaverick.co.za/article/2016-06-07-ethiopias-hailemariam-desalegn-growth-has-to-be-shared-to-be-sustainable/.

[77] See, for example, A. Dijkstra, "Low Wages Draw International Textile Companies to Ethiopia," *Deutsche Welle*, 10 December 2015, https://www.dw.com/en/low-wages-draw-international-textile-companies-to-ethiopia/a-18877027/, for a typical account substantiating starting wages ranging in the monthly 600–800 ETB range at the time. See Central Statistical Agency, *Statistical Report on the 2013 National Labour Force Survey* (Addis Ababa: CSA, 2014), for a more comprehensive breakdown of the incomes of waged workers.

[78] E. Wuilbercq, "L'Ethiopie, Nouvelle Usine du Monde," *Le Monde*, 11 August 2017, https://www.lemonde.fr/afrique/article/2017/08/11/l-ethiopie-nouvelle-usine-du-monde_5171211_3212.html.

[79] World Bank, *Fourth Ethiopia Economic Update: Overcoming Constraints in the Manufacturing Sector* (Washington, DC: World Bank Group, 2015), 55.

Case Study: The Bahir Dar Textile Factory

The Bahir Dar Textile Factory commenced production in 1962. The factory's construction had been financed by Italian war reparations, and its placement in the North-eastern Gojam province was intended to serve as a recognition of the role played by the people of the region in the resistance to the 1936–1941 Italian occupation of Ethiopia. Bahir Dar, however, was a poor provincial city[80] and had an immense shortage of educated personnel. As a result, management staff and skilled workers were recruited from other provinces—particularly the central Shoa region and Eritrea. Meanwhile, the unskilled workforce consisted mainly of locals. This division of labour created tensions in the workforce.

The factory was state-owned until 2017, when it was sold to *Tiret*, a conglomerate established by the EPRDF's regional party—the Amhara National Democratic Movement (ANDM). It has, however, been managed under different arrangements. In its early years, the factory was managed by Yugoslavs. They were later replaced by Indian executive staff—until management was Ethiopianised in the 1970s. Between 1975 and the early 1990s, the factory was integrated into the National Textile Corporation (NTC), before, again, being re-established as a separate state-owned share company. Because of poor profitability, it was leased to Chinese investors in the early 2000s, but the lease was cancelled after only 18 months, and the state resumed management of the enterprise. This state of things came to an end only in 2017.

Despite having been established within an import-substitution regime which granted the textile industry high levels of protection—ranging between 90 per cent and 526 per cent in the 1970s[81]—the Bahir Dar factory was rarely, if ever, profitable. In fact, it has been described as

[80] According to its governor at the time, Gaitachew Bekele, Bahir Dar, in 1961, had no paved road, and only the port administrator's office and residence had piped water and electricity. The imperial government's plans for the city, however, were ambitious, and with the support of West German planners it was expected to grow to become a sizeable and important economic hub. The textile factory was the centrepiece of this plan. Other provisions included the concurrent construction of a referral hospital, a polytechnic institute funded by the Soviet Union, a teacher's training school, and a hydroelectric plant at the nearby Blue Nile Falls. Gaitachew Bekele, *The Emperor's Clothes A Personal Viewpoint of Politics and Administration in the Imperial Ethiopian Government, 1941–1974* (East Lansing, MI: Michigan University Press, 1993), 125–130.

[81] Eshetu Chole "Import Substitution in Practice: The Case of the Ethiopian Textile Industry," (PhD diss., Syracuse University, 1973), 50.

'a financial disaster' which had not avoided losses for a single year by 1973.[82] With the decline in industrial profitability that came with the economic crisis of the subsequent years, it is unlikely that this situation improved much, and when the factory was brought up for privatisation in the early 2000s, its poor profitability discouraged potential investors. It would take more than a decade and additional state investments before a willing and able buyer was found.

As is typically the case, textile production in Ethiopia has been a relatively labour-intensive endeavour. This was one of the reasons textiles had developed into the country's largest manufacturing subsector by the early 1970s—both in terms of the number of workers engaged and the value of output.[83] Women made up the majority of workers in the sector. At the commencement of production, the workforce at the Bahir Dar factory consisted of 1,000 employees. Their number had grown to 1,900 two years later, and reached nearly 2,400 in the late 1960s.[84] The workforce continued to grow in the following decade and remained relatively stable until at least 1991, when the factory employed approximately 2,900 workers.[85] Renewed efforts to achieve profitability, along with the abandonment of overstaffing practices after the fall of the WPE, subsequently reduced the workforce to around 1,500 workers.

The Bahir Dar Textile Factory Workers' Union was registered with the Labour Department of the MNCD in August 1963. It had 550 members. Membership grew to 1,200 in 1964, 1,725 in September 1965, and by 1970, it had reached 2,200 workers.[86] For many years during

[82] Ibid., 53.

[83] Ibid.

[84] International Labour Organization, "Report on Workers' Education in Ethiopia," Report ILO/OTA/Ethiopia/R.6, confidential, ILO, Geneva, 1964, 14; Eshetu Chole "Import Substitution", 54; Demmelash Tebekew, in discussion with the author and Biniyam Negash, 7 May 2015. Former Treasurer, Vice President, Board Chairman, and President of the Bahir Dar textile factory's trade union in the 1960s, and CELU Vice President, Assistant Treasurer and Executive Committee member in the first half of the 1970s.

[85] E. Tarpinian, "Survey of the Ethiopian Textile Industry in Relation to a Title III Program," (report prepared for USAID/Ethiopia, Labat-Anderson Incorporated, 1992).

[86] ILO, "Workers' Education in Ethiopia", 14; Suter, *Labor Law and Practice*, 52; "የኢ.ሠአማን አባል ማኅበሮች እናስተዋውቃላችሁ/Introducing CELU's Affiliates," *Voice of Labour*, Special Issue on the Occasion of the 7th CELU Anniversary and the Inauguration of its New Headquarters (9 April 1970).

the 1960s and early 1970, its president was Workneh Atalai, a native of Gojam. According to various accounts, Workneh purportedly played on regionalist sentiments and divisions within the workforce, while allegedly regarding the union's finances 'as his own'.[87] Accusations of embezzlement would lead to his removal from union office by court order,[88] but having been reinstated by 1970, Workneh developed a relationship with management that was described as 'very harmonious'.[89] The factory union negotiated a first collective agreement with management as early as February 1964.[90] By 1970, three consecutive collective agreements had been concluded. Their provisions included free medical care for workers.[91] They also included stipulations for a check-off system, which greatly benefited the union's finances. As a result, the union was able to establish several facilities and services for the workers. They included a bakery and cafeteria for workers, as well as a school for their children.[92] The union also constructed a three-kilometre road, halving the distance workers residing in the city had to travel from their homes to arrive at the factory.[93]

While workers at the factory suffered from a similar lack of employment security as other workers did in the 1960s and early 1970s, the adoption of the 1975 labour law and the incorporation of the factory into the NTC changed this. Job security was significantly strengthened and the rules surrounding dismissals and transfers became rigid and protective of workers. As a result of this, staff turnover remained very low from the mid-1970s to the early 1990s, and managers in the early 1990s reported

[87] Killion, "Workers, Capital and the State", 511.

His alleged 'regionalism' was an issue also raised by Demmelash Tebekaw, discussion, and Fisschatsion Tekie, interview, Tom Killion Papers; Gebreselassie Gebremariam, interviewed by Tom Killion, 1983, microcassette, Tom Killion Papers.

[88] Killion, "Workers, Capital and the State", 512.

[89] "Introducing CELU's Affiliates", *Voice of Labour*, 50.

[90] The Bahir Dar Textile Factory was the second enterprise in all Ethiopia to conclude a collective agreement with its union, following HVA by only a few days. Stutz, "The Developing Industrial Relations System", 140.

[91] Suter, *Labor Law and Practice*.

[92] "Introducing CELU's Affiliates", *Voice of Labour*, 50.

[93] Report for Period 8 February to 8 August 1966, Pedersen to Secretariat for Technical Cooperation, LO archives.

that absenteeism was low and labour-management relations were good.[94] Although dismissals and retrenchments became permissible again after the adoption of the 1993 labour law and the break-up of NTC, employment security did not deteriorate to the low level of the 1960s.

Despite having entered into collective agreements at a relatively early stage, and despite them containing several beneficial provisions, wages at the factory compared unfavourably with those in other manufacturing establishments in the 1960s.[95] After being integrated into the NTC, the government-set wage policy was strictly applied. All workers were put 'on a fixed pay scale, without regard to production' and without any incentive plans.[96] These pay scales were ungenerous, and were only rarely and marginally revised, regardless of inflation rates. Although this wage-setting policy was abandoned in the 1990s, there were no efforts to improve wages significantly.

The Bahir Dar Textile Factory saw several episodes of labour unrest. Beginning in its early days, workers, according to one of its union leaders, created 'constant disturbances'.[97] Wage and workload-related complaints fuelled near-constant strike activity in the first years of the factory's operation.[98] Although the most acute phase of conflict was brought to an end by the signing of the first collective agreement, unrest never disappeared entirely. Whereas the union refrained from organising any strike over the following years, it repeatedly warned the management that it remained ready to call out the entire workforce.[99] The threat was credible, and was leveraged by the union in the negotiations of the subsequent collective agreements.

In 1966, serious internal infighting erupted *within* the union and among the workers. The union leadership was accused of abusing their power and misusing the union's means. Fissehatsion Tekie, CELU's

[94] Tarpinian, "Survey", 9.

[95] ILO, "Workers' Education in Ethiopia", 10; Ginzberg and Smith, *Manpower Strategy*, 98.

[96] Tarpinian, "Survey", 9.

[97] Demmelash Tebekew, discussion.

[98] Ibid.

[99] Ibid.

general secretary, was dispatched to Bahir Dar to investigate the accusations and mediate a solution. A Danish trade union advisor who accompanied him reported that 'infighting between [the factory's] 2,000 workers' was 'about to develop into chaos'.[100]

> Already at the landing strip in Bahar Dar, we were received by deputations for the aggrieved workers who tried to convince us of the 'actual situation'. The opposition demanded that new elections be held immediately. Groups of workers laid siege to our hotel until late at night to try to convince us of their views, and as if by coincidence one or another polished their pistols during the discussions.
>
> After a week of negotiations, we tried to reconcile the quarreling parties at a meeting at the Nile River. The opposition got so upset that the meeting was overtaken by uproar. They were not interested in establishing guilt or innocence. They have been working to seize power for three months, and have now had enough.
>
> Everyone was shouting and gesticulating with sticks, and no one knew who was carrying a pistol in their pocket. A guard armed with a stick came to protect me. By the time the congregation lost its temper for a third time, we gave up our efforts for the time being.

In addition to the accusations of mismanagement levelled against the union leadership, regionalist sentiments—or, as the Danish advisor put it, 'tribal contradictions'—added explosiveness to the situation. 'There is a strong sense of belonging in the area, and it has always been a problem that the local population wishes to determine the factory's activities and personnel policies. Now it appears the turn has come for trade union matters', the Danish advisor wrote. Later accounts have corroborated the view that the infighting largely stemmed from regionalist sentiments and contradictions between locals and outsiders.[101] This provided for a combustible situation. Unrest spread from the factory and into the city. Since workers of the factory and inhabitants of the city were often armed—one AALC representative was surprised at the frequency of bullets being discharged by union officials and workers to welcome

[100] Report for Period 8 February to 8 August 1966, Pedersen to Secretariat for Technical Cooperation, LO archives.

[101] Killion, "Workers, Capital and the State", 512–13.

him[102]—security forces had to be called in before new union elections could be held. In the aftermath of the elections, the situation was temporarily pacified.

Renewed internal unrest erupted around the time of the revolution, amid accusations that the union leadership was dividing the workers along regional lines. Eventually, the leaders were removed, leading to the election of a new batch of labour leaders more to the liking of the new government. However, that did not put an end to unrest at the factory, as the union became embroiled in the broader struggle over the country-wide labour movement—and the conflict between the militant opposition and the PMAC. The warehouses of the factory were set on fire in late 1974 or 1975,[103] and 'several strikes'[104] took place before repression stamped out the resistance of oppositional workers.[105] To facilitate this, no fewer than 200 workers were enrolled in the factory's Revolutionary Guard[106] militia and equipped with 70 firearms—before being set upon

[102] '[W]hile the people here are friendly enough they don't hesitate to use a gun if they feel it necessary. Feeling it necessary could mean an auditor send in to check their books or a surveyor send in to check the land', John Kilhefner, the AALC representative, wrote. 'During our stay here we were invited to the [union] president's home for dinner. The former president was also invited. During dinner the president suddenly jumped up from the table, pulled out a pistol from a shoulder holster and fired straight at the front door. I found out later that this was a sign of welcome—that he was happy to have us in his home. Later the week more firing took place—all in good fun—they like to "smell bullets"'. "Labor Education Project: Report: Dec. 1968–July 1971," John Kilhefner, AALC Records.

[103] The arson attack occurred sometime in the Ethiopian calendar year of 1967, which overlaps with the last three and a half months of 1974 and the first eight and a half months of 1975 G.C.

[104] However, while the representative of the Bahir Dar textile factory union, Adugna Regassa, signed the 1975 September CELU resolution threatening a general strike, the official *Ethiopian Herald* claimed that the Bahir Dar textile factory workers did not take part in the September 1975 general strike attempt. "Labour Strike in Addis condemned," *Ethiopian Herald*, 3 October 1975.

[105] Demmelash Tebekew, discussion; Killion, "Workers, Capital and the State".

[106] The revolutionary guards—የአብዮት ጥበቃ —organised in workplaces and neighbourhoods was a central instrument of the state-sanctioned violence. In most factories, a guard squad of between 10 and 50 workers, equipped with a dozen rifles, was deemed entirely sufficient. The number of guards and arms at the Bahir Dar Textile Factory is somewhat of an outlier.

dissidents.[107] The chairman of the union and the workers' discussion forum, Seife Asnake, was one of around 10 workers and labour leaders killed in the struggles that followed the revolution.[108] Seife and other workers had been accused of propagating the formation of a 'Provisional People's Government', the EPRP's central demand at the time. Seife's personnel file at the Bahir Dar Textile Factory confirms that he was killed by pro-government actors within the state-sanctioned 'Red Terror' campaign in 1978.[109] Many more were arrested. A second round of purges at the factory targeted around twenty MEISON-affiliated unionists and workers.[110] This purge concluded the phase of open contestation at the factory and ushered in a period of relative tranquillity.

During the mid-1980s, the union developed a number of grievances against the NTC and factory management in the process of bargaining for a new collective agreement. In the absence of any permissible outlet for the increasing frustration of workers, however, the union had no recourse beyond submitting petitions and appeals to the corporation and the Ministry of Industry. These appeals were typically met with rebuttals from the latter. The only major incident of labour unrest within the NTC was the Asmara/Barottolo Textile Factory strike in 1983, and the outcome of that strike left no question as to how the re-emergence of insubordination would be treated.

However, in the 1990s, the factory's union again became involved in contestation. The first episode that attracted outside attention was an alleged act of sabotage in September 1993, conducted by workers who removed key equipment and caused a production shutdown.[111] In late 1993, moreover, the arrest and subsequent disappearance of Abebe Aynekulu, a technician and trade unionist who was alleged to be an EPRP member, caused another bout of unrest at the factory.[112] In response to

[107] "የአብዮት ጥበቃ ኮሚቴዎች የተቋቋሙባቸው ድርጅቶች በ26-1-70 የታጠቁ" memorandum, Revolutionary Guard Provisional Central Committee, 6 October 1977, Confederation of Ethiopian Trade Unions (CETU) archives, CETU, Addis Ababa.

[108] Demmelash Tebekew, discussion.

[109] "Seife Asnake", personnel file, Bahir Dar Textile Factory Archives, International Institute of Social History, Amsterdam.

[110] Negede Gobezie, *ይድረስ ለግንቦት ከየካቲት* (Washington, DC: AESOP Publishers, 2014), 254.

[111] "Factory's Stolen Property Recovered," *Ethiopian Herald*, 21 September 1993.

[112] "Alleged EPRP Members Shot One Youth," *Ethiopian Herald*, 7 May 1994.

Abebe's disappearance, union leaders called on workers to demonstrate and demand that his whereabouts be made known. The workers were intercepted by security forces at the factory gates and dispersed. Forty workers who were accused of sedition were suspended.[113] A final period of contestation occurred in the mid-1990s, as the the factory and its union became involved in the conflict within CETU and between CETU and the government. The union's chairman and an executive committee member were briefly detained in late 1994.[114] They were released a couple of months later, but were not permitted to return to their jobs.[115]

Chart 6.7 below displays the index of average real wages at the factory. It has been calculated from data contained in a randomised sample[116] of personnel files.

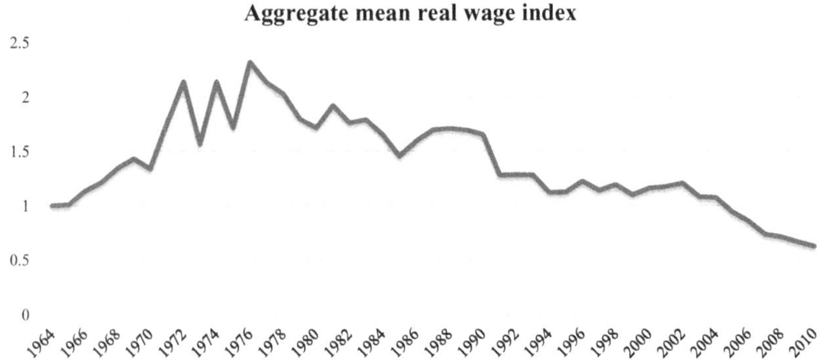

113 Abebe—who had previously been arrested by the government on accusations of being an EPRP militant—never resurfaced. It is likely that he, like several other EPRP militants arrested by the EPRDF government, was extra-judicially executed.

114 Dawey Ibrahim to ICFTU, 14 November 1994, Ministry of Labour and Social Affairs (MoLSA) archives, MoLSA, Addis Ababa.

115 Ibid.

116 The sample from which wages at the Bahir Dar Textile Factory is calculated consists of data harvested from 850 personnel files from the Bahir Dar Textile Factory. The files were randomly selected from 4,221 personnel files digitised by the International Institute of Social History. Real wages were calculated by deflating nominal wages by the computed price index published by the CSA in the annual *Statistical Abstract*.

Chart 6.7 Aggregate mean real wage index from Bahir Dar textile factory sample[117] (*Source* Author's computation of data from Bahir Dar Textile Factory personnel archives sample)

It is apparent from the chart that, much like in the broader manufacturing sector, a sharp and sustained real wage increase occurred during the years between the early 1960s and the mid-1970s. After this, wages at the Bahir Dar Textile Factory—as elsewhere—embarked on a prolonged decline. In the initial years of the decline, the fall was sharp, consuming somewhere between a third and two-fifths of real wages in the eight years that followed the 1976 high-water mark. There was a slight recovery in the second half of the 1980s, again confirming the country-wide trend. However, this episode was followed by another prolonged decline, periodically interrupted by periods of stabilisation.

Nevertheless, there are also variations from the pattern of aggregate sectoral wage movements in the Bahir Dar data. The first deviation is the fact that the wage swings were distinctively sharper at the Bahir Dar Textile Factory than what was the overall case in the manufacturing sector. Real wages at the factory appear to have multiplied by a factor of over 2.3 between 1964 and 1976, only to be reduced to roughly a quarter of that level in the subsequent 34 years. Yet, it took much longer for real wage gains achieved in the 1960s and 1970s to be rolled back at the Bahir Dar Textile Factory than in the sector as a whole. It appears that this reversal was not completed until the first decade of the twenty-first century, while on a national scale the gains from the previous decades had already been depleted by the end of the 1970s. The explanation for this can be derived from the discussion above and relates to the particular wage level at the factory. The sharp upswing of wages in the first phase can probably be explained by the fact that wages at the factory were generally lower than in comparable manufacturing establishments in the 1960s. The comparative levels are illustrated in Chart 6.8 below.

[117] Until 1963, and in some cases afterwards, wages were often recorded in daily terms rather than monthly. When converting daily wages to monthly wages, the 1993 labour proclamation states that 'for purposes of determining the qualifying period of service required for the entitlement of an annual leave, 26 days of service in an undertaking shall be deemed to be equivalent to one month of employment'. For this reason, and since the 48-hour workweek has been constant since the 1963 labour proclamation, 26 work days have been taken to mean one month's pay. "Proclamation No. 42 of 1993: Labour Proclamation," *Negarit Gazeta* 52, no. 27 (20 January 1993).

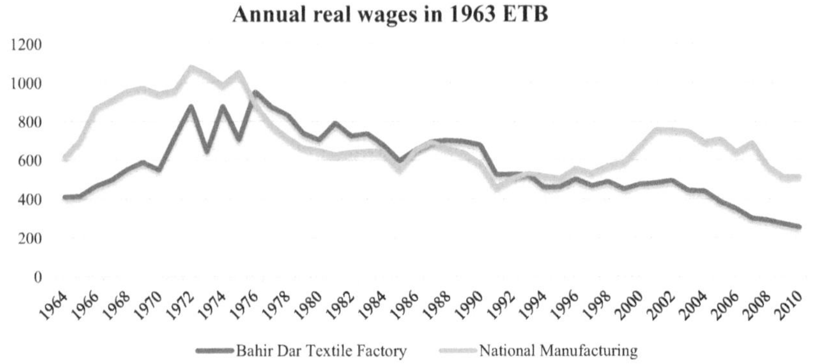

Chart 6.8 Mean annual real wages in 1963 ETB (*Source* Author's computation of data from Bahir Dar textile factory personnel archives sample; CSA's annual *Statistical Abstract* 1963 to 2012/13)

Starting from a significantly lower base, it took over a decade for wages at the Bahir Dar Textile Factory to catch up with the country-wide sectoral average. By 1976, wages at the Bahir Dar Textile Factory had converged with and actually surpassed average wages in the broader manufacturing sector. They remained roughly level until the end of the 1990s. By then, the Bahir Dar plant was no longer at the technological forefront of Ethiopian textile manufacturing. It may be surmised that the emergence of newer, more profitable manufacturing enterprises was a factor that helped stabilise average wages across the aggregate sector, while such stabilisation did not occur at the Bahir Dar Textile Factory. The lowering of protective tariffs in the wake of the EPRDF's deregulation policies also affected the factory negatively. Whatever the relative weight of those factors, the chart illustrates that whereas the Bahir Dar Textile Factory workers were successful in more than doubling their wages through the 1960s and early 1970s, reaching parity with other Ethiopian manufacturing workers, they were unable to secure those wages from collapsing in the years that followed—or even halt their further downward slide in the subsequent decades.

Case Study: The Ethio-Djibouti Railway Enterprise

The Franco-Ethiopian Railway Company (*Compagnie du Chemin de Fer Franco-Ethiopien*, CFE)[118] was established in 1908 to traffic the railway between Djibouti and Addis Ababa, which was under construction at the time and commenced operation nine years later. It was established as a joint venture between French investors, with the Ethiopian government as a minor shareholder. In 1959, however, the Ethiopian state assumed ownership of over half of the stock, securing a majority share. Reflecting this new shareholding balance, the company's head office was moved from France to Ethiopia that same year. In 1981 the company was renamed *Compagnie du Chemin de Fer Djibouto-Ethiopien* (CDE), as the recently independent Djiboutian state took over ownership of French shares, turning it into a joint Ethiopian and Djiboutian state-owned enterprise. In the 1980s and 1990s, however, the CDE entered into a long period of decline, and the rail line fell into disrepair. The creation of a new and separate Ethiopian Railway Corporation in 2007 and the subsequent construction of a new line operated by this corporation signalled its end. The enterprise ceased operation in 2016.

The Dire Dawa depot of the railway enterprise was located midway between Addis Ababa and Djibouti, at the edge of the Eastern Ethiopian highlands. It was selected because of its central location on the line, its proximity to the trading city of Harar, and the relatively cool climate and access to fresh water provided by its location at the escarpment. The area was inhabited mainly by Somali and Oromo Muslims. However, as the city of Dire Dawa developed around the railway, it attracted a distinctly metropolitan population, drawn from all across the country and beyond. In addition to the station and administrative offices, the railway depot also housed supply warehouses, a training centre, a fuelling station, a clinic, and the mechanical workshops of the line.

CDE/CFE was an almost exclusively male workplace, with the majority of the few women employed by the enterprise serving in its clinic.[119] The workforce initially comprised a large proportion of foreign

[118] The CFE was the successor to the *Compagnie Impériale des Chemins de Fer Ethiopiens,* which had begun work on the railway in 1896 but was bankrupted in 1907. It was renamed the CDE in 1981, four years after Djibouti gained independence.

[119] Only 20 out of 2000 CFE employees in 1964 were female. ILO, "Workers' Education in Ethiopia", 10.

workers, but their share gradually declined as management staff and skilled workers were increasingly recruited locally. Racial discrimination was rife in the enterprise and was expressed both in terms of wage differentials and in the hierarchies of authority, with Europeans occupying the management positions in its early years. This began to gradually change in the late 1940s. In the aftermath of the 1974 revolution, the process of Ethiopianising the workforce and management was completed.

Although workers on the line had organised in prior constellations and staged strikes as far back as 1919,[120] the CFE's formal trade union—the *Syndicat des Cheminots,* as it was known—was established in 1946. Its initial aim was to 'protect Ethiopian workers from racial discrimination' by seeking higher wages for Ethiopian workers and the Ethiopianisation of management.[121] The syndicate staged three major strikes—in 1947, 1949, and 1955, before it fell into relative inactivity. Combined with a sharp reduction in traffic and staff—the number of employees fell from 5,000 to 2,000 during the 1950s—this reduced the importance of the syndicate.[122] In 1958, Kenyan labour leader and ICFTU representative Tom Mboya visited Ethiopia and met representatives of the syndicate. He reported that both the syndicate's president and vice-president had died during that year, under what he perceived to be suspicious circumstances, and that they had been replaced by an acting leadership which 'did not seem to know very much about the union'.[123] He noted that the union appeared dormant and weak, organising only some 400 workers.

Nevertheless, in the early 1960s, when the process of establishing a country-wide trade union centre gathered pace, the syndicate was revitalised. It became an important actor in the process, on whose experience, reputation and semi-legal status the broader movement drew. It also achieved formal recognition as a trade union during this period. The syndicate was legally registered in December 1962, and by August 1965

[120] European workers of the enterprise led a series of strikes between 1919 and 1926. See T. Killion, "Railroad Workers and the Ethiopian Imperial State: The Politics of Workers' Organization on the Franco-Ethiopian Railroad, 1919–1959," *International Journal of African Historical Studies*, 3, no. 25 (1992).

[121] "Report on Mission to Ethiopia, 2nd–10th October 1958," Tom Mboya, ICFTU/ITUC archives.

[122] Killion, "Railroad Workers", 603.

[123] "Report on Mission to Ethiopia", Mboya, ICFTU/ITUC archives.

it had a membership of 1,600 workers.[124] Throughout the 1960s and the early 1970s, the union was led by Demena Lemma, who was also a member of CELU's General Council. The head office of the syndicate was located in Dire Dawa, and it operated a branch office in Addis Ababa. It was a relatively well-funded union, whose secretariat employed eight staff members, and could afford to hire external instructors to organise literacy classes for its members. It also owned land and buildings, including a sprawling members' club in Dire Dawa.[125] As one of the largest and most important unions in the country, it was the seventh in order to negotiate a collective agreement, concluding its first such agreement with the railway company in December 1966.[126]

In terms of wages, the workers of CFE/CDE for long constituted a privileged group of relatively well-paid workers: 'a virtual "labour elite" in relation to other Ethiopian industrial workers during the 1960s', according to one scholar.[127] There were several reasons for this. The technological sophistication of the enterprise and the skilled labour force therefore required was one factor. The impact of the high wages paid to European workers—but also Yemeni, Djiboutian and Somali subjects of colonial states—was another factor, as Ethiopian workers fought to close the wage gap. Moreover, the sustained militancy of the organised workers of the enterprise between 1946 and 1955 resulted in repeated wage increments.[128] By the 1960s, the workers on the railway had already secured substantial wage gains and were therefore relatively well-paid. However,

[124] Suter, *Labor Law and Practice*, 52.

[125] "Introducing CELU's Affiliates", *Voice of Labour*; "Mission to Ethiopia 31 August–30 September 1963," H. Robinson, ICFTU/ITUC archives.

[126] Stutz, "The Developing Industrial Relations System", 140.

[127] Killion, "Workers, Capital and the State", 426.

[128] Tom Killion has pointed out how the 'wages and benefits which later were to give the railroad its reputation as the "best paid and most secure employment" in the region did not exist at the end of the world war', but was instead 'won by railroad workers only after a prolonged struggle with French capital' in the subsequent years. One illustrative example is the settlement of the 1947 strike on the railway line, which resulted in general wage increments of between 20 and 40 per cent. Killion, "Workers, Capital and the State", 171–172; "Conciliation Commission (1947) to Settle the 1947 CFE Strike, Yekatit 28 1939 (E.C.)–Megabit (March) 6, 1947 (G.C.)," translation by Awetu Simisso and Tom Killion in "Documents on the History of the Labor Movement in Ethiopia", 1982, Tom Killion Papers.

they were no longer at the forefront of militancy within the Ethiopian labour movement.

The revitalised CFE union staged its first and only major strike in early 1974. By this time it had 1,500 members and was led by Teshome Aberra. The strike led to violence, and six workers were 'seriously wounded' by the police.[129] Unrest along the line during that year also included a demonstration in Addis Ababa and a sabotage of the line outside Dire Dawa.[130] In the immediate aftermath of the revolution, however, the leadership of the union rallied behind the PMAC. It rejected and condemned CELU's September 1974 strike call. Although the city of Dire Dawa was a hotbed of industrial unrest which saw armed repression of the labour movement in the subsequent years, no major strike would occur on the railway again. However, that did not mean that all railway workers were supportive of the union leadership, nor that the union was united in backing the new dispensation. According to a senior EPRP and ELAMA leader who visited Dire Dawa in 1974, 'there was a cleavage, there was a conflict between two major sections of the railway union', which pitted the union leadership and its supporters against the majority of the rank-and-file.[131] The division had both regional and hierarchical aspects, with the union leadership allegedly supported 'mainly [by] French-speaking Ethiopians from the central part of the country'. The two factions were 'at loggerheads with each other', and the opposition was purportedly 'on the verge of calling a strike'.[132] While the railway workers' union was listed as a signatory of a June 1975 multi-union protest note against the 'anti-proletarian' actions of the Dire Dawa office of the labour department,[133] its stamp and its president's signature[134] was conspicuously missing from the document. This was illustrative of the vacillating position of the divided syndicate and the pro-government inclinations of its leadership.

[129] Richard Baurmann to Lester Trachtman, 19 April 1974, AALC Records.

[130] Killion, "Workers, Capital and the State", 429.

[131] Kiflu Tadesse, in discussion with the author, June 15–18, 2014.

[132] Ibid.

[133] Various unions to CELU's Provisional Workers' Committee, 28 June 1975, CETU archives.

[134] It was the only large Dire Dawa union listed in the petition where the stamp and signature of the union chairman—Ali Melew in the case of the railway workers union—was missing.

In 1994, the CDE union became entangled in the renewed conflict within the labour movement and between the movement and the state. Perceived as supportive of CETU's leadership, the CDE union was purportedly an early target of government subversion. The concerned industrial federation allegedly assisted internal dissenters in ousting the union's pro-confederation leadership.[135] The episode marked the definitive end of whatever was left of the railway workers' reputation of militancy.

To summarise, the workers of CFE/CDE played an important role in disseminating the ideas and practices of organisation and collective action among Ethiopian workers. The railway syndicate also provided the Ethiopian labour movement with a key source of militant energy in its earliest phase. Over the subsequent decades, however, this vanguard position was abandoned as the organisation of railway workers increasingly came to favour moderation over militancy.

Chart 6.9 below presents the mean real wage index, calculated from a sample[136] of CFE/CDE personnel files in the Dire Dawa Railway Depot archives. Personnel files from across the Ethiopian section of the line[137] was sent to be stored at the Dire Dawa offices. For this reason, the sample of files from Dire Dawa represents the whole Ethiopian section of the line.

[135] Hailu Ourgessa, in discussion with the author, 28 May 2017.

[136] The sample consists of 300 randomly selected personnel files from the Ethio-Djibouti Railways, digitised by the International Institute of Social History. Ethio-Djibouti Railway, Dire Dawa Hub Archives, International Institute of Social History, Amsterdam.

[137] The Ethiopian and Djiboutian sections of the line were consistently administrated separately, with the Djiboutian headquarters located in Djibouti city after the relocation from Paris. Wages on the Djiboutian section of the line were higher than on the Ethiopian section.

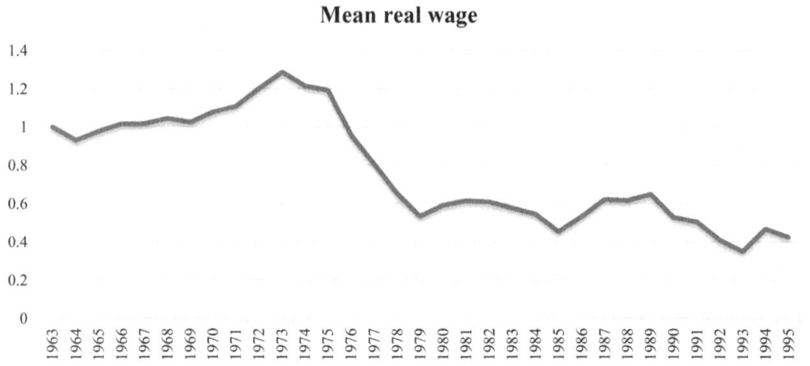

Chart 6.9 Mean real wage index from CFE/CDE sample (*Source* Author's computation of data from CFE/CDE personnel archives sample)

It is apparent from the chart that while the general upward trajectory of Ethiopian real wages in the early 1960s to the mid-1970s lifted wages at the CFE/CDE too, the increase was neither as sharp as in the manufacturing sector as a whole nor, in particular, the Bahir Dar Textile Factory. The downward turn from the mid-1970s onwards was, on the other hand, much sharper than in the aggregate sectoral case. The reason for the former was, in all certainty, that the relatively high wages railway workers had already acquired by the beginning of the 1960s limited the relative weight of subsequent wage gains secured in collective agreements. The wage movements illustrated in the chart began from a significantly higher base. During the downturn, on the other hand, national wage equalisation policies hit the relatively privileged railway workers comparatively harder than lesser-paid workers. A comparison between average real wages on the railway and overall manufacturing wages illustrates this point.

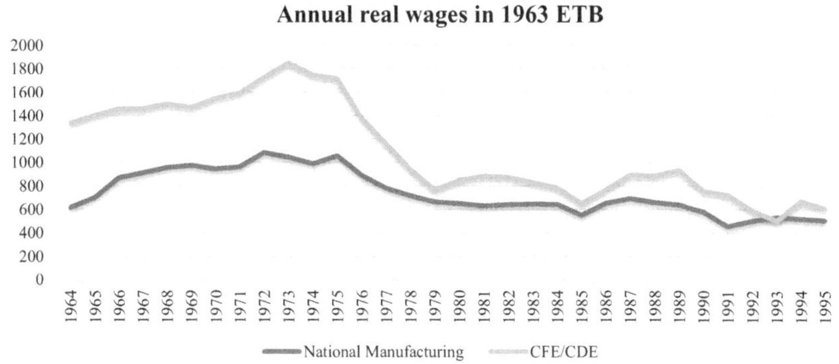

Chart 6.10 Mean annual real wages in 1963 ETB (*Source* Author's computation of data from CFE/CDE personnel archives sample and CSA's annual *Statistical Abstract* 1963 to 2012/13)

Chart 6.10 highlights the comparatively privileged position of CFE workers at the time that the country-wide labour movement came into being. Moreover, the chart illustrates how wage equalisation policies during the rule of the Derg led to a convergence between CFE/CDE wages and manufacturing sector wages, consuming both the wage gains railway workers made prior to the emergence of the country-wide labour movement, and those that had been acquired through collective agreements and contestation in the 1960s and 1970s.

Summary: Wages and Unrest

The shifting level of strike activity in Ethiopia over the past seven decades presents itself in a cyclical pattern. Between the 1960s and 2020, there were three discernable cycles. The first began in the 1960s and reached its crest in the mid-1970s, before abruptly ending amidst heavy repression. The second—much shorter in duration and lesser in intensity—began in the late 1980s and came to an end only a handful of years later. A third cycle began in the mid-2010s and appeared to reach a turning point with the coming of the coronavirus pandemic, civil war, and growing authoritarianism in 2020. The emergence of these cycles has dovetailed with the prevalence of relatively autonomous and assertive trade unionism.

The wage data presented in this chapter reveal two broad trends: a pronounced upward trajectory through the 1960s and early 1970s, followed by a steep and prolonged decline starting in the mid-1970s and lasting into the 1980s. From the mid-1980s to the early 2010s, real wages intermittently stabilised during some periods while continuing to decline during others, but never substantially recovered.

The data presented decisively contradicts the scholarly claim that CELU's leadership's 'gradualist policy [failed] to result in significant material or political gains for Ethiopian workers during the 1960s'.[138] On the one hand, as was discussed in Chapter 2, political gains through the 1960s and early 1970s placed the labour movement in a central position in the political convulsions that followed. This chapter has shown that material gains were also achieved, particularly through the gradual increase in real wages. To be sure, these gains cannot be reduced to mere outcomes of the policies of the leadership. Pressures from the lower ranks of the movement were an important factor propelling these developments. However the standard depiction of the period as one in which workers failed to make meaningful advances does not hold up to scrutiny. Whether because of, despite of, or unrelated to the policies of the leadership, significant advances were made.

The extraordinary gains that Ethiopian workers secured during the long decade preceding the Ethiopian revolution require an explanation. While the political-economic context must be considered, it has been demonstrated that wage outcomes cannot simply be explained by productivity levels. Productivity shifts appear to have been disconnected from the movement of wages throughout most of the period examined. In fact, even the World Bank has acknowledged that 'in Ethiopia, real wages do not reflect productivity levels'—a notable concession from an institution that typically holds the opposite position.[139] Moreover, while relative abundance and scarcity of factors of production may typically help explain wage levels, widespread urban unemployment has been a constant factor, prevailing in Ethiopia throughout this period. Not much has changed in this regard, and as a result, this factor cannot explain the overall wage shifts.

As Samir Amin has noted, wages may not have very much to do with productivity in economies dominated by a peasant-based agrarian

[138] Killion, "Workers, Capital and the State", 476–477.

[139] World Bank, *Why so Idle?*, 51.

sector.[140] In such economies, where only a small proportion of the working population is primarily engaged in wage labour, Amin found the 'political dimension' of wage determination to be far more significant than in industrial economies. In agrarian-dominated economies, there is, according to Amin, 'no obvious relation' between wage movements and the performance of the economy. A low pace of growth can be accompanied by sharp wage increases, while rapid growth may sometimes not result in any wage gains at all. In some cases, he argued, 'there is not the slightest correlation between the movement of wages and the pace of industrialisation, or even the movements of profits'. Amin provides a compelling explanation for this: 'elastic behaviour, upward or downward, in real terms, is only possible, of course, because the problem of wages does not constitute the main axis of income distribution'. In other words, it is because of the relative unimportance of surpluses generated in the waged sectors that the movement of wages appears largely autonomous from the performance of the larger economy.

Similarly, labour historian Tom Killion has argued that 'because the hegemony of the imperial ruling class rested on their control over land and peasants, rather than the capitalist sector', in the Ethiopian case, 'the state was not particularly threatened by the organisation of workers in industries, which were largely foreign-owned'.[141] He appears to have been entirely correct in that respect. The nature of the imperial ruling class—its agrarian roots in particular—provides a plausible explanation for the imperial state's relative laxness towards the labour movement. As it turns out, late imperial Ethiopia was not as consistently inhospitable to the labour movement as the literature has portrayed it.[142] This is probably linked to how the ruling categories perceived their interests—at the apex of the social structure sat a class that relied almost exclusively on agrarian rents rather than industrial surpluses. To this class, the urban unionised sector may largely have seemed irrelevant, functioning as a space for 'modernist' window dressing, mainly performed by and for foreigners. Corroborating this view, a CELU organiser acknowledged

[140] S. Amin, "Income Distribution and the "Privileged" Worker," in *African Social Studies: A Radical Reader*, ed. P.C.W Gutkind and P. Waterman (New York and London: Monthly Review, 1977), 197–199.

[141] Killion, "Workers, Capital and the State", 391.

[142] That having been said, as the numerous dismissals imply, it was not necessarily very hospitable to the individual worker.

that while the government disliked and was suspicious of the labour movement, it 'did not worry very much about it' since most employers who were affected by labour problems were foreigners.[143] The fact that the right to organise was not extended to the agrarian sector—to the day labourers working on the farms of the dominant classes—supports this argument. Ironically—given the egalitarian political rhetoric they espoused—it was the subsequent post-revolutionary governments that intensified surplus extraction in the waged sectors, thereby exacerbating pressure on wages.[144] The collapse of real wages—always prone to political manipulation and never merely the outcome of market factors—and the sharp ascent in the rate of exploitation that followed is linked to this fact.

However, while government policies affected wage movements, the state was not a central actor in the establishment of the series of collective agreements that cumulatively led to the wage hike in the 1960s and early 1970s. The force that propelled this advance was the active pressure from the labour movement, and the numerous conflicts that tended to precede the individual agreements. The most conspicuous historical dynamic was thus the relationship between a combative labour movement and rising wages. Real wages steadily increased during the long decade in which sustained unrest and labour movement activity occurred. They also peaked at the high-water mark of labour movement militancy in the mid-1970s. And they immediately embarked on a sharp downward trajectory when that movement collapsed.

It is not only in hindsight that the correlation, during this period, between the agency of militant workers and the conditions of labour, measured in wages, is evident—it was entirely clear to representatives of Ethiopian employers of the time. Their statements revealed deep concern that successful strikes, resulting in wage gains, fueled more unrest. There are explanations for this in the theoretical literature.

It is well known that strike activity can lead to concrete betterment in the conditions of workers. Strong labour movements engaging in sustained strike activity have frequently 'succeeded in raising wages, improving working conditions, and strengthening workers' rights', labour

143 Emmanuel Fayessa Negesa, interviewed by Tom Killion, 1983, microcassette, Tom Killion Papers.

144 See discussion in Chapter 3.

scholar Beverly Silver has noted.[145] However, successful strikes also tend to have a direct impact on the labour movement itself and its outlook. Labour militancy—expressed in an assertive strategy and willingness to engage in collective action—may not only energise existing structures but result in their expansion through sharp increases in membership.[146] 'Where unions have visibly demonstrated their effectiveness in pursuing, and winning, employee claims and grievances through strike action', industrial relations scholar John Kelly has written, 'non-union workers have been encouraged to join in unusually large numbers'.[147] This, Kelly argued, may set 'a virtuous circle of effectiveness and membership' in motion: 'as the scale of strike activity increased, so did the win rate, and as the win rate increased, bargaining coverage rose, more workers perceived unions to be effective and joined them, which in turn enabled more strikes to be called... and so on'.[148] The obvious corollary is that the reverse is equally possible—that a self-reinforcing cycle of defeat, ineffectiveness, and reduced membership could be set in motion.

Ernesto Screpanti has suggested that a virtuous cycle can also be generated between achievements and assertiveness: 'any consolidated increase in [wage growth] achievements induces expectations of further increases', he has written.[149] 'There is a positive cumulative effect of past experience in relation to actual claims'. This effect could set a somewhat path-dependent cycle of increasing assertiveness, unrest, and achievements in motion.

A reciprocal interrelationship between advances in the position and conditions of labour, on the one hand, and the development of militancy and assertiveness, on the other, can thus emerge, reinforced by expanding ranks of workers attracted by the achievements and inspired by the energies released. Equally, the reverse may occur, resulting in a self-reinforcing cycle of defeat, despondency and docility. Both aspects of this dynamic have been evident at various points in the history of the Ethiopian labour movement.

[145] Silver, *Forces of Labor*, 168.

[146] J. Kelly, *Rethinking Industrial Relations: Mobilisation, Collectivism and Long Waves* (London: Routledge, 1998), 60–64.

[147] Ibid., 62.

[148] Ibid., 101.

[149] Screpanti, "Proletarian Insurgencies", 530.

With regard to the former, the following excerpts from a 1966 memorandum, written by the president of the Ethiopian Employers' Federation (and HVA executive) J.M.J. Prakken, describes how successful collective industrial action inspired and fed into new rounds of unrest:

> Relative calm was disrupted by the illegal strike initiated in 1964 by the workers of EAL [Ethiopian Airlines]. In the second part of 1965 more labour difficulties developed which eventually culminated in an illegal strike at General Ethiopian Transport thus paralysing transport communications in Addis Ababa and all over the Empire of Ethiopia. It is regrettable that apparently no action was taken against the offending strikers concerned who infringed the law, as this seems to have encouraged others considering numerous strikes and slow-downs that erupted in various industries during the past few weeks. In this respect we mention inter alia, a slow-down in A. Besse & Company, a general strike in Debre Berhan Wool Factory and a strike and slow-down in HVA-Ethiopia's Wonji and Shoa Factories, the latter lasting already for more than 15 days. In addition to this, there are reports about an increasing tendency of labour difficulties in many enterprises... The prevailing labour unrest is either a consequence of previous illegal labour actions having remained unpunished, or else that they are incited by agitators intent on embarrassing the Government.[150]

Seven years later, the situation had not improved for employers. New wage gains were fueling further unrest, and vice versa. The president of the employers' federation at the time, Bekele Beshah, lamented that unpunished labour unrest was leading to escalating militancy among workers, new strikes, and, as a result, further wage increases:

> Industrial relations developments in Ethiopia seems to have taken a turn for the worse. The most recent spate of illegal strikes in at least three very important establishments all of which have gone unpunished are in our view a cause for concern. What is even more worrying is the flood of threats, intimidations and coercion that have been directed against the government – and against the responsible officials of the institutions that have been the victims of these illegal acts... It is obvious that there has been a growing misuse of union power which, unless checked by law and its effective and impartial implementation, will jeopardise the future of collective bargaining... Very important issues here, are the costs of such

[150] "Memorandum", Prakken, ICFTU/ITUC archives.

> strikes in loss of production and harm to the economy, and the vulnerability they show of business in general and of the government and public at large to industrial action in key sectors... If organised labour is to play an effective role in the nation's economic endeavour they have to do it as insiders... and not as outsiders pressing their demands and imposing their wishes by brute, naked force of slowdowns and strikes... The irresponsible exercise of trade unionism is not to be taken lightly. If no immediate legal remedies are implemented the chain of events very likely to be created could without any doubt jeopardise economic stability the consequences of which are again quite catastrophic. The submission to pressure, and intimidation as a result of which wages and other conditions of employment may be pushed up will automatically bring in its wake a rise in prices and eventually a spiralling in wages and prices.[151]

When the momentous 1973 bank strikes occurred, a very similar dynamic was predicted by the AALC's representative in Addis Ababa. 'CELU won an impressive victory, which I view as a bench-mark in its history. The high visibility of the battle served to set the power structure to pondering', Jerry Funk wrote after the first successful strike.[152] 'And while the strike can be called a victory, it also opens a new area of concern: how to keep the lid on a potential rash of ill-conceived wildcat strikes. As with all "successes", problems don't go away, they merely shift from one order to another', Funk predicted. His predictions turned out to be entirely accurate. Right after the successful conclusion of the strike at the privately owned Addis Ababa Bank, the more numerous workers of the government-owned Commercial Bank of Ethiopia repeated the feat, securing an even more significant victory. Only a few months later, an unprecedented wave of strikes rolled across the waged economy. 'It has been my projection that subsequent to the successes of the strikes at Addis Ababa Bank and Commercial Bank, strikes here would become more of a fad (the answer to anything) rather than a last, intellectual tool', another AALC official in Addis Ababa wryly noted in January 1974. 'My projection seems to be coming to the fore as strikes are becoming more common and frequent'.[153]

[151] "Speech by Ato Bekele Beshah", ICFTU/ITUC archives.

[152] "Report No. 256: CELU General", Jerry Funk, 23 August 1973, AALC Records.

[153] "Report No. 11", Dick Arnold to AALC/New York, 11 January 1974, AALC Records.

As these pages were written, it was not yet possible to determine whether the upswing in strike activity during the second half of the 2010s had resulted in any aggregate wage gains. However, there was circumstantial evidence that a similar reciprocal relationship between advances in the position and conditions of labour, on the one hand, and the development of militancy and assertiveness, on the other, again prevailed—that achievements again induced expectations of further increases, as Screpanti put it. One aspect of this can be viewed in how successful trade union campaigns created the basis for further advances, as the successful contestation around the 2017 labour bill and the push to pry the industrial parks open for trade union organisers demonstrated. Another aspect of this was discernible in how the successful outcomes of individual strikes appeared to encourage other workers to strike as well. The several waves of emulative strikes that occurred in industrial parks are pertinent examples of this. In the Bole Lemi Industrial Park, researchers found that a nominal wage hike of around 40 per cent was 'most likely due to the increased pressure to raise wages that resulted from the strike wave' that had occurred there.[154] Hawassa Industrial Park saw similar dynamics at play. Moreover, several enterprises outside of the parks were forced to adjust wages by similar ranges in the wake of successful strikes.[155]

However, as important as it is to recognise the reciprocal relationship between the wage gains, increased militancy, and unrest, the reverse dynamic has also been evident. Repression, subjugated structures, and collapsing wages eventually led to a vicious cycle of passivity and defeat beginning in the second half of the 1970s. A negative path dependence that the Ethiopian labour movement, despite repeated attempts, only escaped again in the mid-2010s.

References

Addis Fortune. "CETU Warns of Labour Strike." *Addis Fortune* 18, no. 913 (26 October 2017).

Admasie, S.A. "Dynamics of Assertive Labour Movementism in Ethiopia: Organized Labour, Unrest and Wages in a Socio-Historical Perspective." PhD diss., University of Pavia and University of Basel, 2018.

[154] Schaefer and Oya, *Employment Patterns*, 41.

[155] See, for example, Fasika, "Castel Labour Suspends Strike".

African American Labor Center (AALC) Records. Collection 0547-LBR. Hornbake Library, Special Collections and University Archives, University of Maryland Libraries, College Park, MD.

Amin, S. "Income Distribution and the "Privileged" Worker." In *African Social Studies: A Radical Reader*, 186–200, edited by P.C.W Gutkind and P. Waterman (New York and London: Monthly Review, 1977).

Bahir Dar Textile Factory Archives. International Institute of Social History, Amsterdam.

Bahru Zewde, *Society, State and History: Selected Essays*. Addis Ababa: Addis Ababa University Press, 2008.

Bekure Woldesemait. "The Industrial Labor Force in the Addis Ababa Region Before 1975: Origins, Expectations and Realities." In *Proceedings of the Seventh International Conference of Ethiopian Studies: University of Lund, 26–29 April, 1982*, edited by S. Rubensson, 603–616. Addis Ababa: Institute of Ethiopian Studies; Uppsala: Uppsala University; East Lansing, MI: African Studies Center, Michigan State University, 1984.

Beyene Solomon. የኢትዮጵያ ሠራተኞች አንድነት ማህበር: ውልደት ዕድገት ውድቀት. Self-published, Addis Ababa, 2012.

Blattman, C. and S. Dercon. "Occupational Choice in Early Industrializing Societies: Experimental Evidence on the Income and Health Effects of Industrial and Entrepreneurial Work." Working paper, National Bureau of Economic Research, 2016.

Central Statistical Agency. *Statistical Report on the 2013 National Labour Force Survey*. Addis Ababa: CSA, 2014.

CELU. *3ኛው በየሦስት ዓመት የሚከናወን ጠቅላላ ጉባዔ/3rd Triannual Conference*. Occasional publication. Addis Ababa: Confederation of Ethiopian Labour Unions, 1972.

Confederation of Ethiopian Trade Unions (CETU) archives. CETU, Addis Ababa.

Department of State. *Country Reports on Human Rights Practices for 1985*. Washington DC: Joint Committee Print, 1986.

Department of State. *Country Reports on Human Rights Practices for 1991*. Washington DC: Joint Committee Print, 1992.

Department of State. *Country Reports on Human Rights Practices for 1993*. Washington DC: Joint Committee Print, 1994.

Dijkstra, A. "Low Wages Draw International Textile Companies to Ethiopia." *Deutsche Welle*, 10 December 2015, https://www.dw.com/en/low-wages-draw-international-textile-companies-to-ethiopia/a-18877027/

Eshetu Chole. "Import Substitution in Practice: The Case of the Ethiopian Textile Industry." PhD dissertation, Syracuse University, 1973.

Ethio-Djibouti Railway, Dire Dawa Hub Archives. International Institute of Social History, Amsterdam.

Ethiopian Herald. "Minister Addresses Conference." April 10, 1970.
Ethiopian Herald. "Labour Strike in Addis condemned." October 3, 1975.
Ethiopian Herald. "Factory's Stolen Property Recovered," September 21, 1993.
Ethiopian Herald. "Alleged EPRP Members Shot One Youth," May 7, 1994.
Fasika Tadesse, "Sher on Hot Plate: Heavy Tax, Labour Dispute," *Addis Fortune* 18, no. 911 (8 October 2017).
Fasika Tadesse, "Castel Labour Suspends Strike after Pay Raise Vow," *Addis Fortune* 18. No. 914 (5 November 2017).
Gaitachew Bekele. *The Emperor's Clothes A Personal Viewpoint of Politics and Administration in the Imperial Ethiopian Government, 1941–1974*. East Lansing, MI: Michigan University Press, 1993.
Ginzberg, E. and H.A.S. Smith. *Manpower Strategy for Developing Countries: Lessons from Ethiopia*. New York: Columbia University Press, 1967.
Girma Negash. "The Rise and Rise of Agricultural Wage Labour: Evidence from Ethiopia's South, c.1950–2000." *Africa* 87, no. 1 (2017): 36–52.
ICFTU/ITUC Archives. Collection ARCH0062, International Institute of Social History, Amsterdam.
International Labour Organization. "Report on Workers' Education in Ethiopia." Report ILO/OTA/Ethiopia/R.6, confidential, ILO, Geneva, 1964.
International Labour Organization. *Employment and Unemployment in Ethiopia*. Report of the Exploratory Employment Policy Mission. Geneva: International Labour Office, 1973.
International Labour Organization. "Memorandum to the Government of Ethiopia on Reform of the Wage System: Wage Regulation, Job Evaluation and Payment by Results." Confidential report, ILO, 1983.
Kelly, J. *Rethinking Industrial Relations: Mobilisation, Collectivism and Long Waves*. London: Routledge, 1998.
Krishnan, P. Tesfaye Gebreselassie and S. Dercon. "The Urban Labour Market During Structural Adjustment: Ethiopia 1990–1997." Working paper, Centre for the Study of African Economies, University of Oxford, 1998.
Killion, T. "Workers, Capital and the State in the Ethiopian Region." PhD diss., Stanford University, 1985.
Killion, T. "Railroad Workers and the Ethiopian Imperial State: The Politics of Workers' Organization on the Franco-Ethiopian Railroad, 1919–1959." *International Journal of African Historical Studies*, 3, no. 25 (1992): 583–605.
Landsorganisationen i Danmark (LO) archives. Arbejdermuseet & Arbejderbevægelsens Bibliotek og Arkiv, Copenhagen.
Lefort, R. *Ethiopia: An Heretical Revolution?* London: Zed Press, 1983.
Markakis, J. and Nega Ayele. *Class and Revolution in Ethiopia*. Nottingham: Spokesman Books, 1978.

Mengistu Hailemariam. *Speech Delivered to the Second Congress of the All Ethiopia Trade Union*. Addis Ababa: Provisional Military Government of Socialist Ethiopia/Commission for Organizing the Party of the Working People of Ethiopia, 1982.

Mills, G. "Ethiopia's Hailemariam Desalegn: Growth has to be shared to be sustainable." *Daily Maverick*, 7 June 2016, https://www.dailymaverick.co.za/article/2016-06-07-ethiopias-hailemariam-desalegn-growth-has-to-be-shared-to-be-sustainable/.

Ministry of Labour and Social Affairs. *Labour Statistics Bulletin 1979*. Addis Ababa: MoLSA, 1980.

Ministry of Labour and Social Affairs. *የሥራ ክርክር ሁኔታ ጥናት*. Addis Ababa: Ministry of Labour and Social Affairs, 1987.

Ministry of Labour and Social Affairs (MoLSA) archives, MoLSA, Addis Ababa.

Mulatu Wubneh. "State Control and Manufacturing Labor Productivity in Ethiopia." *Journal of Developing Areas* 24, no. 3 (1990): 311–326.

Mulatu Wubneh and Yohannis Abate. *Ethiopia: Transition and Development in the Horn of Africa*. Boulder, CO: Westview Press, 1988.

Negarit Gazeta. "Proclamation No. 42 of 1993: Labour Proclamation." *Negarit Gazeta* 52, no. 27 (20 January 1993): 268–328.

Negede Gobezie. *ይድረስ ለግንቦት ከየካቲት*. Washington, DC: AESOP Publishers, 2014.

Robinson, D. "Wage Guidelines." In *Socialism from the Grass Roots: Accumulation, Employment and Equity in Ethiopia, Vol II: Working Papers*, 28–42. ILO Jobs and Skills Programme for Africa. Addis Ababa: ILO, 1982).

Samuel Getachew. "Awash suspends production amid workers strike." *The Reporter* (8 September 2018), https://www.thereporterethiopia.com/6344/.

Schaefer, F. and C. Oya. *Employment Patterns and Conditions in Construction and Manufacturing in Ethiopia: A Comparative Analysis of the Road Building and Light Manufacturing Sectors*. IDCEA Research Report. London: SOAS, University of London, 2019.

Screpanti, E. "Long Economic Cycles and Recurring Proletarian Insurgencies." *Review (Fernand Braudel Center)* 7, no. 3 (1984): 509–548.

Senay Likke. *The Ethiopian Revolution: Tasks, Achievements, Problems and Prospects*. Unknown publisher, Addis Ababa, 1976.

Silver, B. *Forces of Labor: Workers' Movements and Globalization Since 1870*. Cambridge: Cambridge University Press, 2003.

Stutz, R. "The Developing Industrial Relations System in Ethiopia." Mimeo. Haile Selassie I University, Addis Ababa, 1967.

Suter, A.C. *Labor Law and Practice in the Empire of Ethiopia*. BLS Report No. 298. Washington, DC: Bureau of Labor Statistics, 1966.

Syoum Gebregziabher. "The Rise of CELU and the EFE Under Haile Selassie's Regime." Mimeo, 2005.

Tarpinian, E. "Survey of the Ethiopian Textile Industry in Relation to a Title III Program." Report prepared for USAID/Ethiopia, Labat-Anderson Incorporated, 1992.

Tesfa Gebremariam. "The Promotion of Collective Bargaining in Ethiopia." In *Collective Bargaining and Security of Employment in Africa: English Speaking Countries: Proceedings of and Documents Submitted To, a Symposium, Victoria Falls, Zimbabwe, 4–8 May 1987*, 147–151. Geneva: International Labour Office, 1988.

Tom Killion Papers. Collection 2017C40, Hoover Institution Library and Archives, Stanford University Stanford, CA.

Voice of Labour. "የኢ.ሠአማን አባል ማኅበሮች እናስተዋውቃላችሁ/Introducing CELU's Affiliates." *Voice of Labour,* Special Issue on the Occasion of the 7th CELU Anniversary and the Inauguration of its New Headquarters (9 April 1970).

World Bank. *Fourth Ethiopia Economic Update: Overcoming Constraints in the Manufacturing Sector*. Washington, DC: World Bank Group, 2015.

World Bank. *Fifth Ethiopia Economic Update: Why so Idle? Wages and Employment in a Crowded Labor Market.* Washington, DC: World Bank Group, 2016.

Wuilbercq, E. "L'Ethiopie, Nouvelle Usine du Monde." *Le Monde*, 11 August 2017, https://www.lemonde.fr/afrique/article/2017/08/11/l-ethiopie-nouvelle-usine-du-monde_5171211_3212.html.

CHAPTER 7

Conclusions

The first six decades of countrywide trade unionism and labour movementism in Ethiopia yielded mixed results. Advances were followed by retreats, surges by collapses, and collapses were followed by new beginnings. In this manner, the history of the Ethiopian labour movement presents itself in the shape of repeated cyclical movements, within which Ethiopian workers have variously developed and acquired; been deprived of and relinquished; and reacquired the collective coherence, organisational resources, autonomy, and militancy required to engage in effective collective action and contestation, capable of alternating the conditions of labour and, occasionally, of commanding influence over broader political affairs. Throughout its history, the movement has been subject to, and has had to overcome, external efforts to subvert, co-opt, control, repress, obstruct, and sometimes eliminate it—emanating from employers and the state. It has also been subject to constraints imposed by international trade union organisations, which have both aided and inhibited its development. Thus far, three cycles are apparent.

The first cycle began as the Ethiopian labour movement emerged countrywide in the late 1950s and early 1960s. Sustained strike activity took place throughout the 1960s, as rank-and-file workers and basic enterprise unions fought to improve conditions. Such wildcat unrest was also the primary reason that the imperial state—lobbied by Western allies weary of the perceived threat of radicalism and Communism—passed legislation

© The Author(s), under exclusive license to Springer Nature Switzerland AG 2025

S. A. Admasie, *The Ethiopian Labour Movement*, Labour in History and Society, https://doi.org/10.1007/978-3-031-72841-9_7

to permit the establishment and registration of trade unions in 1963. The legislation, however, circumscribed this right, excluding large groups of workers, and it also heavily restricted the collective rights of those workers who were included. The imperial state's lack of intention or determination to practically enforce its own labour law—especially its reluctance to protect workers' representatives and trade unionists from harassment and dismissal—left those rights further imperilled. After an early attempt to pressure the imperial state for further concessions failed and triggered repression, the central trade union confederation, CELU, adopted a cautious, incremental strategy, careful not to antagonise the imperial government or to appear too strident towards employers. It was aided and prompted to do so by foreign allies in the international anti-communist trade union movement, who, in return, made substantial financial and organisational resources available to CELU.

CELU's leadership was dominated by a close-knit group of young university graduates with no experience of wage work or rank-and-file unionism. However, they were personally close to the president of the confederation, who himself represented no constituent union and who, in turn, had elevated them from the ranks of unelected staff members to positions of senior officeholders. Through constitutional engineering and subterfuge, a leadership that represented no constituent unions was able to prevail and entrench itself. This group, in turn, created clientelist relationships with constituent union leaders by selectively offering financial and organisational resources made available by foreign allies to those deemed sufficiently loyal and moderate, and denying them to union leaderships that were deemed too radical or untrustworthy. Where this proved insufficient, more direct and forceful methods of ousting militants and opponents in representative positions were resorted to. Both the imperial state and CELU's foreign allies supported the confederation's leadership in doing so and intervened heavily in the unions' internal affairs to create outcomes they considered favourable. The repertoire of practices used to produce such outcomes included flagrant interference in union elections, subversion of majority decisions, illicit use of resources to fund personal campaigns, corruption of officials, as well as the threat and use of repression.

Yet, the portrayal of CELU as a dormant organisation that accomplished very little in terms of improving the conditions of workers is inaccurate. During the long decade that CELU existed, wages grew by leaps and bounds. Collective agreements acquired in a constantly growing number of enterprises—driven by the persistent pressure of rank-and-file strike action—led to workers attaining significantly better conditions. As a result, CELU progressively grew its membership and leverage. By the end of its decade long existence, CELU had repeatedly confronted the imperial state and major employers—and prevailed. Its growing political clout, an observant representative of its North American allies noted, had become 'a recognized factor in Ethiopia'.[1] Rather than merely serving as a passive tool of control over workers, CELU exemplified the dual role of trade unions: on the one hand, functioning as a vehicle for the agency of Ethiopian workers; on the other, acting as a constraint on their militant energies, channeling their efforts into an excessively cautious and submissive strategy, enforced by a thoroughly bureaucratised leadership.

CELU's leadership's cautious approach and reluctance to use its clout more assertively, insistence on centralising power and resources, denial of autonomy to regional branches, rigging of elections and subversion of intra-union democracy, overturning of majority decisions to launch general strikes, and its reliance on external parties—both foreign allies and the Ethiopian state—to maintain its position, were all factors that fueled the increasing opposition and growing rift within the movement. The labour opposition eventually crystallised into a clearly defined camp, distinguished by a considerably greater degree of militancy. For almost a decade, these two strands of the movement—the moderate leadership and allies, and the labour opposition—competed for dominance. CELU's leadership utilised all available resources and external sources of support—including international trade union organisations and the imperial state—to maintain control and restrain the militant strand of the movement. However, the opposition gradually grew stronger, more radical, and eventually became dominant. By 1973, CELU's leadership was struggling to maintain its position and was compelled to sign a truce agreement with the labour opposition. In doing so, it agreed to convene a general congress in which the various constitutional and electoral points of contention would be resolved through majority vote. But before that could occur, a strike wave began, creating a groundswell of militancy

[1] "Report No. 233; Subject: CELU; CONFIDENTIAL for", Jerry Funk to Irving Brown and Patrick O'Farrell, 6 February 1973, African American Labor Center (AALC) Records, collection 0547-LBR, Hornbake Library, Special Collections and University Archives, University of Maryland Libraries, College Park, MD.

among workers and within CELU. In the midst of the Ethiopian revolution that began the following year, the old leadership was ousted. By mid-1975, the opposition had assumed control of the confederation and put it on a radical course, which ended in confrontation with the military government only a few months later.

Scholars have interpreted the outbreak of a strike wave and the radicalisation of CELU in the 1970s as mere products of the revolutionary context or as results of infiltration by cadres from revolutionary movements. This interpretation is built upon false premises that overlook the much longer arc of militancy, radicalisation and unrest, which reaches back far beyond the beginning of the revolutionary upsurge or even the emergence of revolutionary political organisations. The strike wave that occurred around the time of the revolution did not begin with the notable general strike of March 1974, but rather with a series of strikes that began as early as August 1973, when two large and victorious bank strikes occurred, continuing through the remainder of the year. That took place more than a year before the imperial regime was toppled and six months before the February movement of urban unrest even began. Moreover, the militant labour opposition emerged in the 1960s, a time when no radical political organisations existed in Ethiopia. Its leaders were workers' representatives who were politically unaffiliated when the revolution began. 'The overwhelming majority of the leadership [of the labour opposition]', an American ally of CELU's moderate leaders observed in 1973, 'are not radicals'. 'They do have genuine grievances concerning CELU leadership'.[2] 'None of the potential rivals as far [as] visible represent any sort of shift in ideology', he assured his superiors, 'the revolt is personality and ambition oriented, and generally not ideological'.[3] Several members of the labour opposition eventually joined Marxist-Leninist organisations, but this only occurred at a later stage. The long struggle to steer the movement onto a militant and autonomous path was driven by concerns raised by rank-and-file workers and their representatives. It was these workers and their representatives who eventually prevailed, putting CELU on a radical path.

[2] Ibid.

[3] "Report No 234; Subject: Second Half Report 1972", Jerry Funk to AALC, 13 February 1973, AALC Records.

The confrontation between the radicalised labour movement and the military regime ultimately resulted in the complete elimination of the radical strand of the movement and the cessation of strike activity, under violent repression in 1976 and 1977. It also brought an end to the autonomy of the labour movement, which was formally subordinated to the state. In its wake, the conditions of workers in Ethiopia—most notably wages—collapsed. For the following decade, the Ethiopian labour movement remained dormant.

However, in the dying days of Mengistu's WPE regime, new stirrings emerged among the working population and trade unions. Strikes and labour protests began occurring again, and the frequency of such unrest accelerated following the change of government in 1991. As the former trade union confederation was banned by the incoming EPRDF-led government, and as constituent unions were subjected to reorganisation processes, workers and their enterprise-level representatives began to form networks to contend with the state-led process. Eventually, this led to the re-establishment of a relatively autonomous trade union confederation, which, however, soon fell afoul of the authorities and was repressed once again. Another decade of submissive yellow unionism followed, until, in the mid-2010s, the ruling party's control over the unions and workers began to erode, labour unrest resurfaced, and the trade union confederation—CETU—began expanding its autonomy and reclaimed a degree of assertiveness. Coupled with a new wave of strikes that began around the same time, this led to the re-emergence of a vibrant and relatively autonomous labour movement in the final years of the decade.

It is unsurprising that mechanisms of state control over the labour movement began to wither just as the ruling front was thrown into disarray. In his seminal work, *Rethinking Industrial Relations: Mobilisation, Collectivism and Long Waves*,[1] John Kelly brings Charles Tilly's mobilisation theory to bear on workers' collective action.[5] He follows Tilly in outlining the conditions for workers' collective action, which include (i) the social construction and definition of collective interests; (ii) collective mobilisation, which transforms individual workers into

[4] J. Kelly, *Rethinking Industrial Relations: Mobilisation, Collectivism and Long Waves* (London: Routledge, 1998).

[5] C. Tilly, *From Mobilization to Revolution* (New York: Random House 1978).

collective actors; (iii) collective organisation; and, crucially, (iv) opportunity. The opportunity factor—which relates to 'the policies and actions of employers and the state'[6]—encompasses considerations such as the relative balance of power, the costs of repression, and the contingent opportunities available. Employers and the state generally engage in counter-mobilisation, which is 'likely to target all of the dimensions of collectivism',[7] and includes repression. When effective, such counter-mobilisation can restrict opportunities, impose higher costs on collective action, overturn goals and leaders, rearticulate interests, undermine organisations, and demobilise workers.

In Ethiopia, political crises—of the imperial state in the 1970s, the WPE regime in the late 1980s and early 1990s, and the EPRDF in the 2010s—have served as conjunctures in which the Ethiopian labour movement has tended to exercise the greatest relative levels of autonomy. This is because such crises have bolstered the opportunity factor by rendering state and employer counter-mobilisation relatively ineffective. However, in each case, the crises of the state have occurred subsequent to increases in strike activity, labour unrest, and greater trade union assertiveness—in short, *after* heightened workers' collectivisms and mobilisation. Thus, it is not the case that political crises are mechanically determinative of the latter, but rather, a dialectical relationship appears to prevail between, on the one hand, regime efforts to control the labour movement and, on the other, the persistence of labour militancy and autonomous activity. Moreover, it is the collective mobilisation of workers, rank-and-file militancy, and (predominantly wildcat) strike activity that has both created the space for trade union officials to act more assertively, and applied pressure on them to do so.

When considering the impact and effects of the Ethiopian labour movement, the scepticism in much of the scholarly literature has been shown to be somewhat misplaced. There have been episodes, even extended periods spanning many years, during which the Ethiopian labour movement had a significant impact in improving the collective rights, working conditions and wages, and leverage of Ethiopian workers. The prolonged upswing of real wages in unionised sectors from the early 1960s to the mid-1970s is a primary example of this. Such episodes

[6] Kelly, *Industrial Relations*, 37.

[7] Ibid., 128.

of heightened assertiveness and impact have tended to be preceded and accompanied by higher levels of militancy and rank-and-file strike activity. In addition to affecting labour conditions, these episodes have also led to sudden expansions in the membership of trade unions, such as the one that began in the mid-to-late 2010s. In addition, they have enhanced the trade unions' ability to influence broader political affairs.

The Ethiopian labour movement has, at times, substantially impacted the Ethiopian wage labour regime and labour conditions. Through a reciprocal interrelationship, this impact has, in turn, affected the development of the movement. In the general literature on labour movements, it has been observed that militancy—expressed in an assertive outlook and a readiness to engage in collective action to enforce aims—not only energises existing structures but can lead to significant increases in union membership and improvements in the *position* of labour—expressed in the leverage workers exert within the broader political-economic framework.[8] Scholars have noted that, in contexts other than Ethiopia, union membership and 'the expansion of working-class organisational resources seem to have followed intense periods of industrial conflict [and] strike waves in particular'.[9] Strike waves have not only positively impacted trade union membership numbers, but also strengthened 'the full political organisation of the working class and its political position in the national power structure'.[10] That has been the case because confrontational strategies can lead employers to conclude that the 'workers [are] interested in striking for its own sake', thereby '[inducing] employers to provide them with extra wages as a peace payment'.[11] John Kelly has corroborated this point, noting that 'where unions have visibly demonstrated their effectiveness in pursuing, and winning, employee claims and grievances through strike action, then non-union workers have been encouraged to join in unusually large numbers'.[12] This, Kelly has argued, may set 'a virtuous circle of

[8] Kelly, *Industrial Relations*, 60–64.

[9] R. Franzosi, *The Puzzle of Strikes: Class and State Strategies in Postwar Italy* (Cambridge: Cambridge University Press, 2006), 344.

[10] Ibid., 344.

[11] S. Cohn, *When Strikes Make Sense—And Why: Lessons from Third Republic French Coal Miners* (New York and London: Plenum, 1993), 213.

[12] Kelly, *Industrial Relations*, 64.

effectiveness and membership' in motion, as it did in the early twentieth-century United Kingdom. He explained that, 'as the scale of strike activity increased, so did the win rate, and as the win rate increased, bargaining coverage rose, more workers perceived unions to be effective and joined them, which in turn enabled more strikes to be called... and so on'.[13]

Similar to Kelly's argument, Ernesto Screpanti has suggested that a virtuous cycle between workers' achievements and assertiveness can come into being.[14] 'Any consolidated increase in [wage growth] achievements induces expectations of further increases', he has written. 'There is a positive cumulative effect of past experience in relation to actual claims'.[15] This could lead to a virtuous cycle of growing membership, assertiveness and leverage. The obvious corollary is that the reverse also applies: a cycle of successive defeats, linked to the adoption of a submissive approach and strategic unwillingness to engage in militant practices, and accompanied by a shrinking and increasingly passive membership, could equally well be set in motion. Screpanti's thesis holds that, in general, 'claims will change in time in the same direction as achievements, and in such a way that the rate of change of the gap between them will increase (or decrease) as achievements themselves increase (or decrease)'.[16] The cyclical pattern of mobilisation and militant collective activity among Ethiopian workers can largely be explained by this logic.

At the time of writing, the Ethiopian labour movement is in the midst of a third cycle of mobilisation. It is too early to discern what its eventual fate will be—whether it will be sustained in duration as the first cycle, or be cut short like the second; and whether it will have a significant impact on the conditions of labour, as the former did, or fail to result in a discernible effect on the increasing rate of exploitation, as the latter. What

[13] Ibid., 101.

[14] Both John Kelly and Ernesto Screpanti link these processes to economic cycles. However, their role is primarily to trigger the emergence of the virtuous or vicious cycles described. It is thus perfectly possible for virtuous cycles to emerge from significant achievements that break the status quo. The Ethiopian case demonstrates that these reciprocal interrelationships need not be subject to any overarching business-cyclical logic to operate perfectly well.

[15] E. Screpanti, "Long Economic Cycles and Recurring Proletarian Insurgencies," *Review (Fernand Braudel Center)* 7, no. 3 (1984), 530.

[16] Ibid., 531.

is clear is that it has already led to a historic expansion in the membership of trade unions and impact on labour legislation—two aspects that are unlikely to be rolled back readily. In this sense, it has already achieved lasting gains. The basis for any further advances, if past dynamics are any indication, resides in the continued mobilisation of rank-and-file workers and representatives, ready to engage in militant practices. Such militancy has not only repeatedly compelled trade union leaders to make more assertive demands and adopt a more contentious approach, but it has also convinced the state and employers of the advisability of addressing labour's demand, in the process growing the size, momentum, autonomy, and leverage of the movement.

References

African American Labor Center (AALC) Records. Collection 0547-LBR. Hornbake Library, Special Collections and University Archives, University of Maryland Libraries, College Park, MD.

Cohn, S. *When Strikes Make Sense—And Why: Lessons from Third Republic French Coal Miners*. New York and London: Plenum, 1993.

Franzosi, R. *The Puzzle of Strikes: Class and State Strategies in Postwar Italy*. Cambridge: Cambridge University Press, 2006.

Kelly, J. *Rethinking Industrial Relations: Mobilisation, Collectivism and Long Waves*. London: Routledge, 1998.

Screpanti, E. "Long Economic Cycles and Recurring Proletarian Insurgencies." *Review (Fernand Braudel Center)* 7, no. 3 (1984): 509–548.

Tilly, C. *From Mobilization to Revolution*. New York: Random House, 1978.

Index

© The Editor(s) (if applicable) and The Author(s), under exclusive license to Springer Nature Switzerland AG 2025

S. A. Admasie, *The Ethiopian Labour Movement*, Labour in History and Society, https://doi.org/10.1007/978-3-031-72841-9

The manufacturer's authorised representative in the EU is Springer Nature Customer Service Centre GmbH, Europaplatz 3, 69115 Heidelberg, Germany. If you have any concerns regarding our products, please contact ProductSafety@springernature.com

Printed and bound by CPI Group (UK) Ltd, Croydon, CR0 4YY
01/10/2026
02225967-0013